Case Studies

DOLAN'S
CRITICAL CARE
NURSING

Clinical Management
Through the Nursing Process

DOLAN'S
CRITICAL CARE NURSING

Clinical Management
Through the Nursing Process

Second Edition

Susan D. Ruppert, RN, PhD, CCRN, FNP
Associate Professor
The University of Texas—Houston Health Science Center
School of Nursing
Houston, Texas

Jeanette G. Kernicki, RN, PhD, CNS
Clinical Professor
Texas Woman's University
College of Nursing
Houston, Texas

Adjunct Professor of Nursing
The University of Texas
M.D. Anderson Cancer Center
Houston, Texas

Joan T. Dolan, RN, MS, CS, CCRN, CETN, CDE, ANP
Clinical Nurse Specialist
Massapequa General Hospital
Seaford, New York

President, Joan T. Dolan and Associates, Ltd.
Great River, New York

 F. A. DAVIS COMPANY • Philadelphia

F. A. Davis Company
1915 Arch Street
Philadelphia, PA 19103

Printed in the United States of America

Last digit indicates print number: 10 9 8 7 6 5 4 3 2 1

Publisher, Nursing: Robert G. Martone
Nursing Editor: Alan Sorkowitz
Production Editors: Marianne Fithian and Rose Gabbay
Cover Designer: Louis J. Forgione

As new scientific information becomes available through basic and clinical research, recommended treatments and drug therapies undergo changes. The authors and publisher have done everything possible to make this book accurate, up to date, and in accord with accepted standards at the time of publication. The authors, editors, and publisher are not responsible for errors or omissions or for consequences from application of the book, and make no warranty, expressed or implied, in regard to the contents of the book. Any practice described in this book should be applied by the reader in accordance with professional standards of care used in regard to the unique circumstances that may apply in each situation. The reader is advised always to check product information (package inserts) for changes and new information regarding dose and contraindications before administering any drug. Caution is especially urged when using new or infrequently ordered drugs.

Library of Congress Cataloging-in-Publication Data

Dolan's critical care nursing : clincial management through the
    nursing process.—2nd ed. / [edited by] Susan D. Ruppert, Jeanette
    G. Kernicki, Joan T. Dolan.
      p. cm.
    Rev. ed. of: Critical care nursing / Joan T. Dolan. c1991.
    Includes bibliographical references and index.
    ISBN 0-8036-0025-9
    1. Intensive care nursing.   I. Ruppert, Susan D. 1953–.
II. Kernicki, Jeanette. III. Dolan, Joan T. Critical care nursing.
    [DNLM: 1. Critical Care. 2. Nursing Process. WY 154 D8593 1996]
    RT129.I5065 1996
    610.73′61—dc20
    DNLM/DLC
    for Library of Congress   96-5285

To my husband, Mike, and children, Sarah and Michael, for their love, support, and understanding.

S.D.R.

To my family and former teachers who guided me in the pursuit of my educational endeavors.

J.G.K.

To my family, Joe, Joseph, and Mary Krista—my source of strength, my love, my life.

J.T.D.

Foreword

The vision that inspired the first edition of *Critical Care Nursing: Clinical Management Through the Nursing Process* and the effort that went into its success have been refined and enhanced by the collaborative efforts of Doctors Susan Ruppert and Jeanette Kernicki with those of the original editor, Joan Dolan. While maintaining the integral concepts that were the outstanding features of the first edition, they have been able to condense and update its content without sacrificing any of its original richness or brilliance. Thus, this revised second edition will continue to provide a significant contribution to the education and preparation of the critical care nurses of today and tomorrow—nurses who will understand not only the complexities of pathophysiology or the expanding role of technology but also the holistic interactions and disruptions that define the critically ill patient; nurses who will understand the fibers of composition, yet remain cognizant and appreciative of the entire tapestry that is the nursing process. The artful weaving of these components forms the matrix of this text.

The quality of the contributions (and contributors) to this book remains impressive, and readers should feel confident that the up-to-date information is provided by acknowledged nursing experts. Their focused commitment to the dissemination of knowledge pertinent to critical care nursing nobly augments the advancement of the art and science of nursing. Their knowledge and clinical expertise have made explicit what is implicit about the nursing process. We can all be grateful—and, once again, proud.

Elaine Kiess Daily, RN, BS, FCCM
Consultant in Clinical Cardiovascular Research and Education
Madison, Wisconsin

Preface

The tumultuous changes resulting from the ongoing restructuring and redesigning of the health care system herald more demands on the nursing profession. Patients who will be seen in the hospital setting will be more acutely ill, older, and more demanding of nurses' time and energy. Recipients of care will have greater expectations of nurses and will seek out nurses who are highly knowledgeable and competent professionals. Critical care nurses will be greatly in demand, with critical thinking and clinical decision-making abilities a **must** for all health professionals.

The second edition of this text has been designed and written with the goal of providing a text that is "user friendly" for the undergraduate nursing student and that "bridges the gap" as a resource for beginning to intermediate practice in critical care nursing. The book's length has been reduced, and its major focus is on presenting key "need to know" content while maintaining a holistic approach to issues and concepts important to critical care nursing. An effort has been made to include content that will assist the beginning critical care practitioner but not necessarily to duplicate content found in the medical/surgical nursing textbooks currently available. This new edition is appropriate for use by multiple audiences, such as nursing students, novice nurses, and novice critical care nurses. The text also offers a fine review for the experienced nurse wanting to update knowledge in critical care nursing.

Many new figures and tables have been aded to this edition and much material has been set in boxes so that important points are stressed in summary format. All chapters contain appropriate new material. Care plans have been retained, but they have been streamlined to emphasize priority NANDA nursing diagnoses and moved to the ends of chapters to prevent them from breaking the flow of the chapters' text. Measurable care outcomes have been maintained for each nursing diagnosis to assist the nurse in assessing the effects of care delivery. In addition, Chapter 2 now presents a discussion and sample of critical pathways. Case studies allow the student to better understand what is happening to the patient and to recognize inherent problems. Research boxes have been added, and along with the incorporation of research within chapter text, they serve as a means of promoting a strong research-based practice in nursing.

The 60 chapters in this edition are divided into 11 major units, the sequence of which has been rearranged to fit a traditional course structure. These units are as follows:

Unit One	Conceptual Foundations of Critical Care
Unit Two	Cardiovascular System
Unit Three	Respiratory System
Unit Four	Nervous System
Unit Five	Renal/Urinary System
Unit Six	Endocrine System
Unit Seven	Gastrointestinal System
Unit Eight	Immune System
Unit Nine	Hematologic System
Unit Ten	Trauma, Emergencies, and Multisystem Disorders
Unit Eleven	Oncologic Critical Care Nursing

The book begins with the unit Conceptual Foundations of Critical Care, which includes the application of the nursing process to critical care, principles of patient/family teaching and learning, ethical and legal principles, psychosocial implications, and nutritional support. This introductory unit also includes the book's three entirely new chapters—on sleep and sensory alterations, pain and its management, and critical care of the elderly. At the end of the book are a number of appendices containing valuable reference aids and a glossary.

Each unit consists of chapters that have been streamlined for readability and focused on pragmatic content applicable to clinical practice for students and practitioners. A brief review of anatomy and physiology and content on pathophysiology, assessment and monitoring techniques, therapeutic modalities, and nursing management are incorporated into most units. To assist the user, each chapter begins with a list of objectives and a topical outline of the chapter's content. The format for most units includes the following:

- **Anatomy and physiology:** The first chapter of each of these units begins with a thorough review of anatomy and physiology, emphasizing the relationship between structure and function.
- **Assessment:** The second chapter reviews pertinent information on the assessment of the organ system. The discussion of assessment includes the clinical history and the physical examination. A description of pertinent diagnostic tests/studies and implications for nursing care are also included.
- **Monitoring:** This chapter includes information on monitoring techniques including implications for nursing care (e.g., intracranial pressure monitoring, cardiac monitoring, and hemodynamic monitoring).
- **Therapeutic modalities:** The discussion of assessment and monitoring is followed by attention to those therapeutic modalities pertinent to treatment of a disruption/impairment of organ function (e.g., oxygen therapy, suctioning techniques, cardiac pacing and intra-aortic balloon pumping). Sample procedures are provided to assist the nurse to gain further insight into the skills pertinent to critical care nursing.
- **Pathophysiology:** Several chapters in each organ system unit are included to present pertinent, commonly seen pathophysiologic disorders/diseases/syndromes. The discussion of anatomy and physiology provides a basis for understanding the pathophysiology underlying insults to a specific organ system. To assist the reader to appreciate the significance of dysfunction, cross-referencing is provided to illustrations and discussions of normal physiology. Discussions of specific diseases largely include etiology, pathophysiology, clinical presentation, diagnosis, treatment, and nursing management.
- **Nursing management:** The nursing management of specific disease entities is presented through the use of care plans that can be applied clinically by the nurse. They include nursing diagnoses, desired patient outcomes, and nursing interventions and rationales. The use of rationales for nursing interventions enables basic physiologic principles to be integrated with, and provide the basis for, specific nursing actions. Cross-referencing to illustrations and discussions of normal physiology within the same unit, as well as to other units, assists the reader to view the individual as a whole (i.e., in terms of total body processes: physiologic, psychologic, emotional, and social). This educational process is facilitated by cross-referencing between and among care plans throughout the text and to the numerous other tables.

Using the care plan format assists the reader to appreciate the process involved in determining specific nursing diagnoses and shows how these diagnoses relate to desired patient outcomes, nursing interventions, and the language used to define these parameters. Specifically:

○ Each nursing diagnosis is related to specific etiology or etiologies amenable to nursing interventions.
○ Each desired patient outcome is stated in measurable terms and describes the outcome to be achieved by the patient.
○ Nursing interventions are written in terms that reflect specific actions taken by the nurse.
○ Rationales assist to integrate underlying physiologic principles.

- **Case studies:** Case studies of selected pathophysiologic disorders are presented throughout the text. Each one focuses the reader on an actual clinical scenario, thereby integrating the underlying physiologic principles and concepts with the clinical circumstance.

    The sample care plans accompanying most case studies allow the reader to identify the specific assessment data that provide the basis for the nursing diagnoses. The initial nursing diagnoses and their etiologies are listed and developed as part of the sample care plan. Like the comprehensive care plans, the sample care plans include desired patient outcomes, nursing interventions, and rationales. In this way, the language of nursing process is reflected in the nursing care plan. Additional nursing diagnoses and their etiologies based on the assessment data presented in the case study are also listed to enable readers to develop their own care plans.

    This second edition of *Critical Care Nursing: Clinical Management Through the Nursing Process* now offers an excellent package of ancillaries to support the critical care nursing educator. An extensive instructor's guide offers teaching strategies for the classroom, clinical setting, and individual study. It also provides the chapter outlines and objectives from the text, study questions keyed to each chapter's objectives, terminology lists, worksheets for student exercises, and dozens of transparency masters. A computerized testbank offers educators who adopt this text nearly 1200 questions with F. A. Davis's easy-to-use CyberTest software, which lets the educator prepare quizzes and tests of any length needed. A 50-item set of transparencies from the textbook completes the comprehensive ancillary package available to programs adopting the text.

    In today's health care system, where tertiary care settings are increasingly focusing on the care of the very sick patient and the patient's family, the need for critical care nurses capable of providing sophisticated, timely, and humanistic care is greater than ever. Whether in the classroom or at the patient's bedside, it is our hope that this text will help to improve the quality of patient care and contribute to positive outcomes for patients and their families.

Susan D. Ruppert, PhD, RN, CCRN, FNP
Jeanette G. Kernicki, PhD, RN, CNS
Joan T. Dolan, MS, RN, CS, CCRN, CETN, CDE

Acknowledgments

The publication of this second edition reflects the present and past contributions of many. We are indebted to our colleagues who encouraged us along the way as well as to Dr. Patricia Starck, Dean of the School of Nursing, The University of Texas—Houston; Dr. Cheryl Levine, Chairperson, Department of Acute and Continuing Care, The University of Texas—Houston; Dr. Carolyn Gunning, Dean of the College of Nursing, Texas Woman's University; Dr. Carolyn Adamson, Assistant Dean of the College of Nursing, Texas Woman's University—Houston Center; and to Dr. Lenora J. McLean, Dean, School of Nursing, State University of New York at Stony Brook for their strong professional support during the development of this edition.

We are grateful to our colleagues, students, and graduates who inspired the revisions reflected in this edition. Their enthusiasm and motivation in seeking new and expanded knowledge guided the way for us. Our gratitude is extended to the many contributors who so freely shared their expertise and knowledge with respect to the current edition, as well as those who contributed to the first edition.

A special thank you goes to Alan Sorkowitz, Nursing Editor, for his guidance, patience, and fastidiousness throughout the course as well as to the many other individuals at F. A. Davis who assisted in the production of this project. In particular, we wish to thank Herbert J. Powell, Director of Production; Peter Faber, Production Manager; and Marianne Fithian, Production Editor, for their outstanding work in bringing this book to fruition.

Finally, we acknowledge the critical care nurses who touch the lives of so many. Their dedication in shaping a critical care environment that will positively affect their patients and families provides a vision worth admiring.

Susan D. Ruppert
Jeanette G. Kernicki
Joan T. Dolan

Contributors

Cynthia J. Abel, RN, MSN, CEN
Trauma Coordinator
The University of Texas
Medical Branch at Galveston
Galveston, Texas

Mary Amendolari, RN
Nursing Care Coordinator
Intensive Care Unit
Massapequa General Hospital
Seaford, New York

Jackie Anderson, RN, MSN, CCRN
Cardiovascular Outcomes Manager
St. Luke's Episcopal Hospital
Houston, Texas

Roberta H. Anding, MS, RD/LD, CDE
Assistant Professor of Clinical Nursing
The University of Texas—Houston Health Science
    Center
Houston, Texas

Susan Auvil-Novak, RN, PhD
Assistant Professor
Frances Payne Bolton School of Nursing
Case Western Reserve University
Cleveland, Ohio

Lorraine Brown, RNC, MSN
Assistant Director Nursing/Clinical Nurse Specialist
Massapequa General Hospital
Seaford, New York

Michelle Casedonte, RN, BSN
Cardiac Nursing Case Manager
Cleveland Clinic Foundation
Cleveland, Ohio

Christine M. Chmielewski, RN, MS, CNN
Instructor
Division of Nursing
Holy Family College
Philadelphia, Pennsylvania
and
Department of Nursing
Temple University
Philadelphia, Pennsylvania

Marie Clark, RN, MSN
Cardiology Outcomes Manager
St. Luke's Episcopal Hospital
Houston, Texas

Linda Cole, RN, MS, MSN, CCRN
Outcomes Manager/Clinical Nurse Specialist
General Surgery/Digestive Health Service
St. Luke's Episcopal Hospital
Houston, Texas

Adrienne Coppola, RN
Nursing Care Coordinator
Intensive Care Unit
Massapequa General Hospital
Seaford, New York

Elaine Kiess Daily, RN, BS, FCCM
Consultant, Clinical Cardiovascular Research and
    Education
Madison, Wisconsin

Frances Dooley, RN, MS, CNA, CCRN, CDE, ANP
Private Practice
Massapequa, New York

Carol F. Evans, RNC, MS
Administrative Director, Education and Standards
Lower Bucks Hospital
Bristol, Pennsylvania

Anecita P. Fadol, RN, MSN, CCRN, CNS
Clinical Nurse Specialist
The Methodist Hospital
Houston, Texas

Adjunct Faculty
Texas Woman's University
Houston, Texas

Lorraine Fallon, RN, MSN, CEN, CCRN
Staff Nurse, Emergency Department
Memorial Hospital of Burlington County
Mount Holly, New Jersey

Staff Nurse, MICU
Deborah Heart and Lung Center
Browns Mills, New Jersey

Vaunette Payton Fay, RN, PhD, CS
Gerontological Nurse Practitioner
Associate Professor
School of Nursing
The University of Texas—Houston Health Science
    Center
Houston, Texas

Jan Foster, RN, MSN, CCRN
Adjunct Faculty
College of Nursing
Houston Baptist University
Houston, Texas

Doctoral Nursing Student
The University of Texas
Austin, Texas

Marcia Goldstein, RN, MSN, CNN
Clinical Nurse Specialist, Nephrology
Albert Einstein Medical Center
Philadelphia, Pennsylvania

Marc G. Golightly, PhD
Associate Professor of Pathology
Head of Immunology
State University of New York at Stony Brook
Stony Brook, New York

Ginny Wacker Guido, RN, JD, MSN
Professor and Chair
Department of Nursing
Eastern New Mexico University
Portales, New Mexico

Marina Hamilton, RN, MSN, CCRN
Nursing Unit Manager-Otolaryngology
Queen Elizabeth II Health Sciences Centre
Halifax, Nova Scotia

Sandra K. Hanneman, RN, PhD, FAAN
Clinical Professor, Graduate Program
Director of Research
Texas Woman's University
Institute of Health Sciences—Houston
College of Nursing
Houston, Texas

Betty S. Henderson, RN, MN
Assistant Professor
Texas Woman's University College of Nursing
Houston Center
Houston, Texas

Peggy Hollingsworth-Fridlund, BSN, RN
Trauma Coordinator
University of California, San Diego Medical Center
San Diego, California

Susan Houston, RN, PhD
Director, Outcomes Measurement and Research
St. Luke's Episcopal Hospital
Houston, Texas

Karen Sue Hoyt, RN, MN, CEN
NP Clinical Placement Coordinator
University of San Diego
School of Nursing
San Diego, California

Terry L. Jones, RN, MS, CCRN
Critical Care Education Coordinator
Department of Nursing Education
Parkland Memorial Hospital
Dallas, Texas

Sheila M. Keller, RN, MSN
Clinical Instructor
Helene Fuld School of Nursing
Camden, New Jersey

Dorothy M. Kite-Powell, RN, MSN, CCRN
Pulmonary Outcomes Manager
St. Luke's Episcopal Hospital
Houston, Texas

Patricia Smokler Lewis, RN, MS, CCRN
Head Nurse—CCU
The Methodist Hospital
Houston, Texas

Mary Meisel, RN, MS
Surgical Clinical Nurse Specialist
Fairview Southdale Hospital
Edina, Minnesota

Jo-Ann Murray-Schluckebier, MSN, CRNP
Instructor
Holy Family College
Philadelphia, Pennsylvania

Ronald D. Novak, PhD, MPH, MPA
Assistant Professor of Medicine
School of Medicine
Case Western Reserve University
Cleveland, Ohio

Vivian Nowazek, RN, MSN, CCRN, CNS
Instructor of Clinical Nursing
The University of Texas—Houston Health Science
   Center
Houston, Texas

Kristin Kane Ownby, RN, MSN, CS, MPH, OCN
Doctoral Student
Texas Woman's University
Houston, Texas

Deborah Rodzwic Pennypacker, CRNP, MSN, OCN, CS
Family Nurse Practitioner/Oncology
Clinical Nurse Specialist
Atkinson Community Health Center/Brandywine
   Hospital
Coatesville, Pennsylvania

Diane Ragsdale, RN, EdD
Professor
College of Nursing
Texas Woman's University
Houston, Texas

Carol A. Stephenson, RNC, EdD
Associate Professor
Texas Christian University
Harris College of Nursing
Fort Worth, Texas

Cathy J. Thompson, RN, MSN, CCRN, CNS
Assistant Professor
The University of Texas—Houston Health Science
   Center
Houston, Texas

Doctoral Student
Texas Woman's University—Houston Center
Houston, Texas

Deborah M. Thorpe, RN, PhD, CS
Clinical Nurse Specialist
Section of Pain and Symptom Management
The University of Texas
M.D. Anderson Cancer Center
Houston, Texas

Rita Bolek Trofino, RN, MNEd
Burn Nursing Educator and Faculty
Department of Nursing and Allied Health
Indiana University of Pennsylvania
Indiana, Pennsylvania

Merri D. Walkenstein, RN, MSN, OCN
Certified School Nurse
Central Bucks School District
Doylestown, Pennsylvania

formerly Clinical Nurse Specialist
Fox Chase Cancer Center
Philadelphia, Pennsylvania

Wayne C. Waltzer, MD, FACS
Professor of Urology and Surgery
Stony Brook Health Sciences Center
School of Medicine
State University of New York at Stony Brook
Stony Brook, NY

Jeannette Waterman, RN, MSN
Case Manager
VNA Visiting Nurse Service System
Vineland, New Jersey

Janet Donnard White, RN, BSN, CCRN
Fox Chase Cancer Center
Philadelphia, Pennsylvania

Gayle R. Whitman, RN, MSN, FAAN
Vice Chair, Patient Care Operations
Director of Nursing
Cleveland Clinic Foundation
Cleveland, Ohio

Anne W. Wojner, RN, MSN, CCRN
CNS/Outcomes Manager
Neuroscience and Emergency Services
St. Luke's Episcopal Hospital
Houston, Texas

Dolores M. Zygmont, RN, MSN, CCRN
Staff Nurse, CCU
Hospital of the University of Pennsylvania Medical
 Center
Philadelphia, Pennsylvania

Doctoral Candidate
Temple University
Philadelphia, Pennsylvania

Consultants

Linda Baas, RN, PhD, CCRN
Assistant Professor
College of Nursing and Health
University of Cincinnati
Cincinnati, Ohio

Margaret "Mardi" Berkner, RN, MSN
Chairman, Critical Care Nursing
Missouri Baptist Medical Center
School of Nursing
St. Louis, Missouri

Marcia Chorba, RN, MSN
Mercy Hospital
School of Nursing
Pittsburgh, Pennsylvania

Charlene D. Coco, RN, MN
Assistant Professor
Louisiana State University Medical Center
School of Nursing
New Orleans, Louisiana

Margaret R. Colyar, RN, DSN, ARNP
Valdosta, Georgia

Deborah K. Drummonds, RN, MN, CCRN, CEN
Instructor
Valdosta State University
College of Nursing
Valdosta, Georgia

Coleen Fritsche, RN, MS
Assistant Professor of Nursing
Atlantic Union College
South Lancaster, Massachusetts

Alice C. Geissler, RN, BSN, CCRN, CRRN
Director of Nurses
National Medical Care—Home Care Division
Colorado Springs, Colorado

Frank D. Hicks, RN, PhD(c), CCRN
Assistant Professor, Medical-Surgical Nursing
Niehoff School of Nursing
Loyola University
Chicago, Illinois

Alicia M. Horkan, RN, MSN
Instructor
Valdosta State University
College of Nursing
Valdosta, Georgia

Therese M. Lahnstein, RN, MSN, CCRN
Nursing Faculty
Southern Union State Community College
Valley, Alabama

Marilyn Nelsen Pase, RN, MSN
Assistant Professor
School of Nursing
New Mexico State University
Las Cruces, New Mexico

Deborah L. Roush, RN, MSN
Assistant Professor
Valdosta State University
College of Nursing
Valdosta, Georgia

Deborah Sigman, RN, MS
Assistant Professor
Department of Nursing
University of Massachusetts, Lowell
Lowell, Massachusetts

Judith C. Trotti, RN, MSN, CS, CNOR
Clinical Instructor
University of Texas Health Science Center—San
   Antonio
School of Nursing
San Antonio, Texas

Frances B. Wimbush, RN, PhD
Assistant Professor
College of Nursing
University of Delaware
Newark, Delaware

Contents

Abbreviations Used in This Book

$AaDO_2$	Alveolar-arterial oxygen gradient
AAPCC	American Association of Poison Control Centers
a/A ratio	Arterial/alveolar ratio
Ab	Antibody
ABGs	Arterial blood gases
ABO	Blood groups
ACh	Acetylcholine
AChR	Acetylcholine receptor
ACTH	Adrenocorticotropic hormone
ADH	Antidiuretic hormone
ADLs	Activities of daily living
ADP	Adenosine diphosphate
AHA	American Heart Association
AIDS	Acquired immunodeficiency disease (acquired immune deficiency syndrome)
ALG	Anti-lymphocyte globulin
ALS	Amyotrophic lateral sclerosis
ALT	Alanine aminotransferase (SGPT)
AMI	Acute myocardial infarction
An	Antigen
AP	Action potential
ARDS	Adult respiratory distress syndrome
ARF	Acute renal failure
ARF	Acute respiratory failure
AST	Aspartate aminotransferase (SGOT)
ATN	Acute tubular necrosis
ATP	Adenosine triphosphate
BMR	Basal metabolic rate
BSA	Body surface area
BUN	Blood urea nitrogen
CABG	Coronary artery bypass graft
CAD	Coronary artery disease
cAMP	Cyclic AMP (adenosine monophosphate)
CAPD	Continuous ambulatory peritoneal dialysis
CAVH	Continuous arteriovenous hemofiltration
CBC	Complete blood count
CCK	Cholecystokinin

cGMP	Cyclic GMP (guanosine monophosphate)
CHF	Congestive heart failure
CI	Cardiac index
CK (CPK)	Creatinine phosphokinase
CMV	Cytomegalovirus
CNS	Central nervous system
CO	Cardiac output
COPD	Chronic obstructive pulmonary disease
CPAP	Continuous positive airway pressure
CPE	Cardiogenic pulmonary edema
CPP	Cerebral perfusion pressure
CRF	Chronic renal failure
CRH	Corticotrophic releasing hormone
CSF	Cerebrospinal fluid
CT	Calcitonin
CT scan	Computerized axial tomography
CV	Cardiovascular
CVA	Cerebrosvascular accident
CvO_2	Oxygen content of mixed venous blood
CVP	Central venous pressure
CXR	Chest x-ray
DCT	Distal convoluted tubule
DI	Diabetes insipidus
DIC	Disseminated intravascular coagulation
DKA	Diabetic ketoacidosis
DNA	Deoxyribonucleic acid
DPG	2,3-diphosphoglycerate
DTRs	Deep tendon reflexes
DVT	Deep venous thrombosis
ECF	Extracellular fluid
ECG	Electrocardiogram
ECV	Extracellular fluid volume
EEG	Electroencephalogram
EMG	Electromyography
EOMs	Extra ocular movements
ERV	Expiratory reserve volume
ESR	Erythrocyte sedimentation rate
ESRD	Endstage renal disease
f	Respiratory rate (breathing frequency)
FBS	Fasting blood sugar
FDPs (FSPs)	Fibrin degradation products (fibrin split products)
FEV	Forced expiratory volume
FEV_1/FVC	Forced expiratory volume/forced vital capacity
FIO_2	Fraction of inspired oxygen
FRC	Functional residual capacity
FSH	Follicle stimulating hormone
FHF	Fulminating hepatic failure
GCS	Glasgow coma scale

GFR	Glomerular filtration rate
GH	Growth hormone
GHIH	Growth hormone inhibiting hormone
GHRH	Growth hormone releasing hormone
GI	Gastrointestinal
GnRH	Gonadotrophic releasing hormone
GVHD	Graft-versus-host disease
HBD	Hydroxybutyrate dehydrogenase
HCl	Hydrochloric acid
HCO_3^-	Bicarbonate
Hct	Hematocrit
HDL	High-density lipoprotein
HDPM	Hemodynamic pressure monitoring
Hgb	Hemoglobin
HHNK	Hyperglycemic hyperosmolar nonketotic (coma)
HIV	Human immunodeficiency virus
HLA	Human leukocyte antigens
HPI	History of present illness
HPO_4	Phosphate
HR	Heart rate
IABP	Intraaortic balloon pump
IC	Inspiratory capacity
ICF	Intracellular fluid
ICP	Intracranial pressure
ICPM	Intracranial pressure monitoring
ICS	Intercostal space
ICV	Intracellular fluid volume
IDDM	Insulin dependent diabetes mellitus
IDL	Intermediate density lipoprotein
Ig	Immunoglobulin (IgG, IgM, IgA, IgE, IgD)
IL-1, IL-2	Interleukin-1, interleukin-2
IMV	Intermittent mandatory ventilation
IPPB	Intermittent positive pressure breathing
IRV	Inspiratory reserve volume
IVP	Intravenous pyelography (excretory urography)
JGA	Juxtaglomerular apparatus
KCl	Potassium chloride
LAD	Left anterior descending coronary artery
LAP	Left atrial pressure
LBBB	Left bundle branch block
LCX	Left circumflex coronary artery
LDH	Lactic dehydrogenase
LDL	Low density lipoprotein
LH	Leuteinizing hormone
LLQ	Left lower quadrant
LMCA	Left main coronary artery
LMN	Lower motor neuron
LOC	Level of consciousness

LUQ	Left upper quadrant
LVAD	Left ventricular assist device
LVEDP	Left ventricular end-diastolic pressure
LVEDV	Left ventricular end-diastolic volume
LVH	Left ventricular hypertrophy
LVSWI	Left ventricular stroke work index
MAC	Midarm circumference
MAMC	Midarm muscle circumference
MAP	Mean arterial pressure
MASTs	Military antishock trousers
MCL	Mid clavicular line
MCL_1	Modified chest lead (V_1)
MDF	Myocardial depressant factor
mEq	Milliequivalent
MHC	Major histocompatibility complex
MI	Myocardial infarction
mOsm/kg	Osmolality
MOV	Minimal occlusive volume
MR	Mitral regurgitation
MRI	Magnetic resonance imaging
MSH	Melanocyte-stimulating hormone
MVA	Motor vehicle accident
MVO_2	Myocardial oxygen consumption
MVV	Maximal voluntary ventilation
$NaHCO_3$	Sodium bicarbonate
NANDA	North American Nursing Diagnosis Association
NCPE	Noncardiogenic pulmonary edema
NFP	Net filtration pressure
$NH4^+$	Ammonium ion
NIDDM	Noninsulin dependent diabetes mellitus
NIF	Negative inspiratory force
NMJ	Neuromuscular junction
NPO	Nothing by mouth
NSR	Normal sinus rhythm
NTG	Nitroglycerin
$1,25-(OH)_2D$	1,25-dihydroxycholecalciferol
OKT-3	Monoclonal antibody
PA	Pulmonary artery
$PACO_2$	Alveolar carbon dioxide concentration
$PaCO_2$	Arterial carbon dioxide concentration
PAedp	Pulmonary artery end-diastolic pressure
PAO_2	Alveolar oxygen concentration
PaO_2	Arterial oxygen concentration
PAP	Pulmonary artery pressure
PASG	Pneumatic antishock garment
PAW	Pulmonary artery wedge (PCWP)
P_B	Barometric pressure
PCD	Post-cardiotomy delirium

PCO_2	Partial pressure of carbon dioxide
PCT	Proximal convoluted tubule
PCWP	Pulmonary capillary wedge pressure
PEEP	Positive end-expiratory pressure
P_E Max	Maximal expiratory pressure
PERRLA	Pupils equal, round, reactive to light and accommodation
PGE_2	Prostaglandin E_2
pH	Hydrogen ion concentration
PH (PTH)	Parathormone (parathyroid hormone)
PIH	Prolactin inhibiting hormone
P_I Max	Maximal inspiratory pressure
PIP	Peak inspiratory pressure
PMH	Past medical history
PMNs	Polymorphonuclear leukocytes
PND	Paroxysmal nocturnal dyspnea
PNS	Peripheral nervous system
PO_2	Partial pressure of oxygen
PRH	Prolactin releasing hormone
PT	Prothormbin time
PTCA	Percutaneous transluminal coronary angioplasty
PTT	Partial thromboplastin time
$PvCO_2$	Carbon dioxide concentration in mixed venous blood
PvO_2	Oxygen concentration in mixed venous blood
PVR	Pulmonary vascular resistance
Q	Flow
RAP	Right atrial pressure
RAS	Reticular activating system
RBBB	Right bundle branch block
RCA	Right coronary artery
REF	Renal erythropoietic factor
RES	Reticuloendothelial system
RIND	Reversible ischemic neurologic deficit
RLQ	Right lower quadrant
RME	Resting metabolic expenditure
RML	Right middle lobe
RMP	Resting membrane potential
RNA	Ribonucleic acid
ROM	Range of motion
R/T	Related to
RUQ	Right upper quadrant
RV	Residual volume
RVEDP	Right ventricular end-diastolic pressure
RVF	Right ventricular failure
RVH	Right ventricular hypertrophy
RVP	Right ventricular pressure
SaO_2	Percent saturation of hemoglobin
SIADH	Syndrome of inappropriate secretion of antidiuretic hormone
SIMV	Synchronized intermittent mandatory ventilation

SGOT	Serum glutamic oxaloacetic transaminase
SGPT	Serum glutamic pyruvic transaminase
SLE	Systemic lupus erythematosus
SLIDT	Assessment tool (see Table 35–1)
SOB	Shortness of breath
sp.gr.	Specific gravity
SV	Stroke volume
SVCS	Superior vena cava syndrome
SVI	Stroke volume index
SvO_2	Mixed venous blood oxygen tension (saturation)
SVR	Systemic vascular resistance
SVT	Supraventricular tachycardia
T_3	Triiodothyronine
T_4	Thyroxine
TBG	Thyroid binding globulin
TBPA	Thyroid binding prealbumin
TBW	Total body water
TIAs	Transient ischemic attacks
TLC	Total lung capacity
Tm	Maximal rate of mediated transport of a substance across a plasma membrane
TPN	Total parenteral nutrition
TRH	Thyrotrophic releasing hormone
TSH	Thyrotropic stimulating hormone
UMN	Upper motor neuron
$\dot{V}_A$	Alveolar minute ventilation
VC	Vital capacity
$V_D(V_D/V_T)$	Anatomic dead space volume
$\dot{V}_E$	Minute ventilation
VLDL	Very low density lipoprotein
VMA	Vanillylmandelic acid
VSD	Ventricular septal defect
$\dot{V}/\dot{Q}$	Ventilation/perfusion ratio
V_T	Tidal volume
WBC	White blood count
WPW	Wolff-Parkinson-White syndrome

UNIT ONE

Conceptual Foundations of Critical Care

UNIT OUTLINE

CHAPTER 1

Critical Care Nursing: An Introduction

Joan T. Dolan

In the ordinary course of life, the integrity of individual developmental processes and personal interaction with the environment may be disrupted and function may be compromised. Whether the dysfunction springs from a life-threatening crisis or from an exacerbation of a chronic disease, critically ill persons require sophisticated intervention to restore life processes to their dynamic equilibrium. The goal of critical care nursing is to provide essential individualized care directed toward the survival of the person and the achievement of optimal physiologic, psychological, emotional, and social potential. Restoration of individual life processes to dynamic equilibrium requires that the *process that is nursing* promote these life processes in the manner best calculated to achieve desired goals and outcomes.

A major pathophysiologic/psychological insult to individual life processes and functions commonly places an extraordinary strain on the body's normal regulatory mechanisms, undermining the emotional and psychological stability of the affected person and the person's family. It is in this situation that the critical care nurse not only helps to restore those processes vital to life, but also maintains life-sustaining functions until the individual is once more able to assume responsibility for personal interactions with the environment. Pathophysiology is seen within the context of cellular change and the effects of such change on the developmental processes of the individual as a whole and on his or her ongoing environmental interactions.

In approaching the individual as a whole, the critical care nurse bridges the gap between modern technology and the needs of the critically ill. The nurse strives to maintain the integrity of the individual in the face of an increasingly mechanistic environment, recognizing that individual responses to the environment largely reflect such integrity. Skilled nursing interventions aim to assist critically ill individuals and their families to mobilize their resources to support the integrity of individual and interpersonal relationships and to strengthen individual-environment interaction.

The critical care nurse serves as a catalyst in the healing process, making complex and timely judgments and decisions and taking actions for which the nurse remains accountable. The rationale for such decisions is based on a thorough knowledge of the health and behavioral sciences, fully developed skills, and the ability to evaluate one's own responses and limitations. This knowledge base is upgraded continuously by new clinical and educational experiences that reinforce the critical care nurse's professional practice and autonomy.

The nursing process is a scientific approach to decision-making through assessing, diagnosing, planning, implementing, and evaluating. Accurate documentation of the care process facilitates communication among healthcare providers and may also serve as a measure of the quality of the health care given.

With the implementation of prospective payment plans designed to contain healthcare costs and the consequent changes in healthcare delivery, it is essential that the nurse document care in a manner that reflects the appropriateness and effectiveness of skilled nursing interventions. This requires an awareness of the intellectual process involved in providing care, together with an appreciation of the need to document this process in clear, concise language. Thus the critical care nurse defines what is done when care is provided, while also noting whether or not such care brings about a positive change in the patient's responses and clinical outcomes.

Today's critical care nurse is challenged by our ever-expanding knowledge of physiologic, psychological, and sociologic interactions. These advancements, accompanied by complex technologic innovations, require that the critical care nurse function at a highly sophisticated level when caring for the critically ill patient, family, or significant others. Standards of critical care nursing assist nurses to defines their practice because such standards make the profession's expectation regarding quality patient care very explicit.

The American Association of Critical-Care Nurses (AACN), which recognizes the complexity of nursing management of the critically ill, has been innovative in the promotion of competent critical care nursing practice. Through its ongoing activities, the AACN strives to meet the educational needs of critical care nurses to ensure a high standard of care for all patients, their families, and significant others.

Comprehensive care of superior quality is possible only when there are participation and communication among all concerned health professionals. Often, it is the critical care nurse who serves as coordinator and collaborator, encouraging each caregiver to appreciate and to respect the contribution of other team members. This creates a climate in which the team can function with maximum efficiency as reflected by the achievement of desired patient outcomes.

The chapters that follow are designed to assist the critical care nurse to grasp the body of knowledge essential to practice. The study of human systems emphasizes the relationships between structure and function, physiology and pathophysiology, and internal and external environmental interactions. Case studies suggest the application of this knowledge to clinical situations. Nursing care plans based on nursing diagnoses and decision-making rationales demonstrate that clear and concise documentation reflects the actual care process. In this manner, the professional role of the critical care nurse is shown to be vital to the well-being of the critically ill patient.

CHAPTER 2

Application of Nursing Process to Critical Care Nursing Practice

Joan T. Dolan and Anne W. Wojner

LEARNING OBJECTIVES

After completing this chapter, you should be able to:

1. Define nursing.
2. Define nursing process and its essential components.
3. Define nursing diagnosis and its language.
4. Describe the classification of nursing diagnoses developed by the North
   American Nursing Diagnosis Association (NANDA).
5. Analyze the format and language of nursing process.
6. Differentiate criteria for patient outcomes and their documentation.
7. Discuss the characteristics of nursing interventions and implications for
   documentation.
8. Distinguish between independent and collaborative nursing activities.
9. Review Nursing Care Plan: Nursing Diagnoses, Desired Patient Outcomes, and
   Nursing Interventions.
10. Explore the evolution of nursing care delivery systems and the development of
    nursing case management (NCM) and outcomes management (OM) programs.
11. Define the purpose of critical pathways within an NCM and OM program.

NURSING PRACTICE: NURSING PROCESS DEFINED

"Nursing is the diagnosis and treatment of human responses to actual or potential health problems."[1] The fundamental basis of nursing practice is PRO-CESS. Every aspect of practice is affected by an understanding and utilization of nursing process.

Nursing process is an organized approach to problem-solving and decision-making that describes the intellectual activity of the nurse. It is the accepted methodology for nursing practice.

5

NURSING PROCESS: A FIVE-STEP PROCESS

Nursing process involves five steps: assessing, diagnosing, planning, implementing, and evaluating.

Assessing

Assessing involves a thorough, ongoing, comprehensive collection of subjective and objective data of the patient-family-environment interaction. Such data are obtained via history-taking, observation, physical examination, laboratory data, x-rays, and other diagnostic studies. Use of functional health patterns[2] (see Appendices C and D) assists in eliciting information of concern to nursing. The patient's database should reflect those data that form the basis for nursing diagnoses.

Diagnosing

Diagnosing involves the identification of the patient's actual or potential health problem, and the etiology, or cause, of the problem that nurses can independently treat. Nursing diagnosis is a *pivotal* component of nursing process. On the one hand, it is the judgment, conclusion, or decision determined by the nurse as a result of the assessing and problem-solving process. It reflects the process involved in gathering, analyzing, and interpreting the assessment data.

On the other hand, nursing diagnosis provides the basis from which patient outcomes are derived and a plan of appropriate nursing interventions is developed and implemented. In other words, nursing diagnosis emerges from the collection, analysis, and interpretation of assessment data and provides the framework from which the patient's plan of nursing care evolves.

Planning

Planning involves the determination of desired patient outcomes and nursing interventions based on the nursing diagnosis. The nurse supports the individual in self-advocacy for the optimal level of health desired. The nurse motivates the patient, family, or significant others to become actively involved in the "care process." The nurse-patient-family interaction assists in determining priority of nursing diagnoses and setting patient goals and outcomes that clearly communicate the nature of the actual or potential health problem. Ideally, patient outcomes should reflect the patient's input in determining realistic and measurable outcomes.

Implementing

Implementing involves the specific nursing interventions and activities delineated in the patient's care plan and designed to treat the cause of the patient's problem defined in the nursing diagnosis.

Evaluating

Evaluating involves an appraisal of the effectiveness of the nursing interventions in resolving the patient's problem as defined in the nursing diagnosis. A comparison is made of the actual patient outcomes in response to nursing interventions with those outcomes predicted in the patient's care plan.

Reassessment of the patient's status and nursing diagnoses is necessary to determine the effectiveness of nursing interventions. Revisions of the patient's care plan and its implementation are based on the reassessment of the patient and the nursing diagnoses.

KNOWLEDGE: THE RATIONAL BASIS FOR DECISION-MAKING

Nursing diagnoses are formulated based on the analysis of the assessment data obtained. The analysis and interpretation of the assessment data require that the nurse integrate theoretical and experimental knowledge in clinical applications. The integration of such knowledge within the clinical setting provides the *rational basis for decision-making*.

The activities inherent in the care process require that each nurse expand his or her knowledge base and develop more sophisticated skills in assessment, problem-solving, decision-making, and management. The nurse must become disciplined to think through the process, to identify the components of the process as they occur in practice, and to document that process in a language that reflects the functions that are nursing.

NURSING PROCESS: THE LANGUAGE

The language of process is unique because it reflects the nurse's practice; it is used to verbalize what one is doing and why something is being done. Nurses need to communicate the care process to colleagues and fellow healthcare providers as it evolves, and in a precise and concise manner. Language must be clear and consistent so that other healthcare providers will know what to expect of nursing and so that nurses will know what to expect of each other.

Nursing: A Diagnosis-Based Practice

Nursing, as a diagnosis-based practice, demands that nurses become expert at assessing a patient's needs and problems, formulating nursing diagnoses based on that assessment, evolving and implementing a plan of care, and documenting this care process in a manner reflective of the professional, skilled nursing care rendered. Only by documenting nursing activities can professional practice be validated and financially rewarded.

Nursing Diagnosis: Defined

Simply defined, a nursing diagnosis reflects a patient's problem or unhealthful response and the problem's etiology that nurses can treat independently. It is a definitive statement of an actual or potential problem, alteration, or deficit in the life processes (physiologic, psychological, and sociologic) of an individual.

Nursing Diagnosis: A Two-Part Statement

The nursing diagnosis consists of two parts, the problem and its etiology. The *problem* reflects the patient's actual or potential unhealthful response; the *etiology,* if known, reflects the cause of the unhealthful response or problem that is amenable to independent nursing intervention. Use of the phrase "related to" (R/T) suggests a relationship between the patient's unhealthful response and its etiology, or cause. This phrase has been legally recommended because it avoids implying an actual cause-and-effect relationship.

The nursing diagnosis should be specific because it provides the framework for developing the plan of care. The problem portion of the nursing diagnosis predicts what the patient outcomes should be; there is a direct relationship between the patient's problem and the desired outcomes. The etiology portion of the nursing diagnosis dictates what nursing interventions must be implemented if the patient's outcomes are to be achieved and the problem is to be resolved.

Determining the etiology of the patient's problem helps to individualize patient care; that is, no two patients with a similar problem can be expected to have the same underlying etiology or require the same nursing interventions to treat it. It necessitates that interventions required to treat the cause of the patient's problem be within the scope of nursing's independent functions. The nurse must determine whether such interventions can be performed independently.

Nursing Diagnosis: Descriptive Categories

Nursing diagnosis may be described as actual, potential, or possible. An *actual* nursing diagnosis reflects a patient's problem or unhealthful response that is present as indicated by specific signs and symptoms, or defining characteristics. A *potential* nursing diagnosis suggests that a patient's problem or unhealthful response may occur unless preventive nursing measures are initiated. While specific symptomatology or defining characteristics may not be evident, risk factors can usually be identified that suggest the necessity of implementing preventive nursing interventions. A *possible* nursing diagnosis suggests that a patient's problem or unhealthful response may be present, but the symptomatology or defining characteristics may not be apparent or discernible. The nurse must obtain additional information to either confirm or rule out the diagnosis.

Classification of Nursing Diagnoses

For more than 20 years, the efforts of the North American Nursing Diagnosis Association (NANDA)[3] in developing a classification of nursing diagnoses have been highly instrumental in moving the profession of nursing toward the development of a language that communicates its unique functions. As of 1994, NANDA's list contained 128 approved nursing diagnostic categories (see Appendix A), which reflected the patient's actual, potential, or possible problem (i.e., the first part of the two-part nursing diagnosis statement). The addition of the etiology of the problem (i.e., the second part of the nursing diagnosis statement) completes the formulation of the nursing diagnosis and individualizes the diagnosis for the particular patient.

Nurses are encouraged to use these nursing diagnostic categories in their daily practice when formulating nursing diagnoses. Clinical applications and study of these diagnoses must be promoted so that the language of nursing diagnosis and the functions it reflects can be refined and validated.

Nurses need not feel restricted to the use of NANDA's list but rather should be motivated to develop in practice other nursing diagnoses, which can be submitted for possible inclusion in NANDA's list. In this way, nurses are able to share their ideas, experiences, logic, and creativity. The procreation of nursing's language, along with an ever-increasing awareness of the intellectual activity involved in its process and implementation, is every nurse's professional responsibility.

Integration of Knowledge and the Language of Nursing Process

There is another dimension to be considered with respect to the language of nursing process. Often, such terms as "turning and positioning" are used to describe nursing actions. In this regard, the underlying physiologic principle dictating the turning and positioning of the patient is to "maximize mobility to maintain tissue perfusion, decrease the possibility of atelectasis, or prevent a deep venous thrombosis with its concomitant risk of pulmonary embolism." With this latter statement more is communicated than just "turning and positioning." You are *thinking* about what you are doing and you are documenting it. You are integrating your theoretical and experimental knowledge base within the conceptual framework of the interacting whole individual, with respect to both the internal environment (cellular interaction) and the external environment (person-environment interaction). Documentation of such intellectual activities

TABLE 2–1
Criteria for Patient Outcomes

Patient outcomes should:
1. Be written as the patient's behaviors or goals. Patient outcomes reflect those human responses (physiologic, psychological, and emotional) that must occur if the patient's problem is to be resolved. Patient outcomes do not reflect goals that the nurse will achieve. The nurse's role is to support and assist the patient to identify and use his or her capabilities and coping mechanisms more effectively in dealing with the problem.
2. Be written in precise and concise terms using action verbs.
3. Provide direction for care.
4. Specify an appropriate time frame within which the patient is reassessed and the care plan is reevaluated. This serves to determine the effectiveness of the nursing interventions in assisting the patient to achieve the desired outcome(s). (Because time frames need to be individualized for each patient, Nursing Care Plans presented in this text do not incorporate specific time frames.)
5. Be realistic.
6. Be measurable. It is crucial that patient outcomes be stated in measurable terms so that nurses caring for the patient can use the same criteria to evaluate the patient's response to therapy.

TABLE 2–2
Characteristics of Nursing Interventions

1. Determining nursing interventions requires that the nurse have a strong theoretical and experiential knowledge base.
   The nurse must be able to establish appropriate rationales for each nursing intervention implemented.
2. Nursing interventions need to be specific; their implementation is directed toward treating the cause and resolving the patient's problem.
3. Nursing interventions prescribe nursing treatments, that is, what it is the nurse must do to treat the etiology (cause) of the patient's problem. Behaviors described by nursing interventions reflect those of the nurse and not necessarily those of the patient.
   Clear and concise documentation of nursing interventions on the patient's care plan is essential to communicate the activities and behaviors of the nurse to colleagues and other healthcare providers.
4. In writing nursing interventions, the care plan needs to be revised systematically in terms of patient responses and outcomes. Decisions can then be made as to when specific interventions should be revised, updated, renewed, or discontinued. Specific dates and time frames should be documented accordingly. (Note that specific dates and times are not included in the Nursing Care Plans presented in this text because they need to be individualized for the specific patient.)
5. Each documented nursing intervention should be dated and signed by the nurse. The nurse's signature is particularly important in terms of accountability and in the sharing of information (feedback), including clarification of goals and rationales underlying care.

reflects the professional practice of the nurse and becomes the basis for reimbursement of professional service rendered.

Criteria for Patient Outcomes and Their Documentation

Patient outcomes evolve from, and are predicted by, the problem portion (first part) of the nursing diagnosis. Use of precise terminology (language) in formulating and documenting patient outcomes facilitates consistency and continuity in the patient's overall care. It communicates the patient's status to all healthcare providers involved in the patient's care. Criteria for patient outcomes and their documentation are listed in Table 2–1. (Note that because time frames need to be individualized for each patient, such time frames are not incorporated into the nursing care plans presented in this text.)

Characteristics of Nursing Interventions

Nursing interventions evolve from the etiology portion (second part) of the nursing diagnosis. Several characteristics of nursing interventions and their documentation should be noted, and these are listed in Table 2–2. (Note that specific dates and times are not included in the nursing care plans presented in this text because they need to be individualized for the specific patient.)

Nursing Practice: Independent and Collaborative Nursing Functions

Nursing practice involves nursing functions that can be classified as independent or collaborative. *Indepen-*

dent nursing functions include those activities that nurses are licensed to perform. In performing these functions, the nurse has complete autonomy with respect to diagnosing and treating a particular patient problem and does not require the direction of another healthcare provider. The nurse is directly responsible and accountable for decisions made and actions taken.

Collaborative nursing functions are those in which the nurse works together with other healthcare providers (usually physicians) to treat certain pathophysiologic, psychological, and emotional problems. Activities may be performed by the nurse under the direction of another healthcare provider. Although the nurse may be indirectly responsible as a decision-maker, he or she remains accountable for actions taken.

In caring for critically ill patients in the critical care setting, the critical care nurse often engages in many interdependent patient care activities while collaborating with a variety of healthcare providers, including physicians, respiratory therapists, nutritionists, social workers, spiritual advisors, and others.

NURSING CARE PLANS: NURSING DIAGNOSES, DESIRED PATIENT OUTCOMES, AND NURSING INTERVENTIONS

Documentation of the patient's nursing care plan reflects the culmination of the problem-solving/decision-making activities of the professional nurse. Such documentation demonstrates the ability of the nurse to apply nursing knowledge to clinical situations and to integrate this knowledge in the implementation of the components of nursing process.

The nursing care plan format is used throughout this text to afford the reader the opportunity to examine the interrelatedness of the components of process and to appreciate how documentation of the language of process (i.e., nursing diagnoses, desired patient outcomes, and nursing interventions) ultimately reflects those functions and activities within the realm of professional nursing practice.

Nursing diagnoses used in each nursing care plan reflect the two-part nursing diagnosis statement described previously in this chapter; patient outcomes and nursing interventions are written in the manner described in Tables 2–1 and 2–2, respectively. Rationales underlying nursing interventions are included as part of the nursing care plans to assist the nurse to integrate theoretical and experimental knowledge in specific clinical circumstances.

Each nursing care plan included in the text is presented in table form consisting of four sections (see the sample care plan: patient with acute spinal cord injury). The first section lists the most pertinent nursing diagnoses associated with a specific pathophysiologic condition. Nursing diagnoses used throughout the text largely incorporate the diagnostic categories included in NANDA's list (see Appendix A).

The second section of the care plan includes desired patient outcomes predicted by the problem portion (first part) of each nursing diagnosis listed. Nursing interventions to treat the stated etiology (second part) are included in the third section of the care plan format. Appropriate rationales underlying specific nursing interventions are presented in the final section. (Note that specific dates and time frames for desired patient outcomes and nursing interventions are not included in the nursing care plans presented in this text because they need to be individualized for each patient.)

CASE STUDIES

Case studies are also incorporated into the text to provide the reader with the opportunity to apply nursing knowledge to specific clinical situations and to work through the components of nursing process. Nursing diagnoses are formulated based on the assessment data provided, and priority nursing diagnoses are incorporated into the nursing care plan developed for each case study. Sample nursing care plans developed for each case study reflect the language of nursing process, including nursing diagnoses, desired patient outcomes, nursing interventions, and their rationales.

CASE STUDY WITH SAMPLE CARE PLAN: PATIENT WITH ACUTE SPINAL CORD INJURY

RT, a well-nourished, muscular, 21-year-old white man, sustained cervical spinal injury when thrown from his motorcycle while on his way to morning classes at the university, at about 8:45 AM. He was admitted to the emergency room of University Hospital at 9:45 AM, where a diagnosis of transection of the spinal cord at cervical C-6 vertebral level was made. Following stabilization of his condition, Mr. T was taken to the operating room for insertion of tongs.

7/16: 3:00 PM—Upon arrival in the critical care unit, initial assessment reveals the patient on a rotating frame with bed tongs maintained with 15 lb of cervical traction; the patient is aligned appropriately. Mr. T is lethargic, but arousable; oriented to person and place, but not time; pupils equal in size, round, and reactive to light and accommodation (PERRLA). The extremities are flaccid with no sensation or movement.

Vital signs on admission to the unit: blood pressure 90/60, heart rate 56, regular sinus rhythm, rectal temperature 97.6°F. Skin pale, cool, and dry; patient complains of chilling. Intravenous fluid administration of 0.9% normal saline infusing at 100 mL/h. Respiration: patient on room air, breathing shallow at rate of 24/min. Arterial blood gases drawn: PaO_2 80 mmHg, $PaCO_2$ 44 mmHg, pH 7.35. Breath sounds diminished. Gastrointestinal: abdomen soft, nondistended, without bowel sounds. The patient is currently receiving nothing by mouth (NPO). Nasogastric tube to suction. Renal/urinary: straight catheterization in recovery room at 2:30 PM with 400 mL urine obtained. Urine specimen sent for culture/sensitivity. There is no evidence of bladder distention.

Mother at her son's bedside; Mr. T's surgeon spoke briefly with the patient and family, briefing them on the patient's current status and expectations.

Initial Nursing Diagnoses

1. Ineffective breathing pattern: alveolar hypoventilation, related to neuromuscular impairment
2. Ineffective airway clearance, related to compromised cough/gag reflexes
3. Cardiac output, alteration in: decreased, related to loss of systemic vasomotor tone (neurogenic or spinal shock)
4. Urinary elimination, alteration in, related to loss of voluntary control and compromised micturition reflex
5. Skin integrity, impairment of: potential, related to immobility and sensory loss

The above nursing diagnoses are documented on the sample Nursing Care Plan. Additional nursing diagnoses may include:

6. Anxiety, related to unfamiliar environment and disorientation associated with loss of sensory function/perception
7. Bowel elimination, alteration in: constipation,

related to loss of voluntary control and compromised defecation reflex

8. Nutrition, alteration in: less than body requirements
9. Sleep pattern disturbance, related to disrupted motor/sensory function; critical care environment; anxiety
10. Self-concept, disturbance in, related to feelings of powerlessness; dependence on others to satisfy needs

11. Self-care deficit, related to impaired motor/sensory capabilities
12. Coping, ineffective individual/family
13. Knowledge deficit regarding ramifications of catastrophic spinal cord injury and rehabilitation
14. Grieving, related to loss of motor/sensory capabilities
15. Social isolation, related to immobility and prolonged hospitalization

SAMPLE CARE PLAN FOR THE PATIENT WITH SPINAL CORD INJURY

Nursing Diagnoses

Nursing Diagnosis #1
Ineffective breathing pattern: alveolar hypoventilation, related to:
• Altered ventilatory mechanics: hypoventilation associated with paralysis of intercostal and abdominal muscles.

Desired Patient Outcomes

Patient will:
• Demonstrate effective minute ventilation with trend of improving:
  ○ Tidal volume >7–10 mL/kg
  ○ Respiratory rate <25/min
• Achieve a vital capacity of >15–25 mL/kg.
• Verbalize ease of breathing.

Nursing Diagnoses

Nursing Diagnosis #2
Ineffective airway clearance, related to:
• Ineffective cough associated with paralysis of intercostal and abdominal muscles
• Immobility

Desired Patient Outcomes

Patient will:
1. Demonstrate a secretion-clearing cough
2. Maintain arterial blood gas values:
   • PaO_2 > 80 mmHg
   • $PaCO_2$ ~ 35–45 mmHg
   • pH 7.35–7.45

Nursing Interventions

• Perform a comprehensive respiratory assessment:
  ○ Airway patency; rate, rhythm, depth of breathing; chest and diaphragmatic excursion; use of accessory muscles; breath sounds and presence of adventitious sounds.
• Assess neurologic status: mental status, level of consciousness, status of protective reflexes (cough, gag, swallowing).
• Monitor serial pulmonary function tests: tidal volume, vital capacity.
• Assess ability to cough and handle secretions.

  ○ Monitor quality, quantity, color, and consistency of sputum; obtain specimen for culture/sensitivity.
• Implement measures to ensure adequate respiratory function:
  ○ Establish and maintain patent airway.
  ○ Monitor serial arterial blood gases; establish baseline function.
  ○ Initiate oxygen therapy to maintain arterial blood gases within acceptable range.
  ○ Initiate measures to handle secretions; provide humidified oxygen; maintain hydration; nasotracheal suctioning only when necessary.

  ○ Initiate chest physiotherapy when overall condition is stabilized: postural drainage; percussion and vibration; deep breathing and coughing exercises.
  ○ Instruct in use of incentive spirometry.

  ○ Use a calm, reassuring approach: anticipate needs, offer explanations, be accessible to patient/family.

Rationales

• Major goal of airway management is to establish/maintain adequate alveolar ventilation.
  ○ Increased rapid, shallow respirations may signal deterioration of respiratory function.
• Hypoxia may be reflected by changes in mental status or behavior (restlessness, irritability).

• Serial monitoring enables trends to be identified in pulmonary function.
• Loss of intercostal and abdominal muscles compromises the patient's ability to cough effectively.
  ○ Loss of protective reflexes places patient at increased risk of developing aspiration pneumonia.
• Airway obstruction frequently occurs with spinal cord injury or injuries involving head and neck.
  ○ Hypoxemia in the spinal cord–injured patient is most commonly associated with retained secretions.

  ○ Suctioning increases risk of infection; suctioning-associated vagal stimulation may precipitate bradycardia in the spinal cord–injured patient who may already be bradycardic.
  ○ Loosens and dislodges secretions and enhances movement of secretions toward trachea, where they may be accessible to removal by coughing/suctioning.
  ○ Use of incentive spirometry encourages deep breathing, reducing risk of atelectasis.
  ○ Anxiety is a major problem in the spinal cord–injured patient.

SAMPLE CARE PLAN FOR THE PATIENT WITH SPINAL CORD INJURY (*Continued*)

Nursing Diagnoses

Nursing Diagnosis #3
Cardiac output, alteration in: decreased, related to:
• Loss of systemic vasomotor tone (neurogenic shock)

Desired Patient Outcomes

Patient's vital signs will stabilize:
• BP > 90 mmHg systolic (or within 10 mmHg of baseline)
• Heart rate ~ 60/min
• Body temperature 98.6°F

Nursing Interventions
• Assess cardiovascular function and presence of neurogenic (spinal) shock:
  ○ Blood pressure, pulse, body temperature; skin temperature
  ○ Cardiac monitoring for dysrhythmias
  ○ Hydration status
  ○ End-organ perfusion—LOC, U.O., capillary refill
• Implement measures to stabilize cardiopulmonary function:
  ○ Initiate prescribed intravenous and drug therapy ~ 75–100 mL/h.
  ○ Monitor intake and output.
  ○ Initiate measures to minimize orthostatic hypotension: apply antiembolic stockings; abdominal binder.
  ○ Elevate lower extremities at regular intervals.

Rationales
• Spinal cord injury (T_{4-6} and above) precipitates spinal shock with loss of sympathetic autonomic reflexes: loss of systemic tone leads to hypotension; unopposed parasympathetic tone predisposes to bradycardia; interruption of sympathetic innervation underlies hypothermia with impaired temperature regulation.

○ Orthostatic hypotension results from venous stasis associated with impaired vasomotor tone and skeletal muscle paralysis.

Nursing Diagnoses

Nursing Diagnosis #4
Urinary elimination, alteration in, related to:
• Loss of voluntary control of micturition
• Compromised micturition reflex

Desired Patient Outcomes

Patient will maintain:
  ○ Urine output > 30 mL/h
  ○ Weight within 5% of baseline
  ○ Balanced intake and output
  ○ Stable serum electrolytes, blood urea nitrogen (BUN), and creatinine
  ○ Infection-free urinary tract

Nursing Interventions
• Monitor renal and hydration status:
  ○ Specific parameters to assess include body weight (daily), intake/output, serum electrolytes, BUN and creatinine, hematology profile (Hct, Hb).
  ○ Implement straight catheterization protocol using aseptic technique noting amount, color, clarity, and specific gravity of urine.
  ○ Assess for bladder distention at regular intervals and straight catheterize PRN.

Rationales
• Urinary retention predisposes to complications, such as urinary tract infection and autonomic dysreflexia.
• Accurate intake/output and daily weight assist in determining adequacy of renal/urinary function and fluid balance.
• Adequate hydration functions to prevent urinary infection and urinary calculi.
  ○ Adequate renal perfusion maintains filtration and renal function; hemoconcentration may predispose to electrolyte imbalance; increased blood viscosity may cause thromboembolic complications.

Nursing Diagnoses

Nursing Diagnosis #5
Skin integrity, impairment of, related to:
• Immobility
• Sensory loss

Desired Patient Outcomes

Patient will maintain:
• Intact skin with elastic turgor
• Body weight within 5% of baseline

Nursing Interventions
• Maintain skin integrity.
  ○ Assess skin carefully q2h for signs of compromised circulation especially at pressure points.
  ○ Identify potential pressure points specific to the type of bed.

Rationales
• Pressure ulcer develops when there is lack of movement and distribution of weight; pressure is most concentrated between bone and skin surfaces that support body weight.

SAMPLE CARE PLAN FOR THE PATIENT WITH SPINAL CORD INJURY (*Continued*)

Nursing Interventions	Rationales

• Initiate therapeutic regimen:
  ○ Turn/position q2h; document rotation of positions.
  ○ Maintain proper body alignment.
 	
  ○ Initiate passive range-of-motion (ROM) exercises.
  ○ Use footboard, splints, sheepskin or air mattress, elbow/heel pads, special care bed.
  ○ Administer lotion to pressure points.
  ○ Monitor and evaluate response to therapy.
• Consult with nutritionist to initiate necessary nutritional regimen.
• Consult with physical therapy or physical medicine and rehabilitation team.
	• Implementation of therapeutic regimen maximizes tissue perfusion, prevents venostasis and tissue ischemia.
	  ○ Maintenance of proper body alignment prevents further neurologic damage.
	  ○ Passive ROM exercises help to maintain muscle tone and to improve circulation.
	
	• Breakdown of body proteins (gluconeogenesis) impairs tissue healing and places the patient at increased risk of pressure ulcer development and infection.

CRITICAL PATHWAYS

Changes in the healthcare system have directed healthcare providers to deliver not only high-quality but also cost-efficient services. The nursing profession's response to this mandate began taking shape in the mid-1980s with the development of care delivery models that focused on cost awareness and cost-reduction strategies. Nursing case management (NCM) was the first of such models to emerge. NCM evolved from the concepts of primary nursing, embracing characteristics such as continuous, comprehensive (holistic), coordinated, individualized, and patient-centered care delivery.[4,5] NCM delivery systems use nurse case managers to follow up patients from admission to discharge. These staff nurses are responsible for ensuring implementation of cost control measures, the delivery of quality care, and the effective utilization of resources. The NCM delivery model, as its name implies, is a nursing strategy to facilitate comprehensive, coordinated care delivery.

Toward the end of the 1980s, the demands of consumers, insurance companies, and third-party payers created the need for a new multidisciplinary healthcare delivery model with a focus on continuous quality improvement (CQI) and the use of outcomes measures such as length of stay, cost per case, and complication incidence. At the same time, accrediting bodies such as the Joint Commission on Accreditation of Healthcare Organizations (JCAHO) produced standards mandating multidisciplinary CQI. These new definitions for quality measurement fostered the emergence of outcomes management (OM) as a multidisciplinary collaborative healthcare delivery system, which used actual patient outcomes as benchmarks for quality.[6] Figure 2–1 provides an example of intermediate and long-term health outcomes of interest.

Ellwood[7] defined OM as a "technology of patient experience designed to help patients, payers, and pro-viders make rational medical care-related choices based on better insight into the effect of these choices on the patient's life." Simply put, OM empowers consumers to make informed decisions regarding health care through provision of information about the probable effect of healthcare services on patient outcomes. The philosophy of OM is embodied in the American Association of Critical-Care Nurses[7] (AACN) "vision" for a reformed healthcare system. Published in 1992, AACN's vision describes a "patient driven healthcare system" in which critical care nurses make their optimal contribution.[8] OM enables healthcare providers to capture the elements of multidisciplinary CQI, appropriate resource utilization, and cost-efficiency through use of the research process, moving the healthcare system toward provision of patient-driven, holistic care.

Critical pathways, sometimes called clinical pathways, are tools used within both NCM and OM models. Pathways are roadmaps that are directed toward achievement of patient outcomes.[6] In NCM, pathways resemble the format of the nursing care plan and in some institutions have entirely replaced the nursing care plan.

Critical pathways used in an OM model take on a multidisciplinary dimension following the assumption that patient care is a dynamic process based on the contributions of various healthcare providers. Pathways are developed through collaboration with the various healthcare providers involved in moving a specific patient population along the healthcare continuum. Once complete, OM pathways prescribe the healthcare team's actions or processes that will be tested for achievement of specified intermediate or long-term patient outcomes (see sample critical pathway for stroke).[9]

Recall that OM is based on the research process. OM pathways take on an added dimension as data collection instruments and are used to measure the attainment of specified outcomes among the aggre-

Intermediate Outcomes	Long –Term Outcomes
* Hospital length of stay	* Quality of life
* Hospital cost per case	* Functional status
* Postoperative complication rate	* Return to work and leisure activities
* Pain control	* Resource utilization
* Nutritional status	* Mortality and morbidity
* Days on mechanical ventilation	

FIGURE 2–1. Examples of health outcomes of interest.

gate. For example, suppose a team of healthcare professionals managing the care of stroke patients wanted to test an hypothesis that early enteral nutrition improves functional outcomes following stroke. A pathway would be developed outlining the multidisciplinary contributions of each healthcare provider toward ensuring early enteral nutrition. Demographic variables of interest, defined patient variances (or untoward intermediate outcomes), and measures of functional status would be incorporated into the body of the pathway for stroke patients. As patients were managed using the pathway, data would be collected, aggregated, and analyzed to test the hypothesis. Based on the interpretation of the data, the hypothesis would be accepted or rejected and the multidisciplinary care contributions revised as needed. Pathways, then, are never a final design; as science changes, care delivery and research questions change, producing the need for pathway revision. This simple example demonstrates the OM process using critical pathways for data collection. Research of this type fosters the definition of "best" practice for specified patient populations.[9]

Critical pathways may take several forms. They may resemble or replace the traditional nursing care plan in an NCM delivery model, or they may be used to facilitate multidisciplinary outcomes research to determine "best" practice within an OM model. Pathways are unique to a diagnosis and care delivery system. They are intended to suit the care processes for most of the patient population. When utilized optimally, pathways, like nursing care plans, are updated or revised as methods for improvement of patient care are identified through the research process.

CASE STUDY WITH SAMPLE CRITICAL PATHWAY: PATIENT WITH A STROKE

Pathway Day 1

RK, a 79-year-old man, is admitted to the neurology service via the emergency department with sudden-onset right hemiparesis and expressive language dysfunction. Nursing assessment reveals motor strength of 0/5 in the right upper extremity and grade 2/5 in the right lower extremity. Babinski's reflex is present on the right. Sensation is noted to be diminished in the right upper extremity.

A bedside nursing dysphagia assessment identifies the presence of a right facial nerve palsy (cranial nerve VII), resulting in incomplete oral labial closure and drooling. Hypoglossal (cranial nerve XII) function is assessed and movement of the tongue laterally and forward is present, but RK is unable to elevate his tongue against the palate or make an "L" sound. Gag reflex is intact, but assessment of swallow competency with water swallow reveals coughing and choking on 30 mL water, double swallow attempts, and a wet voice.

Although RK is alert, oriented, and able to respond to commands appropriately, his examination also reveals frequent naming errors, incomplete responses, and nonfluent, dysarthric speech. Total admission National Institutes of Health Stroke Scale (NIHSS) score is 15. Electrolytes, blood urea nitrogen (BUN), creatinine, complete blood count (CBC), platelets, prothrombin time/partial thromboplastin time (PT/PTT), and prealbumin are within normal limits, blood glucose is 310. Chest x-ray is clear, and a 12-lead ECG reveals atrial fibrillation. A computed tomography (CT) scan reveals a large area of lucency extending throughout the distribution of the left middle cerebral artery (MCA), and a diagnosis of left cerebral ischemic stroke is made.

By history, RK exhibits several risk factors for stroke: 20-year history of hypertension, type II diabetes, and chronic atrial fibrillation. RK's social history reveals that he has lived alone in a two-story house since his wife's death 5 years ago. RK had been independent in all activities prior to this admission. He has one adult son who lives within an hour's drive; the son is contacted by the social worker.

RK is started on a heparin drip and warfarin before transfer to the stroke unit. Additional orders include a carotid Doppler study, nutritional and social services consultations, application of antiembolic stockings, and a speech and language therapy consultation for assessment of swallowing and language function.

On arrival at the hospital, RK's son is advised of his

ADDRESOGRAPH

ST. LUKE'S EPISCOPAL HOSPITAL

Diagnosis: STROKE
DRG: 14/CD 9:434

Check One:

_____ Hemorrhagic (without craniotomy or coil embolization)

_____ Ischemic

_____ r+PA Study

Dysphagia Assessment Profile

- Dysphagia Diet _____
- Dysphagia Tubefed _____
- Pocketing Food _____
- Audible Swallow _____
- Double Swallow _____
- Cough on H2O _____
- Hx of Frequent U.R.I. _____
- Gag Reflex _____
- Wet voice After Swallow _____
- Dysarthria _____
- VII C.N. Palsy _____
- XII C.N. Palsy _____
- PEG Date _____
- Drooling _____
- Altered Phonation _____

Incomplete Labial Closure _____
"K" Sound _____
"L" sound _____
"M" sound _____

Communication
- Expressive Aphasia _____
- Receptive Aphasia _____
- Global Aphasia _____

Lab Data
- Prealbumin _____

Past Med. History
- Smoker _____
- Diabetic _____
- HTN _____
- Valve Disease _____
- CAD _____
- Atrial Fib. _____
- Previous Stroke _____
- Hx of Estrogen/Oral Contraceptive Prior to Admission _____

Location of Stroke
- Left Cerebellar _____
- Right Cerebellar _____
- Left Cerebral _____
- Right Cerebral _____
- Subcortical _____
- Brain Stem _____

Discharge
- Weight at Discharge _____
- Death _____
- Pre-Hospital Residence _____
- Family Residence _____
- 17 Rehab _____
- Outside Rehab _____
- Skilled Nursing _____

NIH Score at
- Discharge _____
- ICU LOS _____
- Discharge Date _____
- Dischare _____
- Prealbumin _____

DATE	Day +1 ___/___ PCS	Day +2 ___/___ PCS	Day +3 ___/___ PCS	Day +4 ___/___ PCS	Day +5 ___/___ PCS	Discharge
CONSULTS	Neurology CNS (x4455) Social Service Nutritional		PM&R Speech PRN			
DIAGNOSTIC	CXR CT Scan EKG CHEM 7 & 12 PT/PTT; CBC Carotid Doppler	PT/PTT (if on anticoagulant) Swallowing Test PRN				
TREATMENTS	NVS q 1-2 hrs. TED hose I&O Foley PRN Stool Softener Coumadin/Heparin IV	NVS q 1-2 hrs. Orthostatic VS Foley PRN Check BM; bowel program Continency program	NVS q 2-4 hrs. Orthastatic VS D/C Foley	DC IV		
ACTIVITY	Bedrest	Up in chair as tolerated	↑ up in chair Begin self-grooming/feed	- ↑ OOB activity Partial bath		
NUTRITION	RN assessment of swallowing; diet as indicated Weight _____ lbs.	Soft Diet Dysphagia Diet Tube Feed Weight _____ kg			Weight _____ kg	
TEACHING	Unit orientation Stroke booklet Stroke support information		Assess for learning/ reinforcement	Assess for learning/ reinforcement	Discharge	
DISCHARGE PLANNING	SNF/Home Arrangements				Discharge	
N.I.H. STROKE SCALE SCORE	Score = _____ *To be completed by Research Team					

14

Potential Patient Variances:
1. Hemodynamic instability - vasoactive drugs
2. Hemodynamic instability - activity intolerance
3. Decreased LOC
4. Cardiac arrhythmias (specify)
5. Fever ≥ 101°F (specify)
6. Pneumonia diagnosed
7. Atelectasis
8. Other infection diagnosed
9. Inadequate nutrition - underfed
10. Interrupted nutrition (indicate reason)
11. Alteration in GI function (specify, i.e., diarrhea, nausea/vomiting)
12. Skin breakdown - pressure related
13. Ventilator dependency
14. Suspected aspiration
15. Aspiration on modified barium swallow
16. Pulmonary secretions (described)
17. Hyperventilation therapy for cerebral edema
18. Diuretic therapy for cerebral edema
19. Steroid therapy for cerebral edema
20. Disoriented x 1 (time)
21. Disoriented x 2 (time, place)
22. Disoriented x 3 (time, place, person)
23. Seizures
24. Negative family/significant other dynamics
25. Incontinence (any type)

System Variances
1. No bed on 17 Tower.
2. No bed available in outside rehab.
3. No insurance coverage for rehab.
4. No medicare SNF bed available.
5. No medicaid SNF bed available.
5. No insurance coverage for SNF.
6. Delayed insurance verification.
7. Patient/family refuses D/C plan.

Date	Unit	Variances (#)	Action Taken	Other Patient or System Variances	Nurse's Signature

father's current potential for rehabilitation at discharge by the healthcare team. Both RK and his son receive instruction about the stroke process, with emphasis on the rehabilitative phase of care due to the lack of curative processes for stroke. The social worker provides RK's son with a list of rehabilitation centers close to his home and advises him to evaluate these potential discharge sites.

Pathway Day 2

RK is assessed to be at high risk for aspiration by the speech and language therapist; a modified barium swallow study is ordered and confirms potential for aspiration. A nasoenteric feeding tube is inserted, and RK is started on full-strength tube feedings as recommended by the nutrition support dietitian. Speech therapy is started for RK's expressive aphasia.

Nursing assesses RK's neurologic vital signs every 2 hours for changes and begins getting RK out of bed to a chair. He is encouraged to reassume supported participation in activities of daily living. Physical therapy and occupational therapy are started. RK and his son discuss potential rehabilitation centers close to home for discharge.

Pathway Days 3 to 5

RK is now actively participating in care to the best of his ability. He continues to receive daily physical, occupational, and speech/language therapy. He con-

tinues on warfarin, reaching a therapeutic PT level by day 4; heparin therapy is discontinued. RK's weight and prealbumin levels are stable; tube feedings continue, but are changed to a bolus routine to accommodate rehabilitation activities. Both RK and his son demonstrate a strong understanding of the need for rehabilitation, the risk factors for stroke and RK's specific stroke presentation, and RK's individualized multidisciplinary plan of care. No variances are noted on the critical pathway. RK is discharged to the rehabilitation center of his choice on day 5.

REFERENCES

1. American Nurses Association: Nursing: A Social Policy Statement. American Nurses Association, Kansas City, Mo, 1980, p 9.
2. Gordon, M: Nursing Diagnosis Process and Application, ed 3. McGraw-Hill, New York, 1994.
3. North American Nursing Diagnosis Association: Nursing Diagnoses: Definitions and Classifications, Philadelphia, 1994.
4. Marran, G, Barrett, MW, and Bevis, EO: Primary Nursing: A Model for Individualized Care, ed. 2. CV Mosby, St. Louis, 1979.
5. Zander, K: Second generation primary nursing. J Nurs Adm 15(3):18–24, 1985.
6. Hedberg, AM and Wojner, AW: Incorporating Nutrition Care into Critical Pathways for Improved Outcomes. Ross Products Division, Abbott Laboratories, Columbus, OH, 1994.
7. Ellwood, PM: Outcomes management: A technology of patient experience. N Engl J Med 318:1549–1556, 1988.
8. American Association of Critical-Care Nurses. Vision Statement. Aliso Viejo, CA, 1992.
9. Grady, G and Wojner, AW: The good fight. Am J Nursing Suppl November, 31–35, 1994.

C H A P T E R   3

Patient/Family Education: Principles of Teaching and Learning Applied to Critical Care Nursing

Carol A. Stephenson

CHAPTER OUTLINE

LEARNING OBJECTIVES

After completing this chapter, you should be able to:

1. Specify the goal of education of patient and family during the critical phase of illness.
2. State the principles of adult education that facilitate the teaching/learning process.
3. Give examples of how learning can be assessed and evaluated.
4. Identify factors that reduce learning.
5. Describe how the use of the nursing diagnosis ''knowledge deficit'' can be applied clinically.
6. Identify key factors in assessing learning needs.
7. Review the underlying purpose(s) for developing an educational program.
8. Describe the significance of stating specific objectives (goals or patient outcomes) in developing a teaching program.
9. State an objective using measurable terminology.
10. Define the usefulness of contracting as a strategy for patient education.

PHILOSOPHY OF PATIENT AND FAMILY EDUCATION APPLIED TO CRITICAL CARE NURSING

The citizens of our society have come to expect the best and most advanced health care to be available to them when they are ill. As a result, many persons are treated in critical care units. The events that occur in these units, while usually life-saving, can add to the stress of the catastrophic illness for patients and for their significant others. The persons involved are often glad that everything possible is being done for the ill family member, but they have little understanding of exactly what is being done and why. This can lead to unanswered questions, anger, and hostility because of lack of understanding or inappropriate expectations, and to poor cooperation because of not knowing either how or why to cooperate. Education of the patient and family, therefore, becomes a necessity during the critical care experience.

Goal of Education During the Critical Phase of Illness

Education in the critical care area should follow the same principles as education in other areas of health and illness. People use the same learning strategies and have the same barriers to learning when they are critically ill that they have during other times in their lives. However, because of the nature of the crisis, the barriers to learning are often much higher than they are in other situations. Therefore, it is inappropriate to dwell on long-term goals and teaching during catastrophic illness. Teaching in the critical care area should be aimed at what the patients and their significant others need to know at the present moment to cooperate or function and should aim to answer questions and impart basic understandings of the processes and technology involved.

In the critical care area, just as in other areas of patient teaching, the nurse should remember that teaching and learning are not synonymous. Just because the nurse has taught does not mean the patient has learned. Learning can be said to have occurred when a behavior change has occurred as a result of the material that has been taught. It is also important to realize that every instance of information giving is not a teaching/learning experience. If there are no goals for the experience or if teaching is not approached in a way that is optimal for learning, it is not a teaching/learning experience.

Principles of Adult Education

A large porportion of critically ill patients are adults. The parents of children and the significant others of critically ill adults also are usually adults. Therefore, selected principles of adult learning can be applied to teaching in the critical care unit.

Adult Learning: A Volitional Activity

The first consideration with regard to adult learning is that adults consider their learning experiences to be voluntary. Just as is true in any educational setting, patients have a right to choose to learn or not to learn. Even though the healthcare provider knows how much difference the information and resulting behavior changes could make in the health of a patient, there is no way to mandate learning or behavior changes. The nurse may work on motivating strategies to get the patient to want to learn, but the bottom line is that the patient will choose to learn or not to learn and the healthcare provider can do nothing about it. The patient may listen politely as the information is given and even actively participate in the learning experience. In the long run, however, the individual will decide whether to incorporate the information into his or her knowledge base and to act on it. The healthcare provider needs to respect the individual's choices in the matter and not downgrade care or respectful behaviors as a result.

A Trusting Relationship: Basis for Learning

When working with adults, the nurse-teacher has no actual authority over the student. No grades are given, and no deadlines for papers, projects, and the like are set. There is some perceived authority of the healthcare provider over the patient while the patient is in the healthcare setting, but this authority is lost when the patient leaves this setting. The nurse, therefore, must make the development of a collegial, trusting relationship an extremely high priority with regard to patient/family education. It is hoped that having this type of relationship will facilitate the client's learning.

Past Experiences: Impact on Learning

Adult patients bring more maturity and experience to the learning situation than do children and teenagers. This may be a positive or a negative factor in terms of the present learning situation. Past experiences alter the adult patient's expectations of any learning experience and may reduce the patient's expectations that learning can occur. Often, however, past experiences have led a person to have higher expectations of any learning experience than those that a child or a teenager would have. The nurse needs to be certain that the learning encounter is seen by patients as worthy of their time and effort, and that it is productive of useful information or skills.

With regard to maturity, many adults will be better able than youngsters to solve problems and see important concepts and relationships. For some, however, the years of maturing have simply intensified poor interpersonal skills and learning habits. Some adults may be completely closed to new learning experiences, believing they already know what they need to know about a topic. Others may believe they are unable to learn.

Children usually attend school because it is required. They have no specific goal for the educational experience except that of doing exactly what is expected of them. Adults, however, learn better if they have specific goals for learning. They need to know why the learning experience is occurring and what is to be achieved by it. Adults learn even more readily if they participate in stating the goals for the learning experience. In other words, adults define what they want to know or accomplish, and learning is aimed directly at meeting that goal. This leads to much more productive learning than when the nurse is armed with a sheet of paper specifying that "every person with this disease needs to know these things" and provides information without regard for the patient's priorities.

In the critical care area, the nurse should be sensitive to cues from the patient and the family that specify learning goals and should seek information as to the meaning of these cues. For example, when a patient returns from emergency neurosurgery with a bruised and battered face and two black eyes, the family may express concern over the appearance of the patient's face. This can be translated into a goal regarding gaining information about the cause of the altered facial appearance. The nurse can then explain about the frame that supported the patient's face during surgery and about the blood pooling that resulted and can relate these understandings to the altered facial appearance. The nurse can then follow up with information about how and when the bruising might resolve. This type of teaching will achieve the family's immediate goals related to that concern.

Adults may not always seek learning for the sake of learning. They may wish their learning experiences to be practical and meaningful. Before teaching, the nurse should be certain that the information to be given has meaning and practicality for the patient. This can usually be determined by a careful assessment prior to teaching. Information that can be used immediately or can be used to solve problems is usually deemed important by adults.

For some adults, any learning experience is traumatic. If they have had unpleasant educational experiences in the past, they are likely to react to any new learning experience as a traumatic one. The fact that this learning takes place in the presence of a crisis such as critical illness or injury only makes the experience that much more traumatic. The nurse should be alert to verbal and nonverbal cues from the patient and family, which may signal that the learning experience is stressful for them. The teaching approaches should then be modified accordingly.

Computerized Learning

A common method of learning today is through computerized materials. Many adults do not feel comfortable with these materials and do not know how to use computer equipment. Hence, they do *not* learn as well with computerized materials as with other methods. In addition, it is often difficult to individualize computerized materials to match a specific patient's needs. Thus, it is necessary to be certain that the patient can use them without feeling incompetent or threatened and to provide appropriate support during the learning experience if computers are used.

Use of Senses Enhances Learning

The more senses that are involved in learning, the better the patient will learn. A person who hears the concept, sees an illustration or a film of it, and practices and discusses it will retain it much better than one who only hears the concept.

Familiarity Reinforces Learning

Adult learning is more effective when it relates to or builds on familiar concepts. The nurse should get to know patients well enough to be able to use concepts that will be familiar to them and to build on familiar knowledge when teaching new concepts. The nurse who can develop analogies to whatever concepts patients are familiar with will be more successful than the nurse who uses the same explanations for all patients.

Learning Process—Simple to Complex

Learning is enhanced when it proceeds from the simple to the complex. The learning experience should be planned as much as possible so that the simplest concepts are taught first. These concepts can then be used as a base for teaching the more complicated aspects of the topic. Teaching the simpler information first builds success, motivation, and self-confidence.

The teaching/learning environment is important for adult learners, who seem to learn best in a comfortable and informal setting. The situation should be as pleasant as possible. Accommodations should be made as necessary for visual and hearing deficits.

Factors That Reduce Learning

Some of the factors that reduce learning relate directly to the previously described principles of adult learning.

Poor Motivation

If patients see the learning as impractical or unnecessary or if they view it as being in competition with their own belief structure, they will probably be poorly motivated to learn. Adults must want to learn the material and believe it to be valuable.

A nurse once discovered the importance of this while attempting to teach an anemic patient about foods high in iron. The patient was openly hostile to a discussion of iron-rich foods. Finally, the nurse asked why the patient was not interested in the discussion. He explained that he regularly listened to a certain radio program (presented by a food faddist), and from that program, he learned that apples are rich in iron. The evidence presented was the fact that when left open to air, apples turn brown. The faddist explained that the brown is iron. This patient, therefore, ate apples or applesauce daily and was absolutely convinced that he was eating a diet rich in iron!

Low Self-Esteem and Increasing Age

Low self-esteem and increasing age can affect learning. Increasing age tends to reduce openness to new ideas. Some persons believe they are "too old to learn" or that they are incapable of learning. The nurse may be put in the position of having to convince patients that they are capable of learning before they will tackle the learning experience.

The Issue of Literacy

A related problem is literacy. The nurse should not assume that an adult patient can learn with written materials. The patient's reading skills may be so poor that this is not possible. Though the national median literacy level is at the 10th-grade level, 20% of the US population reads at a fifth-grade level or lower.[1]

All written material should be read and discussed. The most important aspects should be pointed out and underlined or highlighted. This is not to say that written materials should not accompany teaching as an aid to recall. Actually, they are invaluable references for almost all patients. However, the nurse should be aware that not everyone will be able to read and understand written materials. In addition, printed materials should be written at a reading level appropriate to the learner. Highly technical language and healthcare provider "jargon" should be avoided. Use of simple pictures or diagrams can augment learning for individuals with poorer reading skills.

Belief Systems

The patient's belief system about whether recommended actions can make a difference is critical to learning. Many persons do not adhere to their therapeutic program simply because they do not believe their actions make a difference or because they do not believe they are at risk. A common example: Few persons today would tell you that they truly do not believe that smoking cigarettes is hazardous to the health of most persons. However, those persons who smoke often say that they do not perceive themselves to be at risk for the known hazards of smoking. They say they have smoked for a given number of years and nothing has happened yet. As a result, they keep on smoking.

Others perceive themselves as victims: They are ill and say they don't know why. They also say that whatever is going to happen will happen whether or not they cooperate with their care, take their medicines, do their exercises, and the like. With this attitude, why bother to buy medicine, cooperate with therapy, or keep appointments?

Anxiety, Fear, Pain, and Medications

Anxiety, fear, discomfort, and medications such as analgesics and sedatives all reduce the individual's ability to pay attention and perceive what is going on in the learning experience. If any of these is present, it can be so overwhelming that the patient may recall nothing else that happened during a given period of time. These factors need to be dealt with and relieved before trying to teach a patient. However, if relieving discomfort involves the use of drugs that reduce perception and cognitive abilities, patients, although they are happier and more comfortable, may be just as unable to learn as they were prior to pain relief. Family members or significant others also experience a lack of attention and the inability to retain information because of the stress of the critical illness event. Information needs to be repeated often and written down.

Self-Pride

Pride is another problem in teaching adults. It is not uncommon for adults to attempt to conceal their lack of knowledge because to admit it would cause "loss of face" or injury to their pride. Such persons would rather do without the knowledge than admit their need for it. The nurse can often deal with this by providing privacy for the learning experience or by presenting a topic in terms such as "a lot of people say this is a problem for them . . . Have you found it to be a problem for you?" Sometimes, group classes help to deal with this problem because one patient will ask a question or admit a problem that another patient may be too proud to admit.

Some persons have developed poor learning skills. They may not have learned how to learn or how to use the resources that are available to them. If the nurse finds this to be the case, it may be necessary to do some remedial teaching about how to learn before teaching the intended content.

Unrealistic Goals or Expectations

Another common poor learning skill is unrealistic goals or expectations. In this event, patients are frustrated when they cannot achieve their self-imposed goals. The nurse will have to assist these patients to revise their goals so as to be realistic. This is often difficult because such revisions may be viewed as a sign of incompetence.

The relationship between the patient and the nurse greatly affects learning. Some patients are openly hostile to the idea of being taught anything. Others simply do not trust the nurse to be able to teach them. A great number of factors contribute to these situations. The nurse must assess and deal with them as well as possible. In some cases, it simply is not possible to teach the patient. In others, teaching is possible only after a rapport has been established. In still others, another person such as a physician or a different nurse may be able to relate better to the patient. Because the ultimate goal is teaching patients what they want and need to know, all possible alternatives should be explored. Certainly, the nurse should approach each patient with an attitude of respect, regardless of his or her individual behaviors.

Nursing Diagnosis: Knowledge Deficit

When doing nursing care plans related to patient education, the accepted nursing diagnosis is "knowledge deficit." The cause of the knowledge deficit varies with the patient. Some may never have had access to the knowledge before or may have forgotten or misinterpreted it. Others may have been taught poorly or at a time when they were not able to learn. Still others may be receiving competing or conflicting information from family, acquaintances, or even healthcare providers. For some patients, the knowledge or related behaviors may be in direct conflict with their belief systems and usual practices.

Some sample information related to this nursing diagnosis is presented in Table 3–1. It is intended only as a starting point for the nurse in preparing nursing care plans. Much individualization will be necessary.

Assessment of Learning Needs

It is very important that patient education not be done on the basis of what the healthcare provider believes the patient needs to know. If formal teaching is to be done, a complete learning assessment should be carried out first.

To accomplish this, the nurse should spend time with the patient and family discussing what they know about the topic and what questions they have. It is very helpful to ask what the patient and family want to know and learn. Teaching may reinforce and build on what they already know. It can also be a time to recognize and reinforce positive health behaviors. It is helpful to attempt to discover what support systems and resources the patient has available, as well as areas in which support or resources are clearly lacking. The nurse should also assess for the presence or absence

TABLE 3–1
Nursing Diagnosis: Knowledge Deficit

Nursing Diagnosis	Desired Patient Outcomes	Nursing Interventions	Evaluation Strategies
Knowledge Deficit Defining characteristics: • Verbalization or performance indicating inadequate knowledge or skill, misunderstandings • Poor utilization of previously taught information • Poor compliance or adherence • Evidence of cognitive impairment • Verbalization of questions or requests for information; complaints about lack of information • Poor knowledge of or utilization of resources • Hostility or unwillingness to participate in learning experience	The patient will: • Correctly complete verbal or written post-test on information that has been taught. • Demonstrate on follow-up visits that information is being used or followed appropriately. • Consistently and correctly perform skills that have been taught. • Verbalize that his or her priorities have been met and questions have been answered. • Verbalize plans to use the material that is taught. • If patient is cognitively impaired, family is taught and verbalizes or demonstrates understanding.	• Assess patient's and family's learning needs carefully; check present knowledge, skills, beliefs. • Adhere to teaching/learning principles. • Include family or significant others in teaching. • Include frequent return demonstrations, post-tests, validation of learning; give support and re-teach PRN. • Use frequent repetition. • Teach by example. • Make appropriate referrals to resource agencies. • Break learning into small parts, which are taught in a logical order and form. • Build success and praise into the experience. • Do not punish for failure. • Save long-term teaching for a time when the situation is no longer critical. • Incorporate learned materials or skills into daily hospital routine. • Use varied but appropriate learning strategies. • If patient is hostile or noncompliant, try to find out why and deal with the problem before teaching; do not force teaching on patient. • If patient is cognitively impaired, limit teaching of patient to what he or she needs to know to function or seems to want to know.	• Give verbal or written post-test. • Conduct an informal follow-up and discussion to check understanding. • On follow-up visits, review understanding, practices, and adherence. • Allow patient and family to do return demonstrations and practice skills frequently. • Ask patient if priorities have been met and questions have been answered. • Teaching of cognitively impaired patient is limited to necessary material; family is taught more. • Ask patient to describe plans to use material. • Note whether the same questions are repeated often or the same unsafe practices are repeated.

of key factors as discussed in the previous section on Principles of Adult Education and for barriers to learning such as lack of motivation, unreadiness to learn, hostility, the presence of pain or anxiety, and the like. These are just as important to deal with as knowledge deficit.

Noncritical Care Setting

In the noncritical care situation, the focus of the assessment may be different from when the patient is critically ill. During the crisis, the patient and family need to focus their energies on coping with the present. This is not the time for long-range planning or discharge teaching. Rather, it is the time for discovering present fears and anxieties as well as what information the patient and significant others want and need during the crisis. After the patient is out of the critical phase of illness, a reassessment can be performed and a new, longer-range teaching plan can be developed. The importance of setting priorities in terms of teaching/learning is illustrated in the following mini-case study.

MINI-CASE STUDY: PATIENT WITH SPINAL CORD INJURY

Mr. H, age 32, is in the ICU 24 hours post-trauma. He has a spinal cord injury without a neurologic deficit. He is on a kinetic bed, which rotates him constantly side to side 60 degrees, and he has tongs to his head. The tongs are attached to traction weights. He is NPO with a nasogastric tube in place. Mr. H is alert and oriented but says very little. He is wide-eyed and appears anxious. He holds his body stiff and clutches the sides of the bed as it turns as if to keep from falling.

Mindy, a senior nursing student, is assigned to care for Mr. H. When she presents her nursing care plan to her instructor, it shows the following:

Nursing Diagnosis. Altered nutrition: excess, related to excess intake, resulting in moderate obesity.

Goal. Within 2 days,
1. Patient will state a specific goal for weight loss.
2. Patient and wife will identify and describe an appropriate diet.

Nursing Interventions
1. Discuss obesity with patient and the need to lose weight.
2. Teach appropriate diet.
3. Help patient set goals for weight loss.

Although the format is acceptable, this nursing care plan has several problems. First, the student (who was quite thin) imposed her priorities on the patient and his wife. Second, even if she did the teaching at this time, the patient and his wife wouldn't hear it. In fact, the student's lack of sensitivity might greatly reduce her rapport with them on a long-term basis.

How much better it would have been if Mindy, after introducing herself, had approached the situation something like this:

Mindy: Mr. H, you don't look very comfortable to me. Is there a problem I can help you with?
Mr. H: No, I'm not comfortable. I hurt all over. I'm afraid I'll fall out of this contraption if I go to sleep.

At this point, Mindy has a choice. She could, as many nurses do, reassure the patient—"Oh, don't be silly. Nobody has fallen out of one of these beds yet. You just relax and let us take care of everything." However, this is not teaching and would do little toward meeting the needs of the patient.

A better choice is to discuss the two problems that have been brought up: pain and fear of falling. The conversation might go like this:

Mindy: Are you having a great deal of pain right now?
Mr. H: I sure am.
Mindy (looking at chart): I see you haven't had a shot for pain for 8 hours. You can have it every 3 hours if you need it.
Mr. H: Nobody told me that.
Mindy: I'll get you a shot now. You tell the nurses when you are hurting so they can try to keep you more comfortable. They need your help to know how you are feeling.
Mr. H: I didn't know I could ask for a shot. I thought the nurses would know what to do and when.
Mindy: No, they need you to tell them what you are feeling and when you need something.

This portion of the interaction is brief, but Mindy has informally taught Mr. H something valuable about communication in the hospital. With this understanding, Mr. H can more readily participate in decision-making regarding his care. It will be relatively easy to evaluate his learning by observing his communication behaviors over the next few days.

After Mr. H is comfortable from the medication, Mindy can then address the fear of falling:

Mindy: Mr. H, you said you are afraid of relaxing because you might fall out of the bed.
Mr. H: I sure am. You must know what you're doing, but this is a scary contraption you've got me in.
Mindy: Would it help if I explain the bed and your traction to you? I can show you why you're on it and how you are protected from falling.
Mr. H: I really need that. Could my wife come in and learn about the bed, too?

Mindy can then call in Mrs. H and explain Mr. H's traction and bed to them in clear, simple terms. She can explain why this bed is necessary, how it is better right now than a "regular" bed, and the bed's safety features. She can later evaluate this discussion in several ways: by asking Mr. and Mrs. H if they have questions after she finishes; by asking them to explain key points back to her; and, most important, by observing whether Mr. H is able to relax and stop clinging to the bed as it rotates. Mindy would then document her teaching and its results in her nurse's notes as follows:

> 16:30—Appears anxious and uncomfortable. Clinging to the bed constantly. Body rigid. In response to questioning, states he is in pain and afraid of falling. Medicated for pain. Discussed the need for him to keep nurses informed of pain and other subjective problems. Explained purpose of traction and bed to patient and wife. Pointed out safeguards to prevent falling. They expressed understanding.
>
> 18:00—Apparently sleeping. Appears relaxed.

Just because Mindy did this teaching today does not mean it won't need repeating tomorrow. As stated earlier, pain, fear, and anxiety reduce perception and information retention. Simple explanations may need to be given on a daily basis or even several times a day. This does not mean the teaching should not be done or is unsuccessful.

Perception is reduced even more if the patient's cognitive abilities are reduced by medication or disease, by trauma, or by surgery. The patient may have the ability to understand simple explanations at the time, but may forget the information within the hour. Major teaching in this case should be done for the family; the patient needs to be taught only what is absolutely necessary for immediate care activities. For example, the family of a patient who has had a cerebral vascular accident (CVA, or stroke) should be taught about what a stroke is, its general treatment, the expectations for rehabilitation, and the like. However, the stroke-injured patient may not have the cognitive abilities to deal with this type of teaching. Teaching should be confined to the patient's immediate needs, such as how to scan the environment to compensate for visual field losses or how to support the affected arm and leg when turning.

PROGRAM DEVELOPMENT

Program Purposes

There are two overall purposes for developing teaching programs. One is to develop a generic program, which includes all the information that a patient with a particular problem is likely to need to know (such as a cardiac rehabilitation program). Once this program is developed, its component parts can be used one at a time with particular patients to supplement knowledge and skills until they have learned what is necessary and essential. This is an excellent way to plan programs to be used on units that have many patients with similar problems (such as cardiac units, diabetic units, orthopedic surgery units, pulmonary medicine units). Patients in these types of units often have similar learning needs. After the program is well developed, it is easy for an individual nurse to adapt it to an individual patient.

This type of program is not always successful in the critical care unit, however. As has been pointed out, the patients and their families are stressed to the point where long-term learning and planning are not possible. It is often more appropriate to plan individual learning programs directed at the particular needs of individual patients and their families.

If the unit is a specialized one that receives many similar patients, it may be helpful to plan *mini-programs* to address common problems of patients and families. If this is done, the nurse does not have to generate a completely new teaching program each time it is needed. For example, a news article on premature infant ICUs focused on one of the parents. It states, "By the time their son was able to come home . . . [the mother] had become an expert on the problems of premature babies. She speaks knowledgeably of transcutaneous oxygen monitors and eye problems that often affect the babies. 'They sent me through a whole medical course,' she says, 'but understanding what was going on was the only thing that saved me.'"[2]

It is conceivable that such a unit might have some prepared materials and simple diagrams or displays regarding such topics as transcutaneous monitors, ventilators, infant hyperalimentation, why a premature infant looks the way he or she does, and parenting needs of premature infants. There would be no point in generating this information from scratch for each parent whose child is admitted to the unit. Individual needs could be added to the teaching plan for each parent. Individualization would also attend to the fact that many other parents might not want or be able to comprehend as much information as this mother did.

Negotiating and Writing Objectives

After the assessment is done, the nurse and the patient can ask, "What does he or she need to know and how will we both know when it is known?" It is critical that the patient be able to specify what learning is important. If nurses teach only what meets their priorities, they may risk losing the patient's desire to learn. Also, by knowing what the patient already knows and does well, nurses can avoid undermining the patient's intelligence and wasting time by re-teaching that material. Teaching the information that is priority knowledge for the patient first increases the desire to learn and ensures patient satisfaction that learning needs are being met. Together, the nurse and patient can set measurable objectives and target dates for their achievement. After that, learning experiences can be planned to meet the objectives.

Evaluation is the last part of the plan and should be based directly on the objectives. Sometimes, the planning may be done formally and the nurse will return at another time to teach. In the critical care unit, however, it is often appropriate to do the teaching as soon as the objective has been stated formally or informally. It is important to know what the objective or goal is so that both nurse and patient know what is to be achieved by the interaction. With a clearly stated objective, both will know when they have achieved it. Without such an objective, they may have differing opinions on what, if anything, was achieved. The objectives will also be a valuable aid to selecting teaching content, strategies, and instructional aids.

Domains of Learning

Objectives can be written in any of the three recognized domains of learning. The *cognitive* or *thinking domain* is concerned with intellectual abilities such as remembering, analyzing, evaluating, and creative thinking. The *affective domain,* which is used less in patient teaching but in some cases may be vitally important, is related to feelings and emotions about the topic in question. Finally, the *psychomotor domain* relates to the performance of skills that require the coordination of body muscles. In other words, this is the doing part of learning.

Statement of the Objective: Specific Components

The statement of the objective has four parts. First, there is a description of the learner. This may simply be "the patient with pulmonary disease" or a like statement. It must be specific enough to distinguish the learner in this case as being different from "anyone, anywhere." The material to be taught is for a person with a specific learning need, not just for anyone. Second, there is a statement about what will be performed or a statement of the behavior to be exhibited if learning has taken place. Third, there is a description of the conditions under which that performance will occur. Finally, there is a standard of accuracy (criterion statement) or how well the performance must be done to be acceptable.

Writing Objectives: Measurable Terminology

The performance statement must be in observable behavioral terms. Often, as healthcare providers, we think we are giving good directions, but in actuality, the patient does not have enough information to accomplish the task or objective. For example, how often do healthcare providers ask patients to "drink plenty of fluids"? For some patients, this may mean four cups of coffee a day; for others, continual fluid ingestion. How much more easily the patient would be able to comply with directions such as "drink eight 8-ounce glasses of fluid a day" or "drink one-half glass of fluid every hour." Terms that cannot be observed or measured are not helpful in aiding the nurse or the patient to know when learning has been achieved.

The statement must be in terms of learner behaviors, not teacher behaviors. For example, a statement such as "to teach the importance of high fluid intake" is a teacher behavior or patient outcome. A statement of learner behavior might be "to list three reasons for

a fluid intake of 2500 mL per day" or "to ingest 2500 mL of fluids per day." Each objective should include only one statement of a behavior.

The performance statement should avoid ambiguous and unmeasurable terms such as:

to know	to understand	to appreciate
to grasp the significance of	to enjoy	to believe
	to have faith in	to want
to perceive	to like	to master
to become	to learn	to feel

The acceptable terms for performance may include many specific terms, only some of which are included here:

to write	to define	to list
to identify	to indicate	to state
to compare	to compute	to contrast
to describe	to differentiate	to discuss
to distinguish	to classify	to apply
to calculate	to demonstrate	to practice
to solve	to use	to analyze
to explain	to summarize	to integrate
to plan	to organize	to assess
to evaluate	to rank	to measure

Stating the conditions under which the performance will take place may includes terms such as the following:

given	using	following
provided with	starting with	beginning with

Finally, the performance standard will describe an acceptable performance. It may include a statement such as "with 80% accuracy," "within 30 minutes," or the like.

Some sample objectives are listed below:
1. Given a diagram of the lungs, the patient will, with 90% accuracy, identify the structures.
2. Provided with a blank injection rotation diagram, the diabetic patient will plan an appropriate site rotation schedule within 30 minutes.

Preparing a Teaching Plan

The nurse can ask several questions when preparing a teaching plan. These include the following:
1. What are the characteristics of the patient?
2. What are the patient's learning priorities?
3. What does the patient need to know?
4. What is my educational purpose?
5. How can I determine if learning has occurred?

The above questions can be used to aid the nurse in developing a set of objectives for the learning experience. The objectives should be as precise as possible so they will be useful as a teaching guide for the nurse and a learning guide for the patient. The following sample objectives might be used in a master teaching plan in a critical care unit where many patients who have emphysema are admitted. It could be individualized according to the learning priorities and prior knowledge of each patient and family.

Given a brief discussion, visual aids, and written

materials, the patient or family member(s) will be able to do the following with 100% accuracy:

1. Identify emphysema by name and general description.
2. Describe the pathology of emphysema.
3. State how the emphysematous lungs differ from normal lungs in terms of structure and function.
4. List the major causes of emphysema.
5. Describe the major symptoms of emphysema and relate these to the client's symptoms.
6. Very generally, describe the care of emphysema. (Care would be taught more specifically at another time when the crisis period is over.)

A simple teaching plan could then be built on these objectives. It would include four columns: the objectives, the content related to the objectives, the teaching strategies and resources, and, finally, the methods of evaluation. See Table 3–2 for an example of a teaching plan.

Evaluation Process

The methods of evaluation would directly relate back to the objectives. In some way, the nurse would evaluate attainment of an objective by asking the patient to do whatever the objective states. For example, if the objective says, "list . . . ," the patient could be asked to list the material verbally or in writing. If the objective asks the patient to "describe . . . ," this could be done verbally during a discussion or in writing. If the objective asks the patient to "perform . . . ," the evaluation would be done by watching the patient perform the task and evaluating it according to accuracy of performance.

In an earlier example of a performance objective, the patient was asked "to ingest 2500 mL of fluids per day." A simple way to evaluate the accomplishment of this objective or goal is to look at the patient's intake sheet for the 24-hour period. If the intake was 2500 mL or more, the goal was accomplished. If the intake was less than 2500 mL, the nurse should seek the reasons why the goal was not accomplished. Perhaps the patient was NPO for several hours for diagnostic tests. In this case, the best route might be to re-evaluate the intake the next day. Perhaps the patient did not understand the teaching or did not like the idea of taking in so many fluids. In this case, the nurse must go back to the original goal and teaching strategies and find another way to motivate the patient to drink; or to help the patient learn why fluids are so important; or how to stagger the intake so he or she is drinking small amounts frequently instead of trying to ingest larger amounts at longer intervals. The evaluation process, therefore, not only helps the nurse to know that teaching has been effective, but is a guide to the need for re-teaching or revision of teaching techniques and strategies.

In addition to all of the teaching principles listed so far, nurses should remember that they teach by example as well as by planned verbal interactions. For example, what is the patient really going to believe if the nurse who is teaching about the hazards of smoking and why it should be stopped has tobacco-stained fingernails and smells heavily of smoke? The nurse who follows a healthy diet and exercise program will teach more by example when discussing these topics than the nurse who is obviously overweight and out of condition. In teaching adults, healthcare providers cannot get by with imparting a message such as "do as I tell you—not as I do."

To summarize the planning of objectives and teaching strategies, an instructional objective should describe the intended learning outcome or behaviors rather than summarizing teaching content. The objectives will be stated in terms of learner behaviors rather than teacher behaviors. For most teaching programs, there will be a series of objectives rather than just one objective. The objective statements should include four parts as previously described. These objective statements then become the guide for selecting teaching content and strategies and for selecting evaluation strategies. Finally, the learner should have a copy of the objectives so that he or she knows what is to be learned. All teaching and the evaluation of its outcomes should be documented in the patient's record.

The teaching plan in Table 3–2 was selected as an example of information that many critically ill patients want and that could be taught relatively easily and quickly. After the assessment has been done and the nurse has found that the patient and his or her significant others do not understand the nature of the illness but would like to do so, the teaching could be done at the earliest opportunity when the patient is awake and relatively comfortable and when interruptions are unlikely. The nurse could take the visual aids and resource materials to the bedside, sit down with the patient and significant others, inform them of what they should understand about the nature of the illness, and encourage them to ask questions.

Nurses should not use the content column of the teaching plan verbatim but should use it as a guide to discuss the disease in their own words. Nurses should allow the patient and significant others time to look at the visual aids and to ask questions. When summarizing the care portion of the teaching, nurses can relate the care back to what has already been said, for example, "there is aminophylline in this IV you are receiving. This drug will open up your airways and help you to breathe more easily. It should relieve some of your shortness of breath and your need to sit up to breathe. It will also help you to clear your airways because they will be more open when you cough."

The nurse can evaluate learning immediately after the teaching presentation or on an ongoing basis for the next few days. For example, when changing the IV aminophylline, the nurse might say, "I have your new bag of aminophylline here. Tell me what you remember about the reason you are receiving it." The client's answer will alert the nurse as to whether re-teaching is necessary.

TABLE 3–2
Sample Teaching Plan: "What Is Emphysema?"

Objective*	Content	Teaching Strategy/Resources	Evaluation Strategy
Identify emphysema by name and general description.	Emphysema and chronic bronchitis are two diseases ordinarily grouped under the title of chronic obstructive lung disease (COPD). Although they often occur together, a person may have predominantly one disease or the other.	Individualize discussion according to the patient's primary disease.	Ask patient to name his or her disease process.
Name the major pertinent respiratory structures and cite the changes in emphysema.	Structure and function of normal lungs: • Purpose of breathing is to get oxygen into the body. • Oxygen provides energy for body functions. • The lungs eliminate the waste product of oxygen use, carbon dioxide. Major pertinent respiratory structures: airways, alveoli, diaphragm • Lungs are elastic spongy tissue. • Airways are hollow, branching tubes like upside-down trees. • Alveoli are air sacs. • Alveoli help keep the airways open during exhalation. • Oxygen and carbon dioxide pass through alveolar walls to and from blood. • Diaphragm is major muscle of respiration. Pathology of emphysema: • Walls of alveoli tear or are destroyed. • There is less area for oxygen exchange. • Airways tend to collapse on expiration. • Airway collapse leads to air trapping and reduced ability to use the diaphragm. • This increases the work of breathing and reduces body oxygen levels.	*Medical Illustrations of Common Disorders of the Respiratory Tract.* Normal airway and lung diagram; emphysema diagram (Lilly publication). An illustration of the diaphragm and its location.	Ask patient to name the pictured lung structures and identify briefly the changes that occur in emphysema.

Describe the general care of emphysema.	The disease can be controlled, not cured.
	• Medications:
	  ○ To open airways (bronchodilators).
	  ○ To reduce inflammation (corticosteroids).
	  ○ To treat infection (antibiotics).
	  ○ To improve oxygenation (oxygen).
	  ○ To reduce water retention if necessary (diuretics).
		As each drug is administered, state briefly what its name is and the major purpose for which it is given.	After the drug has been given and discussed several times, name the drug while administering it and ask the patient to name its purpose.

*Both content and depth should vary according to the patient's condition and ability to learn.

Contracting

Contracting, a strategy for patient education, involves the writing of a contract between patient and nurse. The contract specifies behaviors to be done by the patient and a reward or reinforcer that will be received as a result. The idea of contracting is based on the theory that if a positive reinforcer is received soon after a behavior, the person will be more likely to perform the behavior again.[3] As with any other type of patient education, contracting should be based on a thorough assessment of behaviors, knowledge, and beliefs. It is not finished until the nurse and the

I,_____ , will _____

_____, in return for _____

_____.

Signed _____

Signed _____

Date _____

FIGURE 3–1. A sample contract. (From Steckel,[3] p 44, with permission.)

[*Note:* This part of the page is left blank so that the client and nurse can identify bonuses or future successive approximations. It is also used to record information the client might want, such as blood pressure, weight, diet suggestions, telephone numbers, and so on.]

patient have mutually agreed on the patient's learning priorities.

Contracting can be helpful for a variety of reasons. First, it removes any doubt by the patient as to what behavior is expected. Objectives for the contract are stated very specifically so that both patient and nurse know exactly what the patient is expected to do, under what conditions, and when.

In some cases, patients are more willing and able to adhere to the treatment program if they are working for a reward or a reinforcer. The reinforcer should be meaningful to and, ideally, selected by the patient.

The use of contracts can make the reinforcement of correct behaviors more consistent. Healthcare providers may feel they frequently reinforce patient behaviors by praise, recognition of effort, and the like. Actually this is not usually done systematically, so the patient doesn't expect the praise or other reinforcer to occur every time the behavior is done. With contracting, the nurse and the patient agree on the behavior and the reinforcer ahead of time. Then the reinforcer is given without fail when the behavior is exhibited.

Another advantage of using contracts is to give the patient optimal credit for maintaining his or her health. All too often, the healthcare providers are quick to place blame on the patient when health is not maintained or improved, but if it is improved, the treatment or healthcare providers get the credit.

Contracting also reduces the likelihood that the patient will be scolded or punished as the result of poor health behaviors. If poor behaviors occur, nothing is said. The reinforcer simply is not given.

Writing a Contract. After assessing the patient's beliefs and behaviors, the patient and the nurse should decide on the patient's learning priorities. The learning can then be broken down into smaller bits, each of which can be accomplished rather quickly. The behaviors for the first step will be on the first contract. These are stated so that they are well defined, observable, and measurable. A date by which the behavior will be displayed should be specified. The reinforcer or privilege should be clearly specified, as should a description of what will occur when the con-

tract is not fulfilled (if this is appropriate). In some cases, a bonus clause may be added as a reward for extra accomplishments. Any record-keeping that is to be done should also be specified in the contract. Steckel[3] has developed a very simple contract form (Fig. 3–1).

A Contracting Vocabulary. Definitions of terms pertaining to contracting are presented below, based on Steckel[3]:

Contract: An agreement between a patient and a healthcare provider, which specifies a behavior to be done, a date by which it is to be done, and a reinforcer to be received as a result

Reinforcer: A tangible or intangible consequence that strengthens a behavior

Negative reinforcer: A consequence whose removal strengthens a behavior; not a punishment

Strengthening a behavior: Increasing the chance that behavior will be repeated

Consequence: The result of a behavior

Reward: A pleasant experience but one that does not necessarily strengthen a behavior

MINI-CASE STUDY: PATIENT WITH SEVERE BURNS

MS was a 15-year-old girl recovering from severe burns of her hands and arms. Despite the use of analgesics, physical therapy was very painful for her. As a result, she was so combative and uncooperative that little was being accomplished in the therapy sessions. During a discussion with M and her mother, the nurse discovered that M wanted some cassette tapes of a certain rock star very badly. With that in mind, M, her mother, and the nurse formulated a plan: Each day that M cooperated with the physical therapist rather than fighting, a check would be put on a graph, which was taped to the wall of her room. Five consecutive checks would earn her a tape, to be purchased by her mother. If she missed a day of being cooperative, nothing would be said. Instead, she would start again at the next session to work toward her goal of five consecutive checks.

M's contract would look like this:

I, M_____S_____, will earn five consecutive checks for cooperating with my physical therapy exercises in return for a rock tape of my choice to be purchased by my mother.

Signed—M_____S_____
Signed—CS_____, RN
Date—November 13, 1989

As a result of the contract, M was much more cooperative and began to make progress with her therapy. After using this contract several times, a new contract was written, which required more consecutive checks and which changed the reinforcer to something else M wanted. Notice that the contract did not specify that the physical therapy sessions produce results, only that M cooperate. Whether it is weight loss, respiratory function, or anything else, results are often not predictable enough to use in contracts. Behaviors that would lead to the desired results are more predictable and easier to count. Certainly the behavior should be reinforced, regardless of the results.

Reinforcers do not have to be objects or things. They may be intangibles such as spending time with a special person, discussion of a topic of the client's choice, and reading a story together.

PATIENT EDUCATION RESOURCES

Many resources are available for patient education. The more familiar nurses are with educational principles and materials, the more effective they can be as educators. If nurses are using prepared or purchased materials, they should evaluate them carefully as to appropriateness and usability. The materials should be modified as necessary to meet the needs of the individual patient teaching situation.

A reading list of resources is included at the end of this chapter. This is only a sampling of materials available. Some of the materials may seem old at first glance, but they are classics and can be extremely helpful. Visual aids and pamphlets can often be obtained at low cost or at no cost from drug companies and voluntary agencies such as the American Heart Association, American Lung Association, American Cancer Society, and American Diabetes Association.

SUMMARY

Patient and family education is an integral part of nursing care in every setting. When the educational process is conducted in the critical care setting, the basic principles of teaching and learning apply. Some of the principles become extremely important in such settings. A person's ability to learn and retain information is impeded greatly by anxiety, fear, pain, drugs, and the like. As a result, teaching in the critical care setting should be confined to information that the patient and significant others need to know at the time.

Long-term teaching and plans for care should be delayed until the patient is out of the critical care area. Even when teaching is confined to the urgent learning needs of those in the critical care setting, retention and compliance may be poor. As a result, repetition becomes important. Nurses continually assess critical knowledge and behaviors and should be willing to repeat the teaching of critical material as often as necessary. To aid patient education, it is a good idea for a unit to prepare teaching materials, visual aids, and resources for teaching topics that are used frequently. These can then be easily individualized to any patient situation. Placing simple educational materials in family areas may also be useful. However, this strategy should not be used solely to substitute for personal, individualized teaching.

REFERENCES

1. Redman, BK: The Process of Patient Education, ed 7. Mosby-Year Book, St. Louis, 1993.
2. Sanz, C: The reality behind the miracle babies. Dallas Morning News, Nov 1987, p 10C.
3. Steckel, S: Patient Contracting. Appleton-Century-Crofts, Norwalk, CT, 1982.

SUGGESTED READINGS

Arndt, MJ: Learning style: Theory and patient education. J Cont Ed Nurs 21:28, 1990.
Knowles, M: The Adult Learner: A Neglected Species, ed 3. Gulf Publishing, Houston, 1990.
Mager, RF: Developing Attitude Toward Learning. DF Lake, Belmont, CA, 1984.
Mager, RF: Measuring Instructional Results, ed 2. DF Lake, Belmont, CA, 1984.
Mager, RF: Preparing Instructional Objectives. DF Lake, Belmont, CA, 1984.
Narrow, B: Patient Teaching in Nursing Practice. John Wiley & Sons, New York, 1979.
Rakel, B: Interventions related to patient teaching. Nurs Clin North Am, 27:397, 1992.
Rankin, SH and Stalling, K: Patient Education: Issues, Principles, & Guidelines, ed 2. JB Lippincott, Philadelphia, 1990.
Weilitz, P: The critical care clinical nurse specialist role in patient education. In Gawlinski, A and Kern, L (eds): The Clinical Nurse Specialist Role in Critical Care (pp 120–132). WB Saunders, Philadelphia, 1994.
Whitman, N, et al: Teaching in Nursing Practice: A Professional Model, ed 2. Appleton & Lange, Norwalk, CT, 1992.

CHAPTER 4

Ethical and Legal Principles Affecting Decision-Making in Critical Care Nursing

Ginny Wacker Guido

CHAPTER OUTLINE

LEARNING OBJECTIVES

After completing this chapter, you should be able to:

1. Examine an ethical decision-making model that can be readily applied in clinical settings.
2. Apply ethical principles to everyday nursing practice by describing the practical value of the ethical principle in practice.
3. Distinguish between law and ethics.
4. Examine the various elements of malpractice and negligence and the significance that each element has for the nurse.
5. Discuss intentional and quasi-intentional torts and defenses for each in the professional setting.
6. Analyze the concepts of informed consent, staffing issues, and expanded roles within critical care settings.
7. Discuss specific legal issues with death and dying, including do-not-resuscitate issues, adherence to the patient self-determination act, living wills and natural death acts, durable power of attorney for healthcare, and life-support measures.

Ethical theories and principles as well as legal doctrines guide many of the decisions that critical care nurses make daily in their professional practice. Because nurses have an ever-increasing responsibility and accountability for decision-making, an understanding of ethical principles allows nurses to give order to moral situations and to provide a systematic basis for making nonarbitrary decisions. An understanding of the legal system and laws that regulate nursing practice is essential to ensure that decision-making is consistent with applicable legal principles and to protect nurses from potential legal liability.

SELECTED ETHICAL THEORIES

Many theories have evolved to justify existing moral consensus or particular moral principles. These theories are considered normative, because they are universally applicable theories of right and wrong. Most normative approaches to ethics fall into two broad categories.

Deontological (from the Greek *deon* or "duty") theories derive norms and rules from the duties that human beings owe to one another by virtue of commitments made and roles assumed. Generally, deontologists hold that a sense of duty consists of rational respect for the fulfilling of one's obligations to other human beings. This theory's greatest strength is its emphasis on the dignity of human beings. Deontological ethics look not to the end or consequences of an action, but to the intention of the action. A person's good intentions, the intentions to do a moral duty, ultimately determine the praiseworthiness of the action. Deontological ethics have sometimes been subdivided into situation ethics, in which the decision making takes into account the unique characteristics of each individual, the caring relationship between the person and the caregiver, and what is the most humanitarian thing to do given the circumstances.

Teleological (from the Greek *telos* for "end") theories derive norms or rules for conduct from the consequences of the actions. Right consists of actions that have good consequences, and wrong consists of actions that have bad consequences. Teleologists disagree about how to determine the goodness or badness of the consequences of an action. This theory is frequently termed "utilitarianism" by ethicists in medicine and nursing. The determining factor of whether the act is right or wrong is its usefulness; useful acts bring the greatest amount of good into existence. Another way of viewing this same principle is that the usefulness of an action is determined by the amount of happiness it brings. Utilitarian ethics can then be subdivided into rule and act utilitarianism. *Rule utilitarianism* seeks the greatest happiness for all; it appeals to public agreement as a basis for objective judgment about the nature of happiness. *Act utilitarianism* tries to determine in a particular situation which course of action will bring about the greatest happiness or the least harm and suffering to a single person. As such, act utilitarianism makes happiness subjective.[1]

SELECTED ETHICAL PRINCIPLES

Selected ethical principles actually drive nursing practice much more than do ethical theories. Principles encompass basic premises from which rules are developed. Principles then are the moral norms that nursing, as a profession, both demands and strives to implement in the everyday world of clinical practice. Ethical principles that one considers in ethical decision-making include the following.

Autonomy is personal freedom, individual liberty, and the right to choose what happens to one's person. Components of autonomy are respect for the unconditional worth of the person and respect for individual thought and action as well as respect for persons in general. The legal doctrine of informed consent is a direct reflection of autonomy.

Beneficence is the active promotion of good. In caring for patients, good can be defined in many ways, such as allowing a person to die without advanced life-support systems and promoting comfort measures so that the person can die peacefully. Good may be defined as allowing the infliction of pain for the overall benefit of the individual. An example of the latter definition would be a surgical procedure or placement of an invasive line; pain results from the overall procedure that will allow the individual better health.

Nonmaleficence is the principle of doing no harm. There are many different ways of doing no harm such as not inflicting pain, not killing, and not depriving another of liberty or freedom. This is not an absolute principle, however, and there are times when it is justifiable to cause pain and suffering as with a needed amputation to preserve a person's life.

Veracity is truth telling and incorporates the concept that a person should always tell the whole truth. Nurses use this principle daily when assisting patients to understand the total ramifications of their disease processes, treatments, and potential outcomes. Without veracity, true informed consent is impossible.

Justice is treating people equally and fairly. This principle usually arises in times of short supplies or when there is competition for scarce resources. Justice comes to the forefront in deciding which patient receives an organ transplant when only one organ is available, or which of two patients receives care in a critical care setting when there is only one available bed.

Fidelity is the keeping of one's commitments or promises. Nurses incorporate this principle into their professional practice daily. For example, before promising that the patient will be allowed to die without resuscitation efforts or advanced life-support measures, the nurse must consider what is within his or her control and whether he or she can keep such a promise.

Paternalism is the making of decisions for others and is often seen as a negative or undesirable principle. Actually, applying the principle of paternalism assists patients in making decisions when they do not have sufficient data or expertise to understand the true meaning of the data. Paternalism is used in a positive way when nurses assist patients in making difficult decisions, especially in the area of informed consent and issues concerning death and dying. The difference is that the nurse assists in the decision-making and does not make the decision for the patient.

Respect for others acknowledges the right of individuals to make decisions for themselves and to live by those decisions. Respect for others transcends cultural differences, gender issues, racial concerns, and the like. Nurses positively reinforce this principle daily in their actions with patients, patients' families, peers, and other healthcare providers. Many ethicists feel that respect for others is the highest principle and that it incorporates all other ethical principles.

ETHICAL DECISION-MAKING FRAMEWORK

Ethical decision-making involves reflection on the following: who should make the choices; possible options or courses of actions; available options or alternatives; consequences—both good and bad—of all possible options; rules, obligations, and values that should direct choices; and desired goals or outcomes. When making decisions, nurses must combine all these elements using an orderly, systematic, and objective method. Ethical decision-making models help to accomplish this goal.

There are various models for ethical decision-making. Perhaps the easiest one to remember and to implement in clinical settings is the MORAL model, first developed by Thiroux[2] in 1977 and refined for use in critical care settings by Halloran[3] in 1982. When examined, the model is an outgrowth of the nursing process, and the various steps of both the MORAL model and the nursing process are similar. The letters of the acronym serve to remind nurses of the following ordered steps:

M—Massage the dilemma. Identify and define the issues in the dilemma as seen through the eyes of all the major players in the dilemma. Identify their value systems and ethical principles.

O—Outline the options. Examine all the options, including those less realistic and conflicting. Remember that the only thing being done at this stage is identifying options; do not make a decision at this stage of the process.

R—Resolve the dilemma. Review the issues and options, applying basic principles of ethics to each option. Decide on the best option based on the views of all those concerned in the dilemma.

A—Act by applying the chosen option. This step is best approached through open and honest communication; all members of the healthcare team must continue to support and communicate with one another. Applying the option is usually the most difficult because it requires actual implementation, whereas previous steps have allowed only for dialogue and discussion.

L—Look back and evaluate the entire process, including the implementation. No process is complete without a thorough evaluation. Ensure that those involved are able to follow through on the final option. If not, a second decision may be required and the process must start again at the initial step.

Ethical decision-making endorses possible outcomes and acknowledges that they may not always be the ideal choices. Ethical decision-making is always a process rather than individual steps toward an end. To facilitate the process, use all the available resources, including the hospital ethics committee, and communicate with and support all those involved in the process. Some decisions are easier to reach and support; allow sufficient time for the process so that a supportable option is reached by all involved.

DISTINCTION BETWEEN ETHICS AND LAW

Ethics is subject to philosophical, moral, and individual interpretations. In any healthcare delivery dilemma, there are two systems of interpretation—those of the healthcare providers and those of the healthcare recipients. Ethics is internal in respect to the given person and is based on the values and morals of the given individual. Ethics concerns motives and attitudes and seeks to answer the question of why one acted as one did. Ethics is generally enforced through hospital ethics committees and looks to the good of the individual within a given society.

Laws are founded on rules and regulations of a society and bind the society in a formal manner. Although man-made and capable of being changed, laws provide the general foundation that guides healthcare providers, regardless of the healthcare provider's personal views and values. Laws are thus external to oneself, and they tend to benefit the entire population rather than the individual in society. Laws are enforced through the courts and the legislature. Law can be contrasted to ethics in that laws concern actions and conduct and center on what the individual actually did or failed to do, rather than the reason for acting.

SELECTED LEGAL CONCEPTS

Several key legal concepts may aid the nurse in decision-making in critical care settings. Understanding and applying legal principles protect the nurse from future lawsuits, which are becoming more common among nurses. The legal concepts covered in this chapter are standards of care, nonintentional torts, intentional torts, and quasi-intentional torts.

Standards of Care

Standards of care define the minimum level of care provided by a given profession that is considered adequate. Standards of care are the skills and knowledge commonly possessed by members of a profession.

Standards of care should be incorporated daily in all aspects of healthcare delivery. Standards of care form the basis for high-quality healthcare and serve as criteria for determining whether less than adequate care was actually delivered to a given patient. Thus, the concept of standards of care is a basic legal issue that critical care nurses must understand and apply in everyday practice.

The legal system views standards of care as a pivotal point in a malpractice lawsuit. Nurses have a duty to use reasonable care in interactions with patients. The minimum care that should be given is the care that would be given by a prudent critical care nurse under similar conditions. The question asked is, "How would a reasonably prudent critical care nurse with the same skills, experience, and educational level as the defendant critical care nurse have acted under the same or similar circumstances?" If the reasonably prudent critical care nurse would have acted in the same manner as the defendant critical care nurse did, then the defendant nurse may not be legally liable to the injured party. For the critical care nurse, the current standards of care as published by the American Association of Critical-Care Nurses (AACN) is crucial.

Standards of care are derived from various sources and may be classified into two broad categories: internal and external. *Internal standards* are those set by the nurse's background and role and include the nurse's specific job description and the institution policies and procedures. *External standards* are more global and are set by state nurse practice acts, professional nursing organizations such as the AACN, certification standards, federal guidelines and organizations, current journal articles and textbooks, and precedent court cases.

The most important internal standard is the standard of care set by the practitioner's education and experience. The more education that a nurse possesses and the greater the nurse's professional skills and talents, the more potential liability the nurse has for failure to perform at an acceptable level. The definition of "acceptable care" deepens with increased education and experience.

In the legal system, standards of care are defined during trials by the use of nurse expert witnesses, who aid the judge and jury in determining the acceptable level of care in a given circumstance. These expert witnesses help to interpret the evidence to the judge and jury, explain the actual care given, and establish appropriate standards of care. An expert witness testifying for a critical care nurse must have a thorough understanding of the skills and clinical expertise needed at the time of the alleged malpractice. The expert witness then establishes for the court the standard of care for which the defendant nurse is accountable.

Nonintentional Torts

Malpractice and Negligence

A *tort* is a civil wrong committed against a person or his or her property. Civil law—the body of law dealing with the rights of private individuals—is based on fault: the accountable person either failed to meet his or her responsibility or performed an action below the acceptable standard. Once fault is shown, the person harmed may be awarded compensation by a court of law. Table 4–1 displays the more common torts encountered by the professional nurse.

Most of the lawsuits encountered in clinical practice involve the broad area of nonintentional torts and may be classified as negligence or malpractice. Often used interchangeably, these terms are not synonymous.

Negligence denotes conduct lacking in due care; it is the act or failure to act that leads to the injury of the patient. In its simplest definition, negligence is carelessness. Negligence may be attributed to either a professional or a nonprofessional person. Anyone who fails to perform to the standard of care that a reasonable person would meet in a particular set of circumstances may be guilty of negligence.

TABLE 4–1
Classifications of Torts

Nonintentional Torts
Malpractice or negligence

Intentional Torts
Assault
Battery
False imprisonment

Quasi-Intentional Torts
Invasion of privacy
Defamation

Malpractice is a more specific term and describes the standard of care as well as the professional status of the caregiver. Courts have defined malpractice as any professional misconduct, unreasonable lack of skill or fidelity in professional or judiciary duties, or illegal or immoral conduct (*Napier v Greenzweig*[4] and *Forthofer v Arnold*[5]). Today, malpractice is the failure of a professional person to act in accordance with the prevailing professional standards or failure to foresee consequences that a professional person, having the necessary skills and education, would foresee.

Elements of Negligence and Malpractice. The injured party who brings the lawsuit has the burden to prove six different elements before the professional nurse defendant is found liable for malpractice. These elements are proved in a court of law by the injured party's attorney, and all six elements must be shown before the court will find for the injured party and against the healthcare defendants.

Duty owed the patient is the first element and involves establishing that a professional relationship existed between the nurse and the patient and that the nurse owed the patient a certain level of care. Historically, the relationship between the patient and the nurse is the easiest element to prove in court. Because the nurse works for the hospital and the patient has a contractual relationship between himself or herself and the hospital, a nurse-patient relationship is established. As discussed previously, an expert critical care nurse usually establishes for the court the applicable standard of care.

Breach of duty owed the patient is the second element and involves showing a deviation from the standard of care that was owed the now-injured patient. For example, if the acceptable standard of care involves the taking and recording of vital signs every 5 to 15 minutes, then the taking and recording of vital signs every 30 minutes is below the acceptable standard of care. The nurse has breached the duty owed the patient.

Usually, a deviation from a standard of care is called *ordinary* or *mere negligence,* implying professional negligence either in the action performed or in the omission of a required action. *Gross negligence* or *gross malpractice* may be found when the nurse willingly or consciously ignored a risk known to be harmful to a patient. For example, if the nurse assessed vital signs every 30 minutes after a patient had been placed on potent vasopressors and the patient then incurred a cerebral hemorrhage, the nurse may be considered grossly negligent.

Foreseeability, the third element of malpractice, means that certain events may foreseeably cause specific results. In the previous example, it was foreseeable that elevated blood pressure might result in cerebral bleeding and that potent vasopressors, when unmonitored, could cause such an elevated blood pressure.

Foreseeability is judged on facts at the time of the incident, not in retrospect. In areas of new technology and "cutting-edge" medicine, foreseeability may not yet be shown because healthcare providers are not certain of all of the possible or even probable outcomes.

Causation is the fourth element and requires proof that the resultant injury occurred directly because of the negligent action or omission of the required action. The injury itself is not sufficient proof; the injury must be directly related to the omission or commission of an action. This is true whatever the extent of the patient injury. Unless the injured party can show causation, there is no malpractice.

Because several healthcare providers are generally involved in the care of critically ill patients, the law uses the "substantial factor" test in determining who is potentially liable in the case of an injured person. This test asks the question "Is what I did a substantial factor in what happened to the patient?" If the answer is yes, then the healthcare provider is validly in the lawsuit and the court decides the percentage of liability attributable to that healthcare provider's negligent actions.

Injury must be demonstrated in terms of some type of physical, financial, or emotional injury resulting directly from the breach of duty owed the patient. Generally speaking, courts do not allow emotional injuries unless they are accompanied by physical injuries. For example, pain and suffering is allowed when it accompanies a physical injury, but not allowed when no physical injury can be shown.

Damages, the sixth element, compensates the injured party for the cost of medical care incurred as a result of the injury/negligent care and attempts to restore the patient to his or her original financial state, as far as is possible. Grouped into four general categories, damages are not meant to punish the wrongdoer or to set an example for the profession. Only punitive or exemplary damages are meant to punish the wrongdoer and deter future misconduct, and punitive damages are awarded only when the injured party can show that willful or wanton misconduct was associated with the negligent action. Such willful or wanton misconduct makes the action gross negligence or gross malpractice.

Common examples of malpractice in critical care settings are patient falls, patient medication errors, failing to assess the patient for changes in health status, failing to notify the primary healthcare provider of changes in the patient status, and inadequate patient education and discharge instructions.

Intentional Torts

Intentional torts differ from negligence and malpractice in the following ways. (1) Intent is necessary for an intentional tort. The nurse must intend to do a particular action or appear to intend a particular action that brings about a consequence. (2) For an intentional tort to occur, there must be action against the person. An omission of an action cannot be the basis for an intentional tort. (3) An intentional tort does not have to cause injury or harm. That is, the patient must show that the tort occurred, not that injury or damage occurred.

The most common intentional torts in critical care settings are assault, battery, and false imprisonment. Although assault and battery are usually pled together, they are two distinct torts.

Assault and Battery

An *assault* is any action by one person that makes another person fear that he or she may be touched, without consent or authority, in an offensive, insulting, or physically injurious manner. Actual touching of another is not required; the action or motion alone creates the fear. For example, the nurse approaches the patient with a syringe as if to give an injection without the patient's consent. No contact has occurred, but the patient could successfully show that an assault had occurred.

Battery is a harmful or unwarranted contact with a person without permission. The person so touched need not be injured by the contact, nor does the person need to be aware of the contact. For example, a battery occurs when a patient is touched against his or her consent, even if the patient is not aware of the touching. The contact, not the manner of the contact, results in the commission of the tort.

In most situations, assault and battery are averted because the healthcare provider has consent to proceed with the therapy. Assault and battery do not occur if the patient is confused and unable to understand his or her behavior. Self-defense or defense of others may be a valid defense against a lawsuit for assault and battery. The healthcare provider may use necessary force to prevent patients from either harming themselves or others in the immediate area.

False Imprisonment

False imprisonment is the unjustifiable detention of a person without legal warrant to restrain the person. A nurse falsely imprisons a patient when the nurse confines the patient or restrains the patient in a confined, bounded area with the intent to limit the patient's freedom. Refusing to return clothes, car keys, and personal belongings to a patient may also constitute false imprisonment.

To show liability for false imprisonment, patients must show that they were aware of the confinement and that they requested to be released from the confinement. Confused, disoriented persons who are restrained for their own or others' protection will not be successful in a lawsuit for false imprisonment. Care, caution, and reasonableness are the prerequisites in the use of restraints.

Quasi-Intentional Torts

The law also recognizes what it terms quasi-intentional torts. This type of tort lacks the intent that is so critical to intentional torts, but a volitional action and causation must still be shown so that the tort is more than mere negligence. The two torts in this category that affect critical care areas are invasion of privacy and defamation.

Invasion of privacy is the right to protection against unreasonable and unwarranted interferences with the individual's solitude. This includes the protection of personality as well as the protection against interference with one's right to be left alone. Confidentiality is closely related to this tort and protects the patient's right to privacy of the medical record. This tort is most frequently encountered in critical care settings when confidential data are revealed without permission to someone not entitled to the information. Critical care nurses are encouraged to respect patient privacy rights and guard against the release of such information except to others caring directly for the patient or to those who have a right to the information as patient advocates, subsequent shift members, and authorized medical personnel.

Defamation is the tort of wrongful injury to the reputation of another. This tort involves the written or oral communication to someone other than the person defamed of matters concerning a living person's reputation. A claim of defamation may arise from inaccurate or inappropriate release of medical information or from untrue statements.

Caution is the key word with both of these torts. The nurse should be careful about releasing any information, pictures, or the like about a patient and should be careful about any reference made in charting or oral communications about the patient's actions or reputation. These torts are avoidable if nurses give to patients the same respect and considerations that they give each other and family members.

EXPANDED ROLES AND THE CRITICAL CARE NURSE

As the scope of nursing and the scope of medicine become more intertwined and incapable of exact delineation, critical care nurses have broadened their scope of practice. This is especially true as nurses have become more knowledgeable, more skilled in working with complex technology, and hold either advanced degrees or certification in specific areas of nursing. This broadening of the role of the critical care nurse becomes especially significant in situations that require expert clinical skills and immediate actions.

Today, the law both expects and demands that the nurse act rapidly and appropriately in patient situations.

Several issues must be considered in determining when and to what extent nurses should respond in clinical situations. The courts have long recognized the individual judgment of nurses and have held the nurse accountable to this independent judgment standard (*Fraijo v Hartland Hospital*,[6] 1979 and *Cooper v National Motor Bearing Company*,[7] 1955). More recently, courts have upheld the duty of nurses to act as patient advocates and to ensure that competent care is given the patient by all healthcare providers (*Kirk v Mercy Hospital Tri-County*,[8] 1993).

Second, the state nurse practice act gives guidance for expanded nursing practice and expanding roles. Most state nurse practice acts now allow for nursing diagnoses and nursing treatments. A nurse thus acting in behalf of the patient could be said to be acting in accordance with the legislative act.

Individual hospital policies and protocols also give guidance in such issues. If the acceptable standard of care is that the critical care nurse may institute appropriate measures to alleviate a patient's presenting symptoms in emergency situations, then to do so is within the scope of nursing. These hospital protocols should be established by a joint nursing and medical committee and reviewed and updated as needed. The latter provision allows protocols to remain current in light of changing technology and standards of care.

The Joint Commission for the Accreditation of Healthcare Organizations (JCAHO) and the AACN provide excellent standards of care. These guidelines are unit-specific and nationally based and provide evidence of reasonable nursing care if a subsequent lawsuit is filed.

The presence of an emergency situation may give the experienced critical care nurse more standing to initiate appropriate therapy. Before initiating any standing protocols, the nurse should ensure that (1) this is a true emergency situation and that the patient's life or physical well-being is imminently threatened; (2) the nurse's level of expertise and skills is not exceeded; and (3) a physician is not readily available before proceeding. What is allowable in a true emergency is determined according to whether the nurse acted in a reasonable manner and in accordance with sound nursing principles.

Certification, the process of granting recognition to individuals who have attained a specific level of knowledge and expertise in a given field, may also aid the nurse in proving that he or she had the necessary skills and expertise to act in a specific situation. Advanced certification credentials weigh favorably in the event of a lawsuit if the nurse used the skills appropriately and met standards of care.

INFORMED CONSENT ISSUES

All adult patients have the right to be consulted and to either give or deny consent before healthcare providers proceed with therapies, treatments, and interventions. Informed consent, a concept that evolved in 1957 (*Salgo v Leland Stanford, Jr, University Board of Trustees*[9]) has two elements: "informed" refers to information given the patient about a proposed procedure or treatment, and "consent" refers to the patient's voluntary assent to the procedure or treatment. To be informed, a patient must receive, in terms he or she can reasonably be expected to understand, all the information that a reasonable person would need to either consent or refuse the proposed treatment or procedure.

Information that is given to the patient or designee includes the following: (1) a description of the treatment or procedure, including expected outcomes; (2) the name and qualifications of the person or persons who will perform the treatment or procedure; (3) an explanation of the potential for serious harm or for adverse effects of the procedure or treatment both during and after the treatment or procedure; (4) an explanation and description of alternative treatments or procedures, including the right to no treatment; and (5) an explanation of the risks involved with the procedure or treatment.

The patient has the right to be told all possible effects of not having the treatment or procedure; this concept has come to be known as informed refusal, because the patient must be fully aware of what is being refused and the potential consequences to himself or herself. Like informed consent, the doctrine of informed refusal is based in decisional law (*Truman v Thomas,*[10] 1980).

Informed consent is usually obtained from the patient or legal representative as determined by state law (e.g., a legal guardian for an incompetent adult, a parent or legal guardian for a minor, or an emancipated minor) by the signature on a consent form. Other valid means of obtaining informed consent are verbal, apparent, and implied consent.

Patients in critical care settings often give verbal consent or give their right to sign the consent form to a family member or personal friend. Apparent consent may be used when the patient implies by his or her conduct that consent is being given, for instance, by a nod of the head or the extension of an arm for an injection. More frequently, implied consent is indicated in the critical care setting. In true emergency situations, in which the patient is unable to either give or deny consent and in which a delay in providing care will result in permanent injury to the patient, the law implies consent. Two important factors must be remembered: (1) the treatment or procedure to be performed must be that to which a reasonable person would have consented, and (2) the patient must not have previously refused the procedure or treatment. The latter occurs most frequently with the patient who refuses blood; one cannot wait for the patient to become incompetent and then give the blood.

The responsibility for obtaining informed consent generally rests with the person performing the treatment or procedure, the physician or primary healthcare provider. The role of nursing in this area is still evolving, and most institutions limit or define the nurse's role by policy. Typically, the nurse is responsible for ensuring that the physician or administrator is notified if there is a problem with the patient's informed consent; the nurse is not responsible for obtaining the actual consent.

STAFFING ISSUES

Healthcare facilities often use *floating*, a practice that assigns nurses temporarily to units with which they are unfamiliar, in an attempt to alleviate understaffing. The practice raises questions about the overall competency of the pulled nurse to function within the necessary standard of care. Generally speaking, the nurse who is floated to another unit will be held to the same standard of care to which the experienced nurse working in that unit is held.

There are some things that the float nurse can do to protect himself or herself in this situation. Inform the supervisor and the charge nurse on the unit about expertise and competencies, remembering that most nurses have competencies that are used throughout the institution such as physical assessment skills and ability to take vital signs accurately and perform routine procedures. By the same reasoning, there will be some procedures and medications with which the nurse may not be familiar. Negotiate for procedures that are within the nurse's expertise, and allow someone else on the unit to perform unfamiliar tasks and give unfamiliar medications. Or, negotiate for an assignment on a unit where the nurse has more expertise, and float a second nurse from that unit to the unit that is understaffed.

There are also ways of protecting from potential liability the charge nurse and the supervisor on the unit to which another nurse is floated. Ascertain the float nurse's capabilities and competencies and assign patients accordingly. If a patient becomes more critical during the shift and the float nurse is unable to competently care for the patient, rearrange the patient assignments for optimal care to all patients. Serve as a resource person to the float nurse and ensure that he or she will ask questions before giving care. Also, request that administration cross-train nurses so that nurses can safely be floated from one unit to another and that patient care will not be compromised. The latter suggestion also requires that double pulls be implemented at times so that nurses working in other than their "home" unit will be competent and cross-trained.

LEGAL ISSUES WITH DEATH AND DYING

Several issues face nurses today within the realm of the dying patient. Although there is a concomitant ethical concern, this discussion is limited to the legal aspects and legal decision-making among critical care nurses.

Do-Not-Resuscitate Issues

Cardiopulmonary resuscitation for all patients, unless otherwise noted, has been standardized since the mid-1960s. The issue for nursing has not been whether or not to order a "no code" for a given patient, but whether a verbal order was sufficient and the extent of the code itself.

The best course of action for nursing is to have a written and documented no-code order. Although not dictated by federal or state laws, most hospitals by policy mandate a written order and mandate that the writ-

---

RESEARCH APPLICATION: EFFECT OF DO-NOT-RESUSCITATE ORDERS ON THE NURSING CARE OF CRITICALLY ILL PATIENTS
Henneman, EA, et al. Am J Crit Care, 3(6): 467–472

Purpose: The purpose of this research study was to compare nurses' attitudes about standards of care for critically ill patients with and without do-not-resuscitate (DNR) orders. Because DNR orders can be construed by physicians, nurses, patients, and family members as more than "no cardiopulmonary resuscitation (CPR)," the study was done to discover whether standards of care did differ after the patient became classified as a DNR.

There are few studies to date that have researched this issue. Of those that do exist, some evidence shows that after a patient is classified as a DNR, the aggressiveness of nursing care decreases and more "care and comfort measures" are performed. Because nurses are central in determining the standards of care for critically ill patients, this study was undertaken to see how nurses viewed standards of care when patients had DNR orders compared with those patients who remained a "full code."

Methodology: A quasi-experimental study was conducted in a 500-bed hospital, using the five critical care units in the facility. Two questionnaires were developed by the researchers, each containing a case scenario followed by a list of standards of nursing care. These lists of standards of care represented routine nursing monitoring modalities and interventions, both physiologic and psychological in nature, and included such statements as "allow frequent family visits," "monitor vital signs every 15 minutes," "perform neurologic assessment," "suction every 2 hours and as necessary," and "turn patient every 2 hours." The two scenarios were identical except that the second scenario had a line that read: "The patient has an order that reads do not resuscitate."

Eighty critical care nurses were randomly given either the first or the second questionnaire and asked to complete the questionnaires independently. Forty nurses received the first questionnaire, and 40 received the second questionnaire. The nurses were instructed to read the scenario and, using a five-point Likert scale, to rate how likely they would be to perform the individual interventions.

Results: The demographic data for the two groups showed no differences regarding age, gender, years of critical care experience, or experience with DNR patients. Seventy percent of the nurses (36% of the DNR group and 34% of the non-DNR group) reported that they cared for DNR patients either somewhat or very frequently.

Respondents reported that they would be significantly less likely to perform a variety of physiologic monitoring interventions with DNR patients and that they were more likely to perform psychological interventions such as assessment of spiritual needs and more flexible visiting hours. No statistical analysis was performed between demographic characteristics and nurses' responses because of the small sample size, but the authors concluded that the similarity of the two groups suggests little association.

Practical Implications: The major concern surrounding DNR patients receiving appropriate therapies after the DNR order is written continues to be justified, given the results of this quasi-experimental study. Nurses reported that they were much less likely to perform monitoring modalities and less likely to notify physicians of changes in a patient's condition once the DNR order was written. Consistent with previous studies, this study showed that psychological interventions would be emphasized following a DNR order.

This study supports the concern that a DNR order may well be misinterpreted and extended to other aspects of the patient's care, particularly physiologic aspects, despite the existence of a written policy that DNR refers solely to CPR status and has no implications for other aspects of care. The study may well support the concern that a DNR order equates with enacting a dying patient's protocol of care and comfort measures only.

The authors concluded that the issue of standards of care for patients with limitations on their resuscitation status is significant and requires resolution. Their recommendation is that the letters DNR be avoided and a plan that is collaboratively determined be developed and followed by nursing personnel. Each plan would be unique and developed by collaboration among the multidisciplinary staff, patient, and family.

ten order be re-evaluated, and rewritten if necessary, every 36 to 48 hours. Most hospitals also recognize what has come to be a "chemical" code—a valid order for drug and oxygen interventions and no chest compressions or intubation. These chemical codes often meet the patient's and family's expectations for comfort, but stop short of external massage and actual intubation and ventilation.[11]

What has never been acceptable from a legal perspective is the "little," "slow," or "partial" code. Such a code always falls below the acceptable standard of care because it is predicated on the premise that resuscitation will be done in an ineffective manner. Regardless of the good intent of the "slow" code, such a response opens the nurse and the hospital to a successful malpractice suit for the patient or family members.

Advance Directives

Persons with strong desires to either request or reject aggressive treatment should document their wishes while still competent to do so. A surrogate decision-maker should also be designated while patients are competent so that no doubt exists as to who has the valid informed consent for patients unable to make decisions for themselves.

The Patient Self-Determination Act, effective on December 1, 1991, was passed to ensure that all patients entering healthcare facilities in the United States and its territories would be told of such advance directives and be given the opportunity to enact such advance directives while still competent. Healthcare facilities differ in their enactment of this directive and, in some hospitals and clinics, the burden falls on the nurse to ask the patient about advance directives. No matter its implementation, patients are not required to have such advance directives; this act merely helps to appraise patients of the existence of the directives and assists them in enacting such documents.

Living Wills and Natural Death Acts

Living wills and natural death acts constitute the most popular form of advance directives. Both documents allow competent patients to express in writing their wishes about terminal care, life-support systems, and comfort measures while they are still competent to express their wishes. Living wills have no legislative protection, and natural death acts (sometimes called medical treatment decision acts) are enacted by state legislatures and have provisions to protect healthcare providers when they follow the wishes of the qualified patient or family members. Nurses are cautioned to seek guidance from the institution legal department when such documents are placed on the patient chart to ensure that the document meets state legal requirements before there is a need to rely on its provisions. By seeking legal guidance, if the document does not meet state requirements, the healthcare providers can assist the patient to make a valid document while still competent.

Durable Powers of Attorney for Healthcare

The durable powers of attorney for healthcare are the newer extension of the natural death act in most states. The durable power of attorney for healthcare (called merely a durable power of attorney by some states) allows the competent patient to designate a surrogate decision-maker, who may or may not be a family member, and conveys to that designated surrogate decision-maker the patient's informed consent if the patient becomes incompetent to speak for himself or herself. In addition, the patient has the ability to designate alternative surrogate decision-makers, if the first-listed surrogate is unable or unwilling to serve.

Essentially, durable power-of-attorney documents are "springing" powers of informed consent; the power of consent springs into the designated surrogate when the patient becomes incompetent to make healthcare decisions and springs back into the patient when he or she regains competency. The durable power of attorney for healthcare also designates a specific person to be consulted by the healthcare practitioner, thereby foregoing the need to obtain family consensus (as with living wills and natural death acts). As with the living wills and natural death acts, the durable power of attorney for healthcare must meet specific state provisions; therefore, it is best to seek legal guidance for these documents also when the patient first presents the document.

Withdrawal of Ordinary Care Measures

Withdrawal of ordinary care measures include tube feedings, nutritional and hydration support, and supplemental oxygen therapy. The question of withdrawing ordinary care measures usually concerns the patient who is in a persistent vegetative state, one who does not meet the definition of qualified patient in many state living wills and natural death acts. State courts have usually allowed for the removal of ordinary care measures but still agree that strict guidelines are needed for decision-making in this area. Examples of such guidelines include that the patient be terminal or in a persistent vegetative state, that further treatment would serve only to prolong the dying process, and that all reasonable treatment has been exhausted. In 1983, a presidential commission concluded that no universal treatments exist that a patient must accept, including interventions such as parenteral nutrition or hydration, antibiotics, and transfusions.[12]

NURSING CONSIDERATIONS

To give high-quality, competent care in today's healthcare settings, professional nurses must be as knowledgeable about legal and ethical issues as they are about pathophysiology and technical skills. Nurses are challenged today to care for the entire patient, incorporating a profound regard for humanity and all that such regard encompasses. Professional nursing is high-quality, competent care that addresses the patient's legal rights, ethical concerns, and physiologic considerations.

CONCLUSIONS

This chapter has explored both ethical and legal issues in an effort to assist the professional nurse in effective decision-making in critical care settings. Although the content is divided, there is no such distinction between legal and ethical dilemmas in practice. Having mastered this content, the professional nurse must make his or her own decisions and act accordingly.

CASE STUDY: LEGAL AND ETHICAL ISSUES

Mrs. D, an elderly woman, was discovered in a semiconscious state with multiple fractures, lying in the gutter of a busy street, and was transported via emergency medical transport to a major medical center. Very little medical information could be obtained from the patient, and needed surgery was performed to set her fractures. She was admitted to the surgical intensive care unit for observation and management of hypertension and arrhythmias.

As Mrs. D became more responsive, the staff learned that she lived alone, that she had one sister who was confined to a nursing home in another state, and had no other relatives. Her past medical history included minor surgery in 1950, hypertension dating from the 1960s for which she sometimes took medications, and a myocardial infarction in 1990. She requested that no heroic measures be taken when questioned about the existence of a living will or a durable power of attorney for healthcare and stated that she would like to execute a living will document. Mrs. D further stated that

she had no desire to live longer and had "made her peace with the Lord."

Before the necessary paperwork could be initiated, Mrs. D complained of massive chest pain, an inferior wall infarct was diagnosed on ECG, and she developed severe second degree and third degree heart block. Her mental status at this time wavered between full competency and confusion. The physicians requested that Mrs. D be prepared for an emergency placement of a temporary pacemaker and that the nurses have Mrs. D sign the necessary informed consent documents. When the nurse caring for Mrs. D reiterated to the physician the patient's desire both to execute a living will and for no heroics be done, the nurse was instructed to "do as requested and get the paperwork signed now!"

What are the legal and ethical issues concerning this patient's care and how should the nursing staff proceed at this point?

REFERENCES

1. Guido, GW: Ethical and legal principles affecting decision-making in critical care nursing. In Dolan, J: Critical Care Nursing: Clinical Management Through the Nursing Process. FA Davis, Philadelphia, 1991, p 1409.
2. Thiroux, J: Ethics: Theory and Practice, ed. 4. Macmillan, New York, 1990.
3. Halloran, MC: Rational ethical judgments utilizing a decision-making tool. Heart Lung *11*:566–70, 1982.
4. *Napier v Greenzweig*, 256 F. 196 (2d Cir. 1919).
5. *Forthofer v Arnold*, 60 Ohio App. 436, 21 NE 2d 869 (1938).
6. *Fraijo v Hartland Hospital*, 160 Cal. Rept. 246, 99 Cal. App. 3rd 331 (1979).
7. *Cooper v National Motor Bearing Company*, 136 Cal. App. 2d 229, 288 P. 2d 581 (1955).
8. *Kirk v Mercy Hospital Tri-County*, 851 SW 2d 617 (Mo 1993).
9. *Salgo v Leland Stanford, Jr, University Board of Trustees*, 317 P. 2d 170 (Cal. Dis. Ct. App. 1957).
10. *Truman v Thomas*, 27 Cal. 3rd 285, 611 P. 2d 902 (1980).
11. Olson, CM: The issue of CPR. JAMA *268*:2297–2298, 1992.
12. President's Commission for the Study of Ethical Problems in Medicine and Biomedical and Behavioral Research. Deciding to forgo life-sustaining treatments. Washington, DC: US Government Printing Office, 1983.
13. Guido, GW: Legal Issues in Nursing: A Source Book for Practice. Appleton & Lange, Norwalk, CT, 1988.

CHAPTER 5

Psychosocial Implications in the Care of the Critically Ill Patient and the Family in Critical Care

Susan D. Ruppert and Mary Meisel

CHAPTER OUTLINE

The Critically Ill Patient
□ Critically Ill Patient and Stress
□ Patient Stressors in the ICU
□ Patient Reactions in the ICU
The Family of the Critically Ill Patient
□ Stressors for Families
□ Family Needs
□ Family Reactions
Psychosocial Assessment of Critically Ill
Patients and Their Families

Case Study with Sample Care Plan:
Patient/Family with Psychosocial
Dysfunction with Closed Head Injury
□ Nursing Diagnoses
Case Study with Sample Care Plan:
Patient/Family with Rule-Out
Myocardial Infarction
□ Nursing Diagnoses
References
Suggested Readings

LEARNING OBJECTIVES

After completing this chapter, you should be able to:

1. Define stress and theories of stress.
2. Identify patient stressors in the ICU.
3. Describe patient reactions in the ICU.
4. Identify stressors for families.
5. Describe reactions of families
   to stress.
6. Discuss the needs of the family of the critically ill patient.
7. Define essential components of the psychosocial assessment of critically ill patients
   and their families.
8. List pertinent nursing diagnoses associated with psychosocial function and
   dysfunction.

THE CRITICALLY ILL PATIENT

An intensive care unit (ICU) can be a very intimidating place for a patient. Shrill alarms sound seemingly without reason, lights flash from machines intermittently, and unpleasant odors permeate the air. Although ICU nurses feel comfortable amidst the advanced technology and flashing screens, patients and their families can make little sense of this strange and overwhelming environment. It is difficult for patients and families to know to whom they are talking because all members of the ICU staff are dressed alike in surgical scrub uniforms. Overall, the experience of being admitted to an ICU or having a family member admitted is unsettling and frightening for both patient and family.

The nurse can demystify the ICU for the patient and family by assessing their needs and concerns regarding the ICU environment and by assessing how well the patient and family are coping with the situation. From the assessment, the nurse diagnoses, plans, and intervenes with patients and families to meet their needs and evaluates the effectiveness of these interventions in terms of patient and family outcomes. A nurse who espouses the concept of holistic patient care must include both the patient and the patient's family in that plan of care. Interdisciplinary plans of care should be collaboratively planned and communicated to all members of the team so that family information can be accurately conveyed and consistently verified.

The beginning of this chapter discusses the ICU patient's stressors, reactions to stress, and nursing interventions to facilitate adaptation to that stress. Stressors for families of ICU patients and their reactions are then discussed. A psychosocial assessment of patient and family is presented with case studies.

Critically Ill Patient and Stress

Patients in the ICU have a variety of demographics and different levels of severity of disease and surgical diagnoses. Despite these differences, all ICU patients experience stress as a result of their admission to the ICU. The amount of stress that a patient experiences depends on his or her past experiences with illness, his or her perception of the threat and immediacy of threat of the present illness to self-image and biologic integrity, and the coping methods and support systems available to the patient.

Physiologic Theory of Stress

Various theories of how stress affects people have been proposed. Selye's theory[1] concentrates on the body's physiologic response to stimuli or stressors rather than an individual's psychological response to stress. Selye defined stress as "a state manifested by a specific syndrome which consists of all the nonspecifically induced changes within a biological system"[1] or more simply "the rate of wear and tear in the body caused by life at any one time."[1] A stressor, according to Selye, is that which produces stress. A stressor can be physiologic, psychological, cultural, sociologic, or environmental.

Selye's General Adaptation Syndrome (GAS) describes the individual's adaptation to stressors. The syndrome consists of three stages. The first stage is the alarm stage in which the individual experiences a sudden exposure to a noxious stimulus (stressor) to which he or she is not adapted. The body's defenses are mobilized in this stage. The second is the resistance stage, which involves the person's efforts at adapting to the stressor along with a concurrent decrease in resistance to other stimuli. Effective adaptation to the stressor results in improved physiologic functioning. The final stage, the exhaustion stage, occurs when the stressor is prolonged and severe and all the body's energy is fully exhausted. This stage can result in death because an individual is not infinitely capable of adapting to a stressor.

Selye[1] described the stress response as a "fight-or-flight" reaction associated with release of epinephrine and characterized by an increase in blood pressure, increased cardiac output, increased heart rate and respirations, increased blood glucose, pupillary dilation, decreased renal perfusion, and increased muscle tension in the affected individual. Many of these signs can be observed in newly admitted ICU patients and their families. Prolonged stress can alter an individual's bio-

logic function and has been associated with the development of hypertension, ulcers, asthma, allergies, and cancer.

Psychological Theory of Stress

Lazarus[2] views stress as a transaction between the environment and the person. The person appraises the transaction and interprets the significance of the stress and the effect it may have on the person's well-being. According to Lazarus, individuals cope with the stress by changing themselves or adapting to the environment.

The same stressor does not affect everyone equally. Stress is determined by the person's perception of the stress rather than the stressful situation itself. If patients who are admitted to the hospital to rule out a myocardial infarction perceive themselves to be "well" and do not view hospitalization as a threat, they will not appear to be as stressed as patients who view an ICU admission as a threat to their integrity. The potency of the stressor is related to the perceived imminence of the threat to the individual and the adequacy of the person's coping resources.

Stress and Illness

Stress may increase a person's susceptibility to illness, especially if several stressors are experienced at the same time. Any life event may be stressful if it causes change in and demands readjustment of an average person's normal routine. The individual's chance of becoming ill increases with life events of a high-stress magnitude or when multiple stressors are present.

Individuals who are admitted to an ICU experience many stressors. A major stressor is the life-threatening physiologic alteration that necessitated their ICU admission. Patients also experience a feeling of loss of control of their situation, separation from family and significant others, fear and anxiety related to the overwhelming technical environment of the ICU, and lack of knowledge regarding the diagnosis and the seriousness of their illness and procedures performed on them.

Just as people react differently to the same stressors, so people differ in their reaction to an ICU admission. A person's reaction to illness depends on the type of illness (e.g., whether a stigma is attached) and the nature of the illness (e.g., acute or chronic). The severity of the illness or the prognosis and the course of treatment also influence the reaction. Patients' prior physical and psychological health, availability of support systems, past experiences with illness, sociocultural belief, and personality characteristics all affect their reaction to the present illness.

Patient Stressors in the ICU

The ICU environment provides unique stressors not found in other hospital units. Stressors that affect ICU patients can be physiologic, psychological, emotional, social, and even cultural. A recent study of cardiac surgery patients revealed several of these stressors. Physical stressors such as the presence of oral and nasal tubes, pain, inability to sleep, and thirst were rated as high stressors by the patients. Psychological stressors of not being in control and missing husband or wife were also identified as disturbing.[3] Several common ICU stressors are described.

Communication

Communication between staff members about their personal lives is considered to be a stressor by ICU patients.[3] Patients are also distressed at overhearing conversations between staff members regarding their prognosis and treatment. Patients could misinterpret the conversations and experience emotional distress as a result. ICU staff should refrain from personal conversations among themselves when performing patient care. Equally as distressing is the failure of a nurse to communicate adequately with patients regarding procedures they are undergoing. Concise explanations can ease a patient's fears and help to develop a trusting relationship between patient and staff.

Immobilization

Immobilization and claustrophobia are among the most stressful elements for a surgical ICU patient to cope with.[3] Even patients without actual physical restraints feel tied down by nasogastric tubes, intravenous lines, indwelling catheters, and endotracheal tubes. Patient restraints should be used only when necessary to ensure patient safety. Repeated explanations to patient and family of the function of restraints are necessary to decrease anxiety. Nurses may try to substitute close observation of the patient rather than use physical and chemical restraints.

Depersonalization

Patients also experience stress when the ICU staff depersonalizes care by referring to a patient by diagnosis rather than by name. The patient becomes an object and is not recognized as a thinking, feeling human being. Nurses can enhance a trusting nurse-patient relationship and minimize depersonalization of the patient by introducing themselves by name to the patient and family at the beginning of the shift and addressing the patient by his or her preferred name. Encouraging family members to provide information about the patient as a person (e.g., family, hobbies, work, likes and dislikes, and daily routines) enables staff to personalize care. Family members feel as if they have contributed to that care. Family members should be encouraged to participate actively in providing care (e.g., assisting with feeding, personal hygiene, and range-of-motion exercises) if they are comfortable doing so.

Isolation

Patients may experience a sense of isolation from being physically separated from family and friends. Open or flexible visiting hours can help to decrease this isolation. ICU nurses can make family members feel like welcome participants in the patient's care, physically and emotionally. Some family members may be comfortable in assisting with physical care. Others can participate by providing information about the patient, which allows the nurse to individualize care. This increased time for communication with family members provides an excellent opportunity for teaching and discharge planning. Nurses should encourage family members to touch the patient while being careful of all the "tubes." One study found that the more severely ill an ICU patient is, the greater the number of visitors the patient wanted.[4] Thus, visits should be individualized to patient needs and preferences, not staff desires and convenience. Despite myths that family visitation may be physiologically stressful for the patient, studies have not found significant harmful changes in heart rate, blood pressure, ectopy, or intracranial pressure.[5–10]

Powerlessness

Closely related to control are feelings of powerlessness. Powerlessness is "the perception on the part of the individual of a lack of personal or internal control over events in a given situation."[11] This definition limits feelings of powerlessness to a specific situation and emphasizes that the individual's perception of a lack of control—not the situation itself—leads to feelings of powerlessness.

Patients have very little ability to control their bodies or their environment in the ICU. They *can* experience changes in their body image secondary to the changes in bodily processes and changes in their usual personal and family roles. Being subjected to numerous unfamiliar procedures and often being restrained contribute to feelings of helplessness and loss of control. Intubation often precludes the patient's ability to communicate needs, contributing to feelings of powerlessness. Nurses can intervene by explaining all procedures to patients, listening to patients' concerns and fears, and offering the patient choices when possible.

Patient Reactions in the ICU

A patient's reaction to illness or surgery and to subsequent admission to an ICU depends on past experience with illness and hospitalization, personality characteristics, severity of the illness or injury, whether the illness is an acute episode or a chronic event, the patient's support systems, cultural background, and level of knowledge regarding the illness or surgery. Commonalities in a patient's reaction can be observed despite the variety of factors that influence that reaction. Each reaction is described briefly. Every patient will not demonstrate all these reactions.

Denial

An initial reaction that many ICU patients experience is denial. Denial occurs when a person "refuses to acknowledge or attempts to deny some anxiety-provoking aspect of self, or external reality."[12] A sign of denial is an "inability to appreciate the significance of stimuli" and may include an "insensitivity to changes in body."[13] The person may also distort or minimize meanings to "the point where real meanings are clouded over."[13]

By using denial, a person can control the meaning of an experience by denying that it exists, and thus can decrease or neutralize the anxiety aroused by the experience. An example of denial is a patient experiencing chest pain radiating down the left arm, who delays seeking medical assistance because "I thought the pain would go away" or "I thought it was gas." Avoidance is closely related to denial, but differs in that patients make a deliberate effort not to think about the threat to their health, although they accept the reality of the threat. Patients who change the subject of conversation whenever it touches on their illness may be using avoidance to cope.

Contradicting the patient's view of his or her illness is not an appropriate nursing intervention. The use of denial helps protect the patient from the pain of reality. The nurse must be patient and continually reassess the patient's need for accurate information regarding the diagnosis. Some patients may use denial throughout their entire stay in the ICU.

Anxiety

Anxiety is a common reaction to any stressful situation. It can be defined as an uneasiness due to an impending or anticipated threat, and it can range from mild anxiety to panic. An ICU patient who views hospitalization as a threat will become anxious. An anxious patient may react by fidgeting, being restless, asking the same question repeatedly, talking incessantly, or using inappropriate humor. Some anxious patients may react by withdrawing and limiting conversation. If withdrawal continues, apathy and depression can result. The patient may require counseling to overcome the depression.

Most ICU patients experience anxiety at some level. Nursing interventions for easing a patient's anxiety include providing the patient with explanations regarding treatments and procedures, allowing the patient to verbalize concerns and fears, and listening in a nonjudgmental manner. If necessary, the nurse should discuss with the physician the possibility of using antianxiety medications or should obtain a psychiatric consultation if the patient's anxiety is severe.

Demonstrating a Need for Control

Control is a coping mechanism in which optimal controls "slow down recognition processes and so provide tolerable doses of new information and emotional responses."[13] Control can be viewed as "the tendency to believe and act as if one can influence the course of events."[14] An example of a controlling person is one with a Type A behavior pattern, who wants to conduct business from an ICU bed by telephone, even while experiencing chest pain.

Other patients may try to maintain control over their situation and the ICU environment by asking questions or refusing treatments they do not want or understand. Even the alert patient who deliberately removes an endotracheal tube, intravenous line, or Foley catheter may be trying to demonstrate control over the situation.

The nurse can provide the patient with opportunities to make decisions regarding patient care. If a patient refuses a treatment or medication, the nurse should not attempt to force the issue. Instead, staff should contact the physician and convey the patient's reasons for the refusal. The patient needs a strong advocate, and that advocate is the patient's nurse.

Passivity

Passivity is closely related to powerlessness and the opposite of demonstrating control. A passive response would be observable in the patient who seems to allow events to control him or her, rather than exerts control over the events. An ICU patient who never questions any treatments and follows all directions may be the model of an ideal patient or may be feeling powerless to change the situation and so reacts passively. As with patients who feel a lack of control, allow patients who feel powerless to make decisions about, and participate in, their care and treatment.

Anger

The patient whose reaction to hospitalization is anger may have feelings that malpractice or mistreatment has occurred. A patient who undergoes repeated blood drawing or central line insertion attempts may have reason to be angry if a repeated attempt is required as a result of a practitioner's lack of skill in performing a procedure. The patient is angry at having no control over the situation.

Anger may mask anxiety and act as a release valve for a patient who is "fed up" with treatments and procedures. Anger may also result from a patient's distrust of the ICU staff. Salyer and Stuart[15] found that patients react negatively by demonstrating anger or hostility when a nurse's action is perceived as negative to the patient. An example is the nurse who criticizes a patient or is silent during administration of patient care.

Anger can also mask fear. Patients may fear pain, disfigurement, and death in the ICU. Allow patients to express their anger and try to correct any legitimate complaints voiced. Try not to take the patient's anger personally.

Regression

Patients in an ICU relinquish much of the control over their bodies. A patient may react by regressing to a former level of development. The patient capable of assisting with morning care may want a relative to help brush their hair or feed them. The family needs to understand that the regression is common and temporary, and they should be included in a plan of care that fosters self-care as appropriate.

Humor

Many of the previous patient reactions, such as regression, anger, and denial, have a negative connotation. Some patients' reactions are surprising. Humor can be used effectively as a coping mechanism. Patients may be able to face fear more easily if they can laugh at it. Inappropriate humor, such as sexual comments or innuendo, may be the patient's way of masking fear or perhaps anger at the staff. If the nurse is the recipient of inappropriate humor, a statement such as "Mr. Jones, your remark is inappropriate and offensive to me. Please refrain from that language," is recommended. The nurse can investigate this type of behavior by asking patients if they have any problems or concerns they would like to discuss.

Verbalization

Patients may react to illness by using prayer and clergy for spiritual comfort, and by verbalizing their fears and concerns to sympathetic relatives or ICU staff. Patients sometimes have a need to relive the precipitating event of the hospitalization and a need just to talk. A nurse with an empathetic ear can help a patient by listening and allowing the patient to vent. Some patients may be introverted and not wish to voice their concerns. Nurses need to respect the patient's need for privacy, while also offering support if the patient desires to communicate.

THE FAMILY OF THE CRITICALLY ILL PATIENT

A family is "a basic societal unit in which members have a commitment to nurture each other emotionally and physically."[16] Families can be very diverse and do not always consist only of married or blood relatives. The family has been described as "a system, a complex network of interdependent interactions among family members which fulfills needs and achieves equilibrium."[17]

A family can be viewed as an open system. Any change or disturbance in a part of the system creates a change or disturbance in the whole system.[18] Therefore, any stress on one family member affects the whole family. Illness of a family member is a common situational stress that a family could experience. The family may view a member's illness as a threat to the family's equilibrium and integrity, especially if hospi-

talization is required. Nonhospitalized family members may have to assume the family roles of the sick member.

The illness (stressor) may precipitate a crisis in the family, especially if the stressor is a new stimulus that the family has not dealt with previously. Not all families react similarly to the same stressor. Therefore, every illness and hospitalization may not cause a family to experience a crisis. However, if the family views the illness as a threat to the family's integrity, a crisis can develop.

A crisis occurs when a person is confronted with a problematic situation for which his or her typical way of operating in the world and the usual supports are not sufficient.[18] "A crisis effects a temporary disruption of an individual's normal patterns of living, and is characterized by high levels of tension."[19] The interactional patterns reach a temporary state of disequilibrium in a family crisis. A period of disorganization ensures a period of upset, during which many abortive attempts at solution are made.[20]

The disorganization a family experiences is evidenced in its function and structure. Initially, family members may be immobilized by feelings of disbelief, shock, fear, helplessness, and anxiety.[21–26] The family begins to feel the loss of the predictable functions of the hospitalized relative.[22] Basic emotional and physical needs of the family members may be unmet as they attempt to resolve the disorganization that one member's hospitalization has precipitated. Unmet needs produce additional stress in the family.

If a family's needs are not met, they may be unable to "provide an ongoing social system for the patient during the crisis."[23] The well family members may experience anxiety as their attempts at resolving the disorganization fail because they lack the problem-solving skills to deal with the crisis.

"Interactions between members in a family system are circular. The behavior of one member affects the behavior of another."[24] Family members can transfer their anxiety to the patient, thereby increasing the patient's stress. The patient, especially in the ICU, is struggling to overcome a biologic crisis and does not need the added stress of a family's anxiety. When the stress a family experiences decreases, the amount of support it can offer the patient increases. Cobb[25] stated that "support from the patient's family is crucial to the patient's survival."

Critical care nurses need to be aware of the relation between their patient's recovery and the family members' support. The needs of the family have to be met to reduce the family's stress. The nurse needs to assess the family's potential for crisis and develop interventions that will enable the family to support the patient and regain its equilibrium and continue to grow. During a crisis, a person is more open to suggestions and to help; therefore, nursing interventions have fertile ground in which to work. Successful intervention may help family members regain their previous level of function and perhaps improve their coping ability. The needs of the family may change as time passes, so

RESEARCH APPLICATION: AN EVALUATION OF INTERVENTIONS FOR MEETING THE INFORMATION NEEDS OF FAMILIES OF CRITICALLY ILL PATIENTS
Henneman, E, McKenzie, J, and Dewa, C. Am J Crit Care 1(3):85, 1992.

Purpose: To evaluate the effectiveness of two methods of meeting the information needs of families of critically ill ICU patients; an open visiting-hour policy and a family information booklet.

Methods: A family satisfaction questionnaire that evaluated interventions for meeting information needs was distributed to three family groups; group 1—families with restricted visiting and no information booklet about unit policies and personnel (n = 48); group 2—families who had open visiting but no booklet (n = 50); and group 3—families who had open visiting and were given a booklet (n = 49). The questionnaire also tested families about their knowledge of unit policies and personnel.

Results: The addition of open visiting hours alone significantly increased family satisfaction and knowledge concerning visiting hours and the unit telephone number. No significant differences in satisfaction were found between group 2 and group 3. However, group 3 demonstrated a significant increase in knowledge of specific details of the ICU environment such as the physician's name, the social worker's name, visiting-hour policy, and unit phone number.

Practice Implications: Open or flexible visiting policies allow for more formal and informal information sharing between staff and family members, thus increasing satisfaction. However, open visiting hours alone is no guarantee of communication. Although the addition of a family information booklet did not significantly increase satisfaction, important information was conveyed. Use of written material is especially important, since family members may not be able to recall verbal information given during a period of crisis. Combining intervention strategies further ensures success in meeting family needs and providing family-focused care.

the nurse continually has to reassess the family to plan interventions accordingly.

Stressors for Families

The stressors for families of ICU patients are slightly different from patient stressors. Families experience physical isolation from their relative in ICU. In addition, family members may also experience emotional isolation from other well family members if the family support system is not strong enough or if family members are unable to be together because of physical distances. Families fear death or permanent disability of the ill member, they fear that the injury will cause the relative chronic pain, and they fear the loss of a "healthy" family member. Well members also have to absorb the role responsibilities of the ill member. If the ill member is financially responsible for the family, the illness will take a toll on family finances.

The ICU environment also stresses the family. Members are confronted with machines that alarm seemingly without cause, numerous intravenous lines, and other "tubes." Family members are often overwhelmed by detailed explanations about the technology. Focus is instead placed on familiar and personal aspects of care.[26] If a patient is intubated or in an altered neurologic state, the difficult or impossible communication between patient and family can cause increased stress for the family. Families have to put trust in strangers and hope that the ICU staff is competent. Restricted visiting hours, crowded ICU rooms, and the hurried ICU atmosphere can make families feel unwelcome. Relatives may be reluctant to touch the patient for fear of dislodging a tube or disturbing the patient's sleep.

The ICU waiting room can provide additional stressors if it is crowded, noisy, and located far from eating facilities and restrooms. The family may not want to leave the waiting room to eat for fear of missing the physician's visit or a change in their relative's condition. Since a family's support is vital to an ICU patient's recovery, the ICU staff needs to be aware of these stressors and needs of family members.

Family Needs

When a family member is critically ill, well members concentrate all their energy on the patient at the expense of their own physiologic needs. With the patient's admission to the ICU, families may forego sleep, forget to eat, and push themselves to the point of exhaustion. The well members' primary concern is for the patient to survive the current biologic crisis; all other needs are pushed aside.

Over the past decades research regarding the needs of family members of ICU patients has blossomed. Hampe's[27] pioneer study of the needs of spouses of terminally ill patients revealed that these spouses were able to identify eight personal needs and that the death of their spouse did not change these needs. The eight needs identified by Hampe's subjects were:

1. The need to be with the dying person
2. The need to be helpful to the dying person
3. The need for assurance of the comfort of the dying person
4. The need to be informed of the mate's condition
5. The need to be informed of the impending death
6. The need to ventilate emotions
7. The need for comfort and support of family members
8. The need for acceptance, support, and comfort from health professionals

Breu and Dracup[28] developed a special care plan for the spouses of critically ill coronary care unit (CCU) patients based on the eight needs identified in Hampe's study. The interventions included flexible visiting hours for the spouse, the patient's primary nurse calling the spouse at home twice daily with condition reports, and arranging to meet with the spouse for 15 minutes every day so that the nurse can answer any questions the spouse may have and provide emotional support. The results of their study indicated that spouses who received the special interventions felt that more of their needs were met by the nursing staff than spouses who received the CCU's usual nursing interventions.

Molter's[29] study was another milestone in the identification of family members' needs. In the study, Molter hypothesized that the families of these types of patients may have specialized needs. The subjects included not only the spouse of the patient but also parents, children, siblings, and even a niece. More than one family member per patient was interviewed.

The top 10 ranked needs were:

1. To feel there is hope
2. To feel that hospital personnel care about the patient
3. To have the waiting room near the patient
4. To be called at home about changes in the condition of the patient
5. To know the prognosis
6. To have questions answered honestly
7. To know specific facts concerning the patient's progress
8. To receive information about the patient once a day
9. To have explanations given in terms that are understandable
10. To see the patient frequently

Subjects were also asked to list who they felt were meeting their needs. Results showed that subjects felt that nurses met most of the families' needs overall and that physicians met most of their top 10 needs, including the need for information regarding the patient's prognosis and treatments. The needs that nurses met were related to the physical comfort and emotional support of the patient.

Later studies support Molter's findings. Families consistently identified the following needs to be very important to them: to feel there is hope, to know the prognosis, to be called at home regarding changes in patient's condition, to have questions answered honestly, and to feel that the best possible care was being given to the patient.[23,30–33]

Studies have shown that ICU nurses' assessments of family needs differ significantly from family members' perceived needs.[31,34,35] ICU nurses need to be more knowledgeable regarding the priority needs that families consistently identify, and they must implement interventions to meet these needs. Knowledge of family needs will help the nurse to prioritize interventions.

The literature indicates that family members of ICU patients have specific needs. Among the most important needs are to have honest and consistent information regarding the patient's prognosis and treatment, to feel that the patient is receiving the best care, and to visit the patient frequently. The establishment of good communication and a trusting relationship among patient, family, and ICU team is the first step in meeting these family needs.

Family Reactions

Most families experience shock and fear when a relative is admitted to an ICU. The patient's admission is usually sudden and unexpected and can precipitate a crisis in the family, especially if family members have little experience in dealing with hospitalization. Family members may feel guilty and angry if they feel they are partially responsible for the patient's illness. Like the patient, the family feels physically isolated and powerless. The family has little control over the patient's environment or treatment.

Ruppert[26] found in a study of wives of critically ill patients that the ICU experience was marked by the uncertainty of the situation. These spouses used the processes of keeping a constant vigilance, validating the mate's condition through information and "seeing for oneself," and mobilizing internal and external resources to work toward the return of a normal life.

Families react to their feelings of helplessness and powerlessness differently. Geary[36] identified five common coping mechanisms families used to deal with a relative's hospitalization. According to Geary, a coping mechanism is, "any behavior or mental processes used to attempt to come to terms with illness in the family."[36]

Minimization

Minimization is the first and most prevalent coping mechanism. This mechanism is characterized by reducing or attempting to ignore the significance of an event. An example of minimization is the family who takes on a cheerful demeanor while visiting the patient or talking with the nurse in hopes of reducing the significance of the hospitalization. A family member who does not remember information regarding a patient's condition or cannot understand repeated explanations may be minimizing the patient's situation by ignoring explanations and information.

RESEARCH APPLICATION: EMOTIONAL RESPONSES OF FAMILY MEMBERS DURING A CRITICAL CARE HOSPITALIZATION
Kleiber, C, et al. Am J Crit Care 3(1):70, 1994.

Purpose: To examine emotional responses of family members and their descriptions of supportive behaviors of others during critical care hospitalization.

Methods: Fifty-two subjects with critically ill family members in pediatric, neonatal, medical, surgical, and cardiovascular ICUs kept daily logs of their feelings and the supportive behaviors of others. Major themes were identified through thematic analysis.

Results: Powerful emotions such as fear, worry, anger, and exhaustion were identified during the first 24 hours. However, positive emotions such as relief and happiness also were experienced after the second and third days. Anger and hate emerged in response to technology, other family members, and healthcare providers who conveyed conflicting information. Frustration and helplessness were linked to family members' inability to help the patient during this crisis. Family members continued to ride an emotional roller coaster during the hospitalization.

Subjects identified caring attitudes as the most frequent supportive behavior. The provision of honest and understandable information was also seen as being supportive. Communication with friends, relatives, and other families in the ICU waiting rooms provided needed support.

Practice Implications: To plan and implement appropriate and meaningful family interventions, the nurse must first strive to understand the experience from the family member's perspective. Viewing the experience through such eyes directs the nurse in assessing family coping and planning interventions that recognize emotional responses. Support of family members is critical because they in turn provide the patient with support to overcome the biologic crisis of critical illness.

Intellectualization

Intellectualization is another coping mechanism. Family members who use this mechanism appear overly rational and minimize any feelings they are experiencing. A family member who wants to know every function of a ventilator, but who fails to be concerned about the patient's ventilator dependence, may be using intellectualization.

Repetition

Every ICU nurse has had the experience of a family member repeatedly asking the same questions or repeating the same story over and over. Family members who use repetition as a coping mechanism are reliving the event to decrease their anxiety and may repeat questions to different healthcare personnel to see whether they receive consistent answers.

Acting Strong

An example of this mechanism is the family member who presents a strong, competent attitude. The attitude seems to indicate an ability to deal well with the relative's illness. The family member may be trying to demonstrate that he or she has strong inner resources and can take over the ill member's role if he or she dies or has a long rehabilitation. This role frequently falls to a family member who is a healthcare professional, and the family may rely on that person to be the "expert." This responsibility can heighten the stress of the "expert" family member.

Remaining Near the Patient

Families may react to the patient's illness by keeping a vigil at the patient's bedside or remaining in the waiting room 24 hours a day. Some families feel that leaving the hospital for a while indicates a lack of hope for the patient's recovery, and maintaining hope is a priority need. Ethnic customs and mores can influence a family's reaction to separation from the patient. Some cultures feel that the family's presence either at the patient's bedside or in the waiting room is essential for the patient's recovery. The more critical the illness, the stronger the need is to stay near the patient.

Somatic complaints may be experienced by some family members, including restlessness, interrupted sleep pattern, weight loss, feelings of depression, and diminished appetite. Some family members may increase their smoking or their use of alcohol or other drugs.

Another reaction that family members may demonstrate is turning to others for support, such as friends, relatives, other ICU families, and ICU staff. Families need to feel there is hope for the patient's recovery or, in cases of patients with terminal illnesses, that their relative will not suffer and will die peacefully. Families may consider future events and try to answer the question "What if . . ."

Regardless of the coping methods that a family uses, the family's goal is to manage the stressful hospitalization experience the best that they can. Nurses need to recognize that the family is under stress and trying to cope. The ICU nurse needs to assess how effective a family's coping efforts are and intervene to support or reinforce their coping efforts.

Bowman[23] divided Molter's[29] need statements into three categories: cognitive needs, emotional needs, and physical needs. Nursing interventions for some of the needs in each category were developed. Table 5–1 summarizes nursing interventions to meet the needs of families of ICU patients.

PSYCHOSOCIAL ASSESSMENT OF CRITICALLY ILL PATIENTS AND THEIR FAMILIES

One of the most difficult and often the most neglected patient and family assessment is the nurse's assessment of the patient's and family's psychosocial functioning. The ICU patient is in a biologic crisis, and many times the ICU staff concentrates energy on supporting the patient's physiologic needs and working toward the resolution of the patient's biologic crisis. However, in the center of all the machines, intravenous lines, and various tubes lies a person who is experiencing overwhelming fear and anxiety. The ICU nurse is responsible not only for supporting the patient's physiologic functioning, but also for assessing and supporting the patient's emotional and social needs.

A psychosocial assessment of a patient involves observation of nonverbal behavior. Facial expressions and body language can indicate unvoiced anxiety and fear, depression, and even anger. Signs of anxiety such as facial grimacing, restlessness, picking at bedsheets, clenching hands, and crying can be observed. Fearful and anxious patients may repeat questions, use inappropriate humor, or be silent. Intubated patients may communicate fear through wide-eyed looks and pulling at tubes.

Since the family's support of a patient can help the patient overcome a biologic crisis, it is important for the nurse to assess how supportive a patient's family is and to plan interventions that encourage family support. Observe the quality of the patient and family interactions. Questions regarding the patient's marital status and living arrangements can provide clues to the strength of support systems.

In addition, it is important to gather information about the patient's past hospital experiences (especially past ICU experiences) and the coping methods that helped or did not help the patient and family handle previous hospitalizations. This information can give the nurse clues as to how the patient may react with this hospitalization. Any past history of emotional instability or substance/alcohol abuse by the patient can help the nurse to plan interventions as necessary to protect the patient's safety. Discovering whether the patient or family has recently undergone any major life changes (e.g., divorce, new job, or death of relative) will help in understanding the patient's and family members' current stress level.

The patient's vital signs can also provide clues to emotional status. A patient experiencing emotional distress may exhibit an increased blood pressure and cardiac output, increased pulse and respiratory rate, and dilated pupils as a result of increased epinephrine secretion. Blood glucose and cholesterol levels can also rise.

Specific questions that ICU nurses can ask patients or their families include:

1. Has the patient been hospitalized previously? If yes, what was the experience like? What helped the patient or family deal with the hospitalizations?
2. What are the family living arrangements?
3. What family does the patient have? Where do they live?
4. Who is taking care of home concerns?
5. How close is the family? Who in the family is most affected by patient's hospitalization?
6. What does the family know about the patient's condition?
7. Are there any ethnic, cultural, or spiritual concerns that the family needs assistance with?
8. What questions or concerns does the patient or family have? Is there any need for social services' intervention?

ICU nurses, using these questions as guidelines, can expand their inquiries into potential problem areas. For example, if a mother states that she has a child at home, the nurse can ask who is taking care of the child and determine the need for social services' assistance.

To perform a psychosocial assessment, an ICU nurse needs to use the same skills as those used for any patient/family assessment. Good communication skills are essential for gathering data. Empathetic, objective listening combined with asking open-ended questions are skills that a nurse must possess. Nurses can use their senses of touch, hearing, sight, and smell to gather objective and subjective data. Observing a patient's behavior can provide clues as to how that patient is feeling and coping with illness. The ICU nurse must also understand the importance of the patient's emotional and social status and how the patient's family and support system can positively influence a patient's recovery.

After collecting subjective and objective psychosocial patient data, the nurse formulates a nursing diagnosis based on the data. Examples of nursing diagnoses associated with psychosocial functioning include:

- Adjustment, impaired
- Anxiety
- Body image disturbance
- Communication, impaired, verbal
- Coping, defensive
- Coping, Family: Potential for growth
- Coping, Family, ineffective (specify compromised or disabled)
- Coping, Individual, ineffective
- Denial, ineffective
- Family Processes, altered
- Fear (specify)
- Grieving (specify anticipatory of dysfunctional)
- Hopelessness

TABLE 5–1
Summary of Nursing Interventions to Meet the Needs of Families of ICU Patients

Cognitive Needs
1. To Know Specific Facts About the Patient's Progress.
   - Avoid using generalizations such as "he's much better" or "things are about the same today."
   - Use the same simple terms each day to discuss progress and concerns (e.g., heart rhythm, blood pressure, level of pain, level of oxygen in the blood, not responding/very groggy/sleepy/awake, and so forth). This permits families to focus their attention on the same frame of reference and, when applicable, to put closure on the topic.
   - Relate progress to the illness as you have described it initially.
   - Use nursing care plan to communicate phrases and areas of concern being discussed so that all staff members use the same terminology.
2. To Know the Probable Outcome.
   - Be as realistic as possible, but be aware of family's coping mechanisms (such as denial) as well as their need for hope.
   - Establish short-term goals so that positive change can be identified.
   - If patient's prognosis is poor, allow adequate time to spend with the family so that feelings or questions can emerge. Establish times to meet with the family again.
   - Verbally recognize and accept family's desire for certainty in an ambiguous situation.
3. To Know Exactly What Is Being Done for the Patient (How the Patient Is Being Treated Medically, Why Things Are Being Done for the Patient).
   - Briefly describe each line and/or monitoring device, including IVs, urinary catheters, arterial lines, nasogastric tubes, O_2 devices, and so forth.
   - Encourage questions.
   - Remember that one explanation may not be enough; high anxiety is a barrier to learning.
   - Use simple terminology such as "breathing tube," "cardiogram," or "special intravenous" rather than endotracheal tube, electrocardiogram, or Swan-Ganz catheter.
   - Base explanations of treatment on patient's illness as you have described it initially. Reinforce explanations of pathophysiology as needed.
   - Promote continuity through nursing care plan.
4. To Have Questions Answered Honestly.
   - Be specific; discuss all issues as they relate to the patient as a unique individual.
   - Maintain good communications with physicians so that you are aware of what they have told the family. Discuss with them any information they feel should be withheld to determine rationale.
   - Use nursing care plan for consistency. Families quickly become aware of evasive answers. Consistency decreases anxiety and feelings of dehumanization and promotes cooperation.
5. To Have Explanations Given in Understandable Terms.
   - Assess family's knowledge base and previous experience with patient's condition.
   - Determine family's priority for learning; what do they want to know immediately.
   - Provide basic pathophysiology slowly, allowing time for questions. Repeat pathophysiologic concepts when discussing treatments or progress.
   - Divide informational sessions so that family is not overwhelmed. Establish times at which you will meet with them again to answer questions or provide additional explanations.
   - Remember that high anxiety is a barrier to learning; explanations usually have to be repeated.
   - Respond positively to questions, recognizing their right to understand what is happening.
6. To Have Explanations About the Environment Before Going into ICU for the First Time.
   - Use time before patient arrives on unit to meet with family.
   - Remember that the environment is frightening, not only equipment surrounding patient, but also the equipment used for other patients in the area.
   - While describing equipment, reinforce that much of it is present for prevention and early detection of problems.
   - Verbally recognize family's feelings and reassure them that these are normal and acceptable.
   - Be with family during their first visit to provide additional explanations and support.
   - For planned admissions (e.g., after surgery):
     Establish guidelines in teaching for discussion of environment.
     Provide patient and family tours of ICU if desired.
     Have ICU nurse who will be assigned to patient immediately postoperatively meet with family before surgery.

Emotional Needs
1. To Be Assured That the Best Possible Care Is Being Given to the Patient.
   - Emphasize that nurses and physicians are experienced and have special training to provide expert care.
   - Verbally recognize family's anxiety. Reassure them that such feelings are normal and that they do not have to hide these feelings.
2. To Be Called at Home About Changes in the Patient's Condition.
   - Establish guidelines with family about who is to be called and in what time frame.
   - Always ensure that the family knows about any significant change in patient's status before first visit of the day. If they are not informed about a change for the better, families frequently assume they will not be notified of other changes.
3. To Receive Information About the Patient Once Each Day.
   - Set aside one period during the day, as early as possible, during which progress reports are given.
   - Assess whether this time is adequate and follow up as needed, particularly if patient's condition changes.
   - Be aware if family needs to have physicians' explanations clarified or amplified.
4. To See the Patient Frequently.
   - Review policy for visiting hours to determine if they meet family needs; adjust as permitted by current situation in ICU.
   - If a visit must be delayed, explain reason clearly; make sure that the family does not believe the delay is due to a crisis unnecessarily.
   - Provide time for patient and family to be alone together.

TABLE 5–1
Summary of Nursing Interventions to Meet the Needs of Families of ICU Patients (*Continued*)

Emotional Needs
5. To Feel That Hospital Personnel Care About the Patient.
   • Use information gained during family assessment to anticipate concerns.
   • Listen to family's concerns, demonstrating that staff sees patient as an individual. Seek advice from the family about meeting patient needs.
   • Tell the family what patient communicates.
   • Focus on sensations patient will feel and possibly communicate to the family so that these do not come as a surprise (e.g., sore throat following endotracheal tube, fragility of chest wall after CABG, noisy environment, and so forth).
   • Remember that family members may focus on small details such as patient's position, cleanliness, or bedding because these are within their normal range of control.
   • Remember that family members may take out their feelings of grief, guilt, or anger on nursing staff; be patient.
6. To Talk About the Possibility of the Patient's Death. To Feel There Is Hope.
   • Determine family's perception of situation.
   • Anticipate and recognize signs of anticipatory grieving. Provide open-ended questions to encourage them to express their feelings.
   • Provide concrete information about patient's status slowly, assessing family's response. False reassurance and the opposite extreme, abrupt confrontation with reality, may hinder appropriate coping.
   • Meet jointly with physician and family to discuss use/nonuse of extraordinary measures or advanced life support systems.
   • Be aware of how comfortable you are when discussing a patient's death. If unable to meet family needs by yourself, arrange for another member of the health team to meet with family.
   • If there is no *real* contraindication, allow family to spend additional time with dying patient.

Physical Needs
1. To Help with the Patient's Physical Care.
   • Anticipate that family may be reluctant to touch patient because of equipment and yet want/need to touch him/her for reassurance. Small directed activities meet both these concerns.
   • Allow family to do small things for patient (e.g., providing ice chips, wiping face, washing old blood off hands, and so forth).
   • If there is no *real* contraindication, allow family member to provide parts of morning care.
2. To Visit Anytime.
   • Discuss visiting regulations with family.
   • Be flexible if special arrangements need to be made because of other responsibilities.
   • Recognize that this need will probably diminish over a few days as families become aware that visiting hours are adequate and that they *will* be permitted to see patient frequently.
3. To Have the Waiting Room Near ICU. To Have a Telephone Near the Waiting Room.
   • If these are not available in your hospital, be aware of potential stress for families. Discuss possible alternative arrangements.
   • Discuss the need for family members to get adequate rest so that they will be able to support patient later in hospitalization and to minimize extended stays by family in waiting room.
4. To Have a Place to Be Alone in the Hospital.
   • Direct family to hospital chapel if available.
   • Determine if there is space available nearby, currently being used for another purpose, that could be used by family for periods of privacy.
   • If weather is pleasant, encourage family to exercise outdoors during the day.

Source: Bowman, CC: Identifying priority concerns of families of ICU patients. Dimens Crit Care Nurs 3(5):313, 1984, with permission.

• Personal Identity disturbance
• Powerlessness
• Role Performance, altered
• Self-Esteem disturbance
• Sleep Pattern disturbance
• Social Isolation
• Spiritual Distress

Based on the nursing diagnoses, the nurse plans interventions to achieve the desired outcomes. All interventions need to be evaluated for their effectiveness and revised if outcomes are not achieved.

Family members' needs and concerns should also be assessed by the nurse. The family can provide the nurse with information regarding the patient if the patient is unable to do so. Many times the family is the only source of information. The family can be observed for their methods of coping with their family member's illness and for the amount of support they offer the patient. The nurse can ascertain who in the family fills what roles and which family member has assumed the responsibilities of the sick patient's role or roles. The nurse can gather data about the pa-

tient's family through observation, questioning, and listening.

The following case studies with sample care plans illustrate the use of nursing diagnoses concerned with psychosocial function.

CASE STUDY WITH SAMPLE CARE PLAN: PATIENT/FAMILY WITH PSYCHOSOCIAL DYSFUNCTION WITH CLOSED HEAD INJURY

The Smiths' only child, 19-year-old Cory, sustained a severe closed head injury 2 days ago in a motorcycle accident. Cory is in a deep coma and unresponsive to painful stimuli. His prognosis is grim, and the Smiths have been told that Cory has a minimal chance of regaining consciousness.

Mr. Smith appears calm, but the nurse observed that he has asked more questions about the ventilator and hemodynamic monitoring than about Cory's condition. He states that his wife does not work and that he handles all the financial concerns in the family. "My insurance should easily cover all of Cory's expenses.'' He never touches Cory or sits by the bedside. Mr. Smith's visits are brief and infrequent.

Mrs. Smith insists on sitting by Cory's bed at all times. She leaves the patient's room only when asked to and has slept in the family lounge since Cory's admission. When a nurse suggested she go home and sleep, she stated, ''Cory's all I got and I'm going to stay with him until he wakes up.'' She asks every person that takes care of Cory the same questions, which makes the nursing staff feel as if she is checking up on them. When Mrs. Smith and her husband are in the patient's room together, they rarely converse or touch each other. Mr. Smith leaves the hospital at night. No other relatives have visited Cory or have called.

Nursing Diagnoses

1. Coping: Ineffective, family compromised
2. Anxiety
3. Social Isolation

CASE STUDY WITH SAMPLE CARE PLAN: PATIENT/FAMILY WITH RULE-OUT MYOCARDIAL INFARCTION (p. 52)

CM, a 54-year-old man, experienced acute onset of midsternal chest pain radiating to the left arm while shoveling snow. He was brought to the emergency room (ER) of University Medical Center by ambulance at 10:00 AM.

Mr. M was directly admitted to the coronary care unit (CCU), where he was attached to a cardiac monitor and continued to receive intravenous fluid (IV) at 25 mL/h and oxygen at 3 L/min by nasal cannula. Mr. M received three sublingual nitroglycerin tablets in the ER and 6 mg of IV morphine. His chest pain has subsided.

The CCU nurse completing Mr. M's admission form observes that he answers questions rapidly and repeats phrases several times, such as ''I could not believe I was having chest pain. I thought it was indigestion.'' Mr. M's eyes dart all around the floor, and he makes limited direct eye contact with the nurse. He fidgets with the sheets and keeps folding and unfolding his arms. The nurse records several of Mr. M's statements in the admission note. ''I've never been sick a day in my life. This is the first time I've been in a hospital. I feel so nervous. What is that beeping sound? Is my heart OK? Both my father and my brother died of heart attacks in their fifties. Did I have a heart attack?''

Mr. M's blood pressure is 154/92 mm Hg; pulse, 115 bpm with occasional premature ventricular contractions (PVC), and his respirations are 20. His skin is cool and clammy. His wife is present and sits quietly in a chair by her husband's bed.

Nursing Diagnoses

1. Anxiety
2. Fear of dying, related to familial history of myocardial infarction
3. Potential for ineffective coping: Individual

SAMPLE CARE PLAN: PATIENT/FAMILY WITH PSYCHOSOCIAL DYSFUNCTION WITH CLOSED HEAD INJURY

Nursing Diagnoses	**Desired Patient/Family Outcomes**
Nursing Diagnosis #1 Coping: Ineffective, family compromised, related to sudden catastrophic injury	Patient's parents will: 1. Verbalize questions and concerns regarding son's condition 2. Verbalize knowledge and understanding of illness 3. Verbalize resources within themselves to deal with the situation

Nursing Diagnoses	**Desired Patient/Family Outcomes**
Nursing Diagnosis #2 Anxiety, related to sudden hospitalization, unfamiliar surroundings, and grim prognosis.	Parents will describe decrease in feelings of anxiety and reduce the number of repetitious questions.

Nursing Interventions	**Rationale**
• Exhibit an empathetic attitude; offer to listen, and encourage the family to verbalize concerns when ready to do so.	• The nurse is accessible to the patient's parents and offers a listening ear. This helps to nurture the patient/family/ nurse relationship and develop trust. ○ Family members who intellectualize may do so because they may be unable or unwilling to discuss their feelings with others.
• Assist parents to identify personal strengths. ○ Encourage parents to develop problem-solving skills to deal with son's illness.	• Identifying strengths and problem-solving skills will assist family members in coping.

SAMPLE CARE PLAN: PATIENT/FAMILY WITH PSYCHOSOCIAL DYSFUNCTION WITH CLOSED HEAD INJURY (*Continued*)

- Explain to parents that touching the patient is perfectly okay and offer them the option of assisting with patient's care if they desire.
  ○ Encourage them to sit at bedside and reassure that they will not disturb the patient's equipment or machinery.
- Encourage questions and make necessary explanations.

- Approach patient's mother with concern and state, "It sounds as if you are having a difficult time," after she asks repetitious questions.

- Alert other healthcare providers that asking repetitious questions may reflect the patient's mother's underlying anxiety.
- Explain to patient's parents that when they go home at night, they will be called immediately if there is a change in the patient's condition. (Note: An innovative strategy such as a beeper may be used.)
- Negotiate a set time every day when the nurse will update both Mr. and Mrs. Smith regarding Cory's condition.
  ○ Communicate family information needs to all members of the ICU interdisciplinary team.

- Touching and helping to care for their son may help decrease feelings of powerlessness and anxiety.

- Explanations may correct misconceptions on the part of the patient's parents and provide them with information.
- Patient's mother may be using repetition to mask anxiety; offering to listen may help her verbalize and deal with her anxiety. She may need to "relive" events of son's accident. Verbalizing this can help decrease her anxiety.
- Incorporating this information into the patient's care plan will help to ensure continuity of care.

- The patient's mother may need "permission" to leave the hospital, fearing that by leaving, she shows a lack of hope for her son. As her son's condition stabilizes, she may feel a decreased need to stay at night.
- Providing updates helps keep family informed of patient condition changes.

  ○ This allows for honest and consistent information to be shared with family.

Nursing Diagnoses

Nursing Diagnosis #3
Social Isolation, related to lack of immediate support systems

Desired Patient/Family Outcomes

Patient's parents will:
1. Express feelings of isolation
2. Use family and friends to help with home maintenance and support for themselves

Nursing Interventions
- Provide the family with the ICU telephone number, and encourage calling when they feel apprehensive.
- Explain the need for the parents to take care of themselves, to avoid illness during this time of stress.
- Treat patient and family with respect and demonstrate competence.

- Encourage the patient's mother to visit frequently; provide necessary explanations at those times when she may be asked to leave the patient's room.

- Ascertain whether other relatives or friends are aware of the patient's injury.
  ○ Inquire as to how they are managing in health and home maintenance.
- Encourage patient's parents to use and to share with other family members and friends.
- Advise family of the availability of the hospital chaplain.
  ○ Inquire if they would appreciate a visit from their own minister.
- Reinforce staff support to patient/family.
  ○ Be accessible; listen attentively.
  ○ Take time to care.

Rationales
- Providing an open communication channel eases anxiety and establishes a connection to the patient and staff.
- The family may be unable to provide support to the patient if they themselves are ill.
- By treating patient and family with respect and by demonstrating competence, the parents' anxiety may be eased.
- Allowing mother to visit and providing necessary phone numbers may help to decrease anxiety.
  ○ Providing explanations as to the patient's care may allay anxiety when the patient's mother is asked to leave the patient's room.
- In time of crisis, family members may become disorganized and need support of friends and family to cope with the crisis.

- Many people find comfort in religion and prayer; such activities can provide positive support.

- In a family lacking external support system, the ICU staff and other patients' families can be a source of comfort and support.
- Family members who cannot support each other have limited resources with which to support the patient in this biologic crisis.

SAMPLE CARE PLAN: PATIENT/FAMILY WITH RULE-OUT MYOCARDIAL INFARCTION (MI)

Nursing Diagnoses

Nursing Diagnosis #1
Anxiety, related to sudden illness, unfamiliar surroundings, chest pain, unknown future

Desired Patient Outcomes

Patient will:
1. Verbalize a decrease in anxiety
2. Maintain stable vital signs:
   - BP within 10 mmHg of baseline
   - Heart rate <100/min
   - Respiratory rate/rhythm <25 minutes regular and unlabored
3. Appear relaxed with no nonverbal indications of anxiety

Nursing Interventions

- Encourage patient to verbalize concerns, actively listen.

- Demonstrate an empathic and caring attitude.
  - Provide reassurance; give short, simple explanations.
  - Stay with patient.
- Observe for behavioral clues that anxiety is decreasing (more direct eye contact, less rapid speech, and slower body movements).
- Monitor vital signs: blood pressure, pulse, and respiratory rate and rhythm.

- Monitor response to prescribed analgesia therapy (e.g., morphine, nitroglycerin, or sedatives to reduce and minimize chest pain) and their effectiveness.
  - Antianxiety agents may also be indicated.
- Decrease noise level (e.g., by shutting doors between patient rooms, encouraging a quiet rest period during each shift, and organizing patient care to provide frequent rest periods).
- Orient patient/family to surrounding and protocols.

Rationales

- By verbalizing anxiety, the patient is helped to recognize the existence of anxiety, thus making the anxiety less threatening and easier to deal with.
- An empathic attitude and active listening help demonstrate that the nurse respects the patient, and it helps to develop a trusting nurse-patient relationship.
- Behavior gives clues to underlying anxiety. Body language can be observed for presence of anxiety.

- Somatic signs of the stress response are seen in increased blood pressure, pulse, and cool, clammy skin as epinephrine is released and blood is rerouted to major organs.
- The effectiveness of analgesic and antianxiety medication in relieving pain and anxiety should be carefully monitored.

- The stress response is harmful to the hypoxic (ischemic) heart and could lead to an extension of the infarct.

Nursing Diagnoses

Nursing Diagnosis #2
Fear of death, related to familial history of myocardial infarction

Desired Patient Outcomes

Patient will verbalize concerns and fears and increased emotional comfort.

Nursing Interventions

- Strengthen patient/family/nurse relationship.
  - Exhibit empathic attitude.
  - Listen actively.

  - Encourage patient to verbalize concerns and fears and identify constructive coping methods.
- Consult with patient's physician, sharing familial history ascertained.
  - Share approach to therapy.
  - Jointly inform patient and spouse about diagnosis, course of treatment, and prognosis for recovery.
- Offer patient and family positive information regarding the patient's recuperative progress as patient's condition improves. Avoid offering false reassurance.
- Encourage patient to discuss fears with spouse. Support patient and spouse in reassessing goals and planning beyond discharge.
- Promote use of constructive coping strategies (i.e., relaxation techniques, diversional activities).

Rationales

- An empathic attitude and active listening help to demonstrate that the nurse respects the patient and helps a trusting nurse/patient/family relationship to develop.
  - Verbalization of fear and concerns allows patient to acknowledge fear and thus to begin to deal with it.
- Collegial interaction ensures continuity of care and reassures patient/family.

- Information from members of health team gives facts that patient and family can deal with. This may assist them in handling fears and reassessing lifestyle.
  - Reassurance regarding improvement in patient's condition helps to reduce fear and fosters hope.

- Positive coping may minimize the physiological and psychological effects of stress aid in recovery.

SAMPLE CARE PLAN: PATIENT/FAMILY WITH RULE-OUT MYOCARDIAL INFARCTION (MI) (*Continued*)

Nursing Diagnoses

Nursing Diagnosis #3
Potential for ineffective coping:
Individual, related to
1. Catastrophic illness
2. Necessary changes in lifestyle

Desired Patient Outcomes

Patient will:
1. Discuss impact of illness on lifestyle and feelings regarding this
2. Identify personal strengths
3. Identify previous methods of coping

Nursing Interventions

- Assess patient's present coping status.
- Assist patient to develop problem-solving strategies based on his strengths and personal experience.
- Initiate referrals: e.g., cardiac rehabilitation.

Rationales

- Identification of personal strengths and the development of problem-solving techniques help the patient take control of his situation and motivate needed change in lifestyle.
- Referral to followup services or programs can assist in developing health promotion and disease prevention behaviors.

REFERENCES

1. Selye, H: The Stress of Life. McGraw-Hill, New York, 1956, pp 54, 64.
2. Lazarus, RS: Stress, Appraisal, and Coping. Springer, New York, 1984.
3. Soehren, P: Stressors perceived by cardiac surgical patients in the intensive care unit. Am J Crit Care 4(1):71, 1994.
4. Simpson, T: Critical care patients' perceptions of visits. Heart Lung 20:681, 1991.
5. Hendrickson, S: Intracranial pressure changes and family presence. J Neurosci Nurs 19:14, 1987.
6. Prins, M: The effect of family visits on intracranial pressure. West J Nurs Res 11:281, 1989.
7. Schulte, D, et al: Pilot study of the relationship between heart rate and ectopy and unrestricted vs restricted visiting hours in the coronary care unit. Am J Crit Care 2(2):134, 1993.
8. Simpson, T and Shaver, J: Cardiovascular responses to family visits in coronary care unit patients. Heart Lung 19:344, 1990.
9. Simpson, T and Shaver, J: A comparison of hypertensive and nonhypertensive coronary care patients' cardiovascular responses to visitors. Heart Lung 20:213, 1991.
10. Treloar, D, et al: The effect of familiar and unfamiliar voice treatments on intracranial pressure in head-injured patients. J Neurosci Nurs 23(5):295, 1991.
11. Kobasa, S: The hardy personality: Toward a social psychology of stress and health. In Sanders, GS and Suls, J (eds): Social Psychology of Health and Illness. Lawrence Erlbaum, NJ, 1982, pp 3–32.
12. Haber, J, et al: Comprehensive Psychiatric Nursing, ed 2. McGraw-Hill, New York, 1982.
13. Horowitz, M: Psychological response to serious life events. In Hamilton, V and Warburton, D (eds): Human Stress and Cognition. John Wiley & Sons, New York, 1980.
14. Hackett, TP and Cassem, NH: Psychological management of the myocardial infarction patient. Human Studies 1(3):25, 1975.
15. Salyer, J and Stuart, BJ: Nurse-patient interaction in the intensive care unit. Heart Lung 14:20, 1985.
16. Smilkstein, G: The cycle of family function: A conceptual model for family medicine. J Fam Pract 11:223, 1980.
17. Ruben, HL: Family crisis. Am Fam Physician 11:132, 1975.
18. Parad, HJ and Caplan, G: A framework for studying families in crisis. In Parad, HJ (ed): Crisis Intervention: Selected Readings. Family Services Association of America, New York, 1965, pp 53–72.
19. Umana, RF, Gross, ST, and McConville, MT: Crisis in the Family: Three Approaches. Gardner Press, New York, 1980.
20. Caplan, G: An Approach to Community Mental Health. Grune & Stratton, New York, 1961.
21. Kleiber, C, et al: Emotional responses of family members during a critical care hospitalization Am J Crit Care 3(1):70, 1994.
22. Braulin, J, Rook, J, and Sills, GM: Family in crisis: The impact of trauma. Crit Care Q 5(3):38, 1982.
23. Bowman, CC: Identifying priority concerns of families of ICU patients. Dimens Crit Care Nurs 3(5):313, 1984.
24. Levitt, MB: Nursing and family focused care. Nurs Clin North Am 19:83, 1984.
25. Cobb, S: Social support as a moderator of life stress. Psychosom Med 38:300, 1976.
26. Ruppert, S: Wives' perceptions of situational experiences during critical care hospitalization: A phenomenological study. Dissertation Abstracts International (Microfilms No. 9312904), 1993.
27. Hampe, SO: Needs of the grieving spouse in a hospital setting. Nurs Res 24:116, 1975.
28. Breu, C and Dracup, K: Helping spouses of critically ill patients. Am J Nurs 78:51, 1978.
29. Molter, NC: Needs of relatives of critically ills patients: A descriptive study. Heart Lung 8:332, 1979.
30. Leske, JS: Needs of relatives of critically ill patients: A follow-up. Heart Lung 15:189, 1986.
31. Norris, LO and Grove, SK: Investigation of selected psychosocial needs of family members of critically ill adult patients. Heart Lung 15:194, 1986.
32. Norheim, C: Family needs of patients having coronary artery bypass graft surgery during the intraoperative period. Heart Lung 18:622, 1989.
33. Leske, JS: Overview of family needs after critical illness: From assessment to intervention. AACN Clin Iss Crit Care 2(2):220, 1991.
34. Forrester, DA, et al: Critical care family needs: Nurse-family member confederate pairs. Heart Lung 19:655, 1990.
35. Jacono, G, et al: Comparison of perceived needs of family members between registered nurses and family members of critically ill patients in intensive care and neonatal intensive care units. Heart Lung 19:72, 1990.
36. Geary, MC: Supporting family coping. Supervisor Nurse 10(3):52, 1979.

SUGGESTED READINGS

Artinian, N: Strengthening nurse-family relationships in critical care. AACN Clin Iss Crit Care 2(2):269, 1991.

Bartz, C: An exploratory study of the coronary artery bypass graft surgery experience. Heart Lung 17:179, 1988.

Clark, C and Heidenreich, T: Spiritual care for the critically ill. Am J Crit Care 4(1):77, 1994.

Cochran, J and Ganong, L: A comparison of nurses' and patients' perceptions of intensive care unit stressors. J Adv Nurs 14:1038, 1989.

Danielson, C, Hamel-Bissell, B, and Winstead-Fry, P: Families, Health, & Illness. CV Mosby, St Louis, 1993.

Dracup, K and Bryan-Brown, C: An open door policy in ICU. Am J Crit Care 1(2):16, 1992.

Harvey, M, et al.: Results of the consensus conference on fostering more humane critical care: Creating a healing environment. AACN Clin Iss Crit Care 4(3):484, 1993.

Henneman, E, McKenzie, J, and Dewa, C: An evaluation of interventions for meeting the informational needs of families of critically ill patients. Am J Crit Care 1(3):85, 1992.

Johnson, J and Morse, J: Regaining control: The process of adjustment after myocardial infarction. Heart Lung 19:126, 1990.

Kleman, M, Bickert, A, and Karpinski, A: Physiologic responses of coronary care patients to visiting. J Cardiovasc Nurs 7:52, 1993.

Koller, P: Family needs and coping strategies during illness crisis. AACN Clin Iss Crit Care 2(2):338, 1991.

Marsden, C: Family-centered critical care: An option or obligation? Am J Crit Care 1(3):115, 1992.

Miller, J: Developing and maintaining hope in families of the critically ill. AACN Clin Iss Crit Care 2(2):307, 1991.

Riegel, B and Ehrenreich, D: Psychological Aspects of Critical Care Nursing. Aspen, Rockville, MD, 1989.

Simpson, T: The family as a source of support for the critically ill adult. AACN Clin Iss Crit Care 2(2):229, 1991.

Simpson, T: Visit preferences of middle-aged vs older critical care patients. Am J Crit Care 2(4):339, 1993.

Simpson, T, Armstrong, S, and Mitchell, P: American Association of Critical-Care Nurses demonstration project: Patients' recollection of critical care. Heart Lung 18:325, 1989.

Titler, M, Cohen, M, and Craft, M: Impact of adult critical care hospitalization: Perceptions of patients, spouses, children, and nurses. Heart Lung 20:174, 1991.

Titler, M and Walsh, S: Visiting critically ill adults: Strategies for practice. Crit Care Clin North Am 4:623, 1992.

CHAPTER 6

Being Human
Lorraine Brown and Frances Dooley

CHAPTER OUTLINE

LEARNING OBJECTIVES

At the end of this chapter, you should be able to:

1. Define depersonalization.
2. Describe the process of dehumanization.
3. Discuss interventions to prevent depersonalization and dehumanization in a critical care setting.
4. Identify caring behavior that promotes personalized, humanistic, critical care.

A CASE STUDY IN DEPERSONALIZATION

Depersonalization—the feeling that one is not human, but, rather, an illness to be treated—can occur because healthcare providers are so involved with saving the patient's life that the patient's humanness is ignored.

The sirens roared and the lights flashed as the ambulance raced through the traffic-laden streets of the east side of Manhattan to the Hospital Center. Within minutes I was strapped onto a stretcher, which crashed through two steel doors into a land of mystique and staring eyes. Four white-uniformed personnel mumbled an introduction as they simultaneously attached wires to my four limbs, took my blood, and slapped three round disks to my roughly exposed chest. As my eyes darted around this noise-filled room, the already increasing tightness in my chest was now accompanied by a dry throat and the sweats.

Overwhelmed with fear and anticipation, I lay motionless as my body became the center of various unfamiliar activities. The blurred faces and muffled voices of the doctors and nurses continued around me as I became suddenly aware I had been wheeled into the Heart Room. The lights, beeps, and bells seemed to be penetrating my already overwhelming thoughts of death and fears of the unknown. These white-clothed experts kept referring to me as the new massive MI with occasional PVCs in Room 3.

Two doctors came into my room and immediately focused their eyes on what appeared to be a small TV set, which showed my heart beats. A nurse entered, rambled her name, put a needle in my arm, connected a tube feeding into two bottles, and said this is an IV.

Somehow, I didn't feel like I was part of my body, and I still did not know what was happening to me. The foreign terms, strange noises, and unfamiliar faces made me very nervous and afraid. Several questions paraded through my mind: Was I going to die? Did I have a heart attack? Did anyone call my wife? Should I tell someone I still have that pain in my chest? Does anyone here know my name? What is an EKG? MI? PVC? IV? Why does everyone use initials? Why doesn't someone sit down and tell me what is going on? Why is everyone rushing around to get things done? I just wanted to shout out, "Hey, my name is Joe, I am 48 years old and a New York City fireman, and I am afraid!"

The above account is a patient's assessment of the initial phase of his myocardial infarction within the environment of an emergency room. The critically ill patient arrived in a state of crisis, and the emphasis was placed on the equipment, procedures, and physiologic condition.

As the patient underwent intensive treatment, he appeared to develop an astuteness to what was happening around him. This sensitivity increased when he believed his survival was dependent on equipment and fast-paced personnel. Attachment to machinery provided comfort to the patient who was faced with the threat of death, but it also caused the patient to experience himself as an object who had lost his value as a human being. A setting that will keep the patient feeling human, as well as functioning efficiently, is of great importance when the person is detached from his normal environment.

This environmentally shocked patient was further stressed by the impersonal hustle and bustle of the health professionals. An individual patient such as Joe does not equate himself with his myocardial infarction. If he did, then treating his illness would satisfy his humanistic needs. The caregivers perceived Joe's illness as something he was, not something he had.

The patient was being perceived as a myocardial infarction with presenting ectopic beats instead of as a human being who was ill. Although grateful for the attention given to his physical condition, he was resentful toward those caregivers who had failed to recognize him as a person.

In the initial emergency phase of the illness, Joe is faced with an abrupt alteration in his life. Being unprepared to face this situation renders him helpless and adds to his already overwhelmed emotional state. His feeling of loss of control imposes severe psychological stress, and he submits to treatment in a nonquestioning complacent manner.

This critical situation induced in Joe a state of profound numbness. He experienced a sense of unreality, a strange sensation of being outside of his body. He felt his immediate and familiar presence in jeopardy, and what lay ahead seemed ambiguous to him.

Joe's socioemotional needs were dramatically pushed aside to deal with physiologic needs. The health professionals were so involved with life-saving technical procedures that the humanness of Joe was ignored. The behavioral "me" aspect of Joe as an individual was removed, and he was perceived as an illness rather than a person. Sensation and emotion were nondiscernible for Joe. The numbness and strangeness Joe experienced combine to form a common state shared by many critically ill patients—depersonalization.

A CASE STUDY IN DEHUMANIZATION

Frequently accompanying the state of depersonalization is the process of dehumanization. This process of human reduction begins subtly when the critically ill patient enters the intensive care unit. It continues to increase with the number of healthcare providers perceiving the individual as a patient rather than as a human being. Dehumanization, conscious or unintentional, demotes the person to the level of an object or a thing as seen in the following case study.

> When I first came to, the tubes were everywhere. They were in my mouth, they were in my chest, my neck, my arm, and even in my penis. I hurt all over. There were noises and unfamiliar pieces of equipment all around me. I still didn't know what had happened, and no one cared to tell me. I tried to communicate, but they just kept saying, "Don't worry, you are all right. You are out of the OR. You are in the ICU."

> There were two female nurses by my bed; they were looking at papers and talking about tubes. Suddenly they yanked the sheets down to my knees. They told me that they wanted to check my abdominal dressing and my Foley. They did not introduce themselves or explain things. They didn't even cover my private area. I felt so embarrassed, but I was too afraid to move because my arm was strapped down to a board.

> After examining my exposed body, they said I had to turn on my side. I tried to resist because they were hurting me, but the two of them just pulled and pushed until they were satisfied with my position and assured me that I would be more comfortable.

> The next day the tube in my mouth came out. I thought things were getting better. I started eating spoonfuls of Jello. Suddenly the thought occurred to me, how was I going to go to the bathroom? When I asked the nurse she said, "Don't worry about it."

> Here I was with tubes all over. I knew I couldn't get out of bed, and I needed to answer this worry. Why didn't anyone care? My anger started to rage. Why didn't anyone listen to me? When the time finally came, the nurse said, "Don't worry about it. Just go in the bed if you have to." How could they make me do this? I could not face anyone. I just wanted to sleep. I kept my eyes closed just wanting desperately to be somewhere else.

> That evening when dinner came, I threw the tray on the floor and ordered everyone to leave me alone. I had had enough! I just wanted to shout, "My name is Charlie, I'm only 20 years old and I don't know what happened to me."

This patient is experiencing the process of dehumanization. The high-tech machinery, sophisticated environment, and lack of primary caring and concern on the part of the healthcare providers all help to promote this process. Failure to recognize the patient's beliefs, values, perceptions, and expectations further damaged this already helpless individual. A seriously ill patient hence becomes childlike, with a tendency to look for omnipotence and infallibility in the caregivers. Charlie is seriously ill. He feels damaged and hurt, and no one takes the time to explain what has happened to him. He is not given the opportunity to verbalize his feelings, and he becomes enmeshed in feelings of hopelessness. He begins to experience himself as an object who has lost his value as a human being.

Dehumanization strips the person of human capacity, and it can occur whenever another person or group becomes responsible for making ongoing daily decisions regarding the comfort and welfare of another. The integrity and uniqueness of the individual are lost.

Charlie perceives himself as a helpless child unable to make any decisions regarding even basic activities of daily living. When subjected to this process, Charlie experienced one of the most common emotional responses, anger. Initially, Charlie suppresses his anger for fear of rejection and retaliation by his caregivers. He withdraws into sleep. Charlie is already in a physiologic crisis, and his adjustment is further hampered by a loss of self-identity and a threat of abandonment.

Charlie's caregivers are expected to make things

better for him, but because of their lack of humanistic caring, he becomes more angered and unable to cope with his physiologic crisis. The primary physical care delivered fails to offer satisfaction to Charlie in his time of crisis.

In the scenarios just presented, one can see how the onset of critical illness disrupts the dynamic equilibrium of the individual's life processes. As vividly portrayed in the experiences of Joe and Charlie, the inability of the individual to cope effectively with and to manage a physiologic and emotional crisis is often undermined by the state of depersonalization and the process of dehumanization.

As a result of the incapacitating nature of critical illness, critically ill patients experience a loss of self-worth and self-esteem; they are stripped of their sense of independence and privacy; and they feel isolated from their family and significant others. These patients are dependent on the knowledge, skills, and dedication of the ICU team to meet their complex and intimate needs. Their very lives are entrusted to virtual strangers, which adds to their high level of stress and fear. Patients usually want to experience self-worth and protect their own personal identity and integrity. The nurse must allow patients to resolve these aspects of this human struggle as they face the life-threatening event.

Critical care nurses must be able to recognize clues to these problems, to identify patients at risk, and to be prepared to intervene to alleviate and/or prevent their occurrence. In the discussion that follows, emphasis will be placed on some behaviors the nurse can use in fostering a more personalized and humanistic approach in caring for critically ill patients.

CARING BEHAVIORS

Caring is vital in the achievement of wellness. It is as important as curing and is proclaimed on a national level (i.e., American Nurses Association's Social Policy Statement) as the essential concept underlying nursing practice. The art of caring fosters nursing the "me" quality of patients. Nurses focus on patients as people rather than as illnesses. The thinking, feeling, and sensing human being becomes the central focal point of nursing care.

Personalized humanistic care is provided by the caring behaviors of the caregivers. Along with technologic skills, caring behaviors must be recognized, developed, and integrated into daily practice as professional nurses. These caring behaviors should be incorporated into the care of the critically ill patient on admission to the intensive care setting.

Communicating

A simple yet easily overlooked behavior on the part of the nurse is an introduction, including the nurse's name and a recognition by the nurse of each patient's choice of names. In the process of this social exchange, an extension of hands to affirm the introduction is well received by each individual as a respect for his or her personal worth, and is necessary to establish a nurse-patient bond.

In most critical-care areas, first names are sometimes used by the nurses to foster a close relationship with patients. The admitting nurse initiates the care for the patient and is the professional in whom patients must first place their trust to safeguard their well-being. Time is of the essence in developing a therapeutic relationship to stabilize the patient's disequilibrium brought on by a life-threatening event.

Effective, ongoing communication between nurses and their patients is essential as patients progress through the course of their illness. Communication is the most significant mode of activity through which patients can affect their environment from the supine position. It is vital that the communication be meaningful to the patient. In the first case study, the healthcare professionals used medical jargon, abbreviations, and unfamiliar terms, and failed to offer explanations. Joe's inability to understand and to question his caregivers further overwhelmed him as he faced his physiologic crisis. Likewise in the second case study, Charlie awakens and desperately seeks an explanation as to his present circumstance. The responses of the nurses failed to offer any meaning to him in his confused, fearful state.

The nurses should have attempted to make their communication meaningful. Use of understandable terminology, simple explanations of procedures, and an introduction and orientation to an unfamiliar environment could have assisted both Joe and Charlie in dispelling their fears and confusion.

Touching

As seen in both case studies described previously, nurses failed to establish a therapeutic relationship with their patients. No time was devoted to establishing a personal approach by introducing themselves by name and inquiring from the patients what they wished to be called. A single act of human touch, for example, a warm handshake or gentle squeeze, would have been helpful in establishing a trusting relationship and fostering the personalization of the patient. Personalization reflects a greater sense of one's own identity, and feeling comfortable with oneself and being in touch with one's feelings.

In addition, a warm caring touch of Joe's shoulder or head would have improved the potential for sincere nurse-patient communication. Joe was feeling very nervous and afraid as people hurried around him performing various procedures. A simple touch, which serves to reassure an individual of his self-worth, could have allayed Joe's fears and imparted a sign that someone cared. The distance of the healthcare workers in Joe's case made him sense only blurred faces and muffled voices, and he could not become a part of the experience.

In Charlie's case, the nurses made physical contact

with him, but the contact lacked human touch qualities. Touch should be a deliberate action to convey understanding and acceptance. When possible, touch should be accompanied with eye contact. Touch is a necessary building block in forming a trusting relationship.

Valuing

The development of an interpersonal relationship through communication serves as a basis for nurses to form judgments and make decisions. A recognition of who their patients really are and the patients' right to participate in their own care will enable nurses to be more alert to patients' behavioral cues. Patients need to know that they are valued by the caregivers, and that their behavior and verbalization will be acknowledged as significant to them.

Failure to recognize the person of Joe can clearly be seen in the first example. Who was he? What role did he play in his family, community, and society in general? Joe's identity as an individual, and his feelings, needs, and concerns were pushed aside as the attentions of the caregivers focused on his physiologic instability. Joe, being afraid and isolated from his wife, needed someone to value his feelings, needs, and concerns. If only someone would have called his wife! As for Joe himself, he was so overwhelmed by the activities of his caregivers, he dared not make this request. Upon the initial encounter with Joe, the critical care nurse should have inquired if there was anyone who could be called or contacted on Joe's behalf. In addition, Joe's nonverbal behavior should have alerted the professional nurse to his fear and the need to have a loved one nearby.

Listening

Great emphasis must be placed on listening to patients and responding to their cues and clues. Listening is a sensory skill essential for effective, therapeutic communication. When nurses listen to their patients, they should do so at a conscious level. They should reach out to their patients and become sensitized to their inner world. In caring for patients, nurses voluntarily enter a world of thoughts and feelings that is many times foreign to their own world. Without losing their objectivity, nurses should listen carefully to patients and try to place themselves into their patients' frame of reference.

In reviewing Charlie's experience, it becomes obvious that the nurses failed to place themselves into his world. They failed to realize that here is a 20-year-old youth who has no idea what has happened to him and is frightened by the overwhelming technological and impersonal invasion of his body and person. At first, Charlie cannot verbalize his feelings and misgivings, and the nurses caring for Charlie fail to recognize his

tense, motionless state. From Charlie's perspective, they seem to blatantly disregard his need for modesty and his need to protect his identity and integrity as a man.

Perceiving

Had the nurses truly and consciously listened to Charlie's questions and perceived his feelings, they may have tried to communicate more effectively and diligently with him. They may have encouraged him to express his thoughts and feelings and to formulate realistic expectations about his care and progress. Charlie needed to know what was happening to him. Unable to ask and not given the opportunity to do so, his anticipatory fear led him further into emotional turmoil.

The eruption of anger easily may have been prevented if the nurses had accurately perceived Charlie's reaction to a threatening and perplexing environment. The nurses should have included Charlie in the planning of his care, allowing him to make certain decisions. For example, allowing Charlie to decide which side to be positioned on or seeking his permission to uncover his body to check his dressing and Foley catheter would have helped to maintain Charlie's feelings of control and self-worth.

Involving

For nurses to know a patient well enough to provide individualized care, they must allow themselves to become involved with the patient and his or her world. Involvement is reaching out, touching, and hearing the inner being of another. Nurses obtain knowledge about the patient by recognizing and perceiving that the patient's verbal and nonverbal expressions are reflective of underlying thoughts and feelings, which are in essence the patient's reality. Acceptance of the patient and his or her reality with unconditional positive regard conveys to the patient that he or she is recognized and respected as a separate and distinct person, having the right to his or her own feelings whether or not the nurse agrees with them.

Empathizing

The ability to perceive the feelings of another person accurately is known as empathy. Empathic communication needs to be expressed in the language and feeling tone of patients. When nurses actively respond, patients have a greater sense of being understood. This provides an opportunity for correction of any perceptual errors. Empathic communication is vital in the personalization process.

SUMMARY

As we have seen through the case studies of Joe and Charlie, and the analysis of their experiences, caring behaviors on the part of the nurses might have made a difference in how these patients perceived and reacted to the illness experience. Such behaviors identified in the above discussion included communicating, touching, valuing, listening, perceiving, involving, and empathizing. Through these behaviors, nurses are able to deliver personalized humanistic care and to prevent the state of depersonalization and the process of dehumanization in their patients.

Caring affects both those who care and those being cared for. Thus it is important to demonstrate our caring behaviors to our patients and their significant others. At times, caring can be painful, as well as satisfying, to the nurse who enters the tormented or tragic world of a patient. Cradling a dying infant and sharing the grief of the parents; stroking the forehead of a severely burned victim, hoping it offers some comfort as he writhes in pain from the extensive body dressing changes; having to care for the teenager who has been suddenly paralyzed as a result of a motor vehicle accident and is enmeshed in feelings of hopelessness and despair; all of these certainly challenge the caring nurse who attempts to instill a ray of hope for the future. To fight the battle of AIDS with a patient only to face it over and over again until the struggle becomes futile and death prevails is certainly a heartbreaking experience for the critical care nurse. To be hugged with gratification by the loved ones of a cancer patient who has finally achieved peace in a dignified death is surely a moving experience for the nurse.

We feel with our patients and their loved ones—the pain, the anger, the sorrow, the joy, and hopefully the peace. We cry, we laugh, we touch, and we share a part of ourselves with each other as we face the challenge of critical care nursing. Loretta Zderad[1] summarizes this sensitive caring focus in nursing by her statement:

> To truly treat another as a unique individual, to see him as a subject rather than to look on him as an object, to be able to do with him rather than to him, it is necessary to grasp his perspective, to see his world as he does.

REFERENCES

1. Zderad, L: Empathetic nursing: Realization of a human capacity. Nurs Clin North Am 4(4):655, 1969.

SUGGESTED READINGS

American Nurses Association: Nursing: A Social Policy Statement. American Nurses Association, Kansas City, MO, 1980.

American Nurses Association: Nursing's Social Policy Statement. American Nurses Association, Washington DC, 1995.

Cawley, M: No cure, just care. Am J Nurs 74:2011, 1974.

Hein, E: Listening. Nursing '75, 5(3):93, March 1975.

Kalish, B: What is empathy? Am J Nurs 73(3):1548, Sept 1973.

Qamar, S: The stress-carative model of nursing practice. Focus on Critical Care 13(6):15, 1986.

Roberts, S: Behavioral Concepts and the Critically Ill Patient, ed 2. Appleton-Century-Crofts, Norwalk, CT, 1986.

Roberts, S: Psychological equilibrium. In Kinney, M (ed): AACN's Clinical Reference for Critical Care Nursing. McGraw-Hill, New York, 1981, p 331.

Wright, J: Self-perception alterations with coronary artery bypass surgery. Heart Lung 16(5):483, 1987.

Zderad, L: Empathetic nursing: Realization of a human capacity. Nurs Clin North Am 4(4):655, 1969.

CHAPTER 7

Sharing Feelings

Mary Amendolari and Adrienne Coppola

CHAPTER OUTLINE

Losing a Young Patient
Focusing on the Patient Rather than the
   Equipment

Excellence in Critical Care Nursing
Sharing and Moving on
Suggested Readings

LEARNING OBJECTIVES

At the end of this chapter, you should be able to:

1. Explain how interacting with critically ill patients and their families or significant others impacts on our own feelings, especially regarding death and dying.
2. Explain how we feel about ourselves when we have helped people feel what they need or had to feel.
3. Understand why it is important for critical care nurses to be supportive of one another, particularly when patient outcomes are not always positive.

In caring for critically ill patients and their families, all of whom must try to cope intellectually, emotionally, and physically with what may be a life-threatening illness, critical care nurses themselves experience many moods and emotions. Included among these are feelings of satisfaction and fulfillment that are realized when the patient and family perceive that, as a result of the patient-nurse interaction, a beneficial change has occurred and that the interaction has made a difference in the outcome, be it a return to a quality lifestyle, or to the acceptance of the ultimate outcome, that is, death, with respect and dignity.

Other feelings experienced by critical care nurses include the anxiety and fear that accompanies caring for patients with life-threatening illnesses, whose recovery and eventual return to a quality lifestyle may depend largely on the professional nursing care rendered during the acute phase. Often critical care nurses experience feelings of helplessness, powerlessness, and frustration, when, despite all their effort and that of other healthcare providers, they witness the demise of the patient and the grief of the family with whom they feel a close bond.

In the patient-nurse interactions described in the vignettes that follow, the focus is on the humanness of the critical care nurse, both as a caregiver and as an individual. Through candid sharing of thoughts and feelings experienced by these critical care nurses, one is able to become involved in the intimacy of the patient-nurse interaction and how the process that is

nursing intertwines with the life processes of the patient and family. As a result of these human interactions, there evolves within each individual an ever-increasing awareness and understanding of self and of one's integrity.

LOSING A YOUNG PATIENT

"I have just arrived home after a really busy night in our ICU, a night that has left me physically and emotionally drained. I was called last evening to help out with the workload in what was an especially busy night in the unit. As the Nursing Care Coordinator, that is, the charge nurse in the unit, the staff looked to me for assistance, reassurance, and relief. So I said, OK, and I was on my way.

"As I look back at the events that transpired in the ICU this night, I realized that it was one of those nights when you have mixed emotions and feelings. At one point, I found myself questioning what it was I was doing. I have been a critical care nurse for nearly 11 years now, and I wondered—is it really worth it? Is it really worth all the stress and anguish? Should I do something less stressful and demanding of one's energies? On the other hand, I felt I did my best to help out, to help make people feel what they had to feel and needed to feel. Maybe that's what it's all about, I mean, to experience a fine balance between one's feelings, and when you feel you've got to have a break just to sit back and reflect.

"Let me tell you a little bit about the night. There was a young, handsome guy, about 20 years old, whose name was Peter. He was admitted the day before for a small bowel resection secondary to a bowel obstruction. Clinically, there were many problems. On admission, he had a low hemoglobin, hematocrit, and platelet count. Nevertheless, an exploratory laparotomy with a small bowel resection was performed. Upon his return to the ICU, a pulmonary artery catheter was inserted to assist in monitoring his fluid status. Some difficulty was encountered in stabilizing Peter's vital signs while he was in the recovery room. So it was imperative to monitor his overall status closely, and in particular, his hydration status, postoperatively. In addition, Peter was in a highly agitated state.

"Peter was a tall, strong, rugged guy. If you looked at him, you'd say to yourself, how can this guy be sick? Yet, here he was vented, with a pulmonary catheter and arterial line, and hooked up to a variety of monitors. Anyone looking at Peter would be bewildered by all these lines and equipment.

"When I approached Peter's bedside I found him loosely restrained to prevent him from dislodging his airway or intravenous lines. I went over to him and noticed this look of fear in his expression. I tried to talk softly to him, to explain to him what was going on, why he had the tube in his mouth. I felt very concerned and uncomfortable. I wanted him to relax, but I didn't want to sedate him. I felt it was very important to Peter to know what was going on, because I felt he needed to know. I tried to hold his hand to calm him down. It worked for a while, but we ended up having to give him some Valium. He seemed to relax a bit, and his vital signs remained stable.

"Meanwhile, while I was trying to comfort Peter, the patient in bed 5, Mrs. M, was asking for the bedpan. A woman in her early fifties admitted with a rule-out inferior wall myocardial infarction, she seemed almost apologetic asking for the bedpan, saying, 'You're all so very busy, I hope I'm not bothering you.' I tried not to show my anxiety, which is something difficult to do, especially when the pace is so hectic. While she was probably the least sick of all our patients, I took the time to try to show her that we were there to meet her needs. Inwardly, I recognized that feeling of impatience with her, especially because I was so concerned about Peter. I knew I had to be especially careful not to be abrupt with her, with so many other things on my mind.

"I also realized, however, that I did not want Mrs. M to sense my anxieties because that's something that brushes off on people and patients, especially in an ICU. Allowing patients to sense one's anxieties may, in turn, precipitate other patient problems, as, for example, chest pain in someone of Mrs. M's status. Mrs. M went on to say, 'How can you be running around so quickly, and you're doing so much. It's really busy in here, what's going on with the man next door?' I just told her that he was a young man who

had just had surgery. I reassured Mrs. M, gave her the bedpan and the call bell, and told her to call when she was finished with its use and we would assist her.

"In the meantime, in bed 1, was Ms. T, a woman in her early forties, admitted with an acute anteroseptal wall myocardial infarction. She was in the process of having a pulmonary catheter inserted. She appeared ashen, and her skin felt cool, moist, and clammy. She was also experiencing a lot of chest pain not entirely controlled with morphine. We initiated a nitroglycerin drip, and she seemed to be doing better. However, at that point, we experienced equipment failure with her bedside monitor. The physician was at the bedside agitating about how do we get this monitor to work? The graph wouldn't come on the oscilloscope, and we couldn't get a pulmonary artery pressure reading. I tried fiddling around with the buttons but was still unable to get a reading.

"I placed a call to the evening supervisor who responded immediately. With Ms. T's condition so acute and unstable, it warranted a one-to-one nurse-patient ratio. So I had the nurse caring for Ms. T continue to monitor her closely, while the evening supervisor and I attempted to deal with the equipment failure. We could have moved Ms. T from bed 1 to bed 3, but we felt that she was too unstable to be moved. So we ended up disengaging the patient from the entire system, and with a trusty screwdriver and some logistical maneuvering, we were able finally to hook the patient up to another monitor, and it worked.

"Things went pretty smoothly afterwards, and I had time to reflect on what had transpired. I knew I felt panicky inside. I didn't want to take a chance on moving this patient to another bed because she was so sick. It was kind of hard to deal with the physician at this time. I knew he wanted to get the pulmonary artery catheter inserted as soon as possible. I also sensed the anxieties he was experiencing. I had worked with this physician for quite some time, and when you get to know someone well enough, and this person usually had a mellow-type personality, I just knew by looking at him that he felt panicky and we had to get the job done.

"With Ms. T's condition stabilizing, before I left her bedside, I took the time to reassure Linda, Ms. T's nurse. I briefly reviewed significant events and what could be learned from these events; while also consoling her and verbalizing the anxieties and fears I knew she was experiencing, I let Linda know that it was all right to feel panicky or extremely anxious. We were able to get the job done by working together, as a team.

"I went back to Peter's bedside and was just standing there, kind of helping out with turning and repositioning, when suddenly his eyes rolled back. I quickly looked at the monitor and noted that both his blood pressure and wedge pressure readings were falling. Within moments, Peter went into cardiac arrest and we called a code. While I was resuscitating him with the Ambu bag, I remember thinking to myself that here is a guy but 20 years old. Usually, our patients are much older. Somehow, having such a young patient involved in a code situation just brings about different feelings that ordinarily would not be experienced. Peter is young and such a strong guy—why should this be happening to him? I remember thinking that we *must* bring him back, he has his whole life ahead of him.

"The code team worked on Peter for over an hour, using every therapy at our command. You name it and we tried it. Pharmacologically, we used epinephrine, calcium chloride, dopamine, Levophed, and sodium bicarbonate. A pacemaker wire was inserted, but we couldn't get it to capture. I don't think his heart muscle was intact, and later on, we found out that there were other things involved in his illness.

"As I gazed around and took note of people's expressions, some had tears in their eyes. We all kind of had tears in our eyes. As the code progressed unsuccessfully, the more intense everybody became. My fellow nurses were saying to me, 'We've got to do something else. We need to do *something*.' The physician directing the code, a cardiologist, and one I have high regard for, tried everything possible, but we just weren't getting any results. The expression on everyone's face looked like their very hearts were sinking along with Peter's.

"I remember thinking to myself, maybe there was something else we could do, or perhaps should have done earlier. I began second-guessing myself. Maybe there was something I could have done to prevent this from happening; maybe something else was going on with Peter that I didn't see on the monitor; or maybe we were just so busy and so stressed that we weren't paying closer attention to Peter. So many things were going through my mind. I think down deep inside I felt we did the best we could. But there are just so many mixed feelings.

"Other questions and concerns began to enter my mind. What's going to happen when Peter's mother arrives? The physician called his mother. In the meantime, we all just stood around the bedside as nurses, touching one another, and I guess, you could say we all just stood there, crying. I know I cried. It had really been a long time since I remember crying. But this interaction with Peter, it really upset me.

"Peter's mother arrived about 20 minutes after the physician declared his death. She came into the center of the ICU in front of his curtain. We had closed Peter's curtain and, in so doing, perhaps provided him with a final moment of solitude. The physician explained to his mother that we tried everything humanly possible, but Peter just didn't make it. She suddenly was overwhelmed with the magnitude of this reality, bursting into tears and sobbing uncontrollably with her hands covering her face. She was just sobbing so helplessly.

"As Peter's mother, the physician, and I were standing together, I was thinking to myself, what can I really do to ease her burden, what could I say? Here's a woman who just lost her 20-year-old son. I suddenly found myself putting my arm around her, and I said to her 'I really want you to know that we tried every-

thing we could to save Peter. He was very special to each one of us. I truly wish there was something else that we could do to help you.' I gave her a glass of water and some tissues, and we sat down, my arm around her shoulder.

"Meanwhile, Peter's 18-year-old younger brother came into the unit, and after he saw the closed curtains and his mother crying, he just ran out of the unit. I wanted to run after him, but I realized that it was necessary to let the family handle this burden in their own way. I continued to console Peter's mom, and when his dad arrived, they consoled one another.

"In retrospect, I was comforted by the thought that I was able to comfort Peter's family at least somewhat in their hour of need. As for the staff, we were all drained emotionally, mentally, and physically. My nurses were so drained there was nothing else that they could give of themselves. It's as if they functioned on pure instinct the remainder of the shift. I was also glad that I could be there for my staff, to offer support and to provide reassurance. Having worked with these nurses, being familiar with their personalities, I had a good idea as to how they were feeling. The special bond that exists among critical care nurses, the sharing of feelings—this helps each of us to gain some insight into who we really are, what makes us tick, and, yes, to muster our energies for yet another day.

"We were informed subsequently that, at autopsy, Peter was found to have mitral valve vegetation, some myocardial damage, and severe liver disease. Other factors were identified as possibly contributory to his demise, including a history of drug and alcohol abuse. And so, we laid Peter to rest."

FOCUSING ON THE PATIENT RATHER THAN THE EQUIPMENT

"Let me share with you my interaction with Mr. D, a 60-year-old man with a long-standing history of chronic obstructive pulmonary disease. Mr. D had been hospitalized on numerous occasions with an exacerbation of his disease, and both he and his wife were aware that his emphysema was severe. At this time, it was necessary to intubate Mr. D and initiate mechanical ventilation to ensure adequate alveolar ventilation.

"When I approached Mr. D's bedside I was impressed with the look of fear on both his face, and that of his wife, who was at his bedside. I found myself likewise experiencing some of their fear as I asked myself, how could I help this loving couple? How could I relieve their anxiety? Their anxiety seemed to rub off on everyone. It may have been caused by the alarm on his ventilator, which seemed to be sounding constantly.

"In an ICU, people are especially tuned in to the sounds created by various monitors, ventilators, and other equipment. I found myself thinking as I responded to Mr. D's ventilator alarm, I wonder how many of us tend to concern ourselves more with the equipment rather than directly with the patient? Perhaps, some of us are more comfortable concentrating on the machinery, 'treating' the sounds rather than having to interact with the patient or family. Sometimes you just have so many mixed feelings about caring for patients, especially when you know their prognosis for recovery isn't very positive. I find it's often difficult to deal with these feelings. Perhaps we concentrate more on the equipment rather than on the patient and family as a defense mechanism, as if to insulate our own feelings from surfacing.

"Another mechanism we may employ in caring for patients whose alarms are constantly going off is to sedate these patients, which is what we did with Mr. D. Don't get me wrong, I know that he really needed sedation at this point in time and it did slow down his heart rate a little, but I also know that sedation may not always be necessary. Rather, taking the time to talk to a patient, and touching the patient—holding the patient's hand, placing your hand on the shoulder, or caressing the head—these types of therapies may be sufficiently effective so that there is no need for sedation. This approach can be used even when the patient is experiencing an altered level of consciousness and is unable to respond. They may, nevertheless, hear and feel.

"I remember observing Mr. D's wife on one of her frequent visits, how she took his hand and his eyes closed, and he seemed to relax, if but for a moment. I went over to Mr. D's bedside and introduced myself to both him and his wife and told them I would be taking care of Mr. D during the rest of the evening. I told them that I would stop by to talk with them and would try to anticipate their needs. I suggested to Mr. D that perhaps he could calm down and relax a little bit because this would probably help him with breathing. I rubbed his forehead with my hand, and he seemed comforted by this. I explained to Mr. D that his hands were loosely restrained because he might inadvertently pull out his endotracheal tube while he was sleeping, and he seemed to understand. I did give him some Zanax, which he had been taking at home.

"As I reviewed Mr. D's chart, it was evident that Mr. D's disease was progressive, and his ventilatory and gas exchange capabilities were severely compromised. It occurred to me that perhaps both Mr. D and his wife were concerned that he was going to die and that this, at least in part, underlay their extreme anxiety. I think Mr. D knew that he was really very sick. His wife told me that he had never been intubated so quickly during his previous hospitalizations. She explained that he really stopped breathing at home before the ambulance arrived. She said she was afraid he was going to die.

"The many days I took care of Mr. D, I tried to bring out his feelings. I remember one day in particular when I took his hand and I just said to him, 'I know you're afraid.' I really wanted to say to him that I knew he was afraid that he was going to die. But I guess that I was afraid myself of the thought of him dying. Yet, I knew I had to help him work through what he was feeling. The fear of dying is really something each critical care nurse must work out within himself or herself.

Sometimes it is good just to come out and say it—are you afraid to die? It is important to involve the family in this process if possible, so they can all try to work through their feelings and to deal with them together.

"In retrospect, there was one thing I regret not having done, and this was to give Mr. D the choice of whether or not he wanted to be a Do Not Resuscitate patient. There was time to address this with him earlier in this hospitalization when he was much more alert and oriented. Later on, his condition deteriorated and his level of consciousness became altered. I did bring it up to Mrs. D. I think she wanted this in the beginning, but she never really pursued it with him. I don't think, I really don't know—maybe it's just my feelings of guilt that I didn't emphasize this enough, so that maybe, if I did, Mr. D would have had the choice.

"When Mr. D's time came and he had to be resuscitated, his wife wanted everything to be done. She became almost fanatical about the need to bring him back. I tried to explain to her what the situation was and what we were trying to do. I felt that this was important to her. But, at one point, Mrs. D made me feel as if we weren't doing enough, that there should be other things that we should be doing. When I looked back and thought about Mrs. D, it occurred to me that she was probably using denial to cope. What concerned me was that I may have lost my objectivity in this circumstance and perhaps in so doing did not recognize that Mrs. D was having difficulties resolving the fact that her husband was dying.

"Well, Mr. D did die. He had his wife at his bedside, which I really felt was important to both of them. Caring for Mr. D helped me to deal with some of my own feelings about death and dying, despite the fact that I have been a critical care nurse for over 10 years. I guess there's always a patient who touches you deeply. I guess in caring for Mr. D, some of these thoughts and feelings surfaced. Mr. D, although he was vented, was still alert. He could still choose certain things, or at least be informed of certain things. He was a very intelligent man. It was especially difficult for Mrs. D and the family to accept his death, particularly because Mr. D was only in his early sixties and had so much to live for.

"About a week later, Mrs. D sent all the nurses uniforms and a big box of cookies. She thanked us. Believe it or not, about a year later, she herself was admitted to our ICU with a diagnosis of angina. When I went to her bedside, there was just something about her, I said, 'Mrs. D, how are you doing?' I took care of her that night. I just felt such a close bond with her probably because we did share a lot of inner feelings about her husband."

EXCELLENCE IN CRITICAL CARE NURSING

"As I mentioned earlier, I have been a nurse for about 11 years. I have always worked in an ICU except for a few months early on after graduation from nursing school, when I worked in Med-Surg. But basically, I'm a critical care nurse. I think it's true when it is said that you have to be a special type of person to work in an ICU. I have worked with nurses who came to realize that the tempo and demands of an ICU were not for them. Others I have worked with just burnt out. Still other critical care nurses have worked in an ICU for such a long time, I don't think they have taken the time to think about their feelings, and whether or not they still feel they can function productively and are not just going through the motions.

"Basically, to be an effective critical care nurse, you need to be knowledgeable, you need to really keep up-to-date and on top of things. For myself, I really enjoy attending continuing education offerings, especially when I don't know about something. For example, when thrombolytic therapy with TPA and streptokinase was initiated in our ICU, I realized that this treatment modality was one that I knew very little about. I was able to attend a continuing education program that helped me to learn the essentials of caring for a patient receiving thrombolytic therapy. Now, this therapy is frequently implemented in our ICU.

"It's essential for critical care nurses to seek out information when they are doubtful or uncertain about anything. I especially stress to my nurses that they should consult the policy and procedure manuals initially, and then consult with one of the other nurses, or myself, as the resources in the unit. Critical care nurses also need to use their common sense. Often, one's instincts, experience, and common sense are all that is needed to intervene effectively.

"Psychomotor skills and dexterity are a must for the critical care nurse. Critical care nurses deal constantly with a lot of equipment and instruments. Often, it is necessary to assist physicians with procedures. Even more often, it is the critical care nurse who helps physicians maintain aseptic technique.

"Working with physicians in the ICU can be especially challenging. Over time, you eventually get to know the personalities of the ICU physicians, and this can be very helpful in the day-to-day workings of the ICU. Basically, every physician has his or her own way of performing procedures (e.g., inserting a Swan-Ganz catheter or pacing wire) and of dealing with patients. Often, critical care nurses must be assertive with physicians to ensure that the patient's needs are met. As the patient's nurse, the critical care nurse may be in the best position to determine what the patient's needs are and what type of therapy may be appropriate, and to evaluate the patient's response to therapy. At times, the critical care nurse may not agree that a particular therapy is appropriate for the patient. In the ICU, it is important to bring this to the physician's attention, including the rationales supporting your stance. Critical care nurses, with their level of knowledge essential to caring for the critically ill patient, should not hesitate to question a physician's order if it is felt to be inappropriate. In fact, it is the responsibility of the nurse to do so. It is also the responsibility of each nurse to question another nurse if inappropriate care is being given to a patient.

"An essential characteristic required for nurses to be effective bedside nurses is simply to be caring. Not only caring for patients, but, very importantly, caring for each other as nurses. Some of my most satisfying and fulfilling experiences as a critical care nurse include those when I'm working and interacting with my fellow nurses, knowing that they care. You know they care because everyone is in tune with each other's feelings and, no matter how someone reacts to stress, they can ventilate their feelings knowing someone is listening and really cares.

"Occasionally, in our ICU, one of the nurses becomes really stressed, and she'll suddenly snap at someone. Basically, what I do is to kind of let her be for awhile, give her some space. Eventually, I go to her and say, 'Is there something bothering you? What's going on?' Or I might say, 'How can I help you? Is there something I can do for you?' Or I try to anticipate her needs much as I do with my patients. Often, when I can, I'll go over and tell her to take a break, and I'll monitor her patients for awhile.

"The *esprit de corps* that exists in our ICU is perhaps best illustrated at those times when a patient goes bad, or when we are getting an admission from the Emergency Department, for example. Everyone gets together and pitches in. This togetherness and caring are seen when someone needs a break. Sometimes it is necessary to say to a fellow nurse, 'You look awfully tired, you've really been working a lot. Maybe you need to take a break.' I know there are times when I need a break. I think it occurs at least once a month, I really need a day when I'm totally not thinking of the unit.

"I think my experiences as a critical care nurse have affected my overall view of life. Somehow, when one deals with life and death on a daily basis, when you see people suffering and become cognizant of the terrible problems that beset them, so many things seem trivial in comparison. Having this perspective, you can handle your own life a little better. I know I have become much more organized in my own life. Although, I do know some critical care nurses who are so very organized at work and yet are totally disorganized in their home life. After being a critical care nurse for so long, I believe what you do at your job, how you perform, and how you interact with people are really a reflection of the kind of person you really are. You can't be a phony in an ICU. You have to be down-to-earth, you need to be realistic, you have to deal with problems effectively, and you need to be able to accept criticism as well as other people.

"I think *touch* is a very important component in dealing with people in general, and with patients, in particular. I recently read an article in *Heart & Lung* that discussed how important touch is when performing procedures and caring for patients. It's the way you are with patients, it's a part of caring.

"Let me share my real feelings—how I feel about ICU. I guess I really do love it. I thought about doing other things. I'm sure I probably will in the future. Perhaps I'll attempt to do something different. Of course there have been other occasions when I have thought about this, yet I still end up working in the critical care setting. I think I have gotten the most satisfaction from my practice as a critical care nurse because I go in and care for my patients knowing that, in some small way, I can affect them and can make a difference for them and their families.

"Of course, the most rewarding feeling occurs when you know that the patient is going to improve. Recently, we had a 40-year-old patient admitted with an anterior wall myocardial infarction. He was treated with tPA, and we were able to reverse a lot of the injury to his myocardium. He stopped by to visit us about a month after his discharge. How good it felt to see him, knowing that in some small way we had influenced his life. It's these little things that happen that become meaningful. They recharge the batteries and give us the strength to tackle the next challenge.

"What evolves from experiences in the ICU is that you become a critical care nurse practitioner. You consider what you do to be your practice, rather than just a job. I've become a member of the American Association of Critical-Care Nurses (AACN), the professional organization of critical care nurses. I've tried to encourage my colleagues to join by setting an example. It is such a pleasure observing nurses on their break to be scanning through *Heart & Lung, Critical Care Nurse*, or *American Journal of Critical Care*. Even more satisfying is observing nurses starting to apply new knowledge to patient care. I mean it is just such a good feeling to see other nurses grow as professionals and as individuals. Often, people expect a lot of things in return. As for me, like I said, if you can find satisfaction in these little things—just watching people grow, and you know you've done the best job you can, that's basically all I've ever needed."

SHARING AND MOVING ON

"Elizabeth was a special lady, well-known to us in the ICU. It was just about a year ago that she was brought into the emergency department after having a cardiac arrest. She was intubated and transferred to our unit.

"Elizabeth was under a great deal of stress at the time. She was caring for her husband who was riddled with cancer, and, in addition, she was caught up in the activities, excitement, and tensions of her daughter's wedding. In fact, we didn't know then if Elizabeth would make it, and we all prayed that she wouldn't die before the wedding. Well, she persevered, and, although she remained on the ventilator, Elizabeth did see her daughter dressed in her wedding gown when she came into the ICU. How hard it must have been for the family and for Elizabeth. I couldn't even begin to imagine how they must have felt.

"Although Elizabeth did sustain considerable damage to her myocardium, her condition stabilized and she was discharged on medications, and on limited activity.

"Now, a year later, I again met Elizabeth who was admitted to the ICU, this time with acute congestive heart failure and complaints of chest pain. Her husband had since died, and, on the positive side, she had her first grandson. Knowing that people are especially vulnerable to illness during the first year after a spouse's death, I wondered if perhaps this was true in Elizabeth's case, and I thought about the stress she was experiencing and what she must be going through.

"I requested to care for Elizabeth because I felt close to her, some sort of a bond with her. It was difficult to see her again on the ventilator and the multiple IV drips that were necessary to maintain her. Every day I would tell her how she was doing and try to set goals with her. I knew it was important to be honest and realistic with Elizabeth. I knew she knew how she was doing. So many times, patients just don't know what's going on. Others may be afraid to know. But I feel that if patients aren't informed or don't get any positive feedback, how can they help themselves?

"One day, a few hours after she was extubated, Elizabeth complained of difficulty breathing. Her vital signs were stable, and as I assessed her, I couldn't find any underlying reasons for her respiratory distress, except anxiety, which was causing her to hyperventilate. The results of her arterial blood gases confirmed my suspicions, and I shared the results with Elizabeth. I explained to her that the results of her gases were within normal limits, that she was understandably anxious, but doing quite well off the ventilator. I stayed with her and comforted her until she, herself, believed that she was, in fact, fine.

"As Elizabeth's condition slowly progressed, she was placed on a waiting list for coronary artery bypass surgery at New York University Medical Center. She was of such high risk that this was her only hope.

"Elizabeth's daughters came in to see their mom faithfully, two to three times a day. They were so supportive and caring. I could see that they couldn't bear to think of losing their mother.

"Whenever I had a few moments, I would sit with Elizabeth and hold her hand. We would talk, laugh, and sometimes, cry. She knew her prognosis was guarded, and she worried about what her daughters would do without her. Her face would light up and she had a sparkle in her eyes when she spoke about her little grandson. I made sure Elizabeth got to see him, knowing it was very likely for the last time.

"One day, when I asked her how she really felt she was doing, she said, 'Not so good,' with a sad look in her eyes. I asked her if there was anything I could get for her, and she smiled and said, 'A pastrami on rye with mustard.' She was getting so very weary. Without saying it, Elizabeth knew she wasn't getting any better. As her wait became longer (due to lack of a bed), I found myself becoming more frustrated and angry. This was, after all, her only hope. I became very involved with the family and tried to help them sort out their feelings and to be realistic in their expectations. I tried to prepare them for what no one wanted to face, Elizabeth's death.

"I remember waking her one morning to take her vital signs. She had been in a deep sleep and woke up startled and uneasy. Realizing that something was wrong, I pursued it with Elizabeth. She explained to me that she had been dreaming and she felt 'so tired,' as if she had been 'working all night.' She told me that she dreamed that her daughters were moving furniture in her house and that her husband was breaking down a wall.

"It was at this time that her daughters came to visit their mother, and they told her to stop talking about their father and to stop wanting to be with him. I tried to explain to them that this was a normal part of grieving and that Elizabeth needed to talk about her husband, their father. But I could see that they were uncomfortable with this.

"I, however, found myself being very uncomfortable with Elizabeth's dream. I knew right away that something was going to happen that day. I shared these thoughts with an intern who believed in dreams also, and she confirmed my feelings.

"That night, Elizabeth developed severe chest pain and was put back on multiple IV drips. Her condition steadily worsened, and I could see that she started to withdraw. I tried to comfort her, stroking her forehead and holding her hand, but she continued to get worse. I remember praying that when the time came, and Elizabeth was to die, I didn't want to be there. I felt that I might lose it emotionally. I had gotten so very close to her. I was afraid that, the way I felt about Elizabeth, I wouldn't be able to function.

"My prayers were answered. The day Elizabeth was to die, I was on call and I got called in. As I approached the hospital, one of the nurses informed me that an extra nurse came in by mistake and that I could go home. And so I did. That night Elizabeth coded and died.

"After hearing about Elizabeth's death, I was very upset and tears filled my eyes. After so many years of nursing, it doesn't seem easier—the pain and the hurt are still there when a patient dies, and you feel such a loss.

"Her dream still haunted me, and I was angry with myself for not having looked up its meaning. When I finally did, I sat in disbelief. The dream interpretation was 'being surrounded by loved ones' and 'conclusion of all affairs.' Elizabeth had dreamed her own death!

"For days thereafter, I would look for her in the bed she had occupied for such a long time. I had tried to come to terms with her death, wondering if she needed more time than I had spent with her, to verbalize her fears and feelings. Had I really done enough? So many feelings were awakened in me. Why did I go into nursing? Was it worth it? Was it worth having my emotions played with all the time? But I know deep down that this is my calling in life, and I could never do anything else. Nothing else could give me the sense of satisfaction I feel. I knew that I had helped Elizabeth even if but in some small way. And despite the fact that I kept asking myself if there was something else that I could have done for her, I knew I had touched her heart, just as she had touched mine."

SUGGESTED READINGS

Barker, RK: You made a difference. Focus Crit Care 15(1):38, 1988.

Edwards, LW: Thanks Floyd. Focus Crit Care 12(4):52, 1985.

Estabrooks, C: Touch: A nursing strategy in the intensive care unit. Heart Lung 18(4):392, 1989.

Levine, S, Wilson, S, Guido, G: Personality factors of critical care nurses. Heart Lung 17(4):392, 1988.

Schoenhofer, S: Affectional touch in critical care nursing: A descriptive study. Heart Lung 18(2):146, 1989.

Schunior, C: Close to bull's horns. Focus Crit Care 14(2):19, 1987.

CHAPTER 8

Sleep and Sensory Alterations in the Critically Ill Patient

Susan Auvil-Novak and Ronald D. Novak

CHAPTER OUTLINE

Sleep in the Critical Care Environment
- Universal Requirement for Sleep
- Influence of Biological Rhythms on Sleep
- Sleep Physiology
- Mechanisms of Sleep
- Clinical Measurement of Sleep

Sensory Alterations in the Critical Care Environment
- Environmental Synchronization of Biological Rhythms
- Desynchronization
- Sleep Deprivation
- ICU Psychosis
- Nursing Implications

References

LEARNING OBJECTIVES

After completing this chapter, you should be able to:

1. Discuss the universal need for sleep in humans.
2. Describe the physiologic stages of sleep.
3. Explain the difference between REM and NREM sleep.
4. Identify factors that affect alterations in sensory perceptions in the critical care patient.
5. Describe the impact of alterations in circadian rhythms, environmental synchronizers, and desynchronization on the critically ill adult.
6. Define the short- and long-term consequences of sleep deprivation.
7. List three common causes for sleep deprivation in the ICU setting.
8. Identify interventions to improve sleep and reduce sensory deprivation and sensory overload in the intensive care environment.
9. Describe the effects of commonly prescribed medications on sleep.

SLEEP IN THE CRITICAL CARE ENVIRONMENT

Current practice within the critical care environment remains, for the most part, extremely beneficial to the patient. Innovations in technology, drug therapy, treatment protocols, and the ability to rapidly identify and treat emerging complications, have greatly increased the probability of survival in situations where the opportunity was previously nonexistent. Constant vigilance and numerous interventions by healthcare personnel are required to sustain the individual within the critical care environment. Unfortunately, frequent intercession is not always beneficial to the patient. Much of the technological innovations that has improved survival rates within the critical care

environment has also been related to the debilitating complications that may befall the patient.

The purpose of this chapter is to explore the universal need for and characteristics of sleep. Further, aspects of the critical care environment that impact sleep, sensory deprivation, and sensory overload in the critically ill individual will be identified. Finally, nursing interventions to encourage sleep and prevent sensory deprivation and overstimulation will be described.

Universal Requirement for Sleep

In humans, the need for sleep is universal; however, the range of sleep required by each individual varies significantly. It is well known that some individuals sleep only approximately 3 hours each night without any negative effects, while others require 10 or more hours of sleep per day.[1] Although most individuals require an average of 6 to 8 hours of sleep each 24-hour period, individual sleep requirements usually diminish as a person ages. Sleep is an important activity in life, although its purpose remains unclear. Human existence without sleep (absolute sleep deprivation) is relatively unknown; however, a rare genetic disorder identified as fatal familial insomnia (FFI) and some organic brain diseases do entirely abolish sleep in some individuals. Although the onset of FFI is gradual, survival of these individuals is limited to a few months once absolute sleep deprivation is manifested.

Phenomenon of Sleep

Until approximately 60 years ago, it was commonly believed that sleep was a simple activity that was similar to unconsciousness. This idea changed in the 1930s when it was determined that various stages of sleep existed and could be identified by different patterns in the electroencephalogram (EEG).[2] These stages recur rhythmically throughout the sleep period.

In humans, approximately one third of a person's life is spent in sleep. Because of the enormous time committed to this process by the body, several theories have been postulated regarding the phenomenon of sleep. One of the earliest theories suggests that sleep is a restorative process in which the body regenerates tissue damage that occurred during the waking state.[3]

More recently, it has also been suggested that sleep may be a combination of two phases.[4] The first phase is defined as compulsory or obligatory sleep, which occurs in response to the need for tissue repair and general physiological restitution as a result of normal activity during wakefulness. Obligatory sleep is controlled by the period of prior wakefulness and occurs during the first few hours of the sleep period. The second phase of sleep, described as "facultative" or ancillary sleep, is believed to be under the control of circadian rhythms and other environmental or behavioral factors (such as boredom). Facultative sleep occurs at the end of the sleep cycle. The rest-activity cycle in normal individuals occurs in a fixed circadian pattern, with sleep usually occurring during the night and wakefulness during daylight hours.[4]

The daily alteration between sleep and wakefulness appears to be in synchrony with the earth's rotation and the alteration between natural light and darkness. However, this cyclic behavior is not dependent on the existence of light and darkness, but rather is influenced by it. Cave studies have demonstrated that even people who are isolated from all external time cues exhibit predictable, cyclic patterns of sleep and wakefulness.[5] Thus, it appears that a "biological clock" actually regulates the sleep-wake cycle and is able to maintain time in the absence of synchronizing clues and cues from the environment.

Influence of Biological Rhythms on Sleep

Biological clocks appear to be a normal component of all living beings, from single cellular organisms to humans.[6] The science of chronobiology is relatively new and unfamiliar to most health professionals, although its practice is ancient. Although homeostatic theory has proved useful in understanding basic human physiological function, chronobiology, or the study of biological rhythms, provides greater insight regarding the functioning of biological processes.

In the past, laboratory tests required larger volumes of blood and tissue so that testing once a day or every other day was the only ethical option for critically ill patients. Today, improved technology permits the use of smaller volumes, therefore more frequent sampling is feasible and information regarding changes in physiological parameters throughout the day is now available. It is now known that the physiological and metabolic activities of all living organisms vary predictably over time rather than remain static. In recent years there has been rapid growth in the knowledge and understanding of human biological rhythms. This knowledge is currently being applied to clinical medicine, pharmacology, and nursing.[6]

Circadian Rhythms

Human functions undergo periodic or cyclic alterations during each 24-hour period and result in a predictable variation in human activity and rest. These bioperiodicities are often referred to as circadian rhythms, which are cyclic activities that take approximately 24 hours to complete (circa = about; dian = day). However, these periods are not exactly 24 hours in length and vary between 20 and 28 hours as predetermined by the genetic predisposition of the individual. In addition, the timing of the circadian peaks and troughs of our biological functions is largely determined by the daily scheduling of sleep and activity. In general, changes that delay or advance the initiation of the sleep-wake cycle by more than 2 hours will affect the timing of these cyclic biological functions.[6]

Research suggests that many rhythms are adaptive and serve to adjust organisms to predictable and regular environmental changes. In general, biological cycles can be broken down into three categories: Ultradian rhythms, or those of durations more than 24 hours, the previously mentioned circadian rhythms of 21 to 28 hours in length, and infradian rhythms, or those less than 24 hours. From the beginning of time, life was subjected to repeated periodic changes in the environment. It is probable that this rhythmicity has developed over the eons by living organisms because of continuous exposure to periodic environmental changes.[6]

Sleep Physiology

The sleep state is divided into ultradian stages, which occur repetitively throughout the individual's rest period. There are two distinct phases of sleep: REM (rapid eye movement) sleep, also called paradoxical sleep, and NREM (non–rapid eye movement) sleep, also known as quiet or slow-wave sleep. Figure 8–1 depicts the stages of human sleep. During REM sleep, an increase in eye movement as measured by electro-oculographic (EOG) activity is accompanied by fast potential increases or spikes. In general, muscle activity, as measured by electromyographic (EMG) activity, declines to near-baseline levels and bursts of rapid eye movement begin to appear. The first period of REM sleep usually begins approximately 1 hour to 90 minutes after the onset of sleep but lasts only a very short time.[7] Sleep onset always occurs through NREM sleep.

NREM Sleep

NREM sleep is usually divided into four separate stages based on changes that occur in the recording of the EEG. The progression from stage 1 sleep to stage 4 sleep represents an approximate continuum of increasing depth of sleep.[7] The change from waking state to drowsy (stage 1) sleep (Fig. 8–1) is characterized by a decrease in alpha activity. When activity drops below 50% of the waking level, the epoch is

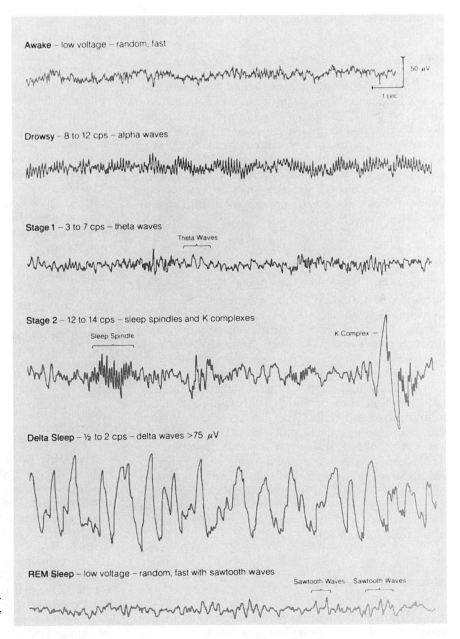

FIGURE 8–1. Stages of human sleep. (Courtesy of Upjohn Pharmaceutical, Kalamazoo, MI.)

scored as stage 1 sleep. Typically, stage 1 sleep is defined by a lack of sleep spindles or K complexes. This stage of NREM sleep lasts only about 1 to 2 minutes. The occurrence of low-voltage EEG activity and the occurrence of sleep spindles and K complexes indicates the arrival of stage 2 sleep. During stage 2 sleep EMG activity is reduced when compared with wakefulness and stage 1 sleep. In young adults, this stage of NREM sleep constitutes approximately 50% to 60% of total sleep time.

When activity includes at least 20%, but not more than 50%, of slow delta waves epochs are scored for stage 3 slow-wave sleep. The final stage of NREM sleep is stage 4, which is characterized by more than 50% delta waves. Stage 4 sleep is often referred to as the deepest level of sleep. Periods of stage 3 and stage 4 sleep last approximately 15 to 30 minutes. These final two stages of NREM sleep, stage 3 and stage 4 sleep, are often referred to as delta sleep or slow-wave sleep.

REM Sleep

REM sleep is usually characterized by a particular type of EEG activation, bursts of rapid EEG activity and muscle atonia. REM sleep is also known as paradoxical sleep because the rapid eye movement and increased cerebral activity resemble the waking state.[8] REM sleep is unique in that it resembles both NREM sleep and the waking state. REM is the only state in which dreams can be experienced. In the past, some societies believed that this "dream sleep" was a third state of consciousness.

Ultradian Sleep Cycles

The cycling of REM and NREM sleep stages are examples of ultradian rhythms, whereas the overall sleep-wake cycle is an example of a circadian rhythm. During the sleep cycle a normal young adult passes through stages of NREM sleep into various stages of REM sleep in a pattern that repeats every 70 to 120 minutes. A typical pattern is as follows: waking, stage 1, stage 2, stage 3, stage 4, stage 3, stage 2, REM. This cycle is followed by further NREM stages 2, 3, 4, 3, 2 followed by another REM period. Over the course of the sleep period each cycle changes in that the amount of NREM sleep decreases and the amount of REM sleep increases. In some persons, particularly the elderly, stage 3 and 4 sleep disappear entirely and are replaced by stage 2 during the NREM portion of the sleep cycle. Although some people complain of not feeling well rested, the impact of these EEG changes is not fully understood.[7]

Mechanisms of Sleep

A great deal of attention has been given to the possible role of the suprachiasmatic nucleus, located in the brain, as a rhythm generator.[9,10] Currently, the results of studies indicate that no single regulator can account for the control of all rhythmic variables.[6] It has been suggested that hormonal secretions from the adrenal cortex are the principal mechanisms that control human adaptation to the daily sleep-wake cycle. Although there have been numerous attempts to locate a single central regulator of circadian and sleep phenomena at the unicellular level, thus far the search has been unsuccessful. Several researchers believe that temporal rhythm control is regulated by the communication between cell membranes.[10]

Hormonal Regulation of Sleep

Various chronobiological studies have also determined that the levels of certain hormones change rhythmically during both the sleep-wake cycle and REM-NREM cycles. Some hormones are believed to be under the control of the sleep-wake cycle, while others may influence the onset of the cycles themselves.[11]

Melatonin is a hormone produced by the suprachiasmatic nucleus (SCN). It is believed that exposure to bright light can influence the production of melatonin via optic nerve stimulation of the SCN.[12-15] Exposure to bright light is also known to alter circadian rhythm adjustment. It is believed that the cycling of melatonin levels is responsible for the initiation of the sleep-wake cycle and a variety of other circadian rhythms. This occurs through the reduction in core temperature (thermoregulation) and the modification of brain levels of other neurotransmitters. It is well known that there is a change in blood levels of melatonin with age and that this factor may help to explain the previously described alteration in the sleep cycle throughout the aging process.[16] Further, it was noted that oral administration of melatonin affects sleep latency, mood, performance, and core body temperature when compared with a placebo. It is believed that the nocturnal surge in plasma melatonin may initiate a significant cascade of events that may induce sleep onset.

Sleep Changes with Age

It is fairly obvious that sleep changes as we age. Infants sleep extraordinary amounts of time when compared with adults. But even after we reach adulthood, the sleep cycle continues to change subtly. In young adults approximately 50% of total sleep time is spent in stage 2 sleep, 25% is spent in REM, 6% is spent in stage 3, 14% in stage 4, and 5% in stage 1. The percentages of the various sleep levels change as a person ages, and total sleep time is reduced after the age of 20. Stage 3 and stage 4 sleep also decrease steadily as a person ages and the amount of stage 1 and stage 2 sleep increase. Figure 8–2 depicts developmental changes in sleep over the lifespan.[1]

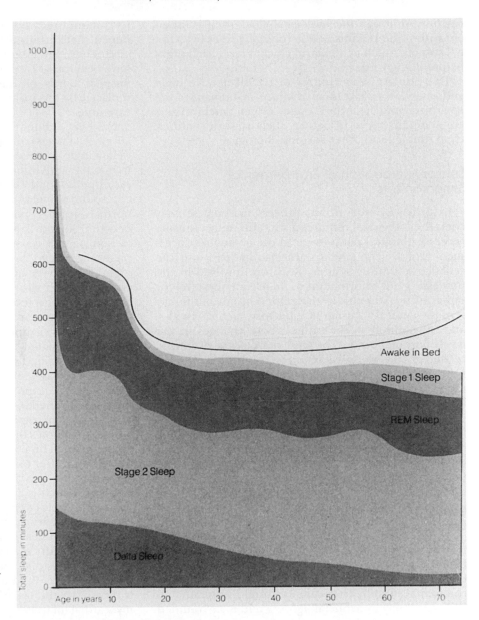

FIGURE 8–2. Developmental changes of sleep throughout the human lifespan. (Courtesy of Upjohn Pharmaceutical, Kalamazoo, MI.)

Clinical Measurement of Sleep

Sleep is still most accurately measured using polysomnographic testing (PST) methods, which were defined and standardized by Drs. Rechtshaffen and Kales.[17] Usually, measures of brain activity through EEG, ocular activity through EOG, and muscle activity through EMG are obtained during the usual sleep period. Information from EEG, EOG, and EMG are used in combination to define sleep stages. Records are primarily read in periods or epochs of 30 seconds duration. NREM sleep is commonly divided into four distinct stages. All are different from each other and from the waking state. While in the waking state, EEG is commonly characterized as containing alpha rhythms and mixed voltage activity. Human sleep stages showing levels of EEG activity are depicted in Figure 8–1.

SENSORY ALTERATIONS IN THE CRITICAL CARE ENVIRONMENT

Environmental Synchronization of Biological Rhythms

Understanding the concept of environmental synchronization is important in understanding the temporal integration of biological rhythms and their resultant impact on individual sleep-wake cycles in the intensive care environment. A synchronizer is a cue or signal from one's environment that serves to reset biological rhythms.[6] The synchronizer is also sometimes referred to as a zeitgeber, or entraining agent. The terms are used synonymously. Synchronizers do not cause and are not the source of biological rhythmicity; however, they do influence certain rhythm characteristics, such as timing of the peak and trough of a given rhythm. Although the biological clock itself is inherent within the organism, it is routinely reset by external stimuli, much as an alarm clock is reset each night before going to sleep.

The primary synchronizer of the sleep-wake cycle and many other circadian rhythms in humans is the environmental light-dark cycle. Other synchronizers are generally social in nature, such as work routines, meal timing, and other sociopsychological cues.[7]

Sensory Perception of Environmental Synchronizers

In order to receive and process external sensory cues, the individual requires a stimulus, intact sensory receptors, neural pathways, and the ability to process such stimuli. The reticular formation (RF) and the reticular activating system (RAS) are involved in the processing of information. The frequency level or power of the stimulus is intercepted by any of the five senses—auditory, gustatory, olfactory, tactile, visual—and transmitted to the brain, where changes in the level of arousal occur. The level of arousal is, of course, related to the sleep-wakefulness continuum. During normal existence, individuals who receive either too much or too little stimulation move to an environment that is more comfortable and offers an adequate or optimum frequency of stimuli.[7] For the critically ill, however, escape from excessive stimuli is frequently impossible, therefore the patient is dependent upon the critical care nurse to serve as advocate in the regulation of environmental stimuli.

Sensory Overload in the Critical Care Environment

Although the critically ill individual greatly benefits from the intensive care setting and the accessibility of technology, the critical care unit is laden with environmental stimuli. The patient is brightly illuminated 24 hours a day by artificial lighting and is surrounded by monitors, ventilators, and various other pieces of equipment that commonly exceed acceptable noise levels.[18,19] Constant lighting and high levels of noise from both machinery and conversation have repeatedly been identified as noxious factors in the critical care unit.[20] Research suggests that 50% of all patients that enter the ICU environment are sleep-deprived within 48 hours.[21]

Sensory overload can be defined as any increase in the intensity of stimuli to greater-than-normal levels or as simultaneous multisensory experiences.[22] In the critical care environment increased vigilance by healthcare providers may frequently result in disruption of the sleep-wake cycle and desynchronization. Although all or any combination of the senses can be routes for sensory overload, hearing and sight are the most frequently abused.

Noise. In general, noise levels of daily living have risen by 1 dB (decibel) over the last 25 years.[23] Bentley[24] monitored the noise levels of ICUs and determined that during the normal sleep period noise is often above an acceptable level. Hospitals in general have become noisy places. The austere silence of the hospital wards of the 1940s and 1950s has been replaced by the turbulence and frenzy of the critical care units.

Noise is defined as audible acoustic energy that adversely affects the physiological or psychological well-being of people.[25] Sound is measured in terms of frequency and intensity. Frequency is measured in cycles per second (Hz) and the intensity or loudness of a sound is measured in decibels (dB). People with normal hearing perceive sounds with frequencies between 20 and 20,000 Hz. The Environmental Protection Agency recommends that noise levels in hospitals not exceed 45 dB during the day and 35 dB at night. Even lower levels have been suggested for the critical care environment. Most hospitals, however, have an average level that is nearly double the suggested evening rate.[23] Some surveys suggest that 50% of all patients complain about hospital noise levels[26] and it is estimated that 40% of patients suffer from noise-based sleep disturbances.[27] Most often, noise in the hospital has been attributed to staff conversation;[18] however, equipment alarms have also been frequently identified as sources of unwanted sound in the critical care environment.

Noise promotes the release of epinephrine and norepinephrine. This endocrine arousal may continue for 1 to 2 hours after exposure to noise.[23] Physiologically, noise or any unwanted sound can elicit a stress response, which is expressed by an increased respiratory rate, general peripheral vasoconstriction, and elevated adrenocortical hormone release accompanied by increases in heart rate.[25]

Patients with essential hypertension experience increases in systolic and diastolic blood pressure with noise exposure[28] and excessive noise may lead to ventricular arrhythmias among patients recovering from myocardial infarctions.[22] In addition, sleeping patients exposed to noise show electroencephalographic signs of arousal. Because older people sleep less deeply than younger people, sound levels that may not awaken a young person may frequently awaken an elderly patient.[25,29] Even noise that is insufficient to awaken an individual may produce evidence of arousal and transitions from various stages of sleep on the EEG.[30] Moreover, if noise levels are high at the normal sleep time, the normal sleep-wake cycle will be disturbed.

Light. Extremely bright light may awaken a healthy sleeping person, and significant light exposure, at a particular time, is believed to alter the phase of particular circadian rhythms.[14] Controlled exposure to bright light is frequently used to improve the condition of individuals with seasonal affective disorder (SAD) and has recently been used to help shift workers adjust their circadian phase.[31] Exposure to bright light and subsequent periods of low light must be carefully controlled, however, or sleep deprivation and/or desynchronization may occur. Originally, several hours of exposure were believed to be necessary; however recent research has shown that single pulses of bright light may also be capable of resetting biological rhythms.[32]

Pain. The common belief that sleeping patients do not experience pain has not been supported by research findings. Traditionally, sleep is considered to be a time of restoration and preparation for the next waking period. During illness, patients are encouraged to stay in bed and attempt to rest, as many nurses believe that the patient's need for sleep is greater during the healing process.[33]

In patients presumed to be sleeping, 61% to 90% reported experiencing pain.[34–36] A study of 100 intensive care patients found subjects ranked pain second only to the "inability to lie comfortably" as the cause of sleep loss.[37] Further, a study of herniorrhaphy patients identified that over 40% of their first two postoperative nights were spent awake due to pain and routine nursing procedures.[38]

Research indicates that postoperative patients are frequently awake during the night. Closs[21] found that of 200 patients on various surgical wards receiving intramuscular analgesics, 170 had their sleep disturbed by pain at some time during their hospital stay. Auvil-Novak[39] noted that the majority of the patients receiving patient-controlled analgesia (PCA) therapy were awake using the PCA pump some time during the normal sleep period. Because it is part of the hospital routine for the nurse to obtain vital signs and give medications during these nighttime hours, it is difficult to ascertain whether the patients awoke due to pain or for treatment. The majority of patients complained to the investigator about being awakened during the night, especially for the first several days postoperatively. However, patients were up at all hours of the night requesting analgesic from the PCA pump. Patients attempted to dose themselves with analgesic as many as 130 times during the first postoperative night.

Sensory Deprivation in the Critical Care Environment

Sensory deprivation is the absence of stimuli that may be perceived by the five senses. Manifestations of sensory deprivation include, performance impairment, restlessness, anxiety, delusions, and visual and auditory hallucinations.[40] Sensory deprivation can result even in the presence of multiple stimuli, if the environmental synchronizers are too infrequent or inappropriately timed. Sensory deprivation can result from the monotony of background noises, isolation from family and staff, or the immobility induced by ICU technology.

Sleep in sensory deprivation situations is also frequently altered, producing greater quantities of slow-wave sleep. One of the potential consequences of sensory deprivation in the critical care patient is desynchronization.

Desynchronization

External Desynchronization

Rhythms in persons in a synchronized state normally have a fixed time relationship. In humans there are many circadian rhythmic functions—including variations in temperature, hormone levels, and enzyme action—that are reset by environmental synchronizers. In the individual's environment, the biological clock is reset daily by environmental synchronizers such as daylight, work routine, television, clocks, and radios. When synchronization does not occur, either because of the absence of these time cues or due to alteration of usual routines through hospitalization, changes occur in the usual relationships between a large number of rhythms. The patient may become externally desynchronized, resulting in free-running rhythms and internal desynchronization.

Free-Running Rhythms

Free-running rhythms develop when the patient receives either too much (sensory overload) or too little (sensory deprivation) stimulation to reset their biological clock in synchrony with external time. In humans, circadian rhythms are generally slightly longer than 24 hours. Individuals dwelling in experimental settings without time cues experience elongated sleep-wake patterns of almost 25 hours.[6] Because the duration of individual cycles is not exactly 24 hours, like a real time clock, individual circadian functions will differ from one day to the next unless reset by environmental synchronizers. In an environment free of synchronizers, or containing too many external cues, clock time no longer can be used by the body to interpret the staging of specific circadian functions. Therefore these circadian functions begin to run freely usually moving ahead 1 or 2 hours a day.

Internal Desynchronization

When patients are isolated from all time cues, certain rhythmic variables, even though they are free-running, remain internally synchronized; that is, they retain the same phase relationship that was demonstrated under the normal synchronized state. On the other hand, some rhythms such as the sleep-activity cycle and body temperature rhythm will become internally desynchronized.[6] This transient state of altered relationships within the circadian system is termed desynchronization.[6] The time relationship of these two rhythmic variables is continuously changing until it is stabilized by the timely introduction of environmental synchronizers. Simply stated, the sleep-wake rhythm can be out of phase with the body temperature

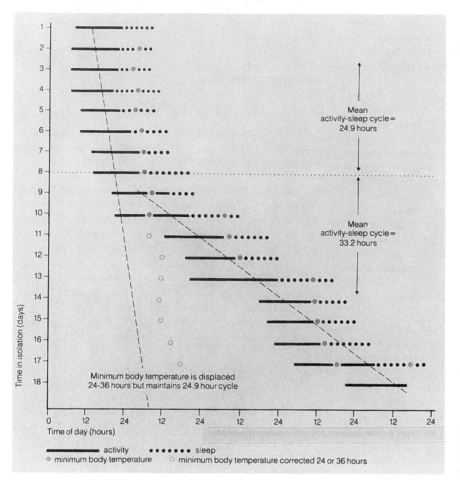

Mean
activity-sleep cycle =
24.9 hours

Mean
activity-sleep cycle =
33.2 hours

Minimum body temperature is displaced
24-36 hours but maintains 24.9 hour cycle

Time in isolation (days)

Time of day (hours)

━━━━━ activity   •••••• sleep
● minimum body temperature   ○ minimum body temperature corrected 24 or 36 hours

FIGURE 8–3. Displacement of circadian rhythms due to desynchronization. (Courtesy of Upjohn Pharmaceutical, Kalamazoo, MI.)

rhythm. If synchronizers are not introduced and the patient continues in the free-running state adverse sequelae, such as psychoses, may result.

The phasing of circadian and other rhythms in human beings is organized temporally to anticipate the different metabolic requirements of activity and rest when adhering to a fixed life routine.[6] This routine is disturbed when the individual's schedule is altered by such events as illness and hospitalization. Some persons seem to be able to adjust to the new routine rather quickly, while others adjust slowly.[6] Individual biological variability makes the estimation of time needed for entrainment or adjustment difficult. Individuals compromised biologically and/or emotionally by disease frequently require more time for adjustment.

During adjustment to a new routine, the rate at which each circadian process shifts may differ for each individual.[6,7] Internal and external desynchronization without nursing intervention will result in decreased biological efficiency. In its mildest form this period of less than optimal biological efficiency is similar to "jet lag," the same phenomenon experienced by travelers and shift workers during the first few days following a sudden change in their sleep-activity routine. This fatigue and general malaise or "sick lag" frequently

occurs in patients in intensive care settings, where normal rhythms have been disturbed by changes or interruptions in scheduling. The elderly in particular tend to be very structured in scheduling their daily routines.[41] Any alteration in synchronizer pattern such as meal- or bedtime routines can be extremely disruptive and may result in rapid desynchronization. When rhythms are desynchronized or uncoupled, it becomes even more difficult for the patient in the intensive care setting to maintain a normal sleep schedule (Fig. 8–3). Changes in the usual sleep-wake schedule result in greater rhythm desynchronization, and a vicious circle results that can further exacerbate the patient's existing health problems. Without intervention, external and internal desynchronization can result in sleep deprivation.

Sleep Deprivation

Some researchers suggest that sleep deprivation can be divided into three classes: total, partial, and selective.[42] Total sleep deprivation is defined as a loss of sleep for a full 24-hour period or more. Partial sleep deprivation is defined as sleeping less than the average 7 to 8 hours each night. This type of deprivation can be initiated in two ways: sleep can be gradually decreased by some fixed period over a preset time (i.e., a loss of 1 hour per month for 4 months), or sleep can be abruptly changed, for example, from 8 hours per night to 4 hours per night.

Sleep deprivation may also be classified as selective, which is artificially created. When a person is evaluated electrophysiologically, specific stages of sleep (i.e., REM sleep) can be reduced or eliminated by waking up the person as they enter that particular stage. Only selective sleep deprivation is artificially induced, although sleep deprivation of all three types can routinely occur in daily life.[42]

Others define sleep deprivation as either chronic or acute. Acute sleep deprivation is analogous to total sleep deprivation, and chronic sleep deprivation is usually assumed to be related to partial sleep deprivation, but may include some selective sleep deprivation as described below. Since REM sleep occurs more frequently at the end of the sleep cycle, waking a few hours earlier than normal will simultaneously produce both partial and selective (REM) sleep deprivation. The distinction between types of sleep deprivation will determine the applicability of the results to the critical care environment. In most cases, sleep disturbances that occur in the critical care units are partial or chronic in nature. Unfortunately, chronic sleep deprivation has been the least actively investigated form of sleep deprivation.

Consequences of Sleep Deprivation

Naitoh et al.[43] suggest that sleep deprivation of all types carries very little risk of health consequences in a normal population. In general, the majority of studies in all types of sleep deprivation have used healthy young subjects consisting of volunteers or military personnel. It has been suggested that the results of these studies are not applicable to middle-aged or elderly populations in poor health or fitness.[43]

Further, the majority of studies have evaluated the results of total sleep deprivation, and few studies have been done to determine the effects of partial sleep deprivation in either healthy or hospital-based populations. Regardless, most ICU patients suffer from chronic or partial sleep deprivation. It is well known that sleep deprivation (initiated by either a change in zeitgeber presentation or lack of zeitgeber presentation) causes a change in the phase of circadian rhythms; however, this finding cannot be carried over to acutely ill populations.

Even in healthy populations, sleep loss may carry a significant risk of injury because of decreased attention and vigilance. Further, combinations of stressors, including sleep loss, may be a factor in increased risk of illness.[42] Signs of sleep deprivation include impaired intellectual functioning, labile affect, anxiety, agitation, depression, confusion; disorientation to time, place, or person; and impaired cognitive func-

TABLE 8–1
Physiologic Consequences of Sleep Deprivation

⇑ Hemodilution	⇑ Blood glucose
⇓ RBC count	⇓ $\dot{V}o_2$
⇓ Hematocrit	⇓ HCO_3^-
⇑ Cortisol	⇓ pH
⇑ T_4	⇓ Maleate dehydrogenase
⇑ T_3, rT_3	⇓ Citrate synthetase
⇑ Insulin secretion	

HCO_3^- = bicarbonate ion; RBC = red blood cell; T_4 = thyroxine; T_3 = tri-iodothyronine; rT_3 = reverse triodothyronine; $\dot{V}o_2$ = oxygen consumption per unit time.

tion.[43] Research has demonstrated that total sleep deprivation in healthy populations can result in decreased aerobic oxygenation capacity and changes in skeletal muscle aerobic capacity,[44] increased plasma volume, reduced hematocrit and erythrocyte count,[45] and a reduction in plasma iron by over one half after 120 hours of sleep deprivation.[46] Further, sleep deprivation for one 24-hour period was found to attenuate ventilatory chemosensitivity by decreasing hypercapnic and hypoxic ventilatory response in healthy individuals.[47] This short period of sleep deprivation is likely to contribute to hypoventilation in acutely ill patients.

It has been demonstrated that 85 hours of total sleep deprivation can cause a metabolic shift from glucose to lipids as the major energy source.[48] The occurrence of a 40% increase in nocturnal insulin clearance in healthy individuals after only 24 hours of sleep deprivation may help to explain this change.[49] Tables 8–1 and 8–2 list common physiological and psychological changes that occur as a result of sleep deprivation.

ICU Psychosis

ICU psychosis or syndrome is believed to result from sleep deprivation and desynchronization. ICU psychosis has been defined in terms of symptoms or behaviors. These include decreased ability to maintain attention, clouding of consciousness, memory problems, disorientation, labile affect. Severe forms exhibit confusion, combativeness, delirium, and neurosis with visual and auditory hallucinations. Research suggests that acute sleep deprivation contributes to the development of ICU psychosis. Sensory overload can con-

TABLE 8–2
Psychological Consequences of Sleep Deprivation

⇑ Sleepiness	⇓ Vigilance
⇑ Stress	⇓ Motivation
⇓ Psychomotor performance	⇑ Agitation
⇓ Mood	

RESEARCH APPLICATION: PILOT STUDY: VALIDATING STAFF NURSES' OBSERVATIONS OF SLEEP AND WAKE STATES AMONG CRITICALLY ILL PATIENTS, USING POLYSOMNOGRAPHY
Edwards, GB and Schuring, LM. American Journal of Critical Care 2:125, 1993

Purpose: The purpose of this research was to validate staff nurses' observations of sleep and wake states among critically ill adult patients using polysomnography.

Methods: The study was conducted in a 10-bed medical ICU in a 540-bed acute care teaching hospital. A convenience sample of 21 patients in the MICU (10 men, 11 women) over 18 years old; oriented to person, place, and time, and of stable physiologic status were used for the study. Study subjects had a variety of diagnoses including renal insufficiency, sleep apnea, cardiac arrest, cardiac arrythmia, pneumonia, asthma, and hypertension. All subjects but one were mechanically ventilated, and 18 of 21 subjects received diazepam and secobarbital sodium. Subjects were evaluated for a 4-hour period (0100 to 0500) via polysomnography while nurses simultaneously evaluated sleep state via a nominal checklist (awake, asleep, could not tell, and no time to observe) for 16 15-minute intervals. A total of 15 nurses spent one or more 4-hour periods with a single subject to evaluate sleep state. Polysomnographic results were retrospectively scored for sleep-wake status for a 2-minute period, during which the checklist for sleep-wake status had been scored. Polysomnographic determination of sleep or wakefulness was then compared with nurse checklist scores.

Results: Analysis suggested that overall nurse evaluation of subject sleep or wakefulness was correct 73.5% of the time, incorrect 16.2% of the time, and inconclusive 10.3% of the time. When conditional probabilities were calculated, nurse observations were correct 69.6% of the time when subjects were awake and correct 87.9% of the time when subjects were asleep.

Practice Implications: The findings of this study reinforce nurses' confidence in their ability to assess patients' sleep and wake states. This confidence can be valuable in the early recognition of potential or actual sleep pattern disturbance. Early recognition may lead to more effective management of a sleep disturbance problem in the ICU. Prevention of sleep disturbance, desynchronization, and sleep deprivation may reduce the frequency of environmentally related ICU psychosis.

tribute to the development of ICU syndrome through the rapid development of acute sleep deprivation and external desynchronization, which results from frequent monitoring, invasive procedures, and excessive light and noise stimulus.[18,50] External desynchronization without intervention results in free-running rhythms, chronic sleep deprivation, and internal desynchronization.

Sensory deprivation provides a slower course for the development of ICU psychosis. Through isolation and immobility, an absence of environmental stimuli results in external desynchronization, free-running rhythms, chronic sleep deprivation, internal desynchronization, and potential ICU psychosis if no intervention reverses the process.

In summary, an optimum level of stimulation exists at which the patient remains synchronized. At levels of low stimulus, time clues and cues are either not presented at all or are presented too infrequently. This sequence of events over time leads to boredom, disorientation, and the development of free-running rhythms in the patient. With isolation, and no longer synchronized by zeitgebers, the individual's biological rhythms separate and become displaced in time (Fig. 8–3). Sleep difficulties and further desynchronization may result in ICU psychosis without nursing intervention. With excessive environmental stimuli, acute sleep deprivation and desynchronization result from inappropriate time cues.

Nursing Implications

Present hospital practice requires physicians to work an 8- or 10-hour day, usually scheduling medical treatment during the work day. Nurses, however, are required to work with the patient throughout the day and night, structuring the patient's therapies to coincide with hospital routines and nurse scheduling patterns over the 24-hour period. Neither discipline is supportive of the temporal orientation of the patient. The rest-activity cycle and sleep-wake patterns, which are very influential in regulating 24-hour rhythms in the individual, are frequently disturbed in an effort to use the nurse's time most efficiently. Patient baths, linen changes, and weights are frequently obtained on the night shift, when patients should be sleeping. Lights are left on in patient rooms at all hours for the convenience of the nurse, rather than the patient trying to sleep. Understanding and identifying the relevance of underlying biologic rhythms will improve the nurse's comprehension of normal sleep physiology and alleviate patient health problems related to sleep deprivation and sleep pattern disorders. With the critical care setting, nurses play a pivotal role in creating an environment that maintains the patient in a state of synchronization and promotes an adequate quantity and quality of sleep.

Nurse's Responsibility for Management of the Intensive Care Environment

Because nurses are not at the bedside 24 hours a day within the hospital setting, the staff nurse is responsible for establishing and maintaining the patient's environment, which in turn influences the patient's rhythms, and thus, patient outcomes.[39,51,52] In an effort to provide holistic patient care, nurses need to structure nursing interventions to maintain an environment that is supportive of the individual's usual sleep-wake patterns. Arranging the timing of therapies is well within the domain of nursing practice.[39] Rest-activity patterns, sleep-wake cycles, treatment times, and analgesic administration are all determined by the nurse caring for the patient.[39]

Nursing Intervention in Sleep Disruption

Nonpharmacologic Interventions. Practices used to create an environment conductive to sleep are referred to as sleep hygiene factors. Sleep hygiene measures that can be utilized by nurses to improve sleep in the healthcare setting are listed in Table 8–3. Providing warm baths approximately 2 to 4 hours prior to the desired sleep time, making sure the patient is not hungry, giving back massages to relax patients, assisting the patient into a comfortable position, and monitoring the peak of the patient's temperature rhythm are basic nursing measures that can be provided to any individual. Ensuring that the patient's room temperature is adequate, supplying

TABLE 8–3
Nursing Interventions in Maintenance of Sleep Hygiene

Keep area quiet—Reduce noise and auditory stimuli (maintain noise level below 35 dB).

Control ambient temperature and humidity–Temperature $\geq 75°F$ disturbs sleep.

Keep area dark—Pulses of bright light may wake patient or induce circadian rhythm changes.

Reduce excessive time in bed—Excessive time in bed is related to fragmented and shallow sleep.

Maintain regular arousal time—to stabilize the individual's sleep-wake cycle.

Increase activity during the daytime and prevent exercise 1–2 hours before bedtime—to prevent temperature rise that will delay sleep.

Give foods containing tryptophan (e.g., milk or turkey)—to promote sleep.

Reduce or eliminate caffeine—to prevent sleep disturbance.

Individual Sleep Hygiene Factors that Should be Assessed by the Nurse
Does the patient prefer quiet or "white noise" environment?
Does the patient have preferences in sleep position?
Does the patient prefer to read before bedtime to help sleep?

extra blankets and pillows as necessary, turning out lights and closing doors if possible, or providing sleep masks and earplugs are all interventions that nurses can provide to prevent sleep pattern disruption.[53,54] Nurses can also control the patient environment through scheduling of treatment and interventions. As 24-hour caregivers nurses can plan patient schedules to minimize unnecessary sleep interruptions from hospital personnel. Medication schedules should be assessed to decrease drug administration during the usual sleep period. Currently, nurses administer drug therapy based on the homeostatic perception that relatively constant doses of an agent given over time is the most effective method to maintain a constant blood level. In fact, the time of therapeutic intervention has traditionally been determined in response to the scheduling patterns, workload assignments and hospital routines of the nurse, which does not consider the temporal structure of physiologic, psychological, or sociological phenomena experienced by the patient.[39] Providing meaningful stimulus to the patient will help combat sensory overload and deprivation. Clocks, calendars, television, cassettes, radios, and family visits help provide meaning in the patient's environment.[55]

If prevention of sleep deprivation is impossible, then alleviation of the causes of sleep deprivation is the most common solution chosen by nurses to resolve the individual's problems. Providing periods of uninterrupted sleep or recovery sleep is one of the most frequent nursing interventions for sleep deprivation. An individual experiencing sleep loss demonstrates a pattern of slow-wave sleep during recovery sleep. In recovery sleep, periods of SWS are prolonged, delaying REM recovery. REM sleep usually rebounds on the 2nd or 3rd night after the recuperation of slow-wave sleep.[7] During periods of REM rebound, healthcare problems normally affected during REM sleep such as angina, arrhythmias, duodenal ulcers, and sleep apnea may be aggravated.[50]

Pharmacologic Interventions. Pharmacologic intervention is also frequently used to reverse the effects of sleep disruption. Hypnotics and sedatives are used to reduce sleep latency, increase total sleep time, and increase arousal thresholds.[7] It may even be possible to hasten the chronobiologic adjustments of sleep-activity routine through the use of special medications called chronobiotics.[6] Examples of potential chronobiotics include the hormones melatonin and serotonin, anesthetics, caffeine, and ethanol.[7] Table 8–4 contains a listing of common medications and their effects on sleep.

Some reports have suggested using fast-acting, short-duration benzodiazepines to alter the sleep-wake cycle.[6,7] None of these hypnotic agents are without unwanted side effects, however, and most hypnotic drugs promote a lightened state of stage 2 NREM sleep. Benzodiazepines are the most commonly used hypnotic agents. During wakefulness, they have little effect on respiration, however, during the sleep cycle some individuals (about 40%) develop increased

TABLE 8–4
Common Medications and Their Effect on Sleep

Drug	NREM Effects	REM Effects	Other Effects
Stimulants			
Xanthines	↓ SWS		↓ Total sleep time
Amphetamines		↓ REM onset, duration	Pemoline and prolintane have minimal effects
Analgesics			
Morphine, heroin, methadone		↓ REM activity	↑ Drowsiness ↓ Performance
Aspirin	↓ SWS, ↑ Stage 2		
Antihistamines			
H$_1$ antagonists (brompheniramine, tripolodine)		Suppress REM activity	↑ Drowsiness ↓ Performance
H$_2$ antagonists (cimetidine)	↑ SWS (Impaired renal function)		
Antidepressants			
Tricyclics, tetracyclics, MAO inhibitors		Suppress REM activity	↑ Drowsiness ↓ Performance
Lithium	↓ SWS	↑ REM latency, ↓ REM sleep	
Cardiovascular			
β adrenoreceptor antagonists (propranolol)		↓ REM sleep	Frequent awakenings, ↑ dreaming, ↑ sleep latency
α adrenoreceptor agonists (clonidine)	↑ Stage 2 sleep	↓ REM sleep	Sedation, ↑ total sleep time
Neuroleptic			
Phenothiazine (chlorpromazine, promazine)	↑ SWS	↓ REM latency	↑ Drowsiness, ↓ performance
Benzodiazepines (diazepam, flurazepam)	↓ SWS	↓ REM (dose-related)	

SWS = slow-wave sleep.

instances of respiratory disturbances.[7] Barbiturates are known to cause an increased number of apneic events in patients with pre-existing sleep apnea disorders and have also been known to decrease both slow-wave and REM sleep.[7]

General anesthetics are powerful central nervous system (CNS) depressants and may also exacerbate pre-existing respiratory difficulties during the sleep cycle. Narcotics are also vigorous CNS depressants and may decrease respiratory response during both sleep and wakefulness.[7]

Because many common hypnotics either cause or exacerbate respiratory difficulty during sleep and may alter portions of the normal sleep cycle, nonpharmacological interventions are generally preferred over pharmacological ones to reduce the risk of engaging the sleep deprivation desynchronization cycle. Maintenance of adequate time cues and clues in the intensive care environment as well as the promotion of good sleep hygiene conditions should be the goal of nurses in the intensive care unit.

REFERENCES

1. Hauri, P: Current Concepts: The Sleep Disorders. Upjohn Pharmaceuticals, Kalamazoo, MI, 1982.
2. Kleitman, N: Sleep and Wakefulness. University of Chicago Press, Chicago, 1963.
3. Canavan, T: The functions of sleep. Nursing 9:321, 1986.
4. Folkard, S and Monk, TH: Hours of Work, Temporal Factors in Work-Scheduling. John Wiley & Sons, Chichester, 1985.
5. Wever, R: The Circadian Systems of Man, Results of Experiments under Temporal Isolation. Springer-Verlag, New York, 1979.
6. Reinberg, A and Smolensky, MH: Biological Rhythms and Medicine: Cellular, Metabolic, Physiopathologic and Pharmacologic Aspects. Springer-Verlag, New York, 1983.
7. Kryger, MH, Roth, T, and Dement, WC: Principles and Practice of Sleep Medicine. WB Saunders, Philadelphia, 1989.
8. Jouvet, M, Michel, F, and Courjon, J: Sur un stade d'activité electrique cerebral rapide au cours, du sommeil physiologique. CR Soc Seances Biol Fil 153:1024, 1959.
9. Reitveld, WJ and Gross, GA: The role of the suprachiasmatic nucleus: Afferents in the central regulation of circadian rhythms. In von Mayersbach, H, Scheving, LE, and Pauly, JE (eds): Biological Rhythms in Structure and Function. AR Liss, New York, 1981, pp. 205–211.
10. Rusak, B and Haddad, G: Neural Mechanisms of the Mammalian Circadian System. Guilford Press, London, 1993.
11. Brandenberger, G: Endocrine ultradian rhythms during sleep and wakefulness. In Lloyd, D, and Rossi, EL (eds): Ultradian Rhythms in Life Processes: An Inquiry into Fundamental Principles of Chronobiology and Psychobiology. Springer-Verlag, New York, 1993.
12. Kripke, DF, Mullaney, DJ, Atkinson, M, and Wolf, S: Circadian rhythm disorders in manic-depressives. Biol Psychiatry 13:335, 1978.
13. Czeisler, CA, Allen, JS, Kronauer, RE, and Duffy JF: Strong circadian phase resetting in man is effected by bright light suppression of circadian amplitude. Sleep Research 17:367, 1988.
14. Czeisler, CA, Allan, JS, and Strogatz, SH: Bright light resets the human circadian pacemaker independent of the timing of the sleep-wake cycle. Science 233:667, 1986.
15. Sack, RL, Lewy AJ, and Hoban TM: Free running melatonin

rhythms in blind people: Phase shifts with melatonin and triazolam administration. In Rensing, L, an den Heiden, U, and Mackey, MC (eds): Temporal Disorder in Human Oscillatory Systems. Springer-Verlag, Berlin, 1987.

16. Dollins, AB, Zdanova, IV, Wurtman, RJ, Lynch, HJ, and Deng, MH: Effect of inducing nocturnal serum melatonin concentrations in daytime, sleep, mood, body temperature and performance. Proc Natl Acad Sci USA 91:1824, 1994.

17. Rechtschaffen, A and Kales, A (eds): A Manual of Standardized Terminology, Techniques and Scoring System for Sleep Stages of Human Subjects. Brain Research Institute, Los Angeles, 1968.

18. Helton, M, Gordon, S, and Nunnery, S: The correlation between sleep deprivation and the intensive care unit syndrome. Heart Lung 9:464, 1980.

19. Wood, AM: A review of literature relating to sleep in hospital with emphasis on the sleep of the ICU patient. Int Crit Care Nurs 9:129, 1993.

20. Hilton, B: Quantity and quality of sleep and sleep disturbing factors in a respiratory intensive care unit. J Adv Nurs 1:453, 1976.

21. Closs, J: Assessment of sleep in hospital patients. J Adv Nurs 13:501, 1988.

22. Baker, CF: Sensory overload and noise in the ICU: Sources of environmental stress. Crit Care Q 6:66, 1984.

23. Grumet, GW: Pandemonium in the modern hospital. N Engl J Med 328:433, 1993.

24. Bentley, S, Murphy, F, and Dudley, H: Perceived noise in surgical wards and in ICU. BMJ 2:1506, 1977.

25. Kryter, KD: The Effects of Noise on Man. Academic Press, Orlando, FL, 1985.

26. Aitken, RJ: Quantitative noise analysis in a modern hospital. Arch Environ Health 37:361, 1982.

27. Soutar, RL and Wilson, JA: Does hospital noise disturb patients? BMJ 292:305, 1986.

28. McLean, EK and Tarnopolsky, A: Noise, discomfort and mental health: A review of the socio-medical implications of disturbance by noise. Psychol Med 7:19, 1977.

29. Sato, T, Kawad, T, Ogawa, M, Aoki, S, and Suzuki S: Effect of some factors on sleep polygraphic parameters and subjective evaluations of sleep. Environ Res 61:337, 1993.

30. Orr, WC and Stahl, ML: Sleep disturbances after open heart surgery. Am J Cardiol 39:196, 1977.

31. Eastman, CI: Squashing versus nudging circadian rhythms with artificial bright light: Solutions for shift work? Perspect Biol Med 34:181, 1991.

32. Dawson, D, Lack, L, and Morris M: Phase resetting of human circadian pacemaker with use of a single pulse of bright light. Chronobiol Int 10:94, 1993.

33. Webster, RA and Thompson, DR: Sleep in hospital. J Adv Nurs 11:447, 1986.

34. Cohen, F: Post-surgical pain relief: Patients' status and nurses' medication choices. Pain 9:265, 1980.

35. Closs, SJ: An exploratory analysis of nurses' provision of postoperative analgesic drugs. J Adv Nurs. 15:42, 1990.

36. Donovan, M, Dillon, P, and McGuire, L: Incidence and characteristics of pain in a sample of medical-surgical patients. Pain 30:69, 1987.

37. Jones, J, Hoggart, B, Withey, J, Donaghue, K, and Ellis, BW: What the patients say: A study of reactions to an intensive care unit. Intensive Care Med 5:89, 1978.

38. Auvil-Novak, SE, Novak, RD, Smolensky, MH, Morris, M, and Kwan, JW: Temporal variation in post-surgical utilization via patient-controlled analgesia. Ann N Y Acad Sci 618:599, 1991.

39. Auvil-Novak, SE: Development and Testing of a Chronobiologic Model for Pain Management in Nursing: Efficacy of Chronotherapeutic versus Traditional Administration of Patient-Controlled Analgesia. University of Texas at Austin, 1992. DAI 53.04B

40. Solomon, P: Sensory Deprivation: A Symposium. Harvard University Press, Harvard, 1961.

41. Kartmann, JL: Sleep and the elderly critical care patient. Critical Care Nurse 5:52, 1985.

42. Naitoh, P, Kelly, TL, and Englund, C: Health effects of sleep deprivation. Occup Med, 5:209, 1990.

43. Naitoh, P, Kelley, T, and Babkoff, H: Sleep inertia: Best time not to wake up? Chronobiol Int 10:109, 1993.

44. Vondra, K, Brodan, V, Bass A, Kuhn, E, Tesinger, J, Andel, M, and Veselkova, A: Effects of sleep deprivation on the activity of selected metabolic enzymes in skeletal muscle. Eur J Appl Physiol 47:41, 1981.

45. Goodman, JM, Plyley, MJ, Lucy, EM, Hart, BPHE, Radomski, M, and Shepard, RJ: Moderate exercise and hemodilution during sleep deprivation. Aviat Space Environ Med 2:139, 1990.

46. Kuhn, E and Brodin, V: Changes in the circadian rhythm of serum iron induced by a 5-day sleep deprivation. Eur J Appl Physiol 49:215, 1982.

47. White, DP, Douglas, NJ, Pickett, CK, Zillich, GW, and Weil, JV: Sleep deprivation and the control of ventilation. Am Rev Resp Dis 128:984, 1983.

48. Radomski, MW, Hart, LEM, Goodman, JM, and Pyley, MJ: Aerobic fitness and hormonal responses to prolonged sleep deprivation and sustained mental work. Aviat Space Environ Med 2:101, 1992.

49. Van Cauter, E, Blackman, JD, Roland, D, Spire, J, Refetoff, S, and Polonsky, KS: Modulation of glucose regulation and insulin secretion by circadian rhythmicity and sleep. J Clin Invest 88:934, 1991.

50. Brewer, MJ: To sleep or not to sleep: The consequences of sleep deprivation. Critical Care Nursing 5:35, 1985.

51. Schactman, M and Greene, J: Rhythm disturbances in the patient with pulmonary disease. Critical Care Nursing 13:40, 1993.

52. Walgenbach, JC: Lullabye and not a good night. Geriatric Nursing 11:278, 1990.

53. Richards, KC and Bairnsfather, L: A description of night sleep patterns in the critical care unit. Heart Lung 17:35, 1988.

54. Littrell, K and Schumann, LL: Promoting sleep for the patient with a myocardial infarction. Critical Care Nurse 9:44, 1989.

55. McGonigal, KS: The importance of sleep and the sensory environment to critically ill patients. Int Crit Care Nurs 2:73, 1986.

CARE PLAN FOR THE SLEEP-DEPRIVED PATIENT

Nursing Diagnosis

Sleep Pattern disturbance, related to:
1. Excessive stimuli from therapeutic regimen
2. Sleep deprivation resulting from excessive pain and discomfort
3. Excessive environmental stimuli resulting from hospitalization

Nursing Interventions

- Assess patient's usual sleep patterns. Identify usual sleep period (e.g., hours of sleep, total sleep time) and attempt to ascertain napping patterns, preferred sleep position, individual's preferred sleep schedule.
- Identify usual sleep preparation routines, sleep promotion, (e.g., reading, listening to music, warm baths, guided imagery, beverages such as warm milk, massage.
- Assess and record temperature q4h, assess for alterations in synchronization; peak temperature to occur at approximately 6 PM ± 2 h in a diurnally active individual.

- Organize tests, procedures, and patient activities to occur within patient's usual waking period.
- Maintain quiet environment or provide earplugs to diminish noise for acutely ill individuals: close door, decrease alarms, telephone rings, and conversation during the usual sleep period.
- Provide 6–8 h *darkness* during usual sleep period. If patient is acutely ill, provide sleep mask.

- For diurnally active individuals, limit napping to early morning to increase REM sleep.

- Bathe patient 1–3 h before desired sleep or nap time.

Desired Patient Outcomes

1. Patient will not experience complications of sleep pattern disturbance, as evidenced by:
   - Patient communicates satisfaction with quantity and quality of sleep.
   - Daily trends in circadian variation in temperature rhythm demonstrates peak from 6 PM ± 2 h.

Rationale

- Patients are generally able to phase advance or delay ± 2 h without affecting their usual sleep pattern. Extensive napping may lead to sleep fragmentation and decreased REM sleep.
- Deviation from familiar environments may affect sleep onset. Attempt to provide usual sleep hygeine factors to relax patient and promote optimal sleep.

- Circadian variation in temperature correlates with sleep-wake cycle. Peak temperature occurs around mid–activity span in diurnally active individuals. Temperature varies from 1°F–2°F in healthy individuals.
- To reduce interruption of normal sleep patterns.

- Excessive environmental noise can lead to arousal from sleep, sensory overload, and resultant sleep deprivation.

- Bright light is a stimulus that may arouse the patient from sleep. Pulses of bright light may phase advance or delay circadian rhythms leading to desynchronization.
- Early morning naps may promote increased REM sleep. However, afternoon or evening naps may delay usual sleep onset.
- Can potentiate sleep onset through precipitous change in temperature. Promotes relaxation.

CARE PLAN FOR THE SENSORY-DEPRIVED PATIENT

Nursing Diagnosis

Sensory/Perceptual alterations related to:
1. Absent or inappropriate environmental cues resulting in sensory deprivation

Desired Patient Outcomes

1. Patient will not experience sensory/perceptual alterations, as evidenced by:
   - Demonstrates appropriate interactions with people and environment.
   - Oriented to time, place, person.
   - Temperature peaks 6 PM ± 2 h, through 6 AM ± 2 h in diurnally active individuals.

Nursing Interventions

- Assess orientation to person, place, time, q4h.
- Display meaningful sensory stimulation in room at all times, e.g., large clocks, calendars, photographs, or other objects from home.
- Leave window blinds open or lights on during usual daylight hours.
- Orient patient to environment, time of day, current events while providing care.
- Encourage significant others to communicate with individual at least daily.
- Explain hospital routines, medical therapies, and equipment to reduce information overload.
- Assess daily sleep-rest patterns for quantity as well as quality of sleep.
- Assess daily trends in temperature rhythm.
- Avoid bursts of bright light during usual sleep period.
- Provide sleep masks during usual sleep period.

Rationale

- To assess reality orientation.
- Regular orientation to environmental stimuli prevents sensory deprivation.
- To maintain environmental synchronization to diurnal sleep-wake cycle and reduce tendency for desynchronization.
- Regular social interaction fosters reality orientation and reduces monotony of hospitalization.
- Fosters sense of security, provides meaningful stimulus, supports reality orientation.
- Decreases environmental stressors, patient fear of unknown, and technological environment.
- For comparison with usual sleep-wake patterns to determine impact of ICU environment on sleep quantity and quality. Prevention of circadian desynchronization is easier than patient resynchronization in the ICU.
- To prevent desynchronization. If peak temperature varies > 2 h or temperature curve disappears, then aggressively promote sleep hygiene factors (Table 8–3).
- Pulses of bright light can desynchronize circadian rhythms.
- To reduce potential for arousal from sleep, and maintain circadian synchronization.

CHAPTER 9

Nutritional Support of the Critically Ill Patient

Roberta H. Anding

CHAPTER OUTLINE

LEARNING OBJECTIVES

After completing this chapter, you should be able to:

1. Explain the mechanisms for energy use in physiologic stress.
2. Identify at least two results of malnutrition in the critically ill.
3. Outline key elements of a nutritional assessment.
4. Discuss the two major therapeutic modalities used in the treatment of patients with an altered nutritional status.

During the initial stages of a critical illness, nutrition is generally not afforded top priority. While this may be appropriate amid life-saving efforts, too often nutrition is the afterthought that could have saved the patient's life. Florence Nightingale recognized the importance of nutrition in 1859. In her book *Notes on Nursing*,[1] she commented that "thousands of patients are annually starved in the midst of plenty." In the 1980s, there still existed a 50% incidence of malnutrition among hospitalized patients.[2,3]

While technology in nursing has increased by leaps and bounds, some basic problems are unresolved. The critical care nurse needs a sound scientific basis from which to assess, deliver, and evaluate nutritional support. This chapter will review the mechanisms of energy use during starvation and stress, nutritional assessment, and therapeutic modalities in the treatment of the patient with an altered nutritional status.

METABOLIC RESPONSE TO STARVATION

Humans, in the absence of injury or stress, are well adapted to starvation. During the early phase of star-

vation, energy needs are met primarily through glycogen. Glycogen, a carbohydrate stored in the liver and muscle, serves as a short-term source of glucose. The amount of glycogen stored is variable, the average being 150 to 200 g. As liver glycogen falls, gluconeogenesis, the production of glucose from noncarbohydrate sources, becomes the sole provider of hepatic glucose production. The central nervous system is the major consumer of the glucose produced and uses approximately 20% of total basal calories. During this time blood glucose levels fall to within a normal fasting, or "fixed hypoglycemic," level. The primary signal for this series of events is a fall in serum insulin level. The low serum insulin level, coupled with a rise in glucagon, initiates gluconeogenesis and maintains blood sugar at this normal fasting level. As starvation progresses, approximately 75 g of skeletal protein is catabolized daily to provide fuel for the brain. Nitrogen excretion increases during the period of rapid gluconeogenesis. Skeletal muscle, or somatic protein, is consumed preferentially and organ protein is spared. Serum proteins, such as albumin, are relatively well preserved. Fat is also being catabolized for energy into free fatty acids and glycerol, with the ultimate con-

TABLE 9–1
Metabolic Changes During Starvation and Stress

Physiologic Characteristics	Starvation	Stress
Metabolic rate	↓	↑ ↑
Gluconeogenesis	↑	↑ ↑ ↑
Insulin level	↓	↑ ↑ *
Blood glucose	↓	↑ ↑
Glucagon level	↑	↑ ↑
Nitrogen excretion	↑	↑ ↑
Serum protein (albumin)	↔	↓ ↓
Body weight	↓ ↓	↓ ↓ †

*Cellular resistance prevents effective insulin utilization.
†Lean body mass is depleted but marked by fluid shifts.

densation of free fatty acids into ketones occurring by approximately the third day of starvation. The brain, heart, and skeletal muscle are able to use ketones as an alternate fuel and decrease the demand for glucose. This process is known as ketoadaptation. During this time, nitrogen excretion decreases and skeletal muscle is conserved. The process of ketoadaptation contributes to long-term survival. During starvation, there is also a decrease in basal metabolic rate, which lowers calorie demand and also contributes to starvation adaptation. Table 9–1 provides a comparison of the physiologic changes during starvation and stress.

METABOLIC RESPONSE TO STRESS

During physiologic stress there is a rapid mobilization of body fuels. Glycogen stores are readily exhausted and provide little caloric support. Protein, through the process of gluconeogenesis, becomes the obligatory source of glucose. Neuroendocrine controls are altered and mediate the dramatic changes in nutritional status. Through the actions of catecholamines, glucagon, and cortisol, an abundance of glucose is produced. Not only does this glucose serve as a preferential energy source for the central nervous system, but a portion of the glucose produced is used anaerobically by fibroblasts, macrophages, and leukocytes in wound healing. Hyperglycemia results and insulin release is stimulated although it is blunted by the action of epinephrine. Cortisol contributes to the cellular insulin resistance and allows the hyperglycemia to persist. This is often referred to as "stress diabetes." The catabolic process of gluconeogenesis is accentuated and loss of protein continues at a greater rate than during unstressed starvation. In this hypermetabolic state, lipolysis mobilizes free fatty acids, which can be oxidized directly as an energy source; however, in contrast to starvation, there is no significant condensation of free fatty acids into ketones to serve as an alternate fuel. During stress, significant ketosis does not develop, probably due to adequate levels of circulating insulin. The brain cannot use free fatty acids generated through lipolysis as an energy source, as they do not cross the blood-brain barrier.

Consequently, during stress, gluconeogenesis continues at a rapid rate at the expense of somatic and visceral (organ) proteins, without significant ketoadaptation. Endogenous protein, therefore, continues to be a major source of calories. This failure to ketoadapt has the greatest clinical implications for the client who is obese.

Obese individuals are often viewed as having ample caloric reserves that are readily accessible; however, the physiologic demand for glucose is met through the process of gluconeogenesis at the expense of body proteins, not fat. An obese person may not be perceived to be at nutritional risk if assessment is based on physical size rather than the degree of physiologic stress. A common misconception is that an obese client is well nourished, whereas obese clients often have multiple nutrient deficiencies and may be predisposed to immunosuppression.[4] In clinical nutrition, the provision of intravenous dextrose, such as D_5W, in the absence of protein, further compromises the process of ketoadaptation by stimulating insulin release.

Specific alterations in protein metabolism occur during stress. Skeletal muscle is catabolized through the action of catecholamines to provide branched chain amino acids, which serve as the substrate for gluconeogenesis, wound healing, and the synthesis of "acute phase" proteins. Acute phase proteins are those synthesized in response to a physiologic insult. Protein synthesis shifts from the production of the proteins of wellness or homeostasis—albumin, transferrin, prealbumin, and retinol binding protein—to the production of these acute phase reactants such as interleukin-1, tumor necrosis factor (cachectin), haptoglobin, complement C3, ceruloplasmin, and clotting factors.[5] The redirection in protein synthesis and protein shift to the interstitial space, coupled with often inadequate nutritional support contributes to the hypoalbuminemia seen in the critically ill, and albumin levels can decline by 1 to 1.5 g/dL within 3 to 5 days as a result of catabolic illness.[6] Alterations in the serum level of visceral proteins of homeostasis can be used as markers to assess the degree of nutritional depletion. Table 9–2 provides a guide to the severity

TABLE 9–2
Guide to Protein Depletion

Indicator	DEGREE OF DEPLETION			
	Normal	Mild	Moderate	Severe
Albumin (g/100 mL)	3.5–5.0	2.8–3.4	2.1–2.7	<2.1
Transferrin (mg/100 mL)	201–260	150–200	100–149	<100
Prealbumin (mg/100 mL)	20–30	10–15	5–9	<5
Retinol binding protein* (mg/100 mL)	4–5	—	—	—

NOTE: To convert albumin (g/100 mL) to international standard units (nmol/L), multiply by 37.06. To convert transferrin (mg/100 mL) to standard international units (g/L), multiply by 0.01.

*Levels of <3 mg/100 mL suggest compromised protein status. The actual degree of depletion (mild, moderate, and severe) has not been defined.

of protein depletion. Further compromising the patient's nutritional status is the characteristic increase in basal metabolic rate. The percent increase in basal energy expenditure depends on the severity of the stress and ranges from a 20% increase for elective surgery to 100% for a severe burn.

RESULTS OF MALNUTRITION IN THE CRITICALLY ILL

Hospital-based malnutrition is referred to as protein calorie malnutrition (PCM) or protein energy malnutrition (PEM). The three subtypes of PCM are: simple starvation or marasmus, stressed starvation also known as hypoalbuminemic malnutrition or kwashiorkor, and a mixed or combination form. Of these subtypes, hypoalbuminemic malnutrition is the most common. It is associated with increased length of stay,[7] a 12-fold increase in the risk of dying,[8,9] and an increase in the incidence of decubitus ulcers.[10] Table 9–3 provides a summary of the distinguishing characteristics of the subtypes of PCM. Additionally, the results of malnutrition may involve any one of the following end-organ effects (Fig. 9–1):

- Delayed wound healing
- Predisposition to intraoperative hemorrhage
- Infection/sepsis
- Cardiac failure unresponsive to inotropic agents
- Difficulty in refeeding, known as refeeding syndrome
- Pneumonia

It is the critical care nurse's responsibility, in conjunction with the dietitian, to assess patients who may be at risk for developing these problems and to plan appropriate interventions.

TABLE 9–3
Subtypes of Protein Calorie Malnutrition

	Distinguishing Characteristics	Serum Proteins
Marasmus	Simple starvation Loss of protein and/or fat	Preserved at expense of somatic proteins
Hypoalbuminemic malnutrition	Secondary to physiologic stress, coupled with poor intake Most common subtype in hospitalized patient Immunosuppression	Decrease in visceral proteins
Mixed	Most serious— marasmic individual with superimposed stress; poor survival Immunosuppression	Significant decrease in visceral and somatic proteins

NUTRITIONAL ASSESSMENT

The process of nutritional assessment consists of a dietary history and evaluation, anthropometric measurements, physical examination, and diagnostic lab studies. One positive finding, such as a decrease in weight, is not conclusive for malnutrition but can provide clues as to the likelihood of developing malnutrition. The components of the nutritional assessment process and the role of the critical care nurse are detailed in the following sections.

Dietary History

It is often not feasible to obtain a dietary history from the critically ill patient. Other sources, such as family and friends, can provide the necessary information. The history often provides clues as to the overall nutritional status and the possibility of pre-existing malnutrition. The registered dietitian (RD) is trained to obtain dietary histories and assess the adequacy of the patient's diet in meeting the recommended dietary allowances (RDAs). Although there is an increased need for calories, protein, vitamins, and minerals, there are no RDAs for the critically ill.

Calorie counts are often employed to evaluate and monitor a patient's intake. Each day, the nurse accurately records all foods and fluids consumed by the patient and specifies type and amount. The registered dietitian or nurse calculates the protein and calories consumed daily and makes recommendations for nutritional support. It is critical to perform calorie counts during weaning from parenteral nutrition or tube feedings to an oral diet. Dietary assessment in the ICU also includes assessment of the adequacy of the nutritional support regimen. The delivery of adequate levels of vitamins and minerals in enteral nutrition support is dependent on the volume of product delivered. The volume of enteral product required to meet the RDA is summarized in Table 9–4.

Anthropometric Measurements

Anthropometry is the measurement of a part or whole of the body. Because weight and body composition depend on nutrition, these measurements are used as one facet of a nutritional assessment. The most commonly used indices are height, weight, tricep skinfold thickness, midarm circumference, and the calculated midarm muscle circumference. Standards exist to compare an individual with a well population but no standards exist for the heterogeneous critically ill population.

Height, serial weights, and change in weight are the most important anthropometric measurements. Table 9–5 provides a guide to the evaluation in change in weight. Preinjury weight is the best baseline of skeletal muscle reserves and serial weights are a crude measure

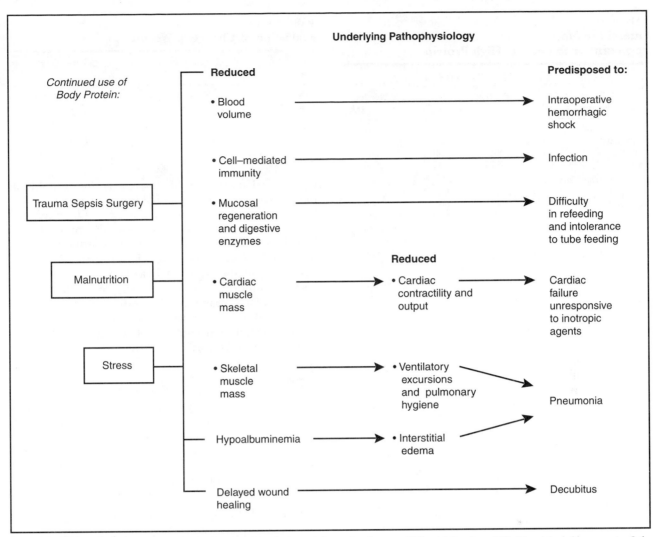

FIGURE 9–1. Results of body protein depletion. (Adapted from Buchanan, RT and Levine, NS: Nutritional support of the surgery patient. Ann Plast Surg 10(2): 159–166, 1983.)

of change in nutritional status. Fluid shifts, which accompany physiologic stress, often mask alterations in body composition thus making interpretation of change in weight difficult. One liter of fluid is equal to approximately 2 lb, therefore fluid shifts can dramatically alter weight. Estimates of ideal or desirable body weight do exist and the Hamwi formula, listed in Table 9–6, is easily utilized. Estimates of ideal body weight, as well as actual body weight whenever possible, are important variables needed to determine the calorie and protein requirements.

Other anthropometric measures, such as skinfold thickness, arm circumference, and midarm muscle circumference are also difficult to interpret. Altered fluid status, differences in skin compressibility, and the lack of appropriate standards for the critically ill are the most common problems. As with weight, serial measurements of the above measures provided the best assessment tool for a particular client.

Physical Assessment

Physical examination is an important component of a comprehensive nutritional assessment. Muscle strength and tone can be a measure of somatic protein reserves and possible protein catabolism. Hand grip strength, an index of protein status, can be measured with a dynamometer and may be useful in predicting postoperative complications.[12] Pre-existing nutrient deficiencies manifested by glossitis and cheilosis or angular stomatis give an index of B vitamin nurtiture. Table 9–7 gives signs and symptoms of vitamin and mineral deficiencies.

Diagnostic Tests

Several diagnostic tests are available to the critical care nurse for the nutritional assessment of critically

TABLE 9–4
Enteral Products
Polymeric, High Calorie, High Protein

Product Name	PRODUCT PARAMETERS			
	cal/mL	Protein g/L	mOsm/kg	Vol Needed to Meet RDA
Ensure Plus HN	1.5	62.6	650	947
Pulmocare	1.5	62.6	490	946
Trauma Cal	1.5	82.4	490	1964
Two Cal HN	2.0	83.7	690	946
Polymeric, High Calorie				
Nutren 1.5	1.5	60	530	1400
Nutren 2.0	2.0	80	800	1000
Resource Plus	1.5	55	600	1600
Sustacal HC	1.5	61	650	1183
Ensure Plus	1.5	54.2	690	1425
Isocal HCN	2.0	74.8	690	986
Magnacal	2.0	70	590	1000
Polymeric, High Nitrogen				
Ensure HN	1.06	44	470	1329
Entrition HN	1.00	44	300	1300
Isocal HN	1.06	44	300	1183
Isosource HN	1.2	53	330	1500
Osmolite HN	1.06	44.4	300	1330
Polymeric with Fiber				
Enrich	1.1	39.7	480	1392
Jevity	1.06	44.4	310	1324
Pro Fiber	1	40	300	1500
Sustacal with Fiber	1.06	46	450	1391
Fibersource	1.2	43	390	1500
Defined/Elemental Diets				
Criticare HN	1.06	38	650	1893
Peptumen	1.0	40	260	2000
Pepti-2000	1.0	40	490	1600
Precision Isotonic	1.0	29	300	1560
Precision HN	1.05	44	525	2850
Reabilan	1.0	31.5	350	2250
Reabilan HN	1.33	58	490	2494
Tolerex	1.0	20.6	550	1800
Traum-AID HBC	1.0	56	760	3000
Travasorb HN	1.0	45	560	2000
Vital HN	1.0	42	500	1500
Vivonex T.E.N.	1.0	38	630	2000
Periative	1.3	67	385	1155
Alitraq	1.0	52.5	575	1500

ill patients. It is important that the nurse be familiar with each of these tests in order to interpret results accurately. The following tests are included in this discussion: anergy testing, total lymphocyte count, serum protein measurements, and urine assays.

Anergy Testing

Immunocompetence is often assessed in clients by using delayed cutaneous hypersensitivity (DCH) to known antigens. Common antigens tested by intradermal injections include mumps, streptokinase-streptodornase, dinitrochlorobenzene, and purified protein derivative. Antigens are injected on the forearm and induration is measured at 24 and 48 hours. The patient is considered anergic, or immunosuppressed, if the level of induration is 5 mm or less.[13] However,

TABLE 9–5
Evaluation of Change in Weight

Time	Significant Weight Loss (%)	Severe Weight Loss (%)
1 week	1–2	>2
1 month	5	>5
3 months	7.5	>7.5
6 months	10	>10

the clinical usefulness of this test is questionable as many factors other than malnutrition can suppress DCH. These include, but are not limited to, advanced age, sepsis, uremia, cirrhosis, hepatitis, inflammatory bowel disease, trauma, general anesthesia, solid tumors, human immunodeficiency virus (HIV) disease, and medications such as steroids, cimetidine, and immunosuppressants.[14] Despite difficulties in obtaining DCH reactions, the finding of anergy is associated with an increase in postsurgical complications.[15] Nutritional support of anergic patients has been shown to restore reactivity.[16]

Total Lymphocyte Count

Total lymphocyte count is a nonspecific measure of protein status. A low count of less than 1500 mm³ may be reflective of protein calorie nutrition. Non-nutritional factors affecting TLC include large wounds and the stress response.[17] A false negative may be seen with this test as well as DCH.

Serum Proteins

The serum proteins of wellness or homeostasis can be used as indicators of nutritional status. Albumin and transferrin are the most commonly used indicators in the clinical setting. The long half-life of albumin (20 days) make it a poor indicator of early protein malnutrition. In the presence of physiologic stress, albumin is also a poor indicator of the response to nutritional support.[18] Many non-nutritional factors can influence albumin levels, such as hydration status, liver disease, infection, sepsis, cancer, and nephrotic syndrome.[19] Transferrin, with a half-life of 8 to 10 days, is a more sensitive marker of protein depletion. Transferrin levels, however, are inversely related to iron stores; they are high with iron deficiency anemia and low when excessive iron is being stored. Prealbumin and retinol binding proteins are short-turnover proteins with half-lives of 1 to 2 days and 10 to 12 hours,

TABLE 9–6
Calculation of Ideal Body Weight

Women	Allow 100 lb for the first 5 ft, add 5 lb for each inch thereafter
Men	Allow 106 lb for the first 5 ft, add 6 lb for each inch thereafter

TABLE 9–7
Vitamins and Trace Elements: Physiologic Function and Clinical Signs of Deficiency*

Trace Element	Physiologic Function	Clinical Signs of Deficiency
A (Retinol) RDA = 1000 μg RE	Retinal function Epithelial tissue Fertility and reproduction Growth Immune function Glycoprotein synthesis	Night blindness Conjunctival xerosis Bitot's spots Corneal xerosis Keratomalacia Xerophthalmic fundus Hyperkeratosis Diarrhea
D RDA = 5 μg	Stimulates intestinal absorption of Ca and P Plays a role in parathyroid hormone bone reabsorption Supports bone growth and mineralization	Bone pain and tenderness Proximal muscle weakness Skeletal deformity Increased serum alkaline phosphatase

E (Tocopherol)
RDA = 10 mg
  α tocopheral
  equivalent (T.E.)
	Antioxidant
	Neutralizes free radicals
	Plays a role in selenium metabolism
	Plays a role in liver microsomal enzyme activity
	Influences neuromuscular function
	Influences biosynthesis of heme products
		Retinal degeneration
		Neuronal axonopathy
		Myopathy
		Decreased serum creatinine

K RDA = 80 μg	Blood clotting Possible role in either bone calcification or demineralization	Bleeding, hemorrhage Prolonged clotting time

B₁ (Thiamine)
RDA = 1.0–1.5 mg
	Cardiovascular, neurologic, and muscular
	  function as precursor of thiamine
	  pyrophosphate; coenzyme in energy
	  metabolism, particularly carbohydrate
	  metabolism
	Plays a role in enzymatic reactions
		Peripheral neuropathy
		Beriberi heart disease
		Wernicke's encephalopathy
		Alcoholic polyneuritis
		Korsakoff's syndrome
		Anorexia
		Fatigue

B₂ (Riboflavin) RDA = 1.5–1.7 mg	Integral part of several oxidative enzyme systems necessary for electron transport	Angular stomatitis Glossitis Seborrheic dermatitis Corneal neovascularization

B₃ (Niacin)
RDA = 19 mg
	Nicotinamide plays a part in coenzymes
	  NAD(H) and NADP(H), which are essential
	  for glycolysis, fat synthesis, energy production
		Pellagra (dermatitis, dementia, diarrhea)

B₅ (Pantothenic acid)
No RDA available
	Vital to all energy-requiring processes within
	  the cell as it is an integral part of coenzyme A
	Plays a role in immunity
		Headache, fatigue
		Impaired motor coordination, paresthesia, muscle
		  cramps
		Intermittent vomiting and cramps
		Decreased antibody formation

B₆ (Pyridoxine) RDA = 2.0 mg	Metabolism of CNS Amino acid metabolism Heme synthesis Involved in glycogen phosphorylase activity	CNS problems Peripheral neuritis Seborrheic dermatitis Glossitis Angular stomatitis Cheilosis
Folic acid (Folacin) RDA = 200 μg	Serves as a coenzyme involved in DNA synthesis	Macrocytic anemia Megaloblastosis of bone marrow Thrombocytopenia Leukopenia Diarrhea Glossitis Weight loss Atrophy of papillae of tongue

B₁₂ (Cyanocobalamin)
RDA = 2 μg
	Essential to the proper functioning of all body
	  cells
	Involved in DNA synthesis
	Serves as a coenzyme in protein, fat, and
	  carbohydrate metabolism
		Pernicious anemia
		Neurologic problems
		GI problems
		Dementia

C (Ascorbic acid)
RDA = 60 mg
	Essential to a variety of biologic oxidation
	  processes
	Role in collagen synthesis
	Essential for normal protein and amino acid
	  metabolism
	Plays a role in carbohydrate metabolism
		Scurvy
		Impaired wound healing
		Capillary fragility
		Muscle pain

TABLE 9–7
Vitamins and Trace Elements: Physiologic Function and Clinical Signs of Deficiency* (*Continued*)

Trace Element	Physiologic Function	Clinical Signs of Deficiency
Iron RDA = 10 mg	Oxygen transport as part of hemoglobin Skeletal muscle function Leukocyte function and host defense Cognitive function and alertness Component of iron metalloenzymes	Pallor Fatigue Exertional dyspnea Tachycardia Headache Paresthesias Burning sensation on the tongue Altered attention span
Zinc RDA = 15 mg	Cell growth and proliferation Sexual maturation and reproduction Dark adaptation and night vision Gustatory acuity Wound healing Host immune defenses Hemostasis	Growth retardation Alopecia Dermatitis Abnormalities of taste and smell Anorexia Diarrhea Mental depression Impaired wound healing Glucose intolerance
Copper ESADDI† = 1.5–3 mg	Erythropoiesis, leukopoiesis Skeletal mineralization Elastin and collagen synthesis Myelin formation Catecholamine metabolism Oxidative phosphorylation Thermal regulation Antioxidant protection Cholesterol metabolism Lymphocyte function Cardiac function Glucose metabolism	Anemia Leukopenia Neutropenia Pallor Depigmentation of hair Glucose intolerance Mental confusion Peripheral neuropathy with ataxia
Manganese	Functions in antioxidant protection and energy metabolism Formation of connective tissue Functions as a cofactor in certain metabolic reactions Fertility and reproduction	Clinical deficiency States have not yet been identified
Selenium RDA = 55–70 µg	Antioxidant	Muscle tenderness Myalgia Cardiac myopathy
Chromium ESADDI = 50–200 µg	Potentiates action of insulin Participates in regulation of lipoprotein metabolism	Glucose intolerance Peripheral neuropathy with ataxia Metabolic encephalopathy

*Based on 1989 RDAs. Reference, man 25–50 years.
†Estimated safe and adequate daily dietary intake.

respectively. These proteins are excellent markers of recent-onset malnutrition and valuable adjuncts to assess the effectiveness of nutritional support.

Urine Assays

Nitrogen Balance. Nitrogen balance is defined as a physiologic condition that occurs when nitrogen intake equals nitrogen excretion. When a client is catabolic, more nitrogen is being excreted than consumed. As the process of anabolism or rebuilding occurs, more nitrogen is consumed than excreted. This is positive nitrogen balance. The significance of a negative nitrogen balance is twofold. A negative nitrogen balance alerts the clinician that catabolism of lean body mass is occurring. There are no stores or reserves of protein, therefore, large losses of nitrogen in the urine imply loss of structural, immunological, or enzymatic function. Secondly, a negative nitrogen balance may signal a need to evaluate the current nutritional support regimen for adequacy. The need for a complete 24-hour urine specimen in nitrogen balance studies may limit its clinical use.

Creatinine Height Index. Creatinine is a metabolic product of the energy source phosphocreatine. It is present in skeletal muscle and can be used as a measure of somatic (skeletal) reserves. The amount excreted is related to the amount of skeletal muscle. As loss of somatic protein occurs, the creatinine excretion decreases. As with other biochemical tests, caution should be used in the interpretation of the values. Severe stress, such as sepsis, can falsely elevate creatinine. As with nitrogen balance, a 24-hour urine collection is required.

TABLE 9–8
Assessment Tools to Determine Likelihood of Malnutrition

Tool	Parameters Included
Prognostic nutritional index (PNI)	Serum albumin Serum transferrin Tricep skinfold Delayed cutaneous hypersensitivity
Nutritional risk index (NRI)	Albumin Current weight Usual weight
Subjective global assessment (SGA)	Comprehensive history Physical exam

Summary

Due to the nonspecific nature of an individual lab study to determine malnutrition or the likelihood of malnutrition, several assessment tools combining different parameters have been developed.[20,21] These are summarized in Table 9–8.

CALORIE AND PROTEIN REQUIREMENTS

Various formulas exist for calculating caloric requirements. The Harris-Benedict equation is the most commonly used formula, although it may often overestimate calorie needs.[22] Additionally, the formula is cumbersome to use and is of limited practical value for critical care nurses. A commonly used estimate of calorie requirements is given in Table 9–9. This formula uses actual body weight unless the client is obese, then ideal body weight is used. Indirect calorimetry is a process of measuring calorie needs for a specific individual rather than an average value. Indirect calorimetry measures oxygen consumed via inhaled gases and the carbon dioxide produced via the oxidation of carbohydrate, protein, and fat. Indirect calorimetry ideally should be performed at rest, and not within 2 hours of stressful procedures. Circulatory indirect calorimetry can be done in clients with a Swan-Ganz catheter and measures oxygen utilization from arterial and mixed venous blood.[23] This method of determining calorie requirements is more precise and reduces the risk as well as the cost of under- or overfeeding. From indirect calorimetry, some clinicians recommend a resting calorie level of

TABLE 9–9
Estimates of Calorie Requirements

Physiologic State	kcal/kg per day
Simple starvation	28
Elective surgery	32
Polytrauma	40
Sepsis	50

TABLE 9–10
Estimates of Protein Requirements

Physiologic State	g/kg of Ideal Body Weight
Healthy adult	0.8
Hemodialysis	1.0–1.2
Trauma	1.0–1.5
Sepsis	1.5–2.0

30 to 35 kcal/kg as the optimal level for the critically ill.[22] Overfeeding is associated with fluid overload, respiratory compromise, hepatic steatosis, and increased cost.[24,25] Calorie requirements are not static in the critically ill and as with other measures should be serially assessed.

Protein requirements can also be estimated using a variety of formulas, but a general rule is to allow 1.5 to 2.0 g protein per kilogram. An estimate of protein needs is summarized in Table 9–10. Organ function, however, often dictates the amount of protein tolerated and delivered. Additionally, the protein content of enteral products varies. Nutritional parameters of various enteral products are summarized in Table 9–4. Critically ill clients require increased intake of protein but may not reach intended levels on low volumes of enteral products. Table 9–11 illustrates an application of the calculation of calorie and protein requirements.

THERAPEUTIC MODALITIES IN THE TREATMENT OF PATIENTS WITH AN ALTERED NUTRITIONAL STATUS

Enteral Nutrition

Persons who are unable to eat a regular diet have two other alternatives: enteral or parenteral support. Enteral nutrition, strictly defined, is nutrition via the gastro-intestinal (GI) tract but generally is interpreted as nutrition via tube feeding into the GI tract. Enteral nutrition has distinct advantages over parenteral support. Enteral nutrition is less expensive[26,27] and more physiologic in that the liver gets the "first pass" at nutrients. If introduced in the early postoperative period, enteral support decreases length of stay,[28] is

TABLE 9–11
Estimation of Protein and Calorie Requirements

C.W. is a 40-year-old man, 5 ft 10 in tall and weighing 210 lb. He is admitted to the trauma unit after sustaining soft tissue injury and multiple fractures in a motor vehicle accident. What are his calorie and protein requirements?

C.W.'s ideal body weight (IBW) is 166 lb or 75 kg. Calorie requirements for polytrauma are approximately 40 kcal/kg. Therefore, estimated calorie requirements are 3000 kcal/d and his protein requirement is 1.5 g protein/kg IBW = 113 g/d. These quick estimates provide a general goal for C.W.'s recovery.

an effective intervention in the prevention of stress ulcers, and decreases the incidence of sepsis.[29] The decrease in the incidence of systemic infection is due in part to enteral nutrition's ability to prevent bacterial translocation. Bacterial translocation is the phenomenon of the migration of bacteria or their endotoxins through the epithelial mucosa to the mesenteric lymph nodes. Normally, the GI tract provides a pH-mediated barrier through the action of hydrochloric acid in the stomach. Additionally, the gut provides a mechanical and immunologic barrier against bacterial and toxin migration. Indeed, two thirds of the immunologic-secreting cells are located in the gut; collectively these are often identified as gut-associated lymphoid tissue (GALT).[30] Thus, the gut can be considered the largest "immune organ" in the body.[31] Failure to provide intraluminal nutrients causes atrophy of mucosal cells and GALT. The bacteria most frequently associated with translocation are *Escherichia coli, Klebsiella pneumoniae, Pseudomonas aeruginosa, Staphylococcus epidermis,* and *Candida enterococcus albicans.*[32] These aerobic bacteria are those often implicated as a cause of sepsis in ICUs. Endotoxins have also been implicated in the development of septic shock. The translocated bacteria and/or endotoxins migrating through the mucosal layer of the gut into systemic circulation, activate macrophages, neutrophils, and the complement system to produce mediators contributing to the development of multisystem organ failure (MSOF).[33] Early aggressive enteral support after traumatic injury may be advantageous, as it helps maintain gut integrity and moderates the elevation of catabolic stress hormones.

Recent research has indicated that glutamine, a nonessential amino acid in the absence of disease, may be a conditionally essential nutrient in the critically ill.[34,35] Glutamine levels dramatically decrease after a major injury due to their use as an oxidative, preferential fuel for the small intestine and the colon. Glutamine depletion, therefore, contributes to gut atrophy. Administration of glutamine can increase jejunal and ileum villus height and help preserve the mucosal barrier.

Additionally, research has indicated that short-chain fatty acids (SCFAs) may play a role in maintaining a functioning gut. Short-chain fatty acids are formed from the fermentation of carbohydrate, particularly fiber. These short-chain fatty acids, in addition to providing energy, have a trophic effect on the intestinal tract. Clinically, SCFAs may be useful in the treatment of intestinal dysfunction such as short bowel syndrome and colitis.[36,37]

Two other enteral components are gaining recognition for their role as immunomodulators. Arginine, another semiessential amino acid, has been shown to promote nutrition repletion and enhance the immune system by increasing the number of helper T cells.[38,39] Omega-3 fatty acids, found in cold-water fish oils and soy oils, enhance the immune response and reduce the prostaglandin-mediated inflammatory response.[40,41]

Barriers to Effective Enteral Delivery

Although enteral nutrition is considered the preferred source of nutritional support, certain prerequisites in the critically ill must be met prior to the initiation of this type of support. Adequate oxygen delivery to the tissues, demonstrated by cardiopulmonary stability is necessary in order to initiate enteral support. Research suggests that the GI tract is the first organ system to be affected by hypoxia. Low cardiac output is the major nonocclusive cause of intestinal ischemia, with malabsorption of protein and carbohydrate usually apparent within 1 hour of the ischemia. Intestinal hypoperfusion can be assessed by monitoring gastric intramucosal pH via gastric tonometry.[42] Gastrointestinal tonometry is a noninvasive and indirect measure of gastric pH. Research suggests that the intramucosal pH decreases with hypoperfusion, and this early, noninvasive marker may be used to predict tolerance to enteral feeding.[43]

Ileus is often cited as a reason to delay or withhold enteral nutrition. Traditionally, the presence of bowel sounds signaled the initiation of enteral support. Ileus commonly occurs in critically ill clients as a result of the underlying pathology or treatment regimens; however, the small intestine, the major absorptive site, usually regains motility within the first 24 hours after insult. The stomach and large intestine frequently take more than 3 days to recover. Therefore, feeding directly into the small bowel, after assessment for mechanical obstruction, represents a viable option.

Diarrhea remains the major physiologic barrier inhibiting the delivery of enteral support. The causes of diarrhea are multifactorial. Depending on the underlying cause, a trial of enteral nutrition may be warranted, or the decision to institute parenteral nutrition may be indicated. Prolonged bowel rest and its subsequent gut atrophy contribute to the diarrhea seen in the critically ill. Causes of diarrhea are summarized in Table 9–12.

The lack of fiber in many feeding products can contribute to diarrhea. Fiber normalizes stooling patterns and provides a source of short-chain fatty acids aiding

TABLE 9–12
Possible Causes of Diarrhea

Prolonged bowel rest
Hypertonic tube feeding
Lack of fiber
Contaminated formula/retrograde
Hypoalbuminemia
Medications
Bacterial overgrowth
Gut failure

in the prevention of diarrhea as well as constipation. Deficiencies in vitamins, such as niacin and vitamin A, can also contribute to the development of diarrhea.

Hypertonic tube feeding is often implicated as a cause of diarrhea and both the osmolality of the enteral product and the location of the tube can contribute. Hypertonic solutions (osmolality > 500 mOsm/kg) cause an osmotic shift resulting in diarrhea. Elemental products, which are predigested, with their higher osmolality are most likely to cause diarrhea. Table 9–4 gives osmolalities of common tube feedings. Tube placement, however, is a major determinant of whether diarrhea develops. When the tube is placed gastrically, the pyloric sphincter controls the rate at which the enteral product is delivered and prevents a dumping syndrome reaction. (Dumping syndrome is the rapid passage of stomach contents into the small intestine. The hyperosmolar chyme draws fluid into the gut causing diarrhea.) On the other hand, feedings directly into the small intestine, while decreasing aspiration risk, increase the risk of diarrhea. In order to minimize the likelihood of diarrhea, feeding directly into the small intestine necessitates the use of continuous feeding using a pump.

Although hypertonic tube feeding is often considered to be a cause of diarrhea, the diarrhea may, in fact, be caused by the exceptionally high osmolalities of many of the medications frequently used. Table 9–13 gives the osmolalities of selected drugs. Many elixirs are formed from a sorbitol base, and sorbitol itself can cause osmotic diarrhea. In addition, broad-spectrum antibiotics attack susceptible species of bacteria and lead to the overgrowth of other pathogenic bacteria species such as *Clostridium difficile*. *Clostridium difficile* bacterium or its endotoxin can contribute to diarrhea, resulting in enterocolitis and toxic megacolon, and can also contribute to intestinal barrier failure. Intestinal barrier breakdown allows other bacteria to translocate and gain access to the systemic circulation.[44]

Hypoalbuminemia can contribute to the development of diarrhea in the critically ill. Colloid osmotic pressure decreases with hypoalbuminemia and results in mucosal edema and impaired absorption. Albumin levels of less than 2.5 g/dL have been reported to increase the likelihood of diarrhea.[45]

H$_2$ (histamine) antagonists and antacids are still prescribed to reduce stress ulceration and bleeding. The buffering of hydrochloric acid reduces the bacteriostatic capabilities of the stomach. Bacterial growth in the stomach occurs when the pH is >3.5 to 4. The growth of the remaining bacteria contributes to the phenomenon of retrograde contamination of the enteral product. The bacteria in the stomach migrate up the feeding tube and can contaminate the enteral product where further multiplication of the bacteria occurs.[46] Contaminated product can contribute to the development or continuation of diarrhea. The use of sucralfate to control stress ulceration may be preferred as it appears to have no effect on intraluminal pH.[47]

The effective delivery of enteral nutrition also requires providing of adequate nutrients, including calories. Many of the products on the market provide approximately 1 kcal/mL. A 70-kg man requiring 40 kcal/kg may need 2.8 L of an enteral product to meet energy needs. Higher calorie (1.5 to 2.0 kcal/mL) formulas do exist and are represented in Table 9–4. Often the volume required to fulfill calorie needs cannot be used with the fluid-restricted patient. Other complications of enteral nutrition exist and are summarized in Table 9–14. The assessment of enteral support includes assessment of prerequisites, barriers, and nutritional adequacy.

Parenteral Nutrition

Venous Access

Parenteral nutrition is administered by a *peripheral* or *central* venous access. The choice for the route of administration depends on such factors as: (1) fluid osmolality, (2) volume to be infused, and (3) available sites. The central route is preferred for the infusion of hypertonic solutions and solutions in large volumes. Superficial peripheral veins are used for short-term therapy of isotonic solutions.

Short, semirigid catheters are used for peripheral veins. The Centers for Disease Control recommend that these catheters have a lifespan of 48 to 72 hours.[48] Central catheters can be used for either short-term or long-term therapy. Access to the central venous system is primarily obtained by the internal jugular and subclavian veins. Fewer complications are associated with the use of these two extremity cannula insertion sites.[48] Materials currently available for catheterization include polyvinylchloride, Silastic, and polyurethane, as well as heparin-coated and antibiotic-impregnated substances. These catheters have a lifespan of 3 to 14 days. Some are available as double- and triple-lumen catheters. The use of the antibiotic or antiseptic catheters reduces bacterial colonization and subsequent sepsis.[49] The benefit of the double- and triple-lumen catheters is that they can be used for the infusion of antibiotics or other intravenous additives.

Long-term therapy (months to years) presents special problems related to catheter infection and displacement. In this case catheters are made of silicone

TABLE 9–13
Osmolalities of Selected Drugs

Drug	Osmolality (mOsm/kg)
Acetaminophen elixir, 65 mg/mL	5400
Cimetidine	5500
Potassium chloride 10%	3500
Digoxin, 50 μg/mL	1350
Furosemide solution, 10 mg/mL	2050

TABLE 9–14
Mechanical Complications Associated with Enteral Feeding Tubes

Mechanical Complications	Cause	Prevention	Treatment
Incorrect tube placement	• Incorrect tube insertion • Inadvertent dislodgement	• Verify tube placement every 4 h. • Anchor tube securely.	• Reposition tube.
Occlusion of feeding tube	• Feeding particles	• Flush feeding tube with 50–150 mL H_2O or 20–50 mL cranberry juice after each feeding. • Thoroughly crush all medications placed down tube and flush tube prior to and after each medication instillation.	• Place a small amount of crushed pancreatic enzyme down the tube, clamp for several hours, then aspirate the contents.
Aspiration of feeding	• Incorrect tube position	• Maintain head elevation at 30 degrees or higher during and 1 h after feeding.	• Early detection of aspiration can be aided by testing pulmonary secretions for the presence of glucose via glucose dipstick.
	• High gastric residuals	• Verify tube placement every 4 h.	• Thorough endotracheal and orotracheal suctioning in the case of witnessed aspiration.
	• Incompetent esophageal sphincter	• Use small-bore instead of a large-bore feeding tube.	• Supportive therapy such as intravenous fluids, close monitoring of vital signs, and positive pressure ventilation as indicated.
	• Decreased ability of glottic closure (endotracheal tube or tracheotomy tube)	• Check gastric residuals every 4 h and treat appropriately. • Feed below the pylorus when possible.	
Tracheoesophageal fistula	• Under pressure on anterior esophageal wall caused by feeding tube along with pressure exerted on the posterior wall of the trachea by a tracheostomy or endotracheal tube	• Use a small-bore instead of a large-bore feeding tube. • Use a gastrostomy or jejunostomy site for feedings.	• Alleviate pressure being exerted on tracheal and esophageal walls where possible.
Acute sinusitis	• Occlusion of sinus tracts by feeding tube	• Use a small-bore instead of a large-bore feeding tube. • Use a gastrostomy or jejunostomy site for feedings.	• Remove of nasal feeding tube. Bed rest. • Apply hot compresses to the face. Administer analgesics.
Otitis media	• Pressure on eustachian tube by feeding tube	• Use a small-bore instead of a large-bore feeding tube. • Periodically change position of a nasal feeding tube to the other nostril. • Use a gastrostomy or jejunostomy site for feedings.	• Remove nasal feeding tube. Bed rest. • Administer antibiotics as appropriate.

rubber (Silastic). They are much longer (approximately 90 cm) than short-term catheters so that they can reach the right atrium and can also be tunneled under the skin of the chest. The major benefit of tunneling is to reduce the likelihood of bacterial migration and thereby decrease the risk of infecting the insertion site.[48] Dacron cuffs are positioned so that they may be placed in the subcutaneous tissues to anchor the catheter in place, and these cuffs may provide a barrier against infection. The most commonly used of this type are the Broviac, Hickman, and Groshong catheters.

Site Care

Although techniques and protocols for site care vary from hospital to hospital, minimizing catheter-related sepsis is apparently successful. Since most infections are cannula-related, the only absolute agreement in methods of site care is that *strict adherence* to *aseptic principles* is essential. Handwashing remains the single most effective measure for the prevention of infection. Initial preparation of the skin must be meticulous. Any disruption of the skin's integrity provides an opportunity for the entrance of bacteria or fungi. Shaving

TABLE 9–15
Commonly Used Antiseptics and Their Mode of Action

Antiseptic	Mode of Action
Isopropyl alcohol 70%	Denaturation of proteins Disinfectant activity—high level
Hydrogen peroxide 3%	Destruction of membrane lipids, DNA, and other cell components Disinfectant activity—high level
Acetone 10%–100%	Loosening of horny layer of epidermis Disinfectant activity—intermittent level
Idophor 1%–2%	Penetration of cell wall of microorganism, with disruption of protein and nucleic acid structure and synthesis Disinfectant activity—intermittent level

Source: Adapted from Forlaw, L and Torosian, MH: Central venous catheterization. In Rombeau, JL and Caldwell, MD (eds): Parenteral Nutrition. WB Saunders, Philadelphia, 1986.

the skin at the catheter insertion site should be avoided because cuts in the skin can occur.

Numerous antiseptics are available for cleansing the skin (Table 9–15). Controversy exists as to whether skin should be defatted by the use of acetone. Until this issue is resolved, many clinicians are hesitant to discontinue the use of defatting agents. Iodophor ointment, because of its antifungal and antibacterial properties, is recommended under transparent or gauze dressings to reduce infection.[50]

Intravenous site dressings serve two purposes: to minimize the risk of infection and to secure the catheter. Several different materials are currently being used, including gauze sponges and transparent semipermeable dressings. The transparent semipermeable dressings gained popularity because they allow direct visualization of the intravenous site, but in order to minimize risk of infection, they need more frequent dressing changes. Gauze is effective in absorbing moisture and protecting the catheter site. It has been recommended that gauze dressing changes be made every 48 to 72 hours on critically ill patients.[48] Although there is not universal agreement in the literature, recent research has indicated that the use of transparent dressings increases the risk of catheter-related sepsis.[51–53] Commercially prepared dressing kits usually contain acetone-alcohol preparation swab sticks, povidone-iodine solution swab sticks and ointment, sterile gauze sponges, sterile gloves, and other dressing materials as the hospital specifies.

Inline Filters and Infusion Devices

The use of filters during the administration of intravenous fluids remains confusing to many. Filters are intended to remove particulate matter and air, reduce

the incidence of phlebitis, and prevent sepsis. It has been recommended that a 0.22-μm filter be used in conjunction with total parenteral nutrition (TPN) and changed every 24 hours.[54] However, the newer 3-in-1 admixtures cannot be filtered through a 0.22-μm filter. These filters can become obstructed by blood and blood products, emulsions, and suspensions. For this reason, all lipid emulsions need to be infused *below* the filter. Additionally, mechanical infusion devices are used to control the infusion rate of the TPN solution thereby avoiding metabolic consequences of delivering a large uncontrolled volume of solution.

Parenteral Solutions

Parenteral nutrition consists of the administration of carbohydrate, protein, lipids, electrolytes, vitamins, and trace elements. These nutritional components are available as combined or single products.

Carbohydrate is supplied in the form of dextrose. Dextrose is available in concentrations ranging from 5% to 70%; however, admixed solutions (those mixed with other substances such as protein or lipids) rarely exceed 50% as a final concentration (Table 9–16). Dextrose solutions greater than 10% require a central vein for administration due to high osmolality and acidic pH. The energy content of dextrose is 3.4 kcal/g.

Protein is supplied in the form of amino acids, which can be used directly for protein synthesis. Newer formulas utilize dipeptides, as well as stabilized glutamine. These formulas contain a combination of both essential and nonessential amino acids. Some solutions even contain premixed electrolytes. Commercially prepared formulas are available in concentrations ranging from 3.5% to 10%, with a final concentration of 3.5% to 5% following admixture. Solutions in the 3.5% range are considered isotonic; higher concentrations are hypertonic. The energy content of amino acid solutions is 4 kcal/g.

Lipid emulsions serve as a source of energy and essential fatty acids. Solutions are prepared from soybean oil or a combination of soybean and safflower oil. Safflower oil contains a greater percentage of the essential fatty acid, linoleic acid (omega-6 family), and

TABLE 9–16
Characteristics of Various Dextrose Solutions

Concentration (%)	Energy Content (kcal/L)	Osmolarity
10	340	505
20	680	1010
50	1700	2525

Source: Adapted from Louie, N and Niemiec, PW: Parenteral nutrition solutions. In Rombeau, JL and Caldwell, MD (eds): Parenteral Nutrition. WB Saunders, Philadelphia, 1986.

RESEARCH APPLICATION: EFFICACY OF HYPOCALORIC TOTAL PARENTERAL NUTRITION IN HOSPITALIZED OBESE PATIENTS: A PROSPECTIVE, DOUBLE-BLIND RANDOMIZED TRIAL
Burge, JC, Goon, A, Choban, PS, and Flancbaum, L (eds). JPEN J Parenter Enteral Nutr 18:203–207, 1994.

Obesity is a major health concern in the United States and affects approximately one third of the population. The calculation of caloric requirements presents a challenge to healthcare providers when the obese individual becomes critically ill. Standard calculations, such as the Harris-Benedict equation underestimate the caloric requirements if an ideal body weight is used and overestimate requirements if the actual weight is used. Indirect calorimetry has allowed clinicians to more closely predict calorie and protein requirements and to allow for studies designed to evaluate the safety and clinical outcomes of hypocaloric feedings. Current research has indicated that providing excess calories can enhance O_2 consumption and increase CO_2 production, thus contributing to ventilatory dependency. Immunosuppression may also be a consequence of aggressive overfeeding. Therefore, there is a renewed interest in the concept of permissive underfeeding. Permissive underfeeding is providing patients with fewer calories than their calculated need in an effort to minimize metabolic alterations.

Purpose: This research was designed to evaluate the clinical efficacy of a hypocaloric total parenteral nutrition solution in mildly to moderately stressed obese clients.

Methods: Sixteen obese hospitalized clients were randomized to either a control group receiving 2942 kcal/d or a hypocaloric regimen containing 1285 kcal/d. The solutions were equal in their protein composition, and supplemented with vitamins, electrolytes, and trace minerals. The control solutions contained twice the amount of dextrose and lipid as the hypocaloric regimen. The average length of time on TPN was 9.6 ± 3.0 days. There were no baseline differences in age, weight, body mass index, initial urinary urea nitrogen (indicator of stress), and caloric needs, or in initial respiratory quotient.

Results: Assessment of nutritional status during the study included the protein status measures of albumin, total iron-binding capacity, and nitrogen balance. Clients were weighed and respiratory quotient (RQ) was calculated. No significant differences were noted between the two groups for the protein status measures indicating the hypocaloric regimen did not have deleterious effects on protein utilizations. Weight loss was not significantly different between the two groups; however, the RQ measures for the hypocaloric group were 0.71 ± 0.09 before intervention and 0.70 ± 0.12 after intervention, and for the control group 0.66 ± 0.09 before intervention and 0.82 ± 0.11 after intervention. These data suggest that the hypocaloric group had RQ values consistent with the fasting state and the control group had RQ values consistent with the fed state.

Practice Implications: The authors conclude that obese clients receiving a hypocaloric regimen determined by indirect calorimetry can achieve positive nitrogen balance. Further research is needed before this data can be extrapolated to the severely stressed client; however, the reduction in the calories, without compromising clinical outcome measures, may provide a significant cost-containment measure.

very little of the other essential fatty acid, linolenic acid (omega-3 family); soybean oil contains a better balance of both fatty acids and is therefore preferred. Lipid formulas are isotonic and may, therefore, be infused by way of a peripheral vein. High levels of linoleic acid are immunosuppressive and research indicates that the omega-3 fatty acids may support immunocompetence.[55]

A test dose of fat emulsions is recommended prior to the full infusion. In adults, 10% fat should be infused at a rate of 1 mL/min for the first 15 to 30 minutes; 20% fat should be infused at a rate of 0.5 mL/min for the first 15 to 30 minutes. Traditionally, 10% solutions are usually infused over 4 to 6 hours, and 20% solutions are infused over 6 to 8 hours. It has recently been suggested that all lipid emulsions be infused over 24 hours to decrease the incidence of fat-overloading syndrome.[56] This can also be prevented by the use of 3-in-1 admixture.

Ten percent lipid emulsions yield a caloric content of 1.1 kcal/mL; 20% solutions yield 2.0 kcal/mL. The administration of a 20% solution has the advantage of supplying twice as many calories per milliliter as the 10% solution. This is of particular importance in the fluid-restricted patient.

Electrolytes are infused either as a component already contained in the amino acid solution or as a separate component. Electrolytes are available in several salt forms (Table 9–17). Their administration is based on the patient's metabolic status.

Malnutrition, specific disease states, and drug therapy may predispose some patients to vitamin deficiencies, for which additional vitamin supplementation is essential. Parenteral multivitamin products and individual vitamins are available to provide additional vitamin therapy.

Trace elements such as zinc, copper, chromium, selenium, and manganese are present routinely in par-

TABLE 9–17
Electrolyte Salt Forms

Sodium chloride
Sodium acetate
Sodium bicarbonate
Sodium lactate
Sodium phosphate
Potassium chloride
Potassium acetate
Potassium phosphate
Magnesium sulfate
Calcium chloride
Calcium gluconate

Source: Reprinted from Louie, N and Niemiec, PW: Parenteral nutrition solutions. In Rombeau, JL and Caldwell, MD (eds): Parenteral Nutrition. WB Saunders, Philadelphia, 1986, p 281, with permission.

enteral solutions. Recommendations for the administration of other elements such as iodide and molybdenum have been made, although required levels are not yet well defined.

Parenteral Nutrition Additives

Many different types of additives are currently being used in parenteral nutrition. It is important that the critical care nurse understand the indications for their use and the degree of *compatibility* with the parenteral solution. Most of the research on drug compatibility has been conducted using the 2-in-1 TPN solution, and this data should not be extrapolated to the newer 3-in-1 solutions. Historically, medications have been added to the TPN solution to minimize fluids, decrease nursing time, and possibly decrease cost. The routine addition of additives to the TPN solution can increase the cost of the solution if the bag needs to be discontinued due to an adverse reaction. Drugs requiring frequent titration such as dopamine should not be added directly to the solution.[57]

Insulin is considered to be chemically stable in parenteral nutrition solutions. Its addition provides a continuous supply of the hormone, an important consideration during glucose administration. It is known that insulin is responsible for the adequate metabolism of carbohydrates. In addition to this, insulin has a lipogenic effect and also increases the muscle's uptake of amino acids.

A certain degree of adsorptive loss of insulin to the solution container, tubing, and filter has been demonstrated in several studies.[58,59] Some have suggested adding albumin to the solution in order to decrease these losses. It has been found, however, that serum glucose levels can be managed adequately without the use of albumin[60] and it is difficult to justify the cost of albumin solely to stabilize insulin content.

Heparin in doses of 1000 to 3000 U/L has been routinely used to decrease the incidence of subclavian vein thrombus, but studies have questioned this practice.[61,62] Larger doses of heparin, perhaps as much as

20,000 U/L, may be needed to reduce the risk of thrombosis. Such doses, however, may carry an increased risk of bleeding complications. Heparin is compatible in parenteral nutrition solutions in amounts up to 20,000 U/L.[63]

Cimetidine, ranitidine, and famotidine are often added to TPN in some hospitals as a prophylactic measure against the development of stress ulcers. It has been found that concentrations of 900 to 1300 mg/L of cimetidine are compatible with parenteral nutrition solutions.[63] Cimetidine may not, however, be compatible with iron, aminophylline, or antibiotics.[64]

Antibiotics added to a parenteral nutrition solution are also beneficial for the fluid-restricted patient. Such a practice would also be helpful in situations in which the availability of intravenous sites is limited. Information, however, is not yet available on several aspects of this practice. It is not known at this time whether: (1) most antibiotics are physically compatible with TPN; (2) 24-hour infusions are stable; (3) a 24-hour infusion is as effective as an intermittent infusion in combatting microorganisms. For these reasons, antibiotic admixture to TPN should be practiced on a limited basis.

Little is currently known regarding the admixture of corticosteroids with parenteral nutrition solutions. The preferred method of administration continues to be intravenous push or co-infusion. The reader should appreciate that examples of drugs used as additives, their dosages, and frequency of administration as discussed in this section reflect only possible approaches to the treatment of patients receiving TPN.

3-in-1 Solutions

A relatively new group of products, 3-in-1 solutions, combines fat, amino acids, and dextrose in one container. Stability of various amino acid and fat solutions and electrolyte and mineral additives is variable. Bacterial and/or fungal growth may be enhanced by the admixture of fat emulsions with dextrose and amino acid solutions, but less than with lipid emulsions alone.[65] This form of nutritional support has been demonstrated to be more efficient and cost-effective than traditional TPN solutions and lipids administered piggyback,[66] and to reduce the complications associated with bolus administration of fat. The rou-

TABLE 9–18
Specialized Parenteral Formulas

Specific Disorder	Parenteral Formulas
Renal failure	Nephramine 5.4% (McGaw)
	Aminosyn RF 5.2% (Abbott)
	Renamin (Travenol)
Liver disease	Hepatamine 8% (McGaw)
Trauma	FreAmine HBC 6%–9% (McGaw)

TABLE 9–19
Complications of Parenteral Nutrition

Complication	Prevention	Treatment
Catheter-Related		
Pneumothorax	• Place patient in Trendelenburg position prior to central line insertion.	• A small pneumothorax may be self-limiting. • Physician inserts a chest tube with underwater seal drainage.
Air embolus	• Place patient in Trendelenburg position prior to central line insertion. • Check the intravenous connections periodically during shift to be certain that they are secure. Tape connections for added protection against disconnection. • Change intravenous tubing during expiratory phase of respiratory cycle. • Apply an occlusive dressing over the site after the catheter has been removed.	• Should a disconnection occur, immediately place a finger over the exposed end of the catheter until the tubing can be reconnected. • Place the patient in a left side–lying Trendelenburg position.
Subclavian vein thrombosis	• Use a catheter that has proved to be the least thrombogenic (silicone). • Administer heparin as ordered by a physician.	• Assist physician with removal of catheter. • Administer heparin as ordered by a physician.
Catheter position displacement	• Securely tape intravenous dressing and tubing in place. • Check dressing at least every 4 h for signs of inadvertent displacement. • Assist with obtaining periodic chest x-rays for visualization of catheter placement.	• Notify physician immediately if catheter is displaced.
Catheter occlusion	• Check intravenous fluid for proper infusion rate at least every 2 h. • Check intravenous tubing for any kinks or bends in the tubing every 2 h. • Do not give blood transfusions through a catheter that is also being used for TPN infusion. • Do not withdraw blood through catheter for blood specimens.	• Have patient cough and/or change body position. • Attempt to aspirate clot with a syringe. • Notify physician if the above measures do not alleviate the problem.
Infection	• Do not add any additives to the TPN solution on the nursing unit. • Avoid the intravenous injection or "piggyback" of any medications to the TPN setup. • Avoid the use of stopcocks. • Tape all connections securely. • Use a biooclusive dressing. • Change dressing and tubing every 48 h.	• Obtain blood cultures. • Administer antibiotics as ordered by a physician. • Assist physician with removal of catheter if necessary. • Send catheter for culture upon its removal.
Metabolic		
Hyperglycemia	• Monitor serum glucose levels frequently. • Do not increase the rate of infusion even if it is behind schedule.	• Administer insulin as ordered by a physician. • Adjust flow rate of infusion as ordered by a physician.
Hypoglycemia	• Monitor serum glucose levels frequently. • Do not discontinue the infusion suddenly.	• Administer dextrose as ordered by a physician.
Allergic reaction	• Administer a test dose of lipid emulsions prior to initiating the infusion at the rate ordered. • Monitor patient closely during the first 30 min of infusion of TPN (allergic reactions have been reported with lipids, iron dextran, heparin, and insulin).	• Administer Benadryl and/or steroids per physician's order. • Avoid the use of TPN products to which the patient demonstrates hypersensitivity.
Burns	• Administer fluids based on patient's clinical status. • Administer electrolytes based on patient's clinical status, especially sodium, potassium, chloride, calcium, magnesium, and phosphorus.	• Destruction of the skin barrier due to thermal injury leads to evaporative water loss. • Electrolytes are depleted along with water via evaporative and renal losses. • Some substances used in burn wound care deplete electrolytes (e.g., silver nitrate, mafenide acetate). • Increased carbohydrate intake necessitates higher quantities of phosphorus.

TABLE 9–19
Complications of Parenteral Nutrition (*Continued*)

Complication	Prevention	Treatment
	Metabolic	
Sepsis	• Administer formulas high in branched-chain amino acids (BCAAs). • Administer lipids as 30%–50% of the total nonprotein calories. • Administer insulin based on patient's clinical status. • Restrict the administration of iron.	• Sepsis increases energy needs. BCAAs supply energy to the heart, liver, and skeletal muscle. • Lipid administration is vital during sepsis as there is an increased breakdown of this substrate. • Hyperglycemia occurs in response to stress. • Insulin may inhibit protein breakdown and stimulate its synthesis. • Iron is essential for the growth of numerous bacteria. • Iron administration during the acute phase of sepsis may increase its severity.

tine addition of medications to this form of TPN may cause a destabilization or separation of the lipid emulsion.[67]

Specialized Parenteral Formulas

As with enteral nutrition, various parenteral formulas have been designed to meet the needs of patients with specific disease states (Table 9–18). Formulas available for use in renal failure contain high amounts of essential amino acids. It is believed that high amounts of essential amino acids increase nephron repair in renal failure.[68] A particular amino acid, L-histidine, appears to enhance amino acid utilization in uremia. Some studies, however, have indicated that solutions high in essential amino acids do not necessarily decrease the need for dialysis or alter the outcome. They have suggested the use of standard formulations in acute renal failure.[69]

Solutions high in branched-chain amino acids (BCAAs) have been formulated for patients with liver disease. Patients with chronic liver disease are often found to have elevated levels of aromatic amino acids and depressed levels of branched-chain amino acids. This disproportion in amino acid levels is believed by some to be an etiologic factor in hepatic encephalopathy.[70] In theory, the administration of formulas high in BCAAs seem to be beneficial; however, clinical studies have not yielded consistent results. The United States Multicenter Trial demonstrated a rapid arousal rate and improved patient survival in clients with advanced liver disease receiving BCAA-enriched nutrition support.[71]

Formulas high in BCAAs have also been recommended in the care of the trauma patient. It is believed that this group of patients has a predilection to catabolize BCAAs in muscles.[72] The administration of BCAAs is thought to replenish those depleted stores; BCAAs are also more easily metabolized than aromatic amino acids.

Complications of Parenteral Nutrition

Much research has been done in the area of parenteral nutrition in the hope of enhancing tolerance and minimizing complications. Advances have been made that have significantly decreased the morbidity associated with this form of therapy. However, it must be emphasized that critically ill clients frequently require a multiple-lumen catheter, for which the infection rate is three times that of single-lumen catheters. Complications may be divided into two groups: *catheter-related* and *metabolic*. Table 9–19[79–82] contains an outline of the various complications along with measures for their prevention and treatment.

SPECIAL CONSIDERATIONS FOR SPECIFIC DISEASE STATES

The preceding sections of this chapter have contained a detailed description of the nutritional requirements of the critically ill patient and the therapeutic modalities available. There are patients, however, with specific conditions who require special nutritional considerations. Specific disease states are presented in Table 9–20,[72–78] along with specially designed treatment plans that are appropriate for clients who are enterally or parenterally fed.

SUMMARY

Nutritional support for the critically ill patient is the foundation from which he or she is able to combat illness and maintain wellness. Because critically ill patients are usually hypermetabolic, and rely on body stores to supply their needs, it is important that nutritional therapy be instituted as soon after admission as possible. Patients who are not able to eat in the usual way are afforded two other methods to receive the needed nutrients, enteral or parenteral nutrition. Methods of delivery and tips for enhancing tolerance

TABLE 9–20
Special Considerations for Specific Disease States

Disease State	Treatment Plan	Rationale for Treatment
Renal failure	• Administer formulas high in essential amino acids (EAAs). • Administer electrolytes based on patient's clinical status. • Restrict fluids based on patient's clinical status.	• Formulas high in EAAs may increase nephron repair. • Electrolyte derangements are a common complication in renal failure. • Fluid overload is a common complication in renal failure.
Liver disease	• Administer formulas high in branched-chain amino acids (BCAAs). • Restrict total protein intake in encephalopathy.	• BCAAs are depressed in severe liver disease; this may lead to encephalopathy. • Protein metabolism is decreased in severe liver disease.
Cardiac disease	• Restrict fluids and sodium based on patient's clinical status. • Provide nutrients in as high a concentration as possible without precipitating fluid overload. • Administer intravenous lipid emulsions cautiously in severe cardiac disease. • Restrict fluids and sodium based on patient's clinical status. • Administer electrolytes based on patient's clinical status, especially potassium and magnesium.	• Fluid overload, including the development of ascites, is a common complication in liver failure. • Protein calorie malnutrition is a common sequelae of severe cardiac disease. • Free fatty acids can be detrimental during periods of acute myocardial ischemia because they have negative inotropic effects and increase heart size. • Fluid overload is a common complication of cardiac disease. • Renal excretion of potassium and magnesium may occur as a result of the potent diuretics commonly used in the treatment of cardiac disease.

Pulmonary disease	• Nonprotein calories should be supplied in the following amounts:
	  ○ Carbohydrates 40%–50%
	  ○ Lipids 30%–50%
	• Administer fluids and sodium cautiously so as not to cause fluid overload.
	• Administer electrolytes based on patient's clinical status, especially phosphorus, magnesium, potassium, and calcium.
		• Carbohydrates supplied in amounts greater than those recommended may lead to the increased production of CO_2. Increased CO_2 levels can decrease respiratory drive.
		• Excess lung water can hamper effective breathing.
		
		• Adequate amounts of these electrolytes are required for normal pulmonary function.

Trauma	• Administer formulas high in BCAAs. • Administer insulin based on patient's clinical status. • Administer fluids and sodium cautiously (after the resuscitation period) so as not to cause fluid overload.	• Trauma causes preferential breakdown of BCAAs in muscles. • Hyperglycemia occurs in response to trauma. • Insulin may inhibit protein breakdown and stimulate its synthesis. • In response to injury, there is an increase in sodium and water retention.
Burns	• Administer higher concentrations of carbohydrates than lipids (e.g., carbohydrates = 60% nonprotein calories; lipids = 40% nonprotein calories). • Administer formulas high in amino acids. • Administer insulin based on patient's clinical status. • Administer fluids based on patient's clinical status. • Administer electrolytes based on patient's clinical status, especially sodium, potassium, chloride, calcium, magnesium, and phosphorus.	• Administration of higher concentrations of carbohydrate than fat in the hypermetabolic burned patient is thought to spare proteins for muscle synthesis. • Formulas high in amino acids accelerate protein synthesis. • Hyperglycemia occurs in response to trauma. • Insulin may inhibit protein breakdown and stimulate its synthesis. • Destruction of the skin barrier due to thermal injury results in evaporative water loss. • Electrolytes are depleted along with water through evaporative and renal losses. • Some substances used in burn wound care deplete electrolytes (e.g., silver nitrate, mafenide acetate). • Increased carbohydrate intake necessitates higher quantities of phosphorus.
Sepsis	• Administer formulas high in BCAAs. • Administer lipids as 30%–50% of the total nonprotein calories. • Administer insulin based on patient's clinical status. • Restrict the administration of iron.	• Sepsis increases energy needs. BCAAs supply energy to the heart, liver, and skeletal muscle. • Lipid administration is vital during sepsis because there is an increased breakdown of this substrate. • Hyperglycemia occurs in response to stress. • Insulin may inhibit protein breakdown and stimulate its synthesis. • Iron is essential for the growth of numerous bacteria. Iron administration during the acute phase of sepsis may increase its severity.

of both parenteral and enteral nutrition have been explored. In the final assessment, the nurse plays a key role in the nutritional support of the critically ill patient.

REFERENCES

1. Nightingale, F: Notes on Nursing: What It Is and What It Is Not. New York, Appleton & Lange, 1860.
2. Bistrain, B: Prevalence of malnutrition in general medical patients. JAMA 235:1567–1570, 1976.
3. Messner RL, Stephens N, Wheeler WE, and Hawes MC: Effect of admission nutritional status on length of hospital stay. Gastroenterology Nursing Spring:202–205, 1991.
4. Methods for voluntary weight loss and control. National Institutes of Health Technology Assessment Conference Statement, March 30–April 1, 1992.
5. Harvey, KB, et al: Biologic measures for the formulation of a hospital prognostic index. Am J Clin Nutr 34:2013–2022, 1981.
6. Patyek, JA and Blackburn, GL: Goals of nutritional support in acute infections. Am J Med 76:81–87, 1984.
7. Reilly, JJ, et al: Economic impact of malnutrition: A model system for hospitalized patients. JPEN J Parenter Enteral Nutr 12:371–376, 1988.
8. Reinhardt, GF, et al: Incidence and mortality of hypoalbuminemic patients in hospitalized veterans. JPEN J Parenter Enteral Nutr 4:357–359, 1980.
9. Apelgren, KN, et al: Comparison of nutritional indices and outcome in critically ill patients. Crit Care Med 10:305–307, 1982.
10. Allman, RM, et al: Pressure sores among hospitalized patients. Ann Intern Med 105:337–342, 1986.
11. Buchanan, RT and Levine, NS: Nutritional support of the surgery patient. Ann Plast Surg 10:159–166, 1983.
12. Webb, AR, et al: Hand grip dynamometry as a predictor of postoperative complications: Reappraisal using age standardized grip strength. JPEN J Parenter Enteral Nutr 13:30–38, 1989.
13. Rose, J, et al: Problems with interpretation of repeat antigen skin tests in the surgical patient. Nutrition Support Services 6(5):14–21, 1986.
14. Dowd, PS and Heatley, RV: The influence of undernutrition on immunity. Clin Sci 66:241–248, 1984.
15. MacLean, LD: Delayed type hypersensitivity testing in surgical patients. Surg Gynecol Obstet 166:285–293, 1988.
16. Hak, LF, et al: Reversal of skin test anergy during maintenance hemodialysis by protein and calorie supplementation. Am J Clin Nutr 36:1089–1092, 1982.
17. Grant, JP: Nutritional assessment in clinical practice. Nutr Clin Prac 1:3–9, 1986.
18. Rosse, RA and Shizgal, HM: Serum albumin and nutritional states. JPEN J Parenter Enteral Nutr 4:450–454, 1980.
19. Doweiko, JP and Nomgleggi, MD: The role of albumin in human physiology and pathophysiology, III: Albumin and disease states. JPEN J Parenter Enteral Nutr 15:476–483, 1991.
20. Buzby, GP, et al: Prognostic nutritional index in gastrointestinal surgery. Am J Surg 139:160–167, 1980.
21. Veteran Affairs' Total Parenteral Nutrition Cooperative Study Group: Perioperative total parenteral nutrition in surgical patients. N Engl J Med 325:525–532, 1991.
22. Hunter, DC, et al: Resting energy expenditure in the critically ill: Estimation versus measurement. Br J Surg 75:875–878, 1988.
23. Williams, RR and Fuenning, CR: Circulatory indirect calorimetry in the critically ill. JPEN J Parenter Enteral Nutr 15:509–512, 1991.
24. Heymsfield, SB, et al: Respiratory, cardiovascular, and metabolic effects of enteral hyperalimentation: Influence of formula, dose and composition. Am J Clin Nutr 40:116–130, 1984.
25. Taplers, SS, et al: Nutritionally associated increased carbon dioxide production: Excess total calories vs high proportion of carbohydrate calories. Chest 102:551–555, 1992.
26. Adams, S, et al: Enteral versus parenteral nutritional support

following laparotomy for trauma: A randomized prospective trial. J Trauma 26:882–891, 1986.
27. Bower, RH, et al: Postoperative enteral vs parenteral nutrition: A randomized controlled trial. Arch Surg 121:1040–1045, 1986.
28. Tkatch, L, et al: Benefits of oral protein supplementation in elderly patients with fracture of the proximal femur. J Am Coll Nutr 11:519–525, 1992.
29. Kudsh, KA, et al: Enteral versus parenteral feeding: Effects on septic morbidity after blunt and penetrating abdominal trauma. Ann Surg 215:503–513, 1992.
30. Brandtzaeg, P, et al: Immunobiology and immunopathology of human gut mucosa: Humoral immunity and intraepithelial lymphocytes. Gastroenterology 97:1562–1584, 1989.
31. Keithley, JK and Eisenberg, P: The significance of enteral nutrition in the intensive care unit patient. Critical Care Nursing Clinics of North America 5(1):23–29, 1993.
32. Alexander, JW: Nutrition and translocation. JPEN J Parenter Enteral Nutr 14:1705–1745, 1990.
33. Marshall, JC, et al: The microbiology of multiple organ failure. Arch Surg 123:309–315, 1988.
34. Smith, RJ: Glutamine metabolism and its physiologic importance. JPEN J Parenter Enteral Nutr 14:945–995, 1990.
35. Souba, WW, et al: Gut glutamine metabolism. JPEN J Parenter Enteral Nutr 14:455–505, 1990.
36. Settle, RG: Short chain fatty acids and their potential role in nutritional support. JPEN J Parenter Enteral Nutr 12:1045–1075, 1988.
37. Koruda, MJ, et al: The effect of a pectin-supplemented elemental diet on intestinal adaptation to massive small bowel resection. JPEN J Parenteral Enter Nutr 10:343–352, 1986.
38. Daly, JM: Immune and metabolic effects of arginine in the surgical patient. Ann Surg 208:512–522, 1988.
39. Kirk, SJ and Barbul, A: Role of arginine in trauma, sepsis and immunity. JPEN J Parenteral Enteral Nutr 14:2265–2295, 1990.
40. Katz, DP, Kuetan, V, and Askanaze, J: Enteral nutrition: Potential role in regulating immune function. Curr Opin Gastroenterol 6:199–203, 1990.
41. Kinsella, JE and Lokesh, B: Dietary lipids, eicosanoids, and immune system. Crit Care Med 18:945–1135, 1990.
42. Doglio, GR, et al: Gastric mucosal pH as a prognostic index of mortality in critically ill patients. Crit Care Med 19:1037–1040, 1991.
43. Clark, C and Gutierrez, G: Gastric intramucosal pH: A non-invasive method for the indirect measurement of tissue oxygenation. Am J Crit Care 1:53–60, 1992.
44. Grube, BJ, Heimbach, DM, and Mariuin, JA: *Clostridium difficile* diarrhea in the critically ill burned patient. Arch Surg 122:655–661, 1987.
45. Brinson, RR and Kolts, B: Hypoalbuminemia as an indicator of diarrheal incidence in critically ill patients. Crit Care Med 15:506–509, 1987.
46. Payne-James, JJ: Retrograde (ascending) bacterial contamination of enteral diet administration systems. JPEN J Parenter Enter Nutr 16:369–373, 1992.
47. Driks, M, et al: Nosocomial pneumonia in intubated patients given sucralfate as compared with antacids or histamine type 2 blockers. NEJM N Engl J Med 317:1376–1382, 1987.
48. Centers for Disease Control: Guidelines for the prevention of intravenous therapy-related infections. Infection Control 3(1):61–72, 1982.
49. Kamal, GD, et al: Reduced intravascular catheter infection by antibiotic bonding: A prospective randomized trial. JAMA 265:2364–2371, 1991.
50. Murphy, LM and Lipman, TO: Central venous catheter care in parenteral nutrition: A review. JPEN J Parenter Enteral Nutr 11:190–198, 1987.
51. Wille, JC, Bluss'e van Oud Albas, A, and Thewessen, EA: A comparison of two transparent film-type dressings in central venous therapy. J Hosp Infect 23:113–121, 1993.
52. Hoffman, KK, Weber, DJ, Samsa, GP, and Rutala, WA: Transparent polyurethane film as an intravascular catheter dressing. A meta-analysis of the infection risks. JAMA 267:2072–2076, 1992.
53. Conly, JM, Grieves, K, and Peters, B: A prospective, randomized

study comparing transparent and dry gauze dressings for central venous catheter. J Infect Dis 159:310–319, 1989.

54. Millan, DA: Final inline filters. Am J Nurs 79:1272, 1979.
55. Robinson, DR, Tateno, S, Patel, BM and Hirai, A: Lipid mediators of inflammatory and immune reactions. JPEN J Parenter Enteral Nutr 12:375–415, 1988.
56. Berge, H, et al: Clearance of fat emulsions in severely stressed patients. NSS 4(12):18–26, 1984.
57. Baptista, RJ, et al: Compatibility of total nutrient admixtures and secondary cardiovascular medications (letter). Am J Hosp Pharm 42:777–778, 1985.
58. Weber, S, Wood, W, and Jackson, E: Availability of insulin from parenteral nutrient solutions. Am J Hosp Pharm 34:353, 1977.
59. Petty, C and Cunningham, N: Insulin adsorption by glass infusion bottles, polyvinyl chloride infusion containers, and intravenous tubing. Anesthesiology 40:400, 1974.
60. Semple, P, White, C, and Manderson, W: Continuous intravenous infusion of small doses of insulin treatment of diabetic ketoacidosis. BMJ 2:694, 1974.
61. Ruggiero, R and Aisenstein, T: Central catheter fibrin sleeve-heparin effect. JPEN J Parenter Enteral Nutr 7:270, 1983.
62. Brismar, B, et al: Reduction of catheter-associated thrombosis in parenteral nutrition by intravenous heparin therapy. Arch Surg 117:1196, 1982.
63. Kobayaski, N and King, S: Compatibility of common additives in protein hydrolysate/dextrose solutions. Am J Hosp Pharm 34:589, 1977.
64. Tsallas, G and Allen, L: Stability of cimetidine hydrochloride in parenteral nutrition solutions. Am J Hosp Pharm 39:484, 1982.
65. Thompson, B and Robinson, LA: Infection control of parenteral solutions. Nutrition in Clinical Practice 6(2):49–54, 1991.
66. Green, BA and Baptista, RJ: Nursing assessment of 3-in-1 TPN admixture. NITA 8:530–532, 1985.
67. Barnett, MI, Cosslett, AG, Duffield, JR, Evans, DA, Hall, SB, and Williams, DR: Parenteral nutrition. Pharmaceutical problems of compatibility and stability. Drug Saf 55:101–106, 1990.
68. Abel, R, Abbot, W, and Fischer, J: Intravenous essential L-amino acids and hypertonic dextrose in patients with acute renal failure. Am J Surg 123:632–638, 1972.
69. Blumendrantz, M, et al: Total parenteral nutrition in the management of acute renal failure. Am J Clin Nutr 31:1831–1840, 1978.
70. Fischer, JE, et al: The effect of normalization of plasma amino acids on hepatic encephalopathy in man. Surgery 80:77–91, 1988.
71. Cerra, FB, et al: Disease specific amino acid infusion (F080) in hepatic encephalopathy: A prospective randomized double blind controlled heal. JPEN J Parenter Enteral Nutr 9:288–295, 1985.
72. Cerra, FB: Branched chain amino acids. I. Stress nutrition. Nutr Supp Serv 5:8–40, 1985.
73. Abel, RM: Nutritional support in the patient with acute renal failure. J Am Coll Nutr 2:33–44, 1983.
74. Maddrey, WC: Branched-chain amino acid therapy in liver disease. J Am Coll Nutr 4:639–650, 1985.
75. Wilson, DO, Rogers, RM, and Hoffman, RM: Nutrition and chronic lung disease. Annu Rev Respir Dis 132:1347–1365, 1985.
76. Armstrong, JN: Nutrition and the respiratory patient. Nutrition Support Services 6(3):8–32, 1986.
77. Krevsky, B and Godley, J: Nutritional support in advanced liver disease. Nutrition Support Services 5(8):8–17, 1985.
78. Wolk, RA, and Swartz, RD: Nutritional support of patients with acute renal failure. Nutrition Support Services 6(2):38–46, 1986.
79. Forlaw, L and Torosian, MH: Central venous catheter care. In Rombeau, JL and Caldwell, MD (eds): Parenteral Nutrition. Philadelphia, WB Saunders, 1986.
80. Ang, SD and Daly, JM: Potential complications and monitoring of patients receiving total parenteral nutrition. In Rombeau, JL and Caldwell, MD (eds): Parenteral Nutrition. Philadelphia, WB Saunders, 1986.
81. Sheldon, GF and Baker, C: Complications of nutritional support. Crit Care Med 8:35–37, 1980.
82. Udall, JN and Richardson, DS: Allergic reactions to parenteral nutrition solutions. Nutrition Support Services 6(4):20–22, 1986.

CHAPTER 10

Pain Management in the Critically Ill Patient

Deborah M. Thorpe

CHAPTER OUTLINE

LEARNING OBJECTIVES

After completing this chapter, you should be able to:

1. Recognize common barriers to effective pain management in critically ill patients.
2. Discuss key aspects of the anatomy and physiology of pain.
3. Identify characteristics of common classifications of pain.
4. Assess pain characteristics and intensity using appropriate patient-specific tools.
5. Discuss safety and efficacy of opioid use in managing pain.
6. Identify nonpharmacologic strategies for managing pain.
7. Discuss appropriate nursing interventions in pain management.

Pain is one of the most common symptoms not only of disease but of many treatments as well. Unfortunately, despite considerable research, new knowledge, and the availability of many treatment options, pain is often significantly undertreated.[1,2] The critically ill patient presents some special challenges in the providing of adequate pain relief, especially when he or she is entubated, in a state of altered consciousness, or cognitively impaired. However, the key principles of pain management apply, regardless of the patient care setting. An overview of basic pain management concepts is provided in this chapter, with emphasis on specific strategies for implementation in the critical care setting.

BARRIERS TO EFFECTIVE PAIN MANAGEMENT

The reasons for persistent undertreatment of pain fall into three broad categories: (1) cultural and attitudinal barriers, (2) knowledge deficits, and (3) governmental and regulatory influences.[3]

Cultural and Attitudinal Barriers

Attitudes, rather than scientific knowledge, are among the most influential forces in assessment and decision making for pain management. Concepts about pain are influenced by a multitude of factors that vary widely among healthcare professionals, patients, and family members. How a patient views pain is derived from cultural and social influences, and the meaning of the pain experience often determines how the patient will respond to and cope with pain. Many patients are naturally stoic and do not complain, despite suffering significant pain. Others express their pain vividly and share their experience with all who will listen. The pain experience for both the stoic and the expressive patient, however, is real. Unfortunately, caregivers often respond to the complaint of pain from their own perspective on pain rather than making an attempt to understand and value the patient's perspective.

Pain is a subjective experience, and there are no truly objective measures to prove that a patient is experiencing pain. Because nurses and physicians are geared toward looking for objective evidence of patient complaints and are given limited training in dealing with subjective phenomena, when a physical cause for a pain complaint cannot be identified and objectively documented, they tend to assume that the pain is not real. Such assumptions contribute to what all too often becomes an adversarial relationship between the patient, who must constantly strive to prove the pain exists to obtain relief, and the caregivers, who do not act unless they believe the pain is real.[4] A significant number of patients continue to suffer unrelieved pain because they accept the belief that their pain is not real or they lack the ability to express their pain in a convincing manner. Others may continue to suffer because they believe that pain is inevitable or because they fear that treatment of the pain—particularly with narcotics—carries with it a significant risk of harm, such as addiction. Because narcotics are generally considered to be "bad" by patients and healthcare professionals, there is a tendency to underuse them. This represents a failure to distinguish between *legitimate* and *illegitimate* uses of narcotics fostered by the pervasive problem of drug abuse in society.[5]

Knowledge Deficits

Few healthcare professionals have had sufficient education in pain management to overcome the influence of the prevailing attitudes about pain and cultural barriers to the effective treatment of pain. In addition, much of what is believed and taught about pain—particularly the use of opioid analgesics (narcotics)—is outdated. In recent years, many advances have been made in understanding pain mechanisms and the pharmacology of opioids. However, these have been only slowly incorporated into curricula, which continue to be influenced by the many myths and misconceptions about opioids. Many of the early opioid drug trials were conducted as single-dose studies in subjects who did not actually have pain; in fact, many

were addict volunteers at federal penal institutions. Years of clinical experience and subsequent studies have demonstrated that the presence of the pain stimulus is a critical factor in the pharmacologic actions of opioids. Scientific advances have also led to a greater understanding of the complex nature of pain mechanisms and the variations in response to treatment, depending on the etiology of the underlying pain. For example, neuropathic or neurogenic pain mechanisms are vastly different from the normal, nociceptive transmission of pain messages that are a part of the natural neurologic defense mechanisms. Nevertheless, clinicians tend to treat all pain in the same way and as a result draw the wrong conclusions when the pain fails to respond to prescribed treatment. The patient who continues to complain of pain despite customary treatment is often labeled an "addict" or "drug seeker," when, in fact, the continued complaint of pain is a result of inadequate or inappropriate treatment.

Mistaken concepts about the action of opioids are still prevalent and contribute significantly to the underuse of this class of drugs. Key among these common misunderstandings are the following.

Myth #1: Narcotic Use Leads to Respiratory Depression

Fear of respiratory depression is one of the most pervasive influences on clinical decision making. Physicians tend to underprescribe and nurses tend to underadminister opioids, which can lead to ineffective relief of pain largely because healthcare professionals do not realize that the pain stimulus itself is a powerful antagonist to the respiratory depressant effects of opioids. Furthermore, tolerance to the respiratory depressant effect (but not the analgesic effect) develops early in the course of opioid use. Narcotics actually have a high margin of safety in use, and in the unlikely event that respiratory depression occurs, it can be easily reversed by the judicious use of the antagonist naloxone.

Myth #2: Oral Narcotics Are Less Effective

Lack of knowledge about the process of biotransformation—metabolic alteration of a drug as it is routed through the hepatic circulation—fosters the conclusion that opioids are less effective when administered orally or, conversely, that they work better when given parenterally. Failure to account for biotransformation results in discrepancies in analgesic effectiveness when changing from one route to another. For example, 10 mg morphine administered parenterally has the equianalgesic potency of 30 mg morphine administered orally. This is because about 66% of the drug administered orally is metabolized and transformed before reaching the opiate receptor binding sites in the central nervous system. Therefore, a larger dose must be given to overcome this biotransformation. If 10 mg parenteral morphine was effective in relieving pain, 10 mg given orally will not produce the same level of analgesia. When inappropriately low doses are given and the patient complains of increased pain, all too often the nurse or the physician concludes that the patient is drug-seeking and is at risk for addiction.

Myth #3: Narcotic Use—Even to Treat Pain—Carries a Significant Risk of Addiction

Lack of knowledge of the characteristics of addiction also contributes to the inadequate use of opioids. Addiction is primarily a psychological and behavioral problem in which drugs are used to attain a psychic effect rather than pain relief. The addict's life is devoted to obtaining and taking drugs, resulting in a pattern in which drug use is the paramount purpose in life—often to the point of sacrificing security, values, and life itself. Conversely, drug use for the relief of pain enables the patient to function better and has positive sequelae. The postoperative patient who has adequate pain relief is able to move and walk earlier and cooperate with coughing and deep-breathing exercises. Effective opioid use and improved pain control have actually been demonstrated to reduce complications and shorten length of hospital stay.[6-8] Few, if any, patients with pain experience the psychic or euphoric effects of opioids that the true drug seeker does because of the antagonizing effects of the pain stimulus. The risk of addiction when opioids are used for medical purposes is *extremely low* in persons who were not addicts *prior* to their medical treatment.[9,10]

Myth #4: Addiction and Dependence Are the Same

Dependence is a physiologic phenomenon in which the nervous system and other physiologic mechanisms adapt to the presence of a drug. If administration of that drug is stopped suddenly, it takes time for various bodily functions to readapt, and the patient experiences an abstinence syndrome, commonly referred to as "withdrawal." Both the addict and the patient who is taking narcotics for pain for more than a few days experience dependence, but the development of dependence does not produce addiction. Withdrawal symptoms are variable and may range from odd feelings that "something is not right" to severe nausea, vomiting, cramping, diarrhea, and diaphoresis. An abstinence syndrome in a critically ill or debilitated patient can have serious consequences. Fear of these unpleasant symptoms may motivate the addict to go out and do whatever it takes to obtain drugs, contributing to the behavioral problems associated with addiction. However, in the patient taking opioids for pain, withdrawal can be prevented by a gradual tapering of the dose if the underlying pain problem is resolved and the drugs are no longer needed.

A phenomenon known as *pseudoaddiction* has been recently recognized as an iatrogenic syndrome in which patients develop behavioral characteristics that are usually associated with psychological dependence or addiction but that are actually a consequence of *inadequate* pain treatment.[11] Pseudoaddiction can occur when medications are used at intervals greater than their duration of efficacy or in doses that are too low or of insufficient potency for the nature and intensity of the pain. It is most often seen with "as-needed" (PRN) dosing when pain is persistent. Consequently, the patient often has to resort to dramatic behavior to prove the reality of the pain or, on his or her own initiative, escalate the dose to the point of pain relief. This may lead to the patient being labeled as "drug-seeking" or "difficult," which in turn leads to an adversarial relationship with members of the healthcare team. The behavioral problems seen in pseudoaddiction are usually resolved once adequate pain control is achieved and trust has been restored.

Governmental and Regulatory Influences

The existence of drug abuse in society makes it necessary to strictly control and regulate the use of opioids. Unfortunately, many of the regulations are vague and ambiguous, and the regulators who enforce them are concerned primarily with numbers rather than clinical outcome when prescribing practices are challenged. In states that require triplicate prescriptions for certain classes of drugs, physicians are acutely aware that their practices are being monitored and as a result may avoid providing patients with quantities greater than those perceived to be acceptable—even though in most states no prescribing parameters are specified by law. In some states, the prescriptions are monitored by police agencies, and this contributes to the perception that it is inherently "bad" or "wrong" to prescribe these drugs. In the hospital setting, nurses must go through rigorous security and administrative procedures to administer controlled drugs. Such procedures may further influence the attitudes of healthcare professionals toward providing these drugs to patients. Although regulations may be necessary to prevent unauthorized use of drugs, nurses must be careful not to let fear of these regulations interfere with sound clinical practice.

It is critical that nurses become aware of the many barriers to pain treatment in order to eliminate their powerful influence on practice. In many states, nurses are taking active roles as advocates for better pain management through participation in their professional organizations and, more recently, state cancer pain initiatives. Cancer patients, who often suffer pain for prolonged periods, have provided a lot of insight and promoted much research that challenges the commonly held beliefs about pain and its treatment. Beginning with the Wisconsin Cancer Pain Initiative, cancer care specialists have taken the lead in promoting awareness of legitimate approaches to pain management by addressing the barriers discussed here. Many states have organized initiatives, and the number is growing annually. In Texas, the state legislature passed The Intractable Pain Treatment Act[12] in 1989, and California has adopted a similar bill. These laws were designed to emphasize the legitimate use of opioids to treat pain and to clarify the ambiguous language of regulations that are often too narrowly interpreted. The intent of these laws is to encourage proper use of narcotics and to reassure physicians that such use will not place their licenses to practice at risk.

All nurses should be familiar with the statutes that regulate controlled substances and the systems established within their states to monitor practice. Nurses should also be encouraged to participate in efforts to inform and educate their state legislators and regulatory boards about the needs of patients in pain.

ANATOMY AND PHYSIOLOGY OF PAIN

There are many complex mechanisms and pathways for the transmission of noxious stimuli and the perception of pain. Pain is the effect of a complex interaction of biochemical, physiologic, and psychological processes.[13] In the past few decades, much progress has been made in developing a greater understanding of these processes; however, much is yet to be learned. The essential structures for pain transmission and the leading theories about pain will be discussed briefly.

Anatomic Structures

Pain originates through stimulation of the peripheral receptors known as *nociceptors;* hence the term *nociception* is often used to describe pain. These receptor sites are stimulated by tissue injury or disease processes. Electrical impulses carry the message through the primary afferent neurons to the somatosensory pathways (including the spinothalamic tract) found in the ventrolateral white matter of the spinal cord. From the spinal tracts, the stimuli are transmitted to the higher centers in the brain, including the thalamus and cerebral cortex where the message is interpreted. At various levels, appropriate motor responses are initiated. For example, when a hand comes in contact with a hot stove, there is a swift and automatic motion to withdraw the hand from the noxious stimulus. Figure 10–1 depicts the primary neural pathways for the transmission of nociceptive messages from the periphery to the brain. For a more thorough understanding of the peripheral, spinal, and brain pathways involved, see Chapter 6, which details the anatomy and physiology of the nervous system.

Nociception is also influenced or mediated by a variety of biochemical factors. Chemical mediators such as serotonin, acetylcholine, histamine, bradykinin, and substance P act at different levels of the pain pathway, either as a neurotransmitter or as a neuromodulator. *Neurotransmitters* are substances involved in the relay of the impulses, whereas *neuromodulators* may act to enhance or inhibit the relay. Other substances, such as prostaglandins, which are released following tissue injury, sensitize the nociceptors to pain and contribute to the inflammatory process.[13]

Endogenous Pain Mechanisms

The discovery of endogenous opioid-like substances produced by the central nervous system has further expanded our understanding of pain mechanisms.[14] Several types of peptide molecules that produce narcotic-like effects have been identified, including endorphin, enkephalin, and dynorphin. The release of endorphins in particular is thought to be involved in producing a placebo response. Some studies have demonstrated that placebo responses are reversible by naloxone. However, there are many underlying mechanisms that are not yet thoroughly understood. Some evidence exists that pain and stress contribute to the release of endorphins; however, the ability to produce endogenous opioids varies significantly. More research is needed to clarify the role of endogenous pain mechanisms and to find ways of activating these systems.

The Gate Control Theory

The most commonly accepted and studied theory of pain is the gate control theory first described by Melzack and Wall[15] in 1965. This theory, depicted in Figure 10–2, represents a comprehensive model for understanding the complex interactions of the biochemical, physiologic, and psychological processes involved in pain. A key aspect of the theory proposes that there is a "gating" mechanism located in the substantia gelatinosa (SG) of the dorsal horn of the spinal cord. This mechanism allows for modulation of the sensory input from the periphery before it reaches the central transmission (T) cells, thus inhibiting the signal from reaching the higher centers in the brain. The mechanism is influenced by the degree of activity from large-diameter (L) A beta and small-diameter (S) A delta and C peripheral nerve fibers. The gating mechanism can also be modulated by descending influences from the brain (cognitive control and descending inhibitory control).

It is thought that stimulation of the small fibers facilitates transmission of pain by opening the gate, whereas stimulation of the large fibers inhibits transmission by closing the gate. Transcutaneous electrical nerve stimulation (TENS) and other physical modalities such as massage and vibration are examples of interventions that capitalize on this gating mechanism. The mildly noxious electrical or mechanical stimuli are thought to activate the large fibers that "close the gate." Cognitive processes such as anxiety and fear are thought to enhance pain by opening the gating mechanism, whereas behavioral interventions such as relaxation techniques may actually diminish pain perception by closing the gate.

Although the gate control theory does not complete our understanding of pain mechanisms, it does pro-

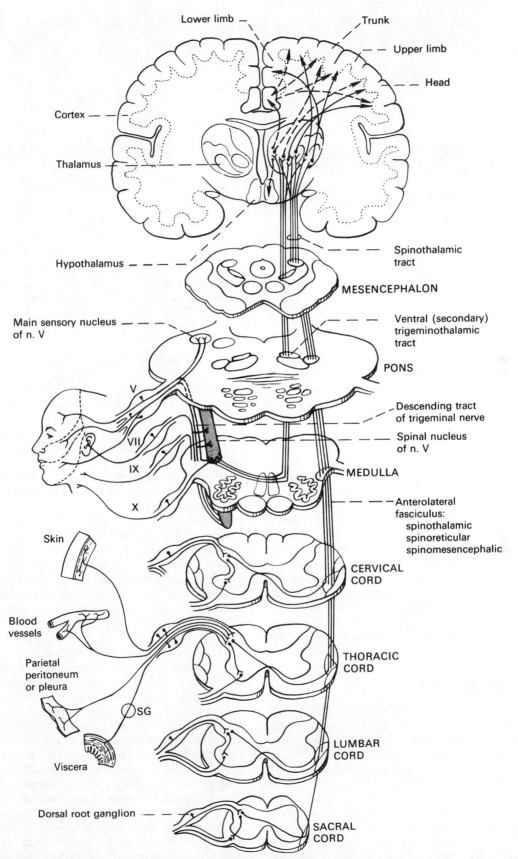

FIGURE 10–1. Primary neural pathways of pain transmission. (From Bonica, JJ: The Management of Pain, Vol. 1. Lea & Febiger, Philadelphia, 1990, with permission.)

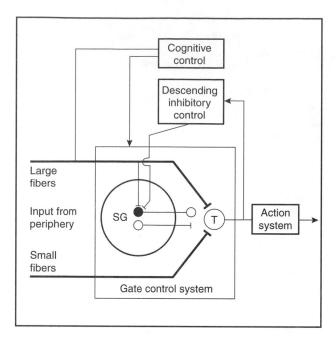

FIGURE 10–2. Schematic diagram of the gate-control theory of pain. (SG = substantia gelatinosa; T = transmission cells.) (Adapted from Melzack, R and Wall, PD: The Challenge of Pain. Basic Books, New York, 1983.)

vide a comprehensive model for understanding the cascade of events that occur with the transmission of pain stimuli. It has served as a model for much of the current research and will undoubtedly continue to evolve as more is learned.

PAIN CLASSIFICATIONS

To adequately assess and manage pain, it is important to be able to recognize the type of pain the patient is experiencing. There are many mechanisms of pain and consequently many ways of describing or classifying pain. Three broad categories of pain are compared and contrasted here: (1) acute versus chronic, (2) benign versus malignant, and (3) nociceptive versus neuropathic. These categories are not mutually exclusive, and patients, particularly the critically ill or those with chronic and progressive illness, may experience several types of pain simultaneously, with each type requiring individual attention and perhaps different interventions.

Acute versus Chronic Pain

Acute pain is short in duration and follows an expected time course, depending on the underlying etiology. A normal defense mechanism, pain often draws attention to a problem and leads the patient to seek medical attention. Severe crushing chest pain associated with myocardial infarction is a classic example. The person experiencing acute pain, whether due to disease or treatment such as surgery, is most likely to present a typical picture of the patient in pain, with characteristic behavioral and physiologic signs. As expected, acute pain may cause the patient to grimace, guard the affected area, and verbalize about the pain. As the nervous and cardiovascular systems respond to

disease or trauma, changes in pulse and blood pressure may be observed or the patient may become diaphoretic. In most acute pain situations, unless the patient is stoic by nature, a diagnosis of pain can be made or validated readily on the basis of the patient's appearance and physiologic parameters. Most patients in acute pain states (e.g., postoperative, trauma, and myocardial infarction) respond readily to predictable doses of analgesics, and such pain is likely to be a result of stimulation of the peripheral nervous system receptors (nociceptors).

Chronic pain is persistent and may continue despite healing of the underlying injury or disease. Although chronic pain is often defined as pain that lasts longer than 6 months, such a set limit is arbitrary. More relevant to the understanding of chronic pain is an awareness of its key characteristics. Chronic pain ceases to function as a warning mechanism; in fact, it often becomes a constant and unpleasant reminder of the underlying problem. Chronic pain becomes less apparent to the observer as physiologic and psychosocial adaptation occurs. Physiologic parameters such as pulse and blood pressure normalize once the body recognizes the pain stimulus as persistent. Likewise, behavior adapts as a result of innate coping abilities or those taught as pain management strategies, such as distraction or relaxation techniques. The patient with chronic pain, particularly one who has adapted well, may not demonstrate any visible signs of pain despite experiencing pain of significant intensity. Unfortunately, because of the lack of objective findings, it is sometimes difficult for the patient experiencing chronic pain to be believed and to receive adequate treatment.[4] Most chronic pain states require multiple interventions, including analgesic medications, with attention to strategies that increase coping and rehabilitation.

Benign versus Malignant Pain

Pain may also be characterized or classified according to the nature of its underlying etiology. *Benign pain* is usually the result of some type of insult such as a surgical procedure or trauma. After the underlying condition is treated or healed, no further damage occurs. Pain in this situation is often the result of structural changes that change the stresses or weight-bearing capabilities of various body parts. Muscle spasm or joint deterioration and chronic, low-grade inflammatory responses may contribute to ongoing pain. Benign pain also may be caused by scar tissue formation, particularly in areas like the spinal column, where delicate nerve roots may become entrapped or compressed against bone. Chronic low back pain is a characteristic example of a benign pain syndrome. Most benign pain syndromes can also be characterized as being chronic.

Malignant pain is associated with an ongoing disease process in which there is persistent new tissue injury and destruction. Metastatic cancer and severe rheumatoid arthritis are examples of malignant pain syndromes. Malignant pain is sometimes characterized as "persistent acute pain" because, although the time course is long and therefore chronic, the features of the pain resemble those of acute pain. Malignant pain syndromes are often accompanied by a significant inflammatory response.

Nociceptive versus Neuropathic Pain

Nociceptive pain is the general characterization for pain that occurs as a result of stimulation of a normal, intact peripheral and central nervous system. The peripheral receptor sites (nociceptors) transmit the noxious stimuli through the spinal cord to the cerebral cortex, where the message is interpreted and appropriate motor responses are initiated (e.g., withdrawal of an extremity from a heat source). Nociceptive pain may also be subcategorized as *somatic*, arising from soft tissue and musculoskeletal structures, or *visceral*, arising from the autonomic fibers of the smooth muscle of the internal organs. Nociceptive pain is characteristically described as dull, sharp, aching, or heavy, or with a variety of other adjectives.

Neuropathic pain is pain in the context of an injury occurring either in a peripheral nerve or anywhere in the central nervous system. Nerves can be injured or damaged by being cut, crushed, compressed, stretched, or exposed to toxic agents such as chemotherapy drugs or viruses. With nerve damage comes a cascade of events resulting in anatomic as well as neurochemical changes in the makeup of the neurons. A cut peripheral nerve may regrow and branch out, covering a wider receptive field than before the injury. Complex changes in the neurotransmitter balance, such as depletion of serotonin and norepinephrine at the synapse, may result in abnormal or aberrant impulse firing. Common examples are postherpetic neuralgia, phantom pain, and peripheral neuropathy.

Neuropathic pain is easy to identify by its characteristic description as "burning." It is also often described in electrical terms such as tingling, shocking, or jolting. Other features include a delay in onset after the precipitating injury and perception of normally mild and nonpainful stimuli (e.g., touch) as being exquisitely sensitive or painful (allodynia). Neuropathic pain may also be accompanied by sympathetic dysfunction. The injured nerve, as it regrows, may become entwined with sympathetic nerve fibers that provide constant input into the peripheral nervous system, as occurs in reflex sympathetic dystrophy, a particularly disabling pain syndrome often associated with crush injuries to an extremity.[16] Compared with nociceptive pain, neuropathic pain is more difficult to treat because the response to opioid analgesics is difficult to predict and may be only partially effective. Other types of drugs, such as the tricyclic antidepressants (useful for their analgesic capability rather than their antidepressant indication) and anticonvulsant drugs and other modalities such as TENS, are usually required.

PAIN ASSESSMENT

Although pain is a subjective phenomenon, there are ways of measuring it that can provide meaningful clinical information and an objective perspective. Assessment of pain, like any other assessment process, involves taking a comprehensive history, performing a physical assessment, and developing a monitoring and documentation plan. The critical care setting offers some unique challenges to the assessment of pain. Patients who are acutely ill—particularly if they are receiving ventilatory support, are heavily sedated, or have cognitive impairments—may have diminished ability to verbalize pain. Unless they have been taught how to rate and communicate their pain in advance of a critical care episode, pain assessment becomes even more subjective. The pain assessment questionnaires and tools most likely to be useful in the critical care setting are discussed in the following sections.

Qualitative Assessment

The qualitative assessment includes basic information about the history and nature of the pain. Key points to assess are the *location* or locations of the pain, *onset* and *duration, characteristics* (e.g., sharp, dull, aching, burning), and *factors affecting the pain* (i.e., what makes the pain better or worse). The words a patient chooses to describe the pain are very helpful indicators. Neuropathic pain especially stands out by the way it is described (see previous section on Pain Classifications). Other words that typify the affective component of pain may reveal the impact pain has on the individual (e.g., horrible, unbearable, exhausting).

100 mm Visual Analogue Scale

NO PAIN _____ WORST PAIN

Directions: Have patient indicate how much pain is experienced by making a mark on the line somewhere between the two extremes. Measure from the left endpoint to the mark to obtain the rating.

Graphic Rating Scale

NO PAIN   0--1--2--3--4--5--6--7--8--9--10   WORST PAIN

Directions: Have patient point to or circle the number that best represents how much pain is experienced.

Verbal Rating Scales

0 = NO PAIN   0 = NO PAIN

10 = WORST POSSIBLE PAIN   10 = WORST POSSIBLE PAIN

Categorical Scale

0 = NO PAIN

1 = MILD PAIN

2 = MODERATE PAIN

3 = SEVERE PAIN

4 = EXCRUCIATING PAIN

FIGURE 10–3. Selected pain assessment tools.

Quantitative Assessment

Quantitative assessment of pain helps the patient to estimate and communicate the intensity of the pain, which can be used as a key monitoring parameter. Of the numerous tools that measure pain intensity, no single tool can be said to be the best or most accurate and therefore applicable in every situation. The most important principle in choosing a tool is to select a tool that the patient can comprehend and use effectively. Figure 10–3 shows some of the commonly used scales. The 0-to-10 scale (or other numerical scales) is used most frequently. A numerical rating system is a commonly understood concept used in a variety of subjective evaluations (e.g., "five-star" restaurants, hotels, or movies). A verbal, numerical scale requires abstract thinking, and some patients may benefit from having a graphic image to accompany the numbers. The faces scale, shown in Figure 10–4, was developed specifically for young children (developmental age 3

years or older); however, it has proved to be useful with adults as well. When there is a language barrier or a functional barrier to communication (e.g., a patient receiving ventilatory support), a more visual tool, such as the faces scale, can be very helpful after it has been properly interpreted and its use demonstrated. If the patient is able to comprehend the purpose of the faces scale, the nurse has only to ask the patient to point (or make another agreed-upon gesture) to the face or number that indicates the intensity of the pain.

The nurse needs to keep in mind two key principles when asking a patient to rate his or her pain. First, *only the patient experiencing the pain can accurately evaluate it.* This requires not only asking the patient about the pain but also believing the patient. Not all patients respond to pain in a predictable or observable manner, and there are no objective methods to validate the patient's complaint. It is the rare patient who is dishonest or deceitful about the nature or intensity of

Faces Pain Rating Scale

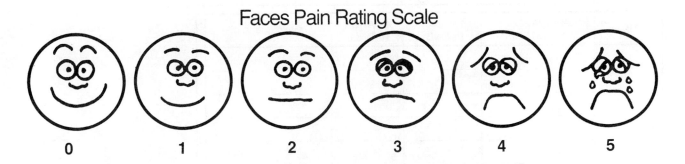

0   1   2   3   4   5

Explain to the person that each face is for a person who feels happy because he has no pain (hurt) or sad because he has some or a lot of pain. **Face 0** is very happy because he doesn't hurt at all. **Face 1** hurts just a little bit. **Face 2** hurts a little more. **Face 3** hurts even more. **Face 4** hurts a whole lot. **Face 5** hurts as much as you can imagine, although you don't have to be crying to feel this bad. Ask the person to choose the face that best describes how he is feeling.

Rating scale is recommended for persons age 3 years and older.

FIGURE 10–4. Pain faces scale. (From Wong, D and Whaley, LF: Clinical Manual of Pediatric Nursing. CV Mosby, St. Louis, 1992, with permission.)

the pain. The nurse's most helpful response is to accept the patient's rating and use it to evaluate, over time, how the pain changes in response to interventions.

Second, *there are no "normal" values.* The ratings that a patient chooses are influenced by a variety of social and cultural factors. If patient A reports a pain intensity of 5 on a scale of 0 to 10 and patient B rates his pain as an 8, the nurse cannot conclude that patient B has more pain than patient A. Between-patient comparisons of pain ratings are not valid. A rating of 5 may represent moderate pain to one patient; yet another may use that number to indicate a pain level that is intolerable. It is helpful for the nurse to clarify the individual meanings of the various ratings that a patient uses to interpret the response accurately. At baseline or when asking the patient to reflect over a period of time, it is helpful to ask for ratings of the *present pain, worst pain* (e.g., over the previous 24 hours), *least pain,* and *tolerable pain.* Pain ratings are most helpful when monitored for change over a period of time in the same patient.

When the patient is unable to communicate information about pain because of cognitive or physical impairments, the nurse must rely on more subjective observations. It is critical to remember that even though a patient is unable to communicate effectively or is comatose, significant pain *can* be a problem. Restlessness, agitation, moaning, and grimacing (particularly with movement) are often signs of pain that can be used to monitor response to interventions.

Pain as a Vital Sign

Systematic assessment of pain is vital to effective pain management, and pain should be considered as a vital sign—equally as important to the well-being of the patient as blood pressure, pulse, oxygen saturation, and other critical parameters. Frequency of assessment, as for any other parameter, depends on the severity and stability of the problem. When pain is acute and not well controlled, assessments should be made and documented often. A postoperative patient awakening from anesthesia should be asked about pain whenever other vital signs are taken. When satisfactory pain control is verbalized, the frequency of the assessment can be decreased. For patients whose pain is well controlled over a period of several days, it may be necessary to ask about pain only when routine vital signs are done (at least once daily.) When pain changes or new pain develops, then the frequency of assessment can be increased until stability is reestablished.

Documentation of the pain assessment is as important as actually doing the assessment. Inclusion of a space for pain ratings on a flow sheet (Fig. 10–5) is critical to recognizing trends and evaluating responses to interventions. It is therefore important to use the same scale each time and to be certain that everyone who reviews the documentation is cognizant of the type of scale used. A rating of 5 on a 0-to-5 scale would be significantly different from a 5 on a 0-to-10 scale. To simplify the interpretation of pain ratings, it is helpful to document them as a fraction with the numerator indicating the rating and the denominator indicating the maximum number of points on the scale. For example, a rating of 5 on a scale of 0 to 10 would be documented as 5/10, whereas a rating of 5 on the faces scale would be documented as 5/5. This method allows for needed flexibility in choosing a scale that the patient is comfortable using while facilitating accurate interpretation of the ratings.

TIME	MEDICATION ADMINISTERED	PAIN RATING	SEDATION RATING	COMMENTS

Pain Scale: 0 = No Pain   OR   0 = No Pain
                   10 = Worst Pain   10 = Worst Pain

Sedation Scale: 0 = Alert, easy to arouse
                    1 = Occasionally drowsy, easy to arouse
                    2 = Frequently drowsy, easy to arouse
                    3 = Sleeping, easy to arouse
                    4 = Somnolent, difficult to arouse
                    5 = Unable to arouse

FIGURE 10–5. Pain flow sheet.

PRINCIPLES OF PAIN MANAGEMENT

Pharmacologic Management with Opioids

Opioids (narcotic analgesics) are the mainstay of pain management, especially in patients with acute and cancer pain. Unfortunately, they are among the most underused and misunderstood categories of drugs (see previous section on "Barriers to Effective Pain Management"). Appropriate use of opioids to relieve pain, however, has been demonstrated to improve outcomes and quality of life.[6,17]

Pharmacology

Opioids produce analgesia by binding to the opiate receptor sites located principally in the brain and spinal cord, although some receptors are located outside the central nervous system. There are three types of opioids: (1) pure agonists, (2) mixed agonist/antagonists, and (3) partial agonists (Table 10–1). *Pure agonists* can be relied on to produce effective analgesia and, except for meperidine, can be given in escalating doses titrated until pain is relieved without reaching a

TABLE 10–1
Opioid Analgesic Classifications

Pure Agonist Opioids
Codeine sulfate (codeine phosphate in Tylenol No. 3 and No. 4)
Fentanyl (Sublimaze)
Hydrocodone (with acetaminophen in Vicodin and Lortab)
Hydromorphone (Dilaudid)
Levorphanol (Levo-Dromoran)
Meperidine (Demerol)
Morphine sulfate (MSIR, Roxanol; controlled release: MS Contin, Oramorph SR)
Methadone hydrochloride (Dolophine)
Oxycodone (Roxicodone) (with acetaminophen in Percocet and aspirin in Percodan)
Oxymorphone (Numorphan)
Propoxyphene (Darvon, with acetaminophen in Darvocet)

Partial Agonists
Buprenorphine (Buprenex)
Dezocine (Dalgan)

Mixed Agonist Antagonists
Butorphanol (Stadol)
Nalbuphine (Nubain)
Pentazocine (Talwin)

ceiling effect. There is no maximum opioid dose for most agonists. Meperidine (Demerol) is limited in its dosing flexibility because one of its metabolites, normeperidine, is toxic and may produce central nervous system excitability (delerium, tremors, or seizures) if used for extended periods or in high doses.[18,19] The toxic effects are enhanced in patients with renal insufficiency or hepatic impairment.

The *mixed agonist/antagonist opioids* possess the ability both to produce analgesia and, paradoxically, to antagonize analgesia. When given alone to a patient who is *not* receiving a pure agonist, a mixed agonist/antagonist drug binds to the opiate receptor sites to produce analgesia. However, in a patient already receiving a pure agonist, the agonist/antagonist acts as an antagonist by displacing the agonist from the opiate receptor sites. This could have significant consequences in the patient who has developed physical dependence (see previous section on Barriers to Effective Pain Management) by precipitating a withdrawal reaction in addition to reversing the analgesia. Withdrawal and exacerbation of pain are to be avoided, particularly in the critically ill and debilitated patient. The mixed agonist/antagonist opioids are also associated with a higher incidence of psychotomimetic side effects; therefore, they cannot be escalated above standard dose levels and are not suitable for long-term use. The action of partial agonists is not yet well understood.

All opioids produce analgesia by means of the same basic mechanism, as previously discussed.[20] The key to effective pain control is titration of the dose to achieve relief of pain. For the pure agonist opioids, there is a great deal of variability in dosage and no maximum dose. Some of the opioids such as morphine and hydromorphone are referred to as "strong" and others such as codeine and hydrocodone as "weak"; however, they are essentially capable of producing equally effective analgesia if given in sufficient doses. The so-called weak opioids are usually combined with aspirin or acetaminophen, and the dose cannot be safely escalated beyond a certain point because of dose-limiting renal and hepatic toxicity associated with the nonopioid drug. Although the milligram strength or potency varies from drug to drug (how much of the drug must be given), the strong opioids can be thought of as being equally effective when given in equianalgesic doses. For example, a dose of hydromorphone requires only 1.5 mg to produce the same degree of analgesia as 10 mg morphine. Likewise, an orally administered drug can be equally as potent in efficacy as a parenterally administered drug if the dose is adjusted to compensate for biotransformation.

When an opioid is administered through the gastrointestinal tract, it is subject to a greater degree of biotransformation because of what is known as the "first-pass effect." The circulation surrounding the upper gastrointestinal tract and, to some degree, the lower tract, routes a significant portion of its blood directly into the hepatic circulation without reaching the systemic circulation. Therefore, a portion of the drug ingested (or administered through a feeding tube or through the rectum) is subject to being transformed into nonanalgesic metabolites. In a patient receiving adequate analgesia from 10 mg morphine sulfate given parenterally, it would take 30 mg orally to achieve the same effect because about 20 mg is metabolized before reaching the systemic circulation. The parenteral-to-oral ratio varies somewhat from drug to drug; therefore, having a conversion chart (Table 10–2) available for ready reference is helpful when a route change is necessitated because of change in status such as bowel obstruction or another contraindication to the oral route. Table 10–3 is designed to facilitate changing from one drug to another. For example, if a patient experiences an intolerable side effect such as persistent nausea, an equianalgesic dose of hydromorphone could be calculated. Morphine is the standard for comparison because it is the most widely used opioid and more is known about its pharmacokinetics. It is also one of the most versatile drugs by virtue of its availability in forms for most routes of administration.

Routes of Administration

The oral route of opioid administration is generally the preferred route because of its simplicity and cost-effectiveness.[14,21] However, opioids are extremely versatile drugs and can be given by numerous routes with

TABLE 10–2
Equianalgesic Dose Conversion Chart

Drug	Parenteral Dose (mg)	Oral Dose (mg)	IV to Oral Conversion Factor	IV-Oral Duration of Action (hours)
Morphine	10	30	3*	3–4
Controlled-release	—	30	—	8–12
Methadone†	10	20	2	4–8
Hydromorphone	1.5	7.5	5	2–3
Fentanyl	100 μg	—	—	1
Meperidine	75	300	4	2–3
Levorphanol‡	2	4	2	3–6
Oxymorphone	1	6	6 §	3–6
Codeine	130	200	1.5	3–4
Oxycodone ‖	—	30	—	3–5
Hydrocodone¶	—	**	—	3–5

*Factor listed is for chronic dosing; single doses may require 6:1 conversion.

†Long half-life; observe for drug accumulation and side effects after 48–72 hours.

‡Same caution as for methadone.

§Available in rectal form only.

‖ Except for Roxicodone, these drugs are combined with aspirin or acetaminophen in doses of 325–750 mg. Note: Dosage must be monitored for safe limits of aspirin or acetaminophen.

¶Same consideration as for oxycodone regarding aspirin and acetaminophen.

**Equivalence data are not substantiated, thought to approximate codeine.

Source: Data from Foley, KM: The treatment of cancer pain. N Engl J Med 212:84–95, 1985, and Portenoy, R: Three-step ladder for management of cancer pain. Anesthesiology News, 1989.

TABLE 10–3
Drug-to-Drug Conversion Table

Oral (to Morphine from)	Factor	Parenteral (to Morphine from)	Factor
Methadone	1.5	Methadone	1
Hydromorphone	4	Hydromorphone	6.7
Meperidine	0.1	Meperidine	0.13
Levorphanol	7.5	Levorphanol	5
Codeine	0.15	Codeine	0.08
Oxycodone	1	Oxymorphone	10
Hydrocodone	0.15	Buprenorphine	25

To Convert From Another Narcotic to Morphine
1. Total the amount of analgesic taken in a 24-hour period that effectively controls the patient's pain.
2. Multiply by the conversion factor shown in the table.
3. Because there is often incomplete cross-tolerance to a change in narcotic, a lower dose than the equivalent may be needed to maintain efficacy. To account for this, divide the above result by 2 to arrive at a *starting* dose. (Note: There is great individual variability; monitor the effect and be prepared to titrate the dose during the first 24 hours.)
4. Divide the calculated 24-hour dose by the appropriate number of doses per day (e.g., six doses for regular, oral morphine at 4-hour intervals or two doses for controlled-release morphine at 12-hour intervals).

EXAMPLE

Mrs. Jones has had good pain control with oral hydromorphone, 4 mg q/3 h. She is to be changed to controlled-release morphine.

(1) 4 mg × 8 doses = 32 mg

(2) 32 mg × 4 (conversion factor) = 128 mg morphine

(3) $\dfrac{128 \text{ mg}}{2}$ = 64 mg every 24 hours (to allow for incomplete cross tolerance)

(4) $\dfrac{64 \text{ mg}}{2 \text{ doses}}$ = 32 mg every 12 hours (Note: Closest tablet size is 30 mg)

---

equivalent efficacy. Choice of route of administration and drug depends on a variety of patient factors, including (1) the nature and stability of the pain, (2) the patient's ability to take oral medications, (3) the functional status of the patient (what regimen he or she is capable of maintaining), (4) the side effects, (5) the dosage forms/availability, and (6) the cost. Selecting the appropriate option also requires an understanding of the process of biotransformation and equianalgesic dosing guidelines. The following are some factors to be considered when selecting a route for opioid administration.[14,18,22]

Oral. The oral route of opioid administration is preferred because it is simple, convenient, well tolerated by most patients, and if doses are adequate, as effective as other routes. Morphine is currently available in controlled or sustained-release (MS Contin, Oramorph SR) pill form, which allows for longer dosing intervals and more sustained pain control. Additional opioids are being developed in sustained-release form, and their future availability will add even greater versatility to the oral route. Another advantage of oral administration is that it is usually the most cost-effective route.

For these reasons, the oral route should be used unless specific patient factors require another route, which is often the case in the critical care setting.

Rectal. The rectal route, although infrequently used, is a simple and cost-effective route when the patient cannot take oral medication and the rectal dose requirement is not very high. Generally, the dose is equivalent to the oral dose. There is some anatomic variability in the degree to which the colorectal circulation is subject to the first-pass effect, so it is important to evaluate patients closely for analgesic efficacy initially and adjust the dose as needed. Note that patients who are neutropenic and immunosuppressed are not suitable candidates for rectal administration because of an increased risk for trauma to the rectal mucosa—and subsequently infection—when this route is used.

Intravenous. The intravenous route of opioid administration provides the most immediate response, with onset of effect within 10 to 15 minutes. However, the duration of effect is usually shorter than with other parenteral routes. Intravenous administration is most suitable in acute care situations in which rapid titration is desirable or oral administration is prohibited (e.g., patients with bowel obstruction or severe nausea and vomiting).

Subcutaneous. The subcutaneous route is often overlooked but is, in fact, one of the more desirable methods of parenteral opioid administration. Subcutaneous injections are less painful and more predictably absorbed than those given intramuscularly. The subcutaneous route is also effective for small-volume, continuous infusion and is often used in the hospice setting when vascular access becomes a problem or is no longer desirable.

Intramuscular. The intramuscular route is the least desirable and reliable route of opioid administration because of injection-related pain and erratic absorption. This route is contraindicated in patients who are thrombocytopenic or immunosuppressed because of its increased risk of infection and bleeding.

Transdermal. The transdermal route is the newest means of opioid administration, and currently only fentanyl (Duragesic) is available by this method. Fentanyl is especially suitable as a transdermal preparation because it is very potent for its molecular weight—100 μg (0.1 mg) equals 10 mg morphine. Therefore, small quantities can be used, allowing for a practical patch size. It takes about 8 hours after initial patch application for the blood level of the drug to reach a steady state; therefore, transdermal administration is most suitable once pain control has been stabilized using another drug such as morphine. Conversion from parenteral morphine to the appropriate transdermal fentanyl dose can be accomplished as outlined in Table 10–4. When discontinuing a patch, it is important to recognize that a reservoir of the drug remains in the subcutaneous tissue and may take 16 hours or longer to be eliminated. Therefore, if a patient has experienced an untoward effect, close monitoring is needed for an extended period.

TABLE 10–4
Transdermal Fentanyl Conversion Table

Parenteral Morphine (mg/24 h)	Transdermal Fentanyl Equivalent (μg/h)
8–22	25
23–37	50
38–52	75
53–67	100
68–82	125
83–97	150
98–112	175
113–127	200

Source: Data from Janssen Pharmaceutica, Clinical Monograph, 1991.

Directions: To Convert to Transdermal Fentanyl (Duragesic):
1. Determine the 24-hour morphine equivalent dose (see Table 10–3).
2. Select the μg/h dose according to the ranges listed above. For doses > 100 μg/h, multiple patches can be used, but the manufacturer recommends no more that 400 μg/h.
3. Duration of action is *usually* 72 hours, but there is individual variability and some patients may require more frequent patch changes. Patients should be monitored closely during the transition period. It may take as long as 14–24 hours to achieve a stable blood level; therefore, anticipate that more frequent PRN dosing may be required for pain control.
4. Patients should have access to a PRN dose of another opioid such as morphine or hydromorphone for breakthrough pain.

Epidural. Originally used primarily for short-term applications (e.g., labor and postoperative pain), the epidural route has become increasingly used in the management of chronic pain. Drugs administered epidurally are mostly absorbed across the dura and circulated in the cerebrospinal fluid to the opiate receptor sites in the brain and spinal cord. Although a small portion of the drug may be absorbed through the epidural capillary circulation, most of the drug is delivered directly to the central nervous system. As a result, very little of the drug is subject to biotransformation, and much smaller doses can be used to achieve the same analgesic effect. This is particularly helpful in patients who require high doses or who have been unable to tolerate opioid side effects such as nausea and sedation. Local anesthetic agents are also used in conjunction with opioids in epidural infusions to enhance analgesia. Patients must be carefully selected for this route when long-term administration is considered. To decrease the risk of infection, catheters can be tunneled under the skin to place the exit port away from the insertion site; however, patients must be capable of managing the techniques and equipment (e.g., infusion pumps, catheter care) necessary to maintain this route. Subcutaneous infusion pumps can be fully implanted and filled with a concentrated drug requiring infrequent refilling; however, the devices are expensive and require a surgical procedure, and they generally are not cost-effective unless the patient is expected to live longer than 3 months.

Intrathecal/Intraventricular. Drugs can be administered directly to the opiate receptor sites *without* being subjected to biotransformation via spinal catheters (intrathecal administration) or an implanted device such as an Ommaya reservoir, which is placed subcutaneously (usually in the frontal region) and connected to a catheter inserted through a burr hole in the skull to give access to the ventricles. These access devices can also be connected to implanted pumps. Consequently, these methods of administration provide the most analgesia for the smallest dose and longer duration of action.

Careful screening of patients for any of the "high-tech" pain management procedures (parenteral, epidural, and intrathecal infusions or implanted pumps) is essential. Other routes that are more cost-effective and carry fewer risks should be explored exhaustively by professionals skilled in pain management before such extraordinary measures are considered for long-term use.

Schedule of Administration

Schedule of administration is another important factor in tailoring drug dosing to meet individual patient needs. Providing medication on a regular rather than PRN basis is the recommended practice, even for short-term, acute pain such as postoperative pain. Studies have shown that it takes less medication to control pain when given on an "around-the-clock" basis compared with a PRN schedule. PRN dosing leads to greater peaks and valleys in analgesic blood levels between doses, especially when patients wait until the pain is severe before requesting medication. PRN administration is most appropriate for supplemental dosing for acute exacerbations or "breakthroughs" of pain, in addition to the scheduled medication or when pain occurs only intermittently and infrequently.[6,14]

Knowledge of expected duration of action of each opioid is essential (see Table 10–2). If a short-acting drug such as hydromorphone (which can be expected to last only 2 to 3 hours) is ordered to be given every 6 hours, the patient will have to endure increasing pain for as long as 3 to 4 hours until another dose is given. A common mistake when attempting to taper or "wean" a patient from an opioid is to increase the interval between doses. Unfortunately, this approach often exacerbates the pain problem. It is better to decrease the dose while maintaining the appropriate interval, according to the expected duration of action of the drug.

The most sensible method of pain control is to give whatever dose it takes to achieve control and to devise a method of management that sustains that control for whatever period of time is needed. When rapid titration is necessary, as in postoperative pain or severe, uncontrolled pain, the patient-controlled analgesia (PCA) pump is ideal. Most pumps are capable of providing a continuous (basal) infusion in combination with a patient-administered (demand) dose on a PRN basis. This allows for highly individualized dosing and sustained analgesia. As the acute problem resolves (e.g., healing takes place) and pain diminishes, the patient requires fewer doses and the drug can be tapered as rapidly as the pain permits. When tapering the dose administered by a PCA pump, it is best to begin by decreasing the basal rate gradually (e.g., 50% every 12 hours). If the number of demand doses the patient requires does not increase significantly, the patient will probably tolerate further dose reduction. If the demand doses required increase, then the basal rate should not be reduced further until the patient is able to tolerate it and requires fewer demand doses. Dose titration always requires frequent assessment of the patient's pain ratings to guide the process.

For those with persistent or chronic pain, it is helpful to draw from the experience of the insulin-dependent diabetic.[23] Diabetes is a chronic condition in which the primary goal is *control* rather than *cure*. When insulin is required, the physician typically selects a long-acting form of insulin that will provide coverage for most of the patient's needs over a 24-hour period. However, blood glucose levels are not steady; they respond to a host of influences, from dietary intake to physical activity. To treat episodic elevations of glucose, a short-acting form of insulin is given, usually on a sliding scale depending on the severity of the problem.

Chronic pain is also a very dynamic state influenced by variables such as activity, positioning, and emotions. Controlled-release pills, continuous infusions, and transdermal delivery systems can be used to provide sustained, baseline analgesia much like long-acting insulin. To continue the analogy, short-acting and rapid-onset forms of opioids (e.g., regular morphine sulfate in pill or liquid form or PCA doses) can be used to treat acute pain exacerbations brought on by movement, treatments, or other factors.

Another important principle is to take a preventive approach to controlling pain. When an event or activity such as coughing, walking, or physical therapy is known to provoke pain, the PRN dose should be given *in advance* of that event, if possible. PRN doses that are preventive or supplemental for breakthrough pain are often referred to as "rescue doses."

Acute Pain Management in the Setting of Chronic Pain

Patients with chronic pain may experience acute episodes of pain when surgery is required or some other traumatic event occurs. When faced with a new pain superimposed on pain that has been managed with opioids, it is critical to recognize that the new pain requires treatment in addition to—not instead of—the pre-existing condition. It should also be anticipated that the doses required to treat the new situation will need to be higher than the standard doses that might ordinarily be ordered. This is in part because of opioid tolerance, as well as decreased tolerance of pain due to the chronic nature of the pain.

CASE STUDY: PATIENT WITH PAIN

Mr. W is a 62-year-old man with a history of sarcoma involving the soft tissues of the right lumbar paraspinal region. The tumor was resected initially in a wide-excision procedure. Mr. W was also treated with postoperative chemotherapy and external-beam radiation therapy. Several months after the surgery, the incision site became infected, resulting in an open draining wound that has failed to heal because of prior radiation to that site. The wound has been a constant source of pain, especially during the daily wound irrigation and dressing procedure. Mr. W was given 180 mg controlled-release morphine in the morning and 120 mg in the evening. In addition, he took 90 mg immediate-release morphine sulfate prior to each dressing change and 30 mg as needed for breakthrough pain. Mr. W also required occasional doses of diazepam, 10 mg, to control intermittent paraspinous muscle spasm. On this regimen, he maintained good pain control for several years, during which time the wound on his back remained open, requiring daily care.

Three years after Mr. W's diagnosis, he developed bilateral pulmonary metastases and was scheduled to have surgery to resect the tumors—first from the right lung and 1 month later from the left lung. The right thoracotomy was performed without complication, and he was admitted to the intensive care unit. Mr. W reported severe pain (10/10), was highly anxious, and could not be extubated when expected. The postoperative pain orders were for morphine sulfate via (PCA) pump at 3 mg/h basal rate with 1 mg every 15 minutes PRN as a PCA demand dose. Mr. W's *preoperative* daily morphine requirement had been about 420 to 480 mg (controlled-release plus PRN doses) per day. The parenteral equivalent of that dose, using the 1-to-3 parenteral-to-oral ratio, would be about 140 to 160 mg. Consequently, Mr. W would have had to press the PCA dose button every 15 minutes for 24 hours just to get the amount of medication he was receiving on a daily basis before the surgery (if he received four 1-mg PCA doses every hour plus the 3 mg/h basal rate, he would get a total of 168 mg). In fact, Mr. W was not using the PCA dose very often because it did not help his pain.

A pain specialist was consulted while the patient was in the ICU because of concern that the amount of morphine was responsible for the difficulty in extubating the patient. After assessing the patient and realizing the patient was actually getting less than his prior daily morphine dose in addition to having undergone major surgery, Mr. W was given sequential 10-mg bolus doses of morphine every 10 minutes until he achieved pain relief. He received a total of 50 mg morphine over the next hour, and his pain went from 10/10 to 6/10, a rating he reported as being tolerable. Mr. W's anxiety had also diminished considerably. At that time, the basal rate of the infusion was increased to 30 mg/h and the PCA dose to 10 mg every 10 minutes PRN. Mr. W was extubated a few hours later and was discharged from the ICU the next morning. Throughout the upward dose titration period, Mr. W's O_2 saturation, pulse, and repiratory rate remained within acceptable parameters. Within 24 hours, the basal rate of the infusion was decreased to 15 mg/h, which Mr. W tolerated well, requiring only occasional PCA doses when he had his respiratory treatments or got out of bed. The following day, his controlled-release morphine was resumed at the preoperative doses and the PCA basal rate was discontinued, leaving only the PCA dose on a PRN basis. At the time of Mr. W's discharge, he was taking about the same amount of morphine as he had prior to surgery.

This case study illustrates the need for individualized and rapid-dose titration to effect pain relief when a patient with chronic pain encounters an episode of acute pain. The doses required to relieve pain in these situations cannot be reliably predicted; therefore, it is essential that the patient be as closely monitored for pain relief as for other vital functions.

Mr. W went on to have his second thoracotomy and in fact had a total of five thoracic procedures over the course of the next few years. After each surgical procedure, he required rapid bolus dosing ranging from 80 to 150 mg morphine to get his pain under control and was subsequently maintained on a PCA pump. In each situation, Mr. W remained on the increased dosage for only a few days and was able to tolerate prompt tapering of the dose back to his baseline daily morphine requirement.

Adjuvant Analgesics

Nonsteroidal Anti-Inflammatory Drugs

Many painful conditions are accompanied by inflammation that triggers the release of prostaglandins, which are thought to cause pain by activating and sensitizing peripheral nociceptors. Nonsteroidal antiinflammatory drugs (NSAIDs) are believed to decrease inflammation and produce analgesia and antipyresis by blocking prostaglandin production. NSAIDs alone may be effective in relieving mild to moderate pain in conditions with an inflammatory component. More often these agents are used in combination with opioids. The peripheral mechanism of prostaglandin inhibition works synergistically to enhance opioid analgesia. Although this classification of analgesic is very useful in relieving pain, judicious use and frequent evaluation for side effects are critical. Most NSAIDs have a significant potential for gastrointestinal, renal, or hepatic toxicity, which may limit their usefulness in some patients. In addition, except for choline magnesium trisalicylate and diflunisal, NSAIDs interfere with platelet aggregation, prohibiting their use in patients receiving chemotherapy or those with blood or bone marrow disease.

Response to NSAIDs is highly variable, and it is difficult to predict which one will be useful in any given patient. The selected drug should be given consistently for 7 to 10 days before it is determined to be ineffective. If a satisfactory response is not achieved with one NSAID, another one from a different class may be effective (Table 10–5).

TABLE 10–5
Nonsteroidal Anti-Inflammatory Drugs

Class	Generic (Trade) Names	Comments
p-Aminophenol derivative	Acetaminophen (Tylenol, Datril, Panadol)	Not anti-inflammatory; no gastrointestinal (GI) toxicity or antiplatelet action Dosage in excess of 6000 mg/d associated with hepatotoxicity
Salicylates	Aspirin	GI toxicity, bleeding
	Choline magnesium trisalicylate (Trilisate)	Minimal GI toxicity, less risk of antiplatelet effect
	Diflunisal (Dolobid)	Less GI toxicity than aspirin
	Salsalate (Disalcid)	Renal and hepatotoxicity at higher doses, less risk of antiplatelet effect
Propionic acids	Diclofenac (Voltaren)	
	Flurbiprofen (Ansaid)	Renal and hepatotoxicity at higher doses
	Ibuprofen (Motrin, Advil)	Available over the counter (OTC)
	Ketoprofen (Orudis)	Renal and hepatotoxicity at higher doses
	Naproxen (Naprosyn, Aleve)	Available OTC
Acetic acids	Indomethacin (Indocin)	Higher GI and CNS toxicity than propionic acids
	Ketorolac (Toradol)	Renal toxicity; available in parenteral form
	Sulindac (Clinoril)	Less renal toxicity
	Tolmetin (Tolectin)	Renal and hepatotoxicity in higher doses
Oxicam	Piroxicam (Feldene)	Peptic ulcer, especially in the elderly
Fenamate	Meclofenamate (Meclomen)	Fairly high GI toxicity
Pyranocarboxylic acids	Etodolac (Lodine)	Low incidence of GI bleeding
Naphthylalkanones	Nabumetone (Relafen)	Low incidence of GI bleeding

Source: Data from Portenoy, RK: Three-step analgesic ladder for management of cancer pain. Anesthesiology News, 1989.

Corticosteroids

Corticosteroids, like NSAIDs, are particularly useful in treating pain in which inflammation is a primary or contributing factor; these drugs also interfere with prostaglandin production. The more potent corticosteroids such as dexamethasone are particularly important in relieving pressure and traction on nerves caused by peritumoral edema associated with bone metastases or trauma to the spine. Other benefits of corticosteroids in patients with metastatic disease are euphoric effects and appetite stimulation, which enhance the patient's sense of well-being. However, corticosteroid use may be limited by a host of side effects such as immunosuppression, gastrointestinal bleeding, myopathy, hyperglycemia, and psychological disturbances.

Tricyclic Antidepressants

Tricyclic antidepressants play several roles in pain management. Although many patients with chronic pain do become clinically depressed and would therefore benefit from antidepressant therapy, the primary indication for a tricyclic agent is for its intrinsic analgesic effect. The mechanism for analgesia is thought to be a neurochemical one through inhibition of serotonin reuptake at the synapse. In neuropathic or deafferentation pain in particular, it is believed that serotonin becomes depleted at the synapse and that blocking reuptake normalizes stimulus transmission. However, newer serotonin-specific antidepressants such as fluoxetine (Prozac) have not been found to be as effective as the older tricyclic antidepressants such as amitriptyline (Elavil), nortriptyline (Pamelor), or desipramine (Norpramin), suggesting that there are additional mechanisms at work in the modulation of pain.[24]

In neuropathic pain syndromes such as postherpetic pain or brachial plexopathy, the tricyclic drugs are considered front-line therapy. Tricyclics may also potentiate analgesia by increasing plasma levels of opioids, thereby enhancing bioavailability of the opioid. Tricyclic-mediated analgesia can be achieved at doses considerably lower than those used to treat clinical depression. For example, 10 to 25 mg amitriptyline may be effective as an analgesic, whereas 100 mg or more is required to treat a significant depression.

Patient education regarding the use of tricyclic antidepressants is especially important. Patients who have experienced attitudes from caregivers that their pain is not real may have their fears that the pain is "psychological" reinforced when given an antidepressant. It should be stressed that the medication is being given for its analgesic effect. The patient should also be informed that because tricyclics work by a different mechanism than do traditional analgesics, the response will also be different. Unlike opioids, tricyclics do not exert a prompt or dramatic analgesia. In fact, the effect may be very subtle, and when questioned about relief, the patient may not be able to discriminate a noticeable change until the does has

been carefully titrated upward. It is helpful for patients to know this so that they do not stop taking the medication on the basis that it is not helping the pain. Because of the potential for dose-limiting side effects of tricyclic antidepressants due to anticholinergic actions, it is wise to start with a low dose and carefully titrate until the desired effect is achieved. It usually takes 7 to 10 days to establish an effective blood level, and the dose may require gradual titration. For pain management purposes, a single dose is usually administered at bedtime.

One side effect of tricyclic antidepressants, which is actually beneficial, is sedation. Sleep disturbances are common in prolonged pain states, and the addition of a tricyclic may restore more normal sleep patterns, often contributing significantly to the patient's sense of well-being. Education is important here as well, because the patient may mistake the tricyclic for a sleeping pill and stop taking it after sleep patterns are normalized. The patient should also be instructed to anticipate feeling "heavy-headed" or drugged in the morning. This commonly occurs when the drug is initiated or the dose is increased, but this effect usually dissipates over time. Other side effects that may be problematic or dose-limiting are dry mouth, cardiac arrhythmias, and postural hypotension. These agents should therefore be used with caution in the elderly or in patients with a history of cardiac abnormalities.

Anticonvulsant Drugs

Anticonvulsants such as carbamazepine (Tegretol), phenytoin (Dilantin), and valproic acid (Depakene) are indicated in the treatment of neuropathic pain, particularly when the pain is characterized by shooting or lancinating qualities. These drugs are believed to work by suppressing the aberrant neuronal firing that occurs with nerve damage. Like tricyclics and NSAIDs, anticonvulsants are associated with significant side effects that require careful evaluation and follow-up. Among the potentially serious side effects are bone marrow depression and hepatic dysfunction. Patients may also experience symptoms of ataxia or diplopia. Regular monitoring of blood counts and liver function as well as careful dose titration and monitoring of blood levels are recommended.

Parenteral and Oral Local Anesthetics

Parenteral infusions of local anesthetics such as lidocaine have shown some usefulness in the management of painful diabetic neuropathy.[25] Trials of the newer sodium channel blocking agents such as mexiletine (Mexitil) that can be given orally have been found effective in neuropathic pain syndromes including diabetic neuropathy and trigeminal neuralgia. More research with this category of drugs is needed.

Psychotropic Drugs

When appropriately used, psychotropic drugs are significant adjuncts in the management of pain. Note,

---

RESEARCH APPLICATION: PARALYZED WITH PAIN: THE NEED FOR EDUCATION
Loper, KA, et al. Pain 37:315-316, 1989.

The practice of inducing neuromuscular paralysis for patients on ventilatory support has often been mistakenly believed to be a calm and painless state. Therapeutic paralysis without benefit of adequate analgesic and anxiolytic medication has been called into question, based on the outcome of several studies and critical examination of the practice.[34–36]

Purpose: The purpose of this study was to survey physician and critical care nurses regarding their knowledge of the analgesic and anxiolytic effects of narcotics, benzodiazepines, and neuromuscular blocking agents.

Methods: A questionnaire survey of 112 medical/surgical house staff and 258 critical care nurses was conducted. Respondents were asked to evaluate medications commonly used in conjunction with patients on ventilators. Narcotics included were fentanyl, meperidine, and morphine. Benzodiazepines included were diazepam, lorazepam, and midazolam. Neuromuscular blocking agents included were pancuronium and succinylcholine.

Results: Although narcotics were correctly identified by the respondents as being analgesic without being anxiolytic, many physicians and nurses *incorrectly* identified the neuromuscular blocking agents as being both analgesic and anxiolytic. Most also endorsed the common misconception that benzodiazepines are analgesic.

Practice Implications: Even under the best of circumstances, the critical care environment is highly stressful for patients. Those on ventilatory support are especially vulnerable to inadequate management of pain and anxiety because of diminished capacity to communicate their needs—a problem magnified many times with the addition of a neuromuscular blocking agent. Patients who have been able to recall their experiences have described them as terrifying.[32] Nurses should be vigilant in their assessment of comfort for these patients. When possible, a careful evaluation of pain and anxiety should be made prior to the induction of paralysis so that appropriate treatment of those symptoms can be initiated and evaluated for efficacy. When feedback from the patient is not attainable, nurses and physicians should anticipate the need for administration of analgesics and anxiolytics for the duration of the period of therapeutic paralysis. Physician and nurse colleagues may hold the misconceptions identified in this study; therefore, the nurse should be prepared to act as the patient advocate and seek appropriate treatment. Institutional policies and quality assurance activities should also be evaluated to address this problem.

---

however, that these agents are *not* substitutes for analgesics. Many practitioners believe that benzodiazepines such as lorazepam (Ativan) and diazepam (Valium) relieve pain. They do not (see Research Application). Inasmuch as anxiety and emotional distress may exacerbate pain or lower tolerance to pain, concurrent treatment of anxiety enhances pain treatment and improves the overall quality of life for the patient. Psychological problems such as anxiety, panic, depression, or other mood disorders should be specifically targeted and treated appropriately with pharmacologic and psychosocial interventions; however, the underlying pain problem also must be adequately addressed and treated. If appropriate analgesics are not provided, neither type of problem is likely to be resolved because continued pain most certainly exacerbates the psychological symptoms.

The benzodiazepines, particularly diazepam, are also useful in the management of muscle spasm, a type of pain that is less likely to respond to analgesics alone. Diazepam (Valium) and clonazepam (Klonopin) in relatively low doses are also helpful in managing myoclonic jerking, a common and sometimes discomforting side effect of opioid therapy.

Phenothiazines have often been promoted as potentiators of analgesia. There is little objective evidence to support this belief,[26] except for methotrimeprazine (Levoprome), which not only is a potent antiemetic but also has been shown to produce analgesia comparable to that of the opioids.[27] Phenothiazines and other antiemetic drugs are best used for their intended purpose, that is, when nausea or vomiting are concurrent problems or side effects of opioid analgesia.

Central Nervous System Stimulants

One of the most common side effects of opioid use, and one that is frequently responsible for self-undermedication by patients, is sedation. Most often, sedation is merely a function of sleep deprivation, which resolves as pain is relieved and normal sleep is restored. In some patients, however, somnolence is persistent and requires targeted therapy with a central nervous system (CNS) stimulant to maintain adequate analgesia. The simplest approach is to encourage the patient to increase caffeine intake, which alone may be enough to counteract the sedating effects of the opioids. A relatively small number of patients may require the addition of a stimulant medication such as dextroamphetamine or methylphenidate (Ritalin). These drugs should be given in the lowest dose that effectively reverses somnolence. They are usually given when the patient awakens in the morning and at noon or in the early afternoon, depending on the patient's activity requirements. Generally, these stimulants should not be given later than 2:00 or 3:00 PM so as not to interfere with normal sleep. CNS stimulants may also enhance analgesia, thus permitting lower opioid doses. Research has shown that the addition of a stimulant contributes to the overall sense of well-being in terminally ill patients by improving not only pain control but activity and appetite as well.[28]

Nonpharmacologic Interventions

Physical Therapy Modalities

Physical therapy modalities play an important role in pain management as primary and adjuvant interventions. Heat, cold, massage, exercise, and TENS are often more effective than analgesics in the treatment of painful muscle spasms associated with vertebral collapse or other skeletal injury. NSAIDs, analgesics, and muscle relaxants are used in the management of muscle spasm; however, for comprehensive management and rehabilitation, aggressive use of physical therapy modalities is essential. For the patient who is critically ill and who may not tolerate an aggressive physical therapy program, simple bedside techniques such as massage and the use of a heating pad may add measurably to patient comfort.

The use of TENS therapy is particularly helpful in situations in which pain is mild and well localized. The presumed mechanism of action of TENS is activation of endogenous pain-modulating pathways through stimulation of peripheral nerves.[29] TENS may also be used to enhance postoperative analgesia using sterile electrodes placed adjacent to the incision at the time of surgery.[30] Although the use of TENS techniques may reduce opioid requirements, which may improve functioning and reduce side effects, there is considerable variability in response among patients, and access to adequate analgesics should always be provided.

Anesthetic Interventions

In addition to providing the expertise for the management of epidural analgesia, anesthesia specialists may be called on to perform nerve blocks in carefully selected patients. Nerve blocks serve a variety of purposes in the management of pain. Blocks can be accomplished using local anesthetic agents, which exert a temporary or short-term effect, or with a neurodestructive agent such as alcohol or phenol, which provides a long-term effect. Blocks are further classified as to whether they are diagnostic, prognostic, preemptive, or therapeutic.[14,31]

Diagnostic blocks are useful in evaluating the nature of the pain and the specific pathways involved. A local anesthetic may be injected in a specific anatomic location so as to discriminate whether the pain source is somatic or visceral or whether there is a sympathetic mechanism.

Prognostic blocks are usually performed with short-acting local anesthetic agents such as lidocaine or bupivicaine prior to injection of a neurodestructive agent or performance of a surgical procedure in order to predict the outcome of the long-term intervention in terms of pain relief and potential side effects such as numbness. Diagnostic and prognostic blocks may be accomplished at the same time; in such situations, it is necessary for the patient to be able to cooperate and to describe the changes that occur to guide the anesthesiologist in placing of the drug and evaluating the outcome.

Preemptive blocks are performed to prevent painful sequelae of procedures that are expected to cause pain, as with dental procedures. Some early evidence suggests that preoperative and perioperative use of epidural analgesia may prevent the occurrence of phantom pain after amputation.[32]

Therapeutic blocks are undertaken to specifically treat painful conditions that are well defined and fit identified criteria. Such blocks are usually accomplished with a neurodestructive agent such as alcohol or phenol. Most therapeutic blocks are performed following a diagnostic or prognostic block using a short-acting local anesthetic.

One of the most effective therapeutic blocks is the *celiac plexus block*, which is indicated in the treatment of upper abdominal pain due to pancreatic cancer or chronic pancreatitis. The celiac nerve plexus is accessible from an anterior or posterior approach. The block is usually performed under fluoroscopic or computed tomography guidance, or it can be done during a surgical procedure.

Therapeutic blocks may provide complete or partial relief from pain for several weeks to several months. If the pain returns, a repeat block can often be performed with equivalent success. As with any procedure that provides a substantial change in pain in a patient who has been receiving opioid analgesics, it is critical that opioids not be withdrawn precipitously. The patient should be put on a dose-tapering schedule and monitored closely for signs of respiratory depression, oversedation, and of opiod withdrawal.

Neurosurgical Procedures

Neurosurgical procedures are usually indicated only when other more conservative and noninvasive treatment options have been exhausted. Patients must be carefully selected for these procedures, which are best performed by an experienced neurosurgeon who specializes in pain management. Neurosurgical techniques may involve procedures that are considered to be *neuroablative*, that is, those that are intended to be neurodestructive, or *neuroaugmentive*, that is, those that are designed to stimulate the nervous system to enhance endogenous pain mechanisms. Neurosurgery may also be indicated as a primary treatment for the underlying cause of pain, as with tumor excision or decompression procedures such as laminectomy or craniectomy.

Percutaneous cordotomy is a neuroablative technique generally indicated for the treatment of pain that is primarily unilateral and somatic in nature. The neurosurgeon creates a thermal lesion (using a radiofrequency generator), usually at the cervical level, to disrupt the pain-conducting tracts in the anterolateral quadrant of the spinal cord. The procedure can be accomplished under local anesthesia and under flouroscopic guidance, making the procedure less invasive and therefore better tolerated by debilitated patients. An open cordotomy may be done; however, it requires a laminectomy and is a more invasive procedure involving all the risks of surgery and general anesthesia.

Commissural myelotomy is a technique known to be effective for the treatment of midline pelvic or perineal pain. The neurosurgeon makes a longitudinal cut in the spinal cord to interrupt the spinothalamic tracts. This procedure is more invasive and requires an open, multilevel laminectomy to expose the desired segments of the lumbar or sacral spinal cord.

Neurosurgical procedures such as cordotomy and myelotomy carry significant risks, and the decision to proceed must be based on careful analysis of the risk-benefit ratio. Possible complications include loss of motor and sensory functions. A person with intact bowel and bladder function risks incontinence and the complications that accompany it. Pain relief may also decay over time, and there is the risk of replacing a somatic pain with a neuropathic pain that may be more difficult to manage. Therefore, these procedures are usually indicated only when life expectancy is limited and the benefits are more likely to outweigh the risks.

Spinal cord stimulation is a neruoaugmentive procedure in which electrodes are implanted to provide electrical stimulation directly to the cord. This approach is based on the same principle as that of TENS. The electrodes are usually placed close to the dorsal columns; hence the common designation as "dorsal column stimulation." The electrodes are sometimes placed via an epidural catheter but may also be placed in an open surgical procedure requiring a laminectomy. These techniques are most often used in the treatment of benign chronic pain syndromes.

NURSING ROLES IN THE MANAGEMENT OF PAIN

By the nature of the close nurse-patient relationship, nurses are in a particularly important position to take an active and assertive role in ensuring pain relief. No other healthcare professional has the same unique perspective from which to assess and evaluate the patient than the nurse at the bedside. It is therefore vital that nurses become skilled in pain assessment, communicating that assessment, advocating for appropriate treatment, and monitoring patient outcomes. A basic guideline for pain management is included in the Nursing Care Plan found at the end of this chapter.

Independent Nursing Interventions

The nurse can do much independently as well as in concert with other healthcare disciplines to manage pain. Psychosocial interventions using cognitive or behavioral techniques such as relaxation, distraction, and imagery can be very effective adjuncts to the management of pain and can be introduced, taught, and coached by nurses who have taken the time and effort to learn these techniques. However, these interventions should not be expected to *replace* other pain treatments. Furthermore, these techniques involve skill development requiring practice, so it is essential that they be introduced early in the course of an illness when patients are more likely to have sufficient strength and energy to exercise the necessary skills.[15] They are rarely effective when introduced during a period of crisis, as is usually the case in the critical care setting. However, if the patient has used cognitive or behavioral techniques in the past, he or she should be encouraged to use them to the extent possible. Keep in mind that a patient who is cognitively impaired is not likely to benefit from such interventions and cannot be relied on to implement them independently. The text by McCaffery and Beebe[33] provides detailed instructions and many practical techniques for independent nursing interventions for the nurse who wishes to develop these skills.

REFERENCES

1. Marks, RM and Sachar, EJ: Undertreatment of medical inpatients with narcotic analgesics. Ann Intern Med 78:173–181, 1973.
2. Melzack, R: The tragedy of needless pain. Sci Am 262(2):27–33, 1990.
3. Hill, CS, Fields, WS, and Thorpe, DM: A call to action to improve relief of cancer pain. In Hill, CS and Fields, WS (eds): Drug Treatment of Pain in a Drug-Oriented Society: Advances in Pain Research and Therapy, vol 11. Raven Press, New York, 1989, pp 353–361.
4. McCaffery, M and Thorpe, DM: Differences in perception of pain and the development of adversarial relationships among health care providers. In Hill, CS and Fields, WS (eds): Drug Treatment of Cancer Pain in a Drug-Oriented Society: Advances in Pain Research and Therapy, vol. 11. Raven Press, New York, 1989, pp 113–122.
5. Foley, KM: The "decriminalization" of cancer pain. In Hill, CS and Fields, WS (eds): The Drug Treatment of Cancer Pain in a Drug-Oriented Society: Advances in Pain Research and Therapy, vol. 11. Raven Press, New York, 1989, pp 5–18.
6. Acute Pain Management Guideline Panel: Acute Pain Management: Operative or Medical Procedures and Trauma. Clinical Practice Guideline. AHCPR Publication No. 92-0032. Agency for Health Care Policy and Research, Public Health Service, US Department of Health and Human Services, Rockville, MD, 1992.
7. Wasylak, TJ, et al: Reduction of post-operative morbidity following patient-controlled morphine. Can J Anaesth 37:726–731, 1990.
8. Wattwil, M: Postoperative pain relief and gastrointestinal motility. Acta Chir Scand 550(Suppl):140–145, 1989.

9. Kanner, RM and Foley, KM: Patterns of narcotic drug use in a cancer pain clinic. Ann NY Acad Sci 362:161–172, 1981.

10. Porter, J and Jick, H: Addiction rare in patients treated with narcotics. N Engl J Med 302:123, 1980.

11. Weissman, DE and Haddox, JD: Opioid pseudoaddiction: An iatrogenic syndrome. Pain 36:363–366, 1989.

12. Texas Acts 1989, 71st Legislature, First Called Session, Ch. 5, Sec. 1, effective November 1, 1989. Codified at Article 4495c Vernon's Civil Statutes.

13. Bonica, JJ: The Management of Pain, vol 1. Lea & Febiger, Philadelphia, 1990, p 28.

14. Basbaum AK and Fields HL: Endogenous pain control systems: Brainstem spinal pathways and endorphin circuitry. Annu Rev Neurosci 7:309–338, 1984.

15. Melzack, R and Wall, PD: Pain mechanisms: A new theory. Science 150:971, 1965.

16. Fields, HL: Pain. McGraw-Hill, New York, 1987.

17. Jacox, A, et al: Management of Cancer Pain: Clinical Practice Guideline No. 9. AHCPR Publication No. 94-0592. Agency for Health Care Policy and Research, US Department of Health and Human Services, Public Health Service, Rockville, MD, March 1994.

18. Armstrong, PJ and Bersten, A: Normeperidine toxicity. Anesth Analg 65:536–538, 1986.

19. Kaiko, RF, et al: Central nervous system excitatory effects of meperidine in cancer patients. Ann Neurol 13:180–185, 1983.

20. Jaffe, JH and Martin, WR: Opioid analgesics and antagonists. In Goodman, LS and Gilman A (eds): The Pharmacological Basis of Therapeutics, ed 7. Macmillan, New York, 1985, pp 532–581.

21. Hill, CS: Oral opioid analgesics. In Patt, RB (ed): Cancer Pain. JB Lippincott, Philadelphia, 1993, pp 129–142.

22. Bruera, E and Ripamonti, C: Alternate routes of administration of opioids for the management of cancer pain. In Patt, RB (ed): Cancer Pain. JB Lippincott, Philadelphia, 1993, pp 161–184.

23. Thorpe, DM: The insulin-dependent diabetic as a model for pain management. Dimensions in Oncology Nursing 4(2):36–38, 1990.

24. Max, MB, et al: Effects of desipramine, amitriptyline, and fluoxetine on pain in diabetic neuropathy. N Engl J Med 326:1250–1256, 1992.

25. Bach, FW, et al: The effect of intravenous lidocaine on nociceptive processing in diabetic neuropathy. Pain 28:69, 1987.

26. McGee, JL and Alexander, MR: Phenothiazine analgesia: Fact or fantasy. Am J Hosp Pharm 36:633, 1979.

27. Lasagna, RG and DeKornfeldt, TJ: Methotrimeprazine: A new phenothiazine derivative with analgesic properties. JAMA 178:887, 1961.

28. Joshi, J, et al: Amphetamine therapy for enhancing the comfort of terminally ill patients with cancer (abstract). Proc Am Soc Clin Oncol 1:C213, 1982.

29. Sjolund, BH and Eriksson, MBE: Endorphins and analgesia produced by peripheral conditioning stimulation. In Bonica, JJ, Liebeskind, DG, and Albe-Fessard, D (eds): Proceedings of the Second World Congress on Pain, Montreal, Quebec. Advances in Pain Research and Therapy, vol 3. Raven Press, New York, 1979, pp 587–592.

30. Hargreaves, A and Lander, J: Use of transcutaneous electrical nerve stimulation for postoperative pain. Nurs Res 38:159–161, 1989.

31. Raj, PP: Prognostic and therapeutic local anesthetic neural blockade. In Cousins, MJ and Bridenbaugh, PO (eds): Neural Blockade in Clinical Anesthesia and Management of Pain, ed 2. JB Lippincott, Philadelphia, 1988, pp 899–935.

32. Bach, S, Noreng, MF, and Tjellden, NU: Phantom limb pain in amputees during the first 12 months following limb amputation, after perioperative epidural blockade. Pain 33:297–301, 1988.

33. McCaffery, M and Beebe, A: Pain: Clinical Manual for Nursing Practice. CV Mosby, St. Louis, 1989.

34. Editorial: Paralysed with fear. Lancet i:427, 1981.

35. Miller-Jones, CMH and Williams, JH: Sedation for ventilation: A retrospective study of fifty patients. Anaesthesia 35:1104, 1980.

36. Vitello-Cicciu, JM: Recalled perceptions of patients administered pancuronium bromide. Focus Crit Care 11:28–35, 1984.

CARE PLAN FOR THE PATIENT WITH PAIN

Nursing Diagnoses

Nursing Diagnosis #1

Alteration in comfort: pain related to trauma, disease process, and/or treatment

Desired Patient Outcomes

Patient will verbalize acceptable degree of pain relief.

Nursing Interventions

- Assist patient in selecting an appropriate rating scale and assess pain regularly with other vital signs, as indicated by the acuity and stability of the pain.
- Evaluate efficacy of current pain medication prescription and discuss needed adjustments with physician, e.g., obtain orders for scheduled administration of an adequate opioid dose, supplemented with PRN order for breakthrough pain.
- Be alert for potential side effects of narcotics, e.g., sedation, constipation, and nausea (see Nursing Diagnoses #2–4). Reassure patient that most side effects dissipate or can be managed effectively.
- Teach appropriate nonpharmacologic methods of pain control such as relaxation or distraction techniques.
- Document effectiveness of pain relief measures (pain ratings) on flow sheet or other appropriate record.
- Teach patient and family members and significant others about pain management strategies.

Rationales

- The patient is the only one who can accurately rate his or her pain.
- The best approach to managing pain is to attain relief and prevent its recurrence.
- Side effects are often responsible for patient reluctance to take pain medications.
- Techniques that patients can implement independently often give a greater sense of control.
- Documentation is essential in identifying trends in response and enhances communication when suggesting changes.
- Teaching is essential to overcoming barriers due to myths and misconceptions about pain treatment.

CARE PLAN FOR THE PATIENT WITH PAIN (*Continued*)

Nursing Diagnoses
Nursing Diagnosis #2
Potential for altered sensorium (sedation), related to opioid effect or sleep deprivation or both

Desired Patient Outcomes
Patient will:
1. Maintain safety while adjusting to opioid medication.
2. Resume normal sleep patterns.

Nursing Interventions
- Teach patient and family that sedation is often transient and should dissipate within 36–72 hours if pain relief is attained and normal sleep pattern is restored.
- Promote normal sleep patterns.
  - Promote a restful sleep environment.
  - Discuss addition of a tricyclic antidepressant as an adjuvant medication with the physician.
- Promote safety measures while the patient is adapting to the opioid.
  - Assistance with ambulation
  - Night lights
  - Side rails
  - Call bell within reach
- Suggest increasing caffeine intake. If sedation persists and pain is controlled, suggest tapering the dosage of pain medication. If patient does not tolerate dose reduction, suggest adding a CNS stimulant medication.

Rationales
- Reassurance that side effects can be managed will encourage patients to continue taking the medications to maintain pain relief.
- Depending on the severity of the sleep deprivation from persistent pain, it may take several days or weeks to correct the problem.

- Caffeine and CNS stimulants counteract the sedating effects of opiods. CNS stimulants may also enhance analgesia.

Nursing Diagnoses
Nursing Diagnosis #3
Potential for altered elimination, related to opioid-induced:
1. Constipation
2. Voiding difficulty or urinary retention or both

Desired Patient Outcomes
Patient will:
1. Maintain normal, comfortable, regular bowel movements
2. Report inability or difficulty with voiding

Nursing Interventions
- Anticipate constipation with opioid medication.
  - Teach patient to monitor bowel movements regularly.
  - Encourage diet including sources of fiber and plenty of fluids.
  - Establish preventive bowel program; most patients require regular doses of a laxative-stool softener, e.g., senna concentrate with docusate sodium (Senekot-S).
- If patient has not had a bowel movement in ≥3 days, check for impaction. Obtain orders for cleansing enemas or the addition of a more potent cathartic such as lactulose or magnesium citrate.
- Teach the patient that difficulty emptying the bladder may occur and that the effect may be transient.
- Instruct the patient to report immediately if urinary retention (inability to empty the bladder) occurs.
- Teach patient techniques to facilitate bladder emptying if difficulty occurs, e.g., running water, placing hand in warm water relaxation techniques.
Note: If urinary difficulties persist, discuss changing to another opioid with the physician.

Rationales
- Constipation occurs in ≥95% of patients taking opioids. This effect can increase discomfort and discourage use of pain medications.

- Hydration and dietary means are usually not adequate to prevent constipation. Bulk agents such as Metamucil may actually contribute to constipation if adequate fluid is not taken with each dose.

- Inability to empty the bladder can add to the patient's discomfort.

- Persistent voiding difficulty may increase risk of urinary infection.

Nursing Diagnoses
Nursing Diagnosis #4
Potential for nausea and vomiting, related to gastrointestinal opioid effects

Desired Patient Outcomes
Patient will implement appropriate measures to manage nausea and vomiting as needed.

Nursing Interventions
- Inform patient that nausea and vomiting are usually transient side effects.

Rationales
- Reassurance that nausea and vomiting can be managed will encourage patient to continue taking the medication to attain and maintain pain relief.

CARE PLAN FOR THE PATIENT WITH PAIN (*Continued*)

- Suggest taking medications with food if nausea is triggered by taking them on an empty stomach.
  - ◦ If patient has a history of heartburn or ulcers, an H₂ blocker may be indicated.
- Obtain an order for an antiemetic medication to be given on a scheduled basis until nausea subsides.
  - ◦ If nausea occurs mostly after meals, schedule the antiemetic for 30 minutes before.
  - ◦ If vomiting interferes with eating or taking the medication, obtain an order for the antiemetic to be given by suppository.
- Assess patient's bowel status and initiate appropriate bowel regimen.
- Assess for other causes of nausea and vomiting, e.g., bowel obstruction, concurrent chemotherapy, antibiotics, or other emetogenic therapies.
- If nausea persists >1 week (assuming bowel function is normal and other causes have been ruled out), discuss changing to another opioid with the physician.

- In some patients, opioids irritate the gastric mucosa.

- Tolerance to the emetic effect of the opiod may develop within a few days to weeks.

- Nausea and vomiting are more likely to occur in the presence of constipation.

- Tolerance to opioids is variable; intolerance to one opioid does not preclude tolerance to another.

CHAPTER 11

Critical Care of the Elderly

Vaunette Payton Fay

CHAPTER OUTLINE

Changing Demographics
Changes Associated With Normal
  Aging
Laboratory Values for Older Adults
Alteration in Presentation of Illness
  ☐ Nonspecific Presentation
  ☐ Infections
  ☐ Acute Confusion or Delirium
  ☐ Maintenance of Homeostasis
Medications and the Older Adult
  ☐ Absorption

☐ Distribution
☐ Binding of Plasma
  Protein
☐ Metabolism
☐ Excretion
Psychosocial Implications
  ☐ Physiologic Changes
  ☐ Autonomy
Nursing Considerations
References

LEARNING OBJECTIVES

After completing this chapter, you should be able to:

1. Describe the physiologic changes that occur in the normal aging process.
2. Discuss the effect that age-related changes may have on the care of older adults in the critical care setting.
3. Discuss the effect that age-related physiologic changes may have on commonly ordered laboratory tests.
4. Describe the typical ways that presentation of acute illness may be modified in older persons.
5. Explain the significance of acute cognitive changes as signs of presenting acute illness.
6. Discuss the effects that normal aging changes have on the pharmacokinetics of medications.
7. Discuss the psychosocial issues that make an impact on the nursing care of older adults in the critical care setting.

In the critical care unit, the nurse is interacting with individuals and families whose lives have been disrupted by acute or chronic illness or a catastrophic event. Critical care beds are being filled more and more by individuals who are 65 years of age and older; yet very few nurses in the acute care setting have received formal or informal education in gerontology and geriatrics. Certain characteristics and issues that are unique to the older adult require special consideration and are frequently overlooked.

In this era of rapid patient turnover and numerous treatments compressed into a short period of time, nurses must expand their knowledge base regarding care of the older adult. It is very important to remember that older adults are a heterogeneous group with great variability in their individual level of wellness and functional abilities. The goal of this chapter is to assist in identifying physiologic changes that occur in aging,

the differences in presenting signs and symptoms of disease in older adults, and some interventions that assist older adults in regaining the highest level of wellness and functioning possible.

CHANGING DEMOGRAPHICS

The most significant demographic factor affecting the American healthcare system is the aging of its population. Adults over the age of 65 years represent 12% of the US population (about 31 million).[1] It is predicted that, by the year 2040, the 65 and over age group will make up at least 20% of the population.[2] The fastest-growing segment of this group is made up of individuals 85 years and older. For example, the life expectancy in 1989 reached a new high of 75.3 years.[3]

Although older adults represent 12% of the population, they constitute 60% of the adult patients on general medical-surgical hospital units[4] and represent 25% of all those with fatal injuries attributed to accidents.[5] Seymour[6] estimates that 50% of patients 65 and older will require surgery at some time during their remaining lifetime.

The improvement of medical care and social living conditions has resulted in increasing growth in the number of older adults. The major health problems that affect the older adult age group are chronic disease or chronic conditions. The National Center for Health Statistics estimated that 80% of older adults have one or more chronic diseases or conditions. As medical technologies have advanced, the number of persons who survive accidents and infectious diseases and reach old age is increasing. Therefore, chronic disease has replaced acute disease as the major health problem for older adults. The most frequently reported chronic diseases or conditions in persons 65 years of age and older are arthritis, hypertension, hearing or visual deficits, heart disease, chronic obstructive lung disease, and cancer.[7] Even though the older adult may be affected by chronic diseases and conditions, certain physiologic changes also occur as part of the normal aging process.

CHANGES ASSOCIATED WITH NORMAL AGING

Physiologic changes that are a normal result of aging occur universally in almost all of the body systems. The amount and rate of change vary markedly from individual to individual and also from system to system within an individual. Table 11–1 summarizes the changes that occur in the various body systems and provides some interventions that the practitioner can use to help the older adult compensate for these changes.

LABORATORY VALUES FOR OLDER ADULTS

A significant task of the critical care nurse is to review and report laboratory values. When reviewing laboratory values of an older adult patient the nurse must question values that are outside the normal ranges to determine whether they reflect normal aging changes or illness. In the older adult patient, the clinical signs and symptoms of illness frequently are vague; therefore, laboratory values are extremely important for diagnosis and monitoring of illness in this age group.

Table 11–2 shows frequently ordered laboratory tests in the critical care setting and their normal value ranges. Note that these values vary from institution to institution, depending on the instrumentation used to perform the tests. The significant changes that occur as part of normal aging are identified, as well as the implications of changes in laboratory values. The list of implications and deviations is not all-inclusive but

serves as a guide for many common deviations seen in older adults in the critical care setting.

ALTERATION IN PRESENTATION OF ILLNESS

Nonspecific Presentation

Older adults with serious acute illnesses often present differently from younger adults. Rather than with the usual classic signs and symptoms of a disease, the older adult may present with vague, nonspecific symptoms. Nonspecific symptoms are problems that cannot be recognized as a marker for a specific disease. The symptoms are usually not specific to or indicative of involvement of one body system. Nonspecific presentations include acute confusion or change in level of dementia, falls, new-onset incontinence (urinary or fecal), change in activity level or functional ability, decrease in appetite or weight loss, and tiredness or apathy (Table 11–3).[8]

Infections

Older adults, especially those 75 years and older, are at higher risk for acquiring an infection. Factors predisposing the older adults to infection are more frequent and longer hospital stays, normal physiologic changes, and chronic disease such as malignancies and diabetes. Urinary tract infection, sepsis, pneumonia, intra-abdominal and soft tissue infections are among the most frequently seen infections in older adults. With the predisposing factors previously noted, the spectrum of pathogens causing common infections in older adults is often different from the pathogens found in younger adults, and the incidence of gram-negative bacilli increases. The infections that occur in older adults are frequently associated with higher rates of morbidity and mortality.[9]

Frail older adults, even with a serious infection, may have no fever at all—only vague symptoms of change in functional status, weakness, confusion, or anorexia. Any temperature elevation in an older adult must be considered a sign of infection unless determined otherwise.[10]

Acute Confusion or Delirium

Kroeger[4] states that between 30% and 50% of hospitalized older adults become acutely confused at some time during their hospital stay. Foreman[11] indicated that up to 80% of hospitalized elderly may be afflicted with acute confusion-delirium states. Multiple factors predispose the older adult to developing delirium in the acute care setting. The early recognition of delirium is extremely important because it is frequently related to other reversible conditions. Schor and associates[12] and Foreman[11] identify some common treatable conditions that can cause acute confu-

TABLE 11–1
Changes Associated with Normal Aging

Normal Aging Changes	Interventions

Overall
Decreased height (stooped posture secondary to increased kyphosis)
Decreased weight
Increased fat-to-lean-body mass ratio
Decreased total body water
Blunted thermoregulatory response

Integumentary Changes
Generalized thinning
Loss of subcutaneous fat
Atrophy of sweat glands
Variation in pigmentation
Increase in size and number of growths
Dry skin (xerosis)

- Monitor closely for skin breakdown.
  - Inspect skin and all pressure points.
  - Avoid friction and shearing.
  - Provide pressure relief devices.
- Increase mobility.
  - Turn frequently.
  - Get patient out of bed as soon as possible.
- Be cautious when applying and removing tape on skin.
- Assess skin for dryness and itching.
  - Use mild nondeodorant soap.
  - Complete bath every other day.
  - Add bath oil to water.
  - Apply moisturizers as needed.
  - Ensure adequate hydration.
  - Offer fluids frequently.

Cognitive Changes
Confusion is not a normal change of aging and should be evaluated and treated.
Increased reaction time
Intelligence—little general decline
Learning—takes longer
Memory—recall of long-past events; impaired recall of recent events
Problem-solving—less effective

- Obtain baseline assessment of mental status.
- Be sure sensory aids are in place.
- Break down the instruction into small units.
- Ask one question or give one instruction at a time.
- Allow time to answer or complete task.
- Include family or caregiver in instructions.
- Provide written material for reinforcement of content when possible.
- Assess for confusion or change in mental status.
- Monitor medications.
- Assess for physiologic cause, i.e., infection, constipation, electrolyte imbalance, dehydration.
- Assess for mental status changes—use Mini-Mental Status tool.
- Assess current medications (a common cause of confusion); note drug interactions. (Drugs have longer half-life in older adults due to ↓ renal and hepatic function and ↑ fat-to-lean body mass ratio.)

Sensory Changes
Touch
Decreased sensitivity to touch
Increased pain threshold

- Assess for safety factors.
- Use touch to communicate.
- Monitor for extreme temperature changes in environment.

Eye and vision
Diminished tear secretion
Decreased pupil size—retina receives less light
Decreased visually acuity
Decreased ability for accommodation (presbyopia)
Increased opacities
Increased sensitivity to glare
Decreased color sensitivity (especially blue-green)
Arcus senilis

- Have glasses available and clean.
- Provide well-lit area.
- Identification of self and environment.
- Decrease glare.

Hearing
Increased threshold sensitivity
Decreased ability to hear (presbycusis)
Decreased ability to hear consonants with high frequency (ch, sh, f, p)
Vowel sounds understood better
Loss of auditory neurons

- Decrease extraneous stimulation.
- Use short, concise sentences.
- Speak in a low-pitched voice.
- Talk slowly and distinctly.
- Focus light on the speaker's face.
- Face person at eye level.
- Have hearing aid in place; check batteries.
- Ask for feedback.

Taste
Increased sensitivity to bitterness
Decreased sensitivity to sweetness and salt
General decrease (70%) in taste buds

- Be aware of aging changes.
- Give options for seasoning other than salt.

Continued

TABLE 11–1
Changes Associated with Normal Aging (*Continued*)

Normal Aging Changes	Interventions
Cardiovascular Changes The elderly person has decreased ability to adapt to stress. The heart has decreased ability to increase its rate when stress occurs, and more time is required for the heart to recover to its normal pulse rate.	

Heart
    Decreased left ventricular compliance
    Increased left ventricular end diastolic pressure
    Thicker and stiffer heart values
    Decreased number of pacemaker cells
    Slowing down of heart's conduction system
    Slowing of electrical impulses through nodal tissue
    Myocardium slower to recover contractility and irritability
    Decreased cardiac reserve
    Resting heart rate (HR) unchanged ↓ in maximum HR that can be achieved with exercise
	• Monitor heart rate and blood pressure (BP); take BP in both arms.
	• Conserve energy.
	• Pace activities.
	• Allow rest periods.
	• Provide ambulation aids.
	• Monitor for activity intolerance.
	• Prevent/eliminate stressors.

Vessels
    Decreased tone and elasticity of aorta and great vessels
    Decreased elasticity leads to increased resistance
    Decreased size of lumen
    Increased systolic BP
    Increased peripheral resistance and pulse pressure
    Baroreceptors less sensitive to pressure change
	• Watch for postural hypotension by taking BP in supine and Fowler position.
	• Assess for carotid bruits.

Pulmonary Changes
Decreased mobility of chest wall
Increased anteroposterior diameter
Decreased vital capacity (17% ↓)
Decreased number of alveoli
Decreased cough response
Decreased PaO_2 + 65–80 mmHg; PCO_2 remains the same
	• Assess lung sounds.
	• Assess for signs and symptoms of hypoxia.
	  ○ Monitor arterial blood gas parameters.
	• Assess for signs and symptoms of infection.
	• Teach deep-breathing exercise and encourage coughing.
	• Prevent immobility.
	  ○ Change position frequently.
	  ○ Get patient out of bed as soon as possible.
	• Ensure adequate fluid intake.

Musculoskeletal Changes
Decreased muscle mass (up to 30% decrease)
Decreased muscle strength; deconditioning occurs rapidly
Bone porous and brittle
Loss of calcium from bone, resulting in osteoporosis
	• Prevent immobility.
	• Get patient out of bed as soon as possible.
	• Request physical therapy consultation for strengthening exercise and early ambulation.
	• Encourage participation in rehab program.
	• Prevent falls.
	  ○ Use assistive devices, if appropriate.
	• For bedridden patients:
	  ○ Provide frequent change in position.
	  ○ Maintain good body alignment.
	  ○ Prevent contracture (passive range-of-motion exercise).
	  ○ Avoid use of restraints.

Gastrointestinal Changes Decreased esophageal peristalsis Delayed esophageal emptying Decreased stomach motility Decreased colonic motility	• Observe for difficulty with swallowing. • Encourage to eat slowly. • Set upright when eating and afterward. • Ensure adequate fluid intake. • Monitor for constipation.

Secretion
    Decreased saliva
    Decreased HCl acid
    Decreased digestive enzymes
	• Offer fluid frequently in patients with restricted oral intake.

Absorption
    Decreased absorption of xylose and dextrose
    Delayed absorption of fat
    Decreased absorption of vitamin B_1 and B_{12}
	• Monitor intake.
	• Obtain a nutritional consultant.
	• Monitor diet for deficiencies.

Renal and Bladder Changes Decreased weight of kidneys Decreased number of nephrons Decreased renal blood flow Decreased glomerular filtration rate Decreased ability to concentrate urine Decreased bladder capacity	• Monitor drugs; provide smaller doses (more susceptible to toxicity from renally excreted drugs). • Monitor electrolytes. • Monitor renal functions closely (drugs that are nephrotoxic should be avoided). • Prevent extremes, i.e., dehydration, overload.

TABLE 11–1
Changes Associated with Normal Aging (*Continued*)

Normal Aging Changes	Interventions
Increased residual urine Increased nocturia, hesitancy and frequency Increased risk of infection	• Assess bladder function. • Assess for distention. • Assess need for presence of indwelling catheter. • Use sterile technique in catheter care. • Remove catheter as soon as possible. • Provide bladder training program, exercises, medication.
Endocrine Changes Shrinkage of thymus gland Decline in natural antibodies Decreased adrenal gland secretion of glucocorticoid Decreased levels of aldosterone Delayed insulin release Reduced peripheral sensitivity to insulin	• Monitor electrolytes. • Observe for early signs of infection. • Monitor for signs of glucose intolerance.
Immune System Changes ↓ T-lymphocyte function ↓ Response to antibiotic therapy Depletion of protein reserves	• Observe for early signs of infection. • Monitor response to antibiotic therapy. • Prevent skin breakdown.
Nervous System Changes Atrophy of brain Increased length of time stimulus response Autonomic and voluntary reflexes are slower Increased pain threshold	• Provide safe environment. See Cognitive Changes.
Neurotransmitter Changes Increased monoamine oxidase and serotonin Decreased norephrinephrine	• Monitor for signs of depression.
Sleep Changes Decreased level 4 stage in sleep Increased arousals during the night Total sleep time slightly reduced	• Encourage consistent sleep patterns. • Allow naps. • Avoid use of sleep medication. • Provide quiet environment. • Avoid stimulants and caffeine.

Self-Concept Changes
Several losses
  Retirement
  Deaths
  Functions losses
  Chronic illness
	• Call person by name.
	• Focus on (+) abilities.
	• Discuss past achievements; reminisce.
	• Give immediate positive feedback.
	• Allow control.
	• Encourage choice-making.
	• Encourage independence.
	• Individualize activities.
	• Use touch.

sion or delirium such as cognitive restrictions (sensory deprivation or overload, transfer to unfamiliar surroundings); physiologic instability (decreased cardiac output, stroke, hypothermia, or hyperthermia); and metabolic instability (e.g., electrolyte abnormalities, hypoxia) (Table 11–4).

Foreman[11] stated that nursing interventions are aimed at identifying the underlying treatable cause of the confusion and treating it. Drugs are a major cause of acute confusion. In a delirious patient, every attempt should be made to discontinue or avoid medications that worsen cognitive functioning. Change in environment, especially a rapid change such as admission to the hospital, can trigger delirium. Placing familiar objects in the room, positioning clocks and calenders in full view, and maximizing sensory input with good lighting and use of patient's sensory aids can help to manage or prevent delirium.[9] See Chapter 8, Sleep and Alterations in the Critically Ill Patient, for further nursing interventions for management of delirium. In elderly patients, fecal impaction and urinary retention are common problems and can have striking effects on cognitive status. Treatment of these problems can produce just as striking a response by changing mental status or clearing confusion.

Maintenance of Homeostasis

The changes that occur as part of the normal aging process occur in multiple organ systems. These changes in turn can make it more difficult for the older adult to maintain homeostasis efficiently. Various homeostatic problems are seen increasingly in older adults. For example, body fluid regulation is less precise, and the geriatric patient may demonstrate a decreased thirst response, even in the presence of hypovolemia or hypernatremia. A reduced cardiovascular reserve makes the geriatric patient susceptible to fluid overload; therefore intravenous fluid challenges

TABLE 11–2
Laboratory Values for Older Adults

Test	Normal Range	Normal Age Change	Implication*
CBC			
Red blood cells (RBC)	4.2–5.9 million/mm³		
Hemoglobin (Hb)	Female: 12–16 g Male: 13–18 g	Slight decrease or unchanged	Hb may decline slightly with age, but do not assume that a low Hct and Hb is normal. If low, look for other sign of anemia and cause.
Hematocrit (Hct)	Female: 37–48% Male: 45–52%		
White blood count	4.3–10.8 mm³	Unchanged or slight decrease	
Differential			
Lymphocytes	20–40%	Increased B cells; decreased T cells	Changes reflect alterations in immune systems and antimicrobial activity seen in older adults; protect from infection Increase Bacterial infection

Neutrophils (polymorphonuclear)	50–60%	Unchanged	Decrease
			  Viral infection
			  Bone marrow damage
			Increase
			  Bacterial infection
			  Pancreatitis
			  Carcinoma
			  Gout

Glucose		Increase	• Decreasing glucose tolerance is well documented in older adults. • Alcohol, monoamine oxidase inhibitors, and β-blockers may contribute to rapid fall in glucose.

Fasting blood sugar
  1 hr postprandial
	60–110 mg/dL
	120–160 mg/dL
		Minimal increase
		Increases 10 mg/dL per decade after age 30
		Average after age 75—200 mg/dL
			Decrease
			  Hyperinsulinism
			  Hypothyroidism
			Increase
			  Diabetes mellitus
			  Hyperthyroidism
			  Infections
			  Thiazide therapy
			  Increase in cranial pressure

2 hr postprandial	<140 mg/dL	Increases up to 100 mg plus age after 40	

Urea nitrogen (BUN)	6–25 mg/dL	Slight increase	A slight elevation may cause no problem unless patient is stressed.
			Decrease
			  Cirrhosis
			  Liver disease
			  Low protein intake
			  Protein malnutrition
			Increase
			  Dehydration
			  GI hemorrhage
			  Acute glomerulonephritis
			  Intestinal obstruction

Creatinine	0.6–1.3 mg/dL	Slight increase	Decrease
			  Anemia
			  Renal failures
			  Leukemia
			Increase
			  Renal dysfunction
			  Chronic glomerulonephritis
			• A high-normal or minimal elevation may indicate substantially reduced renal function.

Creatinine clearance	85–125 mL/min	Decreases by 10% each decade after age 40	• Creatine is a better guide to renal function in older adult due to decreased muscle mass. • Consider creatine and creatinine clearance when giving drugs excreted by kidneys to prevent drug toxicity.

TABLE 11–2
Laboratory Values for Older Adults (*Continued*)

Test	Normal Range	Normal Age Change	Implication*
Electrolytes			
Sodium	134–142 mEq/L	Unchanged	Decrease 　Vomiting 　Diarrhea 　Use of diuretics 　Diabetic acidosis Increase 　Dehydration 　Impaired renal function
Erythrocyte sedimentation rate (ESR)	Female: 0–20 mm Male: 0–13 mm	Increase	Not specific or sensitive for disease in elderly Increase >40 mm/h—investigate further Increase >80 mm/h frequently associated with neoplasm infection or rheumatic disease
Platelet count	150,000–300,000/ mm^2	Unchanged	
Serum Chemistry			
Iron	50–160 mg/dL	Unchanged for young; decreased in old after 74 by 50–75%	Decrease 　Iron deficiency anemia Increase 　Hemolytic anemia 　Pernicious anemia 　Hepatitis 　Hemochromatosis
B$_{12}$	250–1000 mg/mL	Decreases 60–80% in 70+ age group	
Serum folate	2.5–20 mg/mL	May be slightly decreased	Decrease 　Possible malnutrition 　Drug–nutrient interaction
Transferrin	170–369 mg/dL	Unchanged	
Coagulation Tests			
Prothrombin time (PT)	<2 sec deviation from control	Unchanged	Increase 　Anticoagulation therapy 　Liver disease
Partial prothrombin time (PTT)	25–37 sec	Unchanged	
Potassium	3.7–5.1 mEq/L	Increases after sixth decade	Decrease 　Vomiting 　Diarrhea 　Diuretic therapy 　Diabetic acidosis 　Liver disease Increase 　Renal disease 　Tissue breakdown 　Trauma 　Bronchial asthma
Chloride	98–108 mEq/L	Unchanged	Decrease 　Vomiting 　Diarrhea 　Use of diuretics Increase 　Renal failure
Alkaline phosphate	38–126 U/L	Increase	Increase 　Bone fracture 　Liver disease 　Paget's disease 　Renal insufficiency
Lactic dehydrogenase (LDH)	120–300 U/L	1–1½ times higher, especially in females	Increase 　Myocardial infarction 　Hemolytic and macrocytic anemia 　Leukemia and malignancies 　Liver damage
Serum glutamate pyruvate dehydrogenase/ alanine aminotransferase (SGPT/ALT)	1–21 U/L	Very slight increase	Increase 　Hepatitis 　Congestive heart failure 　Shock

Continued

TABLE 11–2
Laboratory Values for Older Adults (*Continued*)

Test	Normal Range	Normal Age Change	Implication*

Serum glutamate-oroloacetic transaminase/aspartate aminotransferase (SGOT/AST)	7–27 U/L	Slight decrease	Increase
			  Myocardial infarction
			  Hepatitis
			  Pulmonary infarction

Total protein	6.5–8.3 g/dL	Slight decrease	Decrease
			  Undernutrition/malnutrition
			  Chronic infection
			  Liver disease

Albumin	3.9–5 mg/dL	Slight decrease	Decrease
			  Liver dysfunction (chronic)
			  Sever malnutrition
			  Burns
			Increase
			  Dehydration

Globulin	2.3–3.5 g/dL	Unchanged	Decrease
			  Altered immune function
			Increase
			  Liver dysfunction

Thyroid Function			

T_4	4.5–12 μg/dL	Unchanged to slight decrease	Decrease
			  Hypothyroidism
			Increase
			  Hyperthyroidism

T_3	75–195 mg/mL	Slight decrease	Increase Hyperthyroidism
Thyroid stimulating hormone (TSH)	0–5 μU/mL	Increases in female 60–89 yrs	Increase Hypothyroidism

Cholesterol	120–220 mg/mL	Gradual increase with age	Decrease
			  Hyperthyroidism
			  Liver disease
			  Malnutrition
			  Pernicious anemia
			  Intestinal obstruction
			Increase
			  Chronic renal failure
			  Hypothyroidism
			  Diabetes mellitus
			  Liver disease
			  Pancreatic dysfunction

Triglycerides	40–150 mg/100 μL	Increases	Increase Diabetes mellitus
Arterial Blood Gases			

P_{CO_2}	34–46 mmHg	Increase or decrease	Increase
			  Metabolic alkalosis
			  Respiratory acidosis
			Decrease
			  Metabolic acidosis
			  Respiratory alkalosis

P_{O_2}	85–95 mmHg	Decrease	Increase
			  Administration of O_2
			Decrease
			  Circulatory disorders
			  Decreased hemoglobin
			  Decreased O_2 supply
			  Poor O_2 uptake and utilization
			  Respiratory exchange problems

Pulmonary Function Studies			
Total lung capacity (TLC)		Unchanged	Decreased lung elasticity a consequence of normal aging Diminished functional reserve Increased prevalence of lung disease
Forced vital capacity (FVC)		Decrease	
Expiratory flow rate		Decrease	Emphysema Increased TLC Increased FRC Increased RV

TABLE 11–2
Laboratory Values for Older Adults (*Continued*)

Test	Normal Range	Normal Age Change	Implication*
Functional residual capacity		Increase	Chronic bronchitis Normal TLC Normal FRC Increase RV
Residual volume (RV)		Increase	
Urinalysis			
Protein	Negative	Slight increase	
Glucose	Negative	Unchanged	
Specific gravity	1.005–1.030 od. (refractometer)	Decrease	

*The implications are not all-inclusive but focus on frequent deviations seen in older adults in the critical care setting.
Sources: Adapted from Ebersole, P and Hess, P: Toward Healthy Aging, ed 4. CV Mosby, St. Louis, 1994; and Melillo, K: Interpretation of laboratory values in older adults. Nurse Pract 18: 59–66, 1993; normal reference range adapted from Melillo, KD: Interpretation of laboratory values in older adults. Nurse Pract 18; 59–66, 1993; and Corbett, JV: Laboratory Tests and Diagnostic Procedures with Nursing Diagnosis, ed 3., Appleton & Lange, Norwalk, CT, 1992.

must be performed with caution because the older adult can easily develop congestive failure. Impairment of cardiovascular responses, decreased elasticity of blood vessels, and increased susceptibility to medications predispose the older adult to have postural hypotension and vasovagal syncope. Thermoregulatory responses are blunted, which can lead to increased susceptibility to hypothermia.[13]

MEDICATIONS AND THE OLDER ADULT

Although older adults represent about 16% of the population of the United States, almost 40% of all medications are prescribed for older adults.[14] Cooper[15] states that as many as one third of all hospital admissions of older adults are associated with drug-related problems, drug reactions, or drug misuse. An estimated 80% of these drug reactions occur with well-known drugs given at the usual dosages. Some of the most common drugs that produce adverse reactions are digoxin, diuretics, coumadin, insulin, antihypertensives, and antidepressants.[13]

Studies suggest that aging is associated with a higher susceptibility to adverse drug effects, which contributes to increased morbidity and mortality in older adults. A number of factors contribute to adverse medication effects in older adults: polypharmacy, prescription of drugs by multiple healthcare providers, errors in administration, self-prescribing including over-the-counter drugs, and noncompliance. Medication therapy may also be affected by the presence of multiple chronic conditions, the aging process, and a variety of social, functional, and economic conditions.[16]

When a patient is admitted to the hospital, a medication history should be obtained. This history should include a list of all medications including prescription drugs, over-the-counter drugs, home remedies and vitamins or supplements from health food stores, and information on how the medications are prescribed (frequency and route); whether the patient is taking the medications as prescribed (if not, why not); and how the medications are taken (time of day, which

TABLE 11–3
Nonspecific Presentation of Disease

Acute confusion
Change in activity level
Worsening of dementia
Falls
Incontinence
Anorexia
Self-neglect
Weight loss

TABLE 11–4
Common Causes of Acute Confusion/Delirium

Cognitive Restriction
Transfer to unfamiliar surroundings
Sensory deprivation or overload
Sleep deprivation

Physiologic Instability
Hypothermia or hyperthermia
Hypoxia
Stroke (cortical)
Infection
Fecal impaction
Urinary retention

Metabolic Instability
Electrolyte abnormality
Acid-base disturbances
Hypercarbia
Azotemia
Hypoglycemia

Decreased Cardiac Output
Volume depletion
Dehydration
Blood loss
Congestive heart failure
Myocardial infarction

Drug or Alcohol Intoxication/Detoxication and Polypharmacy

medications are taken at the same time, and whether they are taken with food). If possible, have the family bring in all the patient's medications. If appropriate, blood levels of medications should be obtained.

The changes associated with the normal aging process in all systems may affect the older adult's response to drugs (Table 11–1). The response to a medication depends on both pharmacodynamic and pharmacokinetic factors. *Pharmacodynamics* refers to the effects of a drug on physiologic processes that mediate or control various bodily functions. *Pharmacokinetics* refers to how the body handles a medication, that is, the movement into, around, and out of the body. The changes that occur in the older adult affect the pharmacokinetic properties of medication.[17]

Absorption

Most drugs are administered orally. The rate and extent of absorption of the medication are dependent on (1) the physical-chemical property of the drug, (2) partial size, and (3) interaction with several segments of the gastrointestinal tract. Changes associated with aging such as decline in gastric acid output, delayed gastric emptying, and changes in intestinal motility can have a variable effect on drug absorption. Of the four factors that affect action of drugs, absorption appears to be the least affected in the elderly. Neither the rate of drug absorption nor the amount of a dose of medication that is absorbed is changed substantially.[18] Aging has perhaps its greatest impact on the transport process (absorption across the gastrointestinal tract), which handles vitamins, nutrients, and minerals.[17]

Distribution

In the systemic circulation, a medication simultaneously undergoes distribution and elimination. Distribution is the process of transferring drug molecules from the blood circulation to other parts of the body. The distribution process involves (1) binding of the drug to circulation cellular elements and fixed tissue macromolecules and (2) partitioning of the drug into fat and cellular and extracellular fluids. Factors that determine drug distribution are (1) body composition, primarily lean body mass, fat, and water content; (2) plasma protein concentration; and (3) local distribution of blood flow to various organs.

Aging is associated with changes in body composition, such as a decrease in total body water, a decrease in plasma albumin concentrations, a reduction in lean body mass, and an increase in the percentage of body fat. Decreases in total body water and lean body mass result in a decrease in the distribution volume for water-soluble medications (e.g., digoxin). Therefore, the loading doses of these medications need to be reduced. Since the percentage of body fat is increased, the distribution volume of lipid-soluble drugs actually increases with age. Medications that are fat-soluble

have a longer half-life, and there is excessive accumulation of the medication in the body of the older adult.

Binding of Plasma Protein

The decreases in serum albumin concentrations and in binding affinity of the albumin contribute to the alteration in protein binding ability in the older adult. These factors increase the older adult's risk of adverse drug reactions. A fundamental principle in pharmacology in that only unbound drugs in the plasma are available to bind with receptors of target organs and tissues. For medications that are usually present in protein-bound form, a decrease in serum albumin and protein binding sites, or a decreased affinity of the binding sites, can contribute to an unintended drug action as a result of drug toxicity or overdose. In other words, there is a lower or narrower therapeutic range, and the interpretation of plasma drug concentrations may be difficult. Careful clinical observation of the older patient is critical because clinical signs of toxicity may occur even when total serum concentration is in the normal range.[19]

Metabolism

The liver is the main site of drug metabolism. The major function of the liver is to transform medications from their parent form to a form that is more readily utilized by the tissues and eliminated. For example, a lipid-soluble form is transformed to a more water-soluble form. This process is known as *biotransformation,* and most drug metabolites are pharmacologically inactive. (However, some metabolites themselves are pharmacologically active.) Hepatic mass, hepatic blood flow, and mixed oxidase enzyme decrease with age. The net effect of these changes is a decrease in the first-pass effect (high hepatic metabolism and extraction during the passage of blood from the portal circulation into the systemic circulation). This can cause an increase in the serum levels and clinical effects of certain drugs or their active metabolites (i.e., propranolol, meperidine, lidocaine, verapamil, nitrates, acetaminophen, and tricyclic antidepressants).

The effect that age-related changes have on the liver's ability to eliminate medications by hepatic metabolism is variable. Unfortunately, routine measurement of liver function is not always a good predictor of drug metabolism. As a result, the need to alter a drug dose is difficult to predict in the absence of overt liver disease. Serum drug levels can be helpful in monitoring potentially toxic drugs.[16,17,19]

Excretion

Many drugs and their metabolites—both active and inactive—are removed from the body by renal excresion. As part of the normal aging process, many changes occur in the kidney: glomerular filtration rate decreases by 30% to 50%, renal plasma flow progressively declines, and nephron loss and reduction of renal mass occur. Drugs such as digoxin, lithium, aminoglycosides, penicillin, and chlorpropamide must be reduced in dosage if creatine clearance is diminished. Drugs that are nephrotoxic must be given cautiously and monitored closely in light of the fact that older adults have decreased renal function.[19]

In the critically ill older adult, a number of factors affect the pharmacokinetics and pharmacodynamics of medications. The physiologic changes that occur as part of the aging process, as well as the effects of acute or chronic conditions, affect the utilization of medications. The critical care nurse must understand the pharmacokinetics and pharmacodynamics of medications and use them to assess the potential risk in administering multiple or potent medications to older adults.

PSYCHOSOCIAL IMPLICATIONS

The critical care area, although very comfortable compared with the intensive care unit (ICU) nurse, is intimidating to the older adult and his or her family. The advanced technologic devices, flashing lights, and noise can contribute to a stressful and overwhelming environment. The older adult is already in a stressful situation because of the current acute illness or problem that has necessitated hospital admission. Therefore, admission to the critical care unit only intensifies this stress. In addition, change of environment and intense stress can cause confusion in the older adult. See Chapter 5, Psychosocial Implications in the Care of the Critically Ill Patient and the Family in Critical Care, for an in-depth discussion of stress and patient needs.

There are additional considerations that make an impact on the psychosocial care of the older adult in the critical care area. The older adult, especially the frail older adult, requires a reasonably stable environment to feel secure. Surroundings that are familiar and calm and maintain a similar routine are the most comfortable. Anxiety, fear, and possibly confusion can result when the older adult is abruptly and often against his or her will moved to an unfamiliar setting.

Physiologic Changes

Physical changes in the sensory systems may cause additional difficulty in processing information from the environment, thus adding to an already stressful situation. See Table 11–1 for changes in the sensory system that make an impact on the ability of older adults to take in information from the environment. Many older adults use assistive devices to aid in this process. The most frequently used assistive devices are hearing aids, glasses, dentures, canes, walkers, and wheelchairs. In the critical care area, ambulatory aids

may seldom be used; however, glasses, hearing aids, and dentures should be in place whenever possible. The nurse should make sure that the patients eyeglasses are clean and that the batteries in the hearing aid work.

The following are nursing diagnoses that may be appropriate in this situation:

Sensory perceptual alteration, related to impaired vision, hearing, kinesthetic ability, or confusion

Social interaction, impaired because of disturbances in perception related to anxiety, altered thought processes, impaired sensory perception, fear, knowledge deficit

Self-care deficit, related to visual impairment, impaired mobility

High risk for ineffective individual coping, related to misinterpretation of the environment

Autonomy

Issues of autonomy are extremely important to the older adult. The healthcare professional who is guided by the principles of respect for autonomy also respects the values and beliefs of the individual. Decisions are based on the preference of the client. The therapeutic plan of care must be patient-based. Nursing interventions should be supportive and provide assistance in problem-solving and decision-making. The older adult and family need to be active participants in the plan of care, especially in goal-setting.

The critical care unit is full of the marvels and miracles of technology. As healthcare providers and patient advocates, the nurse must ensure that technology is not an end unto itself but that it serves the purpose it was designed to perform. The nurse who can make that distinction can then center the nursing care on the person rather than on the machine.

The older adult in the critical care area has entered a healthcare-driven system, which focuses on physiologic diagnosis, treatment, and cure. This older adult, who frequently has multiple chronic diseases, may not fit into the treatment-and-cure focus and may require nursing emphasis on maintenance of self-esteem and control, adaptation, and support. Ethical decisions concerning treatment and the right to a dignified death can be difficult. Refer to Chapter 4, Ethical and Legal Principles Affecting Decision-Making in Critical Care Nursing, for a further discussion.

NURSING CONSIDERATIONS

Caring for the older adult in the critical care unit can be a challenge because of normal physiologic changes, the presence of multiple chronic diseases, and the nonspecific presentation of the disease. Tables 11–1 and 11–2 provide some specific nursing interventions specific to older adults; also, refer to the appropriate chapters in this text for nursing interventions for specific problems or diseases.

The following are the major points to keep in mind when caring for an older adult:

- The patient may have nonspecific disease presentation.
- Older adults may be confused when admitted to the hospital because of altered presentation of illness. This confusion may clear after the metabolic cause or infection is treated. Once individuals are labeled as confused, they continue to be treated as if they are confused and not reevaluated.
- Be sure that sensory aids (including dentures) are in working order and given to the older adult as soon as possible.
- Listen to what the older adult is telling you.
- Avoid the use of restraint, if possible.

REFERENCES

1. US Bureau of the Census, 1990 Census of Population and Housing, Series CPH-L-74.
2. Brock DB, Guralnik, JM, and Brody JM: Demography and epidemiology of aging in the United States. In Schneider, EL and Rowe, JW (eds): Handbook of the Biology of Aging. Academic Press, New York, 1990.
3. National Center for Health Statistics, United States Public Health Service, Hyattsville, MD, 1991.
4. Kroeger, LL: Critical care nurses' perception of the confused elderly patient: Focus on critical care. AACN 18:5, 395, 1991.
5. Rauen, C: The complicated elderly trauma patient: A case study analysis. Crit Care Nurse June, 63, 1993.
6. Seymour, DG: The aging surgical patient—Selective review of areas of recent clinical and research interest. Rev Clin Gerontol 3:231, 1993.
7. US Senate Special Committee on Aging: Aging America: Trends and projections. US Department of Health and Human Services, 1991.
8. Burke, MM and Walsh, MB: Gerontologic Nursing Care of the Frail Elderly. Mosby-Year Book, St. Louis, 1992.
9. Kane, RT, Ouslander, JG, and Abrass, IB: Essentials of Clinical Geriatrics, ed 3. McGraw-Hill, New York, 1994.
10. Yoshikawa, TT: Approach to the diagnosis and treatment of the infected older adult. In Hazzard, WR, et al (eds): Principles of Geriatric Medicine and Gerontology. McGraw-Hill, New York, 1993.
11. Foreman, MD: Complexities of acute confusion. Geriatr Nurs May/June 136–139, 1990.
12. Schor, JD, et al: Risk factors for delirium in hospitalized elderly. JAMA 267:827–831, 1992.
13. Hogstel, MO (ed): Clinical Manual of Gerontological Nursing. Mosby-Year Book, St. Louis, 1992.
14. Pucino, F, et al: Pharmacogeriatrics. Pharmacotherapy 5:6, 1985.
15. Cooper, JW: Reviewing geriatric concerns with commonly used drugs. Geriatrics 44:79–86, 1993.
16. Walker, MK: Drugs and the critically ill older adult. In Fulmer, TT and Walker, MK (eds): Critical Care Nursing of the Elderly. Springer, New York, 1992.
17. Chapron, DJ: Influence of advanced age on drug disposition and response. In Delafuente, JC and Stewart, RB (eds): Therapeutic in the Elderly. Williams & Wilkins, Baltimore, 1988.
18. Shlafer, M: The Nurse, Pharmacology and Drug Therapy. Addison-Wesley, Redwood City, CA, 1993.
19. Ives, TJ: Pharmacotherapeutics. In Ham, RJ and Sloane, PD (eds): Primary Care Geriatrics: A Case-Based Approach. Mosby-Year Book, St. Louis, 1994.

UNIT TWO

Cardiovascular System

UNIT OUTLINE

CHAPTER 12

Anatomy and Physiology of the Cardiovascular System
Patricia S. Lewis

CHAPTER OUTLINE

LEARNING OBJECTIVES

After completing this chapter, you should be able to:

1. Describe the layers of the heart.
2. Discuss the location, structure, and function of the cardiac valves.
3. Describe blood flow through the heart.
4. Explain the coronary circulation.
5. Describe the events of the cardiac cycle and their significance.
6. Identify the principles underlying the concepts of cardiac output and cardiac index and the definition and significance of preload, contractility, and afterload.
7. Differentiate the receptors and actions of the sympathetic and the parasympathetic nervous system.
8. Explain the location and action of the baroreceptor reflex.
9. Describe the structure of arteries and veins.
10. Identify the major arteries of the systemic circulation.
11. Explain the role of the capillaries within the circulation.
12. Describe the dual blood supply to the pulmonary circulation.

ANATOMY OF THE HEART

This chapter discusses the anatomy of the heart, the coronary circulation, the conduction system, and the cardiac cycle. The heart as a pump and regulation of the cardiovascular system is highlighted. In addition, a brief description of the vascular system is included.

The heart is located in the thorax below and to the left of the sternum (Fig. 12–1). The right ventricle is positioned anteriorly, with the left ventricle behind the right ventricle except for the apex of the left ventricle. The heart is positioned on the left dome of the diaphragm and is suspended within the peri-cardial sac by the great vessels (pulmonary artery and aorta).

Layers of the Heart

The heart is composed of three distinct layers: endo-cardium, myocardium, and pericardium (epicardium) (Fig. 12–2). The endocardium is the innermost lining of the heart and is in direct contact with the blood flowing through the heart. It constitutes the smooth lining of the cardiac chambers, the conduction system, the blood vessels, and a muscular network of fibers in the ventricles.

137

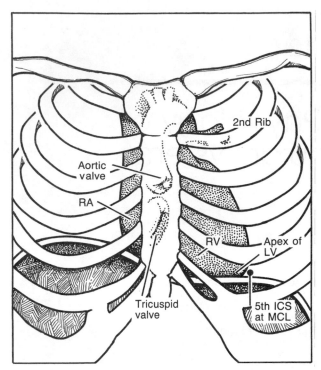

FIGURE 12–1. Position of the heart in the thorax. Note especially heart structures in relation to overlying rib cage: The right atrium (RA) largely forms the right heart border; the body of the sternum overlies the bulk of the right ventricle (RV); the lateral wall of the left ventricle (LV) forms the left heart border; and the apex of the heart is seen at the fifth intercostal space (ICS) at the midclavicular line (MCL). Note also the approximate location of the heart valves and projection of the aorta, details of considerable importance when auscultating heart sounds.

The myocardium is the muscular layer of the heart and is significantly thicker in the left ventricle than the right. This muscular middle layer incorporates the primary contractile elements of the heart.

The outer layer of the heart is called the pericardium. The pericardium is subdivided into the visceral and parietal pericardium, which are separated from one another by a potential space known as the pericardial space. The pericardial space normally contains 10 to 30 mL of pericardial fluid. An acute increase in volume in this area is called cardiac tamponade, while a gradual, chronic increase in fluid in this region is known as a pericardial effusion. The visceral pericardium is also known as the epicardium. The major coronary arteries are located along the epicardial surface of the heart.

Valves of the Heart

The four cardiac valves are located in the fibrous skeleton foundation and are covered with endothelial tissue. The valves do not have a blood supply. The atrioventricular (AV) valves are located between the atria and ventricles, while the semilunar valves are positioned between the ventricles and pulmonary artery and aorta, respectively (Fig. 12–3).

The AV valves are the tricuspid valve, which is located between the right atrium and ventricle, and the mitral valve, which is situated between the left atrium and ventricle. The AV valves look like a parachute. From each of the valve leaflets, there project numerous chordae tendineae, which attach into the papillary muscles that join the muscular network of fibers within the ventricles (Fig. 12–4).

The semilunar valves are structurally different from the AV valves. The semilunar valves are the pulmonic and aortic valves. The pulmonic valve is located

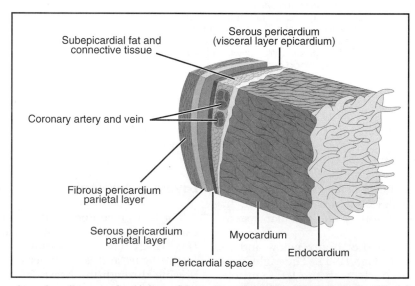

FIGURE 12–2. Cross-section of cardiac muscle. (Adapted from Canobbio, MM: Cardiovascular Disorders. CV Mosby, St. Louis, 1990.)

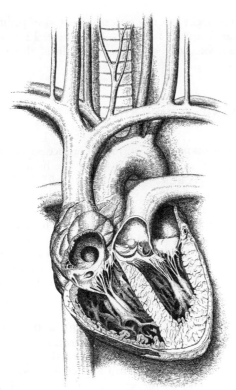

FIGURE 12–3. Cross-sectional view of a portion of the tricuspid, pulmonic, and mitral valves. The aortic valve is positioned posterior to the pulmonic valve and is not visible. (From Wilson, RF: Critical Care Manual: Applied Physiology and Principles of Therapy, ed 2. FA Davis, Philadelphia, 1992, with permission.)

between the right ventricle and the pulmonary artery, while the aortic valve is positioned between the left ventricle and the aorta. To imagine the structure of a semilunar valve, visualize cutting a grapefruit in half

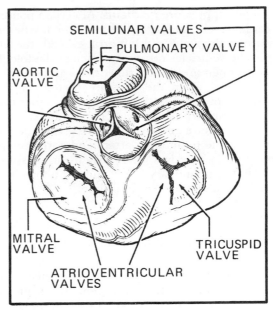

FIGURE 12–5. Posterior view of the semilunar valves and the atrioventricular valves. (From Ahrens, T: Critical Care Certification Preparation and Review, ed 3. Appleton & Lange, Norwalk, CT, 1993, with permission.)

and coring out all the pulp, leaving the inner membrane to form three large sections. No other structures are attached to the semilunar valves as are the chordae tendineae and papillary muscles of the AV valves. The aortic valve has an additional unique feature: The coronary arteries originate from two of the three aortic valve cusps (Fig. 12–5).

Blood flow through cardiac valves occurs as a result

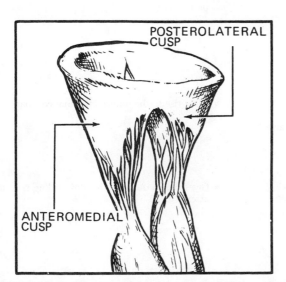

FIGURE 12–4. Side view of the mitral valve. (From Ahrens, T: Critical Care Certification Preparation and Review, ed 3. Appleton & Lange, Norwalk, CT, 1993, with permission.)

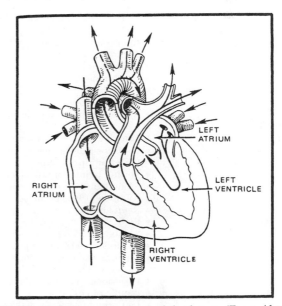

FIGURE 12–6. Four chambers of the heart. (From Ahrens, T: Critical Care Certification Preparation and Review, ed 3. Appleton & Lange, Norwalk, CT, 1993, with permission.)

of changes in pressure gradients. At certain points in the cardiac cycle, all four valves are closed. When the pressure in the right and left atria exceeds the pressure in the ventricles during ventricular diastole, the AV valves open and blood flows from atria to ventricles. Likewise, when the pressure in the ventricles exceeds the pressure in the atria, the AV valves close. A similar response occurs with the semilunar valves. When the pressure in the ventricles is greater than the pressure in the pulmonary artery and aorta, the pulmonic and aortic valves open. When the pressure is higher in the pulmonary artery and aorta than in the ventricles, the semilunar valves close.

Blood Flow Through the Heart

The most important concept to remember about cardiac blood flow is that blood flows simultaneously on each side of the heart. Blood, in a continuous, passive manner, fills the atria. It enters the right atrium from the superior vena cava, inferior vena cava, and coronary sinus. Oxygenated blood from the pulmonary circulation returns blood to the left atrium through four pulmonary veins. From both atria blood flows to the respective ventricles through the tricuspid and mitral valves. Similarly the right and left ventricles eject their contents into the pulmonary artery and aorta, respectively. Figure 12–6 depicts the chambers, valves, and flow of blood through the heart.

CORONARY CIRCULATION

The coronary circulation is composed of arteries and veins; its purpose is to supply the heart with oxygen. The heart utilizes approximately 75% of the oxygen that it receives.

The coronary arteries arise from the cusps of the aortic valve. The three main coronary arteries are the right coronary artery and the left anterior descending (LAD) and circumflex coronary arteries, which arise from bifurcation of the left main coronary artery (Table 12–1). Each of these arteries have further branches. Figure 12–7 demonstrates the coronary artery circulation.

The most notable coronary vein is the coronary sinus. Many veins empty into the coronary sinus, which is located in the posterior aspect of the heart in the AV groove between the atria and ventricles. The coronary sinus drains blood into the right atrium just above the tricuspid valve. Other coronary veins parallel the coronary arteries.

TABLE 12–1
Major Coronary Arteries

Coronary Arteries	Structures and Regions Perfused	Connecting Blood Vessels
Left anterior descending coronary artery (LAD)	• Most of the left ventricle including the anterior wall • Interventricular septum • Anteroapical region • Right bundle branch • Left bundle branch • Left anterior fascicle • Left posterior fascicle • Anterior papillary muscle of the mitral valve	• Gives rise to the diagonal arteries and septal perforators
Circumflex coronary artery	• Left atrium • Lateral wall of the left ventricle • Posterior papillary muscle of the mitral valve • Posterior aspects of the left ventricle • Portion of inferior wall of left ventricle • SA node in 45% of the population • AV node in 10% of the population	• Gives rise to the obtuse marginal coronary artery
Right coronary artery (RCA)	• Right atrium • Right ventricular anterior and lateral walls • SA node in 55% of the population • AV node in 90% of the population • Diaphragmatic or inferior and posterior aspects of the left ventricle • Posterior papillary muscle of the mitral valve • Bundle of His • Left posterior fascicle of the left bundle branch	• Gives rise to the posterior descending coronary artery (PDA)

AV = atrioventricular; SA = sinoatrial.

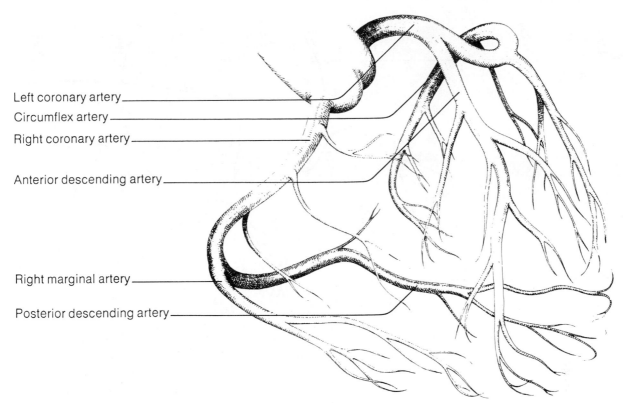

FIGURE 12–7. The distribution of main branches of the coronary arteries. (From Wilson, RF: Critical Care Manual: Applied Physiology and Principles of Therapy, ed 2. FA Davis, Philadelphia, 1992, with permission.)

CONDUCTION SYSTEM

The conduction system is the electrical part of the heart. The heart requires electrical stimulation to achieve mechanical contraction of the cardiac muscle tissues. The conduction system is composed of the following structures: sinus node, AV node, bundle of His, right and left bundle branches, and Purkinje fibers (Fig. 12–8). The electrical impulse originates in the sinus node in the superior aspect of the right atrium. The sinus node possesses the property of automaticity, which means it is able to initiate its own impulse. The electrical impulse travels through the atria to the AV node, where there is a slight delay of the impulse. Then the impulse travels very rapidly through the bundle of His, bundle branches, and Purkinje system, causing electrical depolarization of the heart. Table 12–2 correlates the conduction system with the coronary circulation.

CARDIAC CYCLE

The cardiac cycle is composed of systole and diastole (Table 12–3). Systole is the ejection of blood to the pulmonary and systemic circulation, while diastole is ventricular filling. Diastole encompasses two thirds of each cardiac cycle. As the heart rate increases, diastole is shortened; therefore, as the heart rate increases, one's cardiac output and blood pressure decrease.

Ventricular Diastole

It is important to understand the phases of the cardiac cycle in order to interpret heart sounds and hemodynamic waveforms. Strive to visualize the mechanical events occurring within the heart (Fig 12–9).

Ventricular diastole (ventricular filling) is divided into four phases: isovolumetric relaxation, rapid filling, reduced filling, and atrial kick.

Isovolumetric Relaxation

During isovolumetric relaxation, all four cardiac valves are closed and there is maximal blood volume in the right and left atria. This increases the pressure in the atria so that it exceeds the pressure in the ventricles.

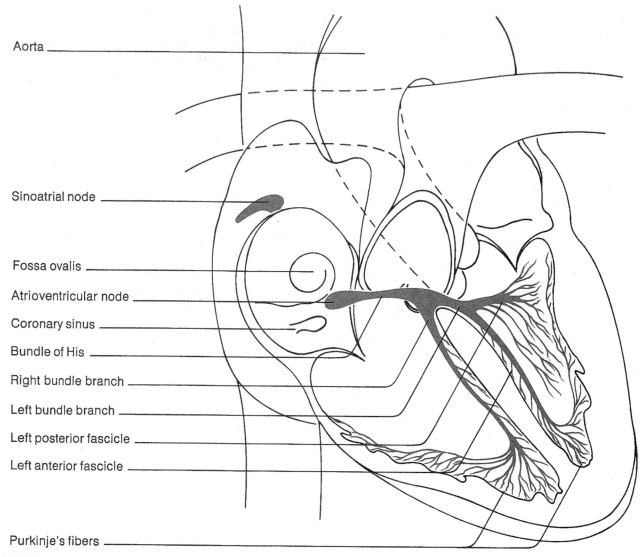

Aorta

Sinoatrial node

Fossa ovalis

Atrioventricular node

Coronary sinus

Bundle of His

Right bundle branch

Left bundle branch

Left posterior fascicle

Left anterior fascicle

Purkinje's fibers

FIGURE 12–8. Conducting system of the heart. The electrical impulses of the heart normally begin in the sinoatrial node, travel over the atria to the AV node, and then down the bundle of His and its branches to the terminal Purkinje fibers. (From Wilson, RF: Critical Care Manual: Applied Physiology and Principles of Therapy, ed 2. FA Davis, Philadelphia, 1992, with permission.)

Rapid Filling

Rapid filling occurs when the AV (tricuspid and mitral) valves open. Blood rushes into the ventricles due to the pressure gradient between the atria and ventricles. Approximately 60% of the total atrial volume of the atria rushes into the ventricles during rapid filling.

Reduced Filling

In the reduced filling phase, 10%–20% of the atrial blood enters the ventricles. The rate is lower due to lessening of the pressure gradient between atria and ventricles.

TABLE 12–2
Blood Supply to the Conduction System

Conduction System Sites	Primary Blood Supply
Sinus node	SA nodal artery: proximal branch of the right coronary artery
AV node	AV nodal artery: branch of the right coronary artery as it becomes the posterior descending coronary artery
Bundle of His	Left anterior descending coronary artery
Right bundle branch	Left anterior descending coronary artery
Left anterior fascicle	Left anterior descending coronary artery
Left posterior fascicle	Dual blood supply: left anterior descending coronary artery and the posterior descending coronary artery of the right coronary artery

TABLE 12–3
Phases of the Cardiac Cycle

Phase	Action	Valve Position
Ventricular Diastole (two thirds of the cardiac cycle)		
Isovolumetric relaxation	Maximum blood volume in right and left atria. The pressure in the atria exceeds the pressure in the right and left ventricles.	All four valves closed.
Rapid filling	60%–70% of the volume of blood from the atria rushes into the ventricles.	Tricuspid and mitral valves opened. Pulmonic and aortic valves closed.
Reduced filling	10%–20% of the volume of blood from the atria continues to flow to the two ventricles.	Same as above.
Atrial kick, contraction, systole	Atrial muscles contract as a response to atrial depolarization. 20%–30% more of the volume of blood from the atria enters the ventricles. This causes the pressure in the ventricles to rise. When the pressure in the ventricles exceeds the pressure in the atria, the AV valves close.	Same as above; tricuspid and mitral valves close.
Ventricular Systole (one third of the cardiac cycle)		
Isovolumetric contraction	Pressure intensifies until the pressure in the ventricles exceeds the pressure in the pulmonary artery and aorta. The right ventricular pressure must reach 20–25 mmHg, while the left ventricular pressure must attain the systolic pressure of the patient.	All four valves closed.
Rapid ejection	This allows the semilunar valves to open, and blood is ejected under pressure to the pulmonary artery and aorta.	Pulmonary and aortic valves open; tricuspid and mitral valves closed.
Reduced ejection	Blood continues to be ejected to the pulmonary artery and aorta until the pressure in the pulmonary artery and aorta exceeds the pressure in the right and left ventricles and the semilunar valves close.	Pulmonic and aortic valves open; tricuspid and mitral valves closed. Closure of pulmonic and aortic valves.

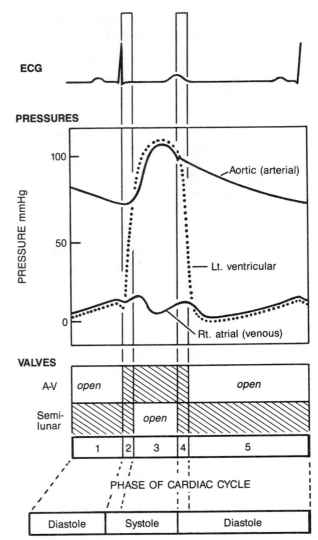

FIGURE 12–9. Phases of the cardiac cycle, illustrating the relationship between electrical (ECG) and mechanical (aortic, left ventricular and right atrial pressures, and valve opening and closure) events in the heart.

Atrial Kick

The last phase of diastole is atrial kick, which is also known as atrial contraction or atrial systole. Atrial kick is an active process whereby the atria contract as a result of atrial depolarization and contribute the remaining 20%–30% of the atrial volume to the ventricles. The atrial contraction accounts for the rise in ventricular pressure. Greater pressure in the ventricles than in the atria causes closure of the AV valves and ends diastole.

This phase is fundamentally important to critically ill patients. Loss of atrial kick can reduce a person's cardiac output by up to 25%–30%. Rhythms associated with loss of atrial kick are atrial fibrillation, junctional rhythms, and ventricular paced rhythms. This is the rationale for striving to achieve sinus rhythm in critically ill patients and why the AV sequential pacemakers were developed to restore atrial kick.

Ventricular Systole

Ventricular systole is normally one third of the cardiac cycle and is composed of three main phases: isovolumetric contraction, rapid ejection, and reduced ejection. Isovolumetric contraction begins when the AV valves close and all four cardiac valves are closed again. This initiates systole. During this phase the pressure in the ventricles is intensifying, until the pressure in the ventricles exceeds the pressure in the pulmonary artery and aorta. The right ventricular pressure must reach 20 to 25 mmHg, while the left ventricular pressure must reach the level of the individual's systolic blood pressure. When the pulmonic and aortic valves open, the rapid ejection phase begins. Palpation of the carotid pulse at this time results in a full, bounding pulsation. Rapid ejection is followed by reduced ejection and then the pressure in the pulmonary artery and aorta exceeds the pressure in the ventricles and the semilunar valves close. This process occurs with every heartbeat.

THE HEART AS A PUMP

The pumping ability of the heart secondary to contractility is known as inotropic action and accounts for the cardiac output. The cardiac output is the amount of blood ejected by the heart with each beat and is recorded in liters per minute. It is the product of heart rate and stroke volume. Normal cardiac output is 4 to 8 L/min. Cardiac output is important because it determines the adequacy of the blood volume supplied to the tissues of the body. A better way to evaluate cardiac output is to consider cardiac index, which is the cardiac output in respect to body surface area (body size). Normal cardiac index is 2.5 to 4.0 L/min per square meter. This is calculated by monitoring system software as well as by the use of the DuBois nomogram.

As stated previously, cardiac output is a product of stroke volume and heart rate. Thus bradycardia and tachycardia may affect cardiac output. In critical care nursing practice, nurses frequently observe tachycardia as a compensatory response. When the heart rate remains greater than 120 beats/min, it will cause a decrease in the cardiac output because of the decrease in ventricular filling time. Tachycardia shortens diastole, decreasing filling time and thus decreasing stroke volume and cardiac output. Bradycardia is usually associated with an increased stroke volume to compensate for the slower heart rate. If the stroke volume is not able to compensate for the slow rate, however, cardiac output will drop. Stroke volume is the amount of blood ejected with each ventricular contraction and is normally 60 to 130 mL/beat. The determinants of stroke volume are preload, contractility, and afterload (Table 12–4).

Preload

Preload reflects the amount of stretch of the muscle fibers, which is determined by the volume of blood filling both ventricles during diastole. The term "preload" refers to left ventricular preload unless it is specified to be the right ventricular preload. The right ventricle receives its preload from the systemic venous circulation. Thus right ventricular preload is the right ventricular end-diastolic volume and is measured by the central venous pressure (CVP) or right atrial pressure (RAP). The left ventricle receives its

TABLE 12–4
Determinants of Stroke Volume

Determinants of Stroke Volume	Definition	How Measured	Normal Range
Preload	Muscle fiber stretch as determined by the volume of blood that fills the ventricle at the end of diastole	Right ventricular preload measured by the CVP or RAP	5–12 mmHg
		Left ventricular preload measured by the PCWP	6–12 mmHg
Contractility	Extent of myocardial fiber shortening	Assessed indirectly by monitoring the preload	
		RV—CVP or RAP	5–12 mmHg
		LV—PCWP	6–12 mmHg
		Ejection fraction	50%–75%
Afterload	Pressure the ventricle must overcome in order to eject its contents	Right ventricular afterload is measured by the pulmonary vascular resistance (PVR)	150–250 dynes sec cm−5
		Left ventricular afterload is measured by the systemic vascular resistance (SVR)	800–1200 dynes sec cm−5

preload from the pulmonary venous circulation. This preload is the left ventricular end-diastolic volume and is measured by the pulmonary capillary wedge pressure (PCWP). Factors that decrease preload include hypovolemia, increased intrathoracic pressure (e.g., in mechanical ventilation, when a patient is on a ventilator with positive end-expiratory pressure [PEEP]); vasodilation due to increased temperature, sepsis, or medications; atrial fibrillation, and cardiac tamponade. Factors that increase preload are hypervolemia and heart failure. Cardiac tamponade is an unusual situation whereby the CVP is increased but the preload (volume of blood in the ventricle at the end of diastole) is decreased. The cardiac tamponade is an increased volume in the pericardial space that is reflected in an increased venous pressure (CVP) but a *reduced* volume of blood in the ventricles because

they are compressed by the pressure in the pericardial space.

Contractility

Contractility is the inherent ability of myocardial muscle to undergo fiber shortening. The greater the myocardial fibers' stretch as determined by preload, the more forceful the strength of contraction within physiologic limits. This principle is known as Starling's law of the heart. Contractility may be assessed indirectly by reviewing the parameters that monitor preload (right ventricle, CVP; left ventricle, PCWP). Factors that decrease contractility thus decrease cardiac output and increase the CVP and PCWP. These factors may include myocardial infarction, left ventricular

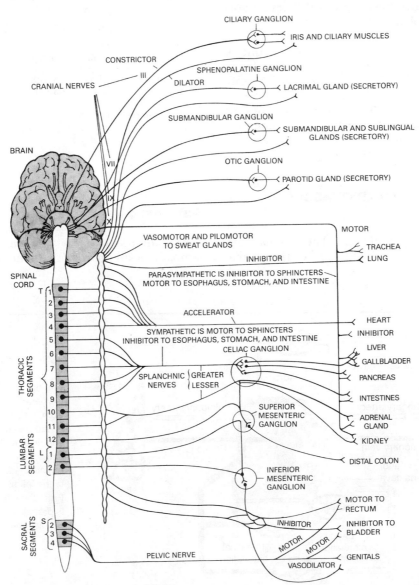

FIGURE 12–10. The sympathetic nervous system. (Modified from Thomas, CL (ed): Taber's Cyclopedic Medical Dictionary, ed 17. FA Davis, Philadelphia, 1993, p 182.)

aneurysm, medications such as beta blockers and calcium channel blockers, cardiomyopathy, and heart failure. Factors that increase contractility are medications (e.g., digoxin, dopamine, dobutamine, amrinone), high-output states (e.g., thyroid storm, pregnancy), and AV fistula.

Afterload

Afterload refers to the pressure the ventricle must overcome in order to eject its contents. Systemic vascular resistance (SVR) is a reflection of left ventricular afterload. Normal SVR is 800 to 1200 dynes sec cm^{-5}. Factors that decrease afterload include sepsis, anaphylactic shock, and vasodilator therapy (e.g., nitroprusside, nitroglycerine, and the intra-aortic balloon pump). Factors that increase afterload will decrease cardiac output and increase the preload. These factors may include hypovolemic shock, cardiogenic shock, hypertension, and heart failure.

The right ventricular afterload is the amount of pressure the right ventricle must achieve in order to eject its volume to the pulmonary circuitry. The pulmonary vascular resistance (PVR) assesses right ventricular afterload. Normal PVR is 150 to 250 dynes sec cm^{-5}. Factors that increase the PVR are pulmonary embolus and pulmonary hypertension. (Refer to Chapter 16, Hemodynamic Monitoring.)

REGULATION OF THE CARDIOVASCULAR SYSTEM

The cardiovascular system is regulated to maintain homeostasis. The two principal means of this regulation are the autonomic nervous system and the baroreceptor reflex.

TABLE 12–5
Effects of Receptor Stimulation*

Receptor	Location	Effect
α_1	Postsynaptic effector cells; primarily arterioles	Vasoconstriction
	Cardiac	
α_2	Presynaptic membranes	Inhibition of NE release
α_{2a}	Platelets	Aggregation
β_1	Myocardium	Increased contractility
	Sinatrial node	Accelerated atrial rate
	Atrioventricular node	Enhanced conduction
β_2	Arterioles	Vasodilation
	Bronchioles	Bronchodilation
β (other)	Adipose cells	Lipolysis
Dopamine$_1$	Renal and mesenteric arteries	Vasodilation
		Natriuresis
		Inhibition of aldosterone
Dopamine$_2$	Presynaptic membrane (?)	Inhibition of NE release

*Additional types of receptors with pharmacologic properties distinct from α, β, and dopaminergic subtypes have also been proposed.
NE = norepinephrine.

Autonomic Nervous System

The autonomic nervous system is divided into the sympathetic and parasympathetic nervous system.

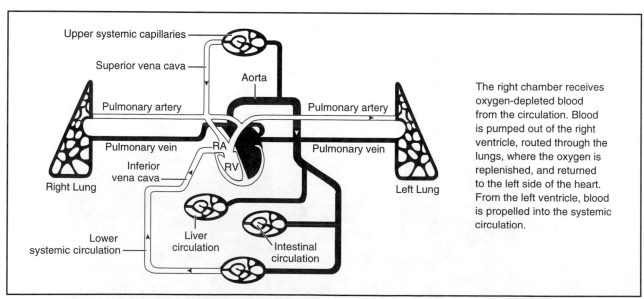

Upper systemic capillaries
Superior vena cava
Aorta
Pulmonary artery
Pulmonary artery
Pulmonary vein
RA
Pulmonary vein
Inferior vena cava
RV
Right Lung
Left Lung
Lower systemic circulation
Liver circulation
Intestinal circulation

The right chamber receives oxygen-depleted blood from the circulation. Blood is pumped out of the right ventricle, routed through the lungs, where the oxygen is replenished, and returned to the left side of the heart. From the left ventricle, blood is propelled into the systemic circulation.

FIGURE 12–11. Circulatory system. (Modified from Canobbio, MM: Cardiovascular Disorders. CV Mosby, St. Louis, 1990.)

Sympathetic Nervous System

The sympathetic nervous system parallels the vertebral column between the second thoracic vertebra (T-2) and the first lumbar vertebra (L-1) (Fig. 12–10). Impulses may travel through sympathetic fibers from the medulla to specific organs or blood vessels. The end fibers of the sympathetic nerve terminal release the neural humoral transmitter norepinephrine. Norepinephrine acts on the receptors of the sympathetic nervous system, which are α and β receptors (α- and β-adrenergic receptors). Activation of α-adrenergic receptors causes peripheral vasoconstriction. The β receptors are subdivided into β_1 and β_2 receptors. Activation of β_1 receptors elicits a cardiac response of positive chronotropic (increased heart rate), positive dromotropic (increased AV conduction), and positive inotropic (increased strength or force of contraction) effects. Activation of β_2 receptors affects the lungs and blood vessels, and leads to bronchodilatation and a mild vasodilating action. Norepinephrine has a very strong affinity for the α receptors and only a minor affinity toward β receptors (Table 12–5).

The adrenal medulla acts as a backup system to the sympathetic nervous system. The adrenal medulla primarily secretes epinephrine and a small portion of norepinephrine. Epinephrine has an equal affinity for α and β receptors.

Parasympathetic Nervous System

The parasympathetic nervous system exerts most of its action through the vagus nerve (cranial nerve X). The neurohumoral transmitter released at the nerve terminals of the parasympathetic nervous system is acetylcholine. The cardiac effects of the parasympathetic nervous system include a negative chronotropic (slowed heart rate) and negative dromotropic (slowed AV conduction) effect.

Baroreceptor Reflex

The baroreceptor reflex allows the body to maintain homeostasis and thus to compensate in the face of critical stressors such as shock. The baroreceptors are located in the carotid and aortic sinuses. The carotid sinus is located at the carotid bifurcation just inside the internal carotid artery, while the aortic sinus is found in the aortic arch. The sinuses are sensitive to stretch and therefore changes in pressure. The reflex occurs when the carotid sinus senses loss of the normal stretch (decreased blood pressure) and sends an impulse to the cardiovascular regulatory center in the medulla. The medulla synthesizes the information and sends a response to the blood vessels and heart. The

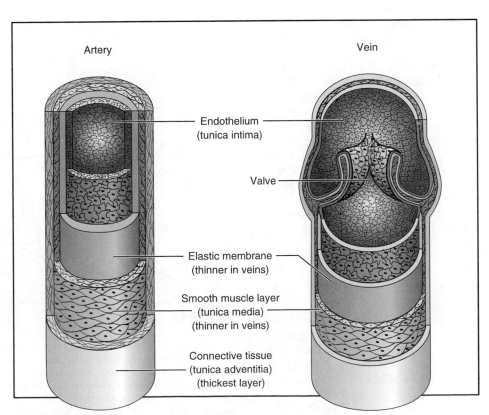

FIGURE 12–12. Structure of arteries and veins. Note thickness of venous walls. (Modified from Thompson, JM, et al: Mosby's Manual of Clinical Nursing, ed 2. CV Mosby, St. Louis, 1989, p 11.)

response is vasoconstriction and an increase in the heart rate to return the body to homeostasis. A corresponding sequence occurs when the carotid sinus senses an increased blood pressure (increased stretch). Impulses travel to the medulla, information is evaluated in the cardiovascular regulatory center, and the response is vasodilatation and a slowing of the heart rate. In clinical practice when a patient develops a rapid atrial tachycardia, the physician may rub (apply gentle pressure to) the carotid sinus in an attempt to create this reflex. The physician is hoping that this intervention will lead to slowing of the heart rate.

THE VASCULAR SYSTEM

The vascular system is composed of the systemic and pulmonary circulation connected in a closed circuit. These systems consist of arteries, capillaries, and veins, which all function to distribute blood to the tissues and return blood to the heart (Fig. 12–11).

Structure of the Arteries and Veins

Arteries and veins are each composed of three layers: intima, media, and adventitia. Arteries have thicker layers than veins. The intima is the inner lining of blood vessels. The media is the smooth muscle layer that constricts or dilates. The adventitia is the outermost layer of arteries and veins. The arteries, and specifically the arterioles, provide resistance in the circulation, while the veins function as capacitance vessels and can accommodate a significant blood volume. There are one-way valves in the veins, especially of the lower extremities, which function to prevent backflow of blood. The valves promote venous return to the heart (Fig. 12–12). At any given time, 75% of the blood volume is within the venous system, 20% is in the arterial system, and 5% is at the capillary level (Fig. 12–13). Figure 12–14 demonstrates the distribution of the arterial circulation.

Capillaries

The capillaries, a single layer of endothelial cells without smooth muscle or elastic tissue, are the only site of gas exchange to the tissues of the body. The diameter of the capillaries permits the red blood cells to travel in single file. The ability of the capillaries to regulate the flow of blood and oxygen to the tissues is governed by hydrostatic and osmotic forces as well as by precapillary sphincters.

Pulmonary Circulation

The main functions of the pulmonary circulation are to perfuse the lungs and facilitate gas exchange between the capillaries and alveoli. Characteristics of the pulmonary circulation include low pressure, low resistance, and a highly capacitive system. Blood travels from the right ventricle to the pulmonary arteries and arterioles, and then to pulmonary capillaries. The blood continues through pulmonary venules to the four pulmonary veins, and then to the left atrium. Bronchial arteries arising from the descending thoracic aorta perfuse lung structures.

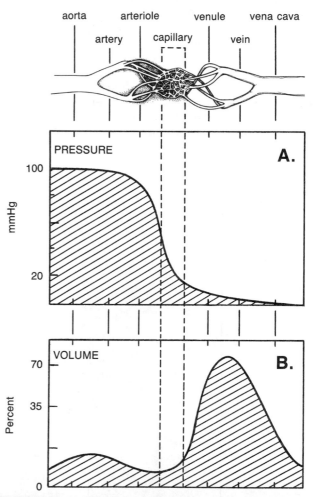

FIGURE 12–13. (*A*) The greatest decrease in systemic blood pressure occurs at the level of the arterioles, also referred to as "resistance" vessels because they offer the greatest frictional resistance to blood flow. Pressure is at its lowest in the venous system. (*B*) At any given moment, the greatest percentage of total blood volume is found within the venous system. These vessels are known as "capacitance" vessels because they can accommodate a large volume of blood with minimal rise in pressure.

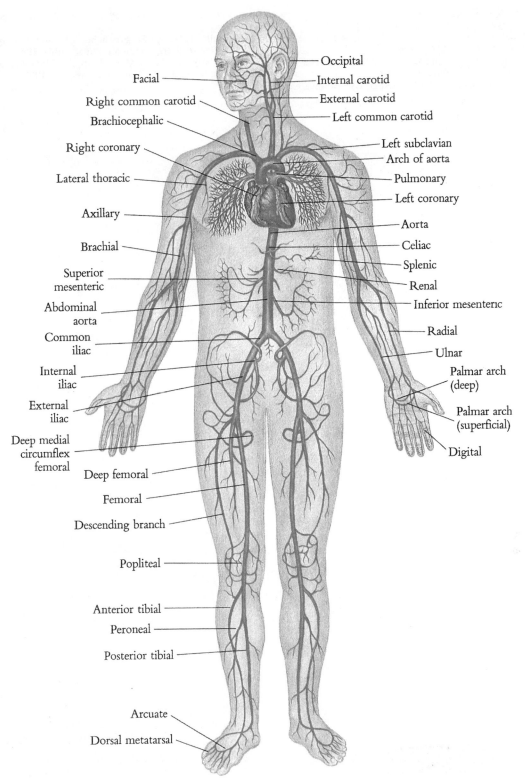

FIGURE 12–14. Arteries of the systemic circulation. (From Scanlon, VC and Sanders, T: Essentials of Anatomy and Physiology, ed 2. FA Davis, Philadelphia, 1995, with permission.)

SUGGESTED READINGS

Ahrens, T: Critical Care Certification Preparation and Review, ed 3. Appleton & Lange, Norwalk, CT, 1993.

Braunwald, E: Heart Disease: A Textbook of Cardiovascular Medicine, ed 4. WB Saunders, Philadelphia, 1992.

Seidel, HM, Ball, JW, Dains, JE, and Benedict, GW: Mosby's Guide to Physical Examination, ed 3. Mosby Year Book, St. Louis, MO, 1995.

Underhill, SL, Woods, SL, Froelicher, ES, and Halpenny, CJ: Cardiac Nursing, ed 2. JB Lippincott, Philadelphia, 1989.

Wilson, RF: Critical Care Manual: Applied Physiology and Principles of Therapy, ed 2. FA Davis, Philadelphia, 1992.

CHAPTER 13

Cardiovascular Assessment
Patricia S. Lewis

CHAPTER OUTLINE

The Clinical History
  □ Cardinal Cardiovascular Signs and Symptoms
  □ Past Medical History
  □ Family History
  □ Lifestyle Health Patterns
Physical Examination
  □ General Survey and Inspection

  □ Examination of the Arterial Pulses
  □ Examination of the Venous Pressure and Pulse
  □ Examination of the Heart
  □ Examination of the Periphery
Case Study: Cardiovascular Assessment of Biventricular Failure
Suggested Readings

LEARNING OBJECTIVES

After completing this chapter, you should be able to:

1. List the cardinal signs and symptoms reflective of cardiovascular dysfunction.
2. Describe the importance of assessing the arterial pulses.
3. Describe the procedure and significance of assessing neck veins (the venous pulse).
4. Identify the locations for auscultating heart sounds.
5. Discuss the information gleaned from inspection and palpation of the precordium.
6. Identify proper use of the diaphragm and bell of the stethoscope.
7. Describe the systematic approach to auscultating heart sounds.
8. Identify helpful hints and techniques for assessing heart sounds.
9. Discuss the assessment of the following heart sounds in relation to clinical significance and correlation to the cardiac cycle: S_1, S_2, S_3, S_4, and pericardial friction rub.
10. State the significance of a murmur.
11. Identify key concepts that relate to murmurs.

The cardiovascular assessment is fundamental in the assessment of any patient due to its link to all body systems. The assessment is divided into the clinical history and the physical examination.

THE CLINICAL HISTORY

The clinical history includes the signs and symptoms that caused the patient to seek medical attention, past medical history, family history, and lifestyle health patterns.

Cardinal Cardiovascular Signs and Symptoms

The cardinal signs and symptoms are the visible observations of the patient's status and the chief complaints voiced by the patient. The initial observation

must be the evaluation of immediate distress. This is usually observed by facial expression, color, and respiratory pattern. If the patient is not in acute distress, a thorough examination may follow. When assessing signs and symptoms, determine the quality, location, frequency, duration, and influencing and/or associated factors.

The cardinal signs and symptoms of cardiovascular problems are chest pain (discomfort), dyspnea, fatigue (weakness), syncope, irregular heart beat, cyanosis, intermittent claudication, and pedal edema. Table 13–1 lists the common signs and symptoms and pertinent nursing observations, assessment, and/or questions.

Past Medical History

The patient's medical history may guide the cardiovascular assessment, as well as provide additional insight into the patient's past and present condition. Information regarding childhood diseases such as mumps, maternal rubella, group A β-hemolytic streptococcal infections, and rheumatic fever has significance. Rheumatic fever, in particular, may lead to valvular heart disease later in life. Additional questions or subjects to ask the patient about are listed in Table 13–2.

Family History

The caregiver should assess the past and present health state of each member of the immediate family: mother, father, siblings, and maternal and paternal grandparents. It is necessary to question the family regarding a history of congenital heart disease, coronary artery disease, hypertension, diabetes mellitus, valvular disease, stroke, obesity, cancer, and hyperlipoproteinemia. In addition, the caregiver should identify family members who have died, and find out their age at death and the cause of death.

TABLE 13–1
Cardinal Cardiovascular Signs and Symptoms

Signs/Symptoms	Nursing Observations/Questions/Assessment
1. Chest pain (discomfort)	1. • Obtain a description of the chest discomfort. *(Don't call it pain).* • Where is the discomfort located? • Identify the severity of the discomfort on a scale of 1 to 10. • What provokes the discomfort? • What alleviates it? Does rest stop the discomfort? • Does the discomfort radiate (move) in any direction? • Is the discomfort sudden or gradual in onset? • What medications is the patient taking?
2. Dyspnea (shortness of breath, breathlessness, uncomfortable awareness of one's sensation of breathlessness)	2. • Obtain a description of the event. • What provokes the dyspnea? • What alleviates the dyspnea? • Does the dyspnea have a sudden or gradual onset? • Does position affect it? • Does time of day affect it?
3. Fatigue (weakness) and syncope	3. • Check blood pressure and pulse. • Review medications patient is taking. • What provokes and alleviates the fatigue?
4. Irregular heartbeat (palpitations)	4. • Observe and identify the rhythm. • Does the patient sense skipped beats or is the heart racing? • Check the blood pressure and heart rate. • Review medications the patient is taking. • What provokes and alleviates the irregular heartbeat?

TABLE 13–1
Cardinal Cardiovascular Signs and Symptoms
(*Continued*)

5. Cyanosis	5. Central cyanosis is best observed by inspecting the mucous membranes of the mouth. Normal oral mucosa is pink and shiny with no relationship to skin color. Central cyanosis signifies shunting of deoxygenated blood to the arterial circulation. Peripheral cyanosis can be observed by assessing the extremities. This is usually associated with cold and is not serious.
6. Intermittent claudication: leg pain that occurs with activity or rest	6. • Assess femoral, popliteal, and pedal pulses. • Assess skin color and temperature of legs. • Locate pain. • What provokes the leg pain? • What alleviates the leg pain? • Assess the severity and quality of the pain.
7. Pedal edema: swelling of the feet and lower legs	7. • Assess femoral and pedal pulses. • Assess skin. • Assess edema. Note the extent of edema in the tissue, i.e., from toes to ankle. To determine pitting edema, gently touch edematous tissue. In 15-second intervals, observe how long it takes the skin to return to a normal state. Thus, 0 to 15 seconds is 1+ edema, 16 to 30 seconds is 2+ edema, 31 to 45 seconds is 3+ edema, and > 46 seconds is 4+ edema. Other sources cite the depth of pitting as the index of 1+ to 4+ edema.

Lifestyle Health Patterns

It is important to evaluate the patient's health beliefs, values, and attitudes. A vital aspect is the patient's perception of having control over his or her own health. Lifestyle health patterns to consider with the patient include, but are not limited to, tobacco intake, caffeine consumption, alcohol consumption, diet, exercise, medications, and use of illegal drugs.

Other areas that may be discussed, if relevant, include sleep and rest habits, elimination patterns, cognitive status, coping abilities, self-concept, sexuality and/or reproductive attitudes, family structure, and support systems.

PHYSICAL EXAMINATION

The physical examination involves fine-tuning all of one's senses—sight (inspection), touch (palpation), and hearing (auscultation). Percussion is not necessary in the cardiovascular assessment. The physical examination section of this chapter is divided into five areas: general survey and inspection, examination of the arterial pulses, examination of the venous pressure

TABLE 13–2
Medical History: Subjects About Which to Question the Patient

Childhood diseases
Rheumatic fever
Previous illness/infections
Previous surgeries
Allergies
Past accidents/injuries
Pulmonary disease
Heart murmur
Hypertension
Hyperlipidemia
Diabetes mellitus
Renal disease
Anemia
Bleeding disorders
Past cardiac problems/chest pain
Past and present medications, including over-the-counter
   medications
Past diagnostic and lab procedures (rationale for the procedure,
   results of the procedure, therapy as a result of the procedure)

and pulse, examination of the heart, and examination of the periphery. Key points to remember are to use an organized, systematic approach; to keep the patient covered for privacy; to inform the patient of what you are doing; and to strive to correlate the examination with underlying tissues and structures within the body.

General Survey and Inspection

The general survey includes a "quick" assessment for signs of distress and the vital signs. The assessment of distress, as stated previously, is performed by observing the facial expression, use of accessory muscles to breathe, and the respiratory pattern. Assessing the vital signs—blood pressure, heart rate and rhythm, respiration rate and pattern, and temperature—may give important clues to direct further evaluation.

The inspection should follow a systematic approach from head to toe. Observation of the patient's nutritional status is evaluated. Is the patient obese? Are signs of cachexia present?

Skin color is assessed to determine if cyanosis is evident. To assess central cyanosis, observe the mucous membranes of the mouth. The mucous membranes should be pink and shiny, irrespective of skin color. Presence of central cyanosis denotes significant arterial desaturation. On the other hand, peripheral cyanosis is generally less serious and is associated with cold extremities. Peripheral cyanosis is generally assessed by observing the fingers and toes, earlobes, nose, and lips. This cyanosis may be due to vasoconstriction; if so, it is usually transient, and improves with warming the area.

Other observations of the skin may include skin texture and hair growth. Frequently patients with diabetes mellitus or atherosclerosis will lack hair growth on the legs and have abnormal thickening of the nails of the toes. Skin texture may vary with aging, diabetes mellitus, and poor nutritional status. The skin must also be assessed for diaphoresis. Diaphoretic skin usually signifies that the body is working to compensate for a reduced cardiac output. Diaphoretic skin is observed in all types of shock, heart failure, myocardial infarction, hypotension, and numerous other conditions.

Inspection of the eyes includes examination for xanthelasmas and arcus senilis. Xanthelasmas are yellow, fatty tissues located on the eyelid that may be associated with hyperlipoproteinemia. Arcus senilis is a light-colored ring around the iris of the eye. This may be normal in the elderly. If arcus senilis is observed in individuals under 40 years old, it may indicate an elevated cholesterol level. Visualization of the eyegrounds using the ophthalmoscope may demonstrate cardiovascular problems such as hypertension and diabetes mellitus. Diagonal bilateral earlobe creases have been said to be associated with coronary artery disease.

Inspection of the arterial and venous pulse will be discussed in subsequent sections. Observation of the thorax is important to evaluate pectoral and vertebral abnormalities that may interfere with the patient's respiratory pattern. The use of accessory muscles to breathe indicates cardiopulmonary problems. In the assessment of the abdomen, it is important to observe for ascites, which may be an indication of right heart failure.

The assessment of the periphery includes observations for edema and clubbing. Edema may be visible in any dependent region. Be sure to assess the occipital area of the head in bedridden patients, the sacrum, and the lower extremities. This peripheral edema may be a result of right heart failure or venous insufficiency. Clubbing is associated with hypoxemia. Remember to assess all of the finger- and toenails. Sometimes clubbing is only visible on two of the five digits. Clubbing is characterized by a loss of the normal angle between the nail and the skin, with an increased curvature of the nail. Clubbing may be observed in patients with cyanotic congenital heart defects and pulmonary disorders. Clubbing does not develop acutely; it occurs gradually in individuals with long-standing hypoxemia and cyanosis.

Examination of the Arterial Pulses

The arterial pulse is initiated with left ventricular ejection and is transmitted throughout the peripheral vascular system, where it can be palpated as pulses. Assessment of the arterial pulses includes determining rate, rhythm, quality, and bilateral equality. To assess the peripheral pulses, use the third and fourth fingertips and palpate with gentle pressure. Using the index fingertip may give the pulse of the examiner (Fig. 13–1). The peripheral pulses the examiner should assess are the carotid, radial, femoral, dorsalis pedis (DP), and posterior tibial (PT). Sometimes the temporal,

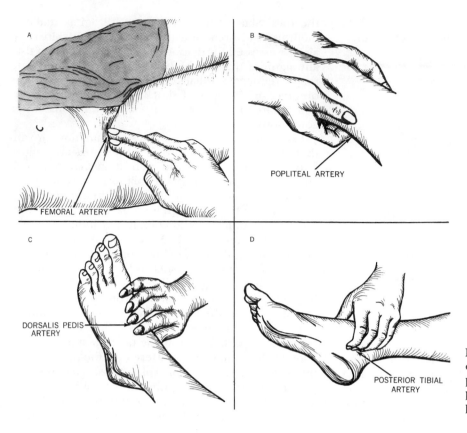

FIGURE 13–1. (*A*) Palpating femoral pulse. (*B*) Palpating popliteal pulse. (*C*) Palpating dorsalis pedis pulse. (*D*) Palpating posterior tibial pulse.

brachial, and popliteal pulses are also palpated. When assessing the pulses, you may use a scale of 0 to 4+ to rate the quality of the pulse.

0   No pulse.

1+ Pulse is thready, weak, easily obliterated with pressure.

2+ This is considered the "normal" pulse, which is easily palpated and does not obliterate with pressure.

3+ This pulse is stronger than a 2+ pulse.

4+ This is the strongest pulse, which is bounding in nature.

Some centers use a 3+ scale in which 2+ is normal. Be sure to note the finding followed by the scale, that is, 2/4 to denote normal. If the examiner feels turbulence with the fingertips when palpating the pulse, this is known as a thrill. Auscultate over the vessel where the thrill is palpated. The swishing noise is called a bruit. The bruit and thrill are produced by a narrowed (stenosed) blood vessel. The narrowed vessel causes turbulence of blood flow, which produces the thrill or bruit.

Pulsus paradoxus is an abnormal arterial pulse that is an exaggeration of a normal phenomenon. Under normal conditions and health, the systolic blood pressure may drop up to 10 mmHg during the inspiratory phase of the respiratory cycle. Therefore, pulsus paradoxus is considered to be a drop in the systolic blood pressure during inspiration of more than 10 mmHg. This problem is associated with cardiac tamponade,

acute asthma attack, and chronic obstructive pulmonary disease. When using a blood pressure cuff, the examiner will hear systole (the first sound of the blood pressure); however, there will be an absence of the sound on inspiration and a reappearance of the sound on expiration. Once the sound is heard on inspiration and expiration, identify this numerical value on the sphygmomanometer. Now subtract this number from the first blood pressure sound. If the difference is greater than 10 mmHg, the patient is described as having pulsus paradoxus. Document the difference in millimeters of mercury (mmHg); this can also be assessed on the arterial waveform in the critical care unit. One would observe a drop in the blood pressure on inspiration and a rise during expiration. Refer to an advanced critical care textbook for information about other abnormal arterial pulse waveforms.

Examination of the Venous Pressure and Pulse

Examining the venous pressure or pulse means assessment of the jugular neck veins. This is performed in order to assess right heart function. When the neck veins are distended, the patient has jugular venous distension (JVD) or increased jugular venous pressure (JVP), which indicate right ventricular failure.

One of the keys to assessing the neck veins is proper

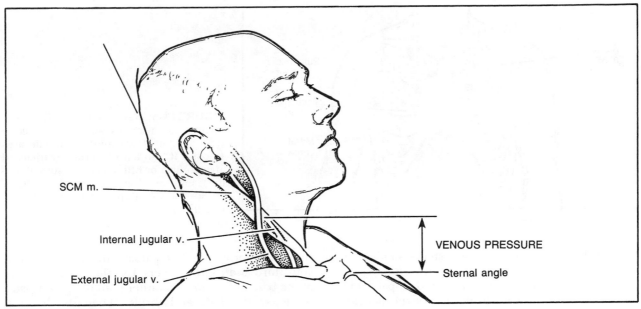

FIGURE 13–2. Measurement of venous pressure. Venous pressure is best estimated from the internal jugular; the external jugular may be used but is less reliable. The level of venous pressure is determined by locating the highest point of pulsation in the internal jugular vein. Because the internal jugular vein lies deep to the sternocleidomastoid muscle (SCM m), use of tangential lighting helps in identifying the pulsations reflected from the internal jugular vein. If the external jugular vein is used, the point above which the external jugular vein appears collapsed is used. The vertical distance between either of these points and the sternal angle (zero point) is recorded as the venous pressure. In order to see the venous pressure level as reflected by the jugular veins, it may be necessary to alter the patient's position. Pressure more than 3 cm to 4 cm above the sternal angle is considered elevated. When discerning pulsations, it is important to be aware that those of the nearby carotid artery must be differentiated.

positioning and normal breathing. The patient must be placed in a 45-degree recumbent position. The examiner should stand on the right side of the patient, with the patient's head turned to the left. The right side of the neck is the preferred side for assessment since the venous flow of blood back to the heart is more direct; however, similar observations should also be apparent on the left side.

Normally, with the patient in a 45-degree position, the jugular veins should not be visible. When the vein is visible, neck vein distension is present, signifying right heart failure. Look for the highest point at which the external jugular vein is visible (Fig. 13–2). This is the best noninvasive method to assess for right heart failure. The invasive method is measurement using the central venous pressure (CVP) or right atrial pressure (RAP) from a triple-lumen catheter or pulmonary artery catheter. (Refer to Chapter 16, Hemodynamic Monitoring.)

Some authors describe sophisticated methods of calculating the number of centimeters for the venous pressure, but this exercise is not necessary. The venous pulse, when visualized directly or by means of a catheter connected to a transducer and monitor, depicts a special curve. The venous pressure consists of an *a* wave and a *v* wave, an *x* descent and *y* descent. Other maneuvers may be elicited to evaluate right heart func-

tion. These include hepatojugular reflux and Kussmaul's sign.

Examination of the Heart

Examination of the heart includes inspection, palpation, and auscultation of the precordium. Use a systematic approach when assessing heart sounds and proceed in an orderly manner to the aortic, pulmonic, tricuspid, and mitral areas (Fig. 13–3). It is in these areas that heart sounds produced by the valves are heard best.

Initially, expose the chest for proper visualization of the precordium. Look for any abnormal pulsations. Table 13–3 lists practical clinical tips for auscultating heart sounds. The two most important things to remember are: Tell the patient what you are going to do, and be patient with your learning of heart sounds.

Locations to Auscultate Heart Sounds

Aortic valve function is assessed by auscultation and palpation at the 2nd intercostal space, to the right of the sternum. If a murmur is auscultated in this region, gradually move the stethoscope toward the right side

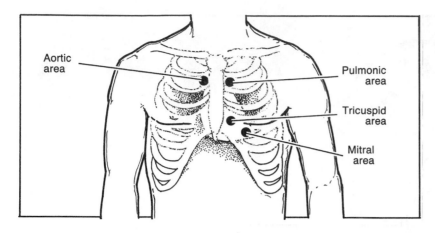

FIGURE 13–3. Auscultatory areas for assessment of heart sounds: aortic area (second ICS to right of sternum); pulmonic area (second ICS to left of sternum); tricuspid area (fourth or fifth ICS at left sternal border); and mitral area (fifth ICS at MCL). (ICS = intercostal space; MCL = midclavicular line.)

of the neck. The murmur of aortic stenosis radiates to the neck.

The pulmonic valve is auscultated and palpated over the 2nd intercostal space, to the left of the sternum. Abnormal pulmonic sounds are more often heard in children.

The tricuspid area or right ventricular area is auscultated and palpated at the 4th intercostal space on the left lower sternal border. Erb's point is located between the pulmonic and tricuspid regions at the 3rd intercostal space, along the left sternal border. Pericardial friction rubs may be auscultated at Erb's point. Additionally, a thrill at Erb's point may be associated with pulmonary hypertension.

The mitral area or left ventricular region is auscultated at the point of maximal impulse (PMI) or apical impulse. Normally this is located at the 5th intercostal space, on the midclavicular line on the left side of the thorax. To locate the PMI, palpate the mitral area with your third and fourth fingers. Use the palmar surface at the base of the fingers, rather than the finger pads, to detect the PMI and thrills. When the heart is enlarged, the PMI may be displaced laterally and downward, for example, the PMI may be located at the 6th intercostal space anterior axillary on the left.

Normal Heart Sounds

The normal heart sounds are the first heart sound (S_1) and the second heart sound (S_2) (Fig. 13–4).

First Heart Sound. The first heart sound (S_1) occurs on closure of the atrioventricular (AV) valves (tricuspid and mitral). Closure of the AV valves correlates with the beginning of systole in the cardiac cycle. When auscultating heart sounds, it is important to visualize and correlate the anatomy below the location

TABLE 13–3
Practical Clinical Tips for Auscultating Heart Sounds in the Critical Care Setting

Use the diaphragm and bell of the stethoscope correctly. To use the diaphragm, apply firm pressure to the auscultatory sites. The bell is applied with no pressure to the skin. Simply set the bell on the chest. Firm pressure with the bell causes it to function as a diaphragm.

Inform the patient about what you are going to do. Tell the patient that a "funny, questioning" face does *not* mean something is wrong; the facial expression demonstrates intense concentration.

Tell the patient that you are practicing to improve your techniques at auscultating heart sounds (a patient is accustomed to someone listening to the chest for about 15 seconds).

Expose the chest. Do not listen through clothing, as clothing will sound scratchy.

For men with hairy chests, use a damp washcloth to moisten the hair to relax it. Hairy chests will cause a scratchy sound.

People with thick chests—obese people, those with barrel-shaped chests, and women with large breasts—may be difficult to auscultate. Do not get frustrated; just be aware of the situation. For women with large breasts, lift the breast and place the stethoscope under the breast in the proper position.

With ventilator patients, suction well prior to auscultating heart sounds.

You may ask the patient to hold his or her breath, in a relaxed manner, to differentiate breathing sounds from heart sounds.

Ask yourself, does the sound change in intensity with respiration? Right-sided sounds are likely to change in intensity with respiration due to changes in intrathoracic pressure. Left-sided sounds do not change in intensity.

Patients with irregular rhythms, like atrial fibrillation and sinus rhythms with frequent premature ventricular complexes (PVCs), are difficult to auscultate for abnormal heart sounds. Again, do not get frustrated. Keep practicing!

To determine where the sound occurs in the cardiac cycle, palpate the carotid pulse as you auscultate the sound. If you hear the sound when you auscultate the pulse, the sound occurs in systole.

Sounds may be easier to discern in different positions. Placing the patient in the left lateral decubitus position (lying on the left side) with the stethoscope positioned over the PMI (mitral area) will cause mitral sounds to be easier to auscultate. Sitting up and leaning forward causes sounds at the base of the heart (aortic and pulmonic) to be louder.

If the patient has a tube to suction, e.g., a nasogastric (NG) tube, turn off the suction during the auscultation of heart sounds. The sounds produced by the suction will interfere with the examiner's ability to distinguish sounds. (Remember to turn the suction on when you finish.)

NORMAL VARIATIONS

AORTIC

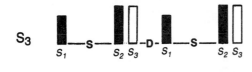

APICAL

EXTRA HEART SOUNDS

S_3

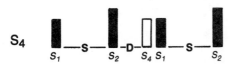

S_4

FIGURE 13–4. Auscultation of heart sounds: normal variations in heart sounds (S_1 and S_2) and extra heart sounds (S_3 and S_4) as heard over the aortic and apical auscultatory areas. (S = systole; D = diastole.)

one is auscultating, as well as to correlate the sound with the phase of the cardiac cycle (Chapter 12) (Fig. 13–5). S_1 is best heard at the apex of the heart (PMI and tricuspid area) with the diaphragm of the stethoscope. S_1 is the "lub" of "lub dub."

Second Heart Sound. The second heart sound (S_2) is heard as a result of closure of the semilunar valves (pulmonic and aortic valves). Thus, S_2 ends systole or initiates diastole. S_2 is auscultated most loudly at the base of the heart at the 2nd intercostal space, to the right (aortic) and left (pulmonic) of the sternum. It is heard with the diaphragm of the stethoscope and is the "dub" of "lub dub."

S_1 and S_2 may be split (lu-lub or du-dub). This means that the examiner can hear closure of the two valves individually (i.e., aortic then pulmonic). S_2 is more often heard as a split sound than S_1 and this is usually normal.

Abnormal Heart Sounds

This section will include the third and fourth heart sounds (S_3 and S_4) (Fig. 13–4), pericardial friction rub, and murmurs.

Third Heart Sound. The third heart sound (S_3) is called a ventricular gallop. When it is heard at the PMI it is a left ventricular gallop, while a right ventricular third heart sound (S_3) is auscultated in the tricuspid area (right ventricular gallop). S_3 is heard with the bell of the stethoscope. The sound is produced by blood rushing into the stiff distended ventricle during the

rapid filling phase of early diastole. Thus S_3 is associated with ventricular failure. S_3 is often heard in children and young adults, and in this setting it is normal. When S_3 is present, there are three heart sounds: S_1, S_2, S_3.

Fourth Heart Sound. The fourth heart sound (S_4) is called an atrial gallop. It is auscultated in the same location as S_3 and with the same part of the stethoscope, the bell. The difference between S_3 and S_4 is related to timing in the cardiac cycle. S_4 is produced by atrial contraction (kick, systole) to a stiff, noncompliant ventricle; therefore it is heard just before the upstroke at the pulse. S_4 is associated with acute myocardial infarction, hypertension, and aortic stenosis (Table 13–4).

Murmurs. Another abnormal heart sound is a murmur. Murmurs are produced as a result of turbulent blood flow through a valve or structure. They are usually best auscultated with the diaphragm of the stethoscope. The intensity (loudness) of the murmur is graded on a scale of 0 to VI. This scale possesses both subjective and objective criteria. Grade 0 is the absence of a murmur. Grade I/VI is a faint murmur that is difficult for the novice to identify. Grade II/VI is louder than grade I and easily discernible. Grade III/VI is louder in intensity than grade II. The novice examiner will easily pick up grade III and some grade II murmurs. Grade IV/VI murmurs are louder than grade III and are associated with a thrill (a palpable vibration due to blood turbulence). Grade V/VI murmurs are louder than grade IV, associated with a thrill, and can be heard with the stethoscope partially off the chest. Grade VI is louder than Grade V, associated with a thrill, and can be heard without a stethoscope.

Murmurs develop as a result of turbulence due to abnormal valve structures. These abnormal valve structures may be associated with stenosis or insufficiency. Stenosis is a narrowed valve opening, which produces the turbulent flow, while insufficiency is produced by an incompetent valve. The valve cannot close as it should. Thus blood flow returns to the area from which it came. Another name for insufficiency is regurgitation.

An important concept to understand is the normal direction of blood flow across a valve. Normal flow across the AV valves (tricuspid and mitral) occurs in diastole, while normal flow through the semilunar valves (pulmonic and aortic) occurs in systole. Stenotic valves are associated with blood flow across the valve in the normal direction of flow. Therefore tricuspid or mitral stenoses are diastolic murmurs, while pulmonic and aortic stenoses are systolic murmurs. The examiner uses the diaphragm of the stethoscope to auscultate in the area over the valve, that is, the aortic area is the 2nd intercostal space to the right of the sternum. Insufficient valves allow blood flow back through the valves in the phase of the cardiac cycle in which there would normally be no flow across the valve. Therefore tricuspid and mitral insufficiencies produce systolic murmurs (normal flow across the valve is in diastole), while pulmonic and aortic insuf-

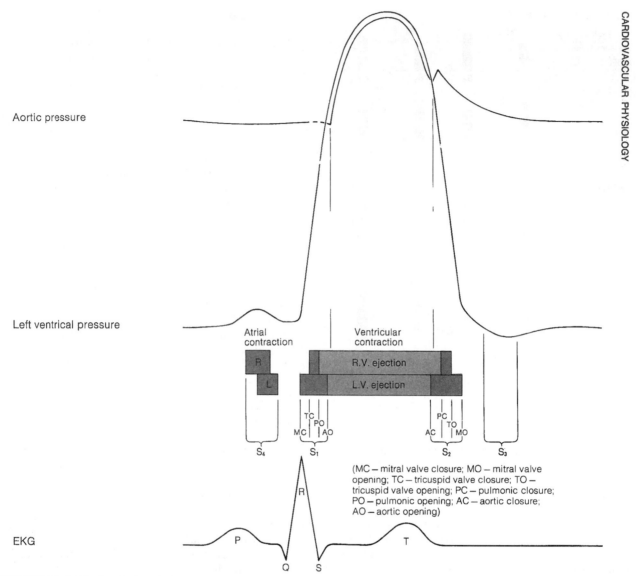

Aortic pressure

Left ventrical pressure

Atrial contraction

Ventricular contraction

R.V. ejection

L.V. ejection

TC
PO
MC | | AO

PC
TO
AC | | MO

S_4 S_1 S_2 S_3

(MC – mitral valve closure; MO – mitral valve
opening; TC – tricuspid valve closure; TO –
tricuspid valve opening; PC – pulmonic closure;
PO – pulmonic opening; AC – aortic closure;
AO – aortic opening)

EKG

P   R   T

Q   S

FIGURE 13–5. Mechanical and electrical correlates of the heart sounds. The first heart sound (S_1) occurs at the beginning of ventricular systole with closure of the mitral and tricuspid valves. The second heart sound (S_2) occurs near the end of systole with the closure of the aortic and pulmonic valves. Note that the left ventricular contraction begins before and ends after right ventricular contraction.

ficiencies cause diastolic murmurs (normal flow across the semilunar valves is in systole). Considering these concepts when auscultating murmurs is more beneficial to the examiner than memorizing that the murmur of aortic stenosis is a systolic murmur.

Murmurs are identified by many descriptive terms based on the quality of the sound and where it occurs in the cardiac cycle. *The novice nurse primarily needs to identify the sound, determine where it is auscultated the loudest, and whether the sound occurs in systole or diastole.* After further practice, the nurse may be able to discern the quality of the sound (musical, harsh); whether the sound is holosystolic, late, early, or mid systolic; and whether the sound is marked by crescendo, decrescendo, crescendo-decrescendo, or is constant in its quality. Clicks, snaps, opening sounds, and ejection

sounds are other sounds that the expert examiner may auscultate. Again, as a novice, do not become frustrated when you do not hear everything you read about right away. Practice, practice, practice! Or rather, auscultate, auscultate, auscultate!

Pericardial Friction Rub. The pericardial friction rub is produced by rubbing of the visceral and parietal pericardia against each other. The friction rub may be intermittent and can be auscultated in any or all phases of the cardiac cycle (systole/diastole). The pericardial friction rub may be easiest to discern at Erb's point (3rd intercostal space, to the left of the sternum). To differentiate a pleural from pericardial friction rub, ask the patient to gently hold his or her breath and listen to the heart sound. If it is a pericardial friction rub, the sound will persist when the per-

TABLE 13–4
Auscultation of Heart Sounds

Heart Sounds	Other Names	Area to Auscultate	Part of Stethoscope to Use	Best Placement of Patient	Relationship to the Cardiac Cycle
S_1	—	Entire precordium, but loudest at apex	Diaphragm	Any position	End of diastole; associated with closure of tricuspid and mitral valves
S_2	—	Entire precordium, but louder at base of heart (2nd intercostal space, to the right and left of the sternum)	Diaphragm	Sitting, leaning forward	End of systole; associated with closure of pulmonic and aortic valves
S_3	Ventricular gallop	Apex; 5th intercostal space, to the left at the midclavicular line	Bell	Supine or left lateral	Early diastole; associated with rapid filling of overdistended, stiff ventricles
S_4	Atrial gallop	Same as S_3	Bell	Supine or left lateral	Late diastole; associated with atrial contraction to stiff, noncompliant ventricles

son holds his or her breath. This sound may be very loud and wet sounding in the patient following open heart surgery. Patients with pericarditis associated with myocardial infarction or infection will demonstrate a softer sound, like leather being rubbed together.

Examination of the Periphery

Assessment of the periphery includes evaluation for capillary refill, skin turgor, and pitting edema, and for signs of thrombophlebitis. Capillary refill of the nails of the fingers and toes should occur in less than 3 seconds. This is performed by applying pressure with your fingers to the nail bed for a few seconds, then releasing the pressure. The color should return in less than 3 seconds. When capillary refill takes longer than 3 seconds, it is said to be sluggish as a result of poor circulation (low cardiac output or atherosclerosis). Skin turgor is assessed by squeezing the skin tissue of the arms and legs to evaluate its ability to return to its normal placement. Elderly people and those with poor nutrition may demonstrate poor skin turgor, with tenting of the skin.

Assessment of pitting edema is important in the evaluation of the periphery. The edema may be due to right heart failure or to venous insufficiency. Inspect and palpate dependent areas such as behind the head, the sacral area, and the legs, ankles, and feet. Pitting edema may be assessed in two ways: how long (in seconds) it takes the pitted tissue to return to a normal state after palpation, and the depth of the pitting edema. The examiner should assess both aspects. Pitting edema may be assessed as 0 to 4+.

1+ indicates pitting lasts for 1 to 15 seconds

2+ indicates pitting lasts for 16 to 30 seconds
3+ indicates pitting lasts for 31 to 45 seconds
4+ indicates pitting lasts more than 45 seconds
The depth of the pitting edema may also be assessed as follows using a small ruler (Fig. 13–6):
1+: 2 mm depth
2+: 4 mm depth
3+: 6 mm depth
4+: 8 mm depth or more
To assess for thrombophlebitis, the foot is gently flexed toward the head (dorsiflexion). If discomfort or pain is noted in the calf, this is known as Homan's sign and is associated with thrombophlebitis.

This chapter has highlighted the clinical history and physical examination as it relates to the cardiovascular system, with emphasis on inspection of the patient; examination of the arteries, veins, and the periphery; and auscultation of the heart.

The following case study demonstrates the importance of a thorough cardiovascular assessment.

CASE STUDY: CARDIOVASCULAR ASSESSMENT OF BIVENTRICULAR FAILURE

OL, an 85-year-old widow, was seen in the clinic because she had trouble catching her breath and had noted that her shoes were tighter than usual. She stated that her lifestyle was sedentary. She lived in a nursing home and walked from her bed to the chair and to the bathroom next door to her room.

A student nurse (SN) assisting the nurse during a clinical rotation performed the initial assessment. The SN learned that OL was a type II diabetic. She

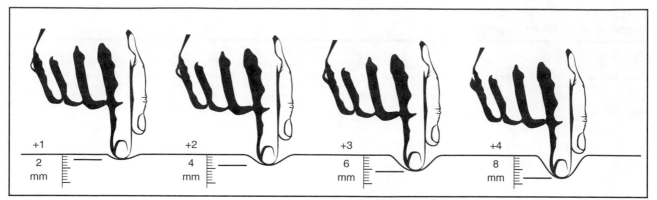

FIGURE 13–6. Assessing for pitting edema. (Modified from Canobbio, MM: Cardiovascular Disorders. CV Mosby, St. Louis, 1990.)

had been diet controlled until 5 years ago, when she was placed on an oral hypoglycemic agent. Since January of this year she has required insulin therapy in place of the oral agent. OL is also receiving a nitrate, a "pill for my nerves," a diuretic, digoxin, and potassium.

The SN asked OL for more information about being short of breath. OL related that she had difficulty catching her breath while sitting in the chair. In addition, she could not get around her room on her own anymore because she was weak, dizzy, and breathless.

The SN took OL's vital signs. Her blood pressure was 102/64 mmHg, heart rate 82 in an irregular rhythm, and her respiratory rate was 24. Placing OL on a monitor, the SN noted OL's rhythm displayed atrial fibrillation. OL was alert and oriented, weak, and frequently shut her eyes during the conversation. Her skin color was dusky. OL's sentences were short and interspersed with periods of rest and taking an exaggerated breath. On inspection, the mucous membrane of OL's mouth displayed a purplish hue.

OL was positioned in a bed with the head elevated at a 45-degree angle. The SN assessed OL's neck veins. Assessing the right side of the neck, the SN had OL turn her head to the left. With adequate lighting, the SN could easily see OL's neck veins. The SN thought she could start an IV in that neck vein. The vein possessed an irregular movement. As the assessment continued, OL's carotid arteries were palpated one at a time and felt to be 1+ to 2+ (weak), with an irregular rate.

Assessment of the thorax was done next to evaluate the heart and lungs. Using the diaphragm of the stethoscope, the SN placed the diaphragm over the 2nd intercostal space, to the right of the sternum (aortic area), followed by the 2nd intercostal space, to the left of the sternum (pulmonic area), followed by the 3rd to 4th intercostal space left lower sternal border (tricuspid area). The SN then palpated for the PMI, which was located at the 6th intercostal space anterior axillary position. To do this, the SN had to lift the left breast upward and place the stethoscope under the breast. At this point, the SN could feel a slight thrill. Upon placing the diaphragm of the stethoscope at the

PMI, she auscultated a "swish" (murmur). She heard the murmur when she palpated the carotid pulse (systolic murmur). The murmur could be also heard to the left, toward OL's left axilla. The SN changed the stethoscope to the bell and auscultated at the PMI. An extra heart sound was heard in early diastole (S_3). No other abnormal heart sounds were heard.

The SN then directed her attention to OL's breath sounds. She auscultated the anterior chest side to side and heard distant but normal breath sounds. OL was asked to lean forward while the SN auscultated the posterior lung fields. Upon auscultation, the SN could hear fine crackles on the right and left lung fields just below the scapula on each side. The crackles did not clear with a cough.

Continuing the assessment, the SN noted femoral, popliteal, and all pedal pulses to be present but weak. Examination of OL's lower legs and feet demonstrated several healing skin tears and pedal edema. OL's feet were enlarged and the edema was above her ankles. Palpating the tissue led to pitting that stayed indented for more than 1 minute.

The SN thanked OL and went to report to her nurse preceptor. The SN stated that OL demonstrated signs and symptoms of biventricular failure. The right heart failure was evident from the neck vein distention and pedal edema. The left heart failure was demonstrated by the weak, thready pulse, irregular rhythm, shortness of breath, rales, displaced PMI, S_3, and systolic murmur. The nurse preceptor confirmed the student's thorough assessment.

SUGGESTED READINGS

Bates, B: A Guide to Physical Examination, ed 6. JB Lippincott, Philadelphia, 1995.

Ignatavicius, D and Bayne, M: Medical-Surgical Nursing: A Nursing Process Approach. WB Saunders Philadelphia, 1991.

Seidel, HM, Ball, JW, Dains, JE, and Benedict, GW: Mosby's Guide to Physical Examination, ed 3. Mosby Year Book, St. Louis, MO, 1995.

Sulzbach, LM: Measurement of pulsus paradoxus. Focus on Critical Care 16:142, 1989.

Yacone-Morton, LA: Perfecting the art of cardiac assessment. RN 54: 28, 1991.

CHAPTER 14

Cardiovascular Diagnostic Techniques

Sheila M. Keller

CHAPTER OUTLINE

LEARNING OBJECTIVES

After completing this chapter, you should be able to:

1. Explain the purpose of specific cardiovascular techniques.
2. Describe cardiovascular diagnostic procedures in terms that the patient and/or family can comprehend.
3. Identify situations for which the procedures would be contraindicated.
4. Discuss interfering factors that may alter proper interpretation of test results.
5. Describe the patient care needed before and after the procedure.
6. Prioritize nursing care measures before and after the procedure.
7. Analyze tests results, identifying abnormalities and their significance in terms of patient outcomes.

The clinical history and physical examination of the cardiac patient are of primary importance in the diagnosis and/or evaluation of cardiovascular disease. These findings are frequently augmented with additional diagnostic studies. Sophistication in testing techniques has greatly increased over the years, with a consequent improvement in the accuracy of diagnostic tests and studies and an ensuing decrease in the morbidity and mortality rates. Nurses must keep abreast of rapid technologic advances in order to provide safe and effective nursing care. To assist the nurse in this regard, specific and pertinent diagnostic tests and studies in current use are discussed in the text that follows. Studies and tests that are in the process of approval and some that are still in the developmental stage are also mentioned. For simplicity and comparison, the purpose, contraindications, normal results, complications, patient preparation, and nursing care implications for each procedure are represented in Table 14–1. The reader is encouraged to refer to this table while reading the text.

TABLE 14–1
Cardiovascular Diagnostic Tests

Diagnostic Test	Purpose	Contraindications	Normal Findings
Chest x-ray	To evaluate and/or detect cardiac disease and abnormalities that change the size, shape, position, and appearance of the heart, lungs, and great vessels To ensure correct positioning of catheters, i.e., pulmonary artery lines, subclavian lines, pacemaker wires, and chest tubes To verify placement of endotracheal tubes, mercury tipped/radiopaque feeding tubes	Pregnancy Young children and infants	Normal size (PA view—the heart is less than 50% of the thoracic diameter) No calcifications No masses No pericardial effusions Lungs clear No pleural effusions No infiltrates
Exercise or stress test (Exercise stress testing may be done within 72 hours of myocardial infarction in some patients.)	To assess cardiac response to increased workload To help diagnose the cause of chest pain to determine the functional capacity of the heart after cardiac surgery, PTCA, or a myocardial infarction To establish readiness for, or set limitations for, an exercise program To identify exercise-related dysrhythmias To evaluate the effectiveness of antidysrhythmics or antianginal drugs	New or changing pain, hypertension, uncontrolled heart failure, acute pericarditis, acute myocarditis, severe anemia, serious dysrhythmias, severe valvular disease, ventricular or dissecting aneurysm, known high-grade left main coronary artery disease Patients severely limited by neurologic, peripheral vascular, or musculoskeletal disease, hyperthyroidism	Little or no change in the ECG rhythm strip after exercise The heart rate increases in proportion to the workload Attainment of the target heart rate Systolic blood pressure increases in proportion to the workload Absence of dysrhythmias with exercise
Thallium stress test	Same as stress test To detect areas of residual ischemia	Same as stress test	Same as stress test Normal perfusion and redistribution

		NURSING CARE	
Complications	**Patient Preparation**	**Pretest**	**Posttest**
None	Explain the procedure and its purpose. Emphasize that the procedure is painless and that there is little radiation given off. Have the patient remove all clothing from the neck to the waist and put on a hospital gown (with ties, not snaps). Have the patient remove all jewelry and other metal objects.	Patient teaching	Review findings. Update nursing care plan.
Dysrhythmias Hypotension Bradycardia Myocardial infarction Cardiac arrest Angina Retinal separation Cardiovascular accident Phlebitis Leg cramps	Explain the procedure and its purpose. Have the consent form signed. Reassure the patient that a physician is available at all times. Avoid stenuous exercise 24 hours before the test. The patient should not eat, smoke, or drink alcohol or caffeine 2–3 hours prior to the test. Continue medications unless the physician specifies otherwise. Wear loose comfortable clothing (shorts or slacks). Men usually do not wear a shirt. Women should wear a soft bra without an underwire and a light, loose, short-sleeved blouse that buttons down the front, or a patient gown with a front closure. Wear comfortable shoes and socks; no slippers. Sneakers are best but any rubber-soled shoes will do.	Patient teaching. Check consent form. Check with the physician concerning cardiac medications. Check for the history and physical. One must be done within 1 week of the test. Check for a baseline 12-lead ECG. Have emergency equipment on standby.	Assist the patient to a chair. Continue monitoring the heart rate, blood pressure, and rhythm strips until parameters return to normal. Monitor for signs of intolerance. Remove all electrodes; clean the sites. Tell the patient to wait 1 hour before taking a *warm* shower (hot water may cause faintness or dizziness). Tell the patient to resume usual diet and activity. Review the findings. Update nursing care plan.
Same as stress test	Same as stress test NPO prior to test NPO or special diet Notify technician and/or physician if patient is tired and cannot go on much longer. Patient must be able to do one more minute of exercise so thallium can be injected before exercise ends. After thallium is injected patient will lie down for 10–40 minutes, during which time he or she must keep the left arm or both arms above head level while the scanning takes place. Patient will return 4 hours after thallium injected for second series of scans.	Same as stress test Check for allergies to shellfish, iodine, or previous contrast. If there is a history of allergy, steroids or antihistamines may be given days before or just prior to test. Check that permit has been signed. Insert heparin lock. Maintain test diet.	Same as stress test. Check for allergic reactions to contrast. Encourage fluids if not contraindicated.

Continued

TABLE 14–1
Cardiovascular Diagnostic Tests (*Continued*)

Diagnostic Test	Purpose	Contraindications	Normal Findings
Pharmacologic stress	Same as stress test	Same as stress test Thallium test History of severe bronchospasm History of recent unstable angina Myocardial infarct (MI) within 5 days Systolic BP <80 mmHg Aminophylline or caffeine within 24 hours of test	Same as stress test
Echocardiogram	To diagnose and evaluate valvular disorders To aid in the diagnosis of hypertrophic and related cardiomyopathies To detect atrial tumors To detect cardiac structural abnormalities To evaluate cardiac function after MI (defects in wall motion, stroke volume, cardiac output, ejection fraction) To detect pericardial effusions, septal defects, and ventricular aneurysms. To evaluate prosthetic valve function To detect presence of bacterial endocarditis	None	Normal motion pattern and structure of the valves Echo-free ventricles No effusions No septal defects Normal prosthetic valve function
Doppler echocardiogram	To identify valve function, septal defects	None	Normal valve function No blood turbulence
Color Doppler flow imaging	Same as echocardiogram	Same as echocardiogram	Same as echocardiogram
Transesophageal echocardiogram (TEE)	To evaluate suspected endocarditis, atrial emboli, atrial tumors, prosthetic valves, aortic dissection, congenital heart abnormalities, thrombi, pericardial effusion To determine size of the cardiac walls, and the size and location of intracardiac shunts	History of esophageal disease, e.g., dysphagia, cancer, surgery, large hiatal hernia Compromised pulmonary status Unstable cervical spine	No abnormalities
Radionuclide studies Thallium imaging (cold spot) Tc-PYP heart scan (hot spot)	To evaluate myocardial blood flow and the status of the myocardial cells To determine ejection fraction and velocity To assess myocardial metabolism To assess myocardial scarring and perfusion To determine whether MI is old or new To evaluate patency of grafts To evaluate the effectiveness of balloon angioplasty To determine the effectiveness of antianginal therapy To diagnose myocardial contusion	Age less than years Pregnancy	Blood flow equal throughout the myocardium Ejection fraction >70% Normal velocity No area of ischemia; no cold spots No hot spots; only the sternum and ribs should be visible. Improved regional perfusion.

| | NURSING CARE | | |
Complications	Patient Preparation	Pretest	Posttest
Same as stress test Allergic reaction to dipyridamole, amminophylline, polyethelyeneglycol, yellow dye, tartaric acid and/or tartrazine	Same as stress and thallium tests. If patient feels symptoms of dipyridamole, notify technician and ask patient to bear with it until scan is done. Aminophylline will be given to counteract symptoms.	Same as stress and thallium tests No aminophylline for 24 hours prior to test	Same as stress and thallium tests
None	Explain the procedure and its purpose. Reassure the patient that the procedure is safe and painless. Explain that some discomfort may be felt due to the amount of pressure needed to keep the transducer in contact with the skin. There is no need to restrict food or fluids. Explain to the patient that it may be necessary to alter breathing patterns or change position.	Patient teaching	Remove the conductive jelly from the patient's chest. Review the findings. Update nursing care plan.
None Same as echocardiogram Esophageal ulceration or rupture (rare) Transient vocal cord paralysis Hypoxia Aspiration Ischemic changes on ECG	Same as echocardiogram Same as echocardiogram Explain procedure. NPO after midnight. If procedure is done as an outpatient, patient will need a ride home because a sedative will be given.	Same as echocardiogram Same as echocardiogram Check allergy to contrast. Ensure consent has been signed. D/C anticoagulants No aspirin for 24 hr. If patient has a prosthetic valve, administer antibiotics as ordered. Have patient remove dentures. Have patient void. Insert large-bore IV in right arm; KVO with NSS.	Same as echocardiogram Same as echocardiogram NPO until gag reflex returns. Administer lozenges or saline gargle for sore throat. Monitor vital signs every 15 minutes, every 30 minutes, and every hour until stable. Have patient sit up or lay on side. Monitor pulse oximetry. Notify physician if patient experiences hemoptysis, pain, or dyspnea. Instruct patient returning home: Nothing to eat or drink for 1 hour, no driving for 12 hours. Review findings. Update nursing care plan.

Continued

TABLE 14–1
Cardiovascular Diagnostic Tests (*Continued*)

Diagnostic Test	Purpose	Contraindications	Normal Findings
Blood-pool imaging (MUGA)	To evaluate left ventricular function To detect aneurysms and other myocardial abnormalities To detect intracardiac shunting To determine the ejection fraction		No aneurysms or muscle wall dysfunction No intracardiac shunting Ejection fraction > 70%
Indium 111 antimysin antibody imaging	To evaluate myocardial function To diagnose MI, i.e., age, size, location To evaluate ventricular function, i.e., left ventricular wall motion, ejection fraction, cardiac output To identify structural abnormalities, i.e., valvular disease, intracardiac shunts To evaluate CAD Prognostic indicator to determine which patients are at risk for future complications	Age less than years Pregnancy	No MI Normal ventricular function Normal ejection fraction Normal valve function No shunts No evidence of CAD
Digital subtraction angiography (DSA)	To analyze ventricular wall motion To calculate ejection fraction To evaluate patency and perfusion of bypass grafts To detect vascular abnormalities, i.e., plaques, tumors, aneurysms, emboli	None	Normal wall motion Patent bypass grafts with good perfusion Ejection fraction >70%. No tumors, plaques, aneurysms, emboli
Computed tomography (CT)	To determine wall thickness To identify ischemia, MI, cardiomyopathies, aneurysms, septal defects To evaluate myocardial perfusion, patency of grafts, and valves To determine pericardial disease, i.e., pericardial effusion, pericarditis, pericardial cysts or masses To identify congenital heart disease and disease of the thoracic aorta	None	Normal wall thickness No MI, myopathies, aneurysms, defects No pericardial disease No congenital heart disease No disease of the thoracic aorta
Positron emission tomography (PET)	To distinguish between viable and nonviable myocardial tissue	Pregnancy	Matched perfusion/metabolism.

	NURSING CARE		
Complications	**Patient Preparation**	**Pretest**	**Posttest**
None	Same as thallium imaging.	Same as thallium imaging.	Same as thallium imaging.
Same as thallium imaging	Same as thallium imaging. Inform patient of need to return for scanning 48 hours after injection.	Patient teaching. Ensure permit signed. Check allergies. For outpatients, handle body fluids with latex gloves, keep fluids away from children and/or pregnant women.	Same as thallium imaging. Coordinate tests so not to interfere with each other. Wear gloves when handling body fluids for next 3 days.
Dysrhythmias Allergic reaction to the contrast medium Bleeding at insertion site Infection	May be done on an outpatient basis. Explain procedure and its purpose. Ensure that consent form is signed.	Patient teaching. Check patient history. Check consent form. Check for allergies.	Monitor vital signs every 15 minutes until stable. Check for bleeding and infection. Force fluids. Discharge teaching should include signs and symptoms requiring immediate medical attention. Review results. Update nursing care plan.
None	NPO if contrast is to be used May take medicines up to 2 hours prior to test. Assure the patient that the procedure is not painful. Head must remain immobile. Patient will be strapped to the table for safety and to ensure immobility. Tell the patient that clicking noises will be heard while in scanner. Patient may wear headphones to help relax. Patient will feel warm and flushed if dye is used. Patient may have salty metallic taste, which usually lasts only 1–2 minutes.	Patient teaching. Ensure that permit is signed. Check for allergies if contrast is to be used. Start a heparin lock if contrast is to be used.	Observe for signs and symptoms if contrast is used. Review findings. Update nursing care plan.
None	Explain procedure and its purpose. Reassure patient that there is no known radiation danger. NPO before test (Some institutions keep patients NPO or on clear liquid diet 4–6 hours prior to the test.) Refrain from caffeine for 24 hours. Refrain from tobacco.	Patient teaching. Ensure that contract is signed. Check blood glucose level. Give insulin or glucose as ordered to maintain blood sugar between 60 and 140.	Monitor vital signs. Monitor glucose. Review findings. Update nursing care plan.

Continued

TABLE 14–1
Cardiovascular Diagnostic Tests (*Continued*)

Diagnostic Test	Purpose	Contraindications	Normal Findings
Magnetic resonance imaging (MRI)	To visualize blood flow To visualize cardiac chambers To visualize the interventricular septum and valvular areas To detect vascular lesions, i.e., abcesses, plaque, tumors, clots, acute and chronic myocardial infarction, vegetations, infections, edema, and hemorrhage	Permanent pacemakers Some metal prosthetics, especially heart valves, nerve-stimulating devices, cochlear implants, metal in the eye, older ferromagnetic intracranial aneurysm clips	No impedance of blood flow. No abnormalities in the interventricular septum Normal valves—no calcification No evidence of tumors, plaques, clots, or MI

Cardiac catheterization	To evaluate cardiac wall action
	To evaluate valve function
	To determine cardiac output
	To determine the presence of cardiac defects and/or abnormalities
	To determine the presence and degree of coronary artery disease
	To determine candidates for balloon angioplasty, fibrinolytic therapy, bypass surgery, heart transplantation, and artificial heart
	To determine the presence of intracardiac shunting
	To evaluate the patency of bypass grafts
		Acute MI
		Acute debilitating conditions.
		Gross cardiomegaly.
		Poor renal function.
		Special conditions—
		• Right-sided catheterization: left bundle branch block (LBBB) unless a temporary pacemaker is inserted
		• Patients with valvular disease: prophylactic antibiotics to guard against subacute bacterial endocarditis (SBE).
		  The following conditions must be corrected prior to the test: severe hypertension, sepsis, hemorrhagic diathesis, prothombin time >10, heart failure, ventricular ectopy.
			Normal wall motion.
			Normal valve movement.
			Coronary arteries smooth, with regular outline.
			Pressures—RA: 0–8 mmHg
			  RV: 15–25 mmHg systolic; 0–8 mmHg diastolic
			  PA: 15–30 mmHg systolic; 8–15 mmHg diastolic
			  LA: 4–12 mmHg
			  LV: 100–140 mmHg systolic; 60–80 mmHg diastolic
			  Ao: 100–140 mmHg systolic; 60–80 mmHg diastolic
			  PCWP: 6–12 mmHg
			Stroke index: 30–65 mL/beat per m^2
			Cardiac index: 2.5–4.0 mL/min per m^2
			Ejection fraction: 70% or greater
			Oxygen saturation:
			Right side: 75% ± 14
			Left side: 95% ± 19
			Valve orifaces:
			Mitral: 5–6 cm^2
			Aortic: 2.5–3.5 cm^2

	NURSING CARE		
Complications	**Patient Preparation**	**Pretest**	**Posttest**
Affects pacemaker function	Explain procedure and purpose. Remove all metal objects, e.g., jewelry, watches, glasses, hair-pins. Do not take credit cards into room (may erase magnetic strip).	Explain that there is no exposure to radiation. Patient teaching. Ensure that consent is signed. Check for removal of metal objects. Check for history of injuries with metal fragments, e.g., shrapnel, flecks of ferrous metal in the eye. Check whether the patient is claustrophobic; if so a sedative maybe needed.	Monitor safety factors if sedative is given. Review results. Update nursing care plan.
General: MI Cardiac tamponade Dysrhythmias Pneumothorax Infection—local and/ or systemic Hypovolemia Pulmonary edema Hemorrhage Hematoma at insertion site Arterial spasm Allergic reaction to the contrast medium Cardiac arrest Left-sided: Arterial emboli Thrombus Cerebrovascular accident Perforation of the aorta, great vessels, or coronary artery Right-sided: Thrombophlebitis Pulmonary emboli Vasovagal reaction	Explain the procedure and its purpose. Ensure that consent form is signed. Restrict foods and fluids 6–12 hours prior to the test (may be allowed to take oral medications with sips of water). Reinforce the need for complete cooperation. Patient must follow orders immediately, e.g., cough. Advise that the patient will be awake throughout the procedure but that a sedative or a tranquilizer will be given. Inform the patient that there will be talking among the staff, and that the staff will call the patient by name when talking to him or her. Patient may wear dentures, glasses, and hearing aid.	NPO after midnight except medications. Check if diuretics to be given. Check history and physical. Weigh patient. Check preprocedure studies: chest x-ray, ECG, coagulation values, cardiac enzymes, CBC, and electrolytes. CHECK FOR ALLERGIES, especially to iodine, seafood, and contrast medium. Check for difficulty in lying flat. Patient teaching. Provide emotional support. Encourage the patient to practice breathing and coughing Administer sedative or tranquilizer as ordered unless the patient has respiratory compromise. Mark peripheral pulses for easier detection after the procedure. Monitor vital signs for baseline parameters. If the patient is on dialysis, it should be carried out that day If the patient is a diabetic, check whether insulin is to be given or the dose altered. Have the patient void and put on a hospital gown before leaving for the procedure. When the procedure is ordered, check about any anticoagulants that the patient is receiving, and whether cardiac drugs are to be given prior to the procedure.	Monitor vital signs every 15 minutes ×4 until stable. Check peripheral pulses every 30 minutes. Observe insertion site for bleeding or hematomas when vital signs are monitored. Have patient wiggle fingers and toes every 30 minutes. Enforce bed rest for 6–8 hours. Apply a sandbag to the insertion site for 6–8 hours if an artery was used. During transfer from the stretcher to the bed, support the extremities and apply pressure during the transfer. Maintain IVs. Monitor for renal failure, i.e., I&O, blood urea nitrogen (BUN), creatinine. Encourage oral fluid intake. If the patient is on dialysis, dialysis should take place after the procedure to prevent fluid overload. Obtain an ECG after the procedure. Review resumption of medications with the physician. Review the test results. Update the nursing care plan. Start discharge teaching.
Prolonged sustained dysrhythmia Phlebitis Pulmonary emboli Thromboemboli Hemmorhage at the insertion site Perforation of the ventricular or septal wall Damage to the tricuspid valve Damage to the catheterized vein (occlusion) Infection: local or systemic Pneumothorax Cardiac tamponade	Explain the procedure and its purpose. Restrict food and fluids for at least 6 hours prior to the procedure. Refer to Cardiac Catheterization.	Patient teaching. Ensure that the consent is signed. Check patient history for ongoing antidysrhythmic therapy. Have emergency equipment on standby. Refer to Cardiac Catheterization.	Refer to Cardiac Catheterization.

RADIOLOGIC TESTING

Chest X-Ray

The chest x-ray[1,2] is one of the most frequently used diagnostic tests, and, in conjunction with other tests, is used to evaluate cardiac and pulmonary diseases. Routinely, posteroanterior (PA) and left lateral views are taken. These provide a sharper and less distorted image of the heart than other views or techniques. If the patient is unable to be transported to the x-ray department, a portable x-ray machine can be used. This technique (portable x-ray) may be used for baseline evaluation or to check placement of endotracheal (ET) tubes, central venous pressure (CVP) lines, pulmonary artery lines, chest tubes, pacemaker leads, or feeding tubes. The portable equipment provides an anteroposterior (AP) view, which may distort the relative size of the heart and great vessels as reviewed and interpreted. Vascular markings in the AP view may appear increased. Other views are the oblique view, which is used to visualize lesions and project them free of overlying structures, and the lateral decubitus, which demonstrates gravitation of pleural fluid and confirms air-fluid levels.[3]

Procedure

The PA view is obtained by having the patient stand erect with the chin resting on top of the cassette holder and the chest and shoulders resting against the holder. The x-ray machine is approximately 6 ft behind the patient. The patient is told to take a deep breath and to hold it until the picture is taken. The technician advises the patient when to breathe again. The patient holds the breath for only a few seconds. Patients who have suffered myocardial infarction should be warned not to bear down (Valsalva maneuver) while holding their breath, as this may precipitate a vagal response that results in bradycardia or other cardiac dysrhythmias. Full cooperation on the part of the patient is necessary for a clear picture.

The AP view is taken by placing the cassette behind the patient's back, with the head of the bed either flat or in a high Fowler's position. The upright position is best, since the patient's diaphragm will not interfere with the visualization of the heart and lungs. The x-ray machine is placed in front of the patient, approximately 2 ft away from the patient's chest. The patient is told to take a deep breath and to hold it until told to breathe again. If patients are unable to hold their breath, the technician times the exposure to take place at the end of inspiration. The AP view is the view obtained when a portable x-ray is desired.

Abnormal Findings

Cardiac enlargement, pericardial effusions, pleural effusions, pericardial tamponade, valve calcification, ventricular and aortic aneurysms, pericardial and mediastinal masses, hiatal hernias, pneumothorax, hemothorax, and coarctation of the aorta arch are some of the abnormalities that can be found on the PA and lateral chest x-ray.[1] Other findings include dextracardia, pulmonary vasculature changes due to cardiac abnormalities, and misplacement of ET tubes, chest tubes, and feeding tubes.

Interfering Factors

Poor technique, inadequate exposure, inability of patients to hold their breath, and patient movement are some of the interfering factors.

EXERCISE (STRESS) ELECTROCARDIOGRAPHY

Exercise tests (stress tests) are utilized to determine electrocardiographic (ECG) changes during periods of increased myocardial oxygen consumption. These changes would not normally be detected on a resting ECG.

Exercise Test/Stress Test

There are a variety of stress tests. The bicycle ergometry test measures the effects of arm and leg exercises applied against a calibrated amount of resistance. The amount of resistance is gradually increased as the patient tries to maintain a constant speed. The patient sits on the bicycle, and the seat and handlebars are adjusted so that the patient is comfortable and able to maintain balance. This test is rarely used today.

The multistage treadmill test measures the effects of graduated exercise at adjusted speeds and inclines. The patient is shown how to step on the treadmill moving at a slow speed and how to use the support rails to maintain balance only. The patient then steps onto the treadmill and continues walking at a slow rate until familiar with the movement pattern; then the speed and incline are gradually increased. The patient is always informed prior to any changes.

Procedure

The day of the test, the patient is not allowed anything to eat for 2 to 4 hours prior to the test in order to prevent nausea or cramps from occuring during exercise.[4] Patients are instructed to avoid stimulants such as coffee, tea, and tobacco because these substances cause increased excitability of the heart's conduction system. Unless otherwise directed, patients should take their regular medications.

In general, the procedure for stress testing or exercise testing includes cleaning (and shaving, if necessary) several areas on the patient's chest and possibly the back. The skin is abraded, and the monitor electrodes are applied in selected leads. (Reassure the patient that no current will be felt from the electrodes.) The electrodes are secured, and the lead cable is placed over the patient's shoulder and secured with tape or pinned to the clothing. A baseline tracing is obtained prior to exercise, as well as a baseline heart rate (HR) and blood pressure (BP). These are obtained in the supine, sitting, and standing positions as well as after a 15-second period of hyperventilating. The patient's heart and lungs are auscultated, noting the presence of extra heart sounds (e.g., S_3 or S_4 gallop) and/or adventitious breath sounds (e.g., rales or crackles). The patient is assessed for pedal edema and the presence of, or change in, chest pain. The test is canceled if any abnormalities are noted. The patient is instructed about what to do and is told to immediately report symptoms of chest pain or discomfort, shortness of breath, fatigue, leg cramps, or dizziness.

Once the test is begun, the patient's ECG rhythm, heart rate, and blood pressure are monitored throughout the test, usually at predetermined intervals. The test level and elapsed time are noted with each set of parameters. The test takes about 30 minutes, although the patient may be in the laboratory for 1.5 hours. The exercise period depends on the patient's physical condition, absence of significant changes in vital signs, heart rhythm, or presence of abnormal symptoms (listed above), but is usually only 10 to 15 minutes.

A patient undergoing a maximal test will exercise until reaching at least 85% of predicted capacity, based on age and measured by the heart rate response.[5] Exercise will continue until the patient becomes fatigued or experiences chest pain or other symptoms. Table 14–2 lists reasons for stopping the test based on subjective and objective data. A patient may undergo a submaximal test, which is used in patients who have suffered a myocardial infarction to reassure them of their ability to perform normal activ-

ities of daily living.[5] Here the test is ended when the patient reaches a certain target heart rate (THR). The target heart rate may vary among institutions. It is usually based upon age and sex; a general rule-of-thumb calculation is 85% of 220 minus the patient's age:

$$(220 - Age) \times 0.85 = THR$$

Upon termination of the test, the treadmill is slowed for several minutes; then the patient is helped off the equipment and into a chair. An ECG is performed, and ECG rhythm strips are obtained at 2- to 3-minute intervals until parameters return to the patient's baseline levels. The blood pressure and heart rate are monitored at 2- to 3-minute intervals, and more frequently if they are abnormal.

Abnormal Results

A positive test consists of a flat or downsloping ST segment (see Chapter 15) of 1 mm. If there is initial depression of the ST segment on the resting ECG, the depression must be −1 mm or greater over the baseline depression during exercise to be of significance. There is controversy concerning the extent of ST segment changes that constitute an abnormal response to exercise, that is, some authorities state that a 2-mm depression is needed for significance. ST depression is significant of ischemia. False positives may occur, especially in women between the ages of 20 and 40. In cases of false positives, further testing may be required.

Interfering Factors

Interfering factors include patient failure to observe pretest restrictions, fatigue, lack of cooperation, the use of β-blockers or digitalis, bundle branch block, Wolff-Parkinson-White syndrome (see Chapter 15), vasoregulatory aesthesia, anemia, hypoxia, electrolyte imbalance, hyperventilation, mitral valve prolapse, and cardiomyopathy.

Thallium Stress Test

Exercise causes an increase in coronary blood flow to a level 1.5 to 3 times that of the normal resting flow. In coronary artery disease (CAD) the increase is absent or not as evident. With the injection of a radionuclide, thallium 201, there is a 75% to 95% chance of detecting CAD.[5] Technitium Tc 99m teboroxime (Cardiotec) and technitium Tc 99m sestamibi (Cardiolite) are new tracing agents that are readily absorbed by the myocardium and therefore reduce imaging time.[5] Indications for thallium stress testing are abnormal resting ECG, digoxin therapy, and atypical angina.

Procedure

The patient undergoes the stress test as mentioned above. Thallium 201, a potassium analogue, is injected intravenously during the last minutes of the stress

TABLE 14–2
Reasons to Terminate Stress Testing

Subjective Data
Chest pain
Extreme fatigue
Extreme weakness
Severe dyspnea
Dizziness or syncope
Ataxia
Claudication

Objective Data
Gallop heart sounds (S_3, S_4)
Valvular regurgitation murmur
Abnormal chest pulsations or heaves
ST-segment elevation or depression of 1 mm or more
Arrhythmias
Target heart rate is reached
Heart rate >80%–85% of maximum rate
Failure of the blood pressure to rise above resting level
Elevation in systolic blood pressure >250 mmHg
Drop in systolic blood pressure >10 mmHg after exercise
Rise in diastolic blood pressure >90 mmHg or >20 mmHg over patient's baseline
Confusion
Cold sweat
Glassy stare
Change in skin color

Source: Adapted from Kenner, CV, Guzzetta, CE, and Dossey, B (eds): Critical Care Nursing: Body-Mind-Spirit. Little, Brown & Co, Boston, 1985.

test.[5] The thallium is absorbed by the myocardium during maximum coronary blood flow. The patient is then placed under a nuclear imaging scanner, where the physiologic distribution of the radionuclide is detected. Three to 4 hours later the patient undergoes another scan to obtain redistribution images.

Abnormal Findings

Areas of light distribution (low radioactivity) indicate decreased or absent perfusion on the initial scan. Perfusion defects that appear on the first scan, but not the second, signify areas of ischemia.[5] A persistent defect in both scans signifies areas of scar tissue from an infarction.[5]

Pharmacologic Stress Test

Pharmacologic stress tests are done if a patient is unable to exercise sufficiently to achieve a target heart rate. Patients with peripheral vascular disease with claudication, mobility defects (e.g., sickness, severe pulmonary disease, those on β-blockers, obesity), and those with poor exercise tolerance would be candidates for the test. The test provides for the assessment of coronary blood flow reserve, where in the normal person there is no oxygen mismatch.[5] Coronary blood flow is increased with pharmacologic agents rather than exercise. Dipyridamole (Persantine) orally or intravenously, or adenosine (Adenocard) intravenously, are the drugs of choice to increase the coronary blood flow (perfusion). Dobutamine (Dobutrex) intravenously also may by used, but instead of increasing perfusion it increases the cardiac output.[5]

Procedure

The patient is sent to the nuclear medicine department. The test is carried out with the patient sitting in a supine position on the table. ECG leads are applied as in a regular stress test. The drug is then given to the patient, and vital signs and symptoms are monitored as the drug takes effect. Some symptoms would include chest pain, nausea, headache, or dizziness.[5] The patient is encouraged to bear with the symptoms until the test is completed. Forty minutes after the oral dose of dipyramidole (Persantine) or 5 minutes after the intravenous dose, thallium 201 will be given. The first scan is done. The patient may then be given a 50- to 125-mg bolus of aminophylline to reverse the action and side effects of the dipyramidole. Two to 3 hours later the patient returns for the second scan. The patient may receive a second dose of thallium to enhance the second set of images.[5]

Abnormal Results

A positive test consists of a flat or downsloping ST segment of 1 mm or more for more than 0.08 second. If there was an initial ST segment depression on the resting ECG, the depression must be −1 mm or greater than the baseline depression during exercise to be of significance. There is controversy concerning the extent of ST segment changes that constitutes an abnormal response to exercise.

In the thallium stress and pharmacologic stress tests, areas of myocardium that demonstrate decreased uptake of the isotope in the first scan only are indicative of a reduction of blood flow, and, therefore, transient or reversible ischemia.[6] Areas with a reduction of 40% or more signify CAD.[7] Areas that demonstrate a decrease or absence of uptake of the isotope in both the first and second scans are indicative of persistent or permanent perfusion deficit at the site of a previous infarction.[7]

Interfering Factors

Accurate interpretation can be difficult when there is inadequate exercise; lack of cooperation from the patient regarding medications, diet, and so on; mitral valve prolapse; sarcoidosis; and cardiomyopathy.[7]

Digital Supine Bicycle Stress Echocardiogram

The digital supine bicycle stress echocardiogram is a new technique for evaluating CAD. It is performed almost exclusively for patients with abnormal results in the maximal treadmill exercise test. The patient performs bicycle exercise in the supine position on a table that has the capability of left lateral tilt and head elevation. The patient's workload is increased, depending upon the patient, by 25 to 50 W every 2 minutes until symptom-limited maximum exercise is achieved. Images are achieved in five views during each stage. This test has been found to be have a sensitivity of 87%, a specificity of 89%, and an accuracy of 88% for disease detection in specific coronary arteries.[8]

ULTRASONOGRAPHY

Echocardiogram

The echocardiogram is a safe, painless, noninvasive, cost-effective procedure that shows the size and movement of cardiac structures, the dimensions of the heart chambers, and cardiac output. Sound waves of high frequency (>2000 Hz second) and short duration (1.9 to 5.0 milliseconds) are directed through the chest wall, which then reflects waves to a transducer and a recording device. The frequency of these waves varies and depends on the density and mobility of the cardiac tissue.[1]

Various techniques are used in performing the procedure. The motion mode (M-mode) involves a thin ultrasound beam striking the heart. This produces a vertical or "ice pick" view of the heart and structures. This mode is especially useful in recording the motion of the intracardiac structures. Frequently, it is done in time-sequence—time-motion mode (TM-mode). This is the best technique for identifying chamber size and valve leaflets.

The other technique, two-dimensional mode (2-D or B mode), involves a rapid sweeping of the ultrasound beam in an arc, thereby producing a cross-sectional or fan-shaped view of the cardiac structures. This mode is useful for recording lateral motion and providing a correct spatial relationship between the cardiac structures.[1,2]

Doppler Echocardiogram

The Doppler echocardiogram records the velocity and direction of moving objects; therefore, it best assesses blood flow through the heart, regurgitant flow through incompetent or stenotic valves, or septal defects. There are two types of directional waves. The continuous wave (CW) measures velocity, whereas the pulsed wave (PW) localizes flow distributions.

Color Flow Doppler Imaging

Color flow Doppler imaging is a superimposed color representation of blood flow onto a black-and-white two-dimensional image of the heart and blood vessels. Cardiovascular blood flow is color coded according to direction and velocity. Blood flowing toward the transducer is coded red; blood moving away is blue. Turbulent blood flow appears green, or as a mix of colors in a mosaic pattern. It is used in the evaluation of specific cardiac chambers and valves.

Procedure

The procedure entails placing the patient in a quiet, darkened room, in a supine position or lying on the left side. Conductive jelly is applied to the chest and a special dime-sized transducer is placed directly over the chest at the acoustic window, that is, the area where bone and lung tissue are absent, at approximately the 3rd to 4th intercostal space to the left of the sternum. The transducer is systematically angled to view different parts of the heart. Patients may be told to change position, breathe slowly, or hold their breath while heart function is being recorded. The procedure usually takes 15 to 60 minutes.

Abnormal Results

Abnormal findings are indicative of valvular disorders, left ventricular hypertrophy, cardiomyopathies, myxomas, ventricular aneurysms, abnormalities in wall motion, or pericardial effusions.

Interfering Factors

Interfering factors include incorrect placement of the transducer, patient movement, and abnormally shaped or thickened chest walls. Technical problems can also arise in patients with small hearts.

Epicardial Echocardiogram

The epicardial echocardiogram (EE) or perioperative epicardial echocardiogram (PEE) offers good-quality films since it is done directly on the heart during cardiac surgery.[9] The echocardiogram is done after the patient is cannulated for cardiopulmonary bypass. It is usually done to assess the results of a valve repair or repair of congenital defects, or to detect micro bubbles in the cardiac cavity after cardiac surgery.

Procedure

Once the heart is cannulated, the transducer is placed directly on the heart over the area to be studied. This is done by trained technicians. Readings can be done at any time during the procedure but cannot be used continuously. Although accurate readings are obtained, certain problems can arise. The transducer must be placed gently over the epicardium; if too much pressure is applied, damage to the myocardium can occur or dysrhythmias can be induced.[9] Pulsations of the heart may interfere with clear images.

Transesophageal Echocardiogram

The transesophageal echocardiogram (TEE) provides a continuous two-dimensional image of the heart and its structures without interference from the chest wall, ribs, and lungs.[9] It is most effective in visualizing structures at the base of the heart, the major vessels, the atria, and the semilunar valves. It can be used in the operating room (PTEE) with relative safety in place of the PEE.

Procedure

The procedure can be done at the bedside. A large-bore IV is started and the patient is given an IV sedative, usually Valium or Midazolam. The patient's pharynx is then numbed with lidocaine and the patient is placed on the left side to decrease the incidence of aspiration. An ultrasonic transducer is mounted on the tip of a flexible gastroscope, which is approximately 9 to 10 mm in diameter. The gastroscope and transducer are then lubricated with a water-soluble gel and advanced through the patient's mouth and down the esophagus. Bite blocks are inserted to prevent damage to the scope and to prevent injury to the physician. The scope is then advanced 30 to 35 cm past the front teeth to view the aortic leaflet. The scope is manipulated to visualize various structures. It is withdrawn 1 cm to view the proximal coronary artery, rotated 30 degrees clockwise and advanced 2 to 3 cm to visualize the mitral valve. It then is withdrawn 2 cm to view the left atrial appendage, which is rarely seen in a transthoracic echocardiogram. The scope then is rotated counterclockwise to view the complete left atrial cavity and interseptum. It then is advanced a few centimeters for a modified four-chamber view. It can be advanced into the stomach (40 to 45 cm from the front teeth) to view the inferior chambers. Throughout the procedure a standard two-dimensional echocardiogram is obtained in conjunction with Doppler and color flow Doppler imaging. The patient's ECG rhythm and vital signs are also monitored. The procedure takes 5 to 20 minutes.[11,12]

Abnormal Findings

Results of the test may show an aortic aneurysm or dissection, thrombi around a valve or in the atria, mitral valve dysfunction, prosthetic valve dysfunction, congenital heart disease, or atrial tumors, to mention a few abnormalities. Intraoperatively it can demonstrate changes in left ventricular function, the adequacy of valve repair or replacement, the presence of air bubbles in cardiac chambers prior to removing the patient from cardio-pulmonary bypass, or monitor the repair of congenital defects, thereby avoiding reoperation due to complications.[11]

Acoustic Quantification

This new advancement in ultrasonography automatically detects blood and tissue interfaces, making real-time quantitative measurement of cardiac function available.[13] A patent is pending.

Intravascular Ultrasound

Intravascular ultrasound,[13] which is currently under development, will be able to provide the physician with highly detailed images of almost histologic value. Insertion of a miniature transducer on the tip of a catheter makes it possible to explore the heart, great vessels, and peripheral vasculature. With this equipment it is possible to distinguish between a soft plaque and a thrombus in a coronary artery. Such information makes it possible to decide on treatment modality, that is, revascularization, percutaneous transluminal coronary angioplasty (PTCA), arthrectomy, or stent placement.

RADIONUCLIDE STUDIES

Thallium Imaging (Cold Spot)

Thallium imaging[14] can be done at rest, in order to detect abnormalities in perfusion, or it can be done in conjunction with stress testing. The radionuclide is rapidly absorbed by healthy myocardial tissue, which appears dark on the scan. Ischemic or necrotic areas do not absorb the radionuclide and appear white or as "cold spots." Within 5 to 20 minutes, absorption is proportional to the regional blood flow so that qualitative information can be obtained concerning left ventricular wall thickness and chamber size. A scan 4 hours after the injection shows the relative distribution of the thallium and indicates myocardial cells that are viable independent of perfusion.[3]

Procedure

The resting thallium test involves the injection of the radionuclide, thallium 201, into a vein. The patient lies supine on the x-ray table. After 3 to 5 minutes, scanning begins. The patient may be repositioned so that the anterior, left anterior oblique, 45- and 60-degree angles, and the left lateral views can be evaluated. The resting thallium test can detect a myocardial infarction within the first few hours of the onset of symptoms. This procedure takes 30 to 40 minutes to complete.

Abnormal Findings

Persistent defects in perfusion indicate a myocardial infarction. Transient defects usually indicate ischemia secondary to CAD.

Interfering Factors

False positives may occur secondary to ventricular aneurysms, metastatic carcinoma, skin lesions, sarcoidosis, myocardial fibrosis, cardiac contusions, apical clefts, coronary spasm; attenuation may be due to soft tissue; and artifacts may be produced by the diaphragm, breast implants, or electrodes. False negatives may be due to insignificant obstruction; delayed imaging; single-vessel disease, especially involving the right or left circumflex arteries; and the presence of collateral circulation. Other interfering factors include mechanical malfunction, technician error, and patient movement.

Technetium Pyrophosphate Imaging

Technetium pyrophosphate imaging (Tc-PYP) is used for patients with a history of chest pain 1 to 3 days prior to admission or seeking medical attention, where the cardiac enzymes may have returned to normal levels. Tc-PYP heart scans involve the injection of technetium Tc 99m pyrophosphate, a radionuclide that is absorbed by damaged or ischemic myocardial cells. Distribution depends on residual myocardial blood flow and the extent of myocardial necrosis. The radionuclide appears as a dark "hot spot" on the film. The Tc-PYP heart scan is helpful in determining the location and age (recent or old) of a myocardial infarction. The test must be performed within 72 hours of the onset of symptoms in order to determine onset of the infarct. The scan can also be performed in conjunction with a stress test to aid in the diagnosis of CAD.

Procedure

The procedure is like that of thallium imaging. The only difference is that scanning must take place 2 to 3 hours after injection of the radionuclide, rather than 3 to 5 minutes after injection, as in the thallium scan. Once the patient returns, 2 to 3 hours after injection of the radionuclide, the test usually takes 30 to 60 minutes to perform, during which time the patient may lie still for 15 to 30 minutes.

Abnormal Findings

Uptake of the radionuclide occurs in areas of valve calcification, necrosis or ischemia of the myocardium, viral myocarditis, and ventricular aneurysm. Images should return to normal within 1 to 2 weeks. Up to 50% of patients continue to have positive scans past this time frame. Patients with persistent positive scans have a higher incidence of persistent angina, recurrent infarctions, congestive heart failure (CHF), and death.[1,14] Patients with positive scans should have additional studies done.

Interfering Factors

Interfering factors include hypotension, scanning done less than 3 hours after injection, previous infarction, subendocardial infarctions, small areas of necrosis (less than 3 g),[4] renal insufficiency, calcification of the aortic and/or mitral valves, cardiac trauma, recent cardioversion, pericarditis, cancer, unstable angina, and patient movement.

Gated Blood Pool Imaging

The gated blood pool scan is a radionuclide test that involves various techniques. These techniques include first-pass scanning, two-framed gated scanning, and multiple-gated acquisition scanning (MUGA), which can be done in conjunction with a stress test (stress MUGA) or with the administration of nitroglycerin (nitro MUGA).[15]

Procedure

These tests involve an intravenous injection of non-radioactive pyrophosphate, which attaches itself to, or "tags," the red blood cells (RBCs). After 30 minutes, an intravenous injection of radioactive technetium is given, which combines with the pyrophosphate on the RBCs, thus creating a radioactive pool. Scintillation cameras record the initial passage of the radionuclide through the heart (first pass). Then, in synchrony with the electrocardiogram, the camera records the left ventricular end-systolic and left ventricular end-diastolic phases for 500 to 1000 cardiac cycles (two-framed gated imaging). This allows visualization of the left ventricle for the presence of akinesia, dyskinesia, or intracardiac shunts.

The MUGA scan records 14 to 64 points of a single cardiac cycle. These sequential images make it possible to evaluate wall motion and calculate the ejection fraction. When done in conjunction with the stress test, the MUGA scan detects changes in the ejection fraction, cardiac output, and wall motion related to exercise or stress. The nitro MUGA is done to evaluate the effect of nitroglycerin on ventricular function, that is, increase myocardial contractility secondary to the increase in myocardial blood flow.[5] The blood pool imaging tests take 60 to 90 minutes to perform.

Abnormal Findings and Interfering Factors

Abnormal findings and interfering factors associated with the MUGA scan are similar to those presented for the Tc-PYP heart scan.

Indium 111 Antimyosin Antibody Imaging

Antimyosin antibody is produced by recombinant DNA technology or in a mouse hybridoma cell line, where human cardiac myosin is injected into a mouse that produces antibodies specific to human cardiac myosin. Antibodies are extracted and labeled with indium 111, a radioactive material.[16] Indium 111 labels necrotic tissue only; therefore, it accurately detects acute myocardial infarctions, both their extent and location. This method is currently awaiting FDA approval.

Procedure

The patient is injected with indium 111 and returns to the lab 24 hours after injection for scanning. Three different views are done so as to visualize all portions of the left ventricle. Some patients return again 48 hours after injection.

Abnormal Findings

Infarcted tissue is seen as bright areas or "hot spots." The scan will be negative if there is only ischemia. As the infarct ages and scar tissue forms, the scan shows progressive decrease in the positive image.

Emerging Technology

Studies are presently being done for the use of indium in the detection of myocarditis and cardiac transplant rejection. Additional studies are exploring the possibility of dual isotope testing, where indium 111 and thallium 201 are used together to distinguish necrosis from ischemia, so that patients at high risk can be identified and more aggressive management strategies implemented.

TOMOGRAPHY

Digital Subtraction Angiography

Digital subtraction angiography (DSA) is a new, relatively noninvasive technique that involves computer-assisted imaging.[3,4,6] It is presently being used to localize regions of peripheral arterial disease; assess ventricular function, including ventricular wall motion and calculation of ejection fractions; identify and quantify intracardiac shunts; visualize coronary artery bypass grafts and congenital cardiac malformations; and evaluate vascular tumors.[3] The scope of DSA as a diagnostic tool is unlimited. It can be used alone or in conjunction with standard arteriographic techniques.

Procedure

There are two methods of employing DSA: the serial or static mode, and the continuous or dynamic mode. The serial or static mode involves obtaining an image of the area to be studied prior to injection of the contrast medium. This is stored in memory as the "mask image." The contrast medium is then power-injected (i.e., machine-controlled to provide consistency in injection) and a second series of images is obtained as the dye passes through the area being studied. A computer subtracts all the background layers such as bone and soft tissue, leaving only the image of the contrast-filled vessels. The images are recorded at a rate of 1 to 4 images per second.

The continuous or dynamic mode is similar to the static mode, but the serial images are obtained at a rapid rate of 30 images per second. Images are stored on a videotape or videodisc, which can be viewed on a screen. Prior to formal interpretation, hard copies are produced for permanent storage.

An advantage of DSA over conventional arteriographic studies is that lower doses of contrast media are required to present consistent images, thereby decreasing the possibility of an allergic reaction to the contrast media.

Abnormal Findings

Abnormal findings include abnormal anatomy or function of the cardiovascular system.

Interfering Factors

Patient movement appears to be the only interfering factor for both modes, thereby reinforcing the need for careful patient education before the procedure. A problem that arises with the continuous mode is the storage of the large quantities of information.

Computed Tomography

Initially computed tomography (CT) scans were used to provide information on brain abnormalities and head injuries.[2] Today a three-dimensional view of various parts of the body can be obtained by combining detailed cross-sectional images. Cardiac CT scans use a high-speed cine CT (50 msec) gated to the ECG. It produces views of the heart in systole and diastole and is used to assess regional and global myocardial function.

Procedure

The patient is placed on a special x-ray table where the electron beams pass over the patient in an arc.[14] The beam of photons generated passes from beneath the patient to the detectors above the patient. Iodine contrast may be used for a greater tissue absorption, therefore, "contrast enhancement."

Abnormal Findings

Some of the abnormal findings that may be evident are aneurysms, masses; hypokinesis, akinesis, dyskinesia; decreased blood flow in the heart and blood vessels and grafts due to thrombi; plaque; pericardial cysts, pericardial fluid, constrictive pericarditis; and congenital heart disease.

Limitations

The cost of the test is prohibitive. The length of imaging time and patient movement also create problems.

Positrom Emission Tomography

Positron emission tomography (PET) has been used for years in the study of neurologic disorders. Currently there is an increase in its use to distinguish between viable and nonviable tissue, thus allowing for a better choice of treatment. The equipment is extremely expensive, and there are only 60 facilities in the United States that perform PET scans.[14] PET has demonstrated a 95% accuracy in the diagnosis of CAD, both symptomatic and asymptomatic.

Procedure

The scan can be done either with the patient in a resting state or in exercise or stressed states. An intravenous line is started and a positron-emitting radionuclide-labeled compound is injected to visualize myocardial perfusion. In a cardiac scan, the compound ammonia N13 ($^{13}NH_3$) is commonly used. Perfusion images are obtained, and the patient is then injected with the second compound, fludeoxy-glucose F 18 (^{18}FDG), to visualize myocardial metabolism, that is, the amount of glucose taken up by the cells. The patient is scanned again to record metabolic uptake. The test takes approximately 1 hour.[14]

Abnormal Findings

The normal myocardium will demonstrate a match between perfusion and metabolism as seen by the areas of red and yellow.[14] Nonviable infarcted tissue shows little or no appearance of the red and yellow, corresponding to the absence or decrease of both perfusion and metabolism. The ischemic myocardium shows a metabolic/perfusion mismatch: There is an increase in the metabolic state (yellow) and a decrease in the perfusion (red). The chance that coronary revascularization will improve heart function is 85% in those patients with metabolic/perfusion match. There is a 78% to 92% probability that revascularization will not be effective in improving heart function in those patients with a metabolic/perfusion mismatch.[14]

Magnetic Resonance Imaging

Magnetic resonance imaging (MRI) is based on the absorption and re-emission of radiofrequency electromagnetic energy by certain nuclei (hydrogen, sodium, carbon, phosphorous, and fluorine)[7] when placed in a strong magnetic field.[2,4,5] This phenomenon is used to generate three-dimensional images in order to diagnose structural and biochemical abnormalities without the risk of ionizing radiation.[3,4,6]

MRI is safe for children and pregnant women. Because of the large magnetic fields, it cannot be used in patients with implants of metal clips because of the danger of displacement. Use of MRI is likewise contraindicated in patients with permanent pacemakers because of the danger of pacemaker reprogramming or switching to the fixed-rate mode.[17,18]

Procedure

The patient is placed in a large supercooled electromagnetic scanner that produces a magnetic field. Normally the protons (i.e., nuclei of hydrogen atoms) are randomly oriented, but when placed inside the magnetic field they become ordered with respect to the field. When an appropriate radiofrequency is applied, some of the protons absorb energy from the radiofrequency wave. These same protons can then re-emit a radio signal that can be detected by an antenna. With the aid of a computer these signals can generate a three-dimensional image. Gadolinium (unrelated to the iodinated contrasts utilized in other studies) is sometimes used to enhance the images. Patient cooperation is of the utmost importance as the body must remain perfectly still during the scanning. Patients with claustrophobia are frequently given a sedative, for example, Valium, prior to the test. Headphones with calming music are frequently provided to help the patient relax.

Abnormal Findings

Abnormal findings may include the following: myocardial infarction (with details of size and age), decreased left ventricular wall motion, decreased ejection fraction, presence of atherosclerotic plaques in proximal coronary arteries, ventricular aneurysms, valvular disorders, pericarditis, hypertrophic cardiomyopathy, vacuolar lesions in dissecting aneurysms, blood clots, and masses and/or tumors.

Interfering Factors

Large moving objects, as, for example, elevators, can interfere with the study. This appears to be the only interfering factor known currently. Disadvantages in using this technique include its expense, the amount of space needed for the equipment, and interference with the operation of other equipment because of the magnetic field.[17,18] Another disadvantage is that nonferrous metals may produce artifacts that degrade the images.

CARDIAC CATHETERIZATION

Cardiac catheterization is a frequently performed invasive technique requiring expert nursing care. Nurses not only have to know what the procedure entails in order to implement patient teaching, but they also need to monitor the patient carefully after the procedure to prevent complications. The mortality rate is 0.1% to 0.2%. Most deaths occur in patients with severe dysfunction or severe CAD, where the mortality rate is 1%.[7,19,20]

Procedure and Nursing Care Implications

The patient is wheeled to the cardiac catheterization laboratory on a stretcher, then placed on a padded x-ray table and strapped in place.[19,20] An intravenous line is started if one does not already exist, and the chart is carefully checked for appropriate consents and for any abnormal results (e.g., laboratory data including electrolytes, liver and/or renal function studies, hematology, prothrombin and partial thromboplastin times, chest x-ray, and ECG). Patients who have any allergies to iodine, fish, shellfish, or contrast medium may be given an antihistamine or steroids to lessen the reaction to the contrast medium. (In some institutions, the patient may be started on steroids or antihistamines a few days prior to the procedure). Electrodes are placed on the patient's extremities to allow for continuous monitoring of the patient's cardiac rhythm during the procedure.

The site to be used for catheter insertion is shaved and cleansed with an antiseptic solution, and a sterile milieu within which to implement the procedure is established and maintained. An antecubital vein is usually used for a right-sided catheterization (the femoral vein is used if a right- and left-sided catheterization is to be done; the femoral artery is the preferred site for left-sided catheterization). When local anesthesia is given, the patient may experience a transient stinging sensation. The catheter can be inserted either by a percutaneous stick or by means of a cutdown. As the artery is entered, the patient may experience a slight "shock" or pain, similar to that experienced when hitting the "funny" bone. As the catheter is advanced under fluoroscopy, the patient may feel slight pressure, but the experience should not be painful. Sometimes the catheter has to be reinserted because of blockage or obstruction in the vessel, anatomical abnormalities, or severe vessel spasms. Once the cathether reaches the heart, pressure readings and blood samples for determining oxygenation are taken from the various chambers and vessels.

Throughout the procedure the patient may be moved into various positions, either physically or by tilting the table, to enhance catheter advancement and visualization. Two frequently used positions are the right anterior oblique, which allows visualization of the anterior, basal, apical, and inferior walls and vessels, and the basal wall segments of the left ventricle; and the left anterior oblique position, which allows visualization of the septum and posterior wall of the left ventricle. The patient may also be asked to breathe deeply, which aids in placement of the catheter into the pulmonary artery. Deep breathing may also aid with catheter placement in the coronary arteries. Visualization may be enhanced by depression of the diaphragm during deep breathing. Throughout the procedure the patient's cardiac rhythm, blood pressure, and heart rate are continuously monitored.

A right-sided or left-sided catheterization can be done singularly, or both sides may be catheterized. If both sides are to be catheterized, the right side is usually done first and the catheter is left in place so that pulmonary artery and pulmonary capillary wedge pressures (as a reflection of left heart pressures) can be monitored and measured simultaneously. The right-sided catheter is subsequently removed.

Cardiac catheterization is usually done in conjunction with angiography, which involves the injection of a radiopaque dye. Various studies can be performed including ventriculography, which is used to assess ventricular contraction; aortography, to assess the ascending aorta and aortic valve function; coronary arteriography, to determine coronary artery patency; levophase angiogram, to evaluate left atrial tumors and ventricular function in patients with prolapsing vegetations of the mitral valve; and pulmonary arteriography, to evaluate the pulmonary artery anatomy and pulmonary valve competence, and to identify the presence of pulmonary emboli.[4] When the contrast medium is injected, the patient may experience a feeling of warmth, flushing, lightheadedness, nausea, or a sudden urge to urinate, due to the vasodilation effect of the contrast medium. This usually occurs when a large amount of contrast is injected into the left ventricle during a ventriculogram. The sensation usually passes within a few seconds.

In response to the injection of the contrast medium, the patient may become hypotensive, exhibit bradycardia, or develop dysrhythmias. Under these circumstances, the patient may be asked to cough deeply to help propel the dye through the heart or coronary arteries. It is important to instruct the patient to cough immediately when asked to do so. If hypotension persists, a pressor agent may be prescribed.

Other drugs may be administered during an angiographic procedure. Nitroglycerin (NTG) may be given sublingually or intravenously, especially if the patient develops chest pain during the procedure. Nitroglycerin is used to eliminate catheter-induced spasms; to assess its effect on coronary artery perfusion, thereby assisting in determining candidacy for coronary artery bypass surgery; and to augment left ventricular contractility.

Ergonovine maleate is another drug that may be used in conjunction with cardiac catheterization. It is valuable in diagnosing variant (Prinzmetal's) or vasospastic angina because its vasoconstrictive action produces coronary artery spasm. Systemic heparin may be administered during left-sided catheterization to decrease the possibility of clot formation at the tip of the catheter. Its effects are reversed with the administration of protamine sulfate.

After the arterial catheters are removed, direct pressure must be applied to the site for at least 15 minutes. A pressure dressing is applied and the patient returned to a regular room. The procedure takes between 1 and 3 hours to complete. (For specific nursing care considerations, refer to the care plan for the patient after cardiac catheterization at the end of this chapter.)

Abnormal Findings

Narrowing or irregularity of the coronary arteries indicates coronary artery disease. A narrowing of greater than 60% is significant, especially in the proximal portion of the left main coronary artery and high in the left anterior descending coronary artery; a narrowing of 75% is significant for the circumflex or right coronary artery. Based on findings from catheterization, a decision can be made concerning the need for revascularization, angioplasty, or fibrinolytic therapy.

Valvular disorders are diagnosed on the basis of differences in pressures on both sides of the valves. The greater the pressure difference (pressure gradient), the greater the degree of stenosis. Incompetent valves are determined by the finding of retrograde blood flow across the valves during systole, as visualized on ventriculography.

Septal defects are confirmed by measurement of the blood oxygen content on both sides of the heart. Elevated blood oxygen on the right is indicative of a left-to-right shunt; a decrease in blood oxygen levels on the left is indicative of a right-to-left shunt.

Ejection fractions under 55% are indicative of myocardial incompetency. Ejection fractions under 35% are generally indicative of a poor surgical prognosis.

(Note: Ejection fraction is defined as the ratio of volume of blood ejected from the left ventricle per beat [stroke volume] to the volume of blood in the left ventricle at the end of diastole. This ratio is expressed as a percent.)

ELECTROPHYSIOLOGIC STUDIES

Electrophysiology of the Bundle of His

Electrophysiologic studies (EPS) constitute an invasive procedure that can supply information about the origin and characteristics of a dysrhythmia, the nature of the conduction pathways, the response of the myocardial cells to external stimuli, and the effectiveness of pharmacologic therapy.[21,22] The study involves the insertion of an electrode-tipped catheter into the right side of the heart in order to record activity of the conduction system, that is, the sinus and atrioventricular (AV) nodes, the bundle of His, and the network of His-Purkinje fibers.

Assessment of the atrioventricular conduction times can be achieved by determining the A–H interval and the H–V interval. The A–H interval reflects the conduction time from the right atrium, through the AV node, to the bundle of His. The A–H interval is measured from the initial deflection of the atrial electrogram to the earliest deflection for the electrogram of the bundle of His. Normally this interval is 45 to 150 milliseconds. The H–V interval reflects the conduction time from the proximal bundle of His to the ventricular myocardium. The H–V interval is measured from the initial deflection for the electrogram of the bundle of His to the initial deflection of the ventricular electrogram. The normal H–V interval ranges between 35 and 55 milliseconds.

Procedure

The procedure involves the same preparation as a right-sided cardiac catheterization. The femoral vein is the usual site for cannulation, although the brachial vein may also be utilized. A series of catheters are advanced under direct visualization. One catheter is placed high in the right atrium near the sinus node, a second crosses the tricuspid valve, and the third catheter is placed at the apex of the right ventricle. The outer ends of the catheters are attached to an oscilloscope that records the intracardiac and ECG wave forms simultaneously.[22]

The catheters are removed, direct pressure is applied for 15 minutes, and a pressure dressing is applied. The procedure takes from 1 to 3 hours to complete.

Abnormal Findings

Abnormal prolongation of the A–H interval (>150 msec) indicates atrioventricular nodal delays as seen in atrial pacing, chronic conduction system disease, carotid sinus pressure, recent myocardial infarction, and antidysrhythmic therapy. Abnormal prolongation of the H–V interval (>55 msec) is indicative of acute or chronic disease of the conduction system.

Interfering Factors

Interfering factors include malfunctioning of the recording equipment, improper catheter positioning, and patient intolerance.

Ventricular Mapping (Programmed Electrical Stimulation)

Ventricular mapping or programmed electrical stimulation (PES)[21,22] is an invasive procedure performed on patients with dysrhythmias refractive to pharmacologic therapy, syncope of unknown etiology, cardiac conduction system disease, and sinus node dysfunction.

Procedure

The procedure is similar to that for electrophysiography of the Bundle of His, but it involves insertion of up to six catheters. The three most common catheter placement sites are high in the right atrium, just below the triscuspid area, and the right ventricular apex.[16] If the dysrhythmia is associated with a pre-excitation syndrome, a catheter may be positioned in the coronary sinus.[16] Catheter position is confirmed by fluoroscopy, and baseline recordings are taken.

The conduction system is stressed by rapidly pacing it or by administering extra stimuli. If a dysrhythmia is induced, its origin (i.e., atrial, supraventricular, or ventricular) is determined by computer analysis. Pharmacologic agents may be administered to control the induced dysrhythmias. If the pharmacologic agents cannot control the dysrhythmia, the situation is evaluated for the possible effectiveness of surgical intervention. Such surgery may involve coronary artery bypass graft for ischemia, ventricular aneurysmectomy if caused by an aneurysm, or surgical ablation of the ectopic focus or re-entrant pathway. In those patients where surgical intervention is successful, their antidysrhythmic therapy may be altered or stopped.

Once the site is identified, the catheter is removed and direct pressure is applied to the cannulated site. The procedure takes 2 to 6 hours to complete. Other types of mapping include epicardial mapping, which is similar to ventricular mapping; and endocardial mapping, which is performed during open heart surgery.

Interfering Factors

Interfering factors include malfunction of the recording equipment, computer malfunctioning, inability to induce the dysrhythmia, or patient intolerance (i.e., cardiopulmonary arrest).

CASE STUDY: CARDIAC CATHETERIZATION

AJ is admitted to your unit for a cardiac catheterization. He is an airplane pilot, who on a routine physical was found to have a positive stress test. He is 42 years old, widowed with three children. He appears very anxious, although he is joking around.

Question 1: What would your precatheterization teaching include?

AJ is scheduled for the cardiac catheterization tomorrow morning at 9:30 AM.

Question 2: What would your precatheterization nursing interventions include? Why?

AJ returns from the cardiac catheterization at 11:00 AM. He had a right- and left-sided catheterization done with the femoral vein and artery cannulated. He has an IV of D_5W running at 100 mL/h.

Question 3: What would your initial assessment of AJ include?

Question 4: What would you teach AJ at this time?

At 12:00 noon: AJ starts getting out of bed to go to the bathroom.

Question 5: What would your nursing interventions be at this time?

Question 6: What additional nursing assessment would you do at this time?

Question 7: What new nursing diagnoses might you formulate at this time?

At 1:00 PM: AJ complains that his feet are cold. You do a peripheral vascular assessment and note that his pedal pulse on the catheterized side is slightly diminished, the extremity is still warm, and there is no change in the color. Capillary refill is 3 seconds.

Question 8: What nursing diagnosis would you formulate at this time?

Question 9: What would your nursing interventions be at this time?

A heparin drip is started on AJ at 900 U/hr. You check his lab values and note that his Hg is 14 g/dL (was 15 g/dL on admission).

Question 10: What additional lab values would you check at this time?

Question 11: What additional nursing assessment would you perform at this time?

At 3:00 PM: AJ voids 100 mL. His last void was at 12:00 noon, at which time he put out 300 mL.

Question 12: What could this possibly signify?

Question 13: What additional nursing assessments would you make at this time?

Question 14: What would your nursing interventions be at this time?

AJ's cardiac catheterization results return. They are:

PA pressure: 6 mmHg   LA pressure: 8 mmHg
RV pressure: 20 mmHg   LV pressure: 120 mmHg
PA pressure: 20 mmHg   PCWP: 9 mmHg
Stroke index: 45 mL/beat/m²
Ejection fraction: 85%
Right coronary artery: 40% occlusion, minimal collateral circulation present
Left main coronary artery: 10% occlusion
Left circumflex coronary artery: <10% occlusion
Left anterior descending coronary artery: 20% occlusion
Normal ventricular motion.
Valves: well-defined openings within normal limits

Question 15: How would you interpret AJ's results? AJ is being discharged today.

Question 16: What would your discharge teaching include?

REFERENCES

1. Come, PC: Diagnostic Cardiology: Non-Invasive Imaging Techniques. JB Lippincott, Philadelphia, 1985.
2. Cahill, M, DiCarlantonio, M, and Leibrandt, T: Diagnostics: Patient Preparation, Interpretation, Sources of Error, Post-Test Care. Intermed Communications, Horsham, PA, 1981.
3. Weeks, LC (ed): Advanced Cardiovascular Nursing. Blackwell Scientific, Boston, 1986.
4. Kenner, CV, Guzzetta, CE, and Dossey, BM (eds): Critical Care Nursing: Body-Mind-Spirit, ed. 2. Little Brown, Boston, 1985.
5. Sergi, N: When your patient needs a stress test. RN 54(3):26–36, 1991.
6. Schwartz, MB and Eisen, HJ: Pharmacologic thallium stress testing. Hospital Practice 26(9A):62–72, 1991.
7. Zorb, SL: Cardiovascular Diagnostic Testing: A Nursing Guide. Aspen, Gaithersburg, MD, 1991.
8. Hecht, HS, DeBord, L, Shaw, R, Dunlap, R, Ryan, C, Stertzer, SH, and Myler, RK: Digital supine bicycle stress echocardiography: A new technique for evaluating coronary artery disease. J Am Coll Cardiol 21:950–956, 1993.
9. Docker, CS, Muthusamy, R, and Balasundaram, SG: Intraoperative echocardiography: An essential tool in cardiac surgery. Journal of the Association of Operating Room Nurses 55(1):167–175, 1992.
10. Weikart, CJ: New eye into the heart. RN 56(10):36–39, 1993.
11. Sullivan-Wutterschein, K, Hussey, and R Perry, M: Using transesophageal echocardiography to assess the heart. Nursing 22(8):62–64, 1992.
12. Beattie, S and Meinhardt, SL: Transesophageal echocardiography: Advanced technology for the cardiac patient. Critical Care Nurse 12(8):42–48, 1992.
13. Robie, BR: Cardiovascular technology. Journal of Cardiovascular Nursing 6(2):36–42, 1992.
14. Velos, JC: A review of cardiac imaging modalities. Nurse Practitioner Forum 2(4):231–238, 1991.
15. Barkett, PA: Cardiac M.U.G.A. scan: Taking first-rate pictures of the heart. Nursing 18(10):76–78, 1988.
16. Cimini, DM: Indium-111 antimyosin antibody imaging: A promising new technique in the diagnosis of M.I. Critical Care Nurse 12(4):44–51, 1992.
17. Engler, MB and Engler MM: Magnetic resonance imaging: An overview and safety considerations. Journal of Emergency Nursing 12(6):360–364, 1988.
18. Steinberg, EP: Magnetic resonance coronary angiography:

Assessing an emerging technology. N Engl J Med 328(12):879, 1993.

19. Perdue, B: Cardiac catheterization—before and after: What the patient should understand. What the nurse needs to know. Advancing Critical Care 5(2):16–18, 1990.

20. Warner, CD, Peebles, BU, Miller, J, Reed, R, Rodriquez, S, and Martin-Lewis, E: The effectiveness of teaching a relaxation technique to patients undergoing elective cardiac catheterization. Journal of Cardiovascular Nursing 6(2):66–75, 1992.

21. Cole, FL: The electrophysiology study. Critical Care Nurse 4(10):112–116, 1984.

22. Monticco, LM and Hill, KM: EP studies: When they're called for, what they reveal. RN 52(2):54–58, 1989.

SUGGESTED READINGS

Anderson, KO and Masur, F: Psychologic preparation for cardiac catheterization. Heart & Lung 18:154–163, 1989.

Apple, S and Thurkauf, GE: Preparing for and understanding transesophageal echocardiography. Critical Care Nurse 12(6):29–34, 1992.

Barta, KJ and Vacek, JL: Transesophageal atrial pacing with stress echocardiography. Focus on Critical Care 16(1):12, 1989.

Cason, CI, Russell, DG, and Fincher, SB: Preparatory sensory information for cardiac catheterization. Cardiovascular Nursing 28(6):41–45, 1992.

Dault, LH, Groene, J, and Herick, R: Helping your patient through cardiac catheterization. Nursing 22(2):52–55, 1992.

DiLucente, L and Gorcsan, J: Transesophageal echocardiography: Application to the postoperative cardiac surgery patient. Dimensions of Critical Care Nursing 10(2):74–80, 1991.

Edelman, RR and Warach, S: Magnetic resonance imaging, I. N Engl J Med 328(19):708–715, 1993.

Fishbach, FT: A Manual of Laboratory Diagnostic Tests, ed 4. JB Lippincott, Philadelphia, 1992.

Hamilton, H (ed): Combating Cardiovascular Disease Skillfully. Intermed Communications, Horsham, PA, 1987.

Hamilton, HK (ed): Nurse's Clinical Library: Cardiovascular Disorders. Springhouse, PA, 1984.

Haughey, CW: Preparing your patient for echocardiography. Nursing 14(5):18–21, 1984.

Hibner, CS, Moseley, MJ, and Shank, TL: What is transesophageal echocardiography? American Journal of Nursing 93(4):74–78, 1993.

Hill, NE, Baker, M, Warner, RA, and Taub, H: Evaluating the use of a videotape in teaching the precardiac catheterization patient. Journal of Cardiovascular Nursing 2(3):71–78, 1988.

Holloway, NM: Nursing the Critically Ill Adult: Applying Nursing Diagnosis, ed. 3. Addison-Wesley, Menlo Park, CA, 1990.

Hudak, CM and Gallo, BM: Critical Care Nursing: A Holistic Approach, ed 6. JB Lippincott, Philadelphia, 1994.

Johnston, BL: Exercise testing for patients after myocardial infarction and coronary by-pass surgery: Emphasis for pre-discharge phase. Heart Lung 13(1):18–27, 1984.

Lamb, JI and Carlson, VR (eds): Handbook of Cardiovascular Nursing. JB Lippincott, Philadelphia, 1986.

LeFever Kee, J: Laboratory and Diagnostic Tests with Nursing Implications. CV Mosby, St. Louis, MO, 1990.

Lewis, SM and Collier, IC: Medical-Surgical Nursing: Assessment and Management of Clinical Problems. McGraw-Hill, New York, 1983.

Loeb, JM: Cardiac electrophysiology: Basic concepts and rhythmogenesis. Critical Care Quarterly 7(2):9–10, 1984.

Manning, WJ, Li, W, and Edelman, RR: A preliminary report comparing magnetic resonance coronary angiography with conventional angiography. N Engl J Med 328(12):823–832, 1993.

McDermott, TJ: Using transesophageal echocardiography to assess the heart. Nursing 22(8):63–64, 1992.

McDonagh, A: Getting your patient ready for a nuclear medicine scan. Nursing 21(2):53–57, 1991.

Peterson, M: Patient anxiety before cardiac catheterization: An intervention study. Heart Lung 20(6):643–647, 1991.

Phipps, WJ, Long, BC, Woods, NF, and Cassmeyer, VL: Medical-Surgical Nursing: Concepts and Clinical Practice, ed 4. Mosby Year Book, St. Louis, MO, 1991.

Porterfield, LM and Porterfield, JG: Radiofrequency ablation of a left-sided free-wall accessory pathway: A case study. Critical Care Nurse 13(2):46–49, 1993.

Sadler, D: Nursing for Cardiovascular Health. Appleton-Century-Crofts, Norwalk, CT, 1984.

Tilkian, A and Daily, E: Cardiovascular Procedures, Diagnostic Techniques and Therapeutic Procedures. CV Mosby, St. Louis, MO, 1986.

Thompson, EJ: Transesophageal echocardiography: A new window on the heart and great vessels. Critical Care Nurse 13(1):55–66, 1993.

Thompson, JM, et al: Clinical Nursing. CV Mosby, St. Louis, MO, 1986.

Tyndall, A: A nursing perspective of the invasive electrophysiologic approach to treatment of ventricular arrhythmias. Heart Lung 12(6):620–630, 1983.

Ventura, B: What you need to know about cardiac catheterization. RN 47(9):24–30, 1984.

Verderber, A, Shively, M, and Fitzsimmons, L: Preparation for cardiac catheterization. Journal of Cardiovascular Nursing 7(1):75–77, 1992.

West, RS (ed): Nursing Photobook: Giving Cardiac Care. Springhouse Corporation, Springhouse, PA, 1981.

Winters, WL and Cashion, WR: Imaging techniques in patients with acute myocardial infarction. Heart & Lung 14(3):259–264, 1985.

Yacone, L: Cardiac diagnostic studies: Nuclear scanning and cardiac catheterization. RN 47(5):129–130, 1984.

CARE PLAN FOR THE PATIENT AFTER CARDIAC CATHETERIZATION

Nursing Diagnoses

Nursing Diagnosis #1
Cardiac Output, decreased (actual and potential): Related to underlying cardiac disease, hemorrhage, cardiac perforation, myocardial infarction, and dysrhythmias.

Desired Patient Outcomes

1. The patient will maintain effective cardiovascular function as measured by:
   a. Stable blood pressure: systolic pressure of 100–145 mmHg, or baseline value for the patient
   b. Regular heartbeat with a rate of 60–100 beats/min, or baseline for the patient
   c. Regular respiratory rate of 12–20 per minute, or baseline for the patient
   d. Absence of angina
   e. Absence of rales or crackles; no distension of neck vein
   f. Minimal bleeding at the catheter site
   g. Optimal cardiac indices including warm, dry skin, usual skin color; brisk capillary refill, <3 sec; patient is alert and oriented, and follows commands

CARE PLAN FOR THE PATIENT AFTER CARDIAC CATHETERIZATION (*Continued*)

Nursing Interventions	Rationales
• Perform a comprehensive cardiopulmonary assessment:	
○ Monitor blood pressure, observing for a drop in systolic pressure, a narrowing pulse pressure, and pulsus paradoxus.	• Changes in blood pressure may reflect reduced cardiac output, possibly related to left ventricular failure, hypovolemia, or cardiac tamponade.
○ Monitor heart rate and regularity.	• Dysrhythmias can compromise cardiac output and increase the risk of life-threatening dysrhythmias.
○ Monitor ECGs and rhythm strips for abnormalities.	• These recordings provide a basis for comparison in the detection of dysrhythmias, ischemia, infarction, or signs of antidysrhythmic toxicity.
○ Monitor heart sounds.	• The presence of S_3 is indicative of heart failure; a murmur indicates valvular dysfunction; and a pericardial friction rub points to pericarditis.
○ Monitor the patient for neck vein distension.	• An increase in neck vein distension warns of increasing heart failure, fluid overload, or cardiac tamponade.
○ Monitor breath sounds.	• The presence of rales is indicative of fluid overload or an increase in ventricular failure. Decreased breath sounds may be indicative of pulmonary emboli or pneumothorax.
○ Monitor the respiratory rate.	• An increase in the respiratory rate may indicate extreme anxiety, pain, hypoxia, or acid-base imbalance.
○ Monitor the amount of bleeding from the catheter site.	• Uncontrolled bleeding would lead to hypovolemia, which would further decrease the cardiac output, increase the workload of the heart, and decrease myocardial oxygenation.
○ Monitor skin and nail beds for changes in strength, color, warmth, and capillary refill.	• These are indices of peripheral vascular perfusion and may be one of the signs of decreased cardiac output.
○ Monitor the presence of angina, evaluating its quality, location, and radiation.	• Immediate medical treatment can be initiated to prevent further complications and deterioration in the patient's condition.
• Institute prescribed therapies and monitor responses:	
○ Maintain intravenous fluids.	• Adequate fluids are necessary to prevent hypovolemia and subsequent renal failure due to the osmotic effect of the contrast medium. If oliguria or anuria occurs, the rate of the infusion may have to be decreased to prevent fluid overload. The IV also provides an access through which emergency drugs can be given.
○ Administer antidysrhythmics, diuretics, and pain medications as prescribed.	• Prompt administration of prescribed medications can help prevent further decrease in cardiac output and prevent cardiopulmonary, neurologic, and renal complications.
• Be prepared to institute emergency treatment:	
○ Have the crash cart available nearby.	• Immediate emergency actions may be necessary to prevent cardiac injury and to treat life-threatening complications, i.e., dysrhythmias.

Nursing Diagnoses	Desired Patient Outcomes
Nursing Diagnosis #2	
Tissue perfusion, altered: Peripheral, related to the insertion of the catheter into an artery and/or vein.	1. The patient will maintain adequate perfusion in the catheterized extremity as evidenced by: a. Warmth of the extremity b. Pink color c. Peripheral pulses equal bilaterally, ≥+2 or at the patient's baseline d. Movement and sensation intact

CARE PLAN FOR THE PATIENT AFTER CARDIAC CATHETERIZATION (*Continued*)

Nursing Interventions

LEFT-SIDED CATHETERIZATION:
ARTERIAL INSERTION

- Monitor pules in the catheterized extremity, distal to the insertion site. Report any changes immediately to the physician.

- Monitor the color and warmth of the extremity, comparing it with the opposite extremity:

  ○ Notify the physician immediately if any signs of decreased perfusion occur.
  ○ Heat may be applied to the opposite extremity. Never apply heat to the affected extremity.

- Administer heparin as prescribed.
- Keep the catheterized extremity straight for 6–8 hours as prescribed.
- Maintain bed rest for 6–12 hours as prescribed.

- Administer pain medication as ordered. Monitor effectiveness in relieving pain.

- Monitor the insertion site for increasing edema and bleeding:
  ○ Apply a sandbag to the femoral insertion site immediately after the procedure.
  ○ Apply direct pressure to the insertion site for moderate to large amounts of bleeding.

  ○ Notify the physician immediately of any active bleeding, excessive swelling, or hematoma formation.

Rationales

- Distal artery can rapidly become thrombotic, and ischemia of the extremity may occur. Arterial spasm may occur in response to the insertion of the catheter. If the thrombosis or arterial spasm is not immediately treated, ischemia can lead to tissue necrosis and possibly the need for amputation.
- Color and warmth are indices of peripheral perfusion. Pale and/or mottled skin indicates a compromised blood supply to the extremity.
  ○ Immediate action must be taken to preserve the circulatory integrity of the affected extremity.
  ○ Heat applied to the opposite extremity will produce a reflex vasodilatation, thereby increasing the blood supply to the extremity. Heat applied to the affected extremity will only further compromise oxygenation of the limb due to enhanced cellular metabolism.
- Heparin will prevent further clots from forming.
- Movement can disrupt the clot at the insertion site and hemorrhage or embolization may occur.
- Bed rest allows the patient to regain strength. It prevents dislodgement of the clot at the insertion site.
- Pain medications will keep the patient comfortable and relaxed. This will break the pain-fear-anxiety cycle that could cause a sympathetic response. This response could precipitate an increase in BP and HR, cause the heart to work harder, and increase the risk of bleeding at the insertion site.
- Enlargement of the limb could indicate bleeding into the soft tissue.
  ○ The weight of the sandbag applies continuous direct pressure to the site, thereby decreasing bleeding.
  ○ Direct pressure slows the blood flow around the insertion site, thereby allowing the normal clotting mechanism to occur.
  ○ Immediate intervention is needed to stop the bleeding, maintain the patient's blood volume, and maintain perfusion to the extremity.

Nursing Interventions

RIGHT-SIDED CATHETERIZATION: VENOUS
INSERTION

- Monitor the pulses distal to the insertion site.

- Elevate the extremity.

- Maintain bed rest for 4–6 hours as ordered.
- Keep catheterized extremity straight for 3–6 hours.
- Monitor insertion site for bleeding or hematoma.

Rationales

- Bleeding from the insertion site into the surrounding tissue can exert pressure against the adjacent structures. This can cause occlusion and compromise circulation.
- Elevation will facilitate venous return and fluid absorption.
- Same as arterial insertion.
- Same as arterial insertion.
- Same as arterial insertion.

CARE PLAN FOR THE PATIENT AFTER CARDIAC CATHETERIZATION (*Continued*)

Nursing Diagnoses

Nursing Diagnosis #3

Fluid Volume deficit, risk for: (refer to Chapter 36).

Desired Patient Outcomes

The patient will:
1. Maintain blood pressure at patient's baseline.
2. Maintain a urinary output >30 mL/hr (for adults).
3. Show no signs of bleeding from the insertion site.
4. Maintain adequate hydration, i.e., moist mucous membranes, supple skin, turgor, serum osmolarity (275–300 mOsm/kg)
5. Maintain a normal hemoglobin (Hb) and hematocrit (HCT):

   Hb   Men: 14–18 g/dL
             Women: 12–16 g/dL

   HCT   Men: 40%–54%
             Women: 37%–47%

Nursing Interventions

- Monitor the blood pressure every hour until stable. Notify the physician of any abnormalities.

- Monitor the urinary output and I & O closely for the first 24 hours.
  - Assess urine specific gravity.

- Monitor for signs of dehydration (dry mucous membranes, poor skin turgor, a decrease in urinary output with a high specific gravity).

- Monitor for bleeding at the insertion site.

- Monitor the hemoglobin and hematocrit.

Rationales

- Timely detection of abnormalities enables timely intervention, thereby reducing the risk of complications, especially bleeding. Nitroglycerin or nifedepine may be ordered to decrease elevated blood pressure, thereby decreasing the risk of bleeding.
- Urinary outputs of less than 30 mL/hr are highly suggestive of hypovolemia or impending renal failure.
  - Renal excretion of contrast dyes requires ample fluid intake to reduce the risk of renal dysfunction. Initial specific gravity determinations will be high, reflecting the presence of the contrast dye in the urine.
- Astute observation for signs of dehydration can prevent the occurrence of renal and/or cardiac complications by identifying the need for fluids. These changes may occur before there is a change in blood pressure.
- Blood loss can cause a decrease in cardiac output because of hypovolemia.
- If the fluid deficit is related to the blood loss, the hemoglobin will be decreased; if it is related to hypovolemia, the hematocrit will be decreased.

Nursing Diagnoses

Nursing Diagnosis #4

Infection, risk for: (refer to Table 56–5: Potential for Infection)

Desired Patient Outcomes

1. The patient will demonstrate no signs of infection as evidenced by:
   a. Maintaining a normal body temperature (98.6°F), or temperature at the patient's baseline.
   b. A clean, dry insertion site, without redness, heat, or exudate.

Nursing Interventions

- Monitor the insertion site for the presence of redness, heat, or exudate every 4 hours.

Rationales

- Redness and heat are the normal responses of the defense system of the body against infection and trauma. They are indicative of infection, especially in the presence of exudate.

CARE PLAN FOR THE PATIENT AFTER CARDIAC CATHETERIZATION (*Continued*)

• Monitor the body temperature every 4 hours.

  ○ Obtain wound and blood cultures if the temperature rises above 101°F and notify the physician.

• Monitor for signs of endocarditis, i.e. high fever, hematuria, and the presence of a new murmur.

• Monitor for signs of pericarditis, i.e., decreased heart sounds, and the presence of a pericardial friction rub.

• Temperature elevation is a normal response of the body's defense system to infection.
  ○ Temperatures above 101°F are indicative of bacterial invasion, and immediate treatment with the appropriate antibiotic is necessary to prevent sepsis. Antibiotic therapy should not be initiated until the appropriate cultures have been obtained.
• Endocarditis is a potential complication of cardiac catheterization and is related to the introduction of a foreign object (the catheter) into the heart, especially in patients with valvular disease.
• Similar to endocarditis. (See above.)

Nursing Diagnoses
Nursing Diagnosis #5
Knowledge deficit

Desired Patient Outcome

1. The patient will verbalize an understanding of prescribed treatment plan including medications, diet, activity level, care of the insertion site, what symptoms require immediate attention, and follow-up care after discharge.

Nursing Interventions
• Provide the patient and family with verbal and written instructions concerning wound care, signs of infection, medications, diet, activity restrictions, medications, and follow-up appointments.
• Discuss the implications of the catheterization, the results, and the physician recommendations. Evaluate the perceptions of patient and family and correct any misconceptions they may have.

Rationales
• Information decreases the patient's anxiety and facilitates participation in self-care; it may help to prevent the occurrence of serious complications.

• Knowledge decreases anxiety. Correcting misconceptions allows the patient greater ability to make objective decisions.

C H A P T E R   15

Electrocardiography: An Overview

Jeanette G. Kernicki

CHAPTER OUTLINE

Cardiac Cell Structure and Function
Myocardial Electrochemical Physiology
□ Membrane Potential
□ Action Potential
□ Conduction System
The Electrocardiogram
□ Leads and Electrodes
□ Components of the
  Electrocardiogram
Sinus Rhythm
□ ECG Criteria of Normal Sinus
  Rhythm
Dysrhythmias
□ Recognition of Dysrhythmia

□ Sinus Abnormalities
□ Atrial Dysrhythmias
□ Atrioventricular Junctional Rhythms
□ Disturbances of Atrioventricular
  Conduction
□ Ventricular Dysrhythmias
□ Miscellaneous Dysrhythmias
**Electrolyte Imbalances and the
Electrocardiogram**
□ Potassium Imbalances
□ Calcium Imbalances
□ Magnesium Imbalances
□ Sodium
References

LEARNING OBJECTIVES

After completing this chapter, you should be able to:
1. Trace the normal pathway of electrical impulses through the heart.
2. Define the following terms:
   a. Transmembrane potential
   b. Action potential
   c. Threshold potential
   d. Refractory period
3. Explain the physiologic principles related to cardiac action, and the role of actin and myosin filaments.
4. List the basic components of the electrocardiogram.
5. Describe the electrocardiographic lead systems.
6. Explain the three methods for determining cardiac rate from the electrocardiographic tracing.
7. Describe the appropriate placement of the electrodes for cardiac monitor leads II, MCL_1, and MCL_6.
8. Interpret certain normal and abnormal ECG readings from specific electrocardiographic tracings.
9. Explain the electrocardiographic findings and course of action taken with each identified dysrhythmia.
10. Identify extracardiac causes of dysrhythmias.
11. Describe the identifying features associated with the extracardiac causes of dysrhythmias.

The efficiency of the heart as a muscular pump is dependent on a well-developed system of propagating the electrical impulse and the coordinated contraction of cardiac muscle. To achieve this purpose, synchronization of the heart's activity must occur. This activity, as well as other hemodynamic parameters, is recorded on the oscilloscope of the bedside cardiac monitor in the form of the electrocardiographic tracing. Understanding what the monitoring tracings reflect is mandatory for the nurse caring for a critically ill patient.

A brief description of the properties of the cardiac

cell, conduction of cardiac impulse, and recording of the electrical activity of the heart will be reviewed.

CARDIAC CELL STRUCTURE AND FUNCTION

From an electrophysiologic view, there are two distinct types of cardiac cells: contractile (muscle) cells and specialized (pacemaker) cells. The contractile cells are responsible for the contraction of cardiac muscle during pumping of the heart. If one were to examine these contractile cells by electron microscopy, striations would become evident. The striations are composed of longitudinal fibers of the proteins actin and myosin. These proteins form the filaments of the sarcomere, which is the contractile unit of the cell.[1] When the cardiac cell receives a stimulus, shortening of the filaments occurs, an action that is essential for pumping blood from the heart chambers to the major vessels. Prior to the actual fiber shortening, many electrochemical activities occur simultaneously.

MYOCARDIAL ELECTROCHEMICAL PHYSIOLOGY

Membrane Potential

Electric currents generated in tissue are referred to as bioelectricity. The external measurement of electric signals of cardiac muscle is the basis of the electrocardiogram. The membrane of cardiac cells (sarcolemma) maintains a voltage difference between the inside and outside of the cell. At "rest" the cell maintains a voltage of -70 to -90 mV (millivolts). The inside of the cell is negative with respect to the outside. This voltage difference is referred to as the transmembrane potential. Electrochemical gradients involving potassium and sodium ions contribute to the transmembrane potential. Potassium ions occupy the inner aspect of the cell and sodium ions the outer aspect. The membrane of the cell is permeable to potassium and impermeable to sodium, which means that potassium ions can readily diffuse out of the cell and leave behind negatively charged proteins, inorganic phosphates, sulfates, and other ions too large to diffuse through the pores of the cellular membrane. This leaves a net negative charge near the interior cell membrane and a positive charge outside the membrane. The charge buildup outside the cell membrane prevents further diffusion of potassium ions.

The large difference in concentration of sodium and potassium across the cell membrane is also the result of an active transport system, the sodium-potassium pump, which is located in the cell membrane. This pump, activated by the enzyme ATPase, actively pumps sodium out of cells and pumps in potassium.[2]

Action Potential

The "resting" potential of a myocardial working cell (fast response) is -90 mV and remains at this level until stimulated. When a stimulus is applied to the cell, its permeability to sodium ions increases and sodium ions rush into the cell, where the sodium ion concentration is lower. This results in a positive shift in transmembrane potential and raises the cell potential from the resting potential to a threshold membrane potential (approximately -60 to -70 mV). The decrease in transmembrane potential indicates that the cell has released some its the stored energy.

Five phases have been used to describe the electrochemical responses of cardiac cells (Fig. 15–1). The initial phase (depolarization) is followed by three phases of repolarization:

Phase 0 (depolarization): There is a rapid influx of sodium ions into the cell interior through fast sodium channels. This movement is so fast that the spike or upstroke of the action potential usu-

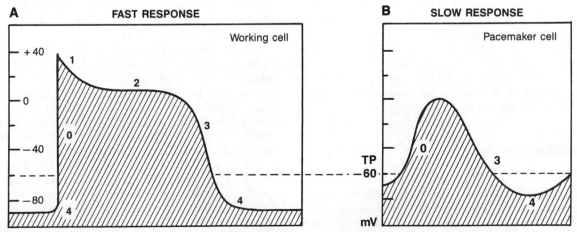

FIGURE 15–1. Myocardial action potentials. (*A*) Myocardial working cell or fast response action potential; (*B*) pacemaker cell or slow response action potential. See text for a description of each phase, and a discussion as to the key differences between fast response and slow response action potentials (TP = threshold potential).

ally peaks at approximately +25 to +35 mV. This is referred to as overshoot (above zero value). Depolarization of the ventricles is depicted at the beginning of the QRS complex on the electrocardiogram.

Phase 1 (early repolarization phase): Rapid closure of fast sodium channels is accompanied by the inward flow of a small number of negatively charged chloride ions.

Phase 2 (plateau phase): There is a slow inward current of calcium (slow calcium channels) and sodium ions. A slowing of the exit of potassium ions also contributes to establishing the plateau. Electrocardiographically, phases 0, 1, and 2 correspond to the QRS complex and include the ST segment.

Phase 3 (late repolarization): The cell becomes increasingly permeable to potassium, so that there is a sharp return of the transmembrane potential to negative values intracellularly (resting membrane potential). Phase 3 corresponds to the T wave of the electrocardiogram.

Phase 4 (diastolic phase; membrane resting potential). To re-establish the electrochemical gradient, the sodium-potassium-ATPase pump actively pumps potassium into the cell and sodium out. The membrane potential is again restored to its high-energy polarized state (resting potential) before another action potential can be generated.

From the beginning of depolarization (phase 0), through phases 1 and 2 or repolarization, the heart is said to be in a state of *absolute refractoriness*, that is, it will not respond to another stimulus, regardless of the strength of the stimulus. Phase 3 is known as the *relative refractory*, or vulnerable, period. A relatively strong stimulus may evoke a response if applied during this phase. If an ectopic focus fires during this vulnerable period (R on T phenomenon), a lethal arrhythmia (ventricular fibrillation) may occur.[3]

Certain cardiac cells have the unique property of automaticity, whereby the cell depolarizes spontaneously and reaches the threshold potential. This critical characteristic is evident in phase 4, diastolic depolarization, and allows automatic pacemaking cells to self-excite. Cells of the sinoatrial node are lacking phase 2 (plateau phase) in the depolarization-repolarization cycle. Ventricular muscle cells have a constant resting membrane potential and do not experience spontaneous phase 4 diastolic depolarization.

Conduction System

The major function of the specialized or pacemaker cells is to generate and conduct the electrical impulse through the conduction system to the myocardial cells, that is, from the sinus node to the atrial and ventricular contractile cells.

The heart has many potential pacemaking or automatic centers, which are situated in the sinoatrial (SA) node, atrioventricular (AV) node, and atria and ventricles. All specialized heart cells have the ability to transmit electrical impulses. It is a fundamental law of cardiac physiology, however, that only the dominant or fastest pacemaker (the one with the highest automaticity) is normally in control of the heart. The intrinsic rate of the SA node is 60 to 80 impulses/min; of the bundle of His is 40 to 60 impulses/min; and of the area below the bundle of His, 15 to 40 impulses/min. The SA node has the fastest inherent heart rate; therefore, it is generally the pacemaker of the heart.

The heart is under the influence of both the sympathetic and parasympathetic divisions of the autonomic nervous system. Sympathetic stimulation affects the properties of conductivity, contractility, and automaticity, and stimulation of the sympathetic fibers results in an increase in sinus rate (positive chronotropic effect), as well as an increase in the strength of contraction (positive inotropic effect). Parasympathetic fiber stimulation causes a decrease in phase 4 spontaneous depolarization of the sinus node (negative chronotropic effect), a decrease in atrial contractility (negative inotropic effect), and a decrease in conduction velocity through the AV node. Normally the heart is under the influence of the parasympathetic division at rest.

If the sinus node pacemaker fails to generate an impulse, subsidiary pacemakers can take over, but the rate of impulse discharge will be slower than that initiated by the normal pacemaker of the heart. Usurpation of pacemaking function can also occur by the subsidiary pacemakers.

As discussed in Chapter 12, in the normal heart, the electrical impulse begins in the SA node, which is situated in the posterior aspect of the right atrium at the junction of the superior vena cava and the body of the right atrium (see Fig. 12–8). The rate of discharge of the sinoatrial node is 60 to 100 impulses/min. A wave of excitation then spreads through the atria by way of the internodal pathways and travels to the atrioventricular node, which is located in the lower posterior part of the interatrial septum near the opening of the inferior vena cava. Depolarization of the atria takes approximately 0.08 second.

To increase the efficiency of the heart, there is a slight delay at the AV node that allows for the atria to complete their systolic phase. The delay is due in part to resistance to current flow as a result of the convergence of internodal tracts and nerve pathways. The delay allows for the sequential contraction of atria and ventricles and also serves to protect the ventricles from abnormally fast heart rates (decremental conduction).

The impulse then travels along the bundle of His, and the right and left bundle branches (fascicles), to the Purkinje network, located just beneath the endocardial surface of the ventricles. The extremely rapid wave of excitation through the Purkinje fibers is essential for the coordinated sequential contraction of the ventricles.[4] There is generally an orderly sequence of events occurring in the heart to bring about the ejection of ventricular contents; that is, impulse conduction, fiber excitation, and cardiac cycle events. This process allows the cells to work as a unit, coordinates the electrical and mechanical events of the heart, and increases the efficiency of the heart as a pump.

THE ELECTROCARDIOGRAM

The electrocardiogram (ECG) is a record of the electrical activity of the heart. The current generated within the heart's conduction system travels to the body surface and is picked up by a machine (galvanometer) that transcribes the information to graph paper. The paper on which the ECG is recorded is divided into 5-mm squares, each subdivided into smaller 1-mm squares (Fig. 15–2). Time is measured horizontally, and voltage or force of contraction vertically. At the usual recording speed of 25 mm/sec, one small square in the horizontal direction represents 0.04 second, and the edge of one large square (5 small boxes) represents 0.20 second. The ECG is usually standardized so that one square in the vertical direction represents 0.1 mV; thus, the edge of one large square represents 0.5 mV and the edge of two large squares represents 1 mV.

Standardization of the ECG enables any part of it to be described in terms of amplitude in millimeters (voltage) and duration in seconds (width). Determining the amplitude and duration of each deflection is essential to meaningful ECG analysis and interpretation.

In addition to amplitude and duration, it is impor-

tant to specify whether a wave or deflection is positive or negative. By convention, an *upward* deflection is called *positive*, a *downward* deflection is called *negative*. Deflections partly above the baseline and partly below it are called *biphasic*. A portion of the trace that lies on the baseline is termed *isoelectric*.

Leads and Electrodes

To measure the heart's electrical activity a routine ECG normally employs 12 leads. They include the 6 extremity leads (standard limb leads I, II, III; augmented leads aVR, aVL, aVF) and 6 chest leads (precordial leads V_1 through V_6).

Standard Limb (Bipolar) Leads

The standard limb leads are shown in Figure 15–3A:
Lead I records the electrical potential between the negative pole on the right arm and the positive pole on the left arm.
Lead II records the electrical potential between the negative pole on the right arm and the positive electrode on the left leg (foot).
Lead III records the electrical potential between the negative pole on the left arm and the positive pole on the left leg.

The standard limb leads form Einthoven's triangle, which was devised by Willem Einthoven. Lead II is frequently used for monitoring because the P wave and QRS complex are more prominent in that lead. Application of electrodes and leads becomes easy if one remembers that the right arm is always negative and the left leg is always positive. The left arm is positive in lead II and negative when recording lead III.

Augmented (Unipolar) Leads

The unipolar leads (aVR, aVL, aVF) are somewhat more narrow in perspective than the standard limb (bipolar) leads. These leads record the electrical activity of the heart from one point: right arm, left arm, or left leg (foot). The letter "a" indicates that the lead is augmented and the letter "V" designates the term vector, representing magnitude and direction of force (Fig. 15–3B).

Precordial (Unipolar Chest) Leads

The precordial leads record the electrical activity of the heart with electrodes at six chest positions (Fig. 15–4A,B):

Lead	Location
V_1	Right sternal margin at the 4th intercostal space
V_2	Left sternal margin at the 4th intercostal space
V_3	Midway between V_2 and V_4

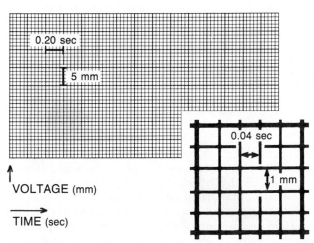

FIGURE 15–2. Electrocardiographic paper is graded paper divided into 1-mm squares. The amplitude of the ECG waves is reflected by horizontal lines occurring 1 mm apart, with each small box equal to 0.1 mV; time (duration) is reflected by vertical lines also occurring 1 mm apart, with each small box equal to 0.04 second. Each larger box is equal to 0.20 second at the usual ECG recording speed of 25 mm/sec. The ECG machine is usually calibrated so that the standardization mark is 10 mm in height.

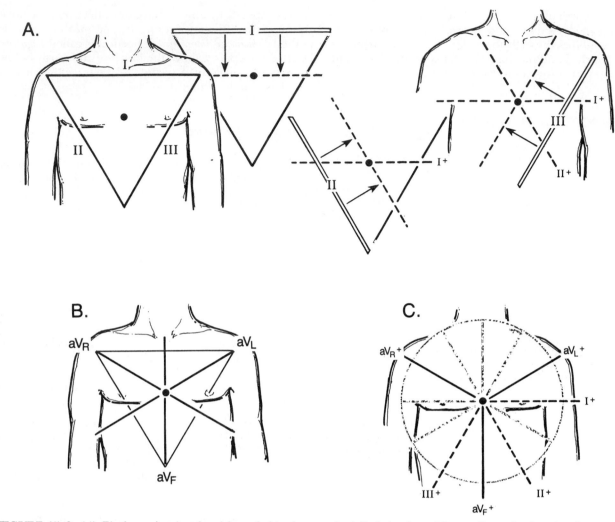

FIGURE 15–3. (*A*) Einthoven's triangle with each bipolar standard limb lead equidistant from the heart at its center. A triaxial figure is produced by shifting the axes of the three standard limb leads (I, II, and III) to the center of the triangle (the center of the heart) where they intersect. The axes of these leads occur 60 degrees apart. (*B*) A triaxial figure reflecting the axes of the unipolar augmented leads can be drawn by intersecting the axis of each lead at the center of the triangle. Each augmented lead (aVR, aVL, and aVF) is drawn from the limb (positive lead) to the center of the equilateral triangle. The axis of each of these leads occur 60 degrees apart. (*C*) When the triaxial figure of the standard limb leads and that of the augmented leads intersect at a common point (taken as the center of the heart) a hexaxial figure is formed. In the hexaxial figure, each augmented lead is perpendicular to standard limb lead. Each lead is labeled at its positive electrode. The hexaxial figure is used to plot mean cardiac electrical forces.

Lead	Location
V_4	5th intercostal space in the midclavicular line
V_5	5th intercostal space in the left anterior axillary line
V_6	5th intercostal space in the left midaxillary line

Figure 15–5 illustrates the use of precordial leads to depict ventricular depolarization. Occasionally in coronary care or telemetry units, recordings are taken from modified chest leads, that is, MCL_1, V_1 (Fig. 15–6); MCL_6, V_6. The use of the modified chest leads is helpful in identifying bundle branch blocks and in distinguishing between a supraventricular rhythm with aberrancy and ventricular ectopy. To record a simulated chest lead, one can place the negative electrode under the left clavicle and positive electrode in the desired precordial (V) position.

Inherent in the application of electrodes (leads) and the monitoring of the heart's electrical activity is the concern that the patient will perceive that something is wrong with the heart. Therefore, prior to the application of electrodes (leads) or recording, it is imperative that the patient and/or family be given an explanation of the purpose of the test and the method used to obtain the recording. One must reassure the patient that there is no danger of an electric shock involved with placement of the electrodes. The monitoring alarm system should be explained, and if

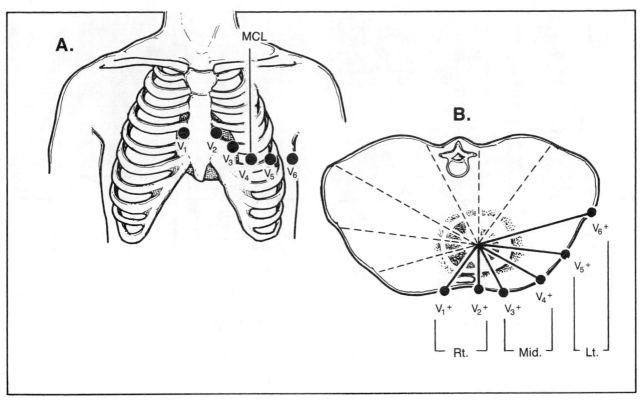

FIGURE 15–4. (*A*) Electrode positions of precordial or chest (unipolar) leads. (*B*) Precordial reference figure: leads V₁ and V₂ are right-sided precordial leads; leads V₃ and V₄ are midprecordial leads; leads V₅ and V₆ are left-sided precordial leads.

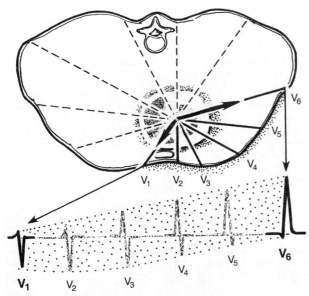

FIGURE 15–5. Ventricular depolarization as recorded by precordial (chest) leads V₁ through V₆. Note the progressive increase in the amplitude of the R waves as one moves from right to left across the chest. This reflects the recording of current flow as the wave of depolarization moves across the chest in the direction of the electrical predominant left ventricle and toward the positive electrodes of the left chest leads. This is referred to as P-wave progression across the precordium.

appropriate, the sound should be reduced. Patient and family members must be cautioned that at no time should the alarm be turned off.

Assessment of the skin for irritation at the site of electrode placement must be performed on each shift. Lead attachment sites should be rotated every 24 hours or according to institution protocol. Additional nursing responsibilities in the care of a patient on a

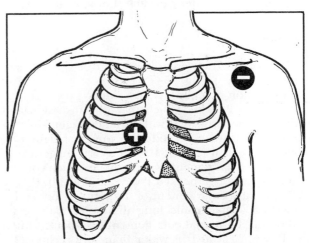

FIGURE 15–6. Modified chest lead (MCL₁).

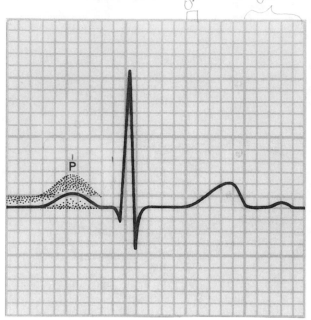

FIGURE 15–7. Normal P wave. It does not exceed 3 mm in height (voltage) and is less than 0.12 second in width (duration).

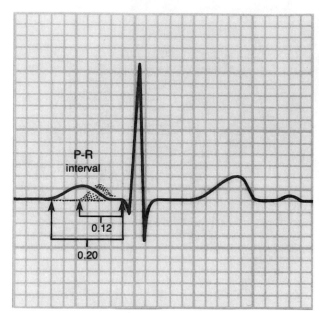

FIGURE 15–8. The PR interval measures between 0.12 to 0.20 second.

cardiac monitoring system are discussed in the care plan at the end of this chapter.

Components of the Electrocardiogram

There are three major components of the ECG tracing: the P wave, the QRS complex, and the T wave. These reflect atrial depolarization, ventricular depolarization, and ventricular repolarization, respectively. Other features of the ECG are the PR interval, QRS duration, QT interval, ST segment, U wave, and artifacts. By convention, capital letters Q, R, and S are used to designate waves of relatively large amplitude; lowercase letters q, r, and s are used to label relatively small waves. The components of the ECG are described in the order in which they appear.

P Wave

The normal P wave corresponds to atrial depolarization-activation (Fig. 15–7). It is recorded as a positive deflection in leads I, II, aVF, and V_4 through V_6.

Abnormal P waves, which may vary in height and width, can be associated with atrial enlargement. For example, a P wave exceeding 3 mm in height (>3 small squares) in leads I, II, and aVF is suggestive of right atrial enlargement. P pulmonale, which consists of a pattern of tall, peaked P waves in leads II, II, and aVF, indicates enlargement of the right atrium and is associated with chronic lung disease or pulmonary embolism.[5] Left atrial enlargement is suspected when the P wave in lead II is wider than 0.12 second (>3 small squares) or there is an abnormally wide, notched

(M-shaped) P wave (P mitrale). P mitrale is associated with mitral valve disease. Suggestions of atrial enlargement can also be seen in lead V_1. Here the P wave is normally biphasic. In right atrial enlargement, the initial part of the biphasic wave is large, while in left atrial enlargement the second component of the biphasic wave is enlarged.

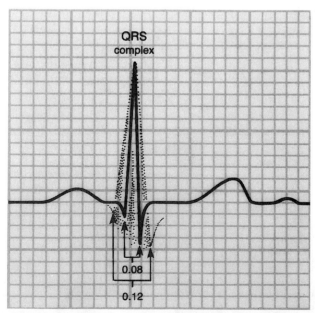

FIGURE 15–9. QRS measurement: normally it is 0.10 second or less in duration; if 0.12 second or greater in duration, a delay in ventricular depolarization is reflected.

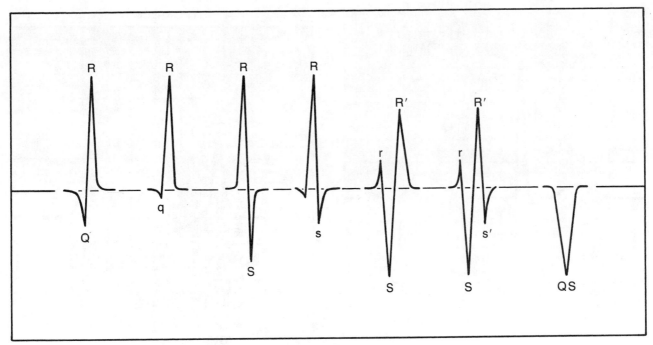

FIGURE 15-10. QRS nomenclature.

Repolarization of the atria is usually obscured by the QRS complex.

PR Interval

The PR interval is measured from the beginning of the P wave to the beginning of the QRS complex (Fig. 15–8). It represents the time it takes for the electrical impulse to travel from the SA node to the ventricles. The normal PR interval time is 0.12 to 0.20 second (at least 2, but nor more than 5, small squares).

QRS Complex

The QRS complex (Fig. 15–9) corresponds to the spread of the electrical impulse down the bundle of His, the bundle branches, and the Purkinje network (ventricular depolarization-activation). The complex includes the Q, R, and S waves; however, not every complex will contain a Q wave, an R wave, and an S wave. Various configurations of the QRS complex may occur, and the term "QRS complex" may be used to described the ventricular complex, regardless of the deflection pattern present (Fig. 15–10).

Q Wave. In the normal QRS complex, the first negative deflection (i.e., below the baseline) is called the Q wave. Normal, small Q waves are seen in leads I, II, III, aVL, AVF, V_5, and V_6.

R Wave. The first positive deflection (above the baseline) is an R wave, which is normally less than 20 mm high in the limb leads and less than 25 mm in the precordial leads. Normally, small R waves are seen in the right precordial leads (V_1 through V_3). The height of the R wave is occasionally examined for evidence of

ventricular enlargement, ventricular hypertrophy, and bundle branch block.

S Wave. The negative deflection following the R wave is an S wave. It is normally quite small, except in the precordial leads. A prominent (deep and wide) S wave occurs in abnormal conditions such as ventricular hypertrophy and bundle branch block.

QRS Duration

The QRS duration represents the time it takes for ventricular depolarization (activation) to occur, that is, from the beginning of the Q wave to the end of the S wave. The normal QRS duration is 0.04 to 0.10 second (1 to 2.5 small squares).

QT Interval

The interval covers the period of ventricular excitation, contraction, and recovery, and extends from the beginning of the QRS complex to the end of the T wave (Fig. 15–11). The normal length of the QT interval depends upon the heart rate. The value of QTc, the QT interval corrected for heart rate, can be calculated from Bazett's formula:

$$QTc = \frac{QR}{\sqrt{R\text{-}R}}$$

where R-R is the interval between successive R waves, that is, the heart rate. The faster the heart rate, the shorter the QT interval. As a rule of thumb, the QT interval is less than half the R-R interval. The normal values for the QT interval are different for men and

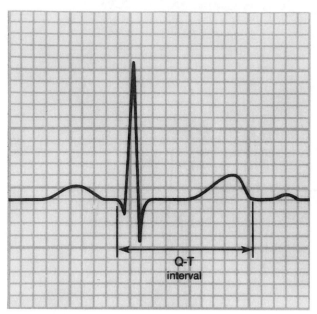

FIGURE 15–11. QT interval measurement.

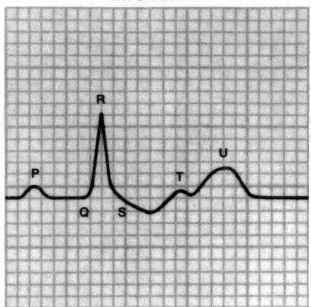

FIGURE 15–13. The U wave.

women. For men the upper limit of QTc is 0.39 second, and for women 0.41 second.

ST Segment

The ST segment is isoelectric (i.e., at baseline) and represents the period during which there is no electrical activity, in other words, when the ventricles have been completely depolarized and are beginning to repolarize. It extends from the end of the QRS complex to the beginning of the T wave (Fig. 15–12). The

point at which the QRS complex meets the ST segment is sometimes known as the J point.

T Wave

The T wave corresponds to ventricular repolarization. Normally, T waves are slightly rounded and asymmetric, the upstroke being longer than the downstroke. The T wave is usually less that 5 mm in height in any standard lead, and less than 10 mm in the precordial leads. For adults, the deflection of the T wave is positive (above the baseline) in leads III, aVL, aVF, V_1, and V_2.

U Wave

A small wave, the U wave, may occasionally be seen following the T wave (Fig. 15–13). It represents increased excitation or repolarization of the Purkinje fibers and is a normal phenomenon in children. The U wave can also be associated with clinical conditions, for example, hyperthyroidism and hypokalemia.

Artifacts

Wave configurations that are not due to electrical currents generated during the cardiac cycle are termed artifacts. These may be due to tremors, standardization, alternating current (AC) interference, lead displacement, and waveforms produced during cardiac resuscitation efforts. Since some of the configurations may resemble broad ventricular beats, the critical care nurse must be able to differentiate what is artifact and what is a waveform reflecting an abnormality in the cardiac electrical current.

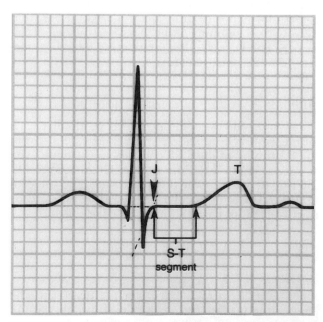

FIGURE 15–12. Characteristics of the ST segment and T wave. The J point marks the beginning of the ST segment; the T wave is normally asymmetrical.

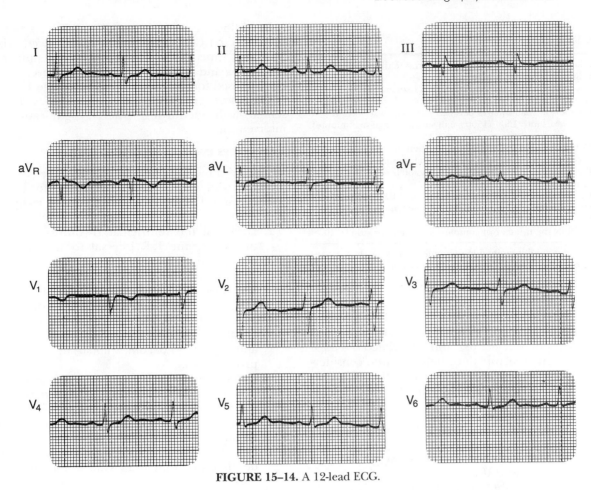

FIGURE 15–14. A 12-lead ECG.

Full 12-Lead ECG

A full 12-lead ECG is shown in Figure 15–14. It can readily be observed that the actual recording of the P Q R S T pattern differs in each lead. Each lead records current from the body in a different direction and reflects the placement of positive and negative electrodes.

SINUS RHYTHM

Activation of the heart by an impulse originating in the sinus node and subsequent activation of the atria, bundle of His, bundle branches, and ventricles, in normal sequence and with normal time intervals, will result in an ECG pattern of sinus rhythm as depicted in Figure 15–15. There is, however, considerable vari-

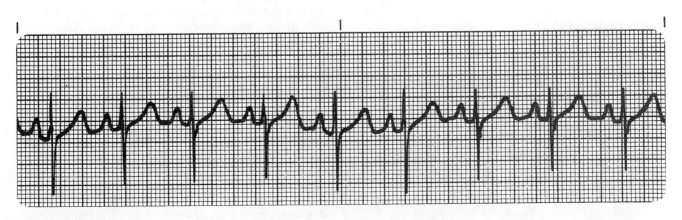

Lead II

FIGURE 15–15. Sinus rhythm.

TABLE 15–1
Heart Rate Determination

The common and simple methods to determine the heart rate are:
1. Slow and regular rhythms (ventricular rate)*
   a. Count the number of small squares (1 square = 0.04 second) between two consecutive R complexes. Divide the number of small squares between the two consecutive R complexes into 1500 (1500 small squares equal one minute).
   or
   b. Count the number of large squares between two consecutive R complexes. Divide the number of large squares between the two consecutive R complexes into 300.
2. Irregular rhythms
   a. Count the number of R-R complexes in a 6-sec strip. (The electrocardiographic paper reflects 3-sec intervals by indicators above the strip.)
   b. Multiply the number of complexes in the 6-sec strip by 10.

*Atrial rates are determined in the same manner by counting the number of boxes between two consecutive P waves.

ation in the normal ECG, depending on the age of the individual, physical status, and associated medical problems. These factors must be taken into consideration when examining and comparing the ECG tracing to that of normal sinus rhythm.

ECG Criteria of Normal Sinus Rhythm

P wave	Positive deflection (above baseline) in lead II
	Height: 3 mm or less
	Width: 0.12 second or less
	Precedes every QRS complex
PR interval	0.12 to 0.20 second
QRS complex	Normal in duration (0.04 to 0.10 second) and configuration
R-R interval	Usually constant, but can vary by 0.04 second
Heart rate	Adults: 60 to 100 beats/min
	Elderly: 50 to 75 beats/min
	Infants: 100 to 150 beats/min. This tachycardia is normal in infants.

DYSRHYTHMIAS

Recognition of Dysrhythmia

Analysis of an ECG strip for dysrhythmia requires consideration of three fundamental aspects of every rhythm:[6]

Anatomic origin	SA node, atria, bundle of His, ventricles
Discharge sequence	Normal inherent, bradycardia, tachycardia, premature, flutter, fibrillation
Conduction sequence	Sinoatrial, atrioventricular, intraventricular

In addition, it is important to establish a systematic approach to ECG interpretation, using the criteria for a normal sinus rhythm to evaluate and compare all waveforms and intervals for normalcy. Several methods are used for rate determination (Table 15–1).

The more commonly seen arrhythmias are presented with identifying criteria, significance, and interventions.

KEY STEPS IN DYSRHYTHMIA DETECTION

1. Determine the rate and compare the calculated rate with what is considered normal for that pacing site. Decide if a bradycardia or tachycardia exists.
2. Decide if the ventricular rhythm is regular by measuring the R-R interval for at least three cycles to determine whether it stays constant.
3. Be sure there is a P wave for every QRS complex. Rhythms where the P wave changes or disappears suggest pacing sites outside the SA node.
4. Measure the PR and QRS intervals for normal duration. Specific forms of block and conduction abnormalities become apparent if there is prolongation.
5. Determine if the T wave is upright or inverted. Is it flat, rounded, or peaked? Is it deflected in the same direction as the QRS complex?
6. Identify whether the ST segment is isoelectric, elevated, or depressed.
7. Look for beats or runs of beats that interrupt the dominant rhythm and create abnormality.

Sinus Abnormalities

Sinus abnormalities are frequently caused by conditions that are not related to heart disease. The heartbeat may be slower than normal for the age group, faster than normal, and/or somewhat irregular.

Sinus Bradycardia

The rhythm strip for sinus bradycardia is much like that of the normal sinus ryhthm, with the exception of the heart rate (Fig. 15–16). As mentioned previously, a slower rate may be "normal" for the elderly, and athletes may have slow heart rates. Additional causes of bradycardia are listed in Table 15–2.

Sinus Tachycardia

A heart rate that exceeds 100 beats/min but otherwise conforms to the criteria for normal sinus rhythm in the average adult population is indicative of sinus origin (Fig. 15–17). The causes of sinus tachycardia vary (Table 15–3).

A sudden drop in blood pressure, or a rise in body temperature, is usually accompanied by an increase in pulse as a compensatory mechanism. For every degree of temperature rise, there is a concomitant rise in pulse rate of approximately 10 to 11 beats/min. Exer-

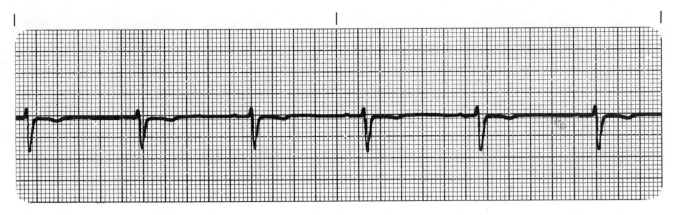

Lead II

FIGURE 15–16. Sinus bradycardia.

cise, pain, emotion, excessive use of stimulants, as well as pathologic factors (sepsis, dehydration) can cause an increase in heart rate. The presence of sinus tachycardia is usually not indicative of heart disease, although it may be.

Sustained sinus tachycardia in the patient who has experienced a myocardial infarction may be hazardous, in that it increases the workload of the heart. Sinus tachycardia may imply that the heart as a pump has become compromised. In that case, therapy for termination of the tachycardia is indicated. In other situations, therapy is aimed at treating the primary problem.

A rhythm strip is necessary at times to differentiate sinus tachycardia from abnormal rhythms such as atrial tachycardia or atrial flutter.

Sinus Dysrhythmia

Irregularity of cardiac rhythm may be related to phases of the respiratory cycle (sinus arrhythmia) or to atrial dysrhythmias, including premature atrial contractions. In sinus dysrhythmia, measurement of the

P-P interval in the recording strip will reveal a variation in the sinus rate that increases on inspiration and decreases on expiration (Fig. 15–18). In such cases, sinus dysrhythmia can be distinguished from atrial fibrillation because, in the former, the heart rate becomes regular when the breath is held. Sinus arrhythmia is most commonly found in children and young people up to 30 years of age, and appears to be a normal phenomenon.

Sick Sinus Syndrome

Sick sinus syndrome (SSS; bradycardia-tachycardia syndrome) comprises several disorders of sinus node and/or atrial disturbances in which cardiac output is compromised. The syndrome occurs more frequently in the elderly population but is not confined to that group. Sick sinus syndrome may appear in one or more of the following forms: episodes of severe, persistent, or recurrent bradycardia; sinoatrial block; sinus arrest with periods of tachydysrhythmias in the form of atrial and junctional tachycardia; atrial fibrillation; and atrial flutter.

Sick sinus syndrome may be caused by abnormalities in sinus node automaticity, SA conduction, or escape mechanism (impulse generation by lower centers such as the AV node). Some individuals experiencing sick sinus syndrome may complain of intermittent episodes of dizziness or light-headedness, while others may be asymptomatic.[8] The episodes of dizziness and light-headedness are thought to be related to inadequate cerebral perfusion.

The most common underlying causes of sick sinus syndrome are:

1. Alterations in blood supply to the sinus node
2. Pathology involving atrial muscle
3. Electrolyte imbalances
4. Drug effects

Documentation of sick sinus syndrome is not always possible by way of the 12-lead ECG; therefore, for persons experiencing the syndrome, a 24-hour Holter monitor recording may be prescribed.

TABLE 15–2
Mechanisms and Causes of Sinus Bradycardia

Mechanism	Cause
Increased vagal tone	Eyeball compression
	Carotid massage
	Endotracheal suctioning
	Valsalva maneuver
Pathologic	Increased intracranial pressure
	Hypothyroidism
	Myocardial infarction
	Hypothermia
Drug-related	Demoral
	Morphine
	β-blocking agents
	Calcium channel blocking agents

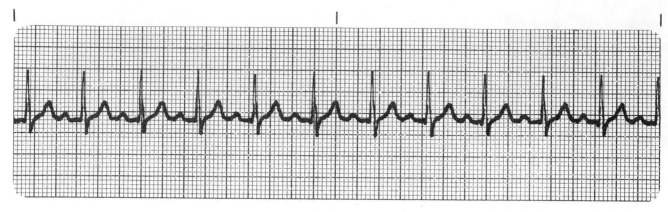

Lead II

FIGURE 15–17. Sinus tachycardia.

TABLE 15–3
Mechanisms and Causes of Sinus Tachycardia

Mechanism	Cause
Compensatory (to increase cardiac output)	Hemorrhage
	Shock
	Anemia
	Congestive heart failure
Physiologic	Maximal exercise
	Pain
	Emotion
	Psychic trauma
	Excessive use of coffee, tea, alcohol
Drug-related	Atropine
	Amphetamines
	Isoproterenol
	Ephedrine
	Theophylline preparations
Pathologic	Infection (febrile illness)
	Sepsis
	Dehydration
	Embolic phenomenon
	Fever
	Hyperthyroidism
	Myocardial infarction (impaired cardiac reserve)
	Neurosis

Atrial Dysrhythmias

Occasionally a focus in the atria becomes the pacemaker of the heart in place of the sinus node. As mentioned previously, cells in the atrial muscle and other areas of the heart have pacemaking properties. Thus the subsidiary pacemaker takes over as a result of failure of the sinus node to fire, or in a process of usurpation. Evaluation of the P wave shows that the shape and size of the P wave differs from that which is normal for a particular lead. Generally, the impulse originating at the sinus node (normal pacemaker) is conducted in a "head-to-foot" direction toward the positive electrode of leads such as II, III, and aVF, and conduction of the atrial impulse shows up as a positive deflection in those leads. With an ectopic focus, however, activation of the atria, and consequently the shape and size of the P wave, may differ from that which is normal for a particular lead. The variation in configuration of the P wave implies that the impulse originated in an area other than the sinus node. If the origin of the ectopic focus is near the site of the sinus node, the variant P wave in monitoring lead II will have a positive deflection (above baseline) and will be

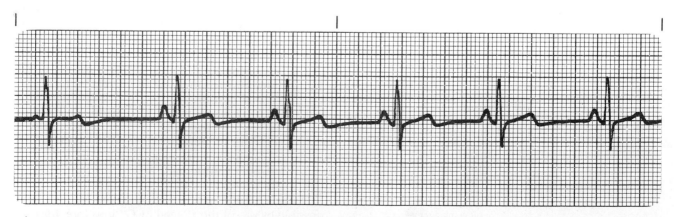

Lead II

FIGURE 15–18. Sinus dysrhythmia.

followed by a normal QRS complex. If the ectopic focus is low in the atria or near the node, activation of the atria will proceed in a retrograde manner; therefore the P wave will be inverted in that lead (i.e., negative deflection).

Premature Atrial Contraction

Premature contractions are the most common of the heartbeat disorders. They do not necessarily indicate cardiac disease but may occur in patients with heart disease, especially cardiomyopathy and coronary artery disease.

A premature atrial contraction (PAC) occurs when an ectopic focus within the atrial muscle usurps the pacemaking function from the sinus node. The ECG then shows a variant P wave occurring prior to the expected sinus P wave.[9] Conduction through the AV node, the bundle of His, and the ventricles progresses in a normal fashion; therefore the QRS complex and the T wave will usually be of normal configuration and duration. The PR interval may be within normal limits, shorter than normal, or longer than normal, depending on the site of the usurping focus (Fig. 15–19).

Premature atrial contractions are usually followed by an incomplete compensatory pause and disturb regular atrial rhythm. If one were to mark off three normal cycles using a strip of paper and then place the first mark of the paper on the normal P wave preceding the variant P wave, the third mark would not fall on the P wave following the premature atrial contraction. This deviation indicates a disturbance in the atrial rhythm. One can also use calipers to determine the presence of a compensatory or noncompensatory pause.

Review of the ECG tracing can make it possible to differentiate premature atrial contraction from that of an escape focus within the atria secondary to failure of the sinus node to initiate an impulse. Measuring a P-P sequence with calipers will reveal that the abnormal P wave occurs later than the expected sinus P wave if it is an escape beat; whereas if it is a premature atrial contraction, the ectopic P wave will occur prior to the expected sinus beat. Depending upon the site of the ectopic pacemaker, the variant P wave may be (1) distorted in configuration; (2) inverted prior to the QRS complex (characteristic of a low abnormal pacemaking site with retrograde activation of the atria); (3) inverted, but follow the QRS complex; or (4) superimposed on the T wave, which is then distorted.[10]

Premature atrial contractions that occur infrequently generally do not cause problems. In this situation, the patient may occasionally be aware of a "skipped" beat or irregularity, or may complain of a disturbing sensation in the chest. If the premature contractions interfere with cardiac output, however, the individual may experience palpitations or manifestations of reduced cardiac output. Recognition and identification of premature atrial contractions is important, since they may be forerunners of atrial fibrillation and atrial flutter.

Treatment measures depend on the condition of the patient. If the premature atrial contractions occur in the presence of known heart disease, antiarrhythmic drugs may be used to prevent further atrial irritability. Additionally, if the premature atrial contractions are distressing to the patient, intervention may be recommended.

Paroxysmal Atrial Tachycardia

Paroxysmal atrial tachycardia, or commonly referred to as supraventricular tachycardia, is characterized by a sudden onset of rapid heartbeat in the range of 150 to 250 beats/min (Fig. 15–20). It is initiated by a premature atrial contraction that assumes the pacemaking function of the heart. The key diagnostic feature of atrial tachycardia is the presence of an abnormal P wave (P′), which precipitates a tachycardia. Frequently the P wave may be buried in the preceding T wave.

Paroxysmal atrial tachycardia usually ends as abruptly as it begins. It is frequently found in normal, healthy people and may be initiated by emotional stress, physical fatigue, stimulants (coffee, tea, tobacco). It is of greater significance in the presence of heart disease since the paroxysm may precipitate congestive heart failure. The rapid ventricular rate reduces coronary artery filling, which may precipitate coronary insufficiency in the individual with pre-existing coronary artery disease.

The more common symptoms associated with par-

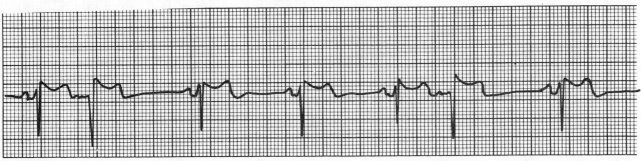

FIGURE 15–19. Premature supraventricular complexes (PACs) (beats two and six). (From Brown, DR and Jacobson, S: Dysrhythmias: A Problem-Solving Guide. FA Davis, Philadelphia, 1988, with permission.)

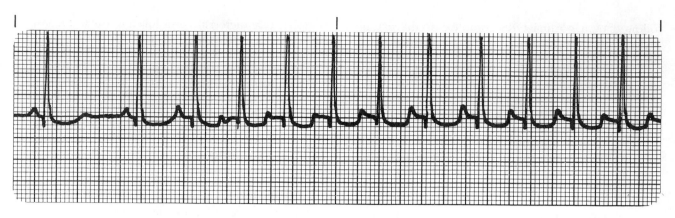

Lead II

FIGURE 15–20. Paroxysmal atrial tachycardia.

oxysmal atrial tachycardia are palpitations, faintness, precordial pain, and anxiety. Other symptoms may be related to the decrease in cardiac output, particularly in those individuals with compromised heart status.

The treatment of the arrhythmia is to increase vagal tone. Reflex vagal stimulation will generally produce sudden cardiac slowing (Table 15–2). Additional treatment measures include sedation, digitalis, preparations, quinidine, beta blocking agents, and calcium blocking agents. Cardioversion, or overdrive pacing, may be indicated if the patient is unresponsive to drug therapy.

Atrial Fibrillation

In atrial fibrillation the atria are essentially "quivering" or fibrillating and are unable to produce an effective contraction. In most but not all cases, the cardiac rhythm is totally irregular, in the range of 100 to 180 beats/min.[11] The rapidity of the atrial beats reaching the AV node is such that the node cannot allow all of the atrial beats to progress to the ventricles (Fig. 15–21); furthermore, not all ventricular beats are transmitted to the radial pulse at the wrist, so that the

ventricular rate at the apex of the heart is greater than the radial pulse. The ECG is marked by total irregularity of the QRS complexes (R-R irregularity), absence of normal P waves before each QRS complex, and the presence of a baseline that undulates variably at a rate of 350 to 600 per minute, indicating fibrillatory activity.[11]

Since the atria are not contracting effectively, the "atrial kick" does not contribute to the volume of blood in the ventricles (20% to 30% of the total ventricular volume) during the latter part of atrial contraction or during end-diastole. Those individuals who may have a "fixed" cardiac output due to abnormalities of heart action are generally reliant upon this extra 20% to 30% of blood provided during the "atrial kick" and may experience problems of a reduced cardiac output.[10] In addition, because the atria do not contract effectively, there is a propensity for clot formation in the atria. When an effective contraction is restored, particles of the clot can break off and travel throughout the body as emboli.

The presence of atrial fibrillation generally indicates disease or streching of the left atrium, for example, coronary artery disease leading to ischemia of

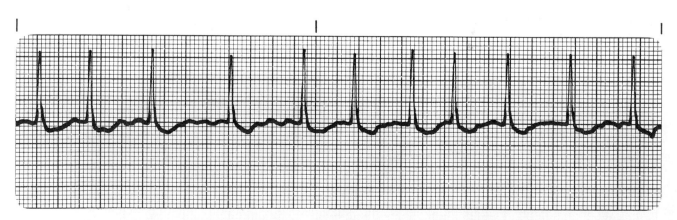

Lead II

FIGURE 15–21. Atrial fibrillation.

atrial muscle, hypertensive heart disease, and mitral stenosis.[11]

Patients who have sustained a myocardial infarction do not tolerate atrial fibrillation well. The rapid ventricular response to atrial fibrillation decreases diastolic filling time. The latter is the period during which most coronary arteries fill; therefore the individual with an already compromised coronary circulation may not tolerate further reduction of blood flow to the myocardium.

Treatment of atrial fibrillation is initiated primarily to decrease the ventricular rate. Drugs such as digoxin, digitalis, and/or verapamil are frequently ordered. Texts on pharmacotherapeutics can be consulted for the mechanism of action.

Atrial Flutter

Atrial flutter is a disorder of cardiac rhythm in which the atria contract rapidly and regularly, often nearly 300 times per minute. This type of arrhythmia is less commonly seen than atrial fibrillation but should be suspected when the ventricular and pulse rates are approximately 150 per minute. In atrial flutter, only every second, third, or fourth atrial impulse is transmitted to the ventricles. Thus if the atria are beating rapidly at 300 times a minute, and every other beat is conducted, the ventricular rate would be 150 beats/min. If every third impulse is conducted, the ventricular rate would be 100 beats/min; if every fourth beat, the rate becomes 75 beats/min. The ratio of conducted beats can vary.[12]

Flutter waveforms have a characteristic appearance on ECG. They are regular and are frequently described as presenting a "saw-tooth" or "picket fence" configuration (Fig. 15–22).

The effect of atrial flutter on body hemodynamics depends on the ventricular rate and the presence of heart impairment. In the absence of heart disease, the individual may experience no symptoms. In the individual with pre-existing coronary disease, however, the rapid heart rate may further compromise blood flow

to the myocardium, in which case the result may be angina or myocardial infarction. Another possible complication of atrial flutter is thrombus formation.

Atrial flutter is usually treated with cardiotonic drugs. Digitalis is the drug of choice, especially in patients who manifest congestive heart failure. Termination of the arrhythmia by direct current (DC) shock may become necessary if drug therapy fails.

Atrioventricular Junctional Rhythms

Atrioventricular junctional tissue possesses automaticity, and hence pacemaking capability. It can assume pacemaking function when there is depression of the SA node or SA block and the sinus rate becomes slower than the inherent rate of the junctional pacemaker, which takes over by default. An increase in automaticity can also result in usurpation of the pacemaking function of the SA node. This phenomenon is manifested electrocardiographically by the early appearance of the ectopic beat. By contrast, an escape pacemaker is identified on the ECG as a beat appearing later than the expected sinus beat. If atrial muscle is activated either by default or usurpation in a retrograde manner, the leads in which the P wave is normally upright (positive deflection) will record an inverted P wave (negative deflection; Fig. 15–23).

Premature junctional contractions occur less frequently than premature atrial or ventricular contractions. They may occur in individuals with heart disease, in healthy subjects, or secondary to digitalis toxicity. If the junctional pacemaker takes over the role of pacing the heart, a junctional rhythm will become evident. A junctional rate faster than the normal inherent rate of junctional tissue will produce junctional tachycardia (Fig. 15–24).[12] In paroxysmal junctional tachycardia the phenomenon begins and ends abruptly (Fig. 15–25). If the individual is symptomatic due to reduced cardiac output secondary to a slow heart rate, atropine may be prescribed or a pacemaker may be inserted.

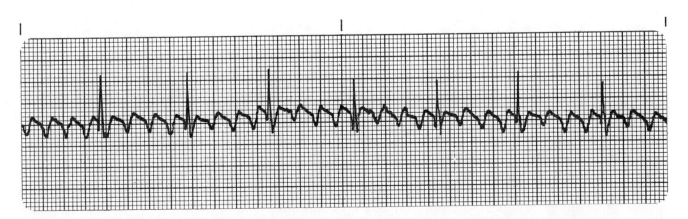

Lead II

FIGURE 15–22. Atrial flutter.

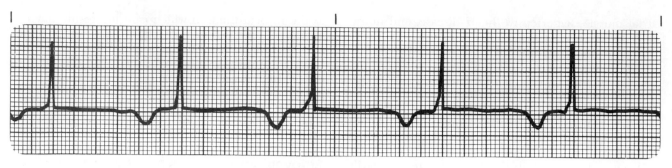

Lead MCL₁

FIGURE 15–23. Junctional rhythm.

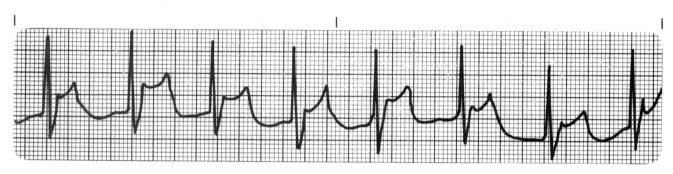

Lead II

FIGURE 15–24. Junctional tachycardia.

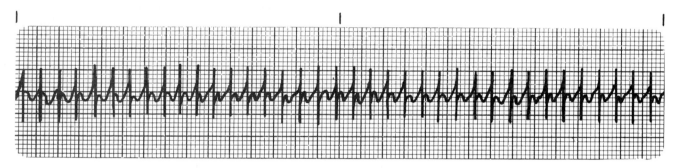

Lead II

FIGURE 15–25. Paroxysmal junctional tachycardia.

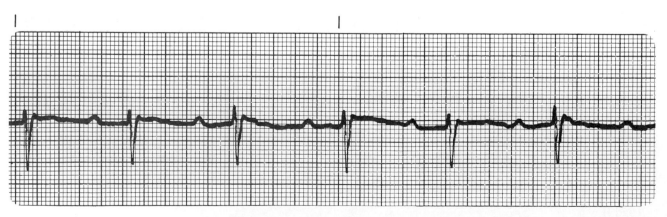

Lead MCL₁

FIGURE 15–26. First-degree AV block.

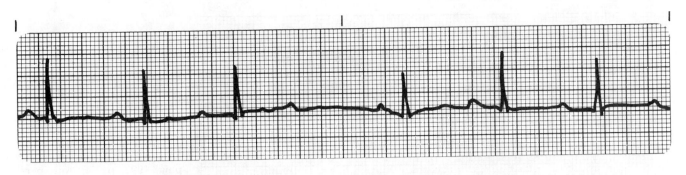

Lead II

FIGURE 15–27. Second-degree AV block (Wenckebach, Mobitz type I).

Disturbances of Atrioventricular Conduction

Atrioventricular Block

A delay in transmission or a blocking of the impulse between the atria and the ventricles causes AV block. The AV blocks are usually classified as first degree, second degree (Mobitz type I [Wenckebach] and Mobitz type II), and third degree, or complete heart block.

The etiology of heart block varies, but it is usually associated with heart disease, cardiac surgery, infections, digitalis toxicity, and electrolyte imbalances.

First Degree AV Block. First degree AV block is characterized by the prolongation of the PR interval beyond 0.20 second, the upper limit of normal. The block reflects a delay in impulse conduction to the bundle of His. Although there is slowing of conduction through the AV node, a ventricular response to each P wave is present (Fig. 15–26).

Treatment of first degree AV block is reserved for individuals whose heart rate is below normal and who are symptomatic. When indicated, the block is treated by administration of atropine.

Second Degree AV Block. There are two types of second degree AV block: Mobitz type I (Wenckebach) and Mobitz type II.

Mobitz Type I (Wenckebach) Block. In Mobitz type I AV block there is a characteristic cycle in which there is progressive lengthening of the PR interval until a beat is dropped as a result of the failure of the impulse to reach the ventricles. After the dropped beat, the sequence is repeated (Fig. 15–27).

Mobitz type I AV block can be caused by:
1. Ischemia of the AV node, possibly due to myocardial infarction
2. Digitalis toxicity
3. Lesions within the conduction system

Treatment is deferred in individuals who are asymptomatic; however, if the conduction problem results in a very slow ventricular rate, atropine is usually prescribed to increase the ventricular rate. Occasionally, the individual who manifests second degree AV block may complain of palpitations, and if the ventricular rate is very slow, dizziness may be experienced. Again, atropine may be ordered to increase the heart rate.

Mobitz Type II AV Block. Mobitz type II block is variously manifested. For example, the P wave and PR interval may appear regular, but some P waves are not followed by a QRS complex. These are nonconducted P waves, that is, P waves that arise in the atria in normal fashion but fail to stimulate the ventricles (Fig. 15–28). The ventricles may respond periodically to every fifth or sixth beat. In another variant of Mobitz type II block, every other impulse to the ventricles may be blocked to give a pattern of 2:1, that is, two P waves for every QRS complex.[12]

For patients with Mobitz type II block, continuous monitoring for progression to third degree AV block is mandatory. Treatment of Mobitz type II AV block includes medications such as atropine and isoproter-

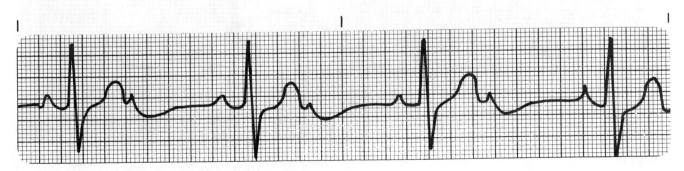

Lead II

FIGURE 15–28. Second-degree AV block (Mobitz type II).

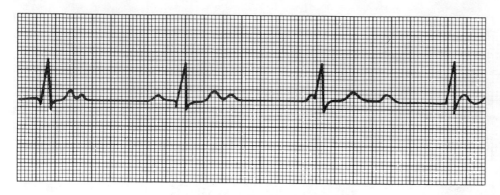

FIGURE 15–29. Complete arteriovenous dissociation with third-degree heart block. (From Wilson, RF: Critical care manual: Applied physiology and principles of therapy, ed 2, FA Davis Company, Philadelphia, 1992, p 156, with permission.)

enol, as well as withholding of digitalis and antiarrhythmics, cardiac pacing, may also be initiated.

Third Degree (Complete) Heart Block. In complete heart block, the atria and ventricles are beating independently. The atria respond to the sinus pacemaker as usual, while the ventricles respond to an impulse originating in the AV node, bundle of His, bundle branches, or Purkinje fibers. The heart rate will be in the range of the inherent rate of the AV node (50 to 60 beats/min). If the ventricles are paced by an impulse originating low in the ventricles, however, the heart rate will be within the range of 20 to 30 beats/min, which is the inherent rate of that site (Fig. 15–29). Individuals who are generally active do not tolerate the slow rate of the ventricular impulse and may experience syncopal episodes. Emergency insertion of a pacemaker may be indicated or temporary pacing with a transcutaneous device can be used. Other treatment modalities may include the administration of atropine or isoproterenol.

A term frequently identified in a discussion of complete heart block is atrioventricular dissociation. In atrioventricular dissociation, as in third degree heart block, two independent pacemakers are present—one to which the atria respond, and another that governs the ventricles. In atrioventricular dissociation, however, the ventricular rate is faster than the atrial rate, possibly due to a functional rather than an organic block. In addition to the fact that impulses of sinus or atrial origin are not conducted to the ventricles, retrograde activation of the atria by a ventricular impulse is impeded due to refractoriness of the conduction tissue. His bundle electrocardiography is frequently used for locating the source and type of heart block.

Ventricular Dysrhythmias

Impulses originating in the ventricles may be life-threatening (ventricular tachycardia and ventricular fibrillation) or life-saving (ventricular escape beat). Even though the heart rate is slow, the ventricular escape beat is crucial when the supraventricular pacemaker defaults. Isolated beats or established rhythms of ventricular origin can generally be distinguished by the wide and bizarre-looking QRS complexes on the ECG tracing, although a supraventricular impulse with aberrant conduction may give a similar QRS complex. The ventricular dysrhythmias include isolated premature ventricular contraction, ventricular tachycardia, and ventricular fibrillation.

Premature Ventricular Contraction

When an ectopic stimulus arising in the ventricular muscle supersedes the normal pacemaker from the sinoatrial node for one beat, it is manifested electrocardiographically as a premature ventricular contrac-

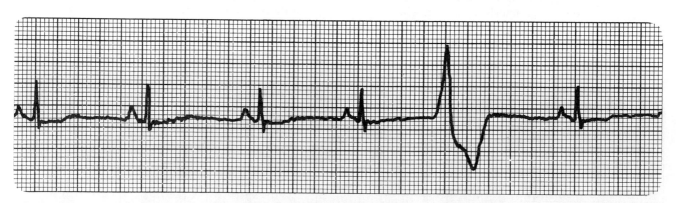

Lead II

FIGURE 15–30. Premature ventricular contraction.

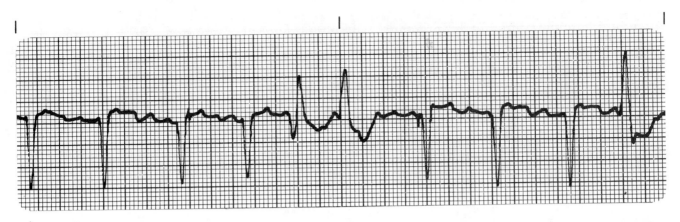

Lead MCL₁

FIGURE 15–31. Multifocal premature ventricular contractions.

tion (PVC; Fig. 15–30). A compensatory pause usually follows an isolated ventricular contraction. The QRS complex of premature ventricular beats is of distinctly abnormal morphology and usually has a width of 0.12 second or more.

The etiology of PVCs is variable. They may occur in a normal heart; in the presence of heart disease; secondary to an irritable focus, as during cardiac catheterization, pulmonary artery insertion, or open heart surgery; in the presence of electrolyte imbalances; or in association with medications. There may be no signs or symptoms associated with premature ventricular contraction. On the other hand, some individuals may complain of palpitation, or a sensation of a "skipped beat," and/or may become anxious.

Premature ventricular contraction may be the result of enhanced automaticity (the ability to initiate an impulse spontaneously) or of re-entry activity, in which unidirectional block of the normally initiated impulse, in conjunction with areas of slow conduction or refractoriness, results in restimulation of ventricular muscle.

Although isolated PVCs may not be troublesome, they can cause a decrease in cardiac output and produce symptoms of congestive heart failure in predisposed individuals. Furthermore, PVCs can herald the onset of more dangerous dysrhythmias such as ventricular tachycardia or ventricular fibrillation.

Examination of the ECG strip (Fig. 15–31) makes it possible to determine whether the premature ventricular contraction has its origin at a single site within the ventricles (unifocal), or at more than one ventricular site (multifocal). It is important to monitor the ECG tracing for increasing frequency of PVCs, as well as changing configuration of the bizarre QRS complex and/or its proximity to the T wave. In the R on T phenomenon, the PVC occurs on the apex of the preceding T wave (Fig. 15–32). This represents a situation where, electrically, the myocardium is especially vulnerable, since the muscle fibers have not completely repolarized but are at varying stages of depolarization and repolarization, and clinically some patients may be at risk of developing ventricular tachycardia or ventricular fibrillation. See Table 15–4 (page 207) for additional terms describing premature ventricular contractions.

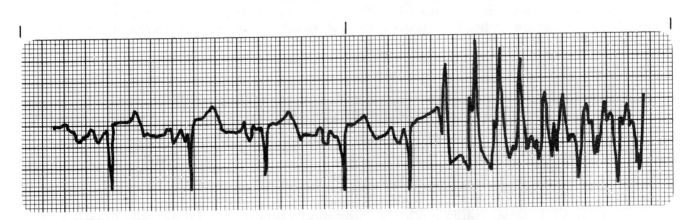

Lead MCL₁

FIGURE 15–32. Premature ventricular contraction: R-on-T phenomenon.

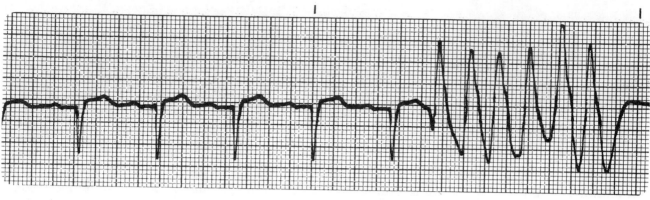

Lead MCL₁

FIGURE 15–33. Ventricular tachycardia.

Ventricular Tachycardia

Three or more PVCs occurring in succession constitute ventricular tachycardia (Fig. 15–33). The normal ventricular inherent rate is 20 to 40 beats/min. In ventricular tachycardia the rate is usually regular and may range from 50 beats/min (indicative of slow ventricular tachycardia) to 220 beats/min (rapid ventricular tachycardia). The ECG shows a widened QRS complex (>0.12 second).

Ventricular tachycardia is a dangerous cardiac arrhythmia and may occur in the presence of ischemic heart disease. It can also be precipitated by drug toxicity or sensitivity, hypoxemia, or electrolyte imbalances. Depending on the prevailing ventricular rate, the arrhythmia can affect cardiac output.[13] Hypotension, loss of consciousness, or congestive heart failure may follow due to the decreased stroke volume. The mechanism of ventricular tachycardia is the same as that of PVCs (enhanced automaticity, re-entry phenomena).

Lidocaine has been used in the treatment of ventricular tachycardia if the patient is hemodynamically stable, but synchronized cardioversion is indicated if the patient becomes hemodynamically unstable. Cardioversion employs the use of electrical energy to convert a dysrhythmia, which produces hemodynamic instability. Synchronization of the electrical shock at a lower wattage (joules) than in defibrillation must coincide with the R wave to avoid countershocking during ventricular vulnerability.

A form of ventricular tachycardia in which the series of bizarre ventricular QRS complexes changes in polarity (i.e., from positive deflection to negative, or vice versa) is called torsades de pointes (twisting of the points).[14] Torsades de pointes is frequently associated with conditions that produce prolongation of the QT interval (electrolyte imbalances, certain antiarrhythmic and psychoactive agents, myocardial disease). The tachycardia is very unstable; it may resolve spontaneously or it may degenerate into ventricular fibrillation. An intravenous infusion of isoproterenol and overdrive pacing with an artificial pacemaker have been used in treatment of the dysrhythmia.

Ventricular Fibrillation

When an ectopic focus in the ventricles becomes so irritable or fires so rapidly that the ventricles cannot respond to it in a unified manner, ventricular fibrillation occurs, that is, the ventricles are quivering and cannot beat effectively, so that there is no cardiac output. The dysrhythmia constitutes a medical emergency and cardiopulmonary resuscitation must be initiated. Defibrillation is the only treatment. During defibrillation, an unsynchronized electrical countershock, is delivered to the heart to terminate the chaotic rhythm.

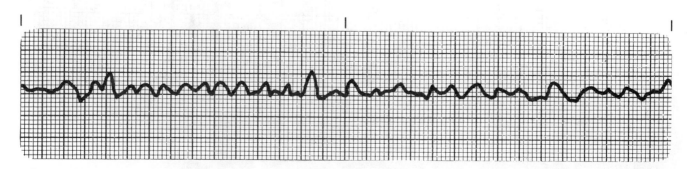

Lead MCL₁

FIGURE 15–34. Ventricular fibrillation: unevenly appearing deflections with no clear-cut P, QRS, or T waves.

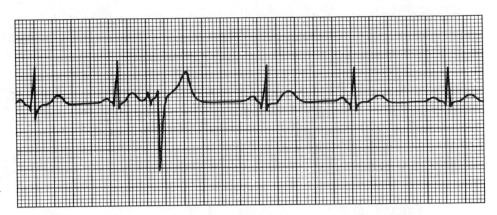

FIGURE 15–35. Premature atrial contraction with aberrant conduction.

The dysrhythmia appears on the ECG in the form of chaotic undulations with no discernible P waves or QRC complexes (Fig. 15–34). Caution must be exercised by the critical care nurse, who must ascertain whether the chaotic complexes are due to ventricular fibrillation or are the result of artifact such as lead displacement. If the patient is responsive, the likely cause of the abnormal waveform is an electrode that has become disconnected.

There are various causes of ventricular fibrillation. Patients who have sustained a myocardial infarction are susceptible to this lethal arrhythmia. Drug toxicity has also been implicated in predisposing individuals to ventricular fibrillation.

Miscellaneous Dysrhythmias

Aberrant Supraventricular/Ventricular Conduction

Aberrant ventricular conduction is the temporary, abnormal intraventricular conduction of a single beat or the constant aberrant conduction found with bundle branch block. Aberrancy occurs when a supraventricular impulse, that is, a premature atrial contraction, arrives at the ventricles before the specialized conduction pathway has completely recovered. Such an impulse produces a widened, bizarre QRS complex

that resembles that of a ventricular ectopic beat (Fig. 15–35). Differentiation between an aberrantly conducted supraventricular beat and a ventricular ectopic beat is important because the clinical significance and therapy required are different (Table 15–5).

Whenever a patient develops a tachyarrhythmia, the first question to be asked is whether the arrhythmia is supraventricular tachycardia (SVT) or ventricular tachycardia (VT). Differential diagnosis can be established, in part, by determining the width of the QRS complexes. A narrow QRS complex on the ECG (0.04 to 0.10 second) reflects normal intraventricular conduction to the ventricles from an impulse above the ventricles; that is, a narrow QRS complex signifies SVT.

A widened QRS complex (>0.12 second), on the other hand, may be due to VT or to SVT with aberration. VT is a life-threatening arrhythmia, which has been discussed in a previous section. SVT with aberration is usually due to either bundle branch block (BBB) or to Wolff-Parkinson-White (WPW) pre-excitation syndrome. Characteristic patterns for each of these make it possible to differentiate SVT with aberration from the more serious VT.

Bundle Branch Block. Intraventricular conduction

TABLE 15–4

Terms Associated with Premature Ventricular Contraction

Term	Explanation
Bigeminy	The PVC alternates with the basic beat.
Trigeminy	Every third beat is a PVC.
Quadrigeminy	Every fourth beat is a PVC.
Multiform	QRS configuration varies from beat to beat, with varying coupling intervals and differing QRS deflections.
Interpolated	A PVC is sandwiched between two sinus beats; therefore a compensatory pause is not observed.
Paired-couplet	PVCs occur in pairs or back-to-back (potential for ventricular tachycardia).

TABLE 15–5

Differentiation of Aberrant Ventricular Conduction from Ventricular Ectopy

Characteristics Favoring Aberrant Ventricular Conduction
Right bundle branch block with R′ > R in V_1
Initial QRS vector same as conducted QRS
QRS duration <0.14 sec
Normal axis (current flowing from base of the heart to the apex)
Preceding premature atrial contractions
Ashman's phenomenon (the second beat is bizarre in a group of beats. The RR cycle, which contains the bizarre QRS complex is shorter than the previous RR cycle)
Characteristics Favoring Ventricular Ectopy
Left axis deviation
QRS >140 msec
Monophasic or diphasic in V_1
Fusion or capture beats
AV dissociation
R > R′ in V_1

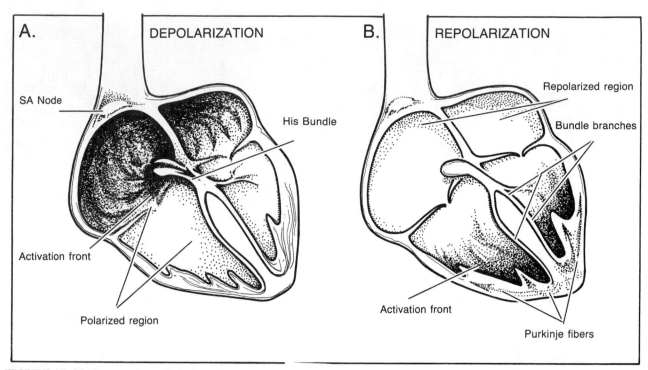

A. DEPOLARIZATION

SA Node

His Bundle

Activation front

Polarized region

B. REPOLARIZATION

Repolarized region

Bundle branches

Activation front

Purkinje fibers

FIGURE 15–36. Propagation of electrical forces within the heart. Upon impulse initiation in the SA node, an activation (a reversal in cellular polarity associated with an inward flow of positively charged sodium ions) is established, and this wave of depolarization (*A*) spreads in all directions, initially throughout the atria and AV node/junction, and subsequently through the His bundle, bundle branches, Purkinje fibers, and throughout the myocardial working cells. As the activation front moves away from the depolarized regions, cellular polarity in these areas is again reversed (there is an outward flow of sodium and potassium ions) resulting in repolarization (*B*).

delay or blockage can occur as a result of interference of impulse transmission along the right or left bundle branches (RBB or LBB). Such a delay will affect the normal sequence of ventricular depolarization (Fig. 15–36). Septal depolarization normally occurs in a left-to-right direction, reflecting the fact that the left bundle branch depolarizes slightly before the right bundle branch. Thus in lead V_1, as current flows toward its positive electrode, a small initial r wave is recorded normally; whereas in lead V_6, as current flows away from its positive electrode, a small s wave is recorded (Fig. 15–5).

With ventricular depolarization, although both ventricles depolarize nearly simultaneously, the left ventricle is electrically predominant because of its greater mass. Therefore, a deep S wave occurs in lead V_1, as the bulk of the current flows away from its positive electrode; whereas in V_6, the flow of current toward the positive electrode is recorded as a tall R wave.

In right bundle branch block (RBBB), septal depolarization remains undisturbed as it normally occurs via the LBB. A small r wave is found in lead V_1, and a small s wave in lead V_6. During the early part of ventricular depolarization, the bulk of the current flows toward the left ventricle, resulting in a deep S wave in lead V_1 and a tall R wave in lead V_6. A RBBB affects mainly the terminal phase of ventricular depolarization. This delayed depolarization of the remaining portion of the right ventricle is reflected by an R′ wave in lead V_1, as current again flows toward its positive electrode, and by an S wave in lead V_6 as current flows away from its positive electrode (Fig. 15–37).

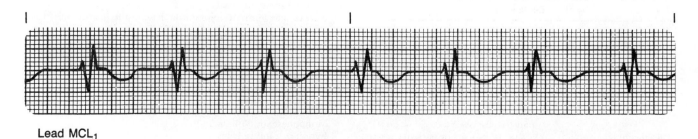

Lead MCL₁

FIGURE 15–37. Right bundle branch block.

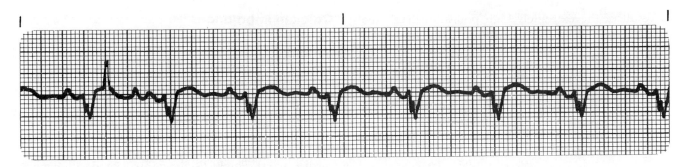

Lead MCL₁

FIGURE 15–38. Left bundle branch block.

Left bundle branch block (LBBB) also produces a pattern with widened QRS complexes. The shape of the QRS complex with LBBB is very different from that of RBBB (Fig. 15–38). The normal pattern of septal depolarization is disrupted and the septum is depolarized from right to left and not from left to right, as it is normally. Thus, there is loss of the septal r wave in lead V_1, and of the q wave in lead V_6. The total time for depolarization is prolonged, resulting in a widened R wave in lead V_6, and a QS complex in lead V_1. As is the case with RBBB, the diagnosis of LBBB can be made by examining leads V_1 and V_6. Lead V_1 shows a widened, entirely negative QS complex, with no septal r wave; while lead V_6 records a tall, widened R wave, without a septal q wave.

SVT with Wolff-Parkinson-White Syndrome. This is a second mechanism underlying tachycardia characterized by a wide QRS complex. An accessory pathway, connecting the atria with either ventricle and bypassing the AV node/junction, is thought to be responsible for Wolff-Parkinson-White pre-excitation. Conduction over the accessory pathway at very high rates may result in a wide QRS complex that may mimic VT. The possible diagnosis of WPW syndrome with atrial fibrillation should be strongly suspected if a tachycardia is encountered with a wide QRS complex and a very high and irregular rate.

There are variants of the WPW syndrome, so that the ECG waveform may vary. Findings on the ECG may include:

1. PR interval <0.12 second
2. Delta wave (distortion of the initial part of the QRS complex)[15]
3. QRS complex >0.12 second

ELECTROLYTE IMBALANCES AND THE ELECTROCARDIOGRAM

The electrolyte imbalances that have a major effect on cardiac action and therefore may affect the ECG tracing are those of potassium, calcium, and magnesium.

Potassium Imbalances

Hyperkalemia

An excess of potassium ion produces a disturbance in transmission of the cardiac impulse at various levels of the specialized conduction tissue. Changes in the ECG may not become evident until the serum potassium level exceeds 6 mEq/L. A symmetric tall T wave is the earliest ECG change associated with hyperkalemia (Fig. 15–39). As the serum level of K increases, subsequent electrocardiographic changes will be noted: an increased depth of the S wave; depression of the ST segment; a prolonged PR interval; absence of a P wave (K^+ = 8 mEq/L); wide QRS complex (K^+ = 10 mEq/L); fusion of QRS, ST segment, T wave (K^+ = 11 mEq/L); followed by ventricular fibrillation or ventricular standstill.[4] The last event is

HYPERKALEMIA

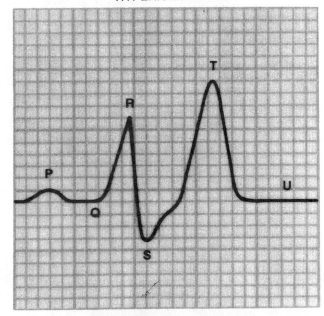

FIGURE 15–39. Hyperkalemia.

a result of the extremely high potassium levels that impede sodium and calcium entrance into the cardiac cell.

Therapeutic intervention to adjust serum levels of potassium are categorized as nonemergency and emergency measures. The drugs of choice as emergency measures include the administration of calcium chloride, sodium bicarbonate, glucose and insulin, as well as cation exchange resin. Additionally, peritoneal dialysis or hemodialysis may be indicated.

Hypokalemia

With serum potassium levels slightly below 3 mEq/L not all individuals will manifest electrocardiographic changes; however, when the serum level falls below 2 mEq/L, more dramatic changes are evident. Frequently observed changes are the shortening and depression of the ST segment, low amplitude or broadening of the T wave, and the appearance of the U wave (Fig. 15–40).

The arrhythmias associated with hypokalemia are premature atrial and ventricular beats that reflect cardiac irritability. In patients who are on a maintenance dose of digitalis, the presence of hypokalemia can potentiate the action of the digitalis. In surgical patients who are on diuretic therapy (e.g., furosemide [Laxis]) the critical care nurse must evaluate the current electrolyte status, particularly the potassium level, prior to administering the diuretic, since a side effect of furosemide is potassium loss. Severe hypokalemia is usually treated by constant infusion of 10 to 20 mEq/L of potassium chloride per hour.

Calcium Imbalances

Hypercalcemia

A consequence of hypercalcemia is decreased muscular contractility as a result of the blockage of sodium entrance into the cell by the increased level of serum calcium. The effects of sodium blockage due to hypercalcemia are shortening of ventricular systole, impairment of intraventricular conduction, and subsequent cardiac arrest. The ECG change associated with hypercalcemia is a shortened QT interval (Fig. 15–41).

Patients who are taking digitalis and become hypercalcemic must be observed carefully for signs of digitalis toxicity, since the high level of calcium increases myocardial sensitivity to digitalis.

Hypocalcemia

Low serum calcium levels result in prolongation of the ST segment and consequently the QTc interval (Fig. 15–42).[7] Although dysrhythmias are rare secondary to low calcium levels, prolongation of the QT interval has received increasing attention because of its relation to torsades de Pointes, and the occurrence of syncopal attacks, particularly when the QT interval is prolonged secondary to the use of certain antidysrhythmic agents such as quinidine, procainamide, and encainide. Hypocalcemia may be seen in hypoparathyroidism, osteomalacia, acute pancreatitis, renal insufficiency, vitamin D deficiency, and magnesium deficiency. See Table 36–10 for additional causes of hypocalcemia.

HYPOKALEMIA

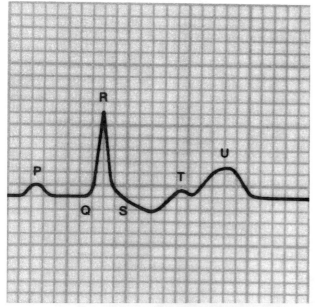

FIGURE 15–40. Hypokalemia.

HYPERCALCEMIA

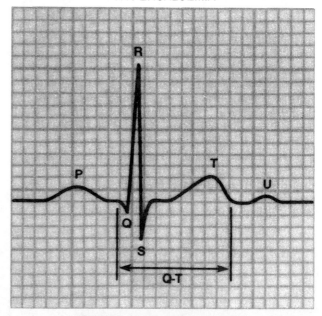

FIGURE 15–41. Hypercalcemia.

HYPOCALCEMIA

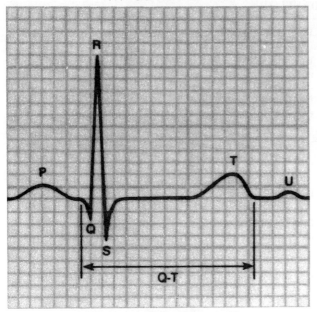

FIGURE 15–42. Hypocalcemia.

Magnesium Imbalances

Magnesium plays an important role in the metabolism of carbohydrates and the synthesis of protein. The effect of imbalances of magnesium on the heart is thought to be related to the electrolyte's influence on adenosine triphosphate breakdown. The latter is essential in providing the energy required for the sodium-potassium pump.

Hypermagnesemia

Since hypermagnesemia frequently occurs in conjunction with other electrolyte imbalances, specific electrocardiographic features are unclear. With excessive use of magnesium therapy administered intravenously, there have been reports of prolongation of the PR interval and QRS duration that result in various degrees of atrioventricular block and premature ventricular contractions.[9,16] Additionally because of the vasodilatory effect magnesium has upon peripheral vessels and consequent hypotension, tachycardia as a compensatory mechanism may be seen in association with its use. Treatment of hypermagnesemia consists of discontinuing magnesium-containing medications (e.g., antacids, laxatives) and correction of the dehydrated state, if present.

Hypomagnesemia

Magnesium deficiency may be associated with gastrointestinal, renal, and endocrine disorders. Additionally, hypomagnesemia may be drug-induced and may occur with burns and sepsis.

Electrocardiographic changes associated with deficiencies in magnesium consist of prolonged PR and QT intervals, widened QRS complexes, ST-segment depression, T-wave inversion, and an increased sensitivity to digitalis.[7,17]

Sodium

Although the role of sodium is vital to maintaining homeostasis of body fluids, the effects of high or low levels of the electrolyte on the electrocardiogram are minimal. When administered intravenously as an adjunct in correcting the problem of intraventricular conduction defects due to hyperkalemia or quinidine, injections of sodium have been found to shorten the duration of the QRS complex.[7]

REFERENCES

1. Ganong, WF: Review of Medical Physiology, ed 15. Appleton & Lange, Norwalk, CT, 1991.
2. Nave, C and Nave, B: Physics for the Health Sciences, ed 3. WB Saunders, Philadelphia, 1985.
3. Dolan, J: Critical Care Nursing: Clinical Management Through the Nursing Process. FA Davis, Philadelphia, 1991.
4. Bayes de Luna, A: Clinical Electrocardiography. Futura Publishing Company, Mount Kisco, NY, 1993.
5. Huang, P: Introduction to Electrocardiography. WB Saunders, Philadelphia, 1993.
6. Schamroth, L: An Introduction to Electrocardiography, ed 7. Blackwell Scientific, Oxford, 1990.
7. Chou, TL: Electrocardiography in Clinical Practice, ed 3. WB Saunders, Philadelphia, 1991.
8. Kernicki, J and Weiler, K: Electrocardiography for Nurses: Physiological Correlates. John Wiley & Sons, New York, 1981.
9. Kuhn, M: Pharmacotherapeutics: A Nursing Process Approach, ed 2. FA Davis, Philadelphia, 1991.
10. Kernicki, J and Weiler K: Electrocardiography for Nurses: Physiological Correlates. John Wiley & Sons, New York, 1981.
11. Fowler, NO: Diagnosis of Heart Disease. Springer-Verlag, New York, 1991.
12. Wharton, J and Goldschlager, N: Interpreting Cardiac Dysrhythmias. Medical Economics Books, Oradell, NJ, 1987.
13. Singh, B, Wellens, H, and Hiraoka, M: Electropharmacological Control of Cardiac Arrhythmias. Futura, Mount Kisco, NY, 1994.
14. Hudak, C and Gallo, B: Critical Care Nursing: A Holistic Approach, ed 6. JB Lippincott, Philadelphia, 1994.
15. Rice, V: The Role of Potassium in Health and Disease. Critical Care Nurse 2(5):62, 1982.
16. Phipps, W, Long, B, Woods, N, and Cassmeyer, C: Medical-Surgical Nursing: Concepts and Clinical Practice, ed. 4. Mosby Year Book, St. Louis, MO, 1991.
17. Wilson, R: Critical Care Manual: Applied Physiology and Principles of Therapy, ed 2. FA Davis, Philadelphia, 1992.

CARE PLAN FOR THE PATIENT WITH A CARDIAC MONITOR

Nursing Diagnoses

Nursing Diagnosis #1
Anxiety

Desired Patient Outcomes

Patient will demonstrate via facial expression, heart rate, and blood pressure a decrease in anxiety level.

Nursing Interventions

- Reassure regarding ease of placing monitor leads, a part of routine care.
- Reassure regarding monitor's electrical safety.
- Administer medication for relief of anxiety as prescribed. Monitor response to therapy.

Rationales

- Alleviating stress decreases sympathetic stimulation, which may in itself promote a tachycardia and/or an ectopic rhythm.

Nursing Diagnoses

Nursing Diagnosis #2
Knowledge deficit

Desired Patient Outcomes

Patient will verbalize an understanding of the cardiac monitor as an adjunct to ICU care.

Nursing Interventions

- Describe the purpose of the monitor and its operational parts.
- Demonstrate function of high-low alarms, muscle artifact, lead displacement, and electrical interference.

Rationales

- Alleviates fear and anxiety regarding equipment.
- Anxiety is decreased with an increased understanding of equipment.

Nursing Diagnoses

Nursing Diagnosis #3
Skin Integrity, impaired, risk for

Desired Patient Outcomes

Patient will demonstrate healthy, intact skin underneath electrode sites.

Nursing Interventions

- Adequately prepare the skin surface by washing, cleansing with an alcohol swab, and shaving hair.
- Replace ECG disks every 24 hr and prn.
- Rotate sites of disks slightly every 24 hr.

Rationales

- Proper skin preparation enhances skin-electrode contact and ensures a good tracing.
- Prepping the skin decreases the chances of entrapping contaminants such as dirt or hair under the disk.
- Rotation of disk sites gives the skin a chance to "breathe" and lessens the opportunities for skin breakdown.

C H A P T E R 16

Hemodynamic Monitoring

Elaine Kiess Daily

CHAPTER OUTLINE

Purpose
Principles and Techniques of Pressure
  Monitoring
  □ Equipment
  □ Preparation
  □ Insertion
  □ Optimization of Hemodynamic
    Pressure Monitoring
Hemodynamic Pressures
  □ Central Venous Pressure (CVP)
  □ Right Atrial Pressure (RAP)
  □ Right Ventricular Pressure (RVP)
  □ Pulmonary Artery Pressure (PAP)
  □ Pulmonary Artery Wedge (PAW)/
    Left Atrial Pressure (LAP)
  □ Systemic Arterial Pressure

Derived Hemodynamic Parameters
Cardiac Output Determination
  □ Principle
  □ Normal Values
  □ Clinical Application
  □ Techniques of Thermodilution
    Cardiac Output Measurement
Continuous Svo_2 Monitoring
Right Ventricular Volume
  Measurements
Nursing Care of the Patient Undergoing
  Hemodynamic Monitoring
References

LEARNING OBJECTIVES

After completing this chapter, you should be able to:

1. State the purpose of hemodynamic monitoring.
2. Identify components of a hemodynamic monitoring system and their functions.
3. Review major nursing care considerations in the preparation, insertion, and implementation of hemodynamic monitoring.
4. Explain the physiologic significance of monitoring hemodynamic parameters.
5. Examine waveforms, normal values, clinical applications, and abnormalities with respect to the following hemodynamic pressures:
   a. Central venous pressure (CVP).
   b. Right atrial pressure (RAP).
   c. Right ventricular pressure (RVP).
   d. Pulmonary artery pressure (PAP).
   e. Pulmonary artery wedge pressure (PAWP).
   f. Systemic arterial pressure.
6. Consider major complications associated with hemodynamic monitoring techniques.
7. Investigate the physiologic significance of cardiac output in terms of cardiac performance and overall tissue perfusion, and methods of determining cardiac output.
8. Explain how continuous monitoring of the oxygen saturation of mixed venous blood (SvO_2) reflects the adequacy of tissue oxygenation.
9. List important hemodynamic parameters that can be derived or calculated using directly measured hemodynamic data.
10. Delineate the nursing process in the care of the patient undergoing hemodynamic monitoring, including assessment, diagnosis, and planning desired patient outcomes and nursing interventions

Invasive hemodynamic monitoring dates back to 1733 when Stephen Hales[1] cannulated the carotid artery of a horse and measured how high the resulting column of blood rose in a brass pipe.[1]

Monitoring blood volume levels in war-injured patients by means of central venous pressure (CVP) was first described by Wilson and associates[2] in 1962. This method gained widespread popularity in the care and management of critically ill patients. In fact, for many years, hemodynamic monitoring of the critically ill consisted of continuous cardiac rate and rhythm monitoring, along with intermittent measurements of blood pressure and CVP.

Hemodynamic monitoring was revolutionized when Drs. Swan and Ganz developed the balloon-tip flotation pulmonary artery (PA) catheter in the late 1960s. This catheter permitted continuous direct measurement of right heart pressures in addition to indirect measurement of the filling pressure of the left side of the heart. Further development of the PA catheter provided the ability to measure cardiac output, perform atrial or ventricular pacing, continuously measure the oxygen saturation of mixed venous blood (SvO_2), and measure the systolic and diastolic volume of the right ventricle.

The usefulness of hemodynamic monitoring in defining pathophysiologic conditions and managing the care of critically ill patients was described by Swan and coworkers[3] in 1970. Since then, bedside hemodynamic monitoring has become an integral part of the care and management of critically ill patients. Hemodynamic parameters are used to assess the response of the cardiovascular system to injury and disease as well as to therapeutic interventions.

PURPOSE

The function of the heart is to pump blood returning from the body to the lungs and into the aorta. This process delivers oxygenated blood and nutrients to the tissues and removes metabolic waste products. How well the heart performs its function is determined primarily by the heart rate, the ventricular end-diastolic volume (preload), the ventricular afterload, and ventricular contractility. The purpose of bedside hemodynamic monitoring is to survey and optimize these determinants by directing appropriate therapeutic interventions for the purpose of providing adequate oxygen delivery to tissues. This is achieved with the aid of data obtained from the balloon-flotation PA catheter and the arterial catheter, which permits direct monitoring of arterial blood pressure. From these measured pressures, various other hemodynamic parameters can be obtained and used to assess the cardiovascular response to injury and disease and to therapeutic interventions.

Critical care nurses are responsible for obtaining accurate, valid hemodynamic data and frequently are responsible for decision-making regarding initiation or titration of certain pharmacologic agents or therapies used to manipulate hemodynamic parameters. This requires not only knowledge of cardiovascular physiology and pharmacology, but a clear understanding of the principles, equipment, and techniques of hemodynamic monitoring. These principles, as well as ways to optimize hemodynamic data collection, interpret hemodynamic waveforms, perform cardiac output measurements, and monitor SvO_2, are discussed in this chapter.

PRINCIPLES AND TECHNIQUES OF PRESSURE MONITORING

Equipment

The measurement of any physiologic signal requires (1) a catheter to relay the signal, (2) a transducer to transform the biophysical event into an electrical signal, (3) an amplifier to energize the transducer and amplify the electrical signal from the transducer, and (4) a monitor screen or paper recorder to display the resultant waveform.

Catheters

Transmission of a pressure signal from the patient to a transducer occurs through a fluid-filled catheter. If the catheter is insufficiently long to provide practical attachment to the external transducer, its length can be extended by the placement of additional fluid-filled tubing. Remember, however, that the closer the transducer is to the physiologic signal, the more accurate the data obtained. Thus, all efforts should be directed toward minimizing all connections (tubing and stopcocks) between the catheter and the transducer.

Catheters used to measure pressures within the right side of the heart are usually multilumened, balloon-tipped, flow-directed catheters made of polyvinylchloride. Inflation of the balloon of the catheter with air allows the catheter to be carried through the heart by the forward flow of blood. Right heart catheters for bedside monitoring are available in sizes 5, 7, or 7.5F with 2, 3, 4, or 5 separate lumens. One lumen provides access to the balloon for inflation or deflation. The balloon capacity varies with the size of the catheter, from 0.5 to 1.5 mL.

The two-lumen catheter has a distal port for monitoring PA or pulmonary artery wedge (PAW) pressures, as well as a lumen for balloon inflation. The three-lumen catheter has an additional lumen whose port is located more proximally, allowing monitoring of right atrial (RA) pressure. The four-lumen catheter has all these features plus a thermistor and computer connecting port for measurement of thermodilution cardiac output measurements. The five-lumen PA catheter has a second proximal port, also terminating in the RA, for infusion of fluids or drugs without interruption during cardiac output measurements.

The addition of fiberoptics to the conventional PA catheter allows continuous monitoring of the oxygen saturation of mixed venous blood (SvO_2) when the catheter is attached to a bedside microprocessor.

A recent modification of the standard PA thermodilution catheter includes the addition of two intracardiac electrodes along with a rapid response thermistor. This modification allows the determination of thermodilution right ventricular volumetric measurements (end-diastolic volume, end-systolic volume, and ejection fraction) in addition to cardiac output determinations. Another recent modification of the PA catheter is the attachment of a thermal filament that delivers sequential bursts of heat, which are measured by the thermistor at the tip of the catheter on a continuous basis. This provides on-line continuous cardiac output measurements.

Although increases in the number of lumens within the PA catheter expand the functional capabilities of the catheter, they also decrease the accuracy of the transmitted pressure waveform and increase the risk of lumen occlusion.

Catheters used for percutaneous arterial cannulation are usually short, Teflon, catheter-over-needle type.

Transducers

Intravascular or intracardiac pressure signals are transmitted via the fluid-filled catheter and tubing to a transducer that converts the mechanical signal to an electrical signal. Most external transducers are strain-gauge transducers wired to form a Wheatstone bridge beneath the diaphragm. When pressure is applied to the diaphragm of the transducer, the wires of the bridge physically change in length and diameter, resulting in changes in the resistance to the flow of current through the wires.

Transducers are electrically energized and are therefore a potential source of current leakage. In addition, defibrillation may damage the diaphragm of these transducers, and therefore they should be changed following defibrillation.

Monitor

Bedside monitoring systems consist of an amplifier (or preamplifier), an oscilloscope, and a digital display or paper recorder.

The purpose of the amplifier is to energize the transducer as well as to amplify, filter, and process the transduced electrical signal. Most transducers produce only about 6 mV (millivolts) when reproducing the systolic arterial pressure, whereas most monitors require a signal of several volts to operate. Therefore, an amplifier is necessary to boost the size of the electrical signal by approximately 1000.

The modified electrical output from the amplifier is intelligible only when it is converted into a readable form and displayed on an oscilloscope or paper recorder. Calibration of the light beam on the oscilloscope, or the ink pen on the paper recorder, allows accurate assessment of hemodynamic pressure values in relation to the respiratory cycle.

Digital displays on monitors provide numerical values of pressure changes during specific times of the cardiac cycle. Selection of systolic, diastolic, or mean pressure values is available on most digital display devices. However, the numerical value displayed on the monitor represents an average of either a certain number of beats or a certain period of time and there-

fore does not reflect the pressure value at a certain point of the respiratory cycle. Accurate measurement of hemodynamic pressures at end-expiration can be obtained only with the use of a calibrated oscilloscope (preferably with a freeze mechanism) or with a calibrated paper write-out.[4]

Preparation

Table 16–1 lists the necessary equipment to be assembled for PA or arterial hemodynamic pressure monitoring.

Initiation of hemodynamic monitoring requires careful preparation and setup of the previously discussed monitoring equipment. Failure to properly prepare the necessary equipment can result in erroneous data and improper patient care and management. Preassembled kits are available, which contain all the necessary equipment for hemodynamic monitoring and therefore minimize the time required for gathering and assembling the equipment.

Disposable Transducer and Flush Solution Assembly

1. If not premixed, heparinize the IV solution in a collapsible bag by adding 1 to 2 units of heparin/mL IV fluid. Label the infusion bag with the date, time, and amount of heparin added.
2. Remove all the air from the infusion bag.
3. Insert IV tubing into the bag, and squeeze the drip chamber to fill about $\frac{1}{2}$ inch. Allow the distal tubing to fill with fluid.
4. Attach the preassembled flush device and disposable transducer to the IV tubing and completely fill with IV fluid by activating the fast-flush device. (To prevent air bubbles, this should not be done while the fluid is under pressure.)
5. If not preassembled, connect the pressure tubing to the stopcock attached to the transducer and fill with IV fluid.

TABLE 16–1
Equipment for Hemodynamic Monitoring

Catheter of choice (balloon-flotation PA catheter or arterial catheter)
Catheter/sheath introducer (for PA catheter)
Catheter sterility sleeve (for PA catheter)
Percutaneous (or cutdown) tray with necessary instruments
Sterile transducer
Heparinized IV solution (nonglucose) in a collapsible bag
IV tubing with pediatric drip chamber
Continuous flush device
Three-way stopcocks
Pressure tubing
Pressurized cuff or pump
Electronic monitor with oscilloscope and paper recorder
Cardiopulmonary resuscitation equipment

6. Carefully check to make sure all air bubbles are removed from the tubing and transducer.
7. Replace all vented stopcock caps with non-vented dead-ender caps.
8. Place the IV bag into a pressure cuff and pressurize to 300 mmHg.
9. Attach the distal IV tubing to the hub of the catheter.
10. Connect the electrical cable of the disposable transducer to the amplifier of the monitor.

Monitor Preparation

Turn on the power on the monitor system, and check the oscilloscope paper recorder to ensure proper function.

Transducer/Monitor Zero and Calibration

To eliminate the effects of atmospheric pressure as well as hydrostatic pressure differences, the monitoring system is "zeroed" to atmospheric air. This is done by positioning the air-reference port of the stopcock at the patient's midchest level (Fig. 16–1) or phlebostatic axis (the presumed level of the catheter tip), opening the side port of the stopcock to air and checking that the digital display on the monitor reads "zero." If necessary, adjust the zero control knob on the monitor to obtain a zero reading. At the same time, adjust the tracing on the oscilloscope or paper recorder to the correct zero position.

The calibration of the monitor should also be checked by pressing and holding the calibration knob on the monitor to read the selected precalibrated value (e.g., 40, 100, or 200 mmHg). Adjust the calibration knob, if necessary, to obtain the correct reading. At the same time, adjust the light beam on the oscilloscope or paper recorder, if necessary. It may, at times, be necessary to also check the calibration and sensitivity of the transducer by applying a known pressure (with either mercury or water) to the transducer and correlating it with the pressure read-out. Special caution must be taken if the calibration check is performed after patient monitoring is instituted to avoid contamination and possible entry of air into the system. Disposable transducers are precalibrated by the manufacturer and usually do not need to be checked prior to use.

All transducers are sensitive to changes in environmental temperature, which can result in some drift of the zero baseline. Re-zeroing should be performed before critical measurement readings are recorded and prior to initiating new therapy, whenever there is a sudden change in a pressure reading or a change in patient position or transducer reference placement.

Catheter Preparation

Under sterile conditions, the PA catheter should be carefully checked before insertion. Faulty PA catheters with either ruptured or inadequately inflated balloons have been found in up to 3% of PA catheters before

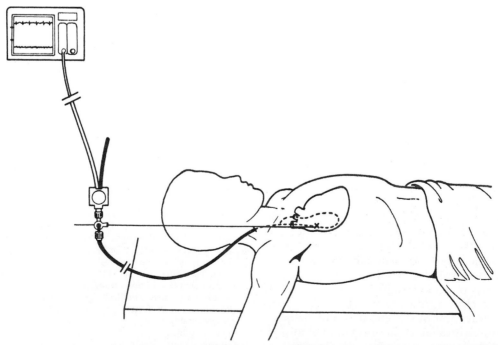

FIGURE 16–1. Illustration showing the proper placement of the air-reference port at the assumed level of the patient's right atrium, which corresponds closely to the patient's midchest. (From Daily, EK and Schroeder, JS: Techniques in Bedside Hemodynamic Monitoring. CV Mosby Co., St. Louis, 1994, with permission.)

insertion.[5] For this reason, the integrity of the balloon should be carefully checked by inflating it with the designated volume of air while immersing the balloon in sterile water to check for any leakage. The thermistor wires of the catheter should also be checked by connecting the cardiac output cable to the thermistor hub of the catheter and depressing the "test" button on the cardiac output computer. If the thermistor wires are damaged, the computer will indicate such information, and a new thermodilution catheter should be used.

Insertion

Catheters for CVP monitoring can be inserted into the internal or external jugular, subclavian, or basilic vein. The tip of the CVP catheter should be advanced to the superior vena cava, just above the right atrium.

The PA catheter can be inserted into the same veins as the CVP catheter. The femoral vein can also be used for PA catheterization, although traversal of the catheter out to the PA is more difficult via this route. Passing the catheter through a sterile sleeve that covers the skin exit portion of the catheter is very useful if later manipulation of the catheter is required. If inserted under meticulous, aseptic technique, catheter sleeves can provide short-term sterility of the PA catheter for 1 to 2 days.[6] Although either catheter can be inserted via a surgical cutdown or percutaneously, the latter method is more common and is associated with fewer infectious complications.

During insertion and manipulation of the PA catheter, the nurse must carefully monitor the patient to determine the chamber location of the catheter according to the waveform and to note the possible occurrence of any arrhythmias. The development of premature ventricular contractions during manipulation of the catheter in the right ventricle (RV) is a common occurrence and usually resolves when the catheter is advanced out to the PA. Occasionally, sustained ventricular tachycardia may develop, necessitating drug therapy or prompt cardioversion. Rarely, ventricular fibrillation may occur, requiring immediate defibrillation. The development of ventricular arrhythmias is more frequently associated with shock states, acute myocardial infarction, hypokalemia, hypocalcemia, hypoxemia, acidosis, and prolonged catheter insertion times.[7] The nurse should be aware of this increased risk and prepared to act accordingly.

The arterial pressure can be measured directly by a short 20- or 22-gauge plastic catheter inserted into a peripheral artery (radial, brachial, or femoral). The smaller the arterial catheter, the less compromise of distal arterial blood flow. In addition, a 22-gauge arterial cannula increases the damping coefficient 260% more than a 20-gauge catheter.[8] This is helpful in reducing arterial pressure overshoot. Arterial catheters are commonly inserted percutaneously but may also be inserted by means of the cutdown technique.

Optimization of Hemodynamic Pressure Monitoring

Accurate measurement of hemodynamic parameters requires careful attention to optimizing the fluid-filled monitoring system. Bedside monitoring systems are generally second-order, underdamped systems with numerous artifacts.[9] To faithfully reproduce the pressure signal, the system should be optimally damped and the natural resonant frequency of the plumbing system should be at least 10 times the fundamental frequency of the signal (the heart rate) being measured.[10,11] This usually can be accomplished by:

1. Minimizing the length of tubing between the transducer and the catheter
2. Minimizing the number of stopcocks used
3. Using very stiff, high-pressure tubing in the system
4. Carefully removing all air bubbles from the system at the time of setup and periodically during the monitoring period
5. Continuously flushing the catheter to discourage formation of blood clots.

In addition to the plumbing and monitoring equipment, certain physiologic factors can affect the accuracy of hemodynamic data and require special consideration. One major factor affecting the recorded hemodynamic pressures is the intrapleural pressure surrounding the heart and great vessels. Measurement of all hemodynamic pressures at end-expiration, when there is no air flow and the intrapleural pressure is unchanging, minimizes the effect of changes in intrapleural pressure on recorded hemodynamic pressures.[12-14] However, determination of the point of end-expiration may, at times, be difficult. Use of a paper printout to identify end-expiration is the most valid way to obtain these data.[4] During spontaneous breathing, hemodynamic pressures decline during

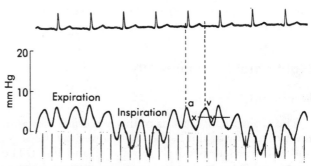

FIGURE 16–2. Normal RA waveform in a spontaneously breathing patient. *Vertical lines* show the *a* wave following the ECG P wave, and the *v* wave following the ECG T wave. *Horizontal line* indicates measurement of the mean right atrial (RA) pressure of approximately 4 mmHg at end-expiration. (From Daily, EK and Schroeder, JS: Techniques in Bedside Hemodynamic Monitoring. CV Mosby Co., St. Louis, 1994, with permission.)

inspiration and rise during expiration. Thus, end-expiratory pressures are measured just prior to the subsequent inspiratory decline on the paper printout (Fig. 16–2). During mechanical ventilation, the pattern reverses, with hemodynamic pressures rising during inspiration and declining during expiration. Thus, end-expiratory pressures are measured just prior to the obvious pressure rise in patients receiving mechanical ventilation. The digital display value is less accurate because most monitors simply average a certain number of beats, regardless of the respiratory phase, and thus do not provide end-expiratory data. However, newer monitoring systems have addressed this issue and now include an algorithm to identify the end-expiratory pressure.[15] The onus of obtaining accurate hemodynamic data falls on the critical care nurse, who must make every effort to ensure that all hemodynamic parameters obtained are as accurate as possible.

Table 16–2 lists problems commonly encountered in hemodynamic monitoring as well as preventive and remedial steps.

HEMODYNAMIC PRESSURES

Central Venous Pressure (CVP)

The CVP measures pressure within the superior vena cava (SVC), which represents pressure in the right atrium. Along with the mean arterial pressure, CVP is an important determinant of both venous return and cardiac output. Monitoring of the CVP is used to assess changes in right ventricular function and the adequacy of vascular volume. The CVP may be measured with a water manometer (in cmH_2O) or with an electronic transducer (in mmHg). To convert cmH_2O to mmHg, simply divide the CVP value (in cmH_2O) by 1.36.

Since CVP represents pressure in the right atrium, the following discussion of the right atrial pressure (RAP) applies to the CVP.

Right Atrial Pressure (RAP)

Waveform

The typical RAP consists of three positive waves, an *a* wave, a *c* wave, and a *v* wave, followed by the *x*, x^1, and *y* descents, respectively (Figs. 16–2 and 16–3). The *a* wave is due to atrial contraction and therefore occurs just after the P wave of the ECG. (This wave is not present in patients with atrial fibrillation and absent P waves on the ECG.) The *x* descent is the subsequent decline in pressure as the atrium relaxes. The *c* wave occurs as a result of tricuspid valve closure. The decline after the *c* wave is termed the *x'* descent. The *v* wave results from an increase in pressure due to an increase in volume as the atrium fills with blood from

the SVC and inferior vena cava (IVC). The *v* wave occurs after the T wave of the ECG (see Fig. 16–2). At the peak of the *v* wave, the tricuspid valve opens and the right atrium rapidly empties into the right ventricle. This decline in volume produces the *y* descent, which immediately follows the *v* wave.

The *a* wave of the RAP waveform is often slightly higher (1–3 mmHg) than the *v* wave. However, because the *a* and *v* waves are similar in value, a mean or average of the two waves is usually recorded.

Normal Value

The normal RA mean pressure is 0 to 6 mmHg.

Clinical Application

The CVP or RAP represents filling of the right side of the heart (preload). As an indicator of the patient's intravascular volume, the CVP or RAP measurement is used as a guide to volume replacement. The response of the RAP to fluid challenges provides important information regarding the patient's volemic and cardiovascular status. If the CVP or RAP is low and increases minimally after a rapid infusion of 200 to 250 mL of fluid, the patient is considered to be hypovolemic and in need of further volume. In contrast, a precipitous rise in CVP or RAP after volume infusion may be considered a reflection of volume overload. However, in the critically ill patient numerous factors other than blood volume influence the CVP and need to be considered when assessing abnormalities in CVP or RAP.

The CVP or RAP is also useful clinically as a reflection of the diastolic pressure of the RV. In RV failure, the CVP or RAP is high because of decreased compliance of the RV requiring higher filling pressures.

Abnormalities

The *a* wave of the RAP may be exaggerated and elevated in any situations that increase resistance to forward blood flow. This includes RV failure, pulmonic stenosis, pulmonary embolus, and pulmonary hypertension.

The *v* wave of the RA waveform becomes dominant and elevated in tricuspid regurgitation due to a reflux of blood backward into the atrium during RV systole. Functional tricuspid regurgitation commonly occurs in patients with RV failure and dilatation. Resolution of the failure is associated with reduction of the size of the *v* wave to more normal levels.

Elevation of both the *a* and *v* waves of the RA waveform occurs with hypervolemia, tamponade, and constrictive pericarditis.

Right Ventricular Pressure (RVP)

When the catheter floats across the tricuspid valve into the RV, the pressure suddenly becomes much

TABLE 16–2
Troubleshooting Intravenous Catheters

Problem	Possible Cause	Prevention	Remedy
Overdamped waveform	Clot at catheter tip	Use continuous flush device. Use heparinized IV solution. Use heparinized catheters. Hand flush occasionally.	Aspirate, then flush catheter with heparin solution (*not* in PA wedge position). Remove catheter if unable to clear.
	Air bubble(s)	Give care and attention to remove all air bubbles during equipment setup, particularly in the pressure transducer. Use macrodrip, not pedidrip.	Flush system carefully (*not* to patient).
	Leak at some connecting point	Use Luer-Lok connectors and stopcocks; tighten securely.	Check all connections and tighten if necessary.
	Kink in catheter	Loosely coil excess catheter. Immobilize arm, if arm insertion. Exercise caution during patient movement.	Straighten kink or replace catheter, if necessary.
	Use of soft, compliant tubing	Use stiff connecting tubing.	Replace soft tubing with stiff connecting tubing.
"Noisy" waveform (with fling)	Use of lengthy tubing	Use no more than 2 or 3 feet of connecting tubing (preferably 18 inches or less). Use stiff connecting tubing.	Decrease tubing length. Use stiff connecting tubing.
	Catheter tip near valve with turbulent blood flow	Position catheter distal to valve.	Check catheter position by radiograph, and reposition if necessary. Use commercial damping device.
	Very rapid heart rate		Slow heart rate, if possible.
Abnormally low or high pressures	Improper air-reference level	Place air reference at midchest level (see Fig. 16–1)	Remeasure phlebostatic axis or midchest and reset air-reference level accordingly.
	Incorrect zero or calibration	Zero and calibrate monitor correctly.	Recheck zero and calibration of monitor.
	Faulty transducer	Calibrate transducer with known pressure; replace if necessary.	Recheck transducer calibration with mercury or water manometer.
"Overwedged" or damped, elevated PAWP	Overinflation of the balloon	Slowly inflate balloon while closely observing waveform; inflate *only* enough to obtain PAWP.	Deflate balloon; reinflate slowly with only enough air to obtain PA wedge waveform.
	Eccentric inflation of the balloon	Check balloon inflation before insertion. Do not inflate 7F catheter with more than 1.0–1.5 mL air.	Deflate balloon; reposition catheter and slowly reinflate.
	Location of catheter tip in zone 1 or 2 of the lung (see Fig. 16–7)	Position catheter in zone 3 below the left atrium. Maintain adequate LA pressure through volume administration. Reduce airway pressure.	Obtain lateral chest film to confirm catheter tip location; if in zone 1 or 2, reposition in zone 3, administer volume, or reduce airway pressure.

Continued

TABLE 16–2
Troubleshooting Intravenous Catheters (*Continued*)

Problem	Possible Cause	Prevention	Remedy
PAWP with balloon deflated	Forward migration of catheter tip due to excessive looping in right ventricle (RV) or RA; inadequate suturing of catheter at insertion site; or excessive arm movement of catheter in antecubital vein	Advance catheter carefully, avoiding excess catheter insertion. Check catheter position on radiograph. Suture catheter securely at insertion site. Insert catheter in vein proximal to shoulder.	Slowly withdraw catheter until PA waveform appears. Obtain chest radiograph to determine excessive looping of catheter in RV or RA.
PA balloon rupture	Overinflation of the balloon Frequent balloon inflations Active balloon deflation by withdrawing air into syringe	Inflate slowly with only enough air to obtain PAWP. Monitor PAEDP as reflection of PAWP and LVEDP. Allow balloon to deflate passively through stopcock. Remove syringe after each inflation.	Remove syringe and apply tape over stopcock to prevent further air injection. Monitor PAEDP.
Drastic change in pressure	Actual change in hemodynamic state	Carefully assess patient.	
	Air-reference or transducer level changed	Maintain air reference at midchest level; re-zero before each reading.	Reposition air reference at midchest level; re-zero.
	Air or blood in transducer dome	Carefully remove all air bubbles during initial setup; maintain adequate pressure (300 mmHg) in infusion bag.	Carefully flush system to remove all air or blood (*not* into patient).
	Change in temperature of environment or IV solution	Use room temperature flush solution.	Re-zero and check calibration.
	Broken transducer cable	Carefully handle transducer and cable.	Check transducer with known pressure of mercury or water; replace if faulty.
No pressure	Power off	Check power.	Turn power on.
	Stopcock open to air	Always turn stopcock off to air after zeroing.	Turn stopcock off to air; open to catheter/transducer.
	Tubing connections loose	Carefully tighten all connections during setup and check periodically.	Tighten all connections.
	Loose cable connections between transducer/monitor/oscilloscope	Carefully and firmly insert all connecting jacks during initial setup.	Check all connecting jacks.
	Transducer attached to wrong module or monitor	Provide careful and accurate transducer and monitor setup.	Attach transducer to appropriate module.
	Gain setting too low	Correctly adjust gain setting of oscilloscope during initial monitor calibration.	Reset gain on the oscilloscope.
	Incorrect scale selection	Select appropriate scale to correspond to the monitored pressure.	Select appropriate scale.
	Faulty transducer	Check transducer with known pressure of mercury or water before patient use.	Check transducer with known pressure of mercury or water; if faulty, replace.

LVEDP = left ventricular end-diastolic pressure; PAEDP = pulmonary artery end-diastolic pressure.
Source: Tilkian, AG and Daily, EK: Cardiovascular Procedures. CV Mosby, St. Louis, 1986, with permission.

higher with a sharp, pointed appearance as displayed on the monitor screen or recorder printout. Ventricular ectopy usually occurs transiently.

Waveform

The RVP reflects the pulsatile, pumping nature of the ventricle with a rapid rise to systolic pressure and falling to or near zero during diastole. The systolic and diastolic phases can be further delineated according to specific cardiac events (see Fig. 16–3*B*). The systolic events include isovolumetric contraction, rapid ejection, and reduced ejection. The diastolic events include isovolumetric relaxation, early diastole, atrial systole (atrial kick), and end-diastole.

Normal Values

RV systolic pressure	20 to 30 mmHg
RV diastolic pressure	0 to 5 mmHg
RV end-diastolic pressure	2 to 6 mmHg

Clinical Application

Because of the risk of arrhythmias, the RVP is not directly monitored at the bedside. However, the RV systolic pressure is indirectly monitored via the PA systolic pressure, which should be the same as the peak RV systolic pressure in the absence of pulmonic stenosis. The RV diastolic, or filling, pressure is also indirectly monitored via the RAP or CVP, which should be the same as the RV diastolic pressure in the absence of tricuspid stenosis. Thus, both the systolic and diastolic pressures of the RV are indirectly monitored at the bedside.

If an RV waveform becomes apparent on the monitor (Fig. 16–4), the balloon of the flotation catheter should be inflated immediately, allowing the catheter to float on out to the PA. It may not float sufficiently far to obtain an acceptable pulmonary artery wedge pressure (PAWP); thereafter, the PA end-diastolic pressure must be used as a reflection of the left ventricle (LV) filling pressure. If the catheter will not float out to the PA, despite balloon inflation, it may be

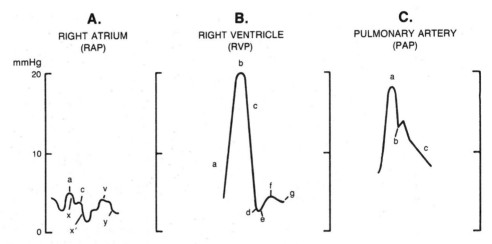

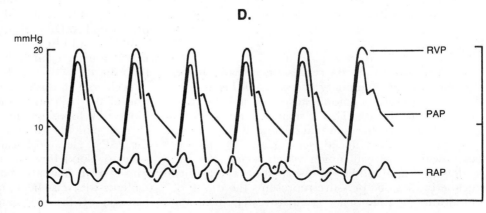

FIGURE 16–3. (*A*) Normal right atrial pressure (RAP) waveform showing an *a* wave, *c* wave, and *v* wave, followed by the *x,x′* and *y* descents. (*B*) Normal right ventricular pressure (RVP) waveform showing isovolumetric contraction (*a*), rapid ejection (*b*), reduced ejection (*c*), isovolumetric relaxation (*d*), early diastole (*e*), atrial systole or atrial kick (*f*), and end-diastole (*g*). (*C*) Normal pulmonary artery pressure (PAP) waveform showing systole (*a*), dicrotic notch (*b*), and end-diastole (*c*). (*D*) Shows all three pressures (RAP, RVP, and PAP) superimposed on one another. All three pressures reflect low-pressure systems of right heart and pulmonary circulation.

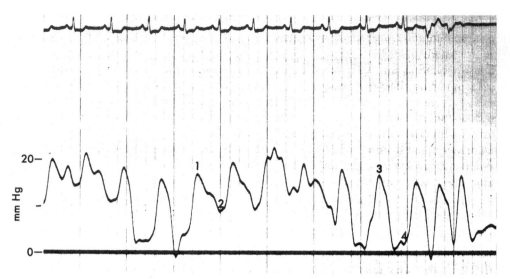

FIGURE 16–4. Pressure tracing obtained from the distal lumen of the PA catheter with the catheter tip moving back and forth across the pulmonic valve, producing intermittent PA and RV pressure waveforms. It is not in a safe location for monitoring purposes (note the occurrence of premature ventricular contractions [PVCs]). It also would be impossible to obtain a PAWP with the catheter tip in this location. Frequently, inflation of the balloon will float the catheter tip distally to the PA, although it may not float distally enough to obtain a PAWP. 1 = PA systole; 2 = PA end-diastole; 3 = RV systole; 4 = RV end-diastole. (From Daily, EK and Schroeder, JS: Techniques in Bedside Hemodynamic Monitoring. CV Mosby Co., St. Louis, 1994, with permission.)

coiled in the RV. In this instance, deflate the balloon and pull the catheter back into the RA. The catheter tip is never allowed to remain in the RV because of the risk of ventricular arrhythmias.

Abnormalities

The RV systolic pressure is elevated in pulmonary hypertension (either primary or secondary), as well as in ventricular septal defects and pulmonic stenosis. The RV diastolic pressure is elevated with RV failure, cardiac tamponade, or constrictive pericarditis.

Pulmonary Artery Pressure (PAP)

Inflation of the balloon of the catheter allows it to float along with the flow of blood from the RV to the PA. This is evidenced on the oscilloscope as a sudden increase in the diastolic pressure, with little or no change in the systolic pressure level.

Waveform

The pressure in the PA represents pulsatile blood flow through the pulmonary artery. Systole begins with the opening of the pulmonic valve and rapid ejection of blood into the PA. This is seen as a rapid rise in pressure followed by a gradual decline as the volume of ejected blood is reduced (see Fig. 16–3C). Diastole begins with the dicrotic notch, which occurs when the leaflets of the pulmonic valve snap shut. The further decline in diastolic pressure represents the runoff of blood into the pulmonary vasculature. The peak sys-

tolic pressure, the end-diastolic pressure, and the mean or average PA pressure are usually recorded.

Normal Values

PA systolic pressure	20 to 30 mmHg
PA end-diastolic pressure	8 to 12 mmHg
PA mean pressure	10 to 20 mmHg

Clinical Application

As mentioned previously, the PA systolic pressure reflects the RV peak systolic pressure (in the absence of pulmonic valve disease). Therefore, the PA systolic pressure reflects the *afterload* of the right side of the heart. At the very end of diastole, when the pulmonic valve is closed and the mitral valve is still open, the pressures in the LV, left atrium (LA), pulmonary veins, and PA essentially equilibrate. Therefore, in the absence of increased pulmonary vascular resistance (PVR) or mitral valve disease, the PA end-diastolic pressure (PAEDP) reflects LV end-diastolic pressure (LVEDP) (within 1 to 4 mmHg).[16] Because of this, many clinicians routinely monitor the PAEDP rather than the PAWP as a reflection of LV filling pressure, or preload.[17] In this way, the risks associated with inflation of the balloon of the catheter and cessation of blood flow to a segment of the PA are avoided. However, in patients with lung disease or increased PVR, the PAP is elevated because of the increase in resistance to blood flow through the pulmonary system. The PAEDP may also be higher than the PAWP in patients with fast heart rates (more than 120 bpm) because of the decreased diastolic filling time.[17]

Therefore, in these patients, it is necessary to obtain a PAWP as a reflection of LVEDP.

The *mean* PAP is used to calculate PVR according to the formula:

$$PVR = \frac{PAm - PAWm \times 80}{CO}$$

where:

PVR = pulmonary vascular resistance
PAm = pulmonary artery mean pressure
PAWm = pulmonary artery wedge mean pressure
CO = cardiac output
80 = conversion factor from mmHg/min/L to dynes sec cm^{-5}

Many clinicians prefer to index both pulmonary and systemic vascular resistance to compare patients of varying body size (particularly pediatric patients).[18] This is done by simply dividing the PVR or systemic vascular resistance by the patient's body surface area.

Abnormalities

The PA systolic pressure becomes elevated (pulmonary hypertension) with any increase in PVR, such as with pulmonary disease, pulmonary embolus, hypoxemia, or primary pulmonary hypertension. Mitral valve disease, as well as LV failure, increase pulmonary venous pressure, which, in turn, increases the PAEDP. Marked increases in pulmonary blood flow, such as in a left-to-right cardiac shunt, also cause an increase in the PA pressure.

Pulmonary Artery Wedge (PAW)/ Left Atrial Pressure (LAP)

Waveform

The PAWP is obtained by inflating the balloon of the PA catheter sufficiently to occlude the branch of the PA in which the catheter tip lies. This blocks off any blood flow and pressure effects from the right heart and allows the catheter tip, which extends beyond the inflated balloon, to sense only the retrograde pressure generated by the LA (Fig. 16–5). (The LAP can also be measured directly in patients undergoing a thoracotomy with placement of a catheter in the LA appendage.) Therefore, the PAWP is an indirect LAP and is morphologically identical with the RAP, consisting of an *a* wave, a *v* wave, and, occasionally, a *c* wave as well as *x* and *y* descents (Fig. 16–6). The *a* wave is produced by LA contraction and is followed by the *x* descent, representing atrial relaxation. The *c* wave that occurs as a result of mitral valve closure may not always be evident on the PAW or LA waveform. The *v* wave is produced by filling of the LA from the pulmonary veins and is followed by the *y* descent, which represents opening of the mitral valve and passive emptying of the LA.

As with the RA waveform, the *a* wave of the LAP or

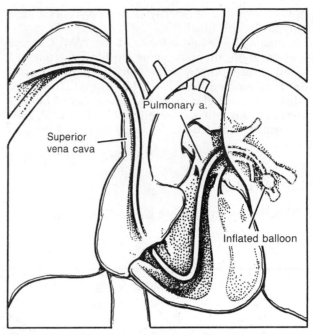

FIGURE 16–5. With the catheter tip in the pulmonary artery, and the balloon inflated to prevent forward flow, the tip of the catheter senses the pressure generated beyond the tip by the left atrium. In the absence of mitral valve disease, this pressure reflects the filling pressure of the left ventricle.

PAWP occurs after the P wave of the ECG, whereas the *v* wave follows repolarization, or the T wave of the ECG. However, because the PAW measures LAP in a retrograde manner, there is a greater time delay between the electrical and associated mechanical event (Fig. 16–6).

Alterations in the contour of the PAW or LA waveform may be related to changes in cardiac rhythm, as with the RAP waveform. The *a* wave is absent in patients with atrial fibrillation and may be exaggerated (cannon *a* waves) with regularity or intermittently in

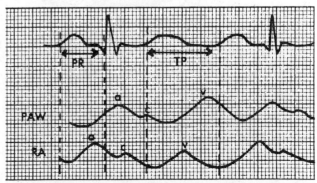

FIGURE 16–6. PAWP and RAP showing the difference in the timing of the waveform components relative to the ECG. Note the later appearance of the PAWP *a* and *v* waves compared with the RAP *a* and *v* waves. (From Daily, EK and Schroeder, JS: Techniques in Bedside Hemodynamic Monitoring. CV Mosby Co., St. Louis, 1994, with permission.)

patients with junctional rhythm or paroxysmal atrial tachycardia with block.

Normally, the *a* and *v* waves of the PAW/LA waveform are about the same value (within a few mmHg), and therefore a mean or average of the two pressure rises is taken (see Fig. 16–6). If, however, the *v* wave is dominant and elevated, the *a* wave should be measured as a more accurate reflection of LVEDP, since the mean will be falsely elevated because of the high *v* wave.

Normal Values

PAW/LA mean pressure is 8 to 12 mmHg.

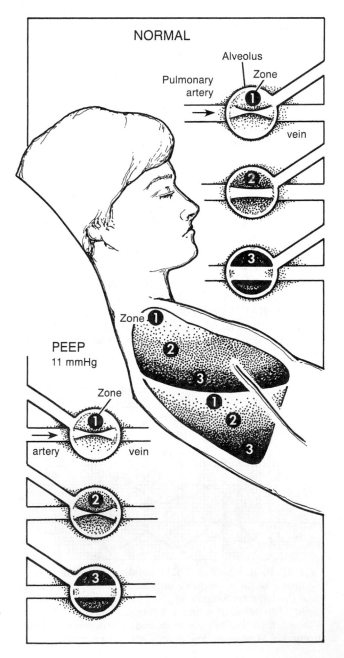

Clinical Application

The LVEDP has traditionally been considered the standard to define the pump function of the left ventricle.[19] In the absence of mitral valve disease, the mean LAP equals LVEDP. Because the PAW is a retrograde measurement of the LAP, it also indirectly reflects LV filling or LVEDP (the preload of the left heart). In most patients, the PAWP correlates closely with the LVEDP over a fairly wide range of filling pressures (5 to 25 mmHg).[20] However, with LVEDP greater than 25 mmHg, the PAWP may underestimate the true LV filling pressure. In contrast, elevations in the LAP or PAWP overestimate the true LVEDP in patients with mitral stenosis or LA myxoma. Decreases in the compliance of the LV alter the relationship between pressure and volume, which also produces an elevated PAWP that does not reflect the volume filling the LV during diastole.[21]

Accurate indirect measurement of LAP via the wedged catheter (PAW) relies on an open continuum between the catheter tip and the LA. This may not be the case when surrounding airway pressure is increased (positive end-expiratory pressure [PEEP], continuous positive airway pressure [CPAP]), when the tip of the catheter lies in zone 1 or 2 of the lung field, or when the LAP is low (Fig. 16–7).[22–25] In these situations, the airway pressure can be greater than the pulmonary venous pressure, resulting in collapse of the microvasculature. The recorded PAWP will be inaccurately elevated (perhaps even higher than the PAP) and will lack the normal contour and characteristics of a PAWP. Placement of the catheter tip below the level of the LA permits the hydrostatic pressure to maintain the vasculature open, and a true PAWP can thus be obtained. Confirmation of the position of the catheter relative to the LA is made via a lateral chest

FIGURE 16–7. Schematic illustration of pressure-flow relationships in zones 1, 2, and 3 of the pulmonary circulation under conditions of normal spontaneous breathing and with positive end-expiratory pressure (PEEP). Zone 1 reflects the physiologic areas of the lung (upper one third) in which alveolar pressure is greater than perfusion pressure and flow is minimal under both normal and PEEP conditions. Balloon inflation in this zone would reflect only alveolar pressures. In zone 2, under normal conditions pulmonary artery pressure is slightly greater than alveolar pressures and flow is increased. However, balloon inflation in this zone interrupting flow is likely to collapse the capillary and the PAWP recorded here would also reflect alveolar pressures. Under conditions of PEEP, the capillary is collapsed by the higher alveolar pressures and only the alveolar pressures would be reflected on balloon inflation. In zone 3, perfusion pressure exceeds alveolar pressure under both normal and PEEP conditions. Balloon inflation in zone 3 most accurately reflects the pulmonary artery pressure and, thus, left atrial pressures. Note the effect of positioning on pressure-flow relationships in the various areas of the lungs. (Adapted from Daily, EK and Schroeder, JS: Techniques in Bedside Hemodynamic Monitoring. CV Mosby Co., St. Louis, 1994.)

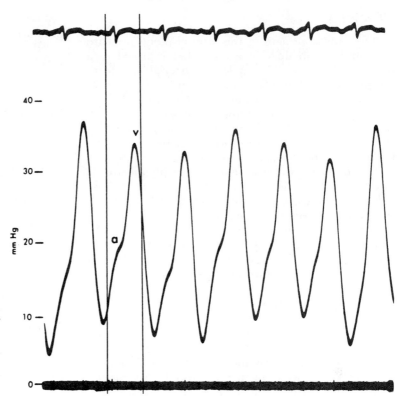

FIGURE 16–8. PAWP waveform with a dominant and elevated *v* wave of 35 mmHg as a result of acute mitral regurgitation associated with papillary muscle dysfunction from an acute myocardial infarction. Note the early appearance of the *v* wave, which almost obscures the minimally elevated *a* wave (18 mmHg). (From Daily, EK and Schroeder, JS: Techniques in Bedside Hemodynamic Monitoring. CV Mosby Co., St. Louis, 1994, with permission.)

film. However, suspicion regarding the possibility of location of the catheter tip in zone 1 or 2 should occur when:

- The mean PAWP value exceeds the PAEDP.
- The PAWP lacks all characteristics of a PAW waveform (i.e., *a* wave, *x* descent, *v* wave, *y* descent)
- The value of the mean PAWP is similar to the level of the PEEP.
- The change in the PAW pressure during positive pressure inspiration is much greater than the corresponding change in the PA pressure.[26]

Some ways to alter the situation and thereby obtain an accurate PAWP include:

- Turn the patient onto the side in which the catheter tip lies (thereby placing the catheter tip below the level of the LA).
- Decrease the airway pressure by reducing the level of PEEP, if possible.
- Increase the LAP via volume administration.
- Reposition the catheter into a zone 3 area.
- Use the PAEDP as a reflection of LVEDP.

Fortunately, because PA catheters are flow-directed, they are most frequently carried out to a zone 3 position, where lung perfusion is the greatest and the most accurate PAWP is obtained.[27]

In patients with cardiac dysfunction, the PAWP is usually optimized between 15 and 18 mmHg to obtain the best stroke volume according to Starling's law. However, the limits to which the PAWP can be raised are dictated by the oncotic pressure. Elevations of the PAWP to levels that cause pulmonary edema, and therefore hypoxemia, can decrease oxygen delivery to the tissues, despite apparent increases in cardiac output.

Abnormalities

The *a* wave of the PAW/LA waveform becomes dominant and elevated in conditions that increase resistance to ventricular filling, such as mitral stenosis or LV failure.

The *v* wave of the PAW/LA waveform becomes exaggerated and elevated with mitral valve regurgitation caused by the reflux of blood into the LA during ventricular systole. A mild increase in the *v* wave of the PAW/LA waveform is commonly seen in patients with functional mitral valve regurgitation secondary to LV failure and dilatation. Acute mitral valve regurgitation due to rupture of the papillary muscle following myocardial infarction is associated with early-appearing, dominant, giant *v* waves (Fig. 16–8). This complication requires prompt treatment to reduce afterload and thereby improve forward cardiac output.

Both the *a* and *v* waves of the PAW/LA waveform are equally elevated in conditions of hypervolemia, cardiac tamponade, and constrictive pericarditis.

Systemic Arterial Pressure

Continuous direct monitoring of arterial pressure is frequently performed in critically ill patients for prompt detection of changes in cardiovascular function and for assessment of arterial blood gases.

Waveform

Direct measurement of the arterial blood pressure is commonly obtained from a catheter placed in a peripheral artery. The systemic arterial waveform resembles the PA waveform in contour, with a pressure value about six times greater than that of the PA. Systole begins with the opening of the aortic valve and rapid ejection of blood into the aorta, producing a sharp upstroke on the waveform (Fig. 16–9). Diastole begins with the closure of the aortic valve, which is evidenced on the downslope of the peripheral arterial waveform by the dicrotic notch. (In the aortic root pressure, systole and diastole are separated by the incisura, which becomes the dicrotic notch in the peripheral arteries.[28]) The decline in pressure following the dicrotic notch represents runoff of blood into the arterial circulation. The peak systolic, diastolic, and mean values of the arterial waveform are recorded.

Because of wave reflection and the tapering diameter of peripheral arteries, the more distal from the aorta the arterial catheter is located, the higher the systolic pressure (by as much as 15 to 30 mmHg) and the lower the diastolic pressure. The mean pressure, however, remains nearly the same.[29] In addition, the more distal the location of the arterial catheter, the sharper the upstroke, the narrower the waveform, and the less defined the dicrotic notch, which virtually disappears into the diastolic pressure in the femoral

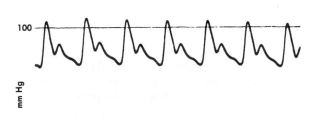

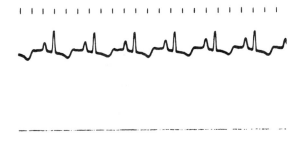

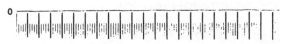

FIGURE 16–9. Normal radial artery waveform. (From Daily, EK and Schroeder, JS: Techniques in Bedside Hemodynamic Monitoring. CV Mosby Co., St. Louis, 1994, with permission.)

artery waveform.[30] These normal changes in systolic pressure account for some of the disparity encountered between cuff blood pressure measured at the brachial artery and direct arterial pressure measured at the radial or femoral artery.[30]

Normal Values

Arterial systolic pressure	100 to 140 mmHg
Arterial diastolic pressure	60 to 80 mmHg
Arterial mean pressure	70 to 90 mmHg

Clinical Application

In the absence of aortic stenosis, the arterial *systolic pressure* reflects the peak pressure generated by the LV. It also reflects the compliance of the large arteries, the total peripheral resistance. In general, the systolic pressure is a clinical indication of the amount of work that the LV generates during systole. The upstroke of the aortic root arterial waveform is often used as an indication of the inotropic state of the ventricle.

The arterial *diastolic pressure* represents the runoff of blood into the arterial system and is determined by the velocity of runoff as well as by the elasticity of the arterial system, particularly the arterioles. The level to which the arterial diastolic pressure falls is also affected by the patient's heart rate, which determines the duration of diastole. The slower the heart rate, the longer the diastolic period, and the greater the fall in the diastolic pressure.

The *mean arterial pressure* refers to the average pressure in the arterial system during systole and diastole. This pressure can be mathematically calculated or, more commonly, is electronically integrated via the bedside monitor, which displays a numerical mean value.

The mean arterial pressure reflects the driving or perfusion pressure and is determined by the volume of blood flow in the arterial system (cardiac output) and the elasticity or resistance of the vessels (SVR). This can be mathematically expressed as:

$$MAP = SVR \times CO$$

where

$$
\begin{aligned}
MAP &= \text{mean arterial pressure} \\
SVR &= \text{systemic vascular resistance} \\
CO &= \text{cardiac output}
\end{aligned}
$$

SVR is primarily determined by the change in radius of the major resistance vessels (arterioles), although other factors such as blood viscosity and vessel length also affect it. SVR cannot be directly measured but can be calculated by rearranging the previous formula:

$$SVR = \frac{MAP}{CO} \times 80$$

More accurate calculation of systemic vascular resistance includes dividing the pressure difference between the proximal and distal ends of the circulatory system (i.e., arterial and venous) by the CO. This is expressed by the following formula:

$$SVR = \frac{MAP - RA\ mean}{CO} \times 80$$

However, since the RA mean pressure is usually low compared with the MAP, it may be eliminated from the calculation of SVR. If, however, the RA mean is significantly elevated, it should be subtracted from the MAP when calculating SVR. SVR is a clinical reflection of the *afterload* of the left side of the heart, that is, the resistance to left ventricular ejection. Afterload levels are manipulated with the use of vasoconstricting or vasodilating agents and therapies.

The MAP determines tissue perfusion. Although some organs can partially autoregulate the amount of blood flow, the myocardium of the LV, which receives most of its blood flow during diastole, requires an arterial driving pressure of 60 to 80 mmHg to maintain perfusion of the coronary arteries. When the MAP falls, coronary blood flow decreases. When the MAP falls to 40 mmHg or less, coronary blood flow virtually ceases, and the coronary arteries collapse.[31] Therefore, in patients with coronary artery disease, every effort is made to maintain coronary perfusion pressure at 60 to 80 mmHg.

The *pulse pressure* refers to the difference between peak systolic and end-diastolic pressures of the arterial pressure. The pulse pressure is primarily determined by the volume of blood ejected with each heartbeat (stroke volume) and the elasticity or compliance of the arterial system. Increases in the arterial pulse pressure occur with increases in the stroke volume, whereas narrow pulse pressures are usually associated with a decreased stroke volume.

Abnormalities

The arterial blood pressure is elevated in the following pathologic conditions:
1. Systemic hypertension
2. Arteriosclerosis
3. Renal failure
4. Aortic regurgitation

The presence of aortic regurgitation is classically associated with a wide pulse pressure (due to a large stroke volume) and an absent dicrotic notch in the arterial waveform (Fig. 16–10).

The arterial blood pressure is reduced in the following conditions:
1. Low cardiac output (from any cause)
2. Aortic stenosis
3. Arrhythmias
4. Vasodilator therapy

It is important to remember that initially the blood pressure is maintained at normal or near-normal levels in the presence of hypoperfusion because of the sympathetic nervous system response. Eventually, however, the blood pressure falls in low cardiac output states.

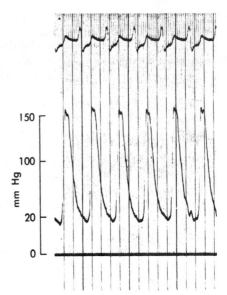

FIGURE 16–10. Arterial pressure waveform in a patient with aortic regurgitation. Note the wide pulse pressure with a high systolic pressure of 150 mmHg and a low diastolic pressure of 20 mmHg, and the absence of a dicrotic notch. (From Daily, EK and Schroeder, JS: Techniques in Bedside Hemodynamic Monitoring. CV Mosby Co., St. Louis, 1994, with permission.)

In aortic stenosis, the arterial pressure waveform exhibits a low pressure with a slow upstroke, poorly defined dicrotic notch, and narrow pulse pressure. Its appearance closely resembles a very damped arterial pressure waveform (Fig. 16–11).

Vasodilator therapy reduces the resistance to ejection of blood, producing a rapid upstroke of the arte-

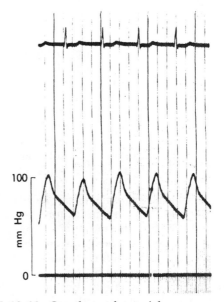

FIGURE 16–11. Overdamped arterial pressure waveform with poor upstroke and loss of dicrotic notch. (From Daily, EK and Schroeder, JS: Techniques in Bedside Hemodynamic Monitoring. CV Mosby Co., St. Louis, 1994, with permission.)

rial systolic pressure, a rapid decline in pressure during the shortened ejection phase, and a smaller change in the pressure during diastole. The degree of these physiologic responses may not be as evident in the peripheral artery pressure waveforms as they are in aortic pressure waveforms.[32]

Regular alternating changes in the value of the arterial systolic pressure may be seen in patients with severe LV failure. This condition, termed *pulsus alternans,* likely represents a regular alternating change in the inotropic state of the ventricle. Pulsus alternans can be felt at the radial artery as a regular pattern of strong, weak, strong, weak pulsations.

During spontaneous inspiration, the arterial systolic pressure normally declines. However, when this physiologic response is exaggerated and the systolic pressure falls more than 10 mmHg during normal spontaneous inspiration, *pulsus paradoxus* is said to exist. Pulsus paradoxus is classically seen in cases of cardiac tamponade but may also be noted in patients with obstructed airway disease and less commonly in those with hypovolemic shock and pulmonary embolism.

DERIVED HEMODYNAMIC PARAMETERS

From directly measured hemodynamic data, other important hemodynamic parameters can be derived or calculated. Appendix F lists the formulas for obtaining certain hemodynamic parameters, as well as the normal values for those parameters.

CARDIAC OUTPUT DETERMINATION

Principle

Cardiac output is the rate at which blood is ejected by the heart and is expressed in liters per minute (L/min). Since blood is ejected with each heartbeat, the CO is a product of the stroke volume (SV) times the heart rate (CO = SV × HR). Although minor discrepancies may occur, the RV and the LV pump the same volume of blood, unless an intracardiac shunt exists. Thus, measurements of blood flow from one ventricle can be assumed to be the same for the other ventricle.

Cardiac output measurements can be made by (1) the Fick method, (2) the indicator-dilution (dye) method, and (3) the thermodilution method. The thermodilution method correlates closely with both the Fick and the dye-dilution methods of determining CO, except in the presence of intracardiac shunts or severe tricuspid regurgitation. Because of this and because of the technical ease with which it can be performed, the thermodilution method is most commonly used at the bedside to measure CO. Discussion here is limited to this method.

Normal Values

Normal resting CO is 4 to 8 L/min. This wide range reflects the variations that can occur from person to person as a result of body size. A more specific measurement is the cardiac index (CI), which individualizes the flow rate by taking into account the patient's body size. The patient's body size or body surface area (BSA) can be obtained from Dubois' height–weight formula (available as a nomogram), and dividing this into the CO value to obtain the CI (CI = CO ÷ BSA). A normal resting CI is 2.6 to 4 L/min/m². This is true for both adults and children over 10 years of age. Because of their increased metabolic and heart rates, children under 10 years of age normally have about a 25% greater CI, that is, 3.4 to 5 L/min/m².[17]

Clinical Application

Tissue function and viability depend on an adequate supply and exchange of oxygen and nutrients from the circulating blood. This supply is dependent on the flow rate (CO) and the content of oxygen in arterial blood. Measurement of CO provides essential information regarding overall cardiac performance in providing adequate perfusion to the tissues.

CO measurement is a reflection of the systolic performance of the ventricle. According to Starling's law, the systolic performance is determined by the diastolic function (preload). This means that the greater the fiber length or stretch during diastole (preload), the greater the fiber shortening and ejection during systole, within physiologic limits. This relationship between the diastolic and systolic function of the ventricle can be graphically plotted to form a ventricular function curve (Fig. 16–12). The LV diastolic measurement of performance (on the horizontal axis) could include LVEDP, LAm, PAWm, or PAEDP. The systolic measurement of performance (on the vertical axis) could include the CO, CI, SV, stroke volume index (SVI), left ventricular stroke work (LVSW), or left ventricular stroke work index (LVSWI). Although flow rates (CO, CI, SV, or SVI) are more commonly used to plot ventricular function curves at the bedside, LVSW or LVSWI provide a more accurate assessment of changes in cardiac performance irrespective of changes in afterload.[18]

A ventricular function curve for the RV can also be plotted and assessed by placing the CVP or RAP (reflecting RV diastolic pressures) on the horizontal axis and the CO, CI, SV, SVI, right ventricular stroke work (RVSW), or right ventricular stroke work index (RVSWI) on the vertical axis.

Normally, the ventricular function curve shows a linear increase in systolic performance as preload increases, up to a certain level (Fig. 16–12). After this level is reached, further increases in preload no longer improve systolic performance. The entire ventricular function curve may be shifted upward and to the left because of increased ventricular contractility, or

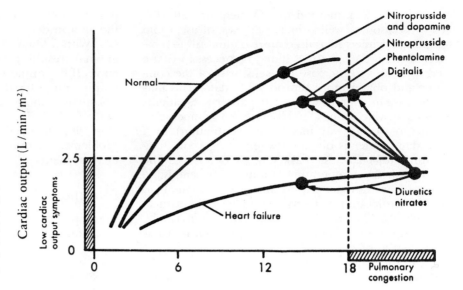

FIGURE 16–12. Ventricular function curves, depicting effects on cardiac output and left ventricular end-diastolic pressure of various agents used for treating heart failure. (Modified from Mason, DT (ed): Congestive Heart Failure. Yorke Medical Book, New York, 1976.)

TABLE 16–3
Conditions Responsible for Low Cardiac Output

Inadequate LV Filling	Inadequate LV Ejection
Tachycardia	Myocardial ischemia or
Arrhythmias	infarction
Hypovolemia	Cardiomyopathy or myocarditis
Mitral stenosis	Aortic stenosis
Tricuspid stenosis	Hypertension
Tamponade or	Mitral regurgitation
constrictive pericarditis	Metabolic disorders
Restrictive cardiomyopathy	Negative inotropic agents
Pulmonary embolus	Ventricular septal defect
Right ventricular failure	
Mechanical ventilation	

downward and to the right because of depressed ventricular function and contractility.

Individual right or left ventricular function curves should be plotted for each patient by the critical care nurse to determine the *optimum* preload (i.e., the filling pressure that produces the maximum cardiac output) for that particular patient. Adjustment of preload levels can be done with administration of volume, diuretics, or nitrate preparations (Fig. 16–12).

Alterations in afterload or the resistance to ejection of blood from the aorta also affect the cardiac output (CO). Conditions that produce vasoconstriction increase the resistance to ejection and thus decrease CO. On the other hand, vasodilatation reduces resistance and increases SV or CO. This is the underlying principle of afterload-reducing therapy with arterial vasodilators or counterpulsation.

Since CO = SV × HR, changes in heart rate also affect CO. CO values are greater with faster heart rates, although SV may remain unchanged. However, at very fast heart rates (more than 130 bpm), the decreased duration of diastole prevents adequate filling, and thus stroke volume falls. Slowing the heart

rate usually improves the stroke volume as well as reducing myocardial oxygen demands. In general, heart rates between 50 and 100 are considered satisfactory in terms of stroke volume and myocardial oxygen demands.

Low CO values can be due to inadequate ventricular filling or inadequate ventricular ejection or both. Table 16–3 lists some of the pathologic conditions responsible for low CO.

High CO values at rest can be seen in hyperdynamic states (postoperatively or with increased thyroid function) or with severe vasodilatory states associated with sepsis or anaphylaxis.

Techniques of Thermodilution Cardiac Output Measurement

The thermodilution CO method was first described by Fegler[33] in 1954. This method applies the indicator-dilution method using a solution of exact known temperature as the indicator. The change in blood temperature produced downstream (from the RA to the PA) is recorded by a thermistor near the catheter tip. The change in temperature over time is inversely proportional to blood flow. A special CO computer analyzes the resultant temperature/time curve and applies appropriate constants to calculate the rate of blood flow through the heart.

Since the indicator used in the thermodilution method consists of a known temperature, it is important that the injectate be different from the surrounding temperature in the PA (at least 12°F or more). Initially, chilled injectates with temperatures close to zero were used to maximize the difference and thus increase the physiologic noise/signal ratio. However, numerous studies have demonstrated that CO determinations obtained with iced injectate and room temperature injectate correlate closely with each other and with the Fick method of CO measurement.[34-36] For this reason, as well as increased ease of use, room temperature injectate is used more commonly to measure CO. However, at times it may be necessary to use iced injectates to increase the sensitivity of the computer and obtain more reproducible data. This may be the case in patients who are hypothermic, patients who have wide swings in baseline PA temperature (which may occur with mechanical ventilation), or if wide data scatter is obtained when using room temperature injectate. An easy way to determine the degree of PA temperature variation is simply to prompt the cardiac output monitor/computer to begin a cardiac output determination, but not to inject any indicator. The resultant baseline variations can be observed on the monitor or paper printout to assess their degree of clinical significance and whether or not iced injectate is necessary.

Whether room temperature or iced temperature injectate is used for CO measurement, the closed system of delivery is recommended to reduce thermal loss and to reduce the risk of contamination or infection.

All CO curves should be visually displayed or recorded on a paper write-out and inspected for accuracy. The upstroke of the CO curve reflects the injection technique and should be smooth and even (Fig. 16–13). Bumps or steps on the upstroke indicate an uneven injection, and the value of such a CO curve should be discarded. The downslope determines the area under the curve, which is inversely proportional to the CO. If the downstroke is rapid (see Fig. 16–13), the area under the curve is small, indicating a high CO. With a low CO, the downslope is very slow and gradual, resulting in an increased area under the curve. If the numerical value displayed by the cardiac output computer does not agree with the displayed CO curve, troubleshooting of the cardiac output computer and equipment should be performed. Table 16–4 lists troubleshooting techniques for various problems encountered with thermodilution CO measurements.

Equipment

Equipment needed for thermodilution CO determinations using room temperature injectate consists of:

- Thermodilution PA catheter
- Sterile IV solution (saline or D_5W) in a collapsible bag
- IV tubing
- 10-mL syringes
- Cardiac output computer (if not included in monitoring system) with connecting cable and temperature probe

Preparation

1. Assemble the injectate solution using a closed system. (Follow manufacturer's directions.)
2. Connect the injectate solution tubing to the

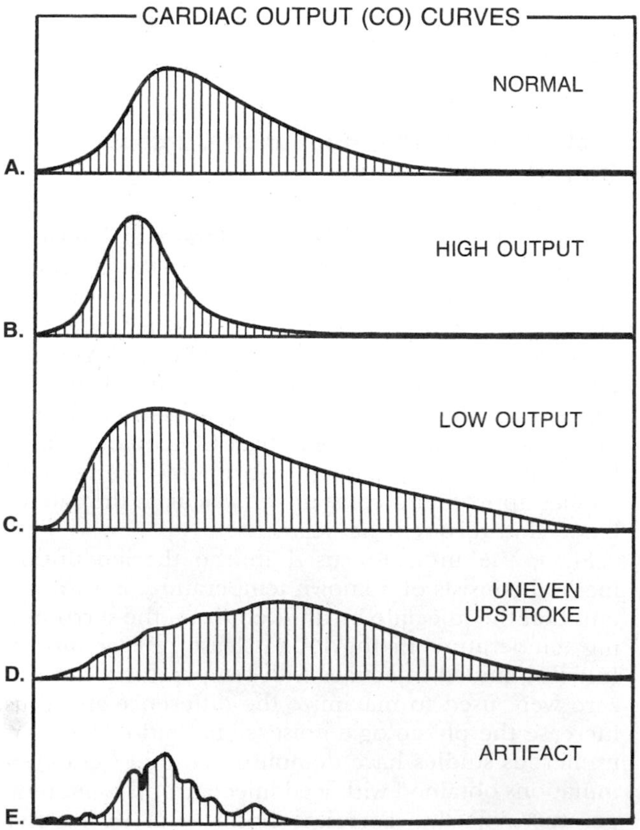

CARDIAC OUTPUT (CO) CURVES

A. NORMAL
B. HIGH OUTPUT
C. LOW OUTPUT
D. UNEVEN UPSTROKE
E. ARTIFACT

FIGURE 16–13. Schematic representation of various thermodilution cardiac output curves. (*A*) Normal cardiac output showing a smooth upstroke; (*B*) small area beneath the curve as seen in patients with high cardiac outputs; (*C*) large area beneath the curve as seen in patients with low cardiac output; (*D*) uneven injection indicated by uneven upstroke on curve; and (*E*) artifact in both upstroke and decline of curve resulting in erroneous cardiac output measurement. (From Tilkian, A and Daily, EK: Cardiovascular Procedures. CV Mosby Co., St. Louis, 1986, with permission.)

TABLE 16–4
Cardic Output Troubleshooting

Problem	Cause(s)	Prevention	Remedy
Cardiac output (CO) reading higher than expected	Inaccurate injectate volume caused by air bubbles or loss of injectate	Carefully check for bubbles and expel, if any.	Check for *exact* volume of injectate before injection.
	Wrong computation constant (CC)	Check appropriate CC on catheter insert and set correctly on computer.	Enter correct CC. For cardiac outputs already done: Correct CO = wrong CO × correct CC ÷ wrong CC.
	Warming of iced injectate in syringe before injection	Handle syringe only briefly.	Perform outputs rapidly with minimal handling of syringe. Use CO-SET with in-line temperature probe.
	Migration of catheter tip toward PA wedge	Ascertain catheter tip position with radiograph. Closely observe PA pressure.	Withdraw catheter a few centimeters.
	Thermistor against wall of artery		Withdraw catheter a few centimeters.
	Uneven injection	Use both hands to deliver fast, even bolus. Use automatic injector.	Use automatic injector. Analyze curve on strip-chart recorder.
	Right-to-left shunt	None	Use another method of cardiac output determination (such as Fick).
	Low stroke volume with long lag time before onset of curve	None	Press START button *after* complete injection of indicator.
Cardiac output reading lower than expected	Inaccurate injectate volume (more than indicated)	Use syringe of size that corresponds to injectate volume. Exercise care in filling syringe.	Check for *exact* volume of injectate before injection.
	Wrong CC	Check appropriate CC on catheter insert and set correctly on computer.	Enter correct CC. For cardiac outputs already done: Correct CO = wrong CO × correct CC ÷ wrong CC.
	Iced injections spaced <1 minute apart	Wait about 1 minute between injections.	Wait about 1 minute between injections.
	Catheter kinked or partially obstructed by clot	Carefully protect catheter during patient movement. Occasionally aspirate and flush manually.	Try to straighten catheter. Aspirate and gently flush catheter. Remove catheter if necessary.
Scattered CO readings (poor reproducibility)	Cardiac arrhythmias (e.g., ventricular ectopic beats, atrial fibrillation)	None	Try to inject during quiet period (i.e., without ventricular ectopic beats). Increase number of determinations (e.g., 5, 6, or 7) and average readings.
	Tricuspid regurgitation	None	Use another method of CO determination (e.g., Fick).
	Wide swings in intrapleural pressure (spontaneous respiration or mechanical ventilation)	Inject at same point in respiratory cycle. Increase number of determinations (e.g., 5, 6, or 7) and average readings. Used iced injectate.	Increase number of determinations (e.g., 5, 6, or 7) and average readings. Use iced injectate.
	Electromagnetic interference	Isolate computer from other electromagnetic sources.	Isolate computer from other electromagnetic sources. Change power source (AC to battery or vice versa).

Continued

TABLE 16–4
Cardic Output Troubleshooting (*Continued*)

Problem	Cause(s)	Prevention	Remedy
	Migration of catheter tip toward PAW or thermistor against artery wall	Ascertain catheter tip location with radiograph. Closely monitor PA pressure	Withdraw catheter several centimeters to position in main PA.
	Catheter looped in RV	Advance catheter carefully, avoiding excessive catheter insertion. Confirm catheter position with radiograph.	Withdraw and reposition catheter.

Source: From Tilkian, AG and Daily, EK: Cardiovascular Procedures. CV Mosby, St Louis, 1986, with permission.

proximal lumen port of the thermodilution PA catheter via a three-way stopcock.

3. Attach the in-line temperature probe and a 10-mL syringe to the side port of the stopcock at the proximal lumen port.
4. Connect the thermistor connector hub of the PA catheter to the cardiac output computer via the appropriate connecting cable.
5. Prepare the cardiac output computer (including entry of the correct constant) according to the manufacturer's directions.

Technique

1. Close the stopcock to the proximal lumen of the catheter and carefully fill the syringe with *exactly* 10 mL from the IV solution bag. (Slow filling of the syringe minimizes the occurrence of any air bubbles, which must be purged before injection.)
2. Activate the CO computer (module) and wait for a READY signal.
3. Check the PA waveform from the distal lumen of the catheter to verify the PA position.
4. Turn the stopcock closed to the IV solution, press the START button on the CO computer, and immediately inject the contents of the syringe into the proximal lumen. The injection must be done rapidly (within less than 4 seconds) and smoothly. The CO reading should be displayed in about 10 to 30 seconds.
5. Check the corresponding CO curve to verify a fast, even injection evidenced by a smooth and rapid upstroke (Fig. 16–13).

Usually at least three successive cardiac output measurements are made and averaged to obtain a mean value. However, if considerable variation among the readings is present, it may be necessary to average five, six, or seven cardiac output measurements. With the use of 10 mL of iced injectate, the first in a series of three sequential thermodilution CO measurements was found to be significantly higher than the following values.[37] This situation, which is frequently observed

in the clinical setting, is often handled by eliminating the results of the first CO determination and averaging the values of three more successive CO determinations. However, this may not be appropriate when fluid restriction is a concern and is not necessary when room temperature injectate is used.

The bolus thermodilution CO technique provides information over a very brief window of time, that is, the few seconds of actual temperature change measurement. This value is used to reflect the patient's flow rate per minute of time. The shorter the time of measurement, the larger the sampling error and the greater the need for precision in the technique of measurement. In addition, any changes in the patient's physiologic parameters (respiratory rate, depth and mode, heart rate and rhythm) can markedly affect the CO values, resulting in wide variations from one determination to the next. Careful inspection of the CO curve is necessary to determine whether variations in CO values are due to faulty technique (as evident on the upslope of the CO curve). In the face of acceptable quality CO curves, the practice of discarding values outside a predetermined variability level cannot be supported. Under strictly controlled in vitro conditions, CO values have been reported to differ from 3% to 13%.[36,38,39] Greater variations occur in patients breathing spontaneously compared with mechanically ventilated patients.[39]

Consistently injecting the solution at a specific point in the patient's respiratory cycle may improve reproducibility of data. However, such data may be erroneously skewed and not reflect the patient's true cardiovascular status.

Continuous Cardiac Output

Thermodilution CO can also be measured on a more continuous basis by a modified PA catheter with specialized filaments that automatically and sequentially provide brief bursts of heat that serve as the indicator. The thermistor of the PA catheter measures the induced temperature changes distally and, by means of cross-correlation, yields an indicator washout curve from which flow is computed.[40] The CO readout is an average of the data collected within the previous 3 to 6 minutes and is updated every 30 seconds.

The theoretic advantages of this technique include the maintenance of a closed system that reduces the risk of infection; reduced administration of fluid; reduced nursing time; elimination of errors associated with injection technique; and the ability to monitor changes in blood flow more immediately. Limited clinical data indicate excellent correlation with standard bolus thermodilution CO values in critically ill patients.[41] Further clinical research is necessary to evaluate the indications as well as the risks, including the cost, of this new technique.

CONTINUOUS SvO_2 MONITORING

The addition of fiberoptic technology to the balloon-flotation PA catheter permits continuous monitoring of the oxygen saturation of mixed venous (PA) blood. Although hemodynamic parameters provide essential information regarding cardiac performance and, in part, oxygen delivery, monitoring the SvO_2 provides information regarding the adequacy of tissue oxygenation.

Principle

Oxygen is taken up in the lungs and delivered to the tissues by the hemoglobin molecules in blood. Each hemoglobin molecule can carry approximately 1.34 mL of oxygen. (Oxygen is also dissolved in the plasma in the amount of 0.003 mL/mmHg partial pressure of arterial blood. Because this amount is so small, it is generally clinically ignored, particularly with the use of trend monitoring.)

The rate of oxygen delivery to the tissues depends on the flow rate, or CO. Thus, the formula for calculation of oxygen delivery is:

Oxygen delivery = CO × hemoglobin × 1.34
× arterial oxygen saturation × 10

Normally, the hemoglobin becomes fully saturated with oxygen, resulting in an arterial saturation of 95% to 99%. Therefore, in a patient with a normal CO of 5 L/min, a hemoglobin of 15 g/dL, and an arterial saturation of 97%, the oxygen delivery would be:

975 mL O_2 delivery = 5 L/min × 15 g/100 mL
× 1.34 × .97 × 10

This represents a normal delivery of oxygen to the tissues and is a commonly used index of the performance of the cardiopulmonary system. However, it does not indicate the adequacy of oxygen delivery in relation to tissue oxygen needs. While low oxygen delivery values are usually associated with tissue hypoxia, normal or even high oxygen delivery values can also be present with tissue hypoxia.[42]

Previously, intermittent mixed venous oxygen saturation samples were obtained to assess the adequacy of tissue oxygenation. When oxygen consumption is constant and arterial oxygen saturation is maintained, SvO_2 varies directly with CO.

Normal Values

The hemoglobin of mixed venous blood in the PA is normally 65% to 77% saturated with oxygen. Venous blood obtained from other sites (RA, RV, peripheral vein) has not adequately mixed and cannot be used as a reflection of overall tissue oxygenation.

Clinical Applications

As mentioned previously, SvO_2 reflects the balance between oxygen supply and demand. Alterations in oxygen supply can be caused by changes in CO, hemoglobin, or arterial oxygen saturation. Anemia or hypoxemia causes an increase in tissue oxygen extraction, which will reduce SvO_2 unless the CO can increase sufficiently to maintain the balance between supply and demand. A reduction in hemoglobin, unless as a result of massive hemorrhage, usually occurs slowly and is less commonly responsible for sudden decreases in SvO_2. Hypoxemia can be evaluated by pulse oximetry or arterial blood gas determination. However, in most clinical situations in which the patient is receiving oxygen therapy or mechanical ventilation, the arterial saturation rarely changes more than 10%.[29]

Low CO is the most common cause of inadequate tissue oxygenation (as reflected by an SvO_2 of less than 60%).[43] Sustained reductions in SvO_2 of 10% or greater for 3 to 5 minutes should prompt an immediate assessment of the patient's cardiovascular status, including cardiac output measurement.[44,45] In this way, CO determinations are performed when hemodynamically indicated, rather than at some preset, routine, or arbitrary time.

Increases in the tissues' demand for oxygen may also result in low SvO_2 readings, despite normal oxygen delivery values. Increases in oxygen consumption may occur with increases in the patient's metabolic rate, temperature, pain, and so forth. However, this is usually evident clinically, and if no apparent increase in oxygen consumption is observed, the components of oxygen supply (CO, hemoglobin, arterial saturation) should be assessed.

Rises in SvO_2 readings to levels above normal (80% to 95%) may be due to distal wedging of the PA catheter in which postcapillary arterialized blood is monitored. This is evidenced by a change in the light intensity on the strip recorder, as well as by the appearance of a PAW waveform from the distal lumen of the catheter. Slight withdrawal of the catheter tip back into the PA corrects such a situation. High SvO_2 values (greater than 77%) may also occur in situations in which tissue oxygen demands are reduced, such as marked hypothermia, induced muscular paralysis, or anesthesia. However, an elevated SvO_2 reading is usually seen in the presence of sepsis in which oxygen

TABLE 16–5
Various Causes of Alterations in SvO$_2$

	SvO$_2$ Reading	Physiologic Alteration	Clinical Causes
High	80%–95%	↓ O$_2$ consumption	Hypothermia Anesthesia Induced muscular paralysis Sepsis
		↑ O$_2$ delivery	Hyperoxia
		Mechanical interference	Wedged catheter Left-to-right shunt
Normal	60%–80%	O$_2$ supply = O$_2$ demand	Adequate perfusion
Low	<60%	↑ O$_2$ consumption	Shivering Pain Seizures Activity/exercise Hyperthermia Anxiety
		↓ O$_2$ delivery	Hypoperfusion (↓ cardiac output) Anemia Hypoxemia

Source: Tilkian, AG and Daily, EK: Cardiovascular Procedures. CV Mosby, St Louis, 1986, with permission

extraction by the tissues is impaired. In fact, a rising SvO$_2$ may be the first indication of a septic condition.[43] Table 16–5 lists pathologic conditions associated with alterations in SvO$_2$.

A normal SvO$_2$ of 65% to 77% represents adequate tissue perfusion and oxygenation, whereas SvO$_2$ readings less than 60% or decreases in SvO$_2$ of 10% or more usually indicate a compromise in at least one of the determinants of oxygen delivery (CO, hemoglobin, or arterial saturation). Since hypoperfusion is the most common cause of decreases in SvO$_2$ in the critical care setting, a CO measurement should be performed immediately to determine and appropriately treat the cause of the reduced oxygen delivery. If the CO is within normal limits, an arterial blood sample should be drawn for blood gas analysis and hemoglobin concentration level. Brief, minor changes in SvO$_2$ readings may be caused by interference. These nonsustained changes are clinically insignificant and likely do not represent changes in CO. Figure 16–14 shows an example of a printout obtained with continuous SvO$_2$ monitoring.[46]

Technique

The SvO$_2$ catheter is a modified 7.5 or 8F PA thermodilution catheter that additionally contains optic fibers that transmit and receive light reflected from the bloodstream. The light signal is converted to an electrical signal and transmitted to a remote data processor that displays the signal on a slow-speed paper recorder or a liquid crystal display (LCD) screen. A digital value is also continuously displayed and updated every 1 to 2 seconds.

Calibration of the light signal should be performed prior to catheter insertion according to each manu-

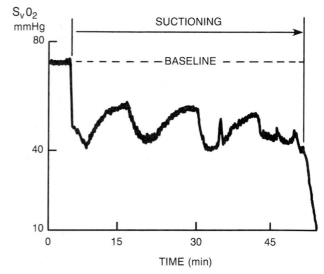

FIGURE 16–14. Example of continuous SvO$_2$ recording showing reductions in SvO$_2$ associated with repeated suctioning. Note that the SvO$_2$ did not return to baseline between suctioning procedures. Ventricular fibrillation occurs as the SvO$_2$ falls to 40% and lower. (From Tilkian, A and Daily, EK: Cardiovascular Procedures. CV Mosby Co., St. Louis, 1986, with permission.)

facturer's directions. After catheter insertion, calibration of the oximeter with a blood sample of a known saturation (determined by the blood gas laboratory) should be performed daily or whenever there are any doubts regarding the displayed SvO$_2$ reading. Calibration with a known oxygen saturation value should be performed at a time when the patient's saturation values are relatively stable, following the manufacturer's directions.

Because of the fiberoptics within SvO_2 catheters, the catheters should be handled with care, avoiding any sharp angles or bends. Breakage of the fiberoptics eliminates the ability to continuously monitor SvO_2; however, the catheter may be continued to be used to obtain routine hemodynamic data.

RIGHT VENTRICULAR VOLUME MEASUREMENTS

Recent modification of the standard PA catheter allows assessment of the systolic and diastolic volume measurements of the RV using the thermodilution technique. In addition to the standard features of a thermodilution catheter, this catheter is equipped with two intracardiac electrodes and a rapid-response thermistor. The proximal and distal electrodes sense the R-wave activity that is necessary for computation of beat-to-beat volume analysis. The thermistor, located near the catheter tip, is a very sensitive rapid-response thermistor, which detects very small temperature changes in the PA.

Principle

The importance of RV function in maintaining circulation has been increasingly recognized and underscores the need to accurately assess both the systolic and diastolic performance of the RV in some patients. Although RV performance can be assessed indirectly using hemodynamic pressure data such as the RAP and the PA systolic pressure, these measurements provide imprecise information regarding ventricular volume. The nonlinear relationship between pressure and volume limits the applicability of pressure measurements as a reflection of preload, or filling volume. In addition, the usual pressure-volume relationship is altered by conditions that decrease ventricular compliance. Such conditions include RV ischemia/infarction, pulmonary disease, pulmonary embolism, or adult respiratory distress syndrome, as well as the use of positive pressure ventilation or PEEP.

One simple expression of RV function is the ejection fraction (the percentage of RV volume ejected each beat), which is influenced by changes in RV preload, afterload, and contractility. The RV volumetric catheter measures thermodilution CO in the standard fashion, while the addition of the two electrodes that sense each R wave during the measurement permits the measurement of the stroke volume. From these values the percent of blood ejected each beat, the *ejection fraction,* is calculated. The computer also calculates the *end-diastolic volume* and the *end-systolic volume* from the stroke volume and ejection fraction.

The accuracy of thermodilution RV volumetric measurements has been evaluated against other measurement techniques such as ventricular angiography, gated and first-pass radionuclide angiography, and two-dimensional echocardiography.[47–49] Whereas the RV ejection fraction measurement has correlated well with that of other techniques, greater variation was observed in end-diastolic and end-systolic volumes.

Normal Values

The normal RV ejection fraction determined by the thermodilution technique is about 40%, which is slightly lower than normal values reported with the use of other techniques.[50] Normal RV end-diastolic volume is 100 to 160 mL, and normal end-systolic volume is 50 to 100 mL.

Clinical Application

Conditions that impair RV function (usually because of increased pulmonary vascular resistance or intrathoracic pressure) limit the ability to assess RV volume status by hemodynamic pressures. In such situations, measurement of end-diastolic volume can be very helpful in guiding fluid administration as well as other pharmacologic interventions.

RV volumetric measurements are not valid in any conditions that prevent homogeneous mixing of the thermal bolus. These conditions include atrial septal defect, ventricular septal defect, tricuspid regurgitation, pulmonic insufficiency, and cardiac arrhythmias such as atrial fibrillation.

Further clinical assessment and investigation are necessary to determine the cost-benefit ratio of this new technology and to define appropriate indications for its use.

NURSING CARE OF THE PATIENT UNDERGOING HEMODYNAMIC MONITORING

Nursing diagnoses, desired patient outcomes, and nursing interventions in the care of the patient undergoing hemodynamic monitoring are presented in the care plan at the end of this chapter.

REFERENCES

1. Hales, S: Statistical Essays: Hemostaticks, ed 3, vol 2. W Innys and R Manby, London, 1978.
2. Wilson, JN, et al: Central venous pressure in optimum blood volume maintenance. Arch Surg 85:563, 1962.
3. Swan, HJC, Ganz, W, and Forrester, JS: Catheterization of the heart in man with the use of a flow-directed balloon-tipped catheter. N Engl J Med 283:447, 1970.
4. Gardner, RM and Hollingsworth, KW: Optimizing the electrocardiogram and pressure monitoring. Crit Care Med 14:651, 1986.
5. Sise, MJ, Hollingsworth, P, and Brimm, JE: Complications of the flow-directed pulmonary artery catheter: A prospective analysis in 219 patients. Crit Care Med 9:315, 1981.
6. Johnston, WE, et al: Short-term sterility of the pulmonary artery catheter inserted through an external plastic shield. Anesthesiology 61:461, 1984.
7. Iberti, TJ, et al: Ventricular arrhythmias during pulmonary artery catheterization in the intensive care unit. Am J Med 78:451, 1985.

8. Scott, WAC: Haemodynamic monitoring measurement of systemic blood pressure. Can Anaesth Soc J 32(3):294, 1985.

9. Boutros, A and Albert, S: Effect of the dynamic response of transducer-tubing system on accuracy of direct blood pressure measurement in patients. Crit Care Med 11:124, 1983.

10. Whalley, DG: Haemodynamic monitoring: Pulmonary artery catheterization. Can Anaesth Soc J 32:1299, 1985.

11. Gardner, RM: Direct blood pressure measurement: Dynamic response requirements. Anesthesiology 54:227, 1981.

12. Bromberger-Barnea, B: Mechanical effects of inspiration on heart functions: A review. Fed Proc 40:2172, 1982.

13. King, EG: Influence of mechanical ventilation and pulmonary disease on pulmonary artery pressure monitoring. Can Med Assoc J 121:901, 1979.

14. Labrousse, J, Tenaillon, A, and Lissac, J: Influence of artificial ventilation on the pulmonary capillary wedge pressure. Chest 74:693, 1978.

15. Ellis, DM: Interpretation of beat-to-beat blood pressure values in the presence of ventilatory changes. J Clin Monitoring 1:65, 1985.

16. Bouchard, RJ, Goult, JH, and Ross, J Jr: Evaluation of pulmonary arterial end-diastolic pressure as an estimate of left ventricular end-diastolic pressure in patients with normal and abnormal left ventricular performance. Circulation 44:1072, 1971.

17. Daily, EK and Schroeder, JS: Techniques in Bedside Hemodynamic Monitoring, ed 5 CV Mosby, St Louis, 1994.

18. Keefer, JR and Barash, PG: Pulmonary artery catheterization. In Blitt, C (ed): Monitoring in Anesthesia and Critical Care Medicine. Churchill Livingstone, New York, 1986.

19. Braunwald, E: On the difference between the heart's output and its contractile state. Circulation 43:171, 1971.

20. Walston, A and Kendall, ME: Comparison of pulmonary wedge and left atrial pressure in man. Am Heart J 86:159, 1973.

21. Calvin, JE, Driedger, AA, and Sibbald, WJ: Does the pulmonary capillary wedge pressure predict left ventricular preload in critically ill patients? Crit Care Med 9:437, 1981.

22. Tooker, J, Huseby, J, and Butler, J: The effect of Swan-Ganz catheter height on the wedge pressure relationship in edema during positive-pressure ventilation. Am Rev Respir Dis 117:721, 1978.

23. Shasby, DM, et al: Swan-Ganz catheter location and left atrial pressure when positive end-expiratory pressure is used. Chest 80:666, 1981.

24. Scharf, SM, et al: Effects of normal and loaded spontaneous inspiration on cardiovascular function. J Appl Physiol 47(3):582, 1979.

25. Berryhill, RE and Benumof, JL: PEEP-induced discrepancy between pulmonary arterial wedge pressure and left atrial pressure: The effects of controlled vs. spontaneous ventilation and compliant vs. noncompliant lungs in the dog. Anesthesiology 51:303, 1979.

26. Teboul, JL, et al: A bedside index assessing the reliability of pulmonary artery occlusion pressure measurements during mechanical ventilation with positive end-expiratory pressure. J Crit Care 7:22–29, 1992.

27. Benumof, JL, et al: Where pulmonary arterial catheters go: Intrathoracic distributions. Anesthesiology 46:336, 1977.

28. Hurst, JS: The Heart: Arteries and Veins. McGraw-Hill, New York, 1982.

29. Gore, M, et al: Handbook of Hemodynamic Monitoring. Little, Brown, Boston, 1985.

30. Bedford, RF: Invasive blood pressure monitoring. In Blitt, C (ed): Monitoring in Anesthesia and Critical Care Medicine. Churchill Livingstone, New York, 1986.

31. Mueller, H, et al: Trans NY Acad Sci, Series II, 34(4):309, 1972.

32. O'Rourke, MF, Kelly, R, and Aviolo, A: The Arterial Pulse. Lea & Febiger, Philadelphia, 1992.

33. Fegler, G: Measurement of cardiac output in an anesthetized animal by the thermodilution method. Q J Exp Physiol 39:153, 1954.

34. Shellock, FG and Reidinger, MS: Reproducibility and accuracy of using room temperature vs. ice temperature for thermodilution cardiac output determination. Heart Lung 12:175, 1983.

35. Daily, EK and Mersch, J: Comparison of Fick method with thermodilution method using two indicators. Heart Lung 16:294, 1987.

36. Stetz, CS, et al: Reliability of the thermodilution method in determination of cardiac output in clinical practice. Am Rev Respir Dis 126:1001, 1982.

37. Kadota, LT: Reproducibility of thermodilution cardiac output measurements. Heart Lung 15:618, 1986.

38. Stevens, JH, et al: Thermodilution cardiac output measurement: Effects of the respiratory cycle on its reproducibility. JAMA 253:2240–2242, 1985.

39. Sasse, SA, et al: Variability of cardiac output over time in medical intensive care unit patients. Crit Care Med 22:225–232, 1994.

40. Gillman, PH: Continuous measurement of cardiac output: A milestone in hemodynamic monitoring. Focus Crit Care 19:155–158, 1992.

41. Yelderman, ML, et al: Continuous thermodilution cardiac output measurement in intensive care unit patients. J Cardiothoracic Vasc Anesth 6:270–274, 1992.

42. Miller, MJ: Tissue oxygenation in clinical medicine: An historical review. Anesth Analg 61:527, 1982.

43. McMihan, JC: Continuous monitoring of mixed venous oxygen saturation. In Schweiss, JF (ed): Continuous Measurement of Blood Oxygen Saturation in the High Risk Patient, vol 1. Beach International Inc, San Diego, 1983.

44. White, KM: Completing the hemodynamic picture: SvO_2. Heart Lung 14:272, 1985.

45. Jaquith, SM: Continuous measurement of SvO_2: Clinical applications and advantages for critical nursing. Crit Care Nurse 5:40, 1985.

46. Tilkian, AG and Daily, EK: Cardiovascular Procedures: Diagnostic Techniques and Therapeutic Procedures. CV Mosby, St Louis, 1986.

47. Vitolo, E, et al: Two-dimensional echocardiographic evaluation of right ventricular ejection fraction: Comparison between three different methods. Acta Cardiol 43:469–480, 1988.

48. Spinale, FG, et al: Right ventricular function computed by thermodilution and ventriculography. J Thorac Cardiovasc Surg 99:141–152, 1990.

49. Starling, RC, et al: Thermodilution measures of right ventricular ejection fraction and volumes in heart transplant recipients: A comparison with radionuclide angiography. J Heart Lung Transplant 11:1140–1146, 1992.

50. Hines, R: Monitoring right ventricular function. Anesth Clin North Am 6:851–863, 1988.

51. Lowenstein, E, Little, JW, and Lo, HH: Prevention of cerebral emobilization from flushing radial-artery cannulas. N Engl J Med 285:1414, 1971.

CARE PLAN FOR THE PATIENT UNDERGOING HEMODYNAMIC MONITORING

Nursing Diagnoses

Nursing Diagnosis #1
Alteration in cardiac output: Decreased

Desired Patient Outcomes

Patient will demonstrate optimal hemodynamic function by:
CI 2.5–4 L/min/m^2
PAEDP/PAWm* or LAm 15–20 mmHg
RAm 4–8 mmHg
MAP 70–80 mmHg
HR 50–100 bpm without ectopy
SVR < 1400 dynes sec cm^{-5}
PVR < 250 dynes sec cm^{-5}
Normal arterial blood gases
Normal hemoglobin level
Urinary output ≥40 mL/h
Oxygen delivery to tissues ≥900 mL/min

Nursing Interventions

- Monitor preload (RA and PAEDP, PAW or LAm) and administer appropriate medications and fluids as prescribed, and monitor response to therapy.
- Measure CO and CI and calculate SVR or PVR or both. Administer appropriate medications as prescribed, and monitor response to therapy.
  ○ Plot ventricular function curves.
  ○ Calculate LVSWI or RVSWI or both. Administer appropriate medications as prescribed, and monitor response.
- Monitor ECG for rate, rhythm, and ectopy, and determine patient's hemodynamic response to changes in rate or rhythm. Treat according to protocol. Implement emergency measures as necessary.
- Physically assess patient (vital signs, heart and lung sounds, skin color and temperature, fluid balance, mentation, jugular vein distention), and report any significant changes.
- Measure arterial blood gases and hemoglobin levels; report significant changes. Administer therapy as prescribed and monitor response.
- Measure hourly urine output and report if <30 mL/h.

- Monitor SvO$_2$ and report reductions >10% for 2–3 minutes, or if <60%.
- Reduce patient's activity and stress.

Rationales

- Optimize preload to increase systolic ejection according to Starling's law.

  ○ High LVSWI or RVSWI indicates increased heart work and myocardial O$_2$ need (M$\dot{V}$O$_2$).

- Very fast heart rates may lower SV by decreasing LV filling. Very low heart rates (<50) may produce inadequate CO (CO = HR × SV). Arrhythmias reduce CO.
- Baseline heart and lung sounds are necessary to determine onset of new sounds associated with cardiac pathology. Decreased mentation or increased restlessness may be early indications of decreased CO.
- Optimize O$_2$ delivery by maintaining CO, arterial saturation, and Hb at normal levels.

- To determine renal perfusion and function and prevent dysfunction due to ischemia.
- Decreases in SvO$_2$ indicate inadequate tissue perfusion. SvO$_2$ <60% is associated with poor prognosis.
- Reduced activity and stress will decrease O$_2$ demands.

Nursing Diagnoses

Nursing Diagnosis #2
Alteration in tissue perfusion (peripheral), related to compromised circulation associated with invasive monitoring

Desired Patient Outcomes

Patient will demonstrate:
1. Optimal skin integrity
2. Normal skin color and temperature
3. Equal arterial pulses in all extremities

Nursing Interventions

- Assess catheter insertion site every other day; cleanse site and apply iodophor ointment and new sterile dressing (as per unit protocol).
- Assess skin color, temperature, and sensitivity in area around catheter insertion site. Report any significant changes.

- Palpate and compare pulses in each extremity. Report any changes.

- Assess catheterized extremity for evidence of edema by measuring the contralateral extremity at the same anatomic location and comparing results from both extremities.

Rationales

- Inflammation at catheter insertion site is associated with infection or thrombophlebitis.

- Alteration in tissue perfusion may result in elevated skin temperature below catheter site. An elevation in skin temperature with pain or tenderness is associated with thrombosis or thrombophlebitis.
- A decrease or loss in arterial pulsation distal to the catheter insertion site is associated with arterial insufficiency secondary to thrombus formation.
- Edema is characteristic manifestation when decreased tissue perfusion is due to venous interference.

CARE PLAN FOR THE PATIENT UNDERGOING HEMODYNAMIC MONITORING
(*Continued*)

Nursing Diagnoses

Nursing Diagnosis #3
Potential for infection related to invasive monitoring.

Desired Patient Outcomes

Patient will be free of infection as demonstrated by:
1. Baseline temperature (normal)
2. Baseline WBC
3. Negative cultures of blood or catheter tip

Nursing Interventions

- Check patient's temperature q4h and prn and report any significant changes.
- Change catheter and catheter site q5 days or as per unit protocol.
- Change IV fluid, tubing, stopcocks, and disposable transducer q48–72 h or as per unit protocol.
- Inspect and cleanse catheter insertion site every other day, and apply iodophor ointment and clean sterile dressing.
- Do not use IV solution containing glucose.
- Place sterile dead-ender caps on all stopcocks.
- Use aseptic technique when withdrawing from or flushing the catheter.
- Carefully remove all traces of blood from stopcock ports after obtaining blood sample from catheter.
- Use sterile plastic catheter sleeve over PA catheter.

Rationales

- Increase in patient's temperature may be associated with an infectious process.
- Risk of infection increases with duration of catheter placement >5 days.
- Static fluid is a potential source for bacterial growth.

- Skin, old blood, and other such substances are potential sources for infection. Iodophor ointment reduces bacterial growth.
- Glucose solutions promote growth of bacteria.
- Open stopcock port allows bacteria to enter.
- Asepsis prevents contamination of system.

- Old blood promotes growth of bacteria.

- Maintain external portion of catheter sterile to permit catheter advancement, if necessary.

Nursing Diagnoses

Nursing Diagnosis #4
Physiologic injury related to:
1. Hemorrhage
2. Thromboemboli
3. Venous air embolism
4. Pulmonary infarction or hemorrhage
5. Cardiac arrhythmias or conduction disturbances

Desired Patient Outcomes

Patient will remain without **hemorrhage** with:
1. Stable vital signs
2. Stable hematology profile

Nursing Interventions

- Keep all catheter connecting sites visible and observe frequently for possible hemorrhage.

- Tighten all catheter connecting sites and stopcocks q4h and prn.
- Restrain patient, if necessary.

- After removal of arterial catheter, apply firm pressure to insertion site for 10 minutes before checking and applying pressure dressing.

Rationales

- Major blood loss can occur without notice from stopcocks or loose connections that are hidden beneath dressings or bed linens.
- Plastic connections become loose over time and leakage can occur.
- A restless or confused patient may pull catheter out or connecting tubing apart.
- This allows clot to form at insertion site to seal vessel opening.

Nursing Diagnoses (See *Nursing Diagnosis #4*)

Desired Patient Outcomes

Patient will remain without **thromboemboli** as evidenced by:
1. Patent catheter
2. Unimpeded infusion or flush
3. Undamped waveform

Nursing Interventions

- Use heparinized IV solution with continuous-flush device to continuously infuse all catheter ports *and* side port of sheath, if used.
- Remove air from IV bag.

Rationales

- Continuous forward flow and use of heparin are associated with decreased thrombus formation at catheter tip or around catheter in sheath.
- Air remaining in bag can diffuse into solution, causing air bubbles and damped waveform.

CARE PLAN FOR THE PATIENT UNDERGOING HEMODYNAMIC MONITORING
(*Continued*)

Nursing Interventions
- Always aspirate and discard the aspirant before gently flushing any catheter. If unable to aspirate, do not flush catheter. Periodically aspirate and manually flush catheter or activate flush device (q4–6h).
- Do not fast-flush arterial catheter for longer than 2 sec; manually flush arterial catheter by gently tapping plunger of flush syringe with no more than 2–4 mL.
- Maintain 300 mmHg pressure on IV cuff.

- Remove all traces of blood from catheter, tubing, and stopcocks after withdrawing blood, and flush completely.

Nursing Diagnoses (See *Nursing Diagnosis #4*)

Nursing Interventions
- Tighten all catheter connecting sites and stopcocks q4h and prn and check frequently.
- Place dead-ender caps on all stopcock ports.
- Keep all connections or possible openings into system below level of heart.

- Remove all air from IV solution bag.
- Have patient hum or suspend respirations when system is opened near or above heart.
- After removal of venous catheter that was in place for a long period of time, apply petroleum jelly and occlusive dressing to site.

Nursing Diagnoses (See *Nursing Diagnosis #4*)

Nursing Interventions
- Continuously monitor PA waveform at distal tip of PA catheter.
- Inflate balloon to wedge catheter briefly (≤20 sec).

- Leave balloon of PA catheter deflated with stopcock open and syringe removed.
- Monitor PAEDP instead of PAW (if closely correlated).

- Check location of catheter tip after insertion and prn via posteroanterior chest film.
- Continuously observe waveform during slow balloon inflation; stop inflation at *first* appearance of PAW waveform. Do not inflate 7F catheter with more than 1.5 mL air.
- Do not inflate balloon with air if resistance is met.

Rationales
- Removal of any fibrin or clot from within or at tip of catheter prevents injection of clot material. Heparinized fluid prevents clot formation.

- Vigorous flushing of arterial catheter with large amounts of fluid (>7 mL) can result in cerebral embolization.[51]

- 300 mmHg or greater are required to maintain flow of heparinized solution via flush device.
- Residual blood in catheter, tubing, or stopcock can form small clots, which can occlude catheter or be injected into patient.

Desired Patient Outcomes
Patient will remain without **venous air embolism**, evidenced by:
1. Absence of pain
2. Arterial blood gases within normal range

Rationales
- Plastic connections become loose over time, permitting intake of air into system.
- Open or vented ports permit intake of air.
- Air intake is more likely to occur through a loose connection or open port when the patient is in an upright position and takes a deep breath.
- Air in bag and solution enters tubing and catheter.
- Air intake through open port occurs during inspiration.

- Air intake can occur through the open track formed by long-dwelling catheter, especially in thin person with little subcutaneous tissue.

Desired Patient Outcomes
Patient will be free of **pulmonary infarction or hemorrhage** as evidenced by:
1. Normal respirations
2. No hemoptysis
3. Normal ABGs

Rationales
- Forward migration of catheter into a wedged position will be evidenced by PAW waveform.
- Brief suflation minimizes cessation in blood flow to reduce risk of pulmonary ischemia or infarction.
- Open stopcock with syringe off permits passive deflation if any air remains in balloon.
- This reduces risks of inflation of balloon and cessation of blood flow in branch of PA.
- Catheter tip may migrate forward along with blood flow into a wedge position (particularly during first 24 h).
- Overinflation of balloon can cause rupture of vessel.

- Catheter may be in a small branch of the PA and already mechanically wedged; or balloon may already be inflated.

CARE PLAN FOR THE PATIENT UNDERGOING HEMODYNAMIC MONITORING
(*Continued*)

Nursing Diagnoses (See *Nursing Diagnosis #4*)

Desired Patient Outcomes

Patient will remain free of life-threatening **arrhythmias or conduction disturbances**.

Nursing Interventions

- Continuously monitor waveform from distal port of catheter.
- Monitor chest film daily.

- If RV waveform appears, quickly inflate balloon of catheter.

- To remove catheter, deflate balloon actively and completely with syringe and quickly remove catheter.
- Follow emergency protocols for occurrence of life-threatening arrhythmias.

Rationales

- Appearance of RV waveform indicates catheter tip has fallen into RV and could cause ventricular arrhythmias.
- Check for coiling of catheter in RV or RA, which could cause arrhythmias.
- Catheter tip in RV can produce ventricular arrhythmias. With balloon inflation, catheter tip is cushioned and catheter should float to PA.
- Rapid removal of catheter with fully deflated balloon should result in few, if any, arrhythmias.

Nursing Diagnoses

Nursing Diagnosis #5
Anxiety, related to fear of technologic equipment and procedures associated with hemodynamic monitoring

Desired Patient Outcomes

Patient will:
1. Verbalize feelings
2. Demonstrate a relaxed manner
3. Verbalize familiarity with hemodynamic monitoring procedures and equipment

Nursing Interventions

- Initiate interventions to reduce anxiety.
  - Assess ability and readiness to learn the following, when appropriate:
    - Reasons for hemodynamic monitoring.
    - Function and purpose of hemodynamic monitoring equipment.
    - Explanation of procedures related to hemodynamic monitoring.
  - Instruct patient in relaxation techniques.
  - Listen attentively, encourage verbalization, and provide a caring touch.

Rationales

- Anxiety interferes with learning.
  - Readiness to learn facilitates meaningful learning and retention of knowledge.
    - Knowing rationale and purpose of hemodynamic monitoring reduces anxiety.

  - Use of energy release techniques helps reduce anxiety.
  - Listening provides reassurance to patient that he or she is not alone.

Nursing Diagnoses

Nursing Diagnosis #6
Sleep pattern disturbance, related to invasive monitoring procedures

Desired Patient Outcomes

Patient will verbalize having restful sleep.

Nursing Interventions

- Do not awaken or reposition patient to obtain hemodynamic parameters.

- Instruct in relaxation techniques.

- Provide quiet, dimly lit environment.

Rationales

- Hemodynamic measurements may be obtained with patient in flat and up to 45-degree semi-Fowler's position as long as air-reference stopcock is adjusted to mid-RA level and transducer is re-zeroed. Lateral positions may be maintained in some patients if significant changes are not observed.
- Energy release techniques help relax patient and aid in sleep.
- Quiet, dark environment is more conductive to sleep.

*PAW (pulmonary artery wedge) pressure is synonymous with PCWP (pulmonary capillary wedge pressure) as used in this text.

C H A P T E R   17

Therapeutic Modalities in the Treatment of the Patient With Cardiovascular Dysfunction

Gayle R. Whitman and Michelle Casedonte

CHAPTER OUTLINE

Goal of Therapeutic Modalities
Cardiac Pacemakers
- Purpose of the Conduction System: Impulse Transmission
- Indications for Artificial Pacing
- Principles of Artificial Pacing
- Methods of Artificial Pacing
- Modes of Artificial Pacing
- Complications of Artificial Pacing
- Nursing Considerations for Artificial Pacing

Intra-Aortic Balloon Pumping
- Goals of Intra-Aortic Balloon Pumping
- Indications for Intra-Aortic Balloon Pumping
- Technique of Counterpulsation
- Principles of Counterpulsation
- Insertion of the Balloon
- Contraindications for Intra-Aortic Balloon Pumping
- Complications of Intra-Aortic Balloon Pumping
- Nursing Considerations

Left Ventricular Assist Device
- Indications for LVAD Therapy
- Insertion of LVAD
- Complications Associated with LVAD Therapy
- Nursing Considerations for Patients with LVADs

Percutaneous Transluminal Coronary Angioplasty
- Goals of PTCA
- Indications for PTCA
- Relative Contraindications
- Technique of PTCA
- Complications of PTCA
- Nursing Considerations

Thrombolytic Therapy
- Goals of Thrombolytic Therapy
- Indications for Thrombolytic Therapy
- Types of Thrombolytic Agents
- Relative Contraindications
- Complications of Thrombolytic Therapy
- Nursing Considerations

Other Interventional Devices: Atherectomy and Stents
- Goals of Interventional Device Therapy
- Indications for Interventional Device Therapy
- Technique of Interventional Device Therapy
- Complications of Interventional Device Therapy
- Nursing Considerations

Suggested Readings

LEARNING OBJECTIVES

After completing this chapter, you should be able to:

1. Identify two indications for artificial pacing.
2. Discuss methods and modes of artificial pacing.
3. Describe nursing interventions in the care of the patient receiving a temporary or permanent pacemaker.
4. Discuss two primary goals of intra-aortic balloon pumping.
5. Review five underlying principles of intra-aortic balloon pumping.
6. Identify three potential complications of intra-aortic balloon therapy.
7. Outline nursing interventions in the care of the patient receiving intra-aortic balloon therapy.
8. Identify two indications for left ventricular assist devices (LVAD).

9. Describe nursing interventions in the care of the patient receiving an LVAD.
10. Identify the major goal of percutaneous transluminal coronary angioplasty (PTCA).
11. Explain the mechanics of the PTCA procedure.
12. Identify three potential complications of the PTCA procedure.
13. Specify nursing interventions in caring for the patient after angioplasty.
14. Identify two major goals of thrombolytic therapy.
15. Explain three criteria for clinical eligibility for thrombolytic therapy.
16. Describe three relative contraindications for treatment with thrombolytic agents.
17. Discuss three common complications encountered with administration of thrombolytic agents for coronary artery disease (CAD).
18. Explain the goals of interventional device therapy.
19. Describe the current indications for interventional device therapy.
20. Identify two major complications of interventional device therapy.
21. Identify two nursing considerations for the patient receiving interventional device therapy.

GOAL OF THERAPEUTIC MODALITIES

The heart is a complex organ that provides the pumping activity necessary to maintain circulation of blood to all the tissues of the body, distributing oxygen and nutrients and removing cellular waste products. Cardiac activity is achieved through integration of electrical and mechanical mechanisms that ensure the forward flow of blood throughout the vasculature. Many conditions occur clinically that impair the heart's intrinsic ability to pump blood and require a variety of therapeutic interventions. These treatment modalities are aimed at supporting the mechanical pumping activity required for adequate tissue perfusion. This chapter highlights the most current interventions that affect both the electrical and mechanical

cardiac activity and examines the goals of treatment, clinical indications, physiologic principles guiding the therapy, relative contraindications, technical aspects of each intervention, potential complications, and nursing considerations.

CARDIAC PACEMAKERS

Purpose of the Conduction System: Impulse Transmission

As previously discussed, the conduction system within the heart is a collection of specialized tissue that transmits impulses throughout the myocardium in a rapid and organized fashion (Fig. 17–1). This causes

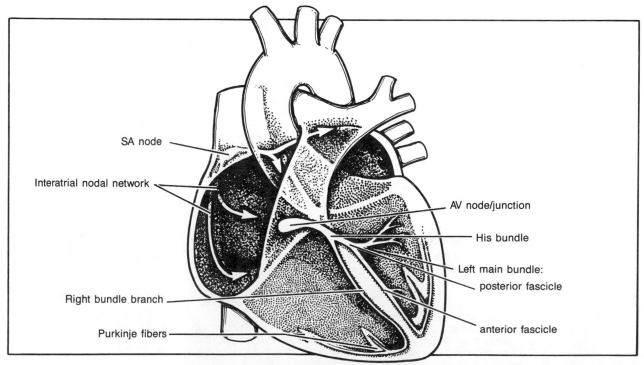

FIGURE 17–1. The conduction system of the heart.

simultaneous depolarization of the atrium and then of the ventricles, which allows for synchronization of contraction and optimal ejection of blood with every beat. Failure of the conduction system to transmit impulses to the ventricle diminishes the heart's ability to maintain adequate tissue perfusion.

The conduction system also possesses the unique property of *automaticity,* which allows the cells to spontaneously depolarize without being stimulated by an outside source. This important property provides a series of back-up mechanisms for pacing the heart if the primary pacemaker—usually the sinus node—fails to discharge impulses at its set rate.

At times, other cells within the myocardium exhibit automaticity and attempt to control the pacing function of the heart (i.e., ectopic pacemakers). If the ectopic pacemaker fires impulses at a rate that exceeds the sinus node discharge rate, the ectopic site then depolarizes the ventricles and assumes the primary pacing function of the heart. Often, depolarization of the ventricles from an ectopic site decreases the ability of the heart to allow for adequate ventricular filling and limits synchronous contractile efforts that normally provide for optimal ejection of blood.

Indications for Artificial Pacing

Artificial pacing is indicated whenever the conduction system fails to transmit impulses from the sinus node to the ventricles, to generate an impulse spontaneously, or to maintain primary control of the pacing function of the heart. Table 17–1 summarizes the primary indications for artificial pacing.

Many pathophysiologic and iatrogenic conditions are encountered clinically that affect the conduction system's ability to function normally, creating circumstances for which pacing is indicated. These conditions, summarized in Table 17–2, may temporarily or permanently impair cellular activity, prohibiting normal generation and transmission of impulses.

Goals of Artificial Pacing

Artificial pacing is intended to provide a physiologic "back-up" for the heart during failure of the conduction system to depolarize the myocardium and main-

TABLE 17–1
Primary Indications for Artificial Pacing

Disruption of the Ability to Generate and Transmit Impulses
Bradyarrhythmias
Heart block
Sick sinus syndrome
Sinus arrest
Asystole

Control of Arrhythmias Related to Ectopic Pacemakers
Atrial tachyarrhythmias
Ventricular tachyarrhythmias

TABLE 17–2
Common Conditions That Impair Cardiac Conduction

Pathophysiologic
Acute myocardial infarction
Myocardial ischemia
Autonomic nervous system failure
Electrolyte imbalance

Iatrogenic
Drug toxicity (antiarrhythmics)
Cardiac, surgery
Ablation

tain an adequate cardiac output. When cardiac output is diminished because of lack of depolarization of the ventricles, artificial pacing will provide the necessary stimulus directly to the ventricles for contraction to occur. If cardiac output is compromised because an ectopic pacemaker is causing the ventricles to depolarize and contract at a rate that does not promote adequate ventricular filling, artificial pacing will compete with the ectopic pacemaker to assume the primary pacing function of the heart.

Principles of Artificial Pacing

The System

An artificial pacemaker provides an external source of energy for impulse formation and delivery and for stimulation of myocardial tissue. In any pacemaker, there are several key components that are integrated within the system: the pulse generator with circuitry, the lead, and the electrode system.

The *pulse generator* is the component that houses the energy source and the electronics that control the pacemaker function. The *lead* is the component that provides communication between the pulse generator and the myocardium. The *electrode* is the component of the pacemaker system that provides direct contact with the myocardial tissue.

The Mechanism

To understand how pacemakers actually work, it is important to reflect on a few basic principles of electricity. First, all tissues of the body are capable of conducting electrical impulses, and it is possible to have positive and negative electrical charges (electrons) present in a system. When this condition occurs, an electrical circuit develops because of the attraction of the electrons from the negative end (or pole) to the positive end. Electrical current, measured in milliamperes (mA), reflects the net electrical energy within the circuit. Next, it is possible to measure the minimal amount of electrical energy that is required to cause depolarization and contraction of the myocardium on a continuous basis. This minimal level of energy is known as the *stimulation threshold.* Finally, the stimulation threshold can be affected by a number of factors, including quality of communication with the myocardial tissue, ability of the tissue to propagate impulses, and the characteristics of the lead itself.

Pacemakers rely on the latter principles in their delivery of energy to the myocardium. Because the goal of impulse delivery is to have electrical energy travel from the lead to the myocardium, there is always a negative pole on the lead itself. The location of the positive pole within the system defines the type of lead configuration used. In a *unipolar* lead system, the positive pole is located outside the myocardium, either on the pulse generator itself or on a positive electrode or on the skin. In this type of system, the energy travels from the lead (negative pole) through the myocardium and thoracic musculature back to the positive electrode. In a *bipolar* system, both the positive and negative poles are located within the myocardium itself, creating an electrical circuit that does not leave the heart. This is by far the most common lead system used.

Methods of Artificial Pacing

There are three major methods of delivering energy to the myocardial tissue for the purpose of artificial pacing: external (transthoracic), epicardial (transthoracic), and endocardial (transvenous). *External* (transthoracic) pacing delivers energy to the heart through the thoracic musculature via two surface electrode patches (Fig. 17–2). Because these electrodes have no direct contact with the heart, large amounts of electrical energy are required to stimulate depolarization of myocardial tissue. This method of pacing is used only when transvenous pacing cannot be used immediately, that is, in emergency resuscitation of a patient in whom a pacing wire has not yet been placed or for whom invasive procedures are contraindicated owing to immunosuppression.

Epicardial pacing is another method of artificial pacing in which the electrical energy travels from an external pulse generator through the thoracic musculature directly to the epicardial surface of the heart via lead wires (Fig. 17–3). This method of pacing is most common during and immediately following open heart surgery, since there is direct access to the epicardium at this time.

The most common method of artificial pacing is by *endocardial* (transvenous) lead wires that are threaded through the large central veins (subclavian, jugular, or femoral) into the right atrium and lodged within the wall of the right ventricle (Fig. 17–3). The electrical energy source for transvenous pacing can arise from an internal or external pulse generator, depending on the nature of the patient's condition.

Artificial pacing can be used for a finite period of time, such as when the disruption of the conduction system is thought to be *temporary,* or the artificial pacer can be implanted as a *permanent* back-up for cardiac function when the disruption of the conduction system is thought to be irreversible.

Modes of Artificial Pacing

An artificial pacemaker can function in a variety of ways to complement the intrinsic electrical activity of the heart. The most basic type of pacemaker fires at a set rate, regardless of the heart's ability to generate

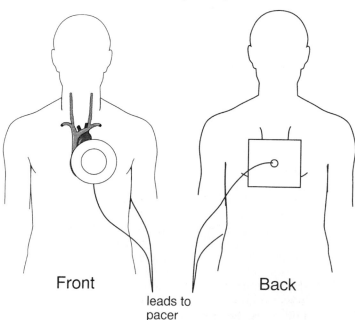

Noninvasive Temporary Pacemakers

Front

leads to pacer

Back

FIGURE 17–2. Example of external (transthoracic) pacing.

Temporary Pacemakers

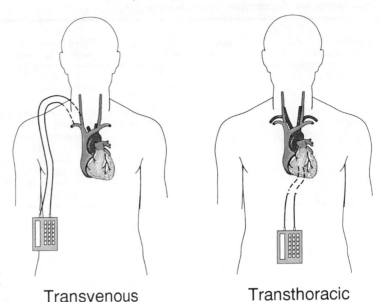

Transvenous   Transthoracic

FIGURE 17–3. Examples of endocardial (transvenous) and epicardial (transthoracic) temporary pacing.

spontaneous impulses. This type of pacemaker is known as an *asynchronous, fixed-rate,* or *nondemand* pacemaker. This mode of pacing is appropriate in the absence of any electrical activity (asystole), but is dangerous in the presence of an intrinsic rhythm because of the potential of the pacemaker to fire during the vulnerable period of repolarization and initiate lethal ventricular arrhythmias.

The more common type of pacemaker senses the natural electrical activity of the heart and fires only when intrinsic activity is not sensed for a predetermined interval of time. This mode of pacing is known as *demand pacing,* because it initiates pacing only when needed.

A pacemaker is also able to pace different chambers of the heart, depending on placement of the lead/electrode system. If the integrity of the conduction system is not impaired through the AV node to the ventricles, it is possible to pace the atria and send impulses normally to the ventricles. This type of pacing would be indicated in the presence of sinus node disease. The electrocardiographic indicator of atrial pacing is a pacer spike followed by a P wave and a normal QRS complex. Atrial pacemakers are beneficial because they preserve the normal synchrony of depolarization and contraction, allowing the atria to contribute to ventricular filling, which can account for 20% to 30% of the total cardiac output.

The ventricles can be stimulated by a pacemaker when a lead wire is placed directly into the right ventricle. This is a common type of pacing seen in critical care, particularly when the pacing is for a temporary situation. Ventricular pacing is indicated when transmission of impulses from the atria is being blocked before depolarization of the ventricles. Electrocardiographic indicators of ventricular pacing include a

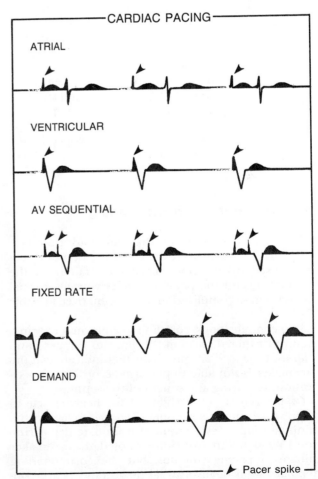

FIGURE 17–4. Electrocardiographic examples of artificial cardiac pacing.

TABLE 17–3
ICHD Code for Pacemaker Identification

First Letter: Chamber Paced	Second Letter: Chamber Sensed	Third Letter: Mode of Response	Fourth Letter: Programmable Functions	Fifth Letter: Tachyarrhythmic Functions
V = ventricle A = atrium	V = ventricle A = atrium	T = triggered (may have energy output triggered)	P = programmable for 1 or 2 functions	B = bursts of pacing
D = dual chamber (both atria and ventricles stimulated)	D = dual chamber (sensing capabilities in atrium and ventricle)	I = inhibited (pacing output inhibited by intrinsic activity)	M = multiprogrammable ability to change functions other than the rate or output	N = normal rate competition
	O = no sensing capability	D = dual chamber (may be either inhibition or triggering of both chambers)		S = scanning

pacer spike followed immediately by a wide QRS complex. Ventricular pacemakers do not permit synchrony of the atrial activity with ventricular contraction and thus result in a loss of the atrial contribution to cardiac output.

Because this synchrony of atria and ventricles is vital in certain patients, pacemakers are available that mimic the physiologic depolarization of the heart by synchronizing an atrial impulse with a ventricular impulse at predetermined intervals. These pacemakers are known as *AV sequential pacemakers*. Examples of artificial pacing on the electrocardiogram (ECG) are depicted in Figure 17–4.

In addition to these capabilities, permanent pacemakers now have special programmable and antitachyarrhythmic functions, which are quite complex. To communicate all the functions of the individual pacemakers, an international code was developed by the Inter-Society Commission for Heart Disease (ICHD). This code is summarized in Table 17–3.

Complications of Artificial Pacing

The many complications that can result from artificially pacing the heart relate to the method and technique used in insertion, mechanical failure of the pacemaker, and the patient's underlying myocardial disease. These complications are summarized in Table 17–4.

Two complications, common to all forms of pacing, require further discussion. "Failure to capture" and "failure to sense" are problems that indicate that the pacemaker is not able to perform according to specification, requiring adjustment of the settings.

Capture refers to the ability of the heart muscle to respond to stimulus output. (*Threshold* refers to the minimal output level required to initiate depolarization.) When failure to capture is noted, the pacemaker initiates a pacing stimulus, but the corresponding depolarization of myocardial tissue (and hence contraction) is absent.

This complication is detected by observing pacing spikes without the associated P wave or QRS complex on the ECG. Increases in stimulus output are commonly needed with fibrosis or dislodgement of the electrode tip, myocardial ischemia or infarction, antiarrhythmic therapy, or electrolyte imbalance. Adjustment of the voltage, current (mA), or pulse duration will correct this problem.

Sensing refers to the ability of the pacemaker to detect intrinsic electrical activity and respond according to the programmed mode. Failure to sense describes a circumstance in which the detection system does not recognize intrinsic electrical activity, responding in ways that might actually compete with

TABLE 17–4
Complications of Artificial Pacing

Method	Complication
External transthoracic pacing	Pain with impulse delivery Skin burns Muscular twitching Psychological reactions Failure to capture* Failure to sense†
Epicardial pacing	Dislodgement of lead Microshock Cardiac tamponade Infection Psychological reactions Failure to capture* Failure to sense†
Endocardial (transvenous) pacing	Myocardial irritability Perforation of chamber or septum Electromagnetic interference Infection Embolism Abdominal twitching Hiccups Pacer-induced arrhythmias Failure to capture* Failure to sense†

*Inability of impulse to initiate a contraction.
†Inability of pacemaker to sense intrinsic electrical activity.

the patient's own rhythm. This is recognized on the ECG by pacemaker spikes falling at intervals that are different from the programmed escape interval (the period of time between the last sensed beat and the paced beat). This condition predisposes the heart to discharge of an impulse during a vulnerable phase of the electrical cycle (i.e., the latter half of the T wave), which might precipitate life-threatening ventricular arrhythmias. Adjustment of the sensitivity setting (decreasing the amplitude at which electrical activity is recognized) or repositioning the catheter may alleviate this complication.

Nursing Considerations for Artificial Pacing

Although the principles for pacing are the same whether temporary or permanent pacing is used, each has distinct nursing implications that should be considered. Areas of focus for the patient receiving a temporary pacemaker include the following:

1. Explanation of the procedure for the patient and family
2. Monitoring the patient's response to the procedure
3. Maintaining electrical safety
4. Monitoring pacing parameters (sensing, capture, threshold)
5. Protecting the patient from injury and infection

Table 17–5 summarizes procedures for checking the threshold of a temporary pacemaker.

The patient receiving a permanent pacemaker also has unique needs on which the nurse must focus. These needs include:

1. Psychological adaptation
2. Patient education
3. Follow-up care
4. Infection

(See the care plans for patients with temporary and permanent pacemakers at the end of this chapter.)

INTRA-AORTIC BALLOON PUMPING

Goals of Intra-Aortic Balloon Pumping

Intra-aortic balloon pumping, or counterpulsation, is a method of providing assistance to the left ventricle during periods of acute cardiac failure.

The intra-aortic balloon pump (IABP) provides support by improving perfusion of the myocardium and reducing the workload of the left ventricle. Major goals of IABP include the following:

1. Improving cardiac output by decreasing myocardial work
2. Decreasing myocardial ischemia
3. Reducing the amount of myocardial damage
4. Providing hemodynamic stability until definitive treatment can be initiated

Indications for Intra-Aortic Balloon Pumping

Intra-aortic balloon pumping can be used in both medical and surgical settings to support the injured myocardium. Table 17–6 summarizes the most common indications for IABP.

TABLE 17–5
Sample Procedure for Checking Threshold

Action	Rationale
1. Make sure pacer is on the demand mode.	1. This prevents competition with the patient's intrinsic rhythm.
2. Turn pacemaker rate up slowly until capture is seen for every beat. (This is evidenced by a pacemaker spike firing at the set rate, followed by a QRS complex for each spike.)	2. The patient has to be pacing continuously to be able to assess the level of energy at which the myocardium is captured by the pacing stimulus.
3. Slowly decrease mA or the current output level until loss of capture is noted. This is demonstrated by pacemaker spikes without associated QRS complexes on the ECG.	
4. Increase mA until capture is noted for every beat.	4. The minimal level of energy necessary to stimulate and depolarize the myocardium with each beat is the threshold.
5. Document this energy level and compare with previous threshold.	5. This monitors for increased tolerance to energy levels. The amount of energy required to depolarize the myocardium is influenced by a number of factors, including electrolyte balance, concurrent drug therapy, and quality of lead contact with the myocardium.
6. Set the mA 1.5–2 points above the threshold.	6. The setting of output should be adjusted to ensure continuous pacing despite changes in the dynamic system of the body.
7. Check threshold daily.	7. Threshold can change owing to fibrosis at lead tip, ischemia, electrolyte balance, and hypoxia.

TABLE 17–6
Indications for Intra-Aortic Balloon Pumping

Clinical Condition	Rationale
1. Preinfarction angina 2. Acute myocardial infarction 3. Cardiogenic shock	To improve coronary perfusion, decrease left ventricular work, and reduce the amount of myocardium that is damaged
4. Refractory ventricular arrhythmias related to ischemias	To improve perfusion to the ischemic area, causing firing of an ectopic focus; to reduce myocardial oxygen demand
5. Severe mitral valve regurgitation 6. Severe ventricular septal defect	To improve left ventricular emptying, encouraging forward flow of blood, and to reduce the severity of regurgitation or shunting
7. Pre–open heart surgery or cardiac transplantation	To support the heart until surgical intervention can ameliorate the underlying problem
8. Intraoperative open heart surgery/weaning from cardiopulmonary bypass 9. Post–open heart surgery	To support the ventricle until it recovers from surgery
10. Low cardiac output syndromes 11. Septic shock	To promote adequate tissue perfusion by assisting left ventricular emptying
12. Prophylaxis	To prevent cardiac decompensation, myocardial damage in high-risk situations (i.e., noncardiac surgeries in the presence of severe left ventricular dysfunction, high-risk PTCA)

Technique of Counterpulsation

The intra-aortic balloon is an oblong, polyurethane receptacle that is attached to a catheter. The catheter may contain a central lumen that communicates directly with the arterial blood in the aorta, providing exact measurements of central aortic root pressures from which balloon inflation and deflation can be timed. The balloon itself is attached to tubing from the pneumatic system, which regulates the shuttling of gas to inflate and deflate the balloon. Two gases are commonly used for balloon pumping: helium and carbon dioxide. The pneumatic drive system is housed in a console, from which all interaction with the balloon occurs.

Principles of Counterpulsation

Intra-aortic balloon pumping must coordinate with the cardiac cycle so as not to impede the ejection of blood. Counterpulsation can be thought of as a completely *diastolic event,* in which inflation of the balloon occurs at the beginning of diastole and deflation occurs just prior to the next systolic ejection.

Because inflation and deflation must coincide with

systole and diastole, a method of *triggering* balloon activity must be selected by the nurse. Most commonly the patient's ECG, or, more specifically, the R wave, is used to signal the beginning of systole. Another triggering mode that can be used is the arterial waveform (see Fig. 16–9), in which the balloon responds to the upstroke of the wave. A third mode of triggering, called *internal trigger,* is used in the absence of any intrinsic electrical or mechanical activity, such as when the patient is on cardiopulmonary bypass. With internal triggering, inflation and deflation occur at a preset rate. This helps to prevent clot formation on a stagnant noninflating balloon.

Although the triggering signal provides the balloon with general information about inflation and deflation, its action must be timed precisely with the mechanical cardiac events to optimize the effects of counterpulsation. Remember that the electrical events reflected on the surface ECG occur before mechanical events are recorded on the arterial tracing. It is therefore essential to monitor a continuous arterial waveform to allow for minute adjustments in balloon inflation and deflation (Fig. 17–5). Ideally, when monitoring an arterial pressure waveform, inflation should occur at the dicrotic notch. The dicrotic notch reflects closure of the aortic valve. Deflation should occur just prior to the next upstroke of the systolic wave, as illustrated in Figure 17–5.

When the balloon inflates at the beginning of diastole, the blood located in that segment of the aorta is forced back into the aortic arch, increasing the amount of pressure with which the coronary arteries are perfused. This increase in aortic pressure during diastole is known as *diastolic augmentation.* Augmentation of coronary perfusion during ischemic events is critical in offsetting the imbalance between oxygen supply and demand. The myocardium is extremely efficient in its extraction of oxygen, such that the *only* way to meet greater metabolic needs is to increase the amount of blood circulating through the tissue. In the presence of occlusive coronary artery disease (CAD), it becomes increasingly difficult to meet these demands.

Upon deflation of the balloon before systole, there is a redistribution of blood away from the aortic root, thereby decreasing the pressure against which the left ventricle must work to open the aortic valve. This reduction in afterload is known as *diastolic unloading.* Diastolic unloading also decreases myocardial oxygen demands significantly, thereby assisting a jeopardized ischemic myocardium from becoming more ischemic.

Insertion of the Balloon

Two techniques are used for initiating balloon pumping: surgical and percutaneous. The surgical technique requires the performance of a femoral arteriotomy and is usually done in the operating room. This method is relatively time-consuming and exposes

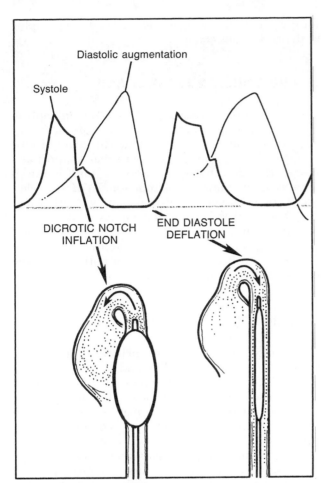

FIGURE 17–5. Intra-aortic balloon pumping and the cardiac cycle reflecting systole and diastole. Balloon inflation and deflation are depicted, with inflation occurring at the dicrotic notch and deflation occurring just prior to the next upstroke of the systolic wave. Diastolic augmentation reflects the increase in aortic pressures afforded by an inflated balloon during left ventricular diastole, thereby increasing coronary artery perfusion pressures.

the patient to greater risks because of the surgical nature of the incision. The advent of the percutaneous technique made balloon pumping a much more attractive treatment modality because of the relative ease with which insertion could occur.

Balloon pumping can occur at a number of frequencies relative to the cardiac cycle, depending on the amount of support required by the left ventricle. The balloon can inflate and deflate with each ejection (1:1 frequency), with every other ejection (1:2), or with every third ejection (1:3). On average, the IABP is used for a period of 2 to 4 days, during which time hemodynamic support with pharmacologic agents is maximized. After the patient's condition has remained stable for a 24-hour period and stable hemodynamic parameters have been achieved, balloon support is withdrawn.

Because the work of the left ventricle has been

assisted for a period of time, it is important to gradually *wean* the patient from the IABP. This is usually accomplished by decreasing the frequency with which balloon pumping occurs (i.e., 1:2, then 1:3).

Clinical parameters used in determining when a patient is capable of being weaned from the IABP include:

1. Evidence of adequate cardiac function
   a. Cardiac index greater than 2.0 L/min per square meter
   b. Pulmonary capillary wedge pressure less than 18 to 20 mmHg
   c. Urine output greater than 30 mL/h
   d. Return of peripheral pulse quality to patient baseline
   e. Absence of subjective complaints of shortness of breath
   f. Breath sounds clear
   g. Skin warm and dry
   h. Mentation returned to baseline
2. Evidence of resolution of myocardial ischemia
   a. Absence of chest pain
   b. Absence of acute ischemia reflected on ECG
   c. Resolution of arrhythmias related to ischemia

During the weaning period, the patient's clinical response must be closely monitored for signs of left ventricular failure or recurrence of myocardial ischemia, since it is possible to develop dependence on the balloon for hemodynamic support and augmentation of coronary perfusion. Once weaning has occurred successfully, the deflated balloon is withdrawn from the aorta along with the introducer sheath and direct pressure is maintained at the femoral site for about 30 minutes.

Contraindications for Intra-Aortic Balloon Pumping

Patient benefit, end goal of treatment regimen, and risks posed by insertion of the balloon catheter must be considered before the IABP is placed. Table 17–7 summarizes these absolute and relative contraindications to IABP therapy.

Complications of Intra-Aortic Balloon Pumping

A number of complications can occur from insertion and maintenance of the IABP in the aorta. Upon insertion, the balloon catheter may dissect any part of the arterial system through which it travels (femoral, iliac, aorta), or it may dislodge a plaque, causing embolization. The placement of the balloon itself may cause problems after it is inserted. If the catheter is too advanced, it can occlude the left subclavian artery, causing diminished flow to the left arm, or it can hinder flow cephalad. If the catheter is not advanced far enough, it can occlude the renal arteries, compromis-

TABLE 17–7
Contraindications for Intra-Aortic Balloon Pumping

Clinical Condition	Rationale
Absolute Contraindications	
Aortic aneurysm	High risk of aortic
Bypass grafting from the aorta to peripheral vessels	dissection
Aortic insufficiency	Inflation of the intra-aortic balloon during diastole will exacerbate the regurgitant flow into the left ventricle
Relative Contraindications	
Peripheral or central atherosclerosis	High risk of vascular compromise distal to the balloon
	High risk of plaque dislodgment
	Inability to pass catheter
Age	Ethical considerations
Severe left ventricular dysfunction	necessary to determine
Multisystem failure	whether there is a
Chronic, debilitating disease	treatment regimen available that will improve the current quality of life before intervention with IABP is instituted
Bleeding disorders	High risk for hemorrhage
History of embolic phenomena	High risk for thromboembolic events with IABP catheter

ing perfusion of the kidneys. It is also possible that, because of severe atherosclerosis, the catheter cannot be threaded at all in some patients.

After the balloon has been placed, possible complications are balloon rupture, embolization, arterial occlusion, mechanical destruction of red blood cells (RBCs) because of pumping, or inability to wean from the pump.

During removal of the catheter, it is again possible to fragment or puncture the intima of the vessel, cause embolization, or cause a hematoma at the insertion site.

Nursing Considerations

The care of the patient requiring intra-aortic balloon support is complex and requires specific training to coordinate all aspects of hemodynamic support. Much attention is centered around monitoring the patient's response to treatment, identifying and treating actual problems, and preventing potential problems. Because of all the equipment and treatments required for the critically ill who need IABP therapy, it is often possible to lose sight of the human factor in care. These patients are usually alert and frightened by the technical support that is required to sustain them. It is imperative for the nurse to provide support and comfort to the patient and family in addition to coordinating other aspects of care. (See the care plan

for the patient requiring intra-aortic balloon pumping at the end of this chapter.)

LEFT VENTRICULAR ASSIST DEVICE

A left ventricular assist device (LVAD) is an implantable, mechanical device used to support or bypass deteriorating myocardial function. The goal of LVAD therapy is to provide temporary cardiac support as a bridge to heart transplantation or until there is improvement in myocardial function. LVADs are electrically or pneumatically driven pumps inserted into the abdominal wall or peritoneal cavity. A cable or pneumatic line extends through the abdominal wall connecting the pump to a power source. The power source is usually contained within a portable console that allows for patient mobility.

Indications for LVAD Therapy

Indications for LVAD use include patients who, despite ample volume loading and maximum inotropic and IABP support, continue to exhibit signs and symptoms of severe left ventricular failure or cardiogenic shock. However, patients may be excluded from LVAD therapy if the following conditions exist: chronic renal failure; severe peripheral vascular, cerebrovascular, hepatic, pulmonary, and hematologic diseases; age greater than 65 years; malignancies with metastasis; or severe infections resistant to therapies. Also, LVADs should be used only in patients with isolated left ventricular failure; they are not appropriate for patients with right ventricular failure.

Insertion of LVAD

Insertion of an implantable LVAD is similar to the procedure in bypass surgery, since cardiopulmonary bypass and a midline incision are required. The left ventricle and aorta are cannulated, and the pump is subcutaneously or preperitoneally inserted into the upper left quadrant of the abdomen. The power cable is tunneled through the abdominal tissue and to the skin surface, where the cable is attached to the console.

Complications Associated with LVAD Therapy

Complications associated with LVADs include acute renal failure, hemorrhage, infection, embolization, adult respiratory distress syndrome, transient ischemic attacks, cerebrovascular accidents, and multisystem failure. Although rare, device failure can also occur secondary to power cable, valve, or console malfunction.

Nursing Considerations for Patients with LVADs

Nursing interventions in patients with LVADs are centered on prevention of complications. Monitoring for signs and symptoms of hemorrhage, infection, arrhythmias, and ventricular failure is critical. Ventricular failure is usually right-sided in LVAD patients and may be treated with medications or, if severe, with a right ventricular assist device. Infrequent premature ventricular contractions (PVCs) are usually tolerated by the patient. However, runs of PVCs and ventricular tachycardia may require treatment with antiarrhythmic medications or cardioversion. To prevent infection, meticulous aseptic technique is vital in LVAD dressing changes, intravenous line, and drainage catheter maintenance. Prophylactic antibiotics are used after insertion. Blood, urine, and sputum cultures are collected when body temperature rises higher than 100.4°F, and antibiotics are initiated when infection is present. Hemorrhage can be life-threatening and is related to the surgical implantation and postinsertion anticoagulation needed for LVAD maintenance. Packed RBCs should always be available until bleeding is controlled.

Psychological support of the patient and family is vital. Patient and family education should include information regarding all procedures and complications associated with LVAD therapy. The patient and family should take part in decision-making, scheduling, and physical care to decrease anxiety and impart a sense of control over their surroundings.

PERCUTANEOUS TRANSLUMINAL CORONARY ANGIOPLASTY

Goals of PTCA

Percutaneous transluminal coronary angioplasty (PTCA) is a nonsurgical method of revascularizing myocardial tissue. Goals of treatment include the following:

1. Prevention of myocardial necrosis
2. Reduction of myocardial ischemia
3. Limitation of myocardial infarct size
4. Improvement of left ventricular function
5. Reduction in morbidity and mortality associated with CAD

Indications for PTCA

PTCA has become a major treatment modality for occlusive CAD. It is indicated for prophylactic treatment of severe CAD before infarction has occurred, in the presence of symptomatic CAD, or during an acute infarction. PTCA is a viable treatment option for stenosis of grafted vessels. It is possible to revascularize multiple vessels at once, but the occlusive lesions must be amenable to dilatation.

Several clinical situations are common indications for resolution of coronary stenosis by PTCA. Single-vessel or multiple-vessel disease associated with recent onset of angina and clinical signs of ischemia with distinct, subtotal lesions not located at the orifice or bifurcation of a coronary artery can benefit from dilatation. Patients with acute evolving myocardial infarctions may be treated with PTCA alone or in conjunction with thrombolytic therapy. Stenotic lesions in bypass grafts may be amenable to dilatation if the lesion is not diffuse and not located in an anatomically difficult location. Many patients who receive angioplasty reocclude and require two or three redilatations. However, benefit to the patient or safety in performing a PTCA cannot be ensured in certain clinical conditions.

Relative Contraindications

PTCA is contraindicated in the setting of severe diffuse coronary atherosclerosis and severe central (i.e., aortic, iliac) and peripheral atherosclerotic diseases.

Technique of PTCA

PTCA is a relatively simple procedure that is performed under fluoroscopy in the cardiac catheterization laboratory. Using aseptic technique, the femoral artery and vein are cannulated with introducer sheaths via a percutaneous approach.

A steerable catheter very similar to the one used for cardiac catheterization with a balloon at the tip is threaded into the coronary artery through the femoral arterial sheath. After the catheter has passed into the coronary artery, it must be positioned so that the balloon is resting at the site of coronary stenosis (Fig. 17–6). The balloon is expanded over the plaque for 10 to 15 seconds to actually compress or flatten the plaque. During this inflation period, blood flow distal to the balloon is compromised. This sequence of inflation and deflation is repeated until improved coronary artery perfusion is noted.

Complications of PTCA

Potential complications of PTCA can be found in Table 17–8.

Nursing Considerations

The patient requiring a PTCA has a disease that is often difficult to accept because of the inability to "see" something wrong. Unless acute symptoms of severe CAD allow the patient to perceive a health threat, it may be hard for the patient to integrate the notion that lifestyle changes are required because of a risk of a severe heart attack. It is a challenge for the

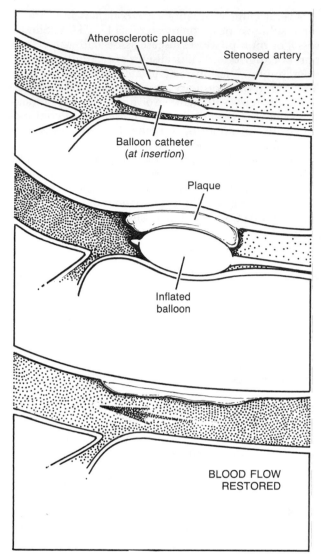

FIGURE 17–6. Technique of percutaneous transluminal coronary angioplasty.

nurse to address these educational issues as well as monitor the patient for actual and potential complications of the procedure. (See the care plan for the patient with percutaneous transluminal coronary angioplasty at the end of this chapter.)

TABLE 17–8
Potential Complications of Percutaneous Transluminal Coronary Angioplasty

Acute coronary occlusion—myocardial infarction
Internal tear of the coronary vessel wall
Dissection of coronary artery
Inability to dilate the stenosis
Embolization of plaque fragments
Restenosis of the coronary artery: acute, chronic
Bleeding/hematoma
Dissection of the aorta, iliac, or femoral arteries
Compromise of peripheral circulation
Arrhythmias

THROMBOLYTIC THERAPY

Goals of Thrombolytic Therapy

Thrombolytic therapy is used for occlusive CAD. A pharmacologic agent is administered for the purpose of dissolving thrombi formed at the site of an atherosclerotic lesion. The major goals of thrombolytic therapy are very similar to those of any other method of revascularization:

1. Improving coronary artery perfusion
2. Limiting the extent of myocardial ischemia/ infarction
3. Improving left ventricular function
4. Limiting arrhythmias related to ischemia
5. Improving morbidity and mortality related to CAD

Indications for Thrombolytic Therapy

Myocardial necrosis can begin within 20 minutes after onset of ischemia and progresses through the myocardial layers within 3 to 6 hours. Thrombolytic therapy is indicated for that patient population in which complete myocardial necrosis has not occurred. The following are indications for thrombolytic therapy:

1. Acute chest pain with clinical presentation of acute myocardial infarction
2. ECG changes that reflect acute myocardial ischemia
3. Lack of relief of chest pain with nitroglycerin administration
4. Initiation of treatment within the first 6 hours after symptom onset

Use of a thrombolytic agent is merely a temporizing measure for reperfusion of the myocardium. Often, more conventional methods of treating the underlying CAD are then required (i.e., coronary bypass grafting or PTCA).

Types of Thrombolytic Agents

Ideally, a thrombolytic agent must be able to specifically dissolve the clot within the coronary artery without disrupting the integrity of the patient's blood clotting system. The two pharmacologic agents currently used for thrombolytic therapy of coronary artery occlusions are streptokinase and tissue-plasminogen activator (tPA).

Streptokinase, an enzyme produced by β-hemolytic streptococci, has been the primary coronary thrombolytic agent used. It acts by stimulating the conversion of plasminogen to plasmin within the circulation, thereby promoting the destruction of fibrin clots.

Tissue-plasminogen activator (tPA or Activase), recently approved for use in the setting of coronary artery thrombosis, is a naturally occurring human enzyme that acts with greater fibrin specificity by converting plasminogen to plasmin *after* it binds to fibrin clots. It is believed to achieve clot lysis more rapidly and with greater efficacy than streptokinase, and its positive effect in salvaging left ventricular function has been conclusively demonstrated in clinical trials.

Relative Contraindications

Thrombolytic agents not only interfere with the blood's ability to form clots, they are also unable to differentiate the offensive coronary artery thrombus from other protective clots that develop in response to vascular injury. In addition, because streptokinase is produced by the β-hemolytic streptococci, it is antigenic to many individuals. Table 17–9 summarizes the conditions that may preclude the use of thrombolytic agents in the treatment of acute myocardial ischemia.

Complications of Thrombolytic Therapy

The nurse caring for the patient receiving a thrombolytic agent must consider the possibility of a number of major complications, including bleeding, allergic response, reocclusion or reinfarction, and reperfusion arrhythmias.

Bleeding is the most common complication encountered during thrombolytic therapy because of the intentional alteration in the patient's blood-clotting ability. The bleeding incidents have ranged from superficial to severe internal hemorrhage.

The most common bleeding complication observed has been oozing or hematoma formation at the catheterization site. Other frequently observed locations for superficial bleeding include venous or arterial puncture sites, gingival bleeding, cuts or abrasions, and ecchymosis from patient manipulation. The more severe, less frequently occurring bleeding incidents include intracranial, gastrointestinal, retroperitoneal, and genitourinary bleeding. Many of these bleeding complications can be minimized or avoided by careful pretreatment assessment of the patient for risk of bleeding.

Because many adults have had prior exposure to the

β-hemolytic streptococcal bacteria, it is very common for a person receiving streptokinase to exhibit some manifestation of an allergic response. (tPA is naturally occurring and nonantigenic.) The severity of this response can range from a mild elevation of body temperature and itching to severe hives and anaphylaxis, depending on the extent of prior sensitization.

There is always a risk of reocclusion of the treated coronary artery following thrombolytic therapy because of the relatively short duration of effect of the therapy. After the clot has been successfully dissolved, a high-degree atherosclerotic lesion may remain, predisposing the patient to recurrence of the occlusion and possible infarction. The risk of reocclusion is greatest within the first 24 hours after recanalization. It has therefore become standard practice to initiate concurrent anticoagulant therapy with heparin to decrease the risk of reocclusion.

Another phenomenon that has been observed following thrombolytic therapy is the occurrence of arrhythmias upon reperfusion of the ischemic myocardium, termed *reperfusion arrhythmias*. The mechanism for these arrhythmias is not clear, but a variety of rhythm disturbances have been manifested, including accelerated idioventricular rhythm, ventricular tachycardia, premature ventricular contractions, sinus bradycardia, and high-grade atrioventricular (AV) blocks.

Nursing Considerations

The patient receiving thrombolytic therapy is at risk for a multitude of actual and potential health problems that the nurse must address in developing a plan of care. Of primary concern is the stabilization of the patient's condition and preservation of myocardial function. Specific nursing diagnoses, desired patient outcomes, and nursing interventions in the care of the patient receiving thrombolytic therapy are presented in the care plan at the end of this chapter.

OTHER INTERVENTIONAL DEVICES: ATHERECTOMY AND STENTS

Coronary atherectomy and intravascular stents are adjuncts to balloon angioplasty that have been developed to overcome the limitations of PTCA. Both procedures are used to increase blood flow to the coronary arteries, thereby reducing myocardial ischemia.

Coronary atherectomy is the excision and removal of atherosclerotic plaque that is restricting coronary artery blood flow (Fig. 17–7). Removal of plaque results in a smoother vessel wall surface. The smoother wall surface reduces the likelihood of platelet aggregation, clot formation, and vessel restenosis.

Intravascular stents are radiopaque stainless-steel mesh, slotted tubes, or coils, which are used to maintain the patency of coronary arteries (Fig. 17–7). The

TABLE 17–9
Relative Contraindications for Thrombolytic Therapy

Traumatic cardiopulmonary resuscitation
Acute trauma
Current anticoagulation
Bleeding disorders
Recent exposure to β-hemolytic streptococci*
Recent intra-arterial or biopsy procedures
Recent aneurysm or cerebrovascular accident
Recent surgery (within 10 days of treatment)
Uncontrolled hypertension (systolic >180 mmHg or diastolic >110 mmHg)

*Specific to streptokinase only.

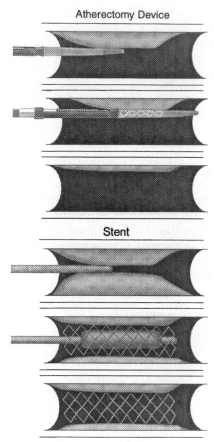

Atherectomy Device

Stent

FIGURE 17–7. Examples of coronary atherectomy and intravascular stent.

stent acts as a scaffolding to support the vessel wall. Over time, endothelial cells begin to layer over the exposed stainless steel to create a smooth vessel wall. Because of the high probability of thrombosis, patients receiving stents are thoroughly anticoagulated until endothelialization is complete. Complete endothelialization can take up to 3 months.

Goals of Interventional Device Therapy

The goals of atherectomy and stenting are to maintain coronary artery blood flow, to decrease myocardial ischemia, and to decrease the incidence of vessel wall dissection and restenosis.

Indications for Interventional Device Therapy

The use of coronary atherectomy is indicated with lesions that are irregular, calcified, or ulcerated. Atherectomy is also indicated for use in vein grafts. Intravascular stents are indicated in acute vessel closure, vessel wall dissection, and restenosis after PTCA with total occlusion of the vessel.

Technique of Interventional Device Therapy

Both procedures are performed in the cardiac catheterization lab. The patient preparation is similar to that of the PTCA procedure. A large groin sheath is inserted to accommodate the large atherectomy and stent catheters. As with PTCA, a series of catheters and guidewires are used to locate the exact position of the lesion within the coronary artery.

The atherectomy catheter is positioned across the plaque and is properly placed when the plaque protrudes into the opening of the catheter. A cutter is then advanced over the lesion to shave off the plaque. The catheter is repositioned, and more plaque is removed until satisfactory results are obtained. The plaque is retrieved at the end of the catheter and is then sent for pathologic analysis.

Intravascular stents are placed over a balloon catheter. The catheter is advanced until it is positioned over the site. When properly positioned, the balloon is inflated and the stent is expanded over the lesion. The balloon is then deflated, the stent left in place, and the catheter removed.

Complications of Interventional Device Therapy

Complications of coronary atherectomy include arterial dissection, arrhythmias, vessel wall perforation, embolization, acute occlusion, and myocardial infarction. Complications of stents are thrombosis, occlusion, coronary artery spasm, restenosis, cardiac tamponade, and migration of the stent.

An increase in femoral artery complications may occur because of the large-sized sheath needed to accommodate the device catheters. Possible complications are hemorrhage, development of pseudoaneurysms, and retroperitoneal bleeding.

Nursing Considerations

Nursing management of interventional device therapy is similar to care of the patient after PTCA. Vigilant inspection of groin status is necessary to identify potential femoral artery complications. Nursing care of patients after stent procedure consists in management of the anticoagulation therapy and careful assessment for bleeding complications.

SUGGESTED READINGS

Alspach, J and Williams, S (eds): Core Curriculum for Critical Care Nursing, ed 3. WB Saunders, Philadelphia, 1985.
Bell, WR, et al: Efficacy of thrombolytic therapy for acute myocardial infarction: A round table discussion. Pract Cardiol 12:51–67, 1986.
Bevans, M and McLimore, E: Intracoronary stents: A new approach to coronary artery dilatation. J Cardiovasc Nurs 7:34–49, 1992.

Bolooki, H: Current status of circulatory support with an intra-aortic balloon pump. Medical Instrumentation 20(5):226–276, 1986.

Bullas, JB: Care of the patient on the percutaneous intra-aortic counterpulsation balloon. Crit Care Nurse 2(4):40–48, 1982.

Crea, F, et al: Percutaneous recanalization of coronary arteries. Lancet, 214–215, July 26, 1986.

Haak, SW: Intra-aortic balloon pump techniques. Dimensions of Critical Care Nursing 2(4):196–204, 1983.

Haywood, DL: Temporary AV sequential pacing using epicardial lead system. Crit Care Nurse 5(3):21–29, 1985.

Mathewson, M and Dusek, JL: DC countershock does not harm today's internal pacemakers. Crit Care Nurse 4(2):48, 1984.

Moroney, DA and Reedy, JE: Understanding ventricular assist devices: A self-study guide. J Cardiovasc Nurs 8:1–15, 1994.

Phibbs, B and Marriott, HJL: Complications of permanent transvenous pacing. N Engl J Med 342:1428–1432, 1985.

Phipps, WJ, et al: Medical-Surgical Nursing: Concepts and Clinical Practice, ed 4. Mosby Year Book, St. Louis, 1991, pp 696–697;1445.

Purcell, JA and Burrows, SG: Pacemakers. Am J Nurs 85:554–568, 1985.

Purcell, JA, Pippin, L, and Mitchell, M: IABP therapy. Am J Nurs 83:776–790, 1983.

Reeder, GS and Vliestra, RE: Coronary angioplasty: 1986. Modern Concepts of Cardiovascular Disease 50(10):49–53, 1986.

Shillinger, FL: Percutaneous transluminal angioplasty. Heart Lung 12:45–51, 1983.

Slusarczyk, SM and Hicks, FD: Helping your patient live with a permanent pacemaker. Nursing '83 13(4):58–63, 1983.

Speroni, R, et al: Coronary atherectomy: Overview and implications for nursing. J Cardiovasc Nurs 7:25–33, 1992.

Spielman, SR: New advances in cardiac pacemaking. In Hakki, AH (ed): Ideal Cardiac Pacing. WB Saunders, Philadelphia, 1984, pp 219–261.

Stevens, L, Redd, R, and Buckingham, T: An alternative to electric countershock for terminating ventricular arrhythmias. Crit Care Nurse 9(3):38, 1989.

Strauss, E and Rudy, EB: Tissue-plasminogen activator: A new drug in reperfusion therapy. Crit Care Nurse 6(3):30–41, 1986.

The ISAM Study Group: A prospective trial of intravenous streptokinase in acute myocardial infarction (I.S.A.M.). N Engl J Med 314:1465–1471, 1986.

Topol, E (ed): Textbook of Interventional Cardiology. WB Saunders, Philadelphia, 1990, pp 563–579; 623–632.

Whitman, G: Intra-aortic balloon pumping and cardiac mechanics: A programmed lesson. Heart Lung 7:1034–1050, 1978.

Whitman, GR: Mechanical assistance for the patient with a failing heart. In Dossey, B, et al (eds): Critical Care Nursing: Body-Mind-Spirit. JB Lippincott, New York, 1992, pp. 261–288.

CARE PLAN FOR THE PATIENT RECEIVING TEMPORARY PACEMAKER THERAPY

Nursing Diagnoses

Nursing Diagnosis #1
Alteration in cardiac output, related to pacer malfunction, arrhythmias

Desired Patient Outcomes

1. Patient will demonstrate clinical behaviors consistent with an adequate cardiac output:
   - Alert and oriented to person, place, and time
   - Systolic blood pressure >90 mmHg
   - Lungs clear to auscultation
   - Capillary refill <2 sec
   - Urine output >30 mL/h
   - Lack of subjective complaints that were verbalized prior to the pacer insertion (e.g., dizziness, fatigue)
   - Strong peripheral pulses
   - Absence of jugular venous distention (JVD)
2. Patient will not demonstrate pacer malfunction as evidenced by ECG analysis.
3. Patient will be free of hemodynamically significant arrhythmias.

Nursing Interventions
- Monitor the pacemaker parameters every shift and document:
  - Sensing ability
  - Capture frequency
  - Threshold (check level every day)
  - Current setting
  - Mode
- Perform comprehensive cardiovascular assessment at least once per shift, including
  - Heart rate, rhythm
  - Quality of peripheral pulses
  - Heart sounds
  - Color, temperature of skin

Rationales
- Failure of the pacemaker in any one of these functions can jeopardize patient safety.
  - Documentation provides baseline data from which trends in condition can be detected.

- Baseline assessment provides data from which comparisons can be made.

  - Development of additional heart sounds may reflect decreased myocardial compliance or incompetence of valves.

CARE PLAN FOR THE PATIENT RECEIVING TEMPORARY PACEMAKER THERAPY
(*Continued*)

Nursing Interventions

- ○ Presence of pulsus paradoxus (a drop of the systolic blood pressure more than the normal 10 mmHg during inspiration)
- ○ Blood pressure
- ○ Quantity of urine output
- ○ Presence of JVD
- ○ Subjective comments
- ○ Level of consciousness
- ○ ECG strip interpretation
- Check pacemaker system every shift including:
  - ○ Integrity of lead connections
  - ○ Battery
  - ○ Pacer generator
  - ○ Pacer settings

- Monitor patient for presence of arrhythmias and document type, patient's response, any associated activity, and pacer activity (i.e., inability to sense).
- Notify physician at onset of any arrhythmias. Keep lidocaine at bedside. Ensure patent IV line is present.

Rationales

- ○ Decreased or muffled heart sounds, JVD, and pulsus paradoxus may reflect tamponade.

- ○ Quality of pulses, urine output, temperature, color of skin reflect tissue perfusion.
- ○ JVD reflects elevation of right-sided heart pressures, which can be associated with tamponade.
- ○ First symptom of decreased cardiac output may be a change in mentation.
- Pacemaker function may be closely assessed through strip analysis.

- ○ Ensure all components of system are functioning appropriately.
- Arrhythmias may or may not be hemodynamically significant or related to pacer activity. The pacemaker may need to be adjusted.
- Physician may want to reposition pacing wire or initiate antiarrhythmic therapy.

Nursing Diagnoses

Nursing Diagnosis #2
Potential for injury from microshock

Desired Patient Outcomes

1. Patient's environment will be free of microshock hazards.
2. Patient will not receive microshock.

Nursing Interventions

- Cover any exposed lead wires with rubber gloves, finger cots, or cellophane tape.
- Wear rubber gloves if handling exposed wires.
- Use only properly grounded equipment, including the electric bed.
- Inspect all electric equipment in room for signs of cord fraying.
- Do not touch patient while handling electrical equipment.

Rationales

- Insulating the lead wires decrease the risk of conduction.
- Improperly grounded equipment poses serious threat to patient safety.

- It is possible for energy to travel from the equipment through the nurse to the patient.

Nursing Diagnoses

Nursing Diagnosis #3
Anxiety, related to invasive procedure, "heart failure"

Desired Patient Outcomes

Patient will demonstrate decreased anxiety as evidenced by:
- Subjective comments
- Decreased restlessness
- Facial expressions
- Nonverbal behavior
- Ability to concentrate

Nursing Interventions

- Assess patient's understanding of situation, reasons for anxiety.
- Provide information in supportive manner.
- Assess patient's understanding of information provided.
  - ○ Observe patient's response.
  - ○ Establish calm, quiet environment.
- Assess past coping.

- Provide sedation if needed.

Rationales

- Pattern interventions to patient's level of comprehension.
- Establishing calm rapport is reassuring to patient.
- Patient's level of anxiety may prevent integration of information.

- Assessing past coping skills helps to develop a more effective plan of care.
- Sedation may be appropriate if nonpharmacologic interventions are ineffective.

CARE PLAN FOR THE PATIENT RECEIVING TEMPORARY PACEMAKER THERAPY
(*Continued*)

Nursing Diagnoses	Desired Patient Outcomes
Nursing Diagnosis #4 Knowledge deficit, related to need for pacemaker, procedure for insertion	Patient/family will verbalize understanding of: • Need for pacemaker • How pacemaker is helping the heart • Procedure for insertion

Nursing Interventions	Rationales

• Assess patient/family's level of knowledge with pacemakers.
• Establish teaching plan, including:
  ○ Need for pacemaker
  ○ How the pacemaker will help
  ○ How long the procedure will take
  ○ Sensations of events expected during insertion
  ○ Post-insertion events
• Provide only necessary information.
• Encourage questions.
	• Assessing prior level of knowledge helps in developing a more effective teaching plan.
	  ○ Including family helps their understanding of events.
	
	• Clarification of questions improves understanding.

Nursing Diagnoses	Desired Patient Outcomes
Nursing Diagnosis #5 Potential for infection, related to invasive line placement	Patient will be infection-free, as evidenced by: • Normal temperature • Lack of redness, heat, swelling, discharge at insertion site

Nursing Interventions	Rationales
• Monitor insertion site every day and document findings. • Monitor patient's temperature q8h; q4h if an elevation is noted. • Change dressing using sterile procedure q24h or per unit protocol. • Change IV solution q24h if a central line is present. ○ Culture any drainage from site, and notify the physician. • Culture all catheter tips if spike in temperature is noted (i.e., central line, pacing catheter). • Do not administer antipyretics for pain.	• Signs and symptoms of infection often begin at local level. • Temperature elevation is a clinical sign of the immune system's activity in combating pyrogens. • Frequent sterile dressing changes can prevent infections by providing an aseptic barrier once the skin integrity has become impaired. • Changes in IV solution decrease medium for bacterial growth. • Identification of organism involved in the infectious process is vital for determining course of treatment. • Antipyretics may mask temperature elevation and signs of infection.

Nursing Diagnoses	Desired Patient Outcomes
Nursing Diagnosis #6 Alteration in comfort, related to invasive line insertion	Patient will verbalize statements of comfort.

Nursing Interventions	Rationales
• Assess patient's level of comfort (by verbal and nonverbal cues). • Reposition patient frequently, using pillows for support. • Rub areas of discomfort with lotion. • Provide medication for pain as needed.	• Patient may not openly admit discomfort. • Repositioning prevents development of pressure areas and fatigue of dependent sites. • Rubbing areas of discomfort promotes relaxation of sore muscle groups and enhances circulation to the area. • Medication can provide analgesia necessary to improve the patient's level of comfort.

CARE PLAN FOR THE PATIENT WITH A PERMANENT PACEMAKER

Nursing Diagnoses

Nursing Diagnosis #1

Alteration in cardiac output, related to:
1. Pacemaker malfunction
2. Pacemaker-induced arrhythmias
3. Electromagnetic interference

Desired Patient Outcomes

1. Patient will demonstrate clinical behaviors consistent with an adequate cardiac output:
   - Alert and oriented to person, place, and time
   - Systolic blood pressure >90 mmHg
   - Lungs clear on auscultation
   - Capillary refill <2 sec
   - Urine output >30 mL/h
   - Lack of the subjective complaints that might have been verbalized before the pacemaker insertion, indicative of low cardiac output (e.g., dizziness, fatigue, nausea)
2. Patient will not demonstrate pacemaker malfunction as evidenced by ECG analysis.
3. Patient will be free of hemodynamically significant arrhythmias.

Nursing Interventions

- Monitor ECG continuously for 24–48 h after pacemaker insertion for:
  - Sensing ability
  - Ability to capture
  - Firing rate that is consistent with settings
  - Frequency of pace-assist
  - Presence of arrhythmias

- Confirm that the pacemaker is firing at the preset rate.

- Cardiovascular assessment same as temporary pacer (see Table 17–7)
- Assess patient's response to arrhythmias and communicate with physician for appropriate treatment regimen.

- Rule out any other potential cause of arrhythmias (i.e., electrolyte imbalance, ischemia, hypoxia).

- If cardioversion/defibrillation is required, do not place sternal paddle directly over pulse generator. Keep current about 10 cm away from pulse generator at all times. Anteroposterior paddle placement is strongly recommended if possible.
- Do not expose patient to any conditions known to cause interference:
  - Nuclear magnetic resonance
  - Cautery
  - Electroconvulsive therapy
  - Electric razors

Rationales

- The pacemaker may "oversense" (i.e., become inhibited by other electrical potential in the body), or it may "undersense" and not recognize intrinsic cardiac activity.
- Conditions may develop that can increase the threshold and decrease the pacemaker's ability to capture (i.e., fibrosis at the pacing catheter tip, hypoxia, dislodgement of pacing catheter, concurrent drug therapy, electrolyte imbalance).
- Determining how frequently the patient's rhythm requires pacemaker assistance provides pertinent clinical information.
  - Foreign object in ventricle can irritate the myocardium and cause arrhythmias.
- The pacemaker-induced arrhythmias may be self-limiting and hemodynamically insignificant, or they might be life-threatening. The physician should be made aware of their occurrence to determine whether therapeutic intervention is warranted.
- Other variables in the patient's clinical picture may be causing the arrhythmias and should be excluded before the pacing catheter is implicated.
- Discharge of high amounts of energy over the electrical circuitry can damage the pacemaker and cause malfunction.

- Electrical and magnetic fields can alter pacer function.

Nursing Diagnoses

Nursing Diagnosis #2

Potential for infection, related to the surgical procedure

Desired Patient Outcomes

Patient will be infection-free as evidenced by:
- Approximation of surgical incision
- Lack of elevation of temperature
- Lack of redness, swelling, discharge, heat at site of incision

CARE PLAN FOR THE PATIENT WITH A PERMANENT PACEMAKER (*Continued*)

Nursing Interventions

- Monitor incision site and document findings.

- Cleanse incision with Betadine daily; keep open to air after 24 h.

- Monitor patient's temperature q8h; q4h, if elevation noted.
- Do not administer antipyretics for pain

Rationales

- Signs and symptoms of infection often begin at local level.
- Washing the wound with antibacterial solution prevents infection. Keeping the incision open to air promotes granulation of tissue.
- Temperature elevation is an accurate clinical sign of the immune system's activity in combating pyrogens.
- Antipyretics may mask temperature elevation and signs of infection.

Nursing Diagnoses

Nursing Diagnosis #3
Alteration in mobility, related to the surgical procedure

Desired Patient Outcomes

Patient will be able to demonstrate full range of motion in affected extremity.

Nursing Interventions

- Encourage patient to perform range-of-motion (ROM) exercises 24–48 h after the insertion to prevent stiffness of shoulder; provide passive ROM if unable.

Rationales

- Stiffness in affected shoulder occurs because of surgical manipulation of large supportive muscle groups.

Nursing Diagnoses

Nursing Diagnosis #4
Anxiety, related to surgical procedure

Desired Patient Outcomes

Patient will demonstrate decreased levels of anxiety as evidenced by:
- Subjective comments
- Decreased restlessness
- Facial expressions
- Noverbal behavior
- Ability to concentrate

Nursing Interventions

- Assess patient's understanding of situation, reasons for anxiety.
- Provide information in calm, supportive manner.
  - Assess patient's understanding of information provided.
    - Observe patient's response.
- Assess past coping behaviors.
- Establish calm, quiet environment.
- Provide sedation if needed.

Rationales

- Pattern interventions to patient's level of comprehension.
- Establishing calming rapport is reassuring to patient.
  - Patient's level of anxiety may prevent integration of information.

- Assessing patient's coping skills helps to develop a more effective plan of care.
- Sedation may be appropriate if nonpharmacologic interventions are ineffective.

Nursing Diagnoses

Nursing Diagnosis #5
Potential disturbance in self-concept after dependence on the pacemaker, related to disfigurement

Desired Patient Outcomes

Patient will verbalize acceptance of the pacemaker as integral part of body.

Nursing Interventions

- Assess patient's level of comfort with the pacemaker. Note comments related to:
  - Dependence on "a machine"
  - Fear of malfunction
  - Insecurity, embarrassment about cosmetic appearance
  - Loss of self-control and independence
- Encourage patient to ventilate concerns; reassure and counsel to dispel misconceptions.
- Assess past coping mechanisms and apply if pertinent.
  - Consult psychiatry if necessary.
- Have patient speak with another recipient of permanent pacemaker.
- Refer to support group (if applicable).

Rationales

- Patients often have difficulty accepting the pacemaker because it is a continual reminder that they have a cardiac condition and because of its limited lifespan.

- Many patients have misunderstandings that promote disturbances.
- Past coping mechanisms indicate adaptive/maladaptive behavior.
- Recognition that problems are not unique provides comfort and strength for recovery.

CARE PLAN FOR THE PATIENT WITH A PERMANENT PACEMAKER (*Continued*)

Nursing Diagnoses

Nursing Diagnosis #6
Knowledge deficit, related to:
1. Indication for permanent pacer
2. How it will function
3. Monitoring pacer function
4. Signs and symptoms of malfunction
5. Return to prior lifestyle
6. Changes in lifestyle
7. Medical alert information
8. Electrical precautions
9. Follow-up care

Desired Patient Outcomes

1. Patient/family will verbalize understanding of:
   • Indication for permanent pacer
   • How it will function
   • Signs and symptoms of malfunction
   • Monitoring pacer function
   • Return to prior lifestyle
   • Changes in lifestyle
   • Medical alert information
   • Electrical precautions
   • Follow-up care
2. Patient or family member will demonstrate how to measure pulse rate with 100% accuracy.

Nursing Interventions

• Assess patient/family level of knowledge regarding pertinent information.
• Develop teaching plan specific to their learning needs.
• Provide written information for reference of the material covered.
• Explain in layman's terms:

   ○ Purpose of conduction system
   ○ Why patient needs pacer
   ○ How it will work to *supplement* the patient's cardiac activity
      □ Signs and symptoms of malfunction (relate to signs/symptoms patient presented with if applicable)
      □ Changes in lifestyle required
      □ Need to carry Medic-Alert card with pacer information at all times—use of bracelet or necklace
      □ Follow-up care
   ○ Electrical precautions:
      □ Magnetic fields (i.e., store theft devices, some microwaves, radar)
      □ Electrical fields (i.e., electric razors, cautery)
• Demonstrate to patient/family how to check pulse.
   ○ Have patient/family do return demonstration with 100% accuracy.

Rationales

• Written materials are helpful references when at home.

• Understanding will improve patient's ability to care for self.
   ○ A common misperception is that the pacer is *replacing* patient's own heart function.
   ○ The patient must be able to identify specifics about pacemaker if it malfunctions.

   ○ Magnetic/electrical fields may cause interference with electrical circuitry; ability of pacemaker to function.

• Patient needs to monitor appropriate functioning of the pacemaker.

CARE PLAN FOR THE PATIENT REQUIRING INTRA-AORTIC BALLOON PUMPING

Nursing Diagnoses

Nursing Diagnosis #1
Potential alteration in tissue perfusion, related to myocardial ischemia, peripheral vascular disease, embolic phenomena

Desired Patient Outcomes

The patient will demonstrate adequate tissue perfusion as evidenced by:
- Absence of angina
- Capillary refill of <2 sec
- Warm extremities
- No change in baseline peripheral pulse quality
- Normal respiratory effort
- Sensorium alert and oriented

Nursing Interventions

- Check peripheral pulse quality, compare with baseline every hour, and document findings.
- Place patient in vascular position (reverse Trendelenburg).
- Monitor patient for complaints of chest pain, shortness of breath, peripheral pain.

- Assess color and temperature of extremities with peripheral pulse checks; compare bilaterally.
- Avoid flexion of patient at hips.

- Monitor left radial pulse quality (or arterial waveform if present), mentation, complaints of dizziness.
- Place a sheet over the leg in which the balloon is inserted for restraint of movement.

Rationales

- Peripheral ischemia or occlusion may occur, caused by embolization or diminished flow distal to the catheter.
- Vascular position promotes blood flow to the peripheral bed.
- Complaints of pain can be indicative of ischemia or embolization.
  - Sudden onset of shortness of breath can indicate development of pulmonary edema or pulmonary embolism.
- The circulation distal to the IABP catheter is most at risk for compromised flow.
- Flexion may cause migration of balloon catheter upward in the aorta.
  - If the balloon catheter migrates forward it will occlude the left subclavian or carotid artery, causing diminished flow to the areas they service.

- This minimizes catheter migration cephalad.

Nursing Diagnoses

Nursing Diagnosis #2
Impaired physical mobility, related to cannulation of femoral artery

Nursing Interventions

- Position patient with head of bed at 30-degree angle.

- Encourage patient to perform ROM exercises in all extremities except the cannulated leg.
- Reposition patient frequently, log-rolling from side to side.

- Have patient continue ankle and foot exercises in affected leg.

Desired Patient Outcomes

Patient will maintain range of motion (ROM) in all extremities except cannulated leg.

Rationales

- A 30-degree angle permits swallowing and performance of some self-care activities. Elevation of head of bed greater than 30 degrees will cause hip flexion and may encourage migration of the IABP catheter.
- Exercises maintain muscular tone.

- Repositioning maintains use of muscle groups. The patient must be log-rolled to maintain alignment of the cannulated extremity.
- Ankle and foot exercises help to maintain full ROM of these areas without jeopardizing catheter placement.

Nursing Diagnoses

Nursing Diagnosis #3
Potential alteration in cardiac output, related to left ventricular dysfunction, arrhythmias

Desired Patient Outcomes

Adequate cardiac output will be maintained as evidenced by:
- MAP 70–90 mmHg
- Urine output >30 mL/h
- Cardiac index >2.0 L/min per square meter
- PCWP <20 mmHg
- SVR 800–1200 dynes sec cm^{-5}

CARE PLAN FOR THE PATIENT REQUIRING INTRA-AORTIC BALLOON PUMPING (*Continued*)

Nursing Interventions

- Monitor the following hemodynamic parameters every 15–30 min:
  - Systolic and diastolic blood pressure, mean arterial pressure, diastolic augmentation
  - Heart rate
  - Pulmonary artery systolic, diastolic, and mean pressures
  - Urine output every hour
  - CVP, PCWP
  - Cardiac output/cardiac index, SVR
- Check balloon timing every hour or more frequently with changes in heart rate +10%.
- Monitor for arrhythmias. Note patient's hemodynamic response.
- If patient is tachycardiac (heart rate >150 bpm), it may be necessary to change IABP frequency to 1:2.
- If cardiopulmonary resuscitation is required, turn balloon to 1:3 frequency and decrease the volume to minimal level.

Rationales

- Ongoing assessment of clinical data is necessary to detect changes in left ventricular function.

- Timing must be precise to optimize effects of IABP.

- Arrhythmias may or may not affect cardiac output.

- At high heart rate, shuttling of gas and ability of IABP to inflate and deflate may be compromised.
- It is impossible to coordinate IABP with resuscitative efforts, but the balloon should never remain still in the aorta because of the risk of thrombus formation.

Nursing Diagnoses

Nursing Diagnosis #4
Anxiety (patient/family) related to invasive procedure

Desired Patient Outcomes

1. Patient/family will verbalize feelings of anxiety.
2. Patient/family will demonstrate relaxed demeanor as evidenced by verbal and nonverbal clues.

Nursing Interventions

- Explain all aspects of treatment or care to patient/family.
- Explain/describe all expected equipment, sounds before they occur.
- Maintain interpersonal contact throughout performance of technical care.
- Approach patient and family with confident, calm, professional behavior.

Rationales

- Understanding of patient care activities minimizes misconceptions and fears.
- Anticipation of sights and sounds helps prepare the patient.
- Recognition of human factor amidst technology is vital.

- Patient/family must have confidence in caregivers.

Nursing Diagnoses

Nursing Diagnosis #5
Potential alteration in sensory perception, related to sensory overload

Desired Patient Outcomes

Patient will demonstrate lucid mentation as evidenced by:
- Appropriate conversation
- Orientation to person, place, and time

Nursing Interventions

- Maintain quiet, soothing environment
- Attempt to preserve day/night sleep cycle.
- Ensure that patient has adequate sleep periods.
- Restrict traffic around patient's bed; coordinate care to minimize disruptions.
- Assess patient's mentation.
- Reorient as necessary.

Rationales

- Interventions are designed to minimize overstimulation, which can contribute to disorientation.

CARE PLAN FOR THE PATIENT REQUIRING INTRA-AORTIC BALLOON PUMPING (*Continued*)

Nursing Diagnoses

Nursing Diagnosis #6
Potential for infection, related to indwelling catheters (see Table 17–7)

Desired Patient Outcomes

Patient will be free of infection as evidenced by:
- Lack of temperature elevation
- Lack of redness, heat, swelling, or discharge at catheter insertion site

Nursing Interventions
- Maintain meticulous handwashing.

- Change femoral dressing with aseptic technique.
  - Observe insertion site for signs and symptoms of infection.
- Monitor temperature q8h.

  - Do not administer antipyretics for pain.

- Maintain meticulous perineal and Foley care.

Rationales
- Handwashing decreases incidence of nosocomial infections.
- Sterile dressings protect site from organisms.

- Temperature elevation is an accurate clinical sign of the immune system's activity in combating pyrogens.
  - Antipyretics may mask temperature elevation and signs of infection.
  - Signs and symptoms of infection often begin at a local site.
- Maintain area free of contamination.

Nursing Diagnoses

Nursing Diagnosis #7
Potential for physiologic injury: Bleeding, related to:
1. Indwelling arterial catheter
2. Concomitant anticoagulation

Desired Patient Outcomes

Patient will not have active bleeding as evidenced by:
- Stable hematocrit, hemoglobin levels
- Guaiac-free stools
- Absence of hematoma, bruising, or ecchymosis
- Stable blood pressure and heart rate

Nursing Interventions
- Monitor laboratory values indicative of bleeding status (PTT, hematocrit, hemoglobin).
- Monitor all stools for presence of occult blood.
- Inspect the patient for oozing and hematoma formation at the catheter insertion site.
  - Inspect the flank area for retroperitoneal ecchymosis. Generally inspect the skin for evidence of bleeding.
- Apply pressure dressing, direct pressure manually or with a C-clamp if bleeding is noted at the insertion site.
- Monitor the patient's blood pressure and heart rate for evidence of diminished intravascular volume.

Rationales
- PTT identifies clotting ability. The hematocrit and hemoglobin identify the level of circulating RBCs.
- Anticoagulation can promote internal bleeding.
- Most common site of bleeding is the catheter insertion site.
  - Retroperitoneal ecchymosis may indicate dissection of the iliac artery upon insertion.
- Stasis of blood can be achieved by application of pressure to the site of bleeding.
- Unexplained drop in systolic pressure with concurrent rise in heart rate may indicate active bleeding.

CVP = central venous pressure; MAP = mean arterial pressure; PCWP = pulmonary capillary wedge pressure; PTT = partial thromboplastin time; SVR = systemic vascular resistance.

CARE PLAN FOR THE PATIENT WITH PERCUTANEOUS TRANSLUMINAL CORONARY ANGIOPLASTY

Nursing Diagnoses

Nursing Diagnosis #1

Anxiety, related to upcoming procedure

Desired Patient Outcomes

Patient will demonstrate decreased anxiety as evidenced by:
- Subjective comments
- Decreased restlessness
- Facial expressions
- Nonverbal behavior
- Ability to concentrate

Nursing Interventions

- Assess patient's understanding of the procedure, any past experiences or misconceptions, and reasons for anxiety.

- Provide information based on assessment in a calm, concise manner.
- Assess the patient's understanding of the information provided, noting nonverbal cues.
- Assess patient's past coping behaviors.

- Establish calm, quiet environment.
- Provide sedation if needed.

Rationales

- Identifying patient's level of comprehension and contributing factors to anxiety allows for clarification through provision of meaningful information.
- Information will be integrated if it is perceived as meaningful.
- Patient's anxiety level may prevent integration of information.
- Assessing patient's coping skills helps to develop a more effective plan of care
- Environmental stimuli can add to anxiety level.
- Sedation may be appropriate to decrease catecholamine release and minimize myocardial oxygen demand if nonpharmacologic interventions are ineffective.

Nursing Diagnoses

Nursing Diagnosis #2

Potential alteration in comfort, related to myocardial ischemia and immobility

Desired Patient Outcomes

1. Patient will remain pain-free as evidenced by lack of verbalization of symptoms of angina.
2. Patient will promptly report any symptoms of angina and will verbalize rapid relief after intervention.
3. Patient will verbalize comfort during period of immobility.

Nursing Interventions

- Instruct patient to report immediately any discomfort. Emphasize the importance of this responsibility.
- Assess the patient for signs and symptoms of angina.
- Assess type of discomfort along with associated symptoms and compare with presenting symptoms.
- Perform stat ECG; note ST-segment changes.
- Notify physician immediately of any complaints of chest pain or changes in condition.
- Administer sublingual nitroglycerin, procardia, or IV nitroglycerin per protocol.
- Instruct patient that although he or she must lie flat during the time interval that the introducer sheaths remain in and for 6 hours after sheaths are removed, measures can be taken to improve his or her comfort level.
  - Place egg-crate or air mattress on bed.
  - Elevate head of bed 30 degrees.
  - Reposition patient on side with pillows. Place rolled towel under small of back.
  - Medicate as necessary.
  - Provide diversional activities.

Rationales

- Many patients are afraid or do not understand the implications of chest pain after the procedure.
- Manifestations of angina may mimic gastric distress.
- It is important to differentiate pain of cardiac angina.

- ECG will reflect changes consistent with ischemia.
  - ECG may need to be repeated procedure.

- Vasodilatation with nitrates and antispasmodic medication is needed to improve coronary perfusion.
- Reassurance that this immobility is limited promotes compliance, tolerance.

  - Interventions are patterned to minimize time lying flat on back.

CARE PLAN FOR THE PATIENT WITH PERCUTANEOUS TRANSLUMINAL CORONARY ANGIOPLASTY (*Continued*)

Nursing Diagnoses

Nursing Diagnosis #3
Potential alteration in tissue perfusion, related to cannulation of femoral artery

Desired Patient Outcomes

Patient will demonstrate adequate tissue perfusion of extremities as evidenced by:
- No change in peripheral pulse quality from baseline
- No change in color, sensitivity, or movement from baseline
- Brisk capillary refill (less than 2 sec)

Nursing Interventions
- Check bilateral pedal pulse quality every 15–30 minutes until sheaths are pulled.
  - After sheaths are pulled, check pulse quality every 30 minutes four times, then every hour for 6 hours. Mark location of pulse with pen.
  - Compare findings with baseline.
- Place patient in mild vascular position (reverse Trendelenburg)
- Remind patient not to bend at waist.

- Instruct patient to report immediately any pain, tingling, or numbness.

Rationales
- The circulation of the extremity distal to the sheath insertion is at high risk for compromise of flow during the period of time that the sheaths remain in and immediately after their removal.

- Vascular position promotes flow to lower extremities.

- Bending at waist could cause puncture of cannulated artery.
- Pain, tingling, or numbness of the cannulated extremity can indicate vascular compromise and decreased tissue perfusion.

Nursing Diagnoses

Nursing Diagnosis #4
Potential for physiologic injury: Bleeding, related to:
1. Cannulation of an artery
2. Concomitant anticoagulation

Desired Patient Outcomes

Patient will evidence no bleeding at site of sheath insertion or retroperitoneal area.

Nursing Interventions
- Check femoral insertion site every 15–30 minutes with pulse checks.
- Assess the integrity of the sheaths. Ensure that the dilator remains within the arterial cannula.

- Assess for oozing, hematoma formation.

- Place 5-lb sandbag over site of insertion.

- Instruct patient to report any warmth in groin or leg area or sharp flank pain.

- Monitor partial thromboplastin time (PTT) levels.

- Assess patient for retroperitoneal ecchymosis. Notify physician immediately if present.
- Place direct pressure over site for 20 minutes, or until bleeding stops.

Rationales
- Bleeding frequently occurs at the sheath insertion site.

- The dilator prevents blood from flowing out of the arterial cannula. If the dilator is not in completely, blood loss can occur.
- Frank oozing can occur around the cannulas, or hematomas can occur within the subcutaneous tissue.
- Sandbag promotes hemostasis at insertion site by providing direct pressure.
- Warmth may indicate unintentional blood flow from the cannulas. Flank pain may indicate iliac dissection, peritoneal bleeding.
- PTT is indicative of clotting ability and will help direct therapy with heparin. The goal of treatment is to prevent reocclusion of the artery that was dilated.
- Ecchymosis may indicate femoral or iliac dissection, internal bleeding.
- Direct pressure prevents blood loss and promotes hemostasis.

CARE PLAN FOR THE PATIENT WITH PERCUTANEOUS TRANSLUMINAL CORONARY ANGIOPLASTY (*Continued*)

Nursing Diagnoses	Desired Patient Outcomes
Nursing Diagnosis #5 Potential alteration in cardiac output, related to: 1. Left ventricular dysfunction 2. Sheath removal 3. Arrhythmias 4. Orthostatic hypotension	Patient will exhibit cardiac output adequate for tissue perfusion as evidenced by: • Systolic blood pressure >90 mmHg • No change in mentation • Brisk capillary refill time <2 sec • Urinary output >30 mL/h

Nursing Interventions	Rationales
• Assess vital signs, rhythm, mentation, capillary refill every 15–30 minutes until sheath removal, then every 30 minutes for 6 hours. Notify physician with status changes.	• Frequent assessment of patient status promotes detection of subtle changes in condition.
• Assess urinary output every hour.	• Urinary output is a consistent noninvasive measure of cardiac output, renal perfusion.
• Assess peripheral circulation with vital signs.	• Vasoconstriction is a compensatory mechanism for decreased cardiac output.
• Assess patient's mentation along with vital signs.	• Mentation is one of the most sensitive indicators of altered tissue perfusion.
• Encourage fluid intake after procedure.	• Fluids are important in maintaining intravascular volume.
• Monitor patient's response to sheath removal, direct groin pressure. Observe for bradycardia, hypotension, complaints of dizziness. Administer normal saline or other rapid volume replacement; place patient in Trendelenburg position and administer atropine, 1 mg IVP, as per protocol.	• It is common to observe a vasovagal reaction to the removal of femoral arterial sheaths.
• Check blood pressures in lying and sitting positions after patient is able to get out of bed, and note decrease in systolic blood pressure >20 mmHg or complaints of dizziness. Return patient to lying position if this occurs.	• Orthostatic changes are common after PTCA because of prolonged bedrest and venodilation with nitrates.

Nursing Diagnoses	Desired Patient Outcomes
Nursing Diagnosis #6 Knowledge deficit, related to coronary artery disease post-PTCA expectations	Patient/family will be able to verbalize an understanding of: • What CAD is • Why this is a problem for the patient • Purpose of PTCA • Immediate post-PTCA care • Risk factors of CAD that the patient can modify • Name, dosage, and purpose of homegoing medications • Follow-up care (appointments) • What to do in an emergency

Nursing Interventions	Rationales
• Determine patient/family understanding of CAD and how it affects them.	• Identification of baseline level of knowledge is necessary in providing individualized teaching.

• Develop comprehensive teaching plan in conjunction with patient and family, based on learning needs.
  ○ Use diagrams and audiovisuals to enhance understanding of CAD.
  ○ Supply patient with written instructions for information pertaining to medications, risk factors, expected behavioral changes, and emergent care.
	• Mutual agreement on what information is needed is helpful in meeting perceived needs and providing meaningful information.
	
	  ○ Levels of anxiety during hospitalization as well as quantity of information communicated necessitate written instructions for clarity.

• Reinforce teaching during care and evaluate level of understanding. • Encourage questions and verbalization of feelings.	• It is important to assess patient's understanding after any teaching to identify any misconceptions.

PTT = partial thromboplastin time.

CARE PLAN FOR THE PATIENT RECEIVING THROMBOLYTIC THERAPY: STREPTOKINASE AND TISSUE PLASMINOGEN ACTIVATOR

Nursing Diagnoses

Nursing Diagnosis #1
Potential for physiologic injury: Bleeding, related to manipulation of clotting cascade

Desired Patient Outcomes

Patient will not have active bleeding as evidenced by:
• Stable hematocrit, hemoglobin levels
• Guaiac-free stools, secretions
• Absence of hematoma, bruising, ecchymosis
• Stable blood pressure
• Stable mentation

Nursing Interventions

• Perform complete assessment of patient at least q4h including:
  ○ Neurologic assessment
  ○ Inspection of skin for areas of discoloration
  ○ Quality of peripheral pulses
  ○ Guaiac results of secretions, excretions
  ○ Evaluation of current laboratory values (hemoglobin, hematocrit, partial thromboplastin time [PTT], fibrinogen levels)

• Monitor vital signs and clinical status every 15–30 minutes until stable, then q24h.
• Inspect insertion sites for bleeding when taking vital signs
• Observe for retroperitoneal ecchymosis and severe lower back pain when taking vital signs.
• Avoid patient care activities that would predispose patient to bleeding or bruising:
  ○ Shaving
  ○ Venipuncture
  ○ Vigorous toothbrushing
  ○ Aggressive patient manipulation
  ○ Use of noninvasive blood pressure cuffs
• Maintain alignment of extremity involved in the procedure and place 5- to 10-lb sandbag over site.
• Coordinate blood work if venipuncture is required, or maintain large-bore IV with saline lock for blood sampling.
• Monitor patient's laboratory work:
  ○ Thrombin time
  ○ Prothrombin time
  ○ PTT
  ○ Fibrinogen split products
  ○ Fibrinogen levels
  ○ Hematocrit
  ○ Hemoglobin
• Alert all personnel that patient is anticoagulated by placing a sign at bedside.
• If invasive procedures are required, avoid noncompressible vessels.
  ○ Subclavian vein
  ○ Internal jugular vein

Rationales

• Complete assessment allows for rapid detection of any possible bleeding complications.

  ○ Hemoglobin and hematocrit determine the volume and oxygen-carrying capacity of RBCs in the circulation. PTT estimates the blood's ability to clot. Fibrinogen estimates the amount of coagulation proteins available to make clots.
• Frequent clinical assessment allows for rapid detection of bleeding.
• Previous sites of clotting frequently are dissolved during administration of thrombolytic agent.
• Catheterization via the femoral artery predisposes patient to iliac or femoral dissection.
• Hemostatic mechanisms are impaired after thrombolytic therapy, preventing rapid resolution of bleeding.

• Movement of extremity may dislodge newly formed clots. Direct pressure promotes hemostasis.
• Maintenance of vascular integrity is critical in preventing uncontrolled bleeding.

• All indicators of clotting are prolonged for 6–12 h after administration of streptokinase.

  ○ Indicators of bleeding should not decrease during postprocedure period.

• Increased communication among healthcare team minimizes risk of complications.
• Predisposes patient to uncontrolled bleeding.

Nursing Diagnoses

Nursing Diagnosis #2
Potential for physiologic injury: Bleeding, related to thrombolytic therapy (diminished clotting ability)

Desired Patient Outcomes

Patient will remain hemodynamically stable and bleeding will be controlled with minimal blood loss as evidenced by:
• No change in blood pressure
• No change in hemoglobin, hematocrit levels

CARE PLAN FOR THE PATIENT RECEIVING THROMBOLYTIC THERAPY: STREPTOKINASE AND TISSUE PLASMINOGEN ACTIVATOR (*Continued*)

Nursing Interventions
- Hold pressure to site for at least $\frac{1}{2}$–$\frac{3}{4}$ hr.
- Notify physician immediately of any bleeding.
- Monitor vital signs and document.

- Be prepared to administer blood products containing clotting factors (fresh frozen plasma, packed RBCs, cryoprecipitate).
- Administer aminocaproic acid as prescribed, and monitor response to therapy.

- Administer fluid and plasma expanders.

Rationales
- Hemostasis is prolonged due to manipulation of clotting cycle.
- Blood pressure will drop and heart rate increase if significant volume loss has occurred.
- Supplementing clotting cycle is effective in maintaining hemostasis.

- Aminocaproic acid is a hemostatic agent used to prevent excessive formation of plasmin. This helps to control bleeding caused by thrombolytic agents.
- Patient may require volume to maintain adequate cardiac output.

Nursing Diagnoses

Nursing Diagnosis #3
Potential alteration in comfort, related to allergic response (specific to streptokinase only)

Desired Patient Outcomes

Patient will not demonstrate discomfort related to manifestations of an allergic response (e.g., itching, musculoskeletal pain, respiratory distress, fever, anaphylaxis).

Nursing Interventions
- Monitor temperature q4h.
  - Inspect skin every 30 minutes–1 hr for 6 hrs then q4h.
  - If febrile, administer medication that does not affect hemostasis (i.e., acetaminophen).
- Monitor patient closely if signs or symptoms of reaction occur and document.

- Be prepared to administer corticosteroids, diphenhydramine, or life-support measures if reaction is severe.

Rationales
- Manifestations of allergic response will occur soon after administration of streptokinase as antigen is encountered.
  - Aspirin may contribute to patient's inability to clot.
- Patient who has recently had exposure to β-hemolytic streptococcal proteins will develop a severe response to thrombolytic therapy.

Nursing Diagnoses

Nursing Diagnosis #4
Potential alteration in cardiac output, related to arrhythmias

Desired Patient Outcomes

Patient will remain hemodynamically stable as evidenced by:
- Maintenance of MAP greater than 70 mmHg
- Lack of signs and symptoms of decreased cardiac output: dizziness, nausea, shortness of breath

Nursing Interventions
- Monitor patient's rhythm continuously, noting and documenting any change from baselines.
- Treat all arrhythmias with standard protocols, noting patient's response.
- Reassure patient that this is not unexpected and signals success of the procedure.

Rationales
- Reperfusion arrhythmias occur frequently after successful thrombolysis.

- Patients often fear that arrhythmias mean the procedure has been unsuccessful.

Nursing Diagnoses

Nursing Diagnosis #5
Potential alteration in tissue perfusion, related to reocclusion of coronary arteries

Desired Patient Outcomes

Patient will remain pain-free or chest pain will be alleviated, with resolution of ECG changes indicative of ischemia or infarction.

Nursing Interventions
- Instruct patient to notify nurse immediately at onset of chest pain; reinforce significance of time.

Rationales
- Patients may not understand the importance of communicating chest pain or are afraid to admit that the problem has not resolved.

CARE PLAN FOR THE PATIENT RECEIVING THROMBOLYTIC THERAPY: STREPTOKINASE AND TISSUE PLASMINOGEN ACTIVATOR (*Continued*)

Nursing Interventions	Rationales

• Observe patient for nonverbal signs of discomfort.
• Obtain a 12-lead ECG with any patient discomfort and observe for ischemic changes.
  ○ Notify physician immediately.
  ○ Administer standard medications for myocardial ischemia.
• Prepare patient for possibility of repeat procedure, emergent IABP, or open heart surgery.
	• ECG indicators of ischemia differentiate true angina from other kinds of discomfort.
	
	• It may be necessary to revascularize the myocardium by more conventional methods if reocclusion occurs.
	  ○ Counterpulsation helps with coronary artery perfusion and minimizes myocardial demands.

MAP = mean arterial pressure.

C H A P T E R   18

Nursing Management of the Patient with Coronary Artery Disease, Angina Pectoris, or Myocardial Infarction

Dolores M. Zygmont

CHAPTER OUTLINE

Coronary Artery Disease
- Pathogenesis
- Atherogenesis
- Risk Factors

Angina Pectoris
- Pathophysiology
- Stable Angina
- Vasospastic Angina
- Unstable Angina
- Assessment of Angina Pectoris

Acute Myocardial Infarction
- Pathophysiology
- Assessment of AMI

Treatment of Coronary Artery Disease
- Pharmacologic Treatment
- Revascularization

Complications Following an AMI
- Electrical Complications
- Hemodynamic Complications
- Mechanical Complications
- Inflammatory Responses

Rehabilitation
- Nursing Care

References

LEARNING OBJECTIVES

After completing this chapter, you should be able to:

1. Identify precipitating causes of coronary artery disease.
2. Define angina pectoris.
3. Discuss pertinent clinical factors that differentiate stable angina from unstable angina.
4. Discuss clinical findings used in the differential diagnosis of chest pain.
5. Describe pathophysiologic mechanisms involved in angina pectoris and myocardial infarction.
6. List pertinent clinical factors involved in making the diagnosis of myocardial infarction.
7. Discuss ECG changes that occur with a myocardial infarction.
8. Identify principles of treatment of myocardial infarction.
9. Describe three main categories of complications associated with a myocardial infarction.
10. Identify specific interventions involved in the management of a patient experiencing a myocardial infarction.
11. Relate pertinent nursing diagnoses, desired patient outcomes, and nursing interventions to the therapeutic goals in the care of the patient with angina pectoris or myocardial infarction.

CORONARY ARTERY DISEASE

Despite major advances in the treatment and understanding of coronary artery disease (CAD), ischemic heart disease still causes about 26% of deaths in the United States, and 1.2 million persons are diagnosed with an acute myocardial infarction each year.[1] Survival following an acute myocardial infarction is directly related to the size of the infarct, that is, the amount of myocardium lost to necrosis. Research in the 1970s focused on identifying ways to decrease myocardial oxygen demand in an attempt to limit infarct size. These results were less than satisfactory, and the focus shifted in the 1980s to identifying ways to increase the oxygen supply to the myocardium in an attempt to limit infarct size.[1] The focus in the 1990s promises further developments in both of these areas. In addition, research currently being done on the atherogenic process seen in CAD and the cellular changes that occur in the myocardium as a result of ischemia promise to increase our understanding and management of CAD, angina, and myocardial infarction.

Pathogenesis

CAD is usually diagnosed when the patient experiences chest pain indicative of myocardial ischemia. Ischemic heart disease is usually the result of a combination of atherosclerotic plaque and thrombus formation.[2,3] The only exception to this may be vasospastic angina,[2] which will be addressed later. Research on the role of the vascular endothelium in plaque and thrombus formation is currently under way and has already contributed to a better understanding of atherogenesis, thrombus formation, and the development of ischemic heart disease.

In individual who do not have CAD, the uninjured endothelium dilates in response to stimuli through the production of endothelial-derived relaxing factor (EDRF) and prostacyclin. In addition, the normal endothelium possesses a defense against platelet deposition by producing a surface that is anticoagulant in nature.[4] If the endothelium is damaged, as seen in CAD and ischemic heart disease, these normal protective functions are lost. The endothelial surface is unable to produce EDRF, and as a result the natural vasodilating ability of the endothelium is lost. The blood vessel then constricts in response to stimuli. In addition, the endothelium becomes prothrombogenic, which increases platelet adhesion and thrombin deposition at the site of the endothelial injury.

Atherogenesis

CAD is believed to be the result of an atherogenic process that begins with injury to the endothelial surface of the coronary artery as a result of risk factors associated with CAD.[3] Monocytes and macrophages migrate to the injured area and penetrate the intimal surface of the artery, where adhesion molecules are present. This forms the early stages of the atherosclerotic plaque.[4] Platelets then interact with the injured endothelium and adhere to its surface. As the platelets accumulate, hormones are released, causing vasoconstriction. Fibrinogen receptors are created as a result of these chemical interactions that enable the platelets to aggregate at the site of endothelial injury.[3] Platelet aggregation then causes the release of platelet-derived growth factor, which results in an increase in smooth muscle cells and fibroblasts. The smooth muscle cells and fibroblasts result in the production of elastin and collagen at the site of injury. This process leads to the development of the fibrous portion of the atherosclerotic plaque.[3]

Lipid accumulation is the final step in the process of atherogenesis. Low-density lipoproteins bind to the fibroblasts and smooth muscle cells at the injured site and are transported into the cell lysosomes. The lipoproteins are stored there until the cells are unable to accumulate any more. At that time, the lipoproteins break up and release cholesterol esters, which are taken up by the adjacent smooth muscle cells.[3] This causes lipid accumulation on the fibrous portion of the atherosclerotic plaque.

Research into the atherogenic process has created a greater understanding of how CAD develops. The current treatment of ischemic heart disease reflects these research developments.

Risk Factors

The risk factors associated with the development of CAD have been shown to directly contribute to the endothelial injury that initiates the atherogenic process. These risk factors can be divided into noncontrollable and controllable risk factors.

Noncontrollable Risk Factors

The most commonly recognized noncontrollable risk factors are gender and genetic predisposition. Men have a much higher incidence of CAD than women. Women are protected from the development of CAD by estrogen until menopause, at which time the incidence of CAD in women increases to three times the rate of menstruating females. Some persons also appear to have a genetic predisposition for developing CAD that is independent of other risk factors. Persons with a strong family history of CAD should be vigilant in their modification of the controllable risk factors.

Controllable Risk Factors

Controllable risk factors are those that can be modified. Commonly recognized controllable risk factors are hypertension, cigarette smoking, elevated serum cholesterol, and hyperglycemia. Other factors that may contribute to the development of CAD are exercise, obesity, and personality type.

Hypertension. Both systolic and diastolic hypertension contributes to the development of CAD by causing injury to the endothelial surface of the coronary artery. Even mild-to-moderate hypertension with systolic blood pressures of 120 to 140 mmHg can double the risk of a person's developing CAD. Individuals with hypertension should be educated about the risk of developing CAD and the importance of continuing treatment.

Cigarette Smoking. Smoking significantly increases the incidence of CAD and increases the mortality rate in persons with CAD. In addition to endothelial injury, the nicotine associated with cigarette smoking increases the heart rate, increases the blood pressure, and causes vasoconstriction of the coronary arteries. This increases the myocardial demand for oxygen and MVO_2 and decreases the supply of oxygen available to the myocardium. Nicotine also limits the amount of oxygen available to the body tissues by shifting the oxyhemoglobin dissociation curve to the left (see Fig. 22–14).

Serum Cholesterol. The link between hyperlipidemia and CAD is well documented. In fact, modification of this risk factor has been shown to decrease the occurrence of myocardial infarction. Both cholesterol and triglycerides are transported in the blood by lipoproteins. The lipoproteins of most concern in the development of CAD are very low-density lipoproteins (VLDL), low-density lipoproteins (LDL), and high-density lipoproteins (HDL).

VLDL is composed primarily of triglycerides and is produced by the liver. Metabolism of VLDL produces LDL, the most atherogenic of the lipoproteins. LDL accounts for about 70% of the total plasma cholesterol and transports cholesterol from the liver to the peripheral tissues, where it is taken up by receptors. Elevations of LDL can be the result of an overproduction of VLDL or an ineffective clearance of LDL. Normal LDL levels are lower than 150 mg/100 mL.

HDL is referred to as the good lipoprotein because of its negative correlation with CAD. High levels of HDL exert a protective effect on the development of CAD by aiding in the transport of cholesterol from the peripheral tissues to the liver for excretion. Individuals should be encouraged to increase the level of HDL to greater than 50 mg/100 mL through weight control, aerobic exercise, and cessation of smoking.

Treatment of hyperlipidemia involves dietary modification alone or in combination with drugs. Dietary modifications include limiting cholesterol and saturated fat intake and increasing polyunsaturated fat intake. The omega-3 polyunsaturated fatty acids found in fish have been found to lower triglyceride levels and should become a major factor in dietary modification.

When dietary modification and exercise alone are unsuccessful in lowering serum cholesterol after 3 to 6 months, antilipemic drug therapy is started. These drugs reduce serum triglyceride or cholesterol levels or both either by reducing their synthesis or by forming insoluble compounds that are excreted in the feces. The drug selected is determined by the lipid profile of the patient. Some commonly used antilipemics are cholestyramine, clofibrate, colestipol, dextrothyroxine, gemfibrozil, lovastatin, niacin, and probucol.

Hyperglycemia. Research has shown that CAD is more extensive and severe in persons with diabetes than in persons without diabetes. Recent studies suggest that tighter glucose control in diabetics may significantly reduce the vascular complications seen in poorly controlled diabetics.

Exercise. A sedentary lifestyle has been associated with the development of CAD for years. Aerobic exercise, three times per week, has been shown to have a positive effect on the development of CAD. In addition to contributing to weight control, it also raises serum HDL levels and lowers the heart rate and blood pressure.

Obesity. Obesity as a risk factor for CAD can most likely be attributed to several other risk factors. For example, increased serum cholesterol and triglyceride levels are common in obese persons because of diets high in fats and refined carbohydrates. These individuals generally lead sedentary lives and frequently have hypertension.

Personality Type. The person with classic type A personality has long been recognized for being at an increased risk for the development of CAD. This type of individual is ambitious, speaks quickly, is competitive, and is constantly striving to achieve more in less time. The link between type A personality and the development of CAD is related to the increased levels of circulating catecholamines that are secreted in response to stress—both environmental and intrinsic. These increased levels of catecholamines increase the heart rate and blood pressure, blood-clotting time, and platelet aggregation. Individuals with type A personality should develop methods of stress reduction through stress reduction programs, biofeedback, and exercise.

ANGINA PECTORIS

Angina is the result of an imbalance between myocardial oxygen supply and oxygen demand. It can be divided into three major categories: stable angina, vasospastic angina, and unstable angina. Despite differences in their clinical presentation, the pathophysiology of angina, regardless of the type, is similar.

Pathophysiology

The chest pain in angina is the result of myocardial ischemia that results from an imbalance in myocardial oxygen supply and demand. Understanding the factors that affect the supply-demand equation contributes to understanding the current treatment of angina.

Increases in myocardial oxygen demand can be related to three factors: (1) heart rate, (2) myocardial contractility, and (3) systolic left ventricular wall tension. These three factors are influenced by increases in afterload, ventricular wall thickness, ventricular volume, and end-diastolic pressure, referred to as preload.[5] Because increases in heart rate, contractility, and systolic left ventricular wall tension increase the workload of the heart, there is an increase in myocardial oxygen demand and myocardial oxygen consumption (MVO_2). The person without CAD can compensate for the increased demand by increasing the oxygen supply through coronary artery dilatation. However, those with CAD are unable to increase the oxygen supply, which contributes to the development of myocardial ischemia.

Myocardial oxygen supply can be increased in persons who do not have CAD through autoregulatory functions of the coronary arteries. The coronary arteries normally extract 70% of the oxygen delivered to the cells. Since this is the maximum amount that can be extracted, the individual without CAD can increase the oxygen supply through the release of EDRF, causing vasodilatation of the coronary arteries. The loss of this vasodilating ability, as found in those with CAD, directly contributes to myocardial ischemia. In addition, the coronary arteries receive most of their blood supply during diastole. Increases in heart rate shorten the duration of diastole, thus decreasing the amount of blood that can flow into the coronary arteries. This also contributes to the risk of myocardial ischemia.

Oxygen supply to the myocardium can be affected by the obstructive coronary artery lesions seen in patients with CAD.[5] The obstructive lesions can be fixed, as seen with plaque deposits and thrombus formation, or they can be dynamic and transient. The dynamic obstructions frequently result from increases in vasomotor tone, causing vasospasm and temporary obstruction of the coronary artery (Fig. 18–1). The presence of either fixed or dynamic obstructive lesions, in combination with the loss of the vasodilating ability of the coronary artery, limits the body's ability to meet the oxygen supply. The increase in blood needed increases the risk of the myocardium to ischemia.

Oxygen supply to the myocardium can also be affected by an inadequate coronary reserve.[5] *Coronary reserve* refers to the heart's ability to increase blood flow up to six times its baseline in response to increased oxygen demand.[6] Inadequate coronary reserve can result from insufficient collateral circulation and decreased subendocardial perfusion as seen with increased left ventricular end-diastolic pressures (LVEDP) or with fixed, obstructive coronary artery lesions. Inadequate coronary reserve limits the ability of the heart to respond to increases in oxygen demand to only two to three times its baseline.[6] This is insufficient to meet the increased oxygen demands of the myocardium and leads to myocardial ischemia and chest pain.

Any process that alters the balance between oxygen supply and demand sufficiently that MVO_2 is compromised will result in myocardial ischemia and chest pain (Fig. 18–2). An indirect measure of MVO_2 is the rate-pressure product (RPP). The RPP is calculated by multiplying the heart rate by the systolic blood pres-

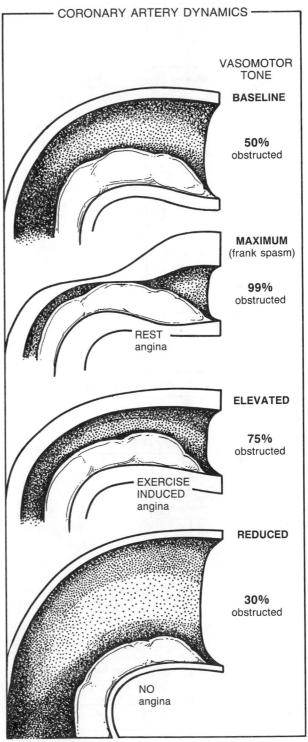

FIGURE 18–1. This schematic demonstrates how the underlying tone of a coronary vessel can influence type of angina in the presence of a 50% obstructive lesion. Rest angina, exercise-induced angina, or no angina may occur as muscle tone varies. (Adapted from Epstein, SE and Talbot, TL: Dynamic coronary tone in precipitation, exacerbation, and relief of angina pectoris. Am J Cardiol 48:797, 1981.)

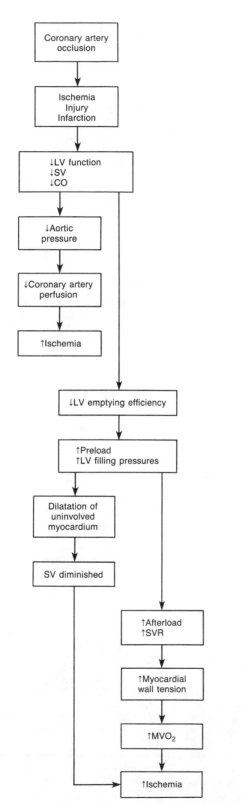

FIGURE 18–2. Hemodynamic consequences prompted by myocardial ischemia associated with coronary artery occlusion.

sure. The RPP is a fairly reliable indicator of when MVO_2 has increased sufficiently to cause chest pain. Stable angina, vasospastic angina, and unstable angina result from an imbalance in the oxygen supply-demand equation.

Stable Angina

Stable angina, frequently referred to as chronic angina or exertional angina, is the result of a fixed, obstructive coronary artery lesion. Chest pain results when the workload of the heart (demand) increases to the extent that the coronary reserve system can no longer compensate (decreased supply). Episodes of chest pain are predictable, such that the individual generally knows what activities are likely to produce chest pain. As a result, persons with stable angina can be taught to avoid activities likely to produce chest pain or to take nitroglycerin prior to engaging in these activities.[7,8]

Because the fixed, obstructive lesion in stable angina limits the heart's ability to increase blood flow in response to increased demand, medical therapy is aimed at increasing the oxygen supply through vasodilatation with nitrates. In addition, attempts are made at decreasing the myocardial oxygen demand through the use of β-blockers and calcium channel blockers to decrease heart rate, contractility, and ventricular wall stress.[9]

Because of its predictability, stable angina can be managed with patient education focusing on modification of risk factors and use of medications. The aim of treatment is to prevent progression of the disease through risk factor modification, control of symptoms, prevention of infarction, and improvement in the quality of life through improved exercise tolerance.[7,8] By adhering to medical therapy and risk factor modification, stable angina can be managed for years with a decreased risk of an acute myocardial infarction (AMI).

Vasospastic Angina

Vasospastic angina is also referred to as variant angina, Prinzmetal's angina, and coronary vasospasm. Unlike stable angina, the obstructive lesion is dynamic and transient in nature, resulting from a local abnormality in the coronary vessel, which causes an increased vasomotor tone and in turn causes coronary vasospasm. This increase in vasomotor tone causes a hyperreactivity in the coronary artery to vasoconstricting stimuli. The resultant vasospasm causes total or subtotal coronary artery occlusion of that vessel. Although the exact cause of the hyperreactivity is unknown, suggested hypotheses are lack of EDRF, the presence of subintimal plaque, and alterations in the underlying arterial smooth muscle or neural mediation.[6] There are no underlying changes in oxygen consumption (MVO_2) in the patient with vasospastic angina. The alteration is strictly in the oxygen supply to the myocardium secondary to coronary artery spasm.

Persons with vasospastic angina may or may not have an underlying atherosclerotic plaque creating a fixed obstructive coronary artery lesion. The chest pain experienced with this type of angina resembles both vasospastic and stable angina. When diagnosis through clinical presentation is equivocal, cardiac catheterization is performed and ergonovine maleate, a potent vasoconstrictor, is administered. When vasospasm is the cause of the angina, ergonovine induces vasospasm and the diagnosis is confirmed.[9]

The chest pain associated with vasospastic angina differs from that associated with stable angina. This individual frequently has pain-free periods lasting days or weeks. When the chest pain occurs, it is frequently in clusters, it commonly occurs during sleep or rest or on arising, and it may be associated with syncope. Although rarely associated with physical exertion, there is some evidence linking emotional stress to the episodes of chest pain.[2,6,9] Vasospastic angina is frequently seen in persons with a history of migraine headaches or Raynaud's phenomenon.[2]

The chest pain caused by vasospastic angina responds to nitroglycerin by causing coronary vasodilatation in the area of the vasospasm. Calcium channel blockers are used to prevent coronary artery vasospasm. The aim of treatment is to control symptoms, prevent progression to unstable angina, prevent infarction, and improve the quality of life.

Unstable Angina

Unstable angina is frequently referred to as preinfarction angina, acute coronary insufficiency, and crescendo angina.[2,10] Unstable angina indicates an active intracoronary process and is frequently the prelude to an AMI. It is considered a medical emergency.

The intracoronary process believed to be responsible for unstable angina is the result of a rupture of the atherosclerotic plaque or a fissure created between the plaque and the endothelial surface. There is no particular triggering mechanism identified for the plaque disruption, but the atherogenic process is initiated after the disruption occurs.[2,6,10,11]

The chest pain associated with unstable angina is generally different from the usual angina pattern. It occurs more frequently and is more severe and more prolonged when compared with the typical angina experienced by the individual. Unstable angina frequently occurs at rest or at unusually low activity levels, and it lasts longer than 30 minutes.

Treatment of unstable angina is aimed at stabilizing and preserving the area of myocardium at risk by interrupting the thrombotic process. Aspirin is given to prevent further platelet aggregation. Heparin is administered to prevent further clot formation. Both interventions are aimed at maintaining vessel patency. Nitroglycerin is given to increase oxygen supply to the myocardium through increased coronary artery vasodilatation. β-Blockers and calcium channel blockers are given to decrease heart rate, contractility, and systolic left ventricular wall tension in an effort to decrease oxygen demand and MVo^2.

Recognition of the related clinical and electrocardiographic changes indicative of increasing ischemia is essential in the evaluation of the effectiveness of medical therapy.[11] Continued evidence of ischemia despite pharmacologic intervention may indicate the need for myocardial revascularization through percutaneous transluminal coronary angioplasty (PTCA), insertion of a coronary artery stent, or coronary artery bypass graft (CABG) (see Chapters 17 and 20).

Assessment of Angina Pectoris

Clinical History of Chest Pain

When a person is admitted to the hospital with chest pain, it is imperative that a complete history be obtained to rule out noncardiac causes of chest pain (Table 18–1). Evaluation should focus on the quality, location, radiation, duration, precipitating factors of the chest pain, and the patient's response to nitro-

TABLE 18–1
Differential Diagnosis of Chest Pain

1. Ischemic heart disease syndromes, including angina pectoris, unstable angina pectoris, acute coronary insufficiency, Prinzmetal's angina (variant angina), or acute myocardial infarction
2. Dissecting aortic aneurysm
3. Mitral valve prolapse
4. Pneumonia
5. Atelectasis
6. Spontaneous pneumothorax
7. Pulmonary embolic disease
8. Pulmonary hypertension
9. Cardiomyopathy
10. Valvular aortic stenosis, idiopathic hypertrophic subaortic stenosis, supravalvular aortic stenosis
11. Aortic aneurysm
12. Costochondritis
13. Chest wall or skeletal trauma, including rib fractures
14. Malignancies resulting in marked marrow packing with neoplastic cells, including multiple myeloma and leukemia
15. Anxiety
16. Carcinoma of the lung
17. Esophageal spasm or hiatal hernia
18. Cervical osteoarthritis
19. Thoracic outlet syndrome
20. Herpes zoster (either before or after the development of skin lesions)
21. Pericarditis

Referred Pain into the Chest
1. Peptic ulcer disease
2. Cholecystitis
3. Pancreatitis
4. Subdiaphragmatic mass or abscess
5. Abdominal aortic aneurysm

Source: Willerson, JT, Hillis, LD, and Buja, LM: Ischemic Heart Disease: Clincal and Pathophysiologic Aspects. Raven Press, New York, 1982, p 115, with permission.

TABLE 18–2
Characteristics of Angina Pectoris

Quality
Sensation of pressure or heavy weight on the chest
Burning sensation
Feeling of tightness
Shortness of breath with feeling of constriction about the larynx
   or upper trachea
Visceral quality (deep, heavy, squeezing, aching)
Gradual increase in intensity followed by gradual fading away

Location
Over the sternum or very near to it
Anywhere between epigastrium and pharynx
Occasionally limited to left shoulder and left arm
Rarely limited to right arm
Limited to lower jaw
Lower interscapular or supracapsular area

Duration
0.5–30 minutes

Precipitating Factors
Relationship to exercise
Effort that involves use of arms above the head
Cold environment
Walking against the wind
Walking after a large meal
Emotional factors involved with physical exercise
Fright, anger
Coitus

Nitroglycerin Relief
Relief of pain occurring 45 seconds to 5 minutes of taking
   nitroglycerin

Radiation
Medial aspect of left arm
Left shoulder
Jaw
Occasionally right arm

Source: Helfant, RH and Banka, VS: A Clinical and Angiographic Approach to Coronary Heart Disease. FA Davis, Philadelphia, 1978, p 48, with permission.

glycerin (Table 18–2). The history should also include the presence of risk factors and a previous history of an AMI.

The quality of anginal pain is frequently described as a heaviness in the chest or a choking feeling. Some patients experience shortness of breath related to a tightness around the chest. The pain usually begins and ends gradually in a crescendo-decrescendo pattern.

Anginal chest pain is typically located in the sternal or retrosternal area. It may radiate to the left shoulder and down the left arm. Occasionally, patients present with an anginal equivalent to chest pain that may be limited to jaw pain, hand pain, or similar, nonfocal locations.

The duration of chest pain is important in the differentiation of the type of angina. Pain associated with stable angina typically lasts from 1 to 5 minutes to a maximum of 10 minutes, whereas the chest pain associated with vasospastic angina can last up to 30 minutes.[6]

The identification of precipitating factors can help differentiate the type of angina. Patients should be questioned about the usual precipitating factors as well as about the differences that might have occurred this time. Questions should focus on the relation of the pain to exercise, emotions, cold temperatures, sex, and meals.

Persons with a history of angina are frequently prescribed nitroglycerin for relief of anginal episodes. They should be asked how many nitroglycerin tablets they took for this episode of chest pain as well as the number of tablets they usually take. If the chest pain was not relieved by nitroglycerin, ask whether they felt a "ping" under the tongue after taking the tablet and whether the tablets were stored in a dark bottle. To maintain potency, nitroglycerin should be stored in a brown bottle without a cotton filler. Cotton absorbs nitroglycerin and decreases its effectiveness. Nitroglycerin tablets should be replaced every 3 months to ensure potency. The ping under the tongue after administration indicates that the tablet has maintained its potency.

Electrocardiographic Changes

A 12-lead electrocardiogm (ECG) is essential in the initial assessment of angina. Persons with stable angina generally demonstrate T-wave inversion or ST-segment depression of 1 mm or greater, measured 0.08 second from the J point in multiple leads during episodes of pain. Vasospastic angina, on the other hand, reveals ST-segment elevation and T-wave changes during chest pain.[12] These changes mimic those seen in an AMI. However, unlike an AMI, in which the changes persist once the pain is relieved, the ECG of a patient with vasospastic angina is normal during pain-free periods. Frequently, when the disease process is limited to discrete anatomic lesions, the ECG is highly indicative of the specific coronary artery involved. It is not uncommon for ECGs to be performed during chest pain and after the chest pain has been relieved. The rationale for these multiple ECGs is to help differentiate among increasing ischemia, progression to an AMI, and the documentation of a vasospastic process that may not be evident on pain-free ECGs.

ACUTE MYOCARDIAL INFARCTION

An AMI occurs when myocardial cells are irreversibly damaged because of prolonged ischemia. During the first hour following an AMI, the myocardial cells are electrically unstable and the patient is most at risk for the development of ventricular tachycardia and ventricular fibrillation. In fact, the highest mortality rate is during this first hour. There has been a progressive decline in the mortality rate associated with AMIs since the 1970s.[13] A major factor in this decline has been the immediate treatment of the lethal arrhythmias—ventricular tachycardia and ventricular fibrillation—with electrical cardioversion and defibrillation. This has been facilitated by the widespread implementation of coronary care units and the use of advanced cardiac life support units within the emergency medical systems.

The most common cause of death following an AMI is related to the severity of left ventricular dysfunction, which presents as congestive heart failure or cardiogenic shock. Since this is directly related to the size of the AMI and the amount of myocardium lost to necrosis, the focus of management is on limiting the size of the infarction through prompt recognition and intervention.

Pathophysiology

An AMI can be viewed as the final stage in the continuum of CAD, beginning with asymptomatic CAD and progressing through stable angina and unstable angina. The underlying disease process in an AMI begins with the atherogenic process described earlier in which the plaque ruptures or fissures occur, causing an increase in the thrombus formation. In fact, research has shown that about 87% of all patients who have an AMI have evidence of thrombus formation.[2,14] The fundamental difference between unstable angina and an AMI is that in the AMI the ischemia is prolonged and significant myocardial necrosis results.[15] The duration of the ischemia has a direct bearing on the actual amount of damage to the myocardium.

In those individuals in whom a thrombus cannot be identified, it is believed that a thrombus did exist and cause the AMI but that the body's intrinsic lytic processes dissolved the clot. Prompt intervention to interrupt the thrombotic process through the use of thrombolytic agents, antiplatalet aggregating drugs, and heparin has been shown to salvage myocardium and limit infarction size.[15]

In addition to the focal changes occurring in the coronary artery, systemic activation of the sympathetic nervous system (SNS) and the renin-angiotensin system (RAS) have been recognized in the early stages of an AMI. This activation is a compensatory mechanism to maintain adequate hemodynamic function and maintain cardiac output.

Stimulation of the SNS results in increased levels of circulating catecholamines, causing significant hemodynamic changes in myocardial function. Heart rate and myocardial contractility increase, thus causing an increase in myocardial oxygen demand and MVO_2. In addition, the increased heart rate limits diastolic filling of the coronary arteries, thus limiting oxygen supply to the ischemic myocardium.

Stimulation of the RAS increases the level of circulating angiotensin II. Angiotensin II causes peripheral vasoconstriction, which increases the arterial blood pressure. The increased blood pressure increase MVO_2 in the ischemic myocardium.

These elevated catecholamine and angiotensin II levels are present during the first several days after an AMI, then gradually subside back to normal levels. However, in patients with left ventricular dysfunction and congestive heart failure following an AMI, these levels have been elevated for up to 1 month after infarction.[16] In fact, the prolonged activation of the SNS and RAS has a significant impact on the morbidity and mortality associated with an AMI by directly contributing to the size of the infarction.[16]

Onset of ischemia, along with stimulation of the SNS and RAS, produces immediate changes in the performance of the left ventricular muscle. The ventricular muscle becomes less elastic, causing a decrease in ventricular compliance. An abrupt increase in left ventricular filling pressures occurs as a result of diastolic alterations in metabolism. These diastolic alterations in metabolism are primarily related to the increased availability of calcium to the contractile elements of the myocardial muscle. The increased amount of calcium limits the amount of diastolic relaxation to the ischemic area. Even though the noninjured areas attempt to compensate for the loss of diastolic relaxation to maintain stroke volume, the net result is increased myocardial work and MVO_2.[17] Without prompt intervention, ischemia is prolonged and the infarction may be increased.

Assessment of AMI

The diagnosis of an AMI is generally made through the clinical history of chest pain, physical examination, ECG changes, and cardiac enzyme changes. The clinical history is initially the most significant indicator of impending myocardial infarction.

Clinical History of Chest Pain

The chest pain associated with a myocardial infarction is frequently described as a heaviness, tightness, or squeezing in the chest. It is usually located in the substernal or retrosternal area of the chest and may radiate to the arm, neck, back, or jaw. Unlike angina, it is frequently associated with nausea, vomiting, and weakness.[14] Some patients may describe the discomfort as indigestion or a burning type of feeling. Patients with a known history of angina report that the pain is different from their usual anginal pain, either in location, duration, intensity, or precipitating events.

Typically, the pain of an AMI lasts longer than 30 minutes and is unrelieved by nitroglycerin. Frequently no clearly identifiable precipitating events cause the infarction, although some patients report a significant emotional trauma prior to the infarction. There does appear to be a relationship between the onset of an AMI and the circadian rhythms. Most AMIs are found to occur in the early morning, and it is hypothesized that the increase in circulating catecholamines that occurs with awakening and ambulation may increase vascular tone in sufficient amounts to cause the plaque rupture or fissures known to initiate the thrombotic process.[15]

Even though chest pain is a primary symptom of an AMI, some patients experience a myocardial infarction without chest pain. Typically, these patients are

RESEARCH APPLICATION: FACTORS INFLUENCING PREHOSPITAL DELAY IN PATIENTS EXPERIENCING CHEST PAIN
Reilly, A, Dracup, K, and Dattolo, J. Am J Crit Care 3(4):300–306, 1994.

Purpose: Mortality and morbidity following an acute myocardial infarction (AMI) are directly related to the amount of time that elapses from onset of symptoms to definitive medical intervention. The purpose of this study was to identify the internal and external motivators that affect a delay in seeking medical care.

Methods: A convenience sample of 77 adult patients from three university affiliated medical centers participated in the study. Study participants were selected according to the following criteria: within 72 hours of admission, diagnosis of suspected or proven myocardial infarction (MI), 35 to 80 years of age, English-speaking, and no other complicating illness of malignancy.

Data were collected using a chart review and the Response to Symptoms questionnaire developed by the Thrombolysis in Acute Myocardial Infarction Trial investigators. The 18-item questionnaire elicits information regarding symptom context factors, such as place and time of day, clinical status and health history, and severity of chest pain, anxiety, and stress levels. One item was added to identify which family member was present at onset of symptoms. Validity and reliability for the instrument were established.

Frequencies, percentages, means, and medians were calculated on the demographic data and delay times. Comparisons were then made between the nondelayers (less than or equal to 3 hours) and the delayers (greater than 3 hours) using *chi*-squared tests for nominal data and independent *t*-tests for interval data.

Results: The mean delay time for the 77 patients was 25.4 hours, with a median delay time of 5 hours. Forty percent of the patients delayed less than 3 hours; 60% delayed more than 3 hours. Patients who experienced symptoms alone had a median delay time of 2 hours, compared with a median delay time of 9 hours when family members were present.

Advanced age, the presence of a family member during symptoms, and the identification of symptoms as not serious were statistically significant in causing a delay in seeking treatment. Demographic variables such as gender, education, ethnicity, work status, and income were not statistically significant, although higher percentages of those with a high school education or less and an annual income of less than $10,000 were seen in the delay group. Although not statistically significant, the severity of chest pain was graded slightly higher in the non-delay group. Anxiety and stress levels had no effect on delay times.

Practice Implications: Despite an increase in the education provided to the lay public regarding the symptoms of an AMI and the need for prompt medical therapy, this study indicates that there has not been a significant impact on symptom recognition and seeking definitive treatment. The authors make three recommendations to healthcare professionals based on the results of this study.

1. Critical care health professionals should target those at high risk for prehospital delay. Individuals 60 years of age or older should be taught how to differentiate cardiac symptoms from symptoms associated with other chronic illness. These patients should also be taught how to access the healthcare system and the importance of seeking help immediately.
2. Critical care health professionals should educate family members about courses of action. Family members should be taught how to recognize the chest pain of an AMI and how and when to call the emergency medical system. They should also be taught how to take control of the situation and not become a part of the denial process in which the patient frequently becomes engaged.
3. The public needs to be educated about the potential negative consequences of prehospital delay. This education should include the symptoms of an AMI, the medical treatment available, and the dangers associated with delayed treatment.

elderly or diabetic or have had heart transplantation.[14] The diagnosis of an infarction in this population is generally made through ECG changes or cardiac enzyme elevation.[18]

Physical Examination

The physical examination of the patient with an AMI varies according to the severity and location of the infarction. During episodes of chest pain, some patients lie quietly with little behavioral evidence that they are experiencing chest pain, whereas others are visibly restless and anxious. Nausea, vomiting, and diaphoresis frequently occur during the AMI.

Patients with an AMI uncomplicated by heart failure or arrhythmias frequently have a normal physical examination. The physical examination of those with large AMIs is often indicative of extensive myocardial muscle damage.

Frequently, patients experiencing an AMI have a sinus tachycardia, which can be the result of pain, anxiety, or SNS stimulation. Sinus tachycardia is also found in patients with extensive muscle damage and congestive heart failure. Paradoxically, patients with an inferior wall infarction commonly experience sinus bradycardia or atrioventricular (AV) nodal heart blocks. This occurs because the sinus node, AV node, and the inferior wall share a common blood supply from the right coronary artery.

Auscultation of the heart may be completely normal in the patient with an AMI. A fourth heart sound, S_4, may he heard as a result of decreased left ventricular compliance following an AMI. However, this finding is not specific for an AMI and can often be heard in healthy, older individuals. A third heart sound, S_3, is heard when extensive myocardial damage has occurred and when congestive heart failure is present. A systolic murmur of mitral regurgitation is heard when the papillary muscle or mitral valve is damaged from ischemia or infarction. This usually occurs with inferior wall infarction.[14]

Auscultation of the lungs reveals clear lungs in an uncomplicated AMI. Rales or wheezes indicate congestive heart failure resulting from an extensive AMI.[14]

Electrocardiographic Changes

Historically, ECG changes associated with an AMI, in particular the development of Q waves, were indicative of the extent of the infarction. Previously, the development of a Q wave indicated a transmural infarction, in which necrosis extended from the subendocardial surface to the epicardial surface. Persons who did not develop Q waves were thought to have had damage to the subendocardial surface of the heart only (subendocardial infarction). The current research suggests that patients with complete coronary occlusion from a thrombus develop Q waves, whereas patients with incomplete occlusions from "smaller" thrombi or spontaneous clot lysis develop non–Q-wave AMIs. Therefore, the newer terminology of Q wave versus non–Q-wave infarct refers to the extent of coronary artery occlusion rather than the extent of myocardial damage.[19] ECG changes associated with non–Q-wave infarcts are frequently inconclusive and can mimic the changes seen in angina. The diagnosis of this type of infarct usually relies on cardiac enzyme changes.[19]

The classic ECG changes associated with Q-wave AMIs reveal ischemia, injury, and necrosis. The area of myocardial involvement is thought of as concentric circles, with the area of necrosis at the center surrounded by the area of injury and then the area of ischemia. Treatment is aimed at restoring blood flow to the ischemic area, thereby limiting the extent of the injured area.

Ischemic changes are reflected in the T wave of the ECG. During the hyperacute phase of the AMI, the T wave has an increased amplitude or peaking. This gradually recedes to symmetric T-wave inversion in which the T wave points away from the ischemic area.[20]

Injury is reflected in changes in the ST segment of the ECG and typically presents as ST elevation.[20] As

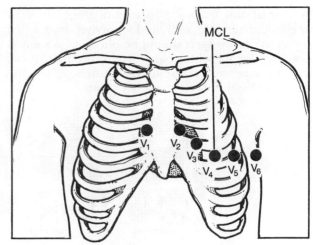

FIGURE 18–3. Twelve-lead ECG. To obtain a 12-lead ECG, attach limb electrodes to the patient's extremities as labeled. Chest electrodes are positioned as follows: V_1 4th intercostal space (ICS), to the right of the sternum; V_2 4th ICS, to the left of the sternum; V_3 halfway between V_2 and V_4; V_4 5th ICS, at the midclavicular line (MCL); V_5 anterior axillary line, halfway between V_4 and V_6; and V_6 5th ICS at the midaxillary line.

the currents of injury subside or necrose, the ST segment gradually returns to baseline.

Q waves reflect myocardial necrosis. Although small Q waves are normally present in leads I, aV_L, V_5, and V_6, the Q waves associated with an AMI are considered pathologic Q waves and are typically greater than 0.04 second in duration. As the Q wave deepens, the R wave facing the infarction loses up to 30% of its amplitude.[20]

Typically, the T-wave changes appear immediately with the onset of myocardial ischemia and can last from several minutes to several hours. The ST-segment changes last for hours to days following the infarct. Q waves usually develop over the first few days of the infarct and last for the life of the individual. However, there have been reports of the disappearance of Q waves, especially after inferior infarctions.[20]

The 12-lead ECG that records cardiac activity from

TABLE 18–3
Location of Infarct by ECG Leads

Infarct Area	ECG Leads	ECG Changes
Anterior wall	V_1–V_6	QS pattern
		Poor R-wave progression
Anteroseptal	V_1–V_3 or V_4	QS pattern
		Poor R-wave progression
Anterolateral	I, aV_L, V_1–V_6	Abnormal Q waves
Inferior wall (diaphragmatic)	II, III, aV_F	Abnormal Q waves
Inferolateral	II, III, aV_F, V_5, V_6	Abnormal Q waves
Posterior wall	V_1, V_2	Tall wide R wave
Posterolateral	V_1, V_2	Tall wide R wave
	I, aV_L, V_5, V_6	Abnormal Q wave
Lateral wall	I, aV_L, V_5, V_6	Abnormal Q waves

the frontal and horizontal planes of the body is an excellent diagnostic tool in identifying myocardial changes (Fig. 18–3). It should be obtained as soon as possible after the chest pain develops, either in the field by emergency rescue personnel or on the patient's arrival in the emergency room.

Localization of Infarction. The ECG changes seen in a patient with an AMI are typically reflected in leads that look directly at the injured surface and indicate the coronary artery involved (Table 18–3).

Inferior wall myocardial infarctions (IWMI), formerly called diaphragmatic infarctions, result from

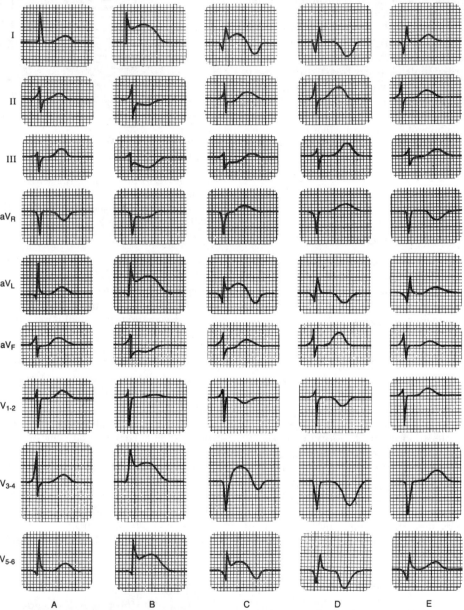

FIGURE 18–4. Diagrammatic illustration of serial ECG patterns in AWMI. (*A*) Normal tracing. (*B*) Early pattern. There is ST-segment elevation in leads I, aV$_L$, and V$_3$ to V$_6$, and ST depression in leads II, III, and aV$_F$ (the ST depression might reflect inferior wall ischemia or reciprocal depression). (*C*) Later pattern (hours to days). Q waves are present in leads I, aV$_L$, and V$_5$ to V$_6$. QS complexes are present in leads V$_3$ and V$_4$, indicating that the major area of infarction underlies the area recorded by leads V$_3$ and V$_4$. ST-segment changes persist but to a lesser degree, and the T waves are beginning to invert in those leads in which ST-segment elevation is present. (*D*) Late (established) pattern (days to weeks). The Q waves and QS complexes persist. The ST segments are isoelectric. The T waves are deeply and symmetrically inverted in the leads that showed ST elevation and tall in the leads that showed ST depression. This pattern may persist for the remainder of the patient's life. (*E*) Very late pattern (months to years). The abnormal Q waves and QS complexes persist, but the T waves have returned to normal. Without the benefit of serial ECGs, it is not possible to determine when myocardial infarction occurred. Therefore, no conclusions should be drawn as to the age of the process on the basis of a single ECG. (Adapted from Goldschlager, W and Goldman, MJ: Electrocardiography: Essentials of Interpretation. Appleton & Lange, Los Altos, CA, 1984, p 89.)

lesions in the right coronary artery. This infarction can be located by looking for ST elevation, T-wave inversion, and Q-wave development in leads II, III, and aV$_F$.[20,21]

Anterior wall myocardial infarctions (AWMIs) can result from lesions in the left main coronary artery or its branches, the left anterior descending coronary artery, and the left circumflex. AWMIs associated with left main coronary artery lesions are extensive and typically cause ECG changes in leads V$_1$ through V$_6$ (Fig. 18–4). This type of infarct is referred to as a massive anterior, anteroseptal, or anteroseptal lateral infarct. Anteroseptal AMIs usually result from lesions in the left anterior descending coronary artery and are seen in leads V$_1$ through V$_4$. Anterolateral AMIs are seen in leads I, aV$_1$, and V$_3$ through V$_6$.[20,21]

Lateral wall myocardial infarctions (LWMIs) usually result from lesions in the left circumflex coronary artery and diagonal branches of the left anterior descending coronary artery. Lateral myocardial infarctions can be subdivided into apical, seen in leads V$_5$ and V$_6$, or high lateral, seen in leads I and aV$_L$. Lateral myocardial infarctions rarely occur alone and are usually associated with AWMIs and occasionally with IWMIs.[20,21]

Posterior wall myocardial infarctions (PWMIs) are associated with lesions in the right coronary artery and occasionally the circumflex branch of the left coronary artery. They typically occur with IWMIs and are much more difficult to diagnose because of their anatomic location behind the anterior myocardial wall. Because there are no leads on the standard 12-lead ECG that look directly at the posterior myocardial wall, ECG evidence of a posterior infarction is indirect. Changes are located in leads V$_1$ through V$_{2-3}$; these are ST depression, tall peaked T waves, and an increased amplitude of the R wave. These changes are the mirror opposites or reciprocal changes of ST elevation, T-wave inversion and Q-wave development (Fig. 18–5).[20,21]

The ability to localize the area of infarct through lead recognition has significant implications in the continuous monitoring of patients. Patients should be monitored on leads that reflect the area of infarct to document changes in the ischemic process and evolution of the AMI. In addition, knowledge of the infarct area indicates the type of complications that can be anticipated and thus guide the care of the AMI patient. Table 18–3 identifies the ECG leads associated with the type and location of myocardial infarction.

Cardiac Enzyme Changes

Cardiac enzyme elevations can be seen with many clinical conditions other than AMI, such as pericarditis, pulmonary embolism, pancreatitis, and myopericarditis. When combined with the clinical history and the ECG, cardiac enzymes are the definitive diagnostic tool in both Q-wave and non–Q-wave AMIs. Cardiac enzymes are elevated as a result of myocardial necrosis. They should be measured on admission in a patient with chest pain and every 12 hours times three (Fig. 18–6). This protocol should be repeated each time the patient experiences new chest pain with the development of congestive heart failure, or arrhythmias.[13]

Total creatinine phosphokinase (CPK) is released from brain, myocardium, and skeletal muscle. Total creatine kinase rises in 6 to 15 hours from onset of infarction, peaks in 24 hours, and remains elevated for

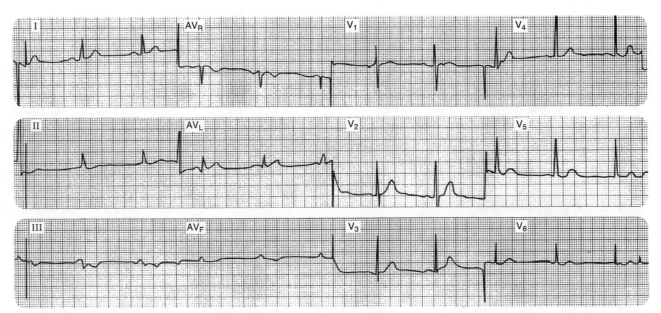

FIGURE 18–5. ECG in posterior myocardial infarction. Note the tall R waves in leads V$_1$ and V$_2$, the upright T wave in lead V$_1$, and flipped T waves in inferior leads III and aV$_F$. (From Cohn, PF: Diagnosis and Therapy of Coronary Artery Disease. Martinus Nijhoff Publishing, Hingham, MA, 1985, p 270, with permission.)

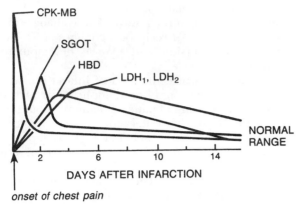

FIGURE 18–6. Evolution of enzyme changes after myocardial infarction.

1 to 4 days. The isoenzyme, CPK-MB, specific for myocardial muscle, is fractionated from the total CPK. Elevation of the CPK-MB occurs within 3 to 15 hours, peaks in 12 to 24 hours, and remains elevated for 1 to 3 days. CPK-MB can also be elevated after cardiac arrest, defibrillation, cardioversion, cardiac contusion, myopericarditis, angioplasty, and prolonged supraventricular tachycardias.[13,14]

Lactate dehydrogenase (LDH) is an enzyme released from cardiac, liver, kidney, and skeletal muscle disease. Total LDH levels rise within 24 hours, peak at 48 to 72 hours, and remain elevated for 7 to 14 days.[13] LDH can also be fractionated into isoenzymes. The isoenzymes for cardiac muscle are LDH_1 and LDH_2. In the normal person, LDH_2 is higher than LDH_1. Following an AMI, this ratio shifts and the LDH_1 is greater than the LDH_2. This inverse, or "flipped," ratio is seen 12 to 72 hours following an AMI.

TREATMENT OF CORONARY ARTERY DISEASE

The ischemic manifestations of CAD can be viewed as being on a continuum, which begins with the atherogenic process and progresses to stable angina, unstable angina, and finally to acute infarction. The similarities in pathogenesis are evident in the similarities in treatment.

Pharmacologic Treatment

Nitrates

The hallmark of treatment for both angina and AMI continues to be nitroglycerin. During chest pain, sublingual nitroglycerin is given every 5 minutes for a total of three doses. If nitroglycerin fails to relieve pain or if chest pain is severe, intravenous morphine in dose increments of 2 to 5 mg is administered.

Intravenous nitroglycerin is used prophylactically on patients admitted with chest pain in whom an AMI is being ruled out. From a starting dose of 5 to 10 µg/min, it is titrated in 5 to 10 µg increments to a maximum of 300 µg/min until the patient is pain-free and maintains a systolic blood pressure of 90 to 100 mm Hg.[13,14]

Nitrates produce both venodilatation and arterial vasodilation, which causes a decrease in both preload and afterload, thus reducing the myocardial oxygen requirement. Evidence suggests that nitroglycerin also inhibits platelet aggregation and limits adhesion of cells to the endothelial surface of the coronary artery.[2,22–24]

When the patient is stable and no longer experiencing acute episodes of chest pain, nitrates are administered in oral form, such as isosorbide (Isordil). Because sustained treatment with nitrates can lead to nitrate intolerance, dosing should allow for an 8- to 12-hour nitrate-free period.[22–24] Antianginal protection during these nitrate-free periods is provided by the concurrent administration of other agents, such as β-blockers or calcium channel blockers.

Morphine

Morphine is administered intravenously in 2- to 5-mg doses when nitroglycerin is ineffective in relieving pain. In addition to pain relief, morphine helps to decrease patient anxiety. It also has beneficial hemodynamic effects by decreasing afterload (SVR) through arterial vasodilatation, thus enabling the ventricle to pump and empty more effectively. Morphine also decreases preload through venodilatation. Reduction in preload results in a decrease in venous return, thus decreasing the workload of the heart.

Thrombolysis

Thrombolysis has been found to limit infarct size, salvage myocardium, and decrease the mortality rate of patients with AMI. Research supports that when thrombolytics are administered within 4 to 6 hours of onset of AMI, the occluded coronary artery is successfully reopened and mortality is decreased.[1,14,15] The advisability of administering thrombolytic agents after 12 hours of onset of chest pain is controversial, although some evidence suggests that these agents have some benefit when persistent ischemia is evident.[14,15] The efficacy of thrombolysis in non–Q-wave AMIs and unstable angina is currently under investigation (see Chapter 17).[15]

Aspirin

Patients admitted with chest pain are treated with aspirin (acetylsalicylic acid [ASA]) to inhibit platelet aggregation and subsequent thrombus formation.[25] If tolerated, ASA is given to the patient immediately on admission to the hospital and daily thereafter. ASA is used as adjunct therapy in patients with stable angina, unstable angina, and AMI, and after the administration of thrombolytic agents. ASA is also used following coronary angioplasties (PTCA) to maintain vessel patency. Dosages as low as 75 to 160 mg/day have been effective in preventing an AMI.[7,8] In the event of contraindications to the administration of ASA, ticlopidine, an alternative antiplatelet drug, can be administered.[2] Dipyrimadole is another drug available to inhibit platelet aggregation. Since an adequate response to dipyrimodole is frequently not achieved for 2 to 3 months, it is usually given in combination with ASA following PTCA and stent placement.

Anticoagulation

Intravenous heparin administration is the standard treatment for preventing further thrombus formation. Administered to patients with unstable angina or AMI, and after angioplasty, heparin has been found to decrease reocclusion rates, relieve ischemia, and prevent infarction.[14,26] Administered as an intravenous bolus and continuous infusion, dosing is aimed at maintaining the activated partial thromboplastin time (aPTT) at 1.5 to 2 times the patient control.[2,14,26] Patients treated with both intravenous nitroglycerin and heparin frequently require larger doses of heparin because of nitroglycerin's antagonistic effect on heparin, which causes resistance to the heparin. Ongoing surveillance of the aPTT with the required dose adjustments in heparin is required.[26]

Magnesium

Magnesium given to a patient with an AMI has been shown to decrease the mortality rate associated with AMI.[27-29] Although the exact mechanism of action has not been firmly established, several hypotheses have been proposed. Some evidence exists that magnesium induces coronary and systemic vasodilatation, inhibits platelet aggregation, exerts an antiarrhythmic effect, and protects the myocardium during ischemia and reperfusion by preventing calcium overload in the cells as well as preserving intracellular adenosine triphosphate.[27-29]

It is not uncommon for serum levels of magnesium to be normal in the AMI patient, despite low intracellular levels. This is because magnesium is an intracellular ion. Magnesium sulfate is given intravenously to the post-AMI patient, regardless of the serum levels. The recommended protocol is magnesium sulfate, 1 to 2 g over 1 hour, followed by 0.5 to 1 g/h over the next 24 hours.[29]

Prophylactic Antiarrhythmics

In the 1970s and 1980s, it was considered standard treatment protocol to administer intravenous lidocaine to patients admitted with a suspected AMI. The rationale for this therapy was that if the most vulnerable period for ventricular arrhythmias is the first 24 hours, prophylactic administration of lidocaine would provide protection against these lethal rhythms and reduce the mortality rate associated with AMI. However, recent research has shown that prophylactic use of lidocaine has no impact on mortality rate and is no longer recommended. Lidocaine and the other antiarrhythmics are reserved for patients with documented arrhythmias.[8,30,31]

β-Blockers

The deleterious effects of SNS activation on MVo_2 with the onset of ischemic chest pain has led to the widespread use of β-blockers in the treatment of angina and AMI. β-Blockers act by binding with the β-receptors, making them unavailable to the circulating catecholamines. The net effect is a decrease in heart rate and a decrease in contractility, which aids in the re-establishment of a balance between oxygen supply and demand. In addition, the decrease in heart rate allows for an increase in the duration of diastole, which increases coronary perfusion. Catecholamine-induced platelet aggregation is also interrupted. Some evidence suggests that the threshold for the development of ventricular fibrillation is raised, thus exerting an antiarrhythmic effect.[2,8,32-34]

β-Blockers can be administered either intravenously or orally. The most commonly used β-blockers are esmolol, administered as a continuous infusion, and metoprolol, administered orally or as an intermittent intravenous injection. When administered within 12 hours of onset of chest pain, β-blockers have been found to reduce the amount of ST elevation, decrease CPK-MB levels, and decrease the size of Q-wave development. A reduction of infarction size has been shown to occur following the administration of β-blockers.[32-34]

Calcium Channel Blockers

Calcium channel blockers exert their effects by inducing coronary vasodilatation, decreasing heart rate, and decreasing afterload. As a result, they increase oxygen supply, decrease oxygen demand, and decrease MVo_2.[35]

Calcium channel blockers are given as a primary treatment for vasospastic angina to prevent coronary artery spasm by limiting the amount of calcium available for contraction.[6,12] There is also evidence suggesting that calcium channel blockers given to patients with a non–Q-wave myocardial infarction improves survival rates by preventing reinfarction.[14,19] Calcium channel blockers have also been found to be effective in controlling the ischemic episodes associated with stable angina when combined with the use of nitrates and β-blockers.[2,8] The most commonly used calcium channel blocker is diltiazem, administered either orally or as a continuous infusion.

Angiotensin Converting Enzyme (ACE) Inhibitors

Following an AMI, there is an increase in ventricular pressure and volume secondary to the increased preload and afterload. The result is a change in the size and shape of the heart through a process known as *ventricular remodeling*. The renin-angiotensin system (RAS), activated following an AMI, increases the preload and afterload as a result of elevated levels of angiotensin II, a vasoconstrictor. Left unopposed, the elevated preload and afterload cause a thinning of the left ventricle, expansion of the infarcted area, and hypertrophy of the uninfarcted segments. These ventricular changes predispose the patient to developing congestive heart failure, ventricular aneurysm, and cardiac rupture. By inhibiting the ACE enzyme, thus preventing the conversion of angiotensin I to angiotensin II, ACE inhibitors decrease the amount of ventricular wall stress. As a result, ACE inhibitors have been found to lower the risk of complications related to left ventricular enlargement.[8,36–38]

Oxygen

The use of oxygen in patients admitted with the chest pain of angina or infarction is controversial. Some evidence suggests that oxygen may increase the systemic vascular resistance and should be avoided unless left ventricular failure is present or the presence of hypoxemia can be demonstrated through arterial blood gases. There is some evidence, however, that patients with AMI are slightly hypoxemic during the first several days; therefore, supplemental oxygen should be administered.[14]

Revascularization

Percutaneous transluminal coronary angioplasty is recommended for stable and unstable angina when medical management is insufficient in controlling symptoms. The current standard of practice following an AMI is to perform a PTCA if thrombolysis is unsuccessful or when postinfarction angina persists.[6,11,15] PTCA has been reported as being successful during the acute phase of the infarction when thrombolysis is contraindicated.[39] Adjunct therapy to PTCA includes atherectomy, in which the plaque is mechanically removed. Intracoronary artery stents can also be used, in which the stent functions as a support for the arterial wall and prevents vascular spasm and restenosis.[40] Stent placement requires long-term anticoagulation with coumadin (see Chapter 17).

COMPLICATIONS FOLLOWING AN AMI

Most complications associated with an AMI can be divided into four main categories: electrical, hemodynamic, mechanical, and inflammatory. Electrical complications are present in the form of rhythm disturbances. Hemodynamic complications are related to the development of congestive heart failure, cardiogenic shock, and right ventricular failure. Possible mechanical complications are papillary muscle dysfunction or rupture, ventricular septal rupture, myocardial rupture, and ventricular aneurysm formation. Possible inflammatory complications are either early pericarditis or Dressler's syndrome.

Electrical Complications

Arrhythmias

Electrical disturbances following an AMI are usually the result of ischemic injury.[14] The incidence of lethal arrhythmias is comparable, regardless of the location of the infarct. The most vulnerable period for the development of ventricular tachycardia and ventricular fibrillation is during the first few hours following an AMI. In fact, most deaths occur during this period following an AMI before the person reaches the hospital. The risk decreases after the first 24 hours.[14] The development of other rhythm disturbances is related to the location of the infarct.

The most common type of arrhythmia following an IWMI is bradycardia. Since the right coronary artery supplies the sinus node and the AV node as well as the inferior wall, rhythm disturbances related to both the sinus node and the AV node are common. These arrhythmias are usually transient and responsive to atropine. The common arrhythmias are sinus bradycardia, sinus blocks, sinus arrests, first degree AV block, and second degree AV block, Mobitz I. Third degree AV block or complete heart block is most likely during the first 48 hours following an IWMI. Despite its ominous appearance, it is usually transient and responsive to atropine, although temporary pacing may be indicated. Escape rhythms originating in the AV node or the ventricle are not uncommon and are related to the ischemic slowing of the sinus node.[14,21]

Anterior infarctions are most frequently associated with atrial ectopy, supraventricular tachycardias, atrial fibrillation, and atrial flutter. These arrhythmias most frequently occur as a result of increased atrial stretch and related congestive heart failure. Because the anterior wall and the ventricular conduction system share a common blood supply in the left main coronary artery and its branches, it is not uncommon for persons with an AWMI to develop right bundle branch blocks, complete left bundle branch blocks, left anterior hemiblocks, and left posterior hemiblocks. Second degree or third degree heart block in patients with AWMI is a poor prognostic indicator. These patients are usually unresponsive to atropine and require temporary pacing.[14,21]

Hemodynamic Complications

Congestive Heart Failure and Cardiogenic Shock

Congestive heart failure and cardiogenic shock are related to the duration of the ischemic episode and the amount of myocardial muscle lost to infarction. These hemodynamic alterations can range from mild pulmonary congestion with basilar rales and slight increases in the pulmonary capillary wedge pressure (PCWP) responsive to diuretics alone to severe hypotension, tissue hypoperfusion, and significant increases in the PCWP requiring vasopressor support.

Chapters 19 and 21 on left ventricular failure and cardiogenic shock provide a detailed description of the pathophysiologic changes and patient management required.

Right Ventricular Infarction

The right coronary artery is the common blood supply for the right ventricle, the inferior wall of the left ventricle, and the posterior wall of the left ventricle. As a result, right ventricular infarctions (RVIs) are most commonly associated with inferior wall infarctions and inferior-posterior wall infarctions. Ischemia of the right ventricle causes a decrease in right ventricular contractility and a subsequent increase in right ventricular end-diastolic pressure, right atrial pressure, and systemic venous pressure. Right ventricular cardiac output decreases, which lowers left ventricular end-diastolic volumes and consequently the systemic caridac output falls. Measure to increase left ventricular output are unsuccessful, since the patient is actually experiencing a relative hypovolemia. The goal of treatment is to re-establish normal pressure gradients within the heart through fluid administration. Fluids increase the right ventricular cardiac output and subsequently increase left ventricular end-diastolic volumes and systemic cardiac output.[41]

RVI is difficult to diagnose using the standard 12-lead ECG, which looks primarily at the left ventricle. Placing the chest electrodes across the right precordium reveals ST-T-wave changes consistent with an AMI. Right precordial leads should be obtained in patients with inferior or inferior-posterior myocardial infarctions with exceptionally high levels of enzymes.[41]

The patient with RVI typically presents with hypotension, neck vein distention, Kussmaul's sign (neck veins distend during inspiration), clear chest x-rays, a wide, split S_2, and a tricuspid regurgitant murmur.[41]

Nitrates and morphine should be used cautiously in patients with RVI because they reduce preload and may further decrease right and left ventricular volume. If volume replacement does not increase the cardiac output, dobutamine may be required. Dobutamine lowers pulmonary vascular resistance (PVR), which facilitates right ventricular ejection.[41]

Mechanical Complications

Acute Mitral Regurgitation

Mitral regurgitation (MR) can occur transiently, as a result of papillary muscle dysfunction from ischemia. Transient MR is relatively common following an AMI and abates when ischemia is relieved. Acute MR occurs when the papillary muscle ruptures, usually following an IWMI. This is an emergency requiring surgical intervention for mitral valve replacement. Papillary muscle rupture occurs anywhere from 2 to 7 days after infarction, and the patient develops acute pulmonary edema with a holosystolic murmur and large v waves on the pulmonary capillary wedge tracing. Inotropic support and the intra-aortic balloon pump (IABP) may be used in an attempt to stabilize the patient temporarily. However, surgery is the only definitive treatment.[14,31]

Ventricular Septal Rupture

Ventricular septal rupture occurs equally in both inferior and anterior wall infarctions. It produces a shunting of blood from the left ventricle to the right ventricle. This increases right ventricular volume. The increased volume causes a rise in right ventricular pressure and pulmonary blood flow. The increased pulmonary blood flow results in increased pulmonary venous return to the left side, causing left ventricular overload. Left ventricular output is impaired and cardiac output falls. Most ventricular septal ruptures occur within 3 to 7 days following an AMI. Such patients present with biventricular failure, an accentuated S_2, and a new pansystolic murmur. Use of inotropic support and the IABP can temporarily stabilize the patient, but surgical correction as soon as possible significantly affects survival.[31]

Myocardial Rupture

About one third of all myocardial ruptures occur within 24 hours of the infarction. The remainder occur within the first 7 days. Rupture is most commonly associated with the elderly, females, those with hypertension, and those following first infarctions. Both subacute ruptures and acute ruptures are possible. With acute rupture, there is rapid development of cardiac tamponade, hypotension, and electromechanical dissociation. In the subacute form, new murmurs and a paradoxical pulse may be identified. Immediate pericardiocentesis and surgical repair are required in both forms of myocardial rupture.[31]

Ventricular Aneurysm

Ventricular aneurysms occur in up to 30% of full-thickness AWMIs. During systole, all the contractile elements of the left ventricle contract in unison in response to electrical stimulation. With the formation of a ventricular aneurysm, the aneurysm becomes a noncontractile segment of the left ventricle, which paradoxically bulges outward during systole. Ventricular aneurysms can be located at the ventricular septum, the anterolateral wall of the left ventricle, or the left ventricular apex.[31]

Often, the first indication of the presence of a left ventricular aneurysm is persistent ST-segment elevation. Patients with ventricular aneurysms almost always have recurrent ventricular arrhythmias. If a significant amount of contractile tissue is lost to aneurysm formation, congestive heart failure results. Because the aneurysm does not contract, blood remains in the aneurysm sac and is likely to form clots. In a small percentage of patients, this can result in systemic emboli.[31]

Treatment for ventricular aneurysms depends on the patient's condition. Those with congestive heart failure are treated with digitalis, diuretics, and ACE inhibitors. Anticoagulation, with heparin initially and coumadin for long-term anticoagulation, is used to prevent or treat systemic embolization. Ventricular arrhythmias are managed through the insertion of implantable defibrillators, endocardial resection, or surgical resection of the aneurysm.[31]

Inflammatory Responses

Pericarditis

Pericarditis, an inflammation of the pericardial lining of the heart, occurs following full-thickness (formerly transmural) infarctions. The area of inflammation occurs in the area surrounding the infarction and is usually accompanied by a pericardial friction rub heard best at the left sternal border. Two forms of pericarditis can be differentiated by the time of occurrence in relation to the AMI: early, also called episternopericarditis, and delayed, also called Dressler's syndrome.

Early pericarditis occurs in 6% to 24% of patients with AMI and usually develops 24 to 96 hours following an AMI. Diagnosis is confirmed by clinical examination and ECG. Some patients are asymptomatic, and diagnosis is made through the identification of a pericardial friction rub. Many patients experience chest pain that may radiate to the upper abdomen, upper arms, or back. This chest pain is distinctly different from the chest pain experienced with ischemia or infarction and is accompanied by a new pericardial friction rub. Persistent ST elevation is seen on the 12-lead ECG in both the symptomatic and asymptomatic patients. Pericarditis is treated with a 3- to 5-day course of nonsteroidal anti-inflammatory drugs.[31,42]

Late pericarditis, Dressler's syndrome, occurs in only 1% to 3% of patients who have AMIs. The exact cause is unclear, but the presence of antimyocardial antibodies in 56% to 83% of these cases suggests an autoimmune process. Dressler's syndrome may develop from 1 week to several months after an AMI and is always associated with a pericardial friction rub. Patients frequently experience chest pain similar to the pain associated with early pericarditis. The chest pain may also be pleuritic in nature. Some patients may have fever, arthralgias, pleural effusions, pulmonary infiltrates, pericardial effusions, and elevations in the erythrocyte sedimentation rate. The ECG reveals diffuse ST-segment changes. Patients with Dressler's syndrome are usually treated with nonsteroidal anti-inflammatory drugs, colchicine, or oral corticosteroids.[31,42]

REHABILITATION

Research has shown that the complications related to prolonged immobility far outweigh the risk of early and progressive activity following an AMI. In fact, early activity has been shown to contribute to both the psychological and physical well-being of the post-AMI patient.

Four phases can be identified in the rehabilitation process following an AMI: phase I occurs in the coronary care unit, phase II occurs during the remainder of the patient's hospitalization, phase III occurs during the patient's convalescence at home, and phase IV involves long-term conditioning.[43]

In an uncomplicated AMI, phase I begins within 2 days of admission. Patients are permitted to perform activities of daily living, range-of-motion exercises, and the use of the commode. The nurse should assess for evidence of exertion or intolerance to the increased activity. Heart rates greater than 20 beats per minute (bpm) over the resting heart rate, or greater than 110 bpm, are indications of activity intolerance. Systolic blood pressures that do not increase with activity or that decrease 20 mmHg also indicate activity intolerance. If either of these signs is present, or if arrhythmias develop, the patient should be instructed to stop the activity and slow the activity progression.[43]

The patient should be instructed to recognize and report signs of overexertion. These include fatigue, shortness of breath, chest pain, dizziness, and palpitations. Patients should also be instructed to stop the activity once these symptoms appear.[43]

During phase II, activity is progressed to include sitting in a chair, ambulating to the bathroom, walking in the hallway, and climbing stairs. Activity intolerance is assessed using the same parameters as in phase I. Prior to discharge, a low-level stress test is frequently performed to determine the activity restrictions that the patient should adhere to at home.[43]

Phase III encompasses the time period from discharge to the patient's return to work or preinfarction lifestyle. Patients should be instructed to walk two to three times per day and should be able to tolerate a pace of about 3 miles in 45 minutes. They can perform light housework but should be instructed to avoid any isometric activities such as carrying heavy objects. Both the patient and the spouse should be told that sexual activity can resume when the patient can climb two flights of stairs without experiencing any symptoms.[43]

The final decision regarding the patient's ability to return to work is usually made 4 to 8 weeks after infarction. In addition to the physical demands of the type of work involved, the psychological and emotional demands of the job should be included in the final determination.[43]

Phase IV is the postconvalescent phase of the rehabilitation process. During this period, the focus is on additional cardiovascular conditioning. Patients should be instructed to perform an aerobic activity three to five times per week for 20 to 30 minutes.

Nursing Care

The care of the patient with ischemic heart disease provides an excellent opportunity for collaborative practice among healthcare professionals. The rapidity with which ischemia progresses and with which complications develop requires a team approach to care and management. There are several principles on which the care of this patient population is based.

1. Relieve chest pain rapidly. Through the use of oxygen, nitrates, and morphine, the ischemic process can be interrupted. Patient response to therapy is assessed with each intervention.

2. Re-establish the balance between oxygen supply and oxygen demand. Through the administration of nitrates, β-blockers, and calcium channel blockers, the myocardial oxygen requirement can be reduced as well as the MVo_2. Tolerance to these agents requires ongoing assessment of relevant clinical data. Bedrest is recommended during the first 24 hours, with activity increased gradually as the patient's condition warrants. A bedside commode can be used.

3. Intervene during the thrombotic process. Through the administration of aspirin, heparin, and thrombolytic agents, dissolution of the existing clot and prevention of further thrombus formation may be obtained. Assess for evidence of reocclusion, reperfusion arrhythmias, continued ischemia, and bleeding.

4. Monitor for evidence of ischemia: bedside monitoring should use leads reflective of the anatomic lesion suspected of causing the ischemia. ST-T-wave changes, with and without chest pain, should be documented and reported. When episodes of chest pain occur, a 12-lead ECG should be obtained, and the ischemia should be treated promptly. Additional enzyme panels should be drawn and evaluated for additional evidence of infarction.

5. Continue to assess heart, lungs, and periphery. Lung fields should be auscultated for the presence or progression of congestive heart failure. Response to diuretics and inotropics should be evaluated. Assess peripheral pulses to determine the presence of embolic phenomenon and tissue perfusion. Obtain hemodynamic parameters of blood pressure, PCWP, and cardiac output as indicated to assess left ventricular function, evaluate response to treatment, and determine the development of complications. Assess heart sounds regularly and during episodes of chest pain for the development of new murmurs, progression of existing murmurs, and extra heart sounds (S_3, S_4).

6. Provide patient and family education and support: the rationale for activity restrictions, dietary restrictions, and treatment should be provided. Answer questions honestly. Provide explanations for the specific drugs being administered. Begin introducing risk factor modification in the critical care unit.

The care of the patient with an AMI warrants critical decision-making and nursing care of the highest quality. See the end of this chapter for a detailed care plan incorporating the nursing process, nursing diagnoses, desired patient outcomes, nursing interventions, and rationales.

REFERENCES

1. Mueller, HS: Management of acute myocardial infarction. In Shoemaker, WC, et al (eds): Textbook of critical care, ed 2. WB Saunders, Philadelphia, 1989, pp 341–353.
2. Theroux, P and Lidon, RM: Unstable angina: Pathogenesis, diagnosis, and treatment. Curr Probl Cardiol 18(3):163–231, 1993.
3. Kottke, BA: Current understanding of the mechanisms of atherogenesis. Am J Cardiol 72: 48C–54C, 1993.
4. Meredith, IT, et al: Role of endothelium in ischemic coronary syndromes. Am J Cardiol 72:27C–32C, 1993.
5. Gorlin, R: Dynamic vascular factors in the genesis of myocardial ischemia. J Am Coll Cardiol 1:897–906, 1983.
6. Maseri, A: Clinical syndromes of angina pectoris. Hosp Pract 24:65–80, 1989.
7. Murphy, K, Vaughan, C, and Fennell, WH: The pharmacologic management of angina pectoris. Irish Med J 86(2):41–42, 1993.
8. Rutherford, JD: Pharmacologic management of angina and acute myocardial infarction. Am J Cardiol 72:16C–20C, 1993.
9. Perchalski, DL and Pepine, CJ: Patient with coronary artery spasm and role of the critical care nurse. Heart Lung 16:392–402, 1987.
10. Smitherman, TC: Unstable angina pectoris: The first half century: Natural history, pathophysiology and treatment. Am J Med Sci 292:395–406, 1986.
11. Stiesmeyer, JK: Unstable angina associated with critical proximal left anterior descending coronary artery stenosis. Am J Crit Care 2(1):48–53, 1993.
12. Matrisciano, L: Unstable angina: An overview. Crit Care Nurse 12(8):30–38, 1992.
13. Lavie, CJ and Gersh, BJ: Acute myocardial infarction: Initial manifestations, management and prognosis. Mayo Clin Proc 65:531–548, 1990.
14. Reeder, GS and Gersh, BJ: Modern management of acute myocardial infarction. Curr Probl Cardiol 18(2):87–155, 1993.
15. Rapaport, E: Overview: Rationale of thrombolysis in treating acute myocardial infarction. Hear Lung, 20(5Pt 2):538–541, 1991.
16. Sigurdsson, A, Held, P, and Swedberg, K: Short and long term neurohormonal activation following acute myocardial infarction. Am Heart J 126:1068–1076, 1993.
17. Calvin, JE and Sibbald, WJ: Applied cardiovascular physiology in the critically ill with special reference to diastole and ventricular interaction. In Shoemaker, WC, et al (eds): Textbook of Critical Care, ed 2. WB Saunders, Philadelphia, 1989, pp 312–326.
18. Granborg, J, Grande, P, and Pederson, A: Diagnostic and prognostic implications of transient isolated negative T waves in suspected acute myocardial infarction. Am J Cardiol 57:203–207, 1986.
19. Lewis, PS: Clinical implications of non-Q-wave (subendocardial) myocardial infarctions. Focus on Critical Care 19(1):29–33, 1992.
20. Rakita, L and Vrobel, TR: Electrocardiography in critical care medicine. In Shoemaker, WC, et al (eds): Textbook of Critical Care, ed 2. WB Saunders, Philadelphia, 1989, pp 353–376.
21. Hanisch, PJ: Identification and treatment of acute myocardial infarction by electrocardiographic site classification. Focus on Critical Care, 18(6):480–488, 1991.
22. Parker, JO: Nitrate therapy in stable angina pectoris. N Engl J Med 316:1635–1642, 1987.
23. Fung, HL: Clinical pharmacology of organic nitrates. Am J Cardiol 72:9C–15C, 1993.

24. Parker, JO: Nitrates and angina pectoris. Am J Cardiol 72:3C–8C, 1993.

25. Byers, JF: The use of aspirin in cardiovascular disease. J Cardiovasc Nurs 8(1):1–18, 1993.

26. Jaffrani, NA, et al: Therapeutic approach to unstable angina. Nitroglycerine, heparin and combined therapy. Am Heart J 126:1239–1242, 1993.

27. Fitzsimmons, L, Verderber, A, and Shively, M: Effects of intravenous magnesium sulfate in acute myocardial infarction. J Cardiovasc Nurs 8(1):80–83, 1993.

28. Woods, KL, et al: Intravenous magnesium sulfate in suspected acute myocardial infarction: Results of the second Leicester Intravenous Magnesium Intervention Trial (LIMIT-2). Lancet 339(8809):1553–1558, 1992.

29. Keller, KB and Lemberg, L. The importance of magnesium in cardiovascular disease. Am J Crit Care 2(4):348–350, 1993.

30. Teo, KK, Yusuf, S, and Furberg, CD: Effects of prophylactic antiarrhythmic drug therapy in acute myocardial infarction. JAMA 270:1589–1595, 1993.

31. Chaterjee, K: Complications of acute myocardial infarction. Curr Probl Cardiol 18(1):7–79, 1993.

32. Jafri, SM and Goldstein, S: Intravenous beta blockers in acute myocardial infarction. Cardiology December, 49:55, 1990.

33. Herlitz, J, et al: Effect of metoprolol on indirect signs of the size and severity of acute myocardial infarction. Am J Cardiol 51:1282–1288, 1983.

34. Herlitz, J, et al: Effect of metoprolol on chest pain in acute myocardial infarction. Br Heart J 51:438–441, 1984.

35. Gill, A, et al: Pharmacology of bepridil. Am J Cardiol 69:11D–16D, 1992.

36. Maxwell, SRJ and Kendall, MJ: ACE inhibition in the 1990's. Br J Clin Pract 47(1):30–37, 1993.

37. Fara, AM: The role of angiotensin-converting enzyme inhibitors in reducing ventricular remodeling after myocardial infarction. J Cardiovasc Nurs 8(1):32–48, 1993.

38. Dickstein, K and Aarsland, T: Effect on exercise performance of enalapil therapy initiated early after myocardial infarction. J Am Coll Cardiol 22:975–983, 1993.

39. Ellis, SG and Topol, EJ: Intracoronary stents: Will they fulfill their promise as an adjunct to angioplasty. J Am Coll Cardiol 13:1425–1430, 1989.

40. Baim, DS: New devises for coronary revascularization. Hosp Pract, 28(10):41–52, 1993.

41. McMillan, JY and Little-Longeway, CD: Right ventricular infarction. Focus on Critical Care 18(2):158–163, 1991.

42. Loveys, BJ: Complications of acute myocardial infarction. In Underhill, SL, et al (eds): Cardiac Nursing, ed 2. JB Lippincott, Philadelphia, 1989, pp 517–526.

43. King, SC and Froelicher, ESS: Cardiac rehabilitation: Activity and exercise program. In Underhill, SL, et al (eds): Cardiac Nursing, ed 2. JB Lippincott, Philadelphia, 1989, pp 739–756.

CARE PLAN FOR THE PATIENT WITH AN ACUTE MYOCARDIAL INFARCTION

Nursing Diagnoses

Nursing Diagnosis #1
Tissue perfusion, alteration in, related to:
1. Coronary artery occlusion resulting in decreased myocardial tissue perfusion
2. Ventricular dysfunction resulting in decreased perfusion to brain, kidneys, lungs, liver
3. Thromboembolism resulting from deep venous thrombosis or mural thrombi

Desired Patient Outcomes

Patient will:
1. Maintain hemodynamic stability:
   - BP within 10 mmHg of baseline
   - HR 60–80/min
   - Absence of arrhythmias
   - Cardiac output 4–8 L/min
   - Brisk capillary refill (within 2 sec)
   - Urine output > 30 mL/h
   - Mental status: alert, oriented
   - Peripheral pulses +2
   - Skin warm and dry
   - Respiration <20
   - Mucous membranes pink
2. Remain without thromboembolic events or, if they occur, thromboembolism will resolve without significant sequelae.
   - Extremities warm to touch; pulses palpable and equal bilaterally
   - Absence of positive Homan's sign
   - Circumference of extremities equal bilaterally

Nursing Interventions
- Initiate rest-promoting activities: bedrest until hemodynamically stable, quiet environment; limit visitors if needed to ensure patient rest.
- Allow bedside commode privileges if hemodynamically stable.

Rationales
- Rest decreases myocardial oxygen consumption.

- Use of bedside commode is associated with less stress than use of a bedpan.

CARE PLAN FOR THE PATIENT WITH AN ACUTE MYOCARDIAL INFARCTION (*Continued*)

Nursing Interventions

- If myocardial infarction (MI) is uncomplicated, patient should be allowed out of bed to the chair for periods of 1–2 hours and should be allowed to use the commode instead of a bedpan from the time of admission.

- For patient with complicated MI, initiate activities to counteract effects of bedrest.
  - Elevate head of bed when possible.
  - Have patient turn frequently in bed.
  - Teach footboard exercises (limit contraction duration to less than 10 seconds when performing these).
  - Apply antiembolism stockings.
  - Consult with physician regarding initiation of minidose heparin (5000 subcutaneously q 8–12 h) if not on heparin infusion.
- Allow to feed self if able and if patient desires.
- Assist with bathing the first day and as needed on subsequent days.

- Monitor for factors that may cause an increase in myocardial oxygen consumption and institute measures to correct these.

- Administer pharmacologic therapy as ordered (nitrates, nitroprusside, β-blockers, calcium channel blockers, vasopressors) to increase myocardial oxygen supply or decrease MVo_2
- Administer oxygen as prescribed.
  - Monitor for possible negative effects of O_2 therapy, including increased HR and systemic vascular resistance.
- Monitor for signs and symptoms of pulmonary embolus, including tachypnea, tachycardia, shortness of breath, anxiety, hypotension, deteriorating oxygenation, pulmonary artery pressure elevation, jugular venous distention.
- Monitor for signs of deep vein thrombosis:
  - Positive Homan's sign
  - Change in color, temperature, or girth of extremity
  - Presence of tenderness or cords

Rationales

- Prolonged bedrest is associated with many complications (fluid shifting, orthostatic intolerance, increased HR, progressive decalcification resulting in osteoporosis and urolithiasis, and thromboembolism). Early ambulation is the most effective means to combat these.
- Footboard exercises may decrease venous stasis. Contractions less than 10 seconds in duration cause no significant detrimental cardiovascular response.

- Self-feeding is less stressful for most patients.
- Bed bathing is associated with insignificant cardiovascular responses in terms of blood pressure, ECG, heart sounds, oxygen uptake.
- Hypotension, hypertension, increased heart rate, increased contractility, pain, fever, anemia, volume depletion, and psychologic stress cause an increase in myocardial oxygen consumption and may increase infarct size.
- Pharmacologic measures to increase myocardial oxygen supply or to decrease demand may help to limit infarct size.

- Oxygen may have negative cardiovascular effects.

- Early detection and treatment of thromboembolic events may aid in more successful recovery.

- Early detection and treatment of thromboembolic events may aid in more successful recovery.

Nursing Diagnoses

Nursing Diagnosis #2
Alteration in cardiac output, related to:
1. Arrhythmias, conduction disturbances
2. Left ventricular dysfunction
3. Hypovolemia
4. Right ventricular infarction

Desired Patient Outcomes

Patient will:
1. Maintain electrophysiologic stability
   - Absence of arrhythmias
   - 12-lead ECG return to baseline
2. Maintain hemodynamic stability
   - HR 60–80/min
   - BP within 10 mmHg of baseline
3 Be normovolemic.
   - Cardiac output 4–8 L/min
   - Brisk capillary refill (2 sec)

Nursing Interventions

- Attach to cardiac monitor as soon as possible.
- Select best lead to monitor based on type of MI patient is having, type of conduction disturbance, and needs of monitor, especially if a computerized arrhythmia detection system is used. Multiple lead monitoring is preferable.

Rationales

- Early detection of arrhythmia allows for early treatment.
- Appropriate lead monitoring allows ECG changes (i.e., ST-segment, T-wave, PR or QRS interval prolongation) to be seen and treated properly.

CARE PLAN FOR THE PATIENT WITH AN ACUTE MYOCARDIAL INFARCTION (*Continued*)

Nursing Interventions	**Rationales**
• Treat lethal arrhythmias immediately (ventricular tachycardia, ventricular fibrillation, asystole) per unit protocols. Nofity physician.	• Prompt treatment of lethal arrhythmias is more successful than delayed treatment
• Be aware of potential significance of warning arrhythmias—VPBs > 6/min, R-on-T VPB, coupling.	• "Warning arrhythmias" may precipitate episodes of ventricular tachycardia, ventricular fibrillation. These arrhythmias may also occur without warning.
• Notify physician and institute treatment of tachyarrhythmias and bradyarrhythmias as soon as possible.	• Bradyarrhythmias and tachyarrhythmias may compromise CO and increase myocardial oxygen consumption.
• Check vital signs (BP, HR, PAP, PCWP, CVP, CO, SVK, CI) with any change in rhythm or conduction.	• Rhythm or conduction changes may be associated with hemodynamic compromise, particularly in a patient with marginal left ventricular function.
• Allow hot or cold beverages in small quantities if patient desires. Elevate head of bed during ingestion.	• Hot or cold beverages in small quantities consumed in a sitting position (at least semi-Fowler's) are not associated with arrhythmias, ECG changes.
• Take oral temperature routinely; rectal temperature if necessary.	• Taking oral temperature is less stressful to the patient; rectal route is not associated with vagal stimulation and thus may be used if necessary.
• Assess for signs and symptoms of left ventricular dysfunction: sinus tachycardia; dyspnea, orthopnea; pulmonary rales; S_3 gallop, pulsus alternans; jugular venous pressure elevation, positive hepatojugular reflex, peripheral or sacral edema; hypotension, elevated PCWP, elevated central venous pressure, decreased cardiac output and cardiac index.	• Myocardial ischemia or infarct predisposes patient to left ventricular dysfunction. • Degree of left ventricular dysfunction is a major determinant of post-MI mortality.

(See Chapter 19 for further discussion of ventricular dysfunction related to cardiogenic shock, mitral valve dysfunction.)

Nursing Interventions	**Rationales**
• Assess for signs of ventricular septal defect (VSD), including a holosystolic murmur heard best at the lower left sternal border; left-to-right shunting; signs of heart failure as above with the degree dependent on the size of the VSD.	• Myocardial damage may result in a defect in the ventricular septal wall.
• Assess patient for signs of hypovolemia. These include hypotension (BP may be increased initially), decreased central venous pressure, decreased PCWP, tachycardia, oliguria, and decreased cardiac output and cardiac index.	• Vomiting, severe diaphoresis, aggressive treatment with diuretics or nitrates may deplete intravascular volume.
• Assess patient for signs of right ventricular infarction. These include hypotension, neck vein distention, Kussmaul's sign (neck veins distend in inspiration), clear chest x-rays, a wide split S_2, and tricuspid regurgitant murmur.	• Right ventricular infarction causes a decrease in right ventricular cardiac output and a subsequent decrease in left ventricular cardiac output.

Nursing Diagnoses	**Desired Patient Outcomes**

Nursing Diagnosis #3
Alteration in comfort: Pain, related to:
1. Myocardial ischemia, necrosis
2. Extension of infarct
3. Pericarditis
4. Dressler's syndrome (late pericarditis)
	Patient will:
	1. Be pain-free
	2. Notify staff immediately of chest pain episodes
	3. Maintain hemodynamic stability:
	  • BP within 10 mmHg of baseline
	  • HR at rest: 60–80/minute without arrhythmias
	  • Mental status: Alert and oriented to person, place, and time
	  • Urinary output >30 mL/h.

Nursing Interventions	**Rationales**
• Have patient describe pain, including location, radiation, associated symptoms (nausea, vomiting, diaphoresis, shortness of breath, palpitations), precipitating factors, quality, duration, relief mechanisms, association with movement, respiration, or palpation.	• Description helps to determine etiology of chest pain. ○ See Table 35–1 for SLIDT tool.
• Have patient rate pain on a scale of 1 to 10, with 10 being most severe.	

CARE PLAN FOR THE PATIENT WITH AN ACUTE MYOCARDIAL INFARCTION (*Continued*)

Nursing Interventions

- Administer nitrates or narcotic analgesia, β-blockers, and calcium channel blockers as needed and monitor response to therapy.

- Monitor vital signs before and per unit protocol after medication administration. Assess for hypotension, bradycardia, tachycardia, and respiratory depression. Assess for relief of pain.
- Obtain 12-lead ECG prior to medication administration, particularly if this is undiagnosed or new-onset chest pain, or recurrence of chest pain in a patient who has been pain-free for 24 hours.
- Obtain cardiac enzymes every 8 hours three times.
- Stay with patient until ischemic chest pain is relieved.

- Assess patient for pericarditis or Dressler's syndrome (depending on time interval after MI) if recurrent MI and infarct extension have been ruled out. Symptoms of pericarditis or Dressler's syndrome may include:
  - Chest pain increased by deep inspiration
  - Chest pain alleviated by leaning forward.
  - Presence of a pericardial friction rub.
  - ECG changes associated with pericarditis (diffuse or localized ST-segment elevation, with upward concavity)
  - Atrial arrhythmias
  - Persistent fever > 101°F (38.3°C)
  - Symptoms of pleuritis, pericardial effusion, or tamponade
  - Response to aspirin or indomethacin
  - If patient is on anticoagulant medication, check with physician about continuation

Rationales

- Nitrates help to relieve pain by means of coronary vasodilatation and both preload and afterload reduction. Narcotics act centrally to relieve pain and also have some afterload-reducing effects. β-Blockers and calcium channel blockers decrease MVO_2.
- Significant change in vital signs (BP decrease > 10 mmHg or <90 mmHg systolic or HR increase > 20 bpm or <50 bpm and respiratory rate of < 10) may necessitate discontinuation of medication.
- Documentation of changes on a 12-lead ECG helps to make the diagnosis of cardiac chest pain (vs other types of chest discomfort), and also helps to diagnose infarct extension, Printzmetal's angina, or pericarditis.

- Presence of caring, supportive, knowledgeable nurse may reduce patient anxiety, which reduces stress response. This causes reduced circulating catecholamines (epinephrine), which help to increase the pain threshold, thereby reducing myocardial oxygen consumption.
- Either condition may occur following MI, particularly Q-wave MIs. Symptoms are similar. Time courses are somewhat similar and overlap does occur, sometimes making it difficult to distinguish between these two syndromes.

  - Anticoagulants may precipitate cardiac tamponade.

Nursing Diagnoses

Nursing Diagnosis #4
Anxiety, related to:
1. Knowledge deficit regarding illness and its prognosis
2. Pain
3. Coronary care environment

Nursing Interventions

- Assess level of understanding of disease process and readiness to learn.
  - Provide patient and family with appropriate information on coronary artery disease and myocardial infarction when patient is ready.
- Orient patient and family to coronary care environment.

Desired Patient Outcomes

Patient will verbalize basic understanding of his/her illness and demonstrate behavior suggesting decreased anxiety, relaxed facies and demeanor.

Rationales

- Fear and anxiety initiate the stress response. This causes increased catecholamine release, which causes increased myocardial oxygen consumption (MVO_2), as well as decreased pain threshold, which further increases MVO_2.

CARE PLAN FOR THE PATIENT WITH MYOCARDIAL INFARCTION

Nursing Diagnoses

Nursing Diagnosis #1
Alteration in comfort, related to myocardial ischemia

Desired Patient Outcomes

Patient will verbalize feeling free of pain

Nursing Interventions

- Assess for presence of chest discomfort

  ○ Have patient rate discomfort on a scale of 1–10, with 10 being most severe.

  ○ Notify physician of any episodes of chest pain and take appropriate actions: obtain vital signs, get a 12-lead ECG.
- Minimize discrepancy between O_2 supply and demand.
  ○ Provide periods of rest
  ○ Regulate activities
  ○ Maintain a quiet environment

Rationales

- Continuous assessment of patient to determine verbal and nonverbal cues of pain episodes is essential as patient may be experiencing denial of his/her condition.
  ○ Patient may not appear to be in distress, but may mask signs of pain as a result of such factors as stoicism and cultural differences. A scaling system is a more objective tool.
  ○ Enhanced sympathoadrenal response associated with pain and anxiety may increase heart rate and oxygen demand, and may provoke myocardial ischemia.
- Goal in treatment is to maximize O_2 supply and minimize O_2 demand.

Nursing Diagnoses

Nursing Diagnosis #2
Potential for anxiety, related to:
1. Coronary environment
2. Newly diagnosed disease

Desired Patient Outcomes

Patient will:
1. Verbalize anxiety and fears
2. Demonstrate behavior suggesting decreased anxiety: relaxed facies and demeanor
3. HR 60–80 bpm
4. Pressure within 10 mmHg of baseline

Nursing Interventionas

- Assess for verbal and nonverbal cues of anxiety.

  ○ Provide patient/family with information regarding diagnosis, diagnostic procedures.

- Orient patient and family to coronary care environment: staff, equipment, visiting hours, when and whom to call for information about the patient's condition.
- Sedate as necessary, and monitor response.

Rationales

- Patient may verbalize he/she is not feeling anxious but may be demonstrating anxious behavior.
  ○ Family members can be helpful in relaxing patient but must be included when giving information regarding care.
- Knowing what to expect assists in coping; family may feel reassured knowing when they can visit or whom to call to get progress reports on the patient's condition.
- Quiet rest and relaxation are essential especially during acute phase when oxygen demands need to be reduced.

Nursing Diagnoses

Nursing Diagnosis #3
Alteration in cardiac output: decresed, related to:
1. Arrhythmias
2. Left ventricular dysfunction

Desired Patient Outcomes

Patient will:
1. Maintain electrophysiologic stability:
   - HR 60–80 bpm
   - Rhythm: regular

Nursing Interventions

- Initiate continuous cardiac monitoring.
  ○ Monitor rate, rhythm.
- Treat serious or warning arrhythmias as per unit protocol.

Rationales

- Early detection of serious arrhythmias allows early treatment and prevention of complications.
- Warning arrhythmias may precipitate episodes of ventricular tachycardia or fibrillation.

CHAPTER 19

Nursing Management of the Patient with Heart Failure

Susan Houston, Marie Clark, and Jackie Anderson

CHAPTER OUTLINE

Compensatory Mechanisms
- Frank-Starling Phenomenon
- Sympathoadrenergic Stimulation
- Myocardial Hypertrophy

Causes and Presentation of Heart Failure
- Abnormal Pressure
- Filling Disorders

- Abnormal Muscle Conditions
- Abnormal Volume Load

Therapeutic Interventions
- Drug Therapy
- Supportive Therapy

Nursing Care
- Therapeutic Goals

References

LEARNING OBJECTIVES

After completing this chapter, you should be able to:

1. Identify the primary hemodynamic alteration associated with heart failure.
2. Differentiate between the signs and symptoms of right heart failure and left heart failure.
3. Describe the normal compensatory mechanisms associated with a fall in cardiac output.
4. Describe the pathologic conditions associated with the development of heart failure.
5. Outline the pertinent clinical assessment and hemodynamic findings of the specific disorders associated with the development of heart failure.
6. Identify the predisposing factors associated with the development of cardiogenic shock.
7. Relate the role of pharmacologic intervention to the treatment and management of heart failure.
8. Discuss the role of supportive care measures in the management of heart failure.
9. Relate pertinent nursing diagnoses, desired patient outcomes, and nursing interventions to the therapeutic goals in the care of the patient with heart failure.

Heart failure occurs when the heart is no longer able to pump blood efficiently enough to meet the metabolic demands of the body. Heart failure may develop slowly, allowing the body time to build compensatory mechanisms to offset the symptoms of failure; at other times, it may present as a rapid deterioration of the body, in which case there is no time for compensatory mechanisms to be set into motion.

Although many factors may contribute to heart failure, the classic outcome of this process is a decrease in cardiac output. Traditionally, factors that lead to heart failure include (1) an increased pressure in the circulatory system, which the heart must pump against, (2) conditons that restrict ventricular filling, (3) interference with the pumping mechanism of the heart, and (4) an increase or decrease in the volume of blood flowing to the heart (Figs. 19–1 and 19–2, Table 19–1). The signs and symptoms of heart failure may also present themselves in people with pre-existing heart conditions who experience an event that requires their heart to pump more efficiently to meet the increased metabolic demands of their body (Table 19–2).[2] This new demand cannot be met by their failing hearts and leads to an acute medical emergency that must be handled by the healthcare team.

When discussing heart failure, it is important to distinguish between right-sided and left-sided failure. These terms denote the primary catalyst responsible for heart failure. Table 19–3 lists the symptoms associated with right-sided and left-sided heart failure. A

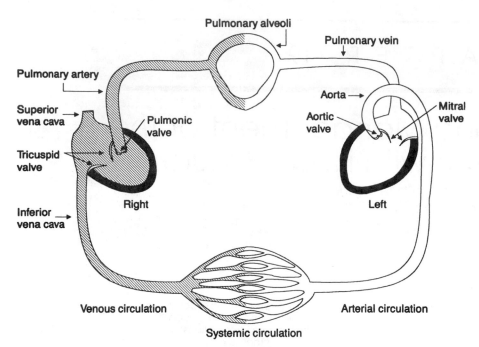

FIGURE 19–1. Normal circulation.

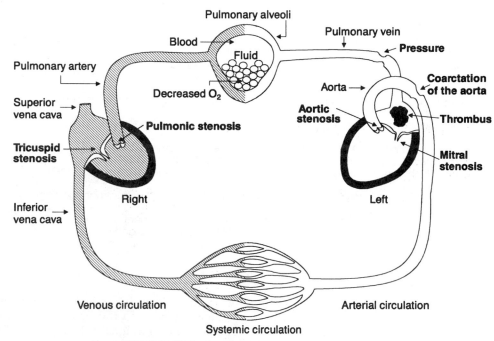

FIGURE 19–2. Causes of congestive heart failure.

TABLE 19–1
Conditions Responsible for the Devleopment of Heart Failure

Abnormal Pressure	Filling Disorders	Abnormal Muscle Conditions	Abnormal Volume
Aortic stenosis	Mitral stenosis	Cardiomyopathies	Valvular imcompetence
Pulmonic stenosis	Tricuspid stenosis	Myocarditis	Left-to-right shunts
Pulmonary hypertension	Atrial myxomas	Myocardial infarction	
Systemic hypertension		Cardiogenic shock	

TABLE 19–2
Precipitating Factors in the Development of Heart Failure

Anemia	Pregnancy
Arrhythmia	Hypervolemia
Infection	Endocrine disorders
Fever	Thyrotoxicosis
Thiamine deficiency	Myxedema
Overexertion	Cushing's syndrome

review of symptoms associated with right-sided heart failure gives the clinician an appropriate picture of a patient who is experiencing an increase in venous pressure. This increase is caused by an increase in blood volume to the right side of the heart that cannot be adequately pumped out of the right ventricle. The back-up of blood leads to an increase in venous pressure as manifested by tachycardia, ascites, and weight gain. On the other hand, left-sided heart failure occurs when the blood volume ejected from the left ventricle is less than the volume delivered to the left side of the heart. As pressure builds on the left side of the heart, the pressure gradient is transmitted into the pulmonary circulation, creating the following symptoms in these patients: anxiety, dyspnea, basilar rales, and a cough. Unfortunately, since the circulatory system is a closed loop, each part is dependent upon the next for the system to work; therefore, if one ventricle cannot sufficiently fulfill its role to pump efficiently, the entire system will be in jeopardy.

Heart failure is a common diagnosis among critically ill patients; therefore nurses must understand the etiology, pathophysiology, and hemodynamic consequences of this disease process. Moreover, heart failure will lead to multiorgan system failure. Prompt recognition of this disease and rapid intervention by the healthcare team are the patient's only hope for survival.

TABLE 19–3
Clinical Presentation of the Patient with Heart Failure

Left-Sided Heart Failure	Right-Sided Heart Failure
Tachycardia	Tachycardia
↑ Pulmonary artery diastolic pressure	↑ Right atrial pressure
↑ Pulmonary capillary wedge pressure	↑ Central venous pressure
Pulsus alternans	Jugular venous distention
Gallop rhythm	Dependent pitting edema
Basilar rales	Ascites
Cyanosis or pallor	Weight gain
Dyspnea	Hepatojugular reflux
Orthopnea	Hepatosplenomegaly
Cough	Jaundice
Nocturnal dyspnea	Complaints of vague abdominal discomfort
Anxiety	Nocturia
Diaphoresis	
Oliguria	
Weakness, fatigue	

COMPENSATORY MECHANISMS

When demand for energy-rich oxygenated blood cannot be met by the heart, three mechanisms are activated to improve the flow of blood from the heart. These mechanisms include the Frank-Starling phenomenon, stimulation of the sympathoadrenergic cycle, and enlargement of the heart muscle itself.

Frank-Starling Phenomenon

When the left ventricle is unable to empty adequately, the volume of blood contained within the ventricle increases. This is referred to as residual volume. Because blood continues to enter the left ventricle at a constant rate, there is an increase in left ventricular end-diastolic volume (LVEDV) and left ventricular end-diastolic pressure (LVEDP). The added volume that exists in the left ventricle causes the walls of the ventricle to distend. This distention will improve the amount of blood ejected from the ventricle during systole and thus maintain a cardiac output adequate to meet the body's needs.[3]

The Frank-Starling phenomenon is clinically represented by a left ventricular curve (Fig. 19–3); the vertical axis represents cardiac output, which is the amount of blood ejected from the left ventricle in 1 minute. The horizontal axis represents pulmonary capillary wedge pressure (PCWP) as a measure of the preload and LVEDP. Preload can be defined as the degree of stretch required in the muscle to accommodate the volume of blood in the ventricle. Left ventricular end-diastolic pressure refers to the amount of pressure that the above quantity of blood exerts on the ventricle. The Frank-Starling phenomenon demonstrates that up to a certain point, as the volume in the left ventricle increases, the amount of blood ejected from the left ventricle will also increase, thus meeting the body's need for oxygen-enriched blood. Optimal ranges for LVEDP are from 12 to 20 mmHg.

Unfortunately, the benefits derived from the above mechanism cannot replace a failing heart. These temporary measures will improve cardiac output for a while; however, the negative effects of this process will only serve to enhance pump failure in the long run. For instance, the improved blood flow back to the heart is beneficial in the early phases of heart failure, but as the cardiac function of the heart continues to deteriorate, the added blood volume leads to systemic pulmonary venous congestion.[2]

Sympathoadrenergic Stimulation

When there is a decrease in cardiac output, impulses received in the brain result in a compensatory sympathetic nerve stimulation of the cardiac and peripheral vasculature. Stimulation of the sympathetic nervous system causes the following effects:

1. Vasoconstriction to peripheral areas of the body (renal, spleen, cutaneous tissues). Vasoconstric-

Ventricular function curve.

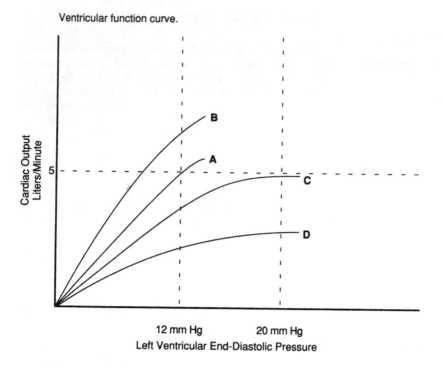

A = normal

B = sympathoadrenergic stimulation

C = compensated heart failure

D = decompensated heart failure

FIGURE 19–3. Left ventricular function curve, plotting cardiac output.

tion of the venous system to the periphery allows for an improved venous return of blood flow to the heart. Vasoconstriction of the arterial system restricts blood flow to the peripheral organs in order to improve blood flow to the vital organs of the body.

2. The release of epinephrine and norepinephrine from the adrenal medulla. These catecholamines lead to an increase in heart rate and contractility, which in turn result in an improved cardiac output.

3. Activation of the renin-angiotensin-aldosterone cycle. As cardiac output decreases, there is a parallel decrease in the renal glomerular filtration rate. This decrease in rate stimulates the renin-angiotensin-aldosterone cycle to increase the tubular reabsorption of sodium and water. This reabsorption of fluid leads to an increase in the volume of blood available in the venous circulation for the heart to pump.

The benefits of activating the sympathoadrenergic system include an increase in heart rate, contractility, and preload; however, prolonged activation of this system will impair cardiac function. For example, persistent tachycardia will decrease the diastolic filling time (i.e., the time necessary to adequately fill the ventricles before systole occurs) and thus decrease cardiac output. Moreover, tachycardia inherently creates a greater demand for oxygen-enriched blood by the

heart muscle itself. This demand cannot be met indefinitely by the heart muscle. Myocardial contractility will decrease as the body depletes its supply of norepinephrine. Finally, the activation of the vasoconstrictive properties of the arterial system lead to heart failure by increasing the pressure that the heart must overcome to open the aortic valve in order to supply blood to the body.

Myocardial Hypertrophy

One of the long-term effects of sustained myocardial workload is the enlargement of the myocardium. This enlargement of muscle mass allows the heart to pump more efficiently. If the muscle outgrows its blood supply, however, ischemic changes may be seen in the tissues that are not adequately perfused.

Concentric hypertrophy occurs when the muscle enlarges without parallel growth in the chambers of the heart. This condition occurs when the heart must pump against elevated afterload pressures (i.e., increases in arterial vasoconstriction). In this situation, higher diastolic filling pressures are required to maintain normal cardiac outputs. Eccentric hypertrophy occurs when the myocardium and chambers enlarge together. This occurs in diastolic volume overload, such as valvular insufficiency, and results in a decrease in the force of myocardial contractility.[2]

CAUSES AND PRESENTATION OF HEART FAILURE

Heart failure is the result of a variety of cardiac conditions that produce a reduced cardiac output. These conditions can be classified according to four main causes: abnormal pressure, filling disorders of the ventricles, abnormal muscle conditions (pumping mechanism), and abnormal volume load.

Abnormal Pressure

The pressure required to adequately empty the ventricles during systole is referred to as afterload. Afterload is assessed through arterial blood pressure measurement and the calculation of systemic valvular resistance (SVR). If the blood flow is impeded by narrowing of the aortic or pulmonic valves, or by an increase in vascular resistance in the peripheral vascular system or the pulmonary vascular system, the heart must contract more forcefully to work against this resistance. Over many years, pressure overload leads to increased intramyocardial wall tension, which allows the heart to pump adequately against the higher pressure. This leads to an increase in left ventricular wall thickness and ventricular hypertrophy. Abnormal pressure disorders with accompanying clinical diagnostic findings and treatment are outlined in Table 19–4.

Aortic Stenosis

Aortic stenosis increases afterload by obstructing the flow of blood from the left ventricle into the aorta during systole. It may be the result of a congenital mal-

TABLE 19–4
Abnormal Pressure Disorders

Clinical Presentation	Physical Assessment	Diagnostic Considerations	Treatment
Aortic Stenosis Angina Syncope during or immediately after physical activity Advanced disease—sign of right and left ventricular failure[4]	Normal arterial blood pressure Advanced disease and decreased systolic pressure and decreased pulse pressure Systolic thrill palpable at base of heart Soft S_1, loud S_4, S_3 present with left ventricular failure Harsh midsystolic ejective murmur, heard best at apex, transmitted along carotid arteries	ECG indicative of left ventricular hypertrophy Chest x-ray reveals left ventricular enlargement and pulmonary congestion Echocardiogram and cardiac catheterization to evaluate LV function; amount of stenosis and presence of other cardiac disease	Digitalis glycosides, diuretics Sodium restriction Activity restriction Prompt surgical replacement for significant stenosis[5]
Pulmonic Stenosis Asymptomatic in mild cases Exercise intolerance in moderate cases May have sudden onset of right ventricular failure	Normal S_1, split S_2 Systolic thrill, palpable at 2nd intercostal space at left sternal border Harsh systolic ejection murmur heard best at upper left sternal border	ECG reveals right axis deviation, right ventricular hypertrophy, right atrial enlargement Chest x-ray normal in mild to moderate stenosis, enlarged right atrium and right ventricle in severe stenosis with dilatation of main pulmonary artery Cardiac catheritization to evaluate severity of stenosis	Digitalis glycosides, diuretics Sodium restriction Pulmonary valve commissurotomy or valvuloplasty[6]
Pulmonary Hypertension Asymptomatic Late in disease process—right heart failure, fatigue, chest pain, exertional dyspnea, and syncope Hoarseness	Increased pulmonary artery pressure, normal PCWP, increased CCVP Atrial gallop at left lower sternal border, narrowly split S_2, ejection click at 2nd intercostal space at left sternal border Palpable right ventricular heave Palpable impulse over main pulmonary artery	ECG reveals right axis deviation and right ventricular hypertrophy Chest x-ray shows cardiac enlargement, especially right-side, dilated pulmonary artery	Diuretics, digitalis glycosides Sodium and water restriction Anticoagulant therapy if pulmonary emboli Oxygen therapy Vasodilator therapy Surgical intervention; heart-lung transplantation
Systemic Hypertension Asymptomatic	Serial (3 or more) blood pressure readings with systolic pressures above 140 mmHg and diastolic pressures above 90 mmHg	ECG reveals left ventricular hypertrophy Chest x-ray may show cardiomegaly	Modify risk factors Sodium restriction Antihypertensive therapy (may include diuretics)

formation above or below the valve, congenital bicuspid valve, rheumatic inflammation, or degenerative calcification and can occur in one of the following locations: valvular, supravalvular, or subvalvular.

The normal aortic valve opening measures 2.5 to 3.5 cm^2. Stenosis is considered clinically significant when the aortic valve opening is reduced to one third its normal size, and is classified as severe when the measured opening is 0.75 cm^2 or less.[4] Calcification, over time, causes the cusps of the aortic valve to thicken and harden. The left ventricle will compensate for the narrower valve opening by increasing wall thickness to generate a higher pressure; the result is left ventricular hypertrophy.

Aortic stenosis may become so severe that, even with an enlarged left ventricle, the cardiac output is fixed. The cardiac output cannot be increased to meet the increased demands of exercise, and the patient may experience dizziness or syncope. The severity of symptoms associated with aortic stenosis is directly related to the amount of stenosis present and the compensatory ability of the left ventricle. Heart failure occurs with moderate to severe disease, and death will often occur within 5 years after the onset of heart failure.

Pulmonic Stenosis

Stenosis of the pulmonic valve is most often a result of congenital disorders but may also be caused by rheumatic heart disease. In pulmonic stenosis, it is the right ventricle that must work harder to overcome the restriction of the pulmonic valve. Right ventricular hypertrophy results from the increased pressure necessary to maintain adequate pulmonary blood flow. Mild pulmonic stenosis may not cause any symptoms. Even in cases of moderate stenosis, the patient may only be symptomatic when a demand for an increased cardiac output occurs. Compromised patients will exhibit symptoms of right ventricular failure.

Pulmonary Hypertension

Pulmonary hypertension is a condition of the pulmonary vasculature that impedes the flow of blood through the lungs and increases the work of the right ventricle. Primary pulmonary hypertension is most commonly seen in women between the ages of 20 and 40 years, and the cause is not well understood. Secondary pulmonary hypertension may be a result of cardiac or pulmonary disease. The causes of pulmonary hypertension are outlined in Table 19–5.[7]

Systemic Hypertension

Systemic hypertension is a common factor in the development of heart failure. Over time, the increase in systemic vascular resistance increases the workload on the left ventricle. As in aortic stenosis, the left ventricle will thicken and gradually hypertrophy in order to compensate for the increased pressure necessary to empty during systole. The increased workload raises

TABLE 19–5
Causes of Pulmonary Hypertension

Diffuse alveolar hypoxia
Obesity
High-altitude hypoxia
Alveolar hypoventilation
Smoke inhalation
Reduction of the pulmonary vascular bed
Recurrent emboli
Widespread interstitial diseases
Cardiac disorders
Mitral stenosis
Atrial myxoma
Congenital heart disease
Left-to-right shunts

the oxygen demands of the myocardium. When the compensatory mechanisms can no longer meet oxygen demands, signs of heart failure develop.

Filling Disorders

A second group of diseases that contribute to the development of heart failure consists of conditions characterized by an inadequate filling of the ventricle from the atrium. This is due to a reduction in the size of the valvular opening. Initially, the heart is able to compensate in order to maintain an adequate cardiac output, but as the compenstory mechanisms fail, the patient will develop signs of heart failure. Abnormal filling disorders with accompanying clinical/diagnostic findings and treatment are outlined in Table 19–6.

Mitral Stenosis

Rheumatic fever is the most common cause of mitral stenosis. The thickening and fusion of the valve commissures produced usually appear after a latent period of 20 years following the initial illness. The normal mitral valve opening is 4.6 cm^2. As the size of the valvular opening is reduced, the left atrium must generate a higher pressure to move blood through the valve into the left ventricle. When the mitral valve opening is reduced to 1.5 cm^2, cardiac output drops and the patient is symptomatic on exertion. As the pressure in the left atrium increases, the pressure in the pulmonary capillaries and pulmonary artery also increases. Eventually, fluid is forced out of the capillaries and into the lung. This results in pulmonary edema.[5]

Tricuspid Stenosis

Tricuspid stenosis is a rare disorder caused by rheumatic fever. It is generally seen in patients with multivalvular disease, most commonly in conjunction with mitral stenosis and combined mitral and aortic stenosis. The obstruction leads to increased right atrial

TABLE 19–6
Abnormal Filling Disorders

Clinical Presentation	Physical Assessment	Diagnostic Considerations	Treatment
Mitral Stenosis Dyspnea Orthopnea and paroxysmal nocturnal dyspnea Cough, dysphagia, hoarseness	Resting tachycardia, increased respiratory rate, and decreased pulse pressure in severe stenosis Jugular venous distention Loud S_1 with patient in left lateral decubitus position Soft, low-pitched diastolic murmur with a rambling quality Atrial dysrhythmias such as atrial fibrillation are common	ECG reveals right axis deviation, right ventricular hypertrophy, left atrial enlargement	Antibiotic prophylaxis Digitalis glycosides, diuretics Sodium restriction Activity restriction Surgical repair by commissurotomy or valvular replacement[5]
Tricuspid Stenosis Fatigue, exercise intolerance	Hepatomegaly, ascites, peripheral edema JVD with clear lung fields Diastolic, rumbling murmur at the left lower sternal border	ECG prolonged PR interval, tall peaked P waves	Antibiotics prophylaxis Digitalis glycosides, diuretics Sodium restriction Surgical repair by commissurotomy

pressure and as the disease progresses, the pressure increase will be reflected in the systemic venous circulation.

Atrial Myxomas

Atrial myxomas are benign cardiac tumors that intermittently block the atrioventricular opening to produce a functional mitral or tricuspid stenosis. The signs and symptoms are the same as those found in mitral or tricuspid stenosis. The myxoma is surgically removed if the patient is symptomatic as a result of the obstruction.

Abnormal Muscle Conditions

The myocardium is able to contract in an organized fashion because of the unique construction of the actin-myosin filaments. When the myocardium is stimulated, actin filaments shorten, allowing the myofibrils to slide together and overlap. This produces a contraction of the muscle. During relaxation the filaments slide back to their original positions. Factors that interfere with this mechanism will affect the contractility of the muscle itself. Contractility may also be altered by manipulations of preload and afterload as evidenced by the Frank-Starling phenomenon.

Cardiomyopathies

Cardiomyopathy refers to disease processes that affect the heart muscle by enlarging the myocardium, with resulting ventricular dysfunction. Cardiomyopathies are divided into groups according to the structural abnormalities present within the myocardium. The three groups of cardiomyopathies and their causes are listed in Table 19–7. Table 19–8 presents

the three types of cardiomyopathies and their associated diagnostic findings and current treatment.

Dilated Cardiomyopathy. Dilated cardiomyopathy is the most common type of cardiomyopathy. It was known as congestive cardiomyopathy in the early 1960s when diagnosis was based on clinical symptoms, which are similar to those of congestive heart failure. However, in dilated cardiomyopathy the four chambers of the heart have become enlarged. This enlargement is a result of the increased volume of blood that remains in the ventricles at the end of diastole. Dilated cardiomyopathy is most often seen in men between the ages of 40 and 60 years of age. Death may occur 6 months to 5 years after the onset of symptoms.[8]

Characteristic symptoms of this process include a decrease in contractility of the heart muscle and a decrease in the systolic ejection fraction. The underlying cause for this decrease in efficiency is an impairment in the ability of the myocardium to obtain the calcium it needs for effective contraction. When the heart cannot pump efficiently, blood flow backs up

TABLE 19–7
Causes of Cardiomyopathies

Hypertrophic Cardiomyopathy
Genetic

Dilated Cardiomyopathy
Alcohol
Peripartum
Viral
Bacterial
Chemotherapy
Hypersensitivity to penicillin, tetracycline, and sulfonamides

Restrictive Cardiomyopathy
Amyloidosis
Sarcoidosis
Hemochromatosis (accumulation of iron in body tissues)
Infiltrative neoplastic disease

TABLE 19–8

Diagnostic Presentation and Treatment of the Cardiomyopathies

Diagnostic Presentation	Treatment
Dilated Cardiomyopathy	
Auscultation Apical impulse displaced laterally	Digitalis, sympathomimetic amines, diuretics, nitrates, anticoagulants Sodium restriction Cardiac transplantation
ECG LV hypertrophy, conduction disturbances, bundle branch block (BBB), atrial/ventricular dysthrythmias	
Catheterization LV impairment, mitral, tricuspid regurgitation, ↓ CO	
Hypertrophic Cardiomyopathy	
Auscultation Crescendo-decrescendo systolic murmur	Surgical Myomectomy with muscle resection Transaortic ventriculomyotomy
ECG LVH, atrial, ventricular dysrhythmia	Medical Antiarrhythmic agents, antibiotics, anticoagulation, β-adrenergic blockers[11]
Catheterization ↓ LV compliance, hyperdynamic systolic function, LV outflow obstruction[11]	
Restrictive Cardiomyopathy	
CXR Mild cardiac enlargement Pulmonary venous hypertension	Same as dilated cardiomyopathy except no vasodilator therapy[10]
ECG High-grade AV blocks, conduction disturbances	
Catheterization ↓ LV compliance, ↑ LVEDP	

into the pulmonary vasculature and patients present with signs of left-sided heart failure.[9] The heart attempts to compensate for this decrease in cardiac output by enlarging the atria and ventricles. The enlarged surface area requires more oxygen-enriched blood and increased ventricular wall tensions, thus limiting its benefits to the cardiovascular system.

Hypertrophic Cardiomyopathy. Hypertrophic cardiomyopathy is transmitted genetically. Classic structural abnormalities include left ventricular hypertrophy, thickening of the mitral leaflets, hypertrophy of the papillary muscles, and thickening of endocardial lining in the overflow tract of the left ventricle. The abnormal appearance of the left ventricle leads to imperfections in the alignment of the papillary muscles. These imperfections manifest themselves in the obstruction of the outflow tract of the left ventricle by the mitral leaflets.

Factors that increase contractility or decrease left ventricular volume further compromise an inefficient pump. Blood volume in the left ventricle increases in hypertrophic cardiomyopathy because of the obstructions in the outflow tract of the ventricle. This increased left ventricular and diastolic volume interferes with the flow of blood from the left atrium and contributes to a decreased cardiac output.[10]

Restrictive Cardiomyopathy. Restrictive cardiomyopathy is caused by disease processes that infiltrate the myocardium, making it more rigid and less flexible during diastole. The noncompliant ventricle leads to an increased diastolic pressure, even with minor changes in blood volume. The abnormal ventricle leads to atrial enlargement as pressures back up in the cardiac system and greater force is needed to overcome the pressure exerted by the noncompliant left ventricle. Further decline in cardiac function eventually leads to left-sided heart failure.

Myocarditis/Endocarditis

Myocarditis is an inflammation of the myocardium. It is usually idiopathic but may be caused by fever, radiation therapy, chemicals, or viruses. The pathologic mechanisms responsible for myocarditis include direct myocardial invasion by causative agents, production of a myocardial toxin, and/or stimulation of antibody production. This disease may lead to focal or diffuse involvement of the heart tissue. Diffuse disease may result in heart failure, whereas focal disease processes may lead to arrhythmias. Treatment plans include antibiotic therapy and supportive measures for heart failure and arrhythmias.

Endocarditis is an inflammation of the endothelial layer of the heart, including valves and septal defects. It may be caused by bacterial or fungal infections. Bacteria are attracted to damaged cardiac structures in chaotic, high-flow areas of the heart. Subsequently, fibrin-platelet complexes may form protective layers around these pathogens, and scarring and structural damage from bacteria may lead to insufficient valve functions. In addition, if the vegetation breaks away it may lead to infarction or abscesses in other areas of the body. Bacteria may also invade the myocardium, causing disturbances in the electrical pathway or abscesses.

Patients may present with infections, fever, weakness, malaise, anorexia, and headaches. Diagnosis is based on blood cultures, but negative cultures may be seen in this disorder as it is difficult to culture fungi. Treatment with antibiotics, antipyretics, or surgery may be necessary.

Myocardial Infarction

Myocardial infarction decreases cardiac output by decreasing the number of functional muscle fibers. This decrease in muscle fibers contributes to a decrease in stroke volume and cardiac output. Chapter 18 outlines the impact of coronary artery disease and myocardial infarction on heart failure.

Cardiogenic Shock

Description. Cardiogenic shock, or heart failure, develops when the myocardium cannot maintain an adequate cardiac output to meet the body's demands. Symptoms include systemic hypotension, arterial vasoconstriction, and impaired tissue and organ perfusion. Cardiogenic shock occurs when 40% of the left ventricle has been destroyed.[12] The mortality associated with shock approaches 85% in the subpopulation of patients who present with an acute myocardial infarction that deteriorates into cardiogenic shock. These patients develop symptoms within the first 24 hours after infarction.

Etiology. Factors contributing to cardiogenic shock are outlined in Table 19–9. The most common cause of shock continues to be a damaged heart muscle that can no longer pump efficiently. The most common culprit is a myocardial infarction. Untreated infarctions lead to necrosis and ischemia of myocardial cells. This damage is most profound when the proximal portion of the left anterior descending artery is involved because this artery supplies the anterior, septal, and apical regions of the left ventricle.

Pathophysiology. Cardiogenic shock occurs when the pumping action of the heart is severely depressed.

TABLE 19–9
Causes of Cardiogenic Shock

Electrical Factors
Bradyarrhythmias
Tachyarrhythmias

Mechanical Factors
Cardiac tamponade
Left ventricular aneurysm
Myocarditis
Dilated cardiomyopathy
Hypertension
Pump failure after cardiac surgery
Myocardial infarction

Structural Factors
Atrial myxomas
Aortic stenosis
Mitral stenosis
Mitral regurgitation
Aortic regurgitation
Ruptured intraventricular system

The inefficient pump cannot deliver enough oxygen-enriched blood to meet the demands of the body. Compensatory mechanisms are activated but cannot replace the failing heart, and circulatory collapse becomes the overriding outcome.

Myocardial compromise is impaired by the body's compensatory mechanisms. For example, the increase in systemic vascular resistance that originally shunted blood to vital organs begins to impede left ventricular ejection and cardiac output. Acidosis from the vasoconstriction of peripheral organs also serves to depress the myocardium. Depletion of norepinephrine and epinephrine interferes with contractility of the myocardium and peripheral vascular tone. Tables 19–10 and 19–11 show the hemodynamic and clinical presentations of patients with shock.[13]

As the body continues to deteriorate, alterations in the performance of organs dependent on consistent blood flow from the heart become more pronounced.

TABLE 19–10
Hemodynamic Profile of Cardiogenic Shock

Hemodynamic Parameter	Value in Cardiogenic Shock	Normal Value
Heart rate	↑	60–90 beats/min
Pulmonary artery pressure	↑	$\left(\frac{20\text{–}25 \text{ mmHg}}{8\text{–}12 \text{ mmHg}}\right)$
Pulmonary wedge pressure	↑	8–12 mmHg
Systemic vascular resistance	↑	800–1200 dynes sec cm^{-5}
Blood pressure	↓	$\left(\frac{100\text{–}120 \text{ mmHg}}{70\text{–}80 \text{ mmHg}}\right)$
Cardiac output	↓	4–8 L/min
Cardiac index	↓	2.5–3.5 L/min/m^2
Stroke volume	↓	50–100 mL/beat
Stroke work index	↓	45–75 g/m^2/beat

TABLE 19-11
**Clinical Presentation of the Patient
with Cardiogenic Shock**

Body System	Signs/Symptoms
Cardiovascular	Systolic blood pressure <90 mmHg
	Tachycardia
	Weak, thready pulses
	S_3, S_4
	Decreased pulse pressure
	Palpitations
	Chest pain
Renal	Urine output ≤30 mL/h
	Decreased urine osmolality
Integumentary	Cool, clammy skin
	Decreased capillary refill
	Peripheral edema
	Pallor or cyanosis
Neurologic	Restlessness, agitation
	Confusion
	Altered level of consciousness
	Dilated pupils
Pulmonary	Tachypnea
	Dyspnea
	Rales
Gastrointestinal	Decreased bowel sounds
	Nausea/vomiting
	Melena
	Hematemesis

The kidney's response to low cardiac output is to (1) decrease glomerular filtration rate, (2) activate the renin-angiotension cycle, and (3) increase aldosterone secretion. These three compensatory mechanisms work against the cardiovascular system in severe cardiac failure by overstretching the heart muscle and lead to inefficient pumping; pulmonary edema, as fluid leaks from capillary beds; and pronounced peripheral edema. The pulmonary system is affected by concomitant vasoconstriction by the release of serotonin and histamines from necrotic pulmonary parenchymal cells. Histamines and serotonin increase pulmonary capillary permeability and vasoconstriction. This intensifies ventilation-perfusion mismatch and aggravates acidosis and hypoxia. Fluid migrates from the pulmonary vasculature into the interstitium, resulting in interstitial edema. Atelectasis develops because the alveoli cannot produce enough surfactant to provide adequate surface tension.[10]

Treatment. Rapid intervention in cardiogenic shock may enhance the patient's chance of survival. Treatment regimens focus on fluid management, provision of sympathomimetic drugs that improve contractility, vasodilator medicines that alter preload and afterload, and mechanical ventilation.

Abnormal Volume Load

The diastolic volume in the heart (preload) is the amount of blood in the ventricle prior to contraction. Preload is determined by the ability of the ventricle to stretch, and by blood volume, venous tone, the condition of the mitral valve, and the timing and force of atrial contraction. Over time, if filling pressures exceed those of the normal heart, the result is a decrease in the strength and quality of ventricular function. Abnormal volume disorders with accompanying clinical/diagnostic findings and treatment are outlined in Table 19-12.

Aortic Regurgitation

Aortic regurgitation can be acute or chronic and occurs most often in men. It may be congenital or may be caused by endocarditis, rheumatic fever, dissecting aortic aneurysm, or connective tissue disorders. Aortic regurgitation is the result of an incompetent aortic valve. Blood pumped into the aorta regurgitates back into the left ventricle through a leaking valve, imposing a volume overload in the resting left ventricle.[14]

In acute aortic regurgitation, the increase in left ventricular volume during diastole increases the pressure in the left ventricle. The left atrium must overcome this measure in order to fill the ventricle adequately. As the left ventricular pressure becomes greater than the left atrial pressure, the mitral valve closes early in diastole to protect the pulmonary circulation. In acute aortic regurgitation, the patient will deteriorate quickly, often requiring emergency surgical intervention.

In chronic aortic regurgitation, the left ventricle will initially compensate by increasing stroke volume and maintaining a normal cardiac output. Over time, the left ventricle will be unable to maintain the contractility necessary, and the pressures in the left side of the heart will begin to rise. As the left ventricular end-diastolic volume (LVEDV) and left ventricular end-diastolic pressure (LVEDP) increase, the pressure is transmitted back into the pulmonary vasculature and eventually to the right side of the heart. Peripheral vasodilation occurs as a compensatory mechanism in chronic aortic regurgitation to decrease afterload and minimize the regurgitant blood flow back through the aortic valve.

Mitral Regurgitation

Mitral regurgitation can be acute or chronic. Acute mitral regurgitation may be caused by a rupture of the chordae and/or papillary muscles or perforation of a mitral valve leaflet. Chronic mitral regurgitation may be the result of rheumatic fever, dysfunction of the papillary muscles, calcification of the mitral annulus, left ventricular dilatation, congenital anomalies, and connective tissue diseases.

Mitral regurgitation results in systolic volume overload in the left atrium. As the left ventricle pumps blood into the aorta, blood also flows back into the left atrium through an incompetent mitral valve. The left atrium dilates and hypertrophies to compensate for the increased volume. The left ventricle also dilates and hypertrophies in an attempt to maintain cardiac output. This is a temporary solution, however, and left ventricular failure develops with progressive dilatation.

TABLE 19–12
Abnormal Volume Disorders

Clinical Presentation	Physical Assessment	Diagnostic Considerations	Treatment
Aortic Regurgitation Sweating, flushing	Corrigan's pulse (water hammer*)[15] Widened pulse pressure—increased systolic, decreased diastolic Diastolic thrill palpable at left lower sternal border S_3 gallop Blowing, high-pitched decrescendo diastolic murmur heard at 2nd right intercostal space and radiating to the left sternal border	ECG reveals left ventricular hypertrophy, left atrial enlargement Echocardiogram Cardiac catheterization may be indicated	Antibiotic prophylaxis Digitalis glycosides, diuretics, vasodilators Sodium restriction Surgical replacement for long-term correction
Mitral Regurgitation Asymptomatic in mild cases Fatigue, exhaustion	Hepatomegaly peripheral edema Atrial fibrillation Systemic embolization Pansystolic murmur heard best at apex Split S_2, S_3 gallop	ECG generally normal Chest x-ray shows left atrial ventricular enlargement Cardiac catheterization to evaluate mitral insufficiency	Digitalis glycosides, diuretics vasodilators Sodium restriction Anticoagulation Antiarrhythmics for atrial fibrillation Surgical intervention—replacement[16]
Pulmonic Regurgitation Symptoms of systemic venous congestion	Early diastolic decrescendo murmur heard best at 4th and 5th intercostal space at left sternal border		Antibiotic prophylaxis, digitalis glycosides, diuretics Sodium restriction
Tricuspid Regurgitation Asymptomatic in mild cases Severe cases of systemic venous congestion	Hepatomegaly, ascites, pleural effusions, edema, JVD Pansystolic murmur heard at 4th intercostal space at left sternal border Atrial fibrillation is common	ECG right bundle branch block	Digitalis glycosides, diuretics Sodium restriction Surgical replacement with stenosis and regurgitation together

*"Water-hammer" pulse is characterized by a rapid rise in arterial pressure during systole followed by a rapid fall in pressure during diastole.

In acute mitral regurgitation, the sudden regurgitant volume causes a rapid, significant increase in left atrial pressure. This is rapidly transmitted through the pulmonary vasculature and leads to the rapid development of pulmonary edema.

Pulmonic Regurgitation

Congenital malformation of the pulmonic valve or the absence of one of the leaflets is the primary cause of pulmonic regurgitation. It may also be acquired from conditions associated with pulmonary hypertension. Pulmonic regurgitation imposes a volume overload in the right ventricle. The right ventricle will dilate and hypertrophy to compensate. Eventually, right ventricular failure occurs, with symptoms of systemic venous congestion and impaired cardiac output.

Tricuspid Regurgitation

Tricuspid regurgitation is the result of right ventricular dilatation, which causes distortion of the chordae tendineae, papillary muscles, and the valvular ring. It may also be caused by endocarditis, trauma, or carcinoid syndrome. As the right ventricle pumps blood to the lungs, regurgitant blood flows back into the right atrium through the incompetent tricuspid valve. This elevation in the right atrial pressure leads to an increase in the pressure in the systemic circulation. Right ventricular dilatation and hypertrophy occur in order to maintain an adequate cardiac output. Tricuspid regurgitation is generally well tolerated. The symptoms in severe cases are related to systemic venous congestion and an inadequate cardiac output.

THERAPEUTIC INTERVENTIONS

The goals of therapeutic intervention in the patient with heart failure are to support cardiac output and enhance emptying of the ventricles. This can be accomplished by drug therapy, dietary restriction of sodium, activity restriction, mechanical circulatory assist devices, and surgical intervention. All these interventions attempt to manipulate one or more of the components of myocardial function. In the critical care setting, the use of bedside hemodynamic monitoring provides necessary diagnostic information and is essential in guiding therapeutic interventions.

Drug Therapy

Diuretics

The goals of diuretic therapy include enhancing the excretion of sodium and water, reducing filling pressures, and reducing the signs of systemic and pulmonary venous congestion. There are five groups of diuretics that accomplish these goals by their actions on specific sites of the nephron:

1. Thiazide diuretics are the diuretics of choice in patients with right ventricular failure and peripheral, dependent edema, and in patients with mild to moderate left ventricular failure.
2. Potassium-sparing diuretics have a long onset of action, thereby limiting their usefulness in the management of acute heart failure; however, they are used successfully in the treatment of chronic heart failure, especially when combined with other diuretics.
3. Carbonic anhydrase inhibitors have limited value in the treatment of heart failure since they have a very small degree of sodium excretion and are frequently used with other diuretics.
4. Osmotic diuretics are used with extreme caution in the heart failure patient. The increased load caused by osmotic diuretics could potentiate a cardiovascular volume overload, and osmotic diuretics are therefore contraindicated in the patient with pulmonary edema.
5. Loop diuretics continue to be the most frequently used diuretics in the acute care setting. They are potent, rapid-acting agents that can be given intravenously or orally. Furosemide possesses vasodilating and diuretic properties that are particularly advantageous in reducing filling pressures in patients with acute left ventricular failure and pulmonary edema.[17]

Two of the main concerns when using diuretic therapy are electrolyte depletion and overdiuresis, which may result in hypovolemia and hypotension. Electrolyte depletion, particularly hypokalemia, is a particular concern in the patient receiving digitalis therapy because this increases the patient's susceptibility to developing arrhythmias.

Inotropic Agents

The decreased contractility seen in heart failure provides the basis for the use of inotropic agents. Digitalis glycosides continue to be the most widely used oral inotropic agents, but their ability to increase the contractile force of the myocardium and improve depressed ventricular function is limited by their modest potency, narrow therapeutic range, and associated toxicities. The hemodynamic effects associated with digitalis administration include a decrease in central venous and pulmonary capillary wedge pressures, an increased stroke volume, and decreased ventricular end-diastolic volume and filling pressures. The increased contractility is associated with an increase in myocardial oxygen requirements; however, this may be offset by the beneficial effects described above. Because digitalis glycosides have a narrow range of therapeutic efficacy and a wide variety of side effects, sympathomimetic agents are more frequently used in the management of the patient with acute heart fail-

ure. Digitalis is commonly reserved for the patient in acute congestive failure precipitated by rapid atrial fibrillation.

Sympathomimetic amines are positive inotropic agents that stimulate sympathetic nervous system (SNS) activity and are used to treat severe low-output failure. The SNS attempts to compensate for a fall in cardiac output by the release of endogenous catecholamines, which cause vasoconstriction and tachycardia. Over time, however, the myocardium develops a resistance to the effects of sympathetic stimulation and requires higher levels of catecholamines to maintain heart rate and contractility. The situation is further complicated by a reduction of endogenous stores of myocardial catecholamines. The combination of these factors contributes to a decrease in the efficiency of the myocardial pumping action. The administration of sympathomimetic amines provides an exogenous method of supporting myocardial function. Although sympathomimetic amines improve myocardial functioning by increasing the heart rate and contractility, there is also an associated increase in myocardial oxygen consumption. An understanding of the response to these drugs makes it possible to manipulate combinations and dosages of these drugs so as to minimize their adverse effects and maximize their therapeutic effects (Table 19–13).

Vasodilators

The goal of vasodilator therapy is to limit venous return, maximize ventricular filling pressures and improve contractility by the Frank-Starling phenomenon, and decrease impedance to left ventricular outflow. This is accomplished by altering the tone of the peripheral vascular system.

An elevated preload, manifested by an increased LVEDP, can be reduced through the administration of venous dilators. This causes a redistribution of the circulating blood volume from the central to the peripheral circulation and results in decreased filling pressures and elimination or reduction of pulmonary venous congestion. On the other hand, venous dilating agents can have deleterious effects in the patient with a normal preload state and can cause hypotension and a further decrease in cardiac output. Venous dilators are most commonly used in patients with left ventricular (LV) failure with pulmonary edema or chronic severe heart failure who are unresponsive to diuretics and digitalis.[17]

Afterload is reduced by the administration of arteriolar dilators, which directly decrease the interference to LV ejection and ultimately decrease intramyocardial wall tension. The result is improved stroke volume, cardiac output, and peripheral perfusion. If there is sufficient improvement in stroke volume, the blood pressure will remain unchanged or fall only slightly, indicating an overall improvement in myocardial pump function.[17]

In addition to the drugs that act on either the venous or arteriolar vascular beds, there is a group of

TABLE 19–13
Sympathomimetic Therapy: A Hemodynamic Comparison

Drug	Receptor Site Stimulated	Hemodynamic Effects					
		HR	MAP	CO	Contractility	SVR	RBF
Dobutamine	β_1, β_2(slight)	O/↑	O/↑	↑	↑	O/↑	
Dopamine							
<2–5 µg/kg/min	β_1 dopaminergic	O	O	↑	↑	O	↑↑
5–10 µg/kg/min	β_1	↑↑	↑	↑	↑↑	↑	↑
	α						
	β_2						
>10 µg/kg/min	α	↑↑	↑↑	↑	↑↑	↑↑	O/↓
Epinephrine	β_1	↑↑	↑	↑↑	↑	↑	↓↓
	α (large doses)						
	β_2 (small doses)						
Isoproterenol	β_1	↑↑↑	O/↑/↓	↑↑	↑	↓↓	O/↑/↓
	β_2						
Norepinephrine	α	↑	↑↑	O	↑	↑↑	
	β_1 (small amount)						
Phenylephrine	α	↓	↑↑	↓	O	↑↑	

HR = heart rate; MAP = mean arterial pressure; CO = cardiac output; SVR = systemic vascular resistance; RBF = renal blood flow; O = unchanged; ↑ = increased; ↓ = decreased; ↑↑↑ = greatest effect; ↓↓↓ = least effect.

drugs that possess both venous and arteriolar dilating properties. The hemodynamic effects of the combined agents are an improved cardiac output and a reduction in cardiac filling pressures. Table 19–14 presents the vasodilator agents and their specific vascular responsiveness.

Morphine sulfate is frequently administered intravenously in small, intermittent doses in the patient

TABLE 19–14
Vasodilator Therapy: A Hemodynamic Comparison

Drug	Receptor Site Stimulated	Hemodynamic Effects							Indications
		HR	SVR	MAP	CO	PCWP	RAP	SV	
Nitroprusside	Arterial and venous vasodilator	O/↑	↓↓	↓	↑	↑	↓	↓↓	Acute left ventricular failure with ↑ pulmonary pressure, ↓ CO
Nitroglycerin	Venous vasodilator	O	O/↓	↓	O/↑	↓↓↓	↓↓↓	↑	Acute left ventricular failure with severe pulmonary congestion and/ or ischemia
Phentolamine	Arterial and venous vasodilator	↑↑	↓↓↓	↓	↑↑	↓↓	↓↓	↑↑	LV failure with low CO; requires high doses for sustained vasodilatation and causes ↑ HR
Hydralazine	Arterial vasodilator	O/↑	↓↓↓	↓	↑↑↑	O/↓	O/↓	↑↑↑	Chronic severe heart failure
Captopril	Arterial and venous vasodilator	O	↓↓	↓↓	↑↑	↓↓↓	↓↓↓	↑↑	Chronic refractory heart failure
Nifedipine	Arterial and venous vasodilator	O/↑	↓↓↓	↓↓	↑↑	↓↓	O/↓	↑↑	Heart failure with coronary vasospasm or acute infarction
Prazosin	Arterial and venous vasodilator	O/↓	↓↓	↓↓	↑↑	↓↓↓	↓↓↓	↑↑	Chronic severe heart failure
Minoxidil	Arterial vasodilator	↑	↓↓↓	↓↓	↑↑↑	O/↓	O	↓↓	Chronic heart failure; hypertension

HR = heart rate; SVR = systemic vascular resistance; MAP = mean arterial pressure; CO = cardiac output; PCWP = pulmonary capillary wedge pressure; RAP = right atrial pressure; SV = stroke volume; O = unchanged; ↑ = increased; ↓ = decreased; ↑↑↑ = greatest effect; ↓↓↓ = least effect.

with acute heart failure. This causes peripheral pooling of blood, with redistribution of the blood away from the congested pulmonary circulation, and results in a decreased preload. Additionally, morphine helps to decrease the anxiety and tachypnea noted in the acute heart failure patient and also helps relax airway smooth muscle to facilitate gas exchange.

Vasodilators are generally not used in the management of valvular stenosis. The hemodynamic consequences of mitral stenosis include an elevation in the left atrial pressure and pulmonary venous pressures. There is a mechanical obstruction to LV filling and little evidence of LV failure; therefore, afterload reduction would have little effect on LV function. In aortic stenosis associated with LV failure, extreme caution must be used with vasodilator therapy. Although cardiac output could be improved by afterload reduction, there is a risk of the vasodilator causing hypotension, which would impair coronary perfusion.

Vasodilator therapy has a limited value in the treatment of right ventricular failure and in the management of pulmonary hypertension because vasodilators have a greater effect on systemic vascular beds than on pulmonay vascular beds. This necessitates the use of high doses of vasodilator agents to achieve a reduction in the interference to right ventricular outflow, and systemic hypotension generally precludes the administration of such high doses.[17]

Supportive Therapy

Oxygen Therapy

Impaired gas exchange develops as a consequence of LV failure due to the movement of fluid from the pulmonary vascular system into the interstitial and alveolar spaces of the lung. Also, a diminished cardiac output leads to impaired perfusion and gas exchange at the cellular level, with resulting tissue hypoxia. Contractility is impaired by hypoxia as the result of an ineffective myocardial cellular metabolism that develops with the shift from an aerobic to an anaerobic state. Supplemental oxygen is provided to reduce the workload of the heart and to support cellular energy requirements.

Dietary Sodium Restriction

Dietary restriction of sodium is also an important part of the management of the patient with heart failure. As a result of sympathoadrenergic stimulation, the renin-angiotensin-aldosterone mechanism results in an increased tubular reabsorption of sodium and water (see Fig. 34–5). In severe cases, the body can retain as much as 10 L of extra fluid and 80 g of sodium. This causes an increase in cardiac workload, increased filling pressures, and contributes to the development of pulmonary edema. The amount of sodium and water retained by the body can be altered by decreasing the amount of sodium ingested in the diet.

Normally, the average American diet contains 2.5 to 6 g of sodium per day. Omitting the use of table salt reduces the sodium intake to 1.6 to 2.8 g per day. However, in cases of severe heart failure, it may be necessary to restrict the sodium intake to 0.2 to 1 g sodium per day. This requires patients to eliminate the use of table salt and salt in cooking, as well as to purchase and prepare foods with a low sodium content.[18]

Activity

The modification of activity is also an important part of the prescriptive plan for patients with heart failure, in order not to place excessive workload demands on the heart. The activity plan is highly individualized, and the degree of restriction is based on the severity of the heart failure. It is generally recommended that the highest level of activity be maintained that does not produce symptoms. Isometric exercises are discouraged since they do not promote cardiovascular conditioning and cause an increase in blood pressure and cardiac workload. Aerobic activities are good for cardiovascular conditioning but must not be too strenuous.

The teaching plan should include assessing the severity of the patient's heart failure and prior activity pattern; teaching the importance of environmental factors on cardiac function; explaining the importance of rest periods and the timing of activity to avoid exercise after a meal or alcohol; and teaching the patient to identify the outcomes of activity intolerance. These usually include the sensation of fatigue, chest discomfort, shortness of breath, palpitations, or a heart rate that exceeds the resting heart rate by more than 25 beats/min.

Mechanical Support

Mechanical support of the failing heart may be fundamental to improving the pumping action of the myocardium and reducing the heart's workload. Mechanical support devices are usually reserved for the treatment of intractable heart failure. The intra-aortic balloon pump (IABP) is the most frequently used device to temporarily support the failing heart and systemic circulation. The beneficial hemodynamic effects anticipated with the use of the IABP include an elevation of the aortic pressure and improved coronary artery perfusion by an increase in arterial diastolic pressure. As the balloon is deflated during contraction, there is a decrease in intra-aortic volume, a diminished resistance to LV ejection, and a decrease in ventricular workload and myocardial oxygen consumption. This is evidenced by an improved cardiac output, increased stroke volume, and a reduction in LVEDP.

The left ventricular assist device (LVAD) is a mechanical device that is used predominantly in postoperative cardiac surgery patients with severe heart failure. The LVAD functions as a reservoir. A pneu-

Purpose: This study examined the perceptions of hospitalized congestive heart failure (CHF) patients and their nurses concerning the importance of specific educational content.

Methods: A survey approach was used to collect data on 30 hospitalized CHF patients and 26 nurses providing their care. A modified learning needs inventory, with established reliability and validity, was used to examine perceptions about learning needs in terms of importance and realism. Learning needs were grouped by the 44-item Likert scale instrument into categories of anatomy and physiology, psychological factors, risk factors, medications, diet, activity, and other. The instrument was completed within 30 minutes by a convenience group of CHF patient subjects and primarily registered nurses.

Results: Mean scores for each information category were obtained for patient and nurse groups. Both nurses and patients rated all information as important to learn and realistic to learn during the patient's hospitalization. Patients rated medication information as the most important to learn, followed by anatomy and physiology, risk factors, other, diet, psychological factors, and activity. Nurses also ranked medication information as the most important category, followed by risk factors and diet. Most of the mean importance and realism scores of patients were slightly higher than those of nurses.

Practice Implications: The predominant finding of this study was that both patients and nurses generally believed that the content areas were important and realistic to learn. The study provides information regarding content areas needed to educate CHF patients. Study findings also suggest that patients value education highly during their hospitalization, a finding which reinforces patient education as a significant nursing intervention.

matically driven pump diverts blood from the left ventricle and pumps it into the ascending thoracic aorta, almost totally relieving the left ventricle of its workload. The beneficial physiologic effects associated with LVAD include a reduction in myocardial wall tension and myocardial oxygen consumption, as a result of a reduction in preload; a reduced afterload is brought about by the mechanical pumping of blood into the aorta and allows a period of rest for the failing heart.[19]

A detailed discussion of mechanical support devices can be found in Chapter 17.

NURSING CARE

Therapeutic Goals

The therapeutic goals listed below provide the framework on which the critical care nurse bases patient care. Implementation of the nursing process with nursing diagnoses, desired patient outcomes, interventions, and their rationales is presented in the care plan at the end of this chapter.

1. Perform a thorough and ongoing assessment.
2. Reduce cardiac workload.
3. Provide hemodynamic support to maintain cardiac output and tissue perfusion.
4. Provide ventilatory support and oxygenation to relieve hypoxia associated with pulmonary venous congestion.
5. Maintain fluid and electrolyte balance.
6. Identify and treat conditions that aggravate the development of heart failure.
7. Maintain nutritional status.
8. Provide emotional and psychological support to patient and family.
9. Initiate patient and/or family health education pertinent to heart failure, clinical manifestations, and treatment regimens.

REFERENCES

1. Canobbio, MM: Cardiovascular disorders. CV Mosby, St. Louis, 1990.
2. Michaelson, CR: Pathophysiology of heart failure: A conceptual framework for understanding clinical indicators and therapeutic modalities. In Michaelson, CR (ed): Congestive Heart Failure. CV Mosby, St. Louis, 1983, p. 45.
3. Guyton, AC: Textbook of Medical Physiology. WB Saunders, Philadelphia, 1986.
4. Cohn, PF: Clinical Cardiovascular Physiology. WB Saunders, Philadelphia, 1985.
5. Cavallo, GAO: The person with valvular heart disease. In Guzzetta, CE and Dossey, BM: Cardiovascular Nursing, Body Mind Tapestry. CV Mosby, St. Louis, MO, 1984, p 631.
6. Walls, JJ, et al: Assessment of percutaneous balloon pulmonary and aortic valvuloplasty. J Thorac Cardiovasc Surg 88:352–356, 1984.
7. Pura, LS and Sam, CS: Underlying causes and precipitating factors in heart failure. In Michaelson, CR (ed): Congestive Heart Failure. CV Mosby, St. Louis, 1983, p 93.
8. Torp, A: Incidence of congestive cardiomyopathies. Postgrad Med J 54:435, 1978.
9. Wingate, S: Dilated cardiomyopathy, part I. Focus 11(4):49–56, 1984.
10. Dossey, BM: The person with cardiomyopathy or myocarditis. In Guzzetta, CE and Dossey, BM: Cardiovascular Nursing, Body Mind Tapestry. CV Mosby, St. Louis, 1984, p 739.
11. Shah, PM: Cardiomyopathies. In Shine, KI (ed): Cardiology. John Wiley & Sons, New York, 1983, p 85.
12. Resnekov, L: Cardiogenic shock. Chest 83:893, 1983.
13. Niles, NA and Wills, RE: Heart failure. In Underhill, SL, et al (eds): Cardiovascular Nursing, ed 2. JB Lippincott, Philadelphia, 1988, p 387.
14. Goldberger, E: Textbook of Clinical Cardiology. CV Mosby, St. Louis, 1981.
15. Brunwald, E: Heart Disease: A Textbook of Cardiovascular Medicine. WB Saunders, Philadelphia, 1992.

16. Rippe, JM and Howe, JP: Acute mitral regurgitation. In Rippe, JM, et al (eds): Intensive Care Medicine. Little Brown, Boston, 1985, p 261.
17. Taormina Paplanus, LM, Strebel, CA, and Michaelson, CR: Drug therapy for congestive heart failure. CV Mosby, St. Louis, 1983.
18. Gawlinski, A: Diet therapy in heart failure. In Michaelson, CR (ed): Congestive Heart Failure. CV Mosby, St. Louis, 1983, pp 354–355.
19. Brannon, PHB and Towner, SB: Ventricular failure: New therapy, using the mechanical assist device. Critical Care Nurse 6(2):76, 1986.

CARE PLAN FOR THE PATIENT WITH HEART FAILURE

Nursing Diagnoses

Nursing Diagnoses #1
Cardiac Output, decreased, related to mechanical factors (contractility, preload, afterload)

Desired Patient Outcomes

Patient will:
1. Demonstrate signs of hemodynamic stability:
   - Cardiac output 4–8 L/min
   - Heart rate <100 beats/min
   - Systolic blood pressure >110 mmHg or within 10 mmHg of baseline
   - Pulmonary capillary wedge pressure 8–12 mmHg (mean)
   - Absence of third and fourth heart sounds (S_3 and S_4)
2. Maintain electrophysiologic stability
   - Absence of arrhythmia

Nursing Interventions

- Ongoing assessment of signs and symptoms of *left* ventricular failure
  - Rales (crackles)
  - Bronchial wheezing
  - Dyspnea
  - Paroxysmal nocturnal dyspnea
  - Nocturia
  - Orthopnea
  - Anxiety, restlessness, disorientation
  - Gallop rhythms
  - Peripheral cyanosis
  - Central cyanosis.
  - Blood-tinged sputum
  - Cheyne-Stokes respirations

- Ongoing assessment of the signs and symptoms of *right* ventricular failure:
  - Jugular venous distention
  - Peripheral edema
  - Weight gain
  - Ascites
  - Hepatojugular reflux

Rationales

- Provides a systematic approach to data collection to determine the severity of the disease and the efficacy of therapeutic intervention.
  - Fluid in alveoli, the result of pressure increases in the pulmonary capillary bed.
  - Bronchiolar constriction from excess fluid
  - Result of elevation in pulmonary interstitial edema.
  - Serum proteins are at lowest level in early morning; redistribution of volume secondary to recumbent position; nocturnal respiratory depression.
  - Increased renal perfusion secondary to postural redistribution of blood flow.
  - Result of increased venous return from postural redistribution of pulmonary blood flow.
  - Decreased cerebral perfusion and cerebral hypoxia.
  - S_3 associated with increased LVEDP, left atrial pressure, and PCWP.
  - S_4 related to decreased ventricular compliance.
  - Secondary to decreased cardiac output and decreased peripheral circulation. Blood stays in the peripheral tissues longer to extract more oxygen, and when blood reaches the distal vascular bed, it has a markedly diminished O_2 content.
  - Results when alveolar edema impairs O_2 diffusion.
  - Ruptures of bronchiolar capillaries due to increased hydrostatic pressure in capillaries.
  - Decreased cardiac output causes prolonged circulation time, which in turn causes the respiratory center in the brainstem to be underperfused and underoxygenated.

  - Result of elevated venous pressures.

  - May gain as much as 10–15 lb of extracellular fluid before edema is readily apparent.
  - Pressure on right upper quadrant compresses liver and acts as a temporary fluid challenge; dysfunctional right heart will show up as a visible increase in pressure in jugular veins; visible increase in pressure with competent right heart.

CARE PLAN FOR THE PATIENT WITH HEART FAILURE (*Continued*)

Nursing Interventions	**Rationales**
◦ Anorexia, nausea, vomiting	◦ Increased pressure in capillaries of abdominal organs results in edema; nausea is secondary to stretching of liver capsule due to edema.
• Administer prescribed medication regimen to maximize effects of preload, afterload, and myocardial contracility. ◦ Cardiac glycosides.	◦ Positive inotropic and negative chronotorpic agent improves cardiac output.

◦ Diuretics:
  □ Monitor I&O; daily weights.
  □ Monitor for side effects of diuretic therapy (hypokalemia, hyponatremia, fatigue, muscle cramps, hypotension, tachycardia).
	◦ Decrease intravascular volume by their direct action on the kidney and by reducing sodium reabsorption, increase venous capacitance, reduce preload to maximize Frank-Starling phenomenon.
	◦ Increased venous capacitance provides beneficial effect in patients with left heart failure and pulmonary edema; in patients with right heart failure with vigorous diuresis, this may be detrimental as it contributes to systemic venous pooling, thereby limiting venous return and right ventricular filling and further contributing to a decreased cardiac output.

◦ Vasodilators: □ Monitor for side effects and efficacy of therapy (headache, dizziness, hypotension, postural hypotension, muscle weakness, syncope; ↓ SVR, ↓ PCWP, ↓ RA pressure, diuresis, increased exercise tolerance, resolution of heart failure symptoms). ◦ Sympathomimetics	◦ Vasodilators increase cardiac output by decreasing SVR and/or reducing LVEDP by decreasing vascular tone. Vasodilators reduce myocardial oxygen demand, which may help minimize ischemia and size of infarction. ◦ Positive inotropic agents increase cardiac output by increasing stroke volume and contractility. The myocardium becomes dependent on circulating catecholamines in heart failure, and sympathomimetic administration provides an exogenous source of catecholamines to support myocardial contractility.

Nursing Diagnoses	**Desired Patient Outcomes**
Nursing Diagnosis #2 Fluid Volume, alteration in, related to: 1. Increased levels of aldosterone 2. Sodium retention 3. Antidiuretic hormone secondary to reduced renal blood flow	Maintain state of normovolemia: ◦ Good skin turgor ◦ Absence of peripheral edema ◦ Absence of jugular venous distention ◦ Absence of rales on auscultation ◦ Stable baseline body weight

Nursing Interventions	**Rationales**
• Monitor fluid balance: ◦ Measure weight daily. ◦ Document fluid intake and output, urine specific gravity. ◦ Maintain fluid restriction as indicated. ◦ Use microdrip or infusion pump for fluid administration. ◦ Prevent volume overload in patients with a compromised cardiac status. • Monitor hemodynamic parameters: ◦ Arterial blood pressure	◦ Daily weights allow practitioners to monitor trends in weight gain/loss, establish baseline for treatment, and evaluate treatment plans. ◦ Accurate intake/output records should correlate with weight gain/loss and allow practitioners to monitor and alter treatment plans. • Provide best indication of patient's response to therapy. ◦ Decreased systolic pressure or narrowed arterial *pulse* pressure indicative of decreased cardiac output; increased diastolic blood pressure indicates increased peripheral vascular resistance.
◦ Pulmonary capillary wedge pressure ◦ Cardiac output and cardiac intake	◦ Pulmonary edema develops when PCWP exceeds plasma osmotic pressure (>28 mmHg).

CARE PLAN FOR THE PATIENT WITH HEART FAILURE (*Continued*)

Nursing Interventions	Rationales
○ Systemic vascular resistance	○ Determines afterload. Increased impedance to left ventricular ejection increases intramyocardial wall tension. As a result of sympathoadrenergic stimulation, increased SVR increases myocardial oxygen requirements and decreases myocardial contractility.
○ Right atrial pressure	○ Elevated in pulmonary hypertension, tricuspid and pulmonic stenosis, tricuspid regurgitation, right heart failure, and hypervolemia.
• Monitor laboratory/diagnostic data:	
○ Arterial blood gases	○ Increased work of breathing secondary to pulmonary congestion leads to hypoxia and hypercapnia, which further depress myocardial contractility.
○ Electrolytes, BUN, creatinine	○ Blood urea nitrogen (BUN) and sodium levels reflect hydration status. Hypokalemia is diuresis-induced; hyperglycemia is secondary to release of stress-related catecholamines.
○ ECG	○ May reveal evidence of ischemia, left ventricular hypertrophy (LVH), RVH, arrhythmia.
○ Chest x-ray	○ Presence of pleural effusion, usually right-sided or bilateral (rarely on the left); interstitial pulmonary edema; enlarged cardiac silhouette.
○ Circulation time	○ Prolonged; secondary to decreased contractility of ventricles, leading to decreased cardiac output.
○ Elevated bilirubin, SGOT, and LDH	○ Result of hepatic congestion in right heart failure.
○ Proteinuria, increased specific gravity, increased BUN and creatinine	○ Indicate renal dysfunction as a result of decreased cardiac output and decreased glomerular filtration rate.
• Implement measures to reduce cardiac workload:	
○ Place patient in semi-Fowler's position if blood pressure allows.	○ Diminishes venous return and promotes adequate lung expansion.
○ Allow for frequest rest periods.	○ Reduces fatigue; decreases myocardial oxygen consumption.
○ Administer oxygen as prescribed.	○ Reduces workload of heart and supports cellular energy requirements.
	○ Correction of hypoxia related to pulmonary congestion.
	○ Myocardial tissue hypoxia predisposes to arrhythmia and further decreases myocardial contractility.
○ Institute measures to allay anxiety (see Nursing Diagnosis #5).	
• Administer medications as ordered:	
○ Diuretics:	○ Decrease intravascular volume by their direct action on the kidney and by reducing sodium reabsorption; increase venous capacitance; reduce preload to maximize position on Frank-Sterling curve.
□ Monitor I&O; daily weights.	
□ Monitor for side effects of diuretic therapy (hypokalemia, hyponatremia, fatigue, muscle cramps, hypotension, tachycardia).	○ Increased venous capacitance provides beneficial effect in patients with left heart failure and pulmonay edema. In patients with right heart failure, vigorous diuresis may be detrimental, as it contributes to systemic venous pooling, thereby limiting venous return and right ventricular filling and further contributing to a decreased cardiac output.
• Assess for hypovolemia (hydration status):	
○ Intake and output including extrarenal (insensible losses; urine output; PCWP; and weight changes).	○ Contraindicated for PCWP >20 mmHg; CVP >12 cmH$_2$O.
○ Keep physician informed of patient's status.	○ Ensures intravascular expansion.
○ Monitor effect of fluid challenge if ordered:	○ End points of challenge are hypotension, PCWP at 20 mmHg, CVP increase by 2 cmH$_2$.
□ Administer fluid challenge (0.9% normal saline) rapidly: 100 mL every 5–10 min.	
□ Determine CVP or PCWP after each bolus.	

CARE PLAN FOR THE PATIENT WITH HEART FAILURE (*Continued*)

Nursing Diagnoses

Nursing Diagnosis #3
Tissue Perfusion, altered (decreased), related to severely impaired myocardial contractility

Desired Patient Outcomes

Patient will:
1. Demonstrate signs of hemodynamic stability:
   - Systolic BP 90 mmHg
   - Diastolic BP 60–90 mmHg.
   - PCWP 8–12 mmHg (mean)
   - Cardiac output 4–8 L/min
   - Heart rate <100 beats/min
   - SVR 800–1200 dynes sec cm^{-5}
2. Maintain adequate tissue perfusion:
   - Patient awake, alert, oriented
   - Urine output >30 mL/h
   - Skin warm and dry
   - Absence of peripheral edema
   - Absence of rales (crackles on auscultation)
3. Maintain electrophysiologic stability
   - Absence of arrhythmia
4. Maintain arterial blood gases within normal limits.

Nursing Interventions

- Identify patients at risk of developing cardiogenic shock (see Table 19–6).
- Assess signs of inadequate tissue perfusion:
  - Cardiovascular
    - Blood pressure

    - Heart rate
    - Cardiac output/cardiac index

    - SVR

    - Mean arterial pressure (MAP)

    - Right atrial pressure
    - Pulmonary artery pressure (PAP), PCWP

  - Renal:
    - Measure urine output hourly; notify physician if <30 mL/h.
    - Measure intake and output.
    - Monitor BUN and creatinine.
    - Assess for increased tolerance to diuretic therapy.
- Monitor for and document arrhythmia.
  - Maintain continuous ECG monitoring.
  - Administer treatment to correct arrhythmia (may include pacing, antiarrhythmics, and/or cardioversion).
- Administer medications as prescribed.

  - Monitor medications for efficacy and toxicity.

  - Monitor hemodynamic parameters to assess efficacy of pharmacologic therapy.
  - Monitor arterial pH.

Rationales

- Early recognition and intervention are crucial determinants to patient survival.

  - Decreased pulse pressure, increased diastolic blood pressure, systolic pressure < 90 mmHg—indicative of increased SVR and decreased cardiac output.
  - Compensatory tachycardia.
  - Decrease in heart failure; indicator of tissue perfusion.
  - Measurement of afterload; increased secondary to sympathetic nervous system stimulation.
  - Decreased MAP and increased LVEDP (PCWP) result in decreased coronary artery perfusion with potential to result in myocardial ischemia and necrosis.
  - Measurement of adequacy of central venous return.
  - Increased secondary to impaired myocardial contractility; maintained slightly higher than normal to maximize response on Frank-Starling curve; serial measurements to evaluate left ventricular function and response to therapy.

  - Decreased cardiac output results in decreased renal perfusion and function: the afferent arterioles vasoconstrict and glomerular filtration decreases, which results in a decreased ability of the kidneys to filter, excrete, and reabsorb.
- Increased irritability of myocardium predisposes patient to arrhythmia.
  - Bradyarrhythmias may decrease cardiac output secondary to decreased stroke volume
  - Tachyarrhythmias reduce diastolic filling time and increase myocardial oxygen consumption. Loss of atrial kick contributes to a decreased cardiac output.
  - Hypotension, redistribution of blood volume, and impaired renal and hepatic perfusion may impair absorption and metabolism.
  - Best indices to LV function and systemic perfusion.

  - Most vasoactive therapy has decreased efficacy in an acidotic or alkalotic environment.

CARE PLAN FOR THE PATIENT WITH HEART FAILURE (*Continued*)

Nursing Interventions

- Prepare for use of mechanical circulatory assistance if above measures are ineffective in restoring tissue perfusion.
- Institute measures to allay anxiety.
- Assess neurologic status: level of consciousness; restlessness, agitation, confusion, and somnolence; response to verbal and tactile stimuli; extraocular motions (EOMs) and pupillary responses.

- Assess capillary refill.
- Assess warmth, color, and moistness of skin.

- Assess quality of peripheral pulses.

- Monitor bowel sounds.
- Assess for abdominal discomfort.

Rationales

- Decreases afterload during systole and increases perfusion by increasing aortic pressure during diastole.

- See Nursing Diagnosis #5, below.
- Decreased cardiac output causes diminished carotid and vertebral artery blood flow. Blood flow to medulla remains normal until late in the stages of shock; midbrain, cerebellum, and cerebral cortex are underperfused.

- Cool, moist skin indicates decreased perfusion secondary to redistribution of blood flow to central circulation.
- Weak, thready peripheral pulses are indicative of vasoconstriction.
- Indicative of decreased perfusion and ischemia to splanchnic area secondary to a profound decrease in cardiac output.

Nursing Diagnoses

Nursing Diagnosis #4
Gas Exchange, impaired, related to alveolar capillary changes due to increased pulmonary capillary pressure

Desired Patient Outcomes

Patient will:
1. Demonstrate signs of adequate cerebral oxygenation:
   - Alert mental status
   - Oriented to person, time, and place
2. Demonstrate normal respiratory effort:
   - Rate <25/min
   - Pattern eupneic
3. Maintain optimal arterial blood gases:
   - pH 7.35–7.45
   - PaO_2 >60 mmHg
   - $PaCO_2$ 35–45 mmHg
4. Maintain breath sounds clear to auscultation
5. Demonstrate clear lung fields on chest x-ray
6. Maintain effective cardiovascular function:
   - HR 60–80/min
   - Cardiac output 4–9 L/min

Nursing Interventions

- Perform ongoing mental status assessment: confusion, restlessness, anxiety, stupor, loss of consciousness.
- Monitor respiratory function on ongoing basis:
  ○ Respiratory rate and rhythm

  ○ Dyspnea
  ○ Orthopnea

  ○ Cough
  ○ Status of weakness and fatigue

  ○ Secretions: quality, quantity, presence of blood (frequently pink and frothy secretions)
  ○ Cyanosis, pallor

  ○ Auscultation of lungs for presence of adventitious sounds: rales, bronchial wheezing

- Monitor diagnostic tests and studies:
  ○ Arterial blood gases

Rationales

- Hypoxemia may predispose to cerebral tissue hypoxia.

  ○ Reflects work of breathing: increased work of breathing increases oxygen consumption and myocardial oxygen demand.
  ○ Secondary to increased pulmonary interstitial edema.
  ○ Increased venous return secondary to postural redistribution of pulmonary blood flow.
  ○ Usually nonproductive, periodic, and nocturnal.
  ○ Secondary to decreased perfusion to skeletal muscles. Increased work of breathing further fatigues the patient and predisposes to alveolar hypoventilation with hypercapnia and respiratory acidemia.
  ○ Result of capillary hydrostatic pressure exceeding pulmonary capillary oncotic pressure, which allows fluid to leak into pulmonary interstitium; when this cannot be reabsorbed via the pulmonary lymphatic system, fluid fills the alveoli.
  ○ Frequent assessments allow for early intervention, minimizing deleterious effects of respiratory compromise

  ○ Reflect effectiveness of gas exchange. Decreased PaO_2 is the result of alveolar flooding; $PaCO_2$ initially decreases secondary to hyperventilation; then it elevates secondary to patient fatigue.

CARE PLAN FOR THE PATIENT WITH HEART FAILURE (*Continued*)

Nursing Interventions

- ○ Chest x-ray

- ○ ECG
- Assess cardiovascular function frequently:
  - ○ Heart rate

  - ○ Hemodynamic parameters;
    - ▫ Systemic blood pressure

    - ▫ Cardiac output
    - ▫ PCWP

    - ▫ Jugular venous distention; peripheral edema, sacral edema; presence of S$_3$, S$_4$, gallop rhythm; pulsus alternans; palpitation, chest pain
- Implement measures to increase gas exchange:
  - ○ Administer oxygen as prescribed and monitor response to therapy.

  - ○ Reassure patient concerning the need for oxygen and that the need is temporary.
  - ○ Administer positive pressure as needed.

  - ○ Assess hemodynamic parameters meticulously during positive pressure therapy (PEEP).
  - ○ Initiate intubation and mechanical ventilation as necessary.
  - ○ Initiate intubation and mechanical ventilation as necessary.
- Implement measures to decrease preload and afterload.
  - ○ Place patient in high Fowler's position with dependent lower extremities if blood pressure allows.
  - ○ Administer morphine sulfate IV.

    - ▫ Monitor for respiratory depressant effects; have morphine antagonist at bedside.
    - ▫ Monitor blood pressure for hypotension.

  - ○ Administer intravenous vasodilators such as nitroprusside and nitroglycerin. Carefully monitor arterial blood pressure while administering these drugs.
  - ○ Administer intravenous diuretics as ordered (usually potent loop diuretics such as furosemide and ethacrynic acid). Carefully monitor for hypotension and tachycardia, and check for signs of hypokalemia.

  - ○ Apply rotating tourniquets as ordered (automatic tourniquet machine) following appropriate procedures:
    - ▫ Connect to upper portion of arms and legs; only three cuffs should be inflated simultaneously.

Rationales

- ○ Butterfly distribution of pulmonary infiltrates; may take 24 h after symptoms develop to become apparent on chest x-ray.
- ○ May reflect signs of myocardial ischemia.

- ○ Initial tachycardia is the result of sympathetic nervous system stimulation; return of heart rate to baseline may be indicative of resolving pulmonary edema.

  - ▫ Hypertension may result from sympathetic stimulation.
  - ▫ Reflects tissue perfusion.
  - ▫ Increased LVEDP reflected back to pulmonary capillary bed, increasing pulmonary intravascular hydrostatic pressure; PCWP >20 mmHg.
  - ▫ Affords noninvasive evaluation of changes in venous pressure.

- ○ O$_2$ is given to raise PaO$_2$ above 60 mmHg when there is hypoxemia without hypercapnia.
- ○ Hypoxia enhances likelihood of arrhythmia development, depresses myocardial contractility, and causes pulmonary vasoconstriction, which increases the workload of the right side of the heart; elevating the PaO$_2$ will minimize and/or reverse these processes.
- ○ Most patients tolerate administration of oxygen by mask poorly and frequently fear suffocation.
- ○ Increases mean lung volume (functional lung capacity), allowing more alveoli to participate in gas exchange.
- ○ Positive pressure can impede venous return, thereby decreasing cardiac output.

- ○ See Tables 32–7 and 32–9.

- ○ Dilates peripheral arteries and veins and causes venous pooling, thereby decreasing venous congestion.
- ○ Reduces patient's anxiety, decreases tachypnea, causes peripheral pooling of blood, decreases preload and afterload.
  - ▫ Respiratory depression occurs in approximately 7 min.
  - ▫ Hypotension, the result of baroreceptor vasoconstrictive reflexes, is inhibited by morphine.
- ○ Reduce vascular hydrostatic pressure and reduces PWCP. These drugs have systemic venous and arterial vasodilatory properties.

- ○ Reduce total blood volume and increase venous capacitance.
- ○ Cause reduction in sodium reabsorption in loop of Henle; direct effect on arterial and venous dilatation.
- ○ Evidence of circulatory intolerance and potassium wasting is associated with use of these diuretics.

CARE PLAN FOR THE PATIENT WITH HEART FAILURE (*Continued*)

Nursing Interventions

- □ Inflate blood pressure cuffs to 10 mmHg below the diastolic pressure.

- □ Check for presence of peripheral pulses, warmth, and color of extremities.
- □ Make certain tourniquets rotate every 15 min.
- □ When discontinuing tourniquet, remove one by one in a counterclockwise direction every 15 min.
- ○ Assess patient's tolerance to discontinuance of treatment.
- Implement measures to improve left ventricular contractility.
  - ○ Administer cardiac glycosides as prescribed.
  - ○ Administer dopamine, dobutamine in low doses as prescribed.
  - ○ Administer aminophylline as prescribed (observe for hypotension, arrhythmia).

Rationales

- □ Higher pressures will cause fluid loss into the patient peripheral extravascular spaces.
- □ Should not occlude arterial blood flow.
- □ Pulse should be palpable with cuff inflated.

- □ Avoids excessive increase in venous return.

- Increased myocardial contractility leads to increased cardiac output with a reduction in LVEDP and PCWP.
  - ○ Stimulate myocardial β-receptors to enhance contractility.

  - ○ Bronchodilator; also increases myocardial contractility and enhances diuresis.

Nursing Diagnoses

Nursing Diagnosis #5
Anxiety, related to:
1. Potential for lifestyle modification
2. Powerlessness (see Chapters 5 and 6)
3. Intensive care setting
4. Uncertainty related to illness and diagnosis

Desired Patient Outcomes

Patient will:
1. Verbalize anxieties and fears
2. Verbalize feeling less anxious
3. Demonstrate a relaxed demeanor

Nursing Interventions

- Obtain baseline assessment of anxiety level and coping patterns from patient, family members, or significant others.

- Assess level of anxiety; include heart rate, blood pressure, increased muscle tension, increased startle response, a change in sleeping patterns, nightmares, irritability, diaphoresis, nausea, diarrhea, repetitive behaviors.
- Ascertain what the patient or family member is experiencing; eliminate a physiologic basis of symptoms
- Determine what the individual's needs are and what resources can be mobilized to decrease feelings of anxiety; provide positive reinforcement when appropriate.
- Implement therapeutic measures to decrease anxiety.
  - ○ Encourage the patient and/or family to verbalize anxieties and concerns; encourage them to ask questions; listen attentively; provide a caring environment.
  - ○ Explain procedures and limitation to patient/family. Relate to nature of heart disease.
  - ○ Familiarize patient with ICU staff, routines, equipment
  - ○ Mobilize appropriate resources:
    - □ Consult with social services, chaplaincy program, financial advisor, or other such services, as appropriate.
    - □ Modify the environment to decrease anxiety; modify the policy regarding visitors; increase or decrease environmental stimuli as indicated; increase frequency of nurse-patient contacts.
  - ○ Involve patients in their own care within physical limitations.

Rationales

- Baseline data are essential in evaluating the effectiveness of therapeutic interventions and the patient's ability to cope.
  - ○ Assists in determining the underlying cause of anxiety and provides a basis for intervention.
- Hypoxemia, hypercarbia, decreased cardiac output, and pain precipitate and intensify feelings of apprehension and anxiety.

- Positive feedback helps nurture confidence.

  - ○ Helps to create a trusting relationship; reassures patient he or she is not alone.

  - ○ Knowing what to expect will help to reduce anxiety.
  - ○ Removal or modification of precipitating factors may reduce anxiety; social interaction helps modify feelings of depersonalization that accompany hospitalization (see Chapter 6).

  - ○ Will decrease anxiety by re-establishing sense of control and purpose.

CARE PLAN FOR THE PATIENT WITH HEART FAILURE (*Continued*)

Nursing Diagnoses

Nursing Diagnosis #6
Activity Intolerance, risk for, related to compromised cardiac reserve

Desired Patient Outcomes

Patient will:
1. Maintain normal muscle tone
2. Maintain highest level of activity that does not produce symptoms of myocardial dysfunction
3. Identify end-points of activity tolerance

Nursing Interventions

* Perform assessment of activity and exercise tolerance:

  ○ Age

  ○ Weight
  ○ Gender

  ○ Cardiovascular disorder

  ○ Previous activity and motivation

* Initiate gradual activity progress in the critical care setting.

  ○ Encourage patients to participate in activities of daily living (feed self, wash hands, shave, active range of motion).
  ○ Maintain bedrest with commode privileges during acute phase of heart failure.

  ○ Prevent complications of immobility.
    □ Assist with frequent position change.
    □ Provide frequent back care and skin care.
  ○ Encourage hourly deep breathing while awake.
  ○ Maintain in semi-Fowler's position.

* Assess tolerance to activity progression by checking blood pressure, heart rate, and respiratory rate 1 min and 4 min after the activity. Indicators of poor tolerance include dyspnea, syncope, angina, diaphoresis, cyanosis, fatigue, weakness, arrhythmia. Heart rate should return to baseline within 4 min. Heart rate should not exceed 20 beats/min above resting heart rate and it should not exceed 100 beats/min.
  ○ Monitor systolic blood pressure.

* Assess readiness to learn and instruct regarding indicators of activity intolerance, as noted above:
  ○ Teach patient how to take own pulse.
  ○ Isometric exercises should be discouraged.

  ○ Encourage gradual resumption of aerobic activity when free of heart failure.
  ○ Reemphasize to patient that activity will progress gradually and will be supervised during the initial states; provide positive reinforcement when appropriate; gradually transfer supervision of tolerance from healthcare personnel to patient and family.

Rationales

* Initial assessment provides pertinent data that will guide individualized activity prescription from acute to rehabilitative phase.
  ○ Physical endurance decreases with age; older patients will tolerate less activity.
  ○ Obesity increases myocardial burden.
  ○ Women have more endurance; men can tolerate workload of higher intensity due to the increased ratio of muscle mass to total body weight.
  ○ Cardiovascular history may influence the attitude of the patient to activity (e.g., if angina or palpitations developed in exertion, this may influence the patient's attitude toward exercise.).
  ○ Identifies patients who may need encouragement to exercise.
* Minimizes the deleterious efforts of deconditioning, which include a decreased work capacity, tachycardia, orthostatic hypotension, venous thrombosis, and feelings of hopelessness and dependency.
  ○ Such activities improve circulation and help to prevent phlebitis or thromboembolism

  ○ Physical activity redistributes blood from viscera and kidneys to the skeletal muscle and skin. Bedrest allows for a limited cardiac output and decreases myocardial oxygen demand; however, myocardial oxygen consumption is greater when a patient uses bedpan than during commode use.

    □ Maintenance of skin integrity and muscle tone.

  ○ Minimizes development of atelectasis.
  ○ Reduces venous return to the heart; increases ability to expand lungs during deep-breathing exercises.
* Physical activity increases venous return to the heart, increases myocardial workload, and increases metabolic heat production, i.e., one fifth of cardiac output is shunted to skin in thermoregulation and the patient with impaired myocardial function cannot compensate for this with a tachycardia or increased contractile force; symptoms of pulmonary venous congestion and decreased cardiac output intensify.
  ○ Fall of 20 mmHg below resting level and failure of systolic blood pressure to increase above the resting level suggest poor exercise tolerance.
* Readiness to learn facilitates meaningful learning.

  ○ Isometrics result in increased blood pressure and cardiac workload; do not improve cardiovascular conditioning.
  ○ Increases functional capacity and cardiovascular conditioning.
  ○ Builds and reinforces self-confidence; helps minimize deleterious effects of psychophysiologic responses to stress (increased myocardial oxygen consumption).

CARE PLAN FOR THE PATIENT WITH HEART FAILURE (*Continued*)

Nursing Diagnoses

Nursing Diagnosis #7
Knowledge deficit, related to underlying heart disease, treatment, and follow-up

Desired Patient Outcomes

Patient will:
1. Describe underlying disease process and relationship to heart failure
2. Identify his or her own risk factors or precipitating conditions that require modification
3. Identify the importance of follow-up care and symptoms requiring medical intervention
4. Describe the importance of medications, diet, and activity to the overall treatment plan
5. Identify signs and symptoms of activity intolerance
6. Identify indications of endocarditis prophylaxis (if patient is in high-risk profile)

Nursing Interventions
- Assess knowledge of heart failure, underlying disease process, and expectation of disease progression.

  ○ Encourage verbalization of patient and/or family concerns and their learning needs.

- Assess readiness to learn.
- Implement teaching plan, which should include:
  ○ Explanation of normal heart function, heart failure, and underlying disease process.
  ○ Explanation of signs and symptoms and appropriate action regarding their development.
  ○ Explanation of risk factors and factors that will aggravate the symptoms of heart failure and methods to modify these factors.
  ○ Explanation of medication regimen (including name, dosage, frequency, action, and side effects).
  ○ Activity prescription and signs and symptoms of activity intolerance.
- Assist patient and/or family in identifying family strengths and resources.
- Initiate referral to appropriate resources if indicated (social services; community resources).

Rationales
- Readiness to learn varies because of differences in general educational background, intellectual ability, and motivation. Assessment establishes baseline data from which to build, or determines need to alter misconceptions.
- Fosters establishment of open, trusting relationship. Learning is enhanced when patient participates in goal setting. Heart failure affects patient and his or her lifestyle and affects the entire family to varying degrees.
- Readiness facilitates more effective learning.
- Patient and family have a right to receive information about the disease, treatment, and prognosis; understanding enhances compliance; knowledge allays anxieties and the adverse effects associated with psychophysiologic stress.

- Engenders self-confidence.

- It is reassuring to have support services available.

Nursing Diagnoses

Nursing Diagnosis #8
Nutrition, altered, less than body requirements, related to impaired absorption of nutrients due to decreased cardiac output (CO)

Desired Patient Outcomes

Patient will:
1. Demonstrate absence of malnutrition
2. Describe the importance of maintaining nutritional state

Nursing Interventions
- Observe patient daily for signs of malnutrition and cardiac cachexia.

  ○ Evaluate laboratory data.

  ○ Determine patient's baseline weight. Weigh daily: upon rising, after voiding, with same clothing.

  ○ Maintain diet as ordered; consult with dietitian as indicated.
  ○ Supplement meals with high-caloric feedings.
  ○ Carry out measures to improve appetite.

Rationales
- Nutritional deficits occur as a result of (1) the body's inability to absorb nutrients because of poor tissue perfusion, and (2) hypermetabolic state that occurs in heart failure. Patient's intake and malabsorption make patient unable to meet increased demand.
  ○ Malnutrition and protein depletion are reflected as low levels of serum transferrin and lymphocytes.
  ○ To assess actual weight loss and to obtain consistent and accurate body weight, which will assist in determining caloric needs.
  ○ To ensure that diet will meet required caloric needs.

  ○ To maintain minimum required caloric intake.
  ○ Environmental and psychosocial factors affect appetite.

CARE PLAN FOR THE PATIENT WITH HEART FAILURE (*Continued*)

Nursing Interventions	Rationales
○ Offer small, frequent meals.	○ Enlarged liver, ascites, GI hypomotility, and delayed gastric emptying can contribute to feeling of fullness as well as nausea and vomiting.
○ Permit patient to choose foods. Where possible, encourage family to bring food from home and assist with feedings.	○ Psychosocial support is enhanced by encouraged participation in meals and by providing involvement by support systems.
○ Remove unsightful and odorous items from room during mealtime.	○ To reduce noxious stimuli, which may contribute to nausea.
○ Arrange medication schedule so it does not interfere with meals.	○ Side effects of certain medication may contribute to loss of appetite, e.g., bitter taste of medication, dry mouth.
○ Administer antiemetics and/or analgesics before meals.	○ To ensure patient comfort and improve appetite.

SGOT = serum glutamic oxaloacetic transaminase; LDH = lactic dehydrogenase; PEEP = positive end-expiratory pressure.

CHAPTER 20

Nursing Management of the Cardiac Surgical Patient

Sheila M. Keller

CHAPTER OUTLINE

Myocardial Revascularization:
  Coronary Artery Bypass Graft
    □ Preoperative Anxiety: Clinical
      Significance
    □ Preoperative Nursing Management
    □ Preoperative Teaching
    □ Procedure
    □ Postoperative Nursing
      Management
    □ Postoperative Teaching
Cardiac Myoplasty
    □ Indications
    □ Procedure
Valvular Surgery
    □ Approaches to Valvular Surgery
    □ Types of Prosthetic Heart Valves
    □ Complications of Valve
      Replacement
    □ Nursing Care in Valve Replacement

Ventricular Aneurysms
Artificial Hearts and Ventricular Assist
  Devices
Heart Transplantation
    □ Criteria for Heart Transplant
      Candidacy
    □ Donor Procurement
    □ Surgical Approaches
    □ Postoperative Nursing
      Management
Case Study: Myocardial
  Revascularization
Case Study: Cardiopulmonary Bypass
Case Study: Mitral Valve Prolapse
Case Study: Cardiac Transplantation
References
Suggested Readings

LEARNING OBJECTIVES

After completing this chapter, you should be able to:

1. List indications and contraindications for myocardial revascularization.
2. Describe the significance of anxiety in terms of postoperative complications.
3. Identify major aspects of preoperative teaching for the cardiac surgical patient.
4. Identify major aspects of the postoperative assessment in the immediate postoperative period and implications for nursing care.
5. Prioritize postoperative nursing care for the cardiac surgical patient.
6. Delineate the nursing process in the care of the cardiac surgical patient including assessment, nursing diagnoses, patient outcomes, and nursing interventions.
7. Describe indications for cardiac myoplasty.
8. Identify common causes of valvular defects in the adult patient.
9. Describe the types of artificial heart valves.
10. Identify possible complications of valvular surgery.
11. List nursing implications for the patient after valvular surgery.
12. Formulate a postoperative teaching care plan for the patient with a cardiac valve replacement.
13. Describe the nursing implications for a patient with a ventricular aneurysm.
14. Identify modalities of treatment for ventricular aneurysms.
15. Describe the nursing care considerations unique to the patient with an artificial heart.
16. Describe the nursing care considerations unique to the heart transplant patient.
17. Discuss the quality of life for patients with myocardial revascularization, prosthetic heart valves, cardiac myoplasty, ventricular aneurysm repair, artificial hearts, and transplanted hearts.

Cardiac surgery has long been associated with the repair of congenital defects, largely in infants and children. More recently, surgical procedures have been developed to repair acquired defects including repair of ventricular-septal defects, ventricular aneurysms, pericardial defects, and valvular defects. Other surgical procedures developed include myocardial revascularization, cardiac myoplasty, heart transplantation, and the implementation of the artificial heart.

The development and expansion of cardiovascular nursing have accompanied these advances in cardiac surgical techniques, and nursing has become an integral component in the care of the cardiac surgical patient. Preoperative and postoperative teaching, so vital to the successful outcome of the cardiac surgery, is largely the responsibility of the patient's nurse.

In this chapter, an attempt is made to briefly examine specific cardiac procedures, with emphasis on myocardial revascularization, mainly the coronary artery bypass graft (CABG). The discussion of nursing care of the patient having a CABG may serve as a template for the care of the cardiac surgical patient in general. The chapter includes nursing care plans concerned with the preoperative and postoperative care of the cardiac surgical patient.

Protocols and procedures for care of the cardiac surgical patient differ among hospitals nationwide. With this in mind, only generalizations regarding nursing care are presented. Since the text that follows is limited to the adult patient, readers interested in the care of the pediatric cardiac surgical patient are referred to an appropriate pediatric text.

MYOCARDIAL REVASCULARIZATION: CORONARY ARTERY BYPASS GRAFT

During the past three decades the CABG has been the most common type of cardiac surgery (Fig. 20–1). In this procedure, a blood vessel, usually the saphenous vein or the internal mammary artery, is anastomosed to a coronary artery distal to the point of occlusion, and to the ascending aorta (if the saphenous vein is used), thereby bypassing the obstruction and reestablishing coronary artery perfusion. Advantages of the CABG include better treatment of global ischemia, more complete revascularization, and easier accessibility to reperfusing distal obstructions.[1] The mortality rate for CABG is 1% to 2%; in an evolving myocardial infarction (MI), 4% to 6%; and in emergency procedures, 4% to 5%.[1] Mortality rates in women are slightly higher, 8.8%.[2] The 1-year graft patency rate is 80% for men, whereas women have a lower 1-year patency rate of 66%.[2] This lower rate is thought to be due to the

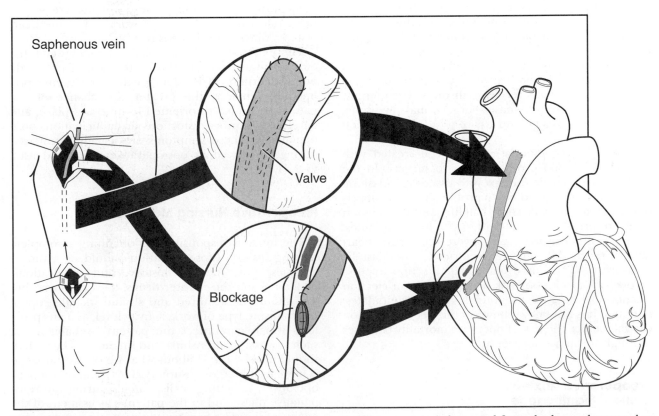

FIGURE 20–1. Coronary artery bypass graft surgery: a section of saphenous vein is harvested from the leg and reversed so that it can be used as an arterial graft to bypass blockage in a coronary artery. (Adapted from Black, JM and Matassarin-Jacob, E: Luckmann and Sorensen's Medical-Surgical Nursing: A Psychophysiologic Approach, ed. 4, WB Saunders, Philadelphia, 1993.)

fact that women have a thinner-walled saphenous vein, fewer grafts, smaller vessels, and greater complications.[2] After CABG, 90% of the patients demonstrate improvement in cardiac function, and 60% demonstrate elimination of anginal episodes.[1] Allen records that 70% to 90% of CABG patients attain relief from angina, of which 60% to 70% attain complete relief and 20% to 50% attain improved maximum exercise performance.[3] Positive results for women tend to be lower, since women have smaller distal coronary arteries, a greater incidence of diabetes, and reduced graft patency.[2]

The purpose of the CABG is to relieve angina, prevent ischemia, prolong life, and preserve myocardial function.[2,4] Indications for CABG are: chronic and preinfarction angina, angina or ischemia unresponsive to medical therapy, and triple vessel disease. Emergency CABG surgery also can be done for an evolving MI within 6 hours of the onset of symptoms or for an evolving MI when thrombolytic therapy or percutaneous transluminal coronary angioplasty (PTCA), or both, have been unsuccessful.[1]

The questions as to what type of patient should have a CABG and what lesions should be grafted remain controversial. The consensus seems to be that life expectancy is increased when the procedure is performed on patients with left main coronary artery disease or severe triple vessel disease. The obstruction should be greater than 70% of the diameter of the artery, with good distal runoff. Surgery should not be performed on only one vessel unless it is the left main coronary artery, or possibly an obstructed high-grade proximal left anterior descending coronary artery.[1,4,5]

Bypass surgery is contraindicated in patients with an acute cerebral vascular accident (CVA) and bleeding disorders. In patients receiving thrombolytic therapy, for example, streptokinase, surgery may be done, although there is a greater risk of postoperative blood loss.[1]

Underlying coagulopathy should be treated with appropriate blood products prior to surgery. In the case of thrombolytic therapy with tissue-type plasminogen, there appears to be no problem postoperatively due to plasminogen's short half-life, and coagulation levels return to normal within 30 to 40 minutes. Patients with cardiomegaly, severe congestive heart failure, recent MI, high left ventricular end-diastolic pressure (LVEDP), and inadequate ejection fraction below 35% are a poor risk. Patients with an ejection fraction below 20% are very high risk candidates, although it is not known how low the ejection fraction can fall before the risk of operative mortality becomes too high to carry out surgery.[1]

Preoperative Anxiety: Clinical Significance

A patient may wait 1 to 6 days for surgery to be scheduled and/or performed. Normally there is some degree of preoperative anxiety associated with the psy-

chological adjustment to and/or acceptance of the necessity of the procedure.[4,6] Depression, a low self-esteem, and withdrawal are not uncommon in patients about to have heart surgery. As the waiting period increases, so does the intensity of the adjustment difficulties. Frequently the patient must draw upon inner strengths and coping mechanisms that have proved reliable in the past. A thorough assessment of the patient's functional health patterns may assist the patient and family to identify their strengths and to cope more effectively.

Prior to surgery, some patients appear to cope best by seeking information. Members of the health team can become highly supportive and helpful in this regard. Individuals who have had similar surgery can be helpful, especially if the surgery has been effective for them.

Other patients become more anxious if they perceive that they are being bombarded with information regarding details of the upcoming surgery. These patients may prefer not to know what to expect, or what is expected of them. They may experience more adjustment difficulties when they receive more specific information, and this, in turn, may complicate the postoperative phase of care.

Excessive preoperative anxiety can have a negative influence on the patient's postoperative recovery. Anxiety stimulates the sympathetic nervous system and causes an increase in circulating catecholamines (norepinephrine and epinephrine), which increase the heart rate and, therefore, the workload of the heart just at a time when it needs to rest.[6]

There is also a direct relationship between the amount of anxiety and the occurrence of postcardiotomy delirium (PCD). The greater the patient's preoperative anxiety, the greater the chance of the patient becoming disoriented to time and place, and developing sensory distortions or hallucinations postoperatively. These symptoms are usually manifested during the immediate postoperative period and last 2 to 3 days.[6]

Preoperative Nursing Management

The nurse is responsible for obtaining a complete nursing history. Close attention should be given to allergies, past medical history, and medications, including over-the-counter drugs. A psychosocial history should be acquired and should include coping mechanisms, type of work, activity level, and any problems which may affect the patient's rehabilitation, such as work, relationships, and finances.[7] The patient should also be asked about what he or she hopes to achieve by undergoing surgery. This is important postoperatively in setting realistic goals during the rehabilitative phase and in the patient's assessment of the quality of life. The family also needs to be included in the data collection process.

The nurse needs to establish baseline measurements of the patient's blood pressure, heart rate and rhythm, and pulses (pedal pulses should be marked with a permanent marker if saphenous veins are to be used so that postoperatively they can be easily located). Other assessment measurements include respiratory rate and rhythm, and the presence of adventitious sounds or abnormal chest shapes, that is, kyphosis, scoliosis, funnel chest, or barrel chest, which could result in abnormal breathing patterns or pulmonary dysfunction in the postoperative phase.

The nurse needs to make sure that the permit is signed, the laboratory studies have been completed, and the results are on the chart. Any abnormal results should be immediately reported to the physician.

Other areas of importance include making sure that the patient takes nothing by mouth, has a Betadine shower, and that the chest and legs (if the saphenous veins are being used) are shaved and cleansed with betadine if ordered. The nurse is also responsible for administering any medications ordered. Usually antianginal medications will be continued until the surgery is performed. The nurse should inquire concerning other medications the patient is currently taking. Most of all, the nurse is responsible for teaching what the patient needs to expect and to do preoperatively and postoperatively.

Preoperative Teaching

The preoperative teaching of the cardiac surgical patient should follow an individualized plan geared to the patient's specific needs.[8] Sadler[9] identifies four areas of preoperative teaching: (1) teaching the patient about the normal function of the heart; (2) providing a description of the disease process and risk factors that have necessitated surgery; (3) providing a description of the surgery and the preoperative physical preparation; and (4) preparing the patient and family for the postoperative course.

Teaching the patient about the normal function of the heart should include the specific areas of the heart that are to be repaired: for CABG, this includes how the heart is nourished by the coronary arteries; in patients having valve replacement surgery, the function of the heart valves; in patients undergoing surgery for congenital defects, what is normal and how their anatomy differs.

The description of the disease process that has necessitated the myocardial revascularization surgery should include risk factors associated with heart disease. Among these risk factors are hypertension, smoking, high serum cholesterol and triglyceride levels, obesity, stress, and diabetes.[9] (Refer to Chapter 18 for an in-depth explanation of the risk factors in coronary artery disease.)

The description of the surgery to be performed should be simple and easy for the patient and family to understand. The nurse's presentation should take into account the patient's overall outlook on the surgery and readiness to learn. Since the surgery is not a cure, it is important that the patient and family learn

as much as possible to adjust their lifestyles to minimize the underlying pathophysiologic process. Discharge planning and teaching begin upon admission and are carried through even after the patient goes home.

Preparation for the patient and family includes attention to several factors. The role of each member of the surgical team should be described and the patient should understand that consultants from the cardiology and anesthesia departments will be visiting them. These physicians are responsible for evaluating their status to assure a stable preoperative condition. The patient is instructed that consents for the operative procedure and transfusions must be obtained. It should be explained that laboratory technicians will be coming in to acquire numerous blood samples that are needed to evaluate their present status and for comparison during the surgery. Some of the blood studies ordered will be a complete blood count (CBC), coagulation studies, arterial blood gases, chemistry profile, and possibly drug levels. Other tests may be ordered by the physicians, such as a chest x-ray, pulmonary function tests, and so on.

The nurse should explain to the patient the physical preparations that will be made for surgery:

1. Skin preparation
   a. Removal of hair to decrease the risk of postoperative infection. The physician may order a shave to be done the night before surgery, or may opt to do it in the operating room. Alternatively, a depilatory cream may be used in place of a shave to avoid nicks in the skin that could be ports for infection.
   b. A shower with Betadine or other antibacterial soap may be used to decrease the number of organisms on the skin and thus reduce the risk of infection.
2. GI preparation
   a. No eating or drinking after midnight on the day of surgery except for sips of water with medications. This ensures that the stomach will be empty prior to surgery.
   b. A laxative and/or enema may be given to empty the lower bowel in order to avoid a bowel movement early in the postoperative period.
3. Removal of effects. On the day of surgery, dentures should be removed (unless the anesthesiologist requests that they be left in place), as should prostheses and nail polish. All the patient's effects may be given to the family to take home if storage space is not available.
4. Preanesthesia medications
   a. A sleeping medication may be given the evening before surgery to help the patient get a good night's sleep.
   b. Medication is given immediately prior to the move to the operating room to help the patient relax.
   c. Nasal oxygen may be prescribed to enhance the effects of the preoperative medication.

As part of the preoperative teaching, the ICU routine should be described, including the average length of stay, the monitoring equipment, and intensive nursing care. This is usually done by one of the ICU nurses, usually the nurse who is going to be taking care of the patient in the ICU. Family members are made aware of the visiting hours, the number of visitors allowed, and the telephone extension to use to call for information on the patient's condition. In some institutions the patient and/or family may visit the ICU prior to the surgery.

Specific instructions should be provided regarding the various invasive lines. These include an arterial line, which will be used to monitor blood pressure and to provide easy access for blood sampling; a pulmonary artery catheter, which will be used to measure the heart function; and a number of IV lines, which may be in the neck and/or arms.

The patient's respiratory status should be discussed in detail so that the patient will know what to expect in terms of respiratory care and what he or she needs to do to maintain optimal respiratory function.

Both patient and family need to know that:
1. In the operating room an endotracheal tube will be inserted after the patient is asleep to provide a patent airway through which the patient will be assisted with breathing while under anesthesia. It also serves as a conduit through which accumulated secretions can be removed via suctioning.
2. Speaking is not possible while the endotracheal tube is in place, so that a system of communication must be established prior to surgery, for use while the patient is intubated. This must be documented for the ICU nurses to follow.
3. Extubation occurs when the patient is able to breathe without assistance, usually the night after surgery. Hoarseness and a sore throat may be experienced after extubation.
4. Active patient participation is essential postoperatively. The patient should practice the necessary activities prior to surgery:
   a. Coughing to promote mobilization and removal of secretions
   b. Deep-breathing exercises
   c. Use of the incentive spirometer to promote lung expansion and aeration

Another important aspect in preoperative teaching of the cardiac surgical patient concerns incisions. A midsternal incision is routine for CABG. When the saphenous vein(s) are used as the grafts, there will also be an incisional line along the inner aspect of one or both legs from the ankle to the knee or thigh, or from the knee to the thigh. Teds or Ace bandages are usually applied for these patients. Teds are applied to the entire leg in patients having valve replacement.

Patients should be instructed regarding the presence of pleural or mediastinal tubes, and their function in draining blood and fluid that has accumulated during and after surgery. Chest tubes are attached to an underwater seal drainage (see Figs. 26–1 to 26–3), with 20 to 40 cmH$_2$O suction.

An indwelling urinary catheter is inserted in the operating room and left in place during the early postoperative period to assist in monitoring renal function. Hourly urine outputs are closely monitored, Infrequently, a perioperatine hypotensive episode may precipitate prerenal failure.

A temporary cardiac pacemaker may be used in patients having valve replacement surgery and in certain bypass surgical patients. Two epicardial atrial pacing wires are inserted at the conclusion of the operation and removed 1 to 2 days prior to discharge. Edema of the skeletal ring associated with valve placement may impinge on the atrioventricular (AV) node located therein, predisposing the patient to arrhythmias, that is, bradycardia and heart block. If the heart rate becomes too slow, the pacemaker can be activated to assure an optimal heart rate. The atrial epicardial wire may also be used to obtain an atrial electrocardiogram, which can aid in detecting the foci of a arrhythmia.

The patient and family should be advised that blood transfusions may be provided to offset a lowered blood count, which sometimes occurs after surgery. Patients can have family and friends donate blood prior to the surgery. Autotransfusion is another option that can be discussed with the patient.

Finally, the patient should be assured that pain medication is available and should be encouraged to request it as needed. The patient may experience chest pain but should be informed prior to surgery that the pain is usually incisional or bone pain and does not necessarily mean that the surgery was unsuccessful. Pain medication helps the patient to cooperate in coughing, deep breathing, use of the incentive spirometer, and moving in the early postoperative period. The nurse should closely monitor the degree of discomfort and the effectiveness of the analgesic therapy in relieving the patient's pain. Any complaints of chest pain need immediate investigation, followed by appropriate interventions.

In general, the preoperative teaching protocol should be modified to meet the individual needs of the patient and family. The patient's nurse needs to be sensitive to the feelings of the patient and family, and closely monitor their tolerance of stress. Refer to the preoperative care plan for the cardiac surgical patient at the end of this chapter.

Procedure

The actual and sequential events occurring within the operating room (OR) may vary from center to center, but overall, the approach to cardiac surgery is quite similar. The patient is placed on the operating table, cardiac monitor electrodes and pads/electrodes are applied, and intravenous and arterial lines are inserted. A narcotic anesthesia and a paralyzing agent are usually administered and the patient is immediately intubated. A flow-directed pulmonary artery catheter or some other central line access is inserted at this time and baseline data are established. The skin is prepared and a midline sternotomy is performed, splitting the sternum and separating the ribs to allow full visualization of the heart. The pericardium is then opened fully to expose the heart.

While the chest is being opened, another surgical team works on the legs, harvesting the superficial saphenous vein. The saphenous vein is used because there are collateral veins available in the leg to return blood to the heart and the saphenous vein is accessible to surgical removal. The length of the vein excised is determined by the number of grafts to be done and the condition of the saphenous vein. Once removed, the veins are checked for patency, and for the presence of disease. Side channels to other vessels are tied off and the vessel is tested for leakage. Sometimes it is necessary to remove the saphenous vein from both legs. If the internal mammary artery is to be used rather than the saphenous vein, it is localized and prepared at this time.

While the veins are being harvested, preparations are made to place the patient on the cardiopulmonary bypass machine (Fig. 20–2). The function of the bypass machine is to provide oxygenation, circulation, and hypothermia during induced cardiac arrest.[3,7] It also provides a bloodless field for the surgeons to work in. The bypass machine is initially primed with lactated Ringer's solution or another electrolyte solution, thereby reducing the need for transfusions. This helps to reduce the risk of transfusion reactions and transmission hepatitis and human immunodeficiency virus (HIV).

The bypass machine is connected to the patient via venous and arterial cannulae. The venous cannula is inserted into the ascending aorta or femoral artery. As the blood enters the machine, heparin is administered to prevent clot formation. The blood travels through the tubing to the oxygenator, where it receives oxygen as carbon dioxide is removed. While the blood is pumped through the bypass machine, formed elements (including red blood cells [RBCs], white blood cells [WBCs], and platelets) and unformed elements (e.g., plasma proteins) of the blood are traumatized by direct contact with the surface of the pump, its mechanical and consequent turbulent flow, and by the intracardiac suction system. The free hemoglobin released in conjunction with trauma to the RBCs is eventually cleared by the kidneys. Administration of mannitol and furosemide facilitate the clearance process. Patients usually tolerate this disturbance postoperatively as long as the bypass time is under 3 hours.

The oxygenated blood then travels to the heart exchanger, where it is cooled to 25°C to 30°C. Prior to returning to the patient, the blood travels through a filter or bubble trap where the blood is filtered of clots, fat, debris, air, and other particulate matter. The blood then returns to the patient through an arterial cannula placed in the femoral or iliac artery or, commonly, the ascending aorta. The mean arterial pressure is maintained by adjusting the rate of perfusion and blood flow through the bypass machine, or by administering vasopressors.[7]

Complications related to the use of cardiopulmonary bypass usually include: blood dyscrasias leading to loss of clotting factors or thromboembolism; reduction in pulmonary surfactant leading to pulmonary edema and atelectasis; and showers of microemboli to the brain causing cerebral hypoxia and strokes.

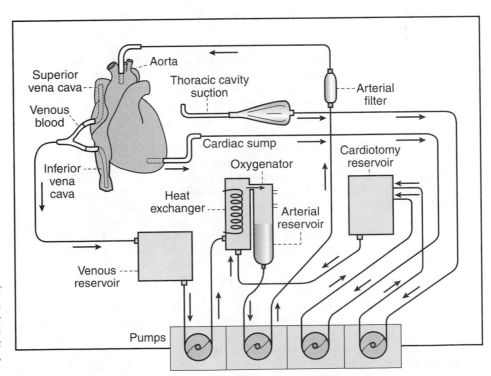

FIGURE 20–2. Circuitry of pump oxygenator. (Adapted from Luckmann, J and Sorensen, KC: Medical-Surgical Nursing: A Psychophysiologic Approach, ed. 3. WB Saunders, Philadelphia, 1987.)

The bypass begins with the cross-clamping of the aorta, and the heart is cooled by an infusion of cold, potassium-rich cardioplegia solution into the aortic root or coronary artery ostia, causing the heart to stop in diastole. To further lower the temperature of the myocardium, the pericardium may be filled with lactated Ringer's solution at 4°C. This induced hypothermia reduces the oxygen requirements of the body as well as the myocardium. In some cases an additional catheter in inserted into the left ventricle to prevent ventricular distention. Once the heart is arrested, grafting begins. The saphenous vein is inverted, with the proximal end anastomosed to the aorta, and the distal end anastomosed to the coronary artery distal to the point of occlusion. The grafts are measured for flow rates. The basal flow rate should be greater than 40 mL/min and peak flow rates should be greater than 80 to 100 mL/min.[10]

Upon completion of the grafting, the heart is slowly rewarmed and the cardioplegia solution is flushed from the heart and mediastinum. As the blood circulates through the heart, the heart muscle regains its rate, rhythmicity, and strength of contraction. If this does not happen spontaneously, defibrillation of the heart may be needed. The blood is rewarmed and the rate of return from the cardiopulmonary bypass machine is decreased. As the patient is weaned from the machine, the grafts are assessed for leakage at the suture sites and for patency, before the patient is removed from the bypass machine. Protamine sulfate is given to counteract the effect of the heparin as weaning occurs. Once satisfactory arterial pressure and cardiac function are achieved, the patient is taken completely off the bypass machine and the cannulae are removed.

The pericardium may be left open to prevent tamponade should postoperative bleeding occur. Mediastinal chest tubes are placed and connected to water seal drainage. Atrial and ventricular pacemaker wires may be sewn to the epicardium if electrical malfunctioning of the heart is anticipated in the immediate postoperative period. This is a special consideration for patients who have valvular repair or replacement surgery because of the anatomic proximity of the AV node to the tricuspid and mitral valves.

The sternum is closed with stainless steel wire and the chest closed with sutures. A sterile dressing is applied. The patient is then transferred to a postoperative bed and accompanied to the recovery room or ICU by the anesthesiologist, the surgeon, and possibly an OR nurse.

There are some cases in which the sternum will not be closed: for example, with complications that cause edema and dilatation of the heart secondary to injury and/or noncompliant lungs secondary to prolonged cardiopulmonary bypass; myocardial ischemia where cardiac size increases; and excessive intraoperative bleeding.[11] By closing the sternum, significant increase in the intrathoracic pressure would be applied, causing cardiac tamponade and resulting hemodynamic instability. In such cases the sternum is left unsutured, the incision is covered with an elliptical patch of impermeable rubber latex (rubber dam; Fig. 20–3), which is sutured to the skin edges, and an iodine-soaked gauze is placed on the patch and skin edges.[11] The rubber dam makes it possible to assess the site for tamponade due to excessive postoperative bleeding, as well as for an accumulation of blood or clots in the mediastinal cavity. Multiple sternotomies can thus be avoided and there is easy access for initiation of internal cardiac massage if the patient goes into cardiac arrest.[11]

Throughout the operative procedure, close monitoring of the patient's vital signs, heart rhythm, arterial blood gases, serum electrolytes, coagulation values, and urinary output is performed. Bypass time is also closely monitored and kept to a minimum (less than 3 hours) since the longer the patient is on bypass, the greater the risk of complications. Uncommonly, some patients are difficult to wean from the bypass machine and require the assistance of the intra-aortic balloon pump (refer to Chapter 17) to augment left ventricular function.

Postoperative Nursing Management

Immediately upon return from the operating room, the patient is connected to various types of bedside monitoring equipment: cardiac monitor, hemodynamic monitors, thoracic suction, intravenous infusion pumps, and mechanical ventilator. A portable chest x-ray is obtained to check the placement of the endotracheal tube and provide a baseline cardiac silhouette in case of cardiac tamponade. Pulmonary, cardiovascular, neurologic, and abdominal assessments are performed. Blood is drawn for baseline laboratory studies, including arterial blood gases, serum electrolytes, complete blood count, hematology profile, cardiac enzymes, and coagulation studies. Baseline hemodynamic values are obtained: arterial blood pressure, central venous pressure or right atrial pressure, pulmonary artery pressure, pulmonary capillary wedge pressure, and left atrial pressure. Cardiac rhythm, body temperature, and urine outputs are closely monitored.

Therapeutic Goals

The goals of care for the cardiac surgical patient include the following: (1) maintain adequate cardiac output and tissue perfusion; (2) prevent complications; (3) assist the patient and family to initiate rehabilitative activities.

Cardiac Output. To maintain adequate cardiac output and tissue perfusion the nurse must constantly analyze assessment data—identifying trends, and initiating timely and appropriate interventions. It is often necessary to manipulate the determinants of cardiac output—preload, afterload, contractility, and heart rate—to maintain an optimal cardiac output without undue strain on the heart. A low cardiac output syn-

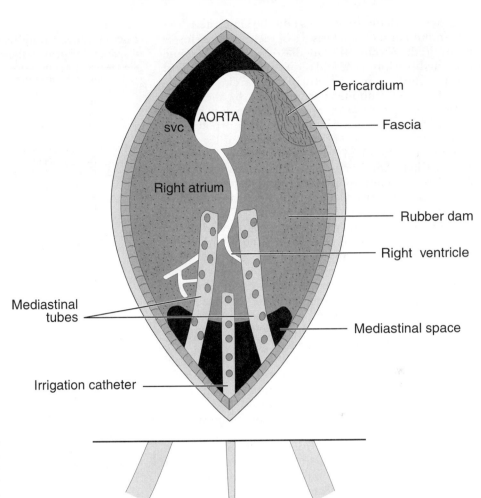

SVC

AORTA

Pericardium

Fascia

Right atrium

Rubber dam

Right ventricle

Mediastinal
tubes

Mediastinal space

Irrigation catheter

FIGURE 20–3. Rubber dam. (Adapted from Zellinger, M and Leinberger, TPL: Use of the rubber dam after open heart surgery. Crit Care Nurs 11:25–27, 1991.)

drome is reflected by systemic hypotension, peripheral vasoconstriction (cool, clammy, pale, or mottled skin), oliguria, and neurologic changes (mental status and orientation). After cardiac surgery, the low cardiac output in most patients is associated with hypovolemia, that is, reduced preload, and responds well to fluid volume expansion and/or replacement. If the hematocrit or hemoglobin is low, part of the fluid volume expansion can be achieved by transfusion of blood or blood products.

A state of low cardiac output may also be caused by an increase in afterload; it is characterized by increased systemic vascular resistance and arterial hypertension. Reduction in afterload is accomplished with rewarming or with vasodilator therapy, that is, nitroprusside, providing the preload is adequate. Patients who have received β-adrenergic blockers (e.g., propranolol) prior to surgery may experience depressed cardiac contractility postoperatively. These patients are usually responsive to dopamine. If pharmacotherapeutics are successful in improving the cardiac output, the intra-aortic balloon pump (IABP) may be used. The purpose of the IABP is to decrease the afterload and increase the coronary artery and tissue perfusion.

Cardiac arrhythmias may also cause a low cardiac output. Bradyarrhythmias and AV blocks are frequently associated with valve replacement surgery. These abnormalities may be responsive to chronotropic therapy. More commonly, atrial-ventricular sequential pacing is the therapy of choice, as the "atrial kick," that is, the volume of blood delivered to the ventricles with atrial contraction just prior to ventricular systole, is preserved. Tachyarrhythmias are usually controlled with antiarrhythmic agents. It is essential to monitor serum electrolytes and the acid-base status as premature ventricular contractions (PVCs) may evolve into lethal arrhythmias in the presence of hypokalemia and acidosis. Replacement potassium chloride is added to the intravenous therapy, or potassium challenges may be given to maintain the serum potassium level >4.0 mEq/L. Abnormalities in serum potassium may arise from hemodilution, nasogastric suction, diuretic therapy, and from the overall response of the body to the stress of the surgery.

Hemorrhage. A major postoperative complication is hemorrhage. Excessive bleeding may occur at the site of the surgery, that is, the graft suture lines. This may be associated with insufficient reversal of heparin with protamine sulfate or be caused by a decrease in clotting factors. Mediastinal tubes must be kept patent and the amount and characteristics of the drainage closely monitored. Should the mediastinal tubes become occluded by clots, accumulation of blood and fluid in the pericardial sac may precipitate cardiac tamponade. Cardiac tamponade is reflected by the classic signs of rising central venous pressure with neck vein distention, falling arterial pressure with hypotension and a narrow pulse pressure, and muffled heart sounds. This triad of symptomatology is known as Beck's triad. Another sign of cardiac tamponade is that of pulsus paradoxus. Timely and aggressive intervention is imperative. Patients with the rubber dam are assessed for movement of the dam.[11] Normally the dam retracts when negative pressure is applied to the chest tube. With accumulation of fluid in the chest, the dam will bulge outward when negative pressure is applied to the mediastinal tube. Postoperatively, the cardiac surgical patient is at risk for developing pulmonary emboli, pneumonia, and fluid overload. Frequent position changes, range of motion exercises, and early ambulation help in preventing thromboembolic episodes. Ace bandages or antiembolic stockings applied to the lower extremities help to promote venous return and prevent venous stasis. In patients where the saphenous vein was harvested, elastic bandages applied along the entire suture line (i.e., toe to knee or toe to thigh) prevent oozing from the incisional site and hematoma formation.

Pulmonary Status. The patient's pulmonary status must be evaluated at frequent intervals. Serial arterial blood gases, continuous monitoring of arterial blood saturation with oxygen (SaO_2), and chest x-rays help to monitor the pulmonary function. Coughing, turning, and deep breathing are essential in raising secretions and preventing atelectasis. Splinting of the chest incision assists the patient in coughing by decreasing the pain somewhat and by giving the patient psychological reassurance that the chest will not split open while performing these activities. Once extubated, incentive spirometry is used to support deep breathing. Special attention to these details helps to prevent pulmonary complications. (Refer to Table 20–1 for additional potential postoperative complications.)

Infection. Infection is another primary concern. Depending upon the surgery performed, the patient may have one or more incisions. These must be assessed every shift for signs of redness, swelling, drainage, and increased pain or discomfort. Usually after the first 24 hours, the incisions will be left open to air. Wound care may be ordered specifically by the physician, or there may be protocols followed by different institutions.

If the patient has a rubber dam in place, astute assessment is necessary so that complications of mediastinitis, osteomyelitis of the sternum, and sepsis do not occur.[11] Strict aseptic technique is used for daily dressing changes, the first of which is performed by the surgeon. Minimal pressure is applied to the area being cleaned. A small irrigation catheter may have been inserted when the chest tubes were positioned.

TABLE 20–1
Postoperative Complications in the Cardiac Surgical Patient

1. Cardiovascular dysfunction
   a. Low cardiac output syndrome
      1) Reduced preload
         Hypovolemia
         Hemorrhage
         Surgical site
         Overheparinization
         Depleted clotting factors
      2) Increase afterload
         Increased systemic vascular resistance
         Arterial constriction
         Hypothermia
         Dehydration
      3) Cardiac arrhythmias
         Bradyarrhythmias
         Tachyarrhythmias
         Conduction defects
   b. Congestive heart failure
   c. Cardiogenic shock
   d. Cardiac tamponade
   e. Acute myocardial infarction
   f. Electrolyte disturbances
      1) Hypokalemia
         Extracorporeal circulation
         Hemodilution
         Diuretic therapy
         Nasogastric decompression
2. Pulmonary dysfunction
   a. Pneumothorax
   b. Hemothorax
   c. Atelectasis
   d. Pneumonia
   e. Pulmonary edema (cardiogenic vs. noncardiogenic pulmonary)
   f. Pulmonary embolism
3. Renal dysfunction
   a. Prerenal failure
4. Gastrointestinal dysfunction
   a. Stress ulcer
   b. Paralytic ileus
5. Neurologic dysfunction
   a. Postpericardiotomy syndrome (postcardiotomy delirium associated with cardiopulmonary bypass and manifested by behavioral changes, ranging from confusion to psychosis)
6. Infection
   a. Endocarditis
   b. Mediastinitis
   c. Sepsis
7. Miscellaneous
   a. Thromboembolic disorder
   b. Disseminated intravascular coagulation (DIC)

Antibiotic irrigations may be ordered if the operating time was long or if emergency sternal opening was performed.[11] The solution can be warmed, but strict asepsis must be adhered to. Strict intake and output control must be performed to prevent excess accumulation of irrigation solution in the mediastinal cavity. The nurse needs to monitor the drug levels of the antibiotic to prevent toxicity and assure therapeutic levels.

Rubber Dam. Patients with the rubber dam in place should be kept supine at all times except when giving skin care. They are not turned, only tilted to a maximum of 30 degrees. Support must be given to the chest to prevent detachment of the rubber dam, but undue pressure should be prevented because of the unstable sternum. The head of the bed should be elevated no more than 20 degrees.[11] Chest physiotherapy and extubation should be delayed until after the sternum is closed. The patient may need to be sedated, if anxious or restless, to prevent dislodging of the rubber dam or tubes, or damage to the chest and organs.

Rehabilitation. Following the stabilization of the patient in the immediate postoperative period, the focus of nursing care becomes the patient's rehabilitation and discharge. It is at this time that the rapport and support systems established preoperatively assist the patient and family during the recuperative period, when there is the adjustment of moving from the ICU setting to a step-down unit or to a general postoperative floor. This move can be an experience fraught with anxiety for both the patient and family. The patient who does not experience a dramatic improvement in overall body function may become depressed. It should be emphasized that each case is different and that it sometimes takes from 3 to 6 months for an individual to experience any significant improvement in overall physical and psychological status. The achievement of strength, stamina, and optimal well-being may take longer than the patient had anticipated before the operation.[12]

Nursing Diagnoses, Patient Outcomes, and Nursing Interventions

For pertinent nursing diagnoses, patient outcomes, and nursing interventions in the postoperative care of the cardiac surgical patient, refer to the care plan at the end of this chapter.

Postoperative Teaching

Postoperative teaching serves to reinforce information presented to the patient regarding preoperative activities and to expand on those factors essential to postoperative recuperation and home health maintenance. It is necessary to assess patients and their support systems to gain a clear understanding of the patient and family members as individuals, singularly and collectively, the environment in which they live and work, as well as health management concerns and rehabilitation. Assessment of functional health patterns enables this data to be identified, explored, and mutually acted upon.[10]

In addition to the information presented in preoperative instruction, postoperative teaching is concerned with expectations of the recuperative phase and overall rehabilitation. Areas of particular importance include the patient's emotional status, activities of daily living, exercise, diet, sexual activity, prevention of infection, medication regimen, follow-up care, and instruction regarding the underlying disease process that necessitated the surgery. Teaching that has taken place while in the hospital needs to be reinforced after the patient goes home, since research has shown that a patient's ability to retain information during hospitalization is limited.[10]

Postoperatively, it is not unusual for patients to feel anxious, irritable, and depressed. Often these feelings are related to concerns regarding changes in body image and the fear of the "chest opening." Sleep disturbances after surgery are not unusual, and they may last for as long as 4 to 6 weeks. Appropriate explanation and reassurance can defuse some of these feelings and assist the patient to form more realistic expectations of the healing process.[10]

Immediate and long-term progression of activity is an essential factor in the patient's recuperation and needs to be addressed in the postoperative instruction.[13] Immediately after surgery, the patient can be expected to change position while in bed. By the second and third day after surgery, the patient should progress to sitting in a chair and then walking. The nurse should encourage the patient to perform leg exercises that assist in returning blood to the heart, and the patient should elevate the legs while sitting in a chair to minimize fluid accumulation. To ensure adequate circulation the legs should not be crossed. Support stockings should be worn during the first few weeks after surgery to help improve circulation and prevent fluid accumulation and venous stasis.

Prior to discharge, the patient should be able to verbalize the expected activity and limitations. Cardiac surgical patients should avoid driving for 4 to 6 weeks after surgery, until the sternum has healed. When riding for longer than an hour, frequent rest stops should be planned to allow ambulation. This promotes venous return and increases circulation to the legs. Commercial air travel is allowed, but unpressurized air cabins should be avoided. If the trip is longer than 1 hour, again the instruction is to walk around. At the airport, the chest wires may activate the metal detector.[14] If airport personnel are informed about the heart surgery, they will use the hand wand.

Gradually the patient can return to household chores and recreational activities as directed by the surgeon. Frequent rest periods and an afternoon nap should be planned. Excessive visitors should be avoided as extensive socialization causes fatigue. Lifting objects over 10 lb or straining is to be avoided to prevent separation of the sternum. Sports which involve too much arm movement should also be avoided during this period.[14]

Regularly planned exercise is necessary to promote cardiovascular fitness. Slow progressive ambulation is recommended. The patient may walk 1 block the second week, gradually increasing the distance to 1 mile as tolerated. The patient should avoid extremes of outside temperatures and refrain from exercise for 30 minutes to 2 hours after meals to prevent competition for oxygen needs between the gastrointestinal organs and muscle.[7] Ideally, the patient would participate in a cardiac rehabilitation program to optimize physical and psychological recuperation.

In conjuction with a planned progressive exercise program, the patient and family should receive appropriate diet instruction. Such instruction should take into consideration who in the family shops and prepares meals. Alcohol consumption should be minimal (less than 1 to 2 ounces daily). The patient's weight should be obtained daily. Any weight gain of 5 lb (2 lb over a few days) should be reported to the physician, as should any swelling of the hands or ankles; the latter is indicative of water retention and needs immediate attention.

Usually, after the first week, any steady pain should be gone. Brief stabbing chest pains may occur occasionally for up to several months.[14] It is very common to experience muscle aches throughout the chest, upper back, shoulders, and neck. A heating pad or shower massage may be useful.[14]

After CABG, patients need to be taught how to care for their leg incisions in order to prevent infection and separation of the incision edges.[15] The patient should wash the incision daily with a nondetergent soap and water, and leave it open to the air. No creams, ointments, or powders should be applied to the incision unless ordered by the physician,[15] and any scabs that may be present should not be removed. The patient should inspect the incision daily for the presence of redness, swelling, and drainage. A diary should be kept of body temperature, weight, incision appearance, drainage, pain, and distance walked,[15] and the physician should be notified immediately if there is an increase in the amount of redness, swelling, drainage, pain, separation of the incision edges, or a change in the color or odor of the drainage. If there is an infection prior to discharge, the patient will need to be taught how to do dressing changes (if ordered), and it should be explained that if antibiotics are ordered, all the medicine should be taken as ordered. Again patients should be encouraged to keep their legs elevated when sitting, to gradually increase their walking distances, to do their ankle exercises, and to take their prescribed medications for pain.[15] Patients should also be encouraged to wear their elastic stockings/antiembolic stockings during the day, washing them out thoroughly at night and allowing them to air dry.

Following cardiac surgery, the patient's medication regimen frequently changes. After CABG, patients are often placed on aspirin or persantine; patients with valve replacement may be placed on long-term coumadin therapy. The patient and family should be instructed regarding the specific medications, their names, purpose, dosage, schedule, and side effects. Special instructions may be necessary. For example, patients placed on coumadin therapy must appreciate the importance of ongoing follow-up care. They should know to contact the physician immediately should any of the following signs or symptoms be noted: black or tarry stool, pink or red urine, excessive bruising or unexplained swelling, severe headaches, abdominal pain, coffee-ground vomitus, epistaxis (nosebleed), or heavier than usual menses. The patient should be instructed to use a soft toothbrush and an electric razor. Only prescribed medications should be taken, and over-the-counter drugs should be avoided, unless otherwise ordered. The patient should always carry a card listing all medications, including doses and time of administration. Patients should also be encouraged to wear a Medic-Alert tag.

Patients with valve replacements are at high risk of infection, that is, bacterial endocarditis. These patients should contact their physician regarding the need for prophylactic antibiotics when dental work, surgery, invasive procedures, or self-injection of drugs is anticipated.

The patient's return to work should be discussed with the physician. Depending upon the type of work, for example, clerical work versus manual labor, the patient may be able to resume work within 4 to 6 weeks. The patient and family should be encouraged to verbalize their concerns regarding livelihood and changes in lifestyle. The nurse should assist patient and family to identify effective coping mechanisms and support systems. Instruction in relaxation techniques may be initiated early on in the postoperative phase.[10]

Finally, for the patient who has had CABG, it is essential to teach the patient and family about the underlying disease process and risk factors associated with heart disease. The function of the heart as a pump, the significance of coronary artery perfusion, and the nature of the atherosclerotic process should be discussed. Patients should be able to identify risk factors for heart disease and their own risk factors. Physical conditions and living habits that contribute to the process of coronary artery disease should be discussed, as well as modifications in lifestyle needed to control some of the risks identified, for example, stress management, diet, weight reduction, and exercise.

Patients are generally discharged 4 to 7 days after surgery. Discharge teaching is very important to help ease the transition from hospital to home. Some hospitals offer a callback system where patients and their families can call for advice if they are experiencing difficulties or have questions. Nurses also call the patients to see how they are doing and if they are experiencing any problems. This system not only helps ease the psychological transition to home, but it also helps prevent severe complications by advising the patient to seek medical assistance in a timely manner.

Much research has been done on the improvement in the quality of life in the objective sense in patients receiving CABGs verses other treatment modalities. A patient's perception of an improvement in the quality of life is mainly based on subjective factors.[16] Many things affect this perception, such as length of time the patient had angina and its severity prior to the surgery, exercise tolerance, activity limitations, symptoms, side effects of the medications, the ability to return to work, anxiety, depression, fatigue, the feeling of well-being, and family, social, and sexual satisfaction. Nurses can help their patients to develop a greater sense of well-being and to gain control over their future by offering support and reassurance. Follow-up support needs to be incorporated into the total plan of care extending into the postdischarge phase. Much emphasis has been placed on teaching to prepare the patient for discharge and lead a healthy life, but research has shown that many patients do not retain much of what was taught in the hospital. This is due to many factors, such as anxiety, pain, fear, preoccupation with their condition, and anticipation of going home, to name a few. Teaching and support must continue after discharge, to help the patient accept his or her condition and modify behavior. Family involvement is especially important, for illness evolves out of the total interaction between the individual, the family, and significant others. Nurses need to consider how they may affect the patient-family-environment interaction so that when a patient is discharged, adequate support is available and the patient can make adjustments in lifestyle. Enrollment in support groups and in a cardiac rehabilitation program is of utmost importance.

CARDIAC MYOPLASTY

For the past 50 years, experiments have been carried out on the use of skeletal muscle in cardiac surgery for irreversible congestive heart failure, ventricular aneurysms, in the improvement of collateral circulation of the myocardium, and after the removal of myocardial tumors.[17] There was much hope that one day failing hearts could be made stronger, prolonging a patient's life. In later experiments the skeletal muscle was stimulated in synchrony with the heart, thereby increasing the diastolic and mean aortic pressure. These experiments, however, ended with little success due to the muscle's susceptibility to fatigue under conditions of intensive use.

Continued research has been done in basic muscle physiology to help look for a possible solution for muscle fatigue. Although cardiac and skeletal muscle are composed of the same contractile proteins (sarcomeres), which are similar in structure and orientation, there are significant differences that lead to an explanation of the muscle fatigue observed in the skeletal muscle experiments. These include differences in periods of contraction versus rest, the number of mitochondria, the type of metabolism, and the use of energy. Skeletal muscle was noted to be able to be "conditioned" with bursts of stimuli so that it fatigued less frequently and was able to augment the natural heart pumping function. Muscles used in the research were the latissimus dorsi, pectoralis, rectus abdominus, and the diaphragm.

Indications

Indications for skeletal muscle augmentation include: disease associated with irreversible and extensive loss of cardiac muscle contractility such as ischemia, cardiomyopathy, dilated cardiomyopathy, myocarditis, and dysplastic myocardial disease.

Procedure

There are two ways in which skeletal muscle is used in cardiac surgery. In the first method skeletal muscle is used to construct a separate skeletal muscle chamber, or SMV. This method is still in the experimental phase, but it has many potential outcomes.

The second method is that of wrapping skeletal muscle around the heart, cardiac myoplasty, which is presently in the clinical trial phase. The latissimus dorsi muscle is used because its removal causes little physical impairment, due to the fact that the surrounding muscles compensate for its loss. Moreover, it is easily freed from its position and moved near the heart; and it has its own single blood and nerve supply. Although the other aforementioned muscles can be used, the latissimus dorsi is the preferred muscle.

The surgical procedure consists of making two incisions, one in the left lateral chest and the other a midline sternotomy. Through the lateral incision, the latissimus dorsi muscle is freed from the iliac crest, the spine, the inferior scapular angle, and the 9th to 12th rib attachments. A 6-cm segment of the anterior portion of the second rib is removed to allow for transportation of the graft into the thorax. The graft is carefully pushed through the opening where the rib was removed. The muscle is sutured to the 1st or 3rd rib. Care is taken not to twist the neurovascular pedicle because of the blood and nerve supply. Extreme care must be taken not to compress the lung and cause a decrease in pulmonary function. The skeletal muscle is then wrapped around the heart (Fig. 20–4).[17] Two pacing wires are implanted in the proximal portion of the muscle for long-term stimulation. Two sensing

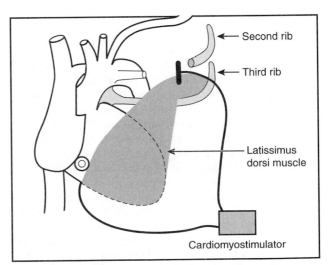

FIGURE 20–4. Cardiomyoplasty. (Adapted from Koroteyev, A, et al: Skeletal muscle: New techniques for treating heart failure. AORN 53:1010, 1991.)

leads are placed on the heart, and a cardiomyostimulator is placed beneath the rectus abdominous muscle. The procedure takes 4 to 6 hours in the absence of complications.[17]

How the procedure works no one knows for sure. Although the initial improvement in the symptoms of heart failure and the ejection fraction is slight, the patient feels much better later in the postoperative course, when the muscle is stimulated. It is thought that the skeletal muscle provides an accessory contractile layer that assists in the ejection of blood. Other hypotheses suggest that the graft prevents the heart from further dilatation and that the blood supply is increased by the collateral circulation of the skeletal muscle graft.[17]

Early postoperative care is the same as for the patient with a CABG. The muscle is allowed to rest for 2 weeks, then stimulation begins. The graft is progressively put into use, slowly increasing the burst frequency pattern. After approximately 4 months, the skeletal muscle can be stimulated at a synchronous ratio of 1:1 or 1:2 with the heart.

If these procedures continue to be developed, there may be hope for those who are not candidates for a heart transplant or those awaiting a donor heart.

VALVULAR SURGERY

Over the past three decades significant advances have been made in the treatment of valvular defects. Common causes of valvular dysfunction include rheumatic fever and endocarditis. Additional causes include cardiomyopathies, myomatous degeneration of the mitral valve, myocardial infarction, congenital defects, and trauma.[18]

The valvular disorders most frequently treated surgically include aortic stenosis, aortic regurgitation, mitral stenosis, and mitral regurgitation. Stenotic lesions often require urgent treatment, while regurgitation can be tolerated by the heart for a longer period.[18] Breathlessness is the main presenting symptom of valvular dysfunction. Patients with aortic stenosis may present with chest pain, syncopal attacks, and embolic problems. Eventually all valvular lesions lead to left ventricular failure or right ventricular failure secondary to pulmonary hypertension. Bacterial infection of the diseased valves can complicate the signs and symptoms with systemic or pulmonary emboli, which can cause rapid deterioration.[18]

Collaborative diagnosis of valvular dysfunction can be made by physical assessment, history, chest x-ray, resting 12-lead electrocardiogram (ECG), echocardiogram, and cardiac catheterization. Color flow Doppler imaging is the most useful study and makes cardiac catheterization unnecessary in most cases.[18] The transesophageal echocardiogram provides essential information in the assessment of mitral valve function.

Patients with valvular dysfunction are treated initially with a medical regimen of inotropic agents and diuretics. Antiarrhythmics and anticoagulants may be prescribed for patients with atrial arrhythmias, particularly atrial fibrillation. Valvular surgery is performed when medical management is no longer effective in controlling heart failure and the formation of thromboemboli.

Approaches to Valvular Surgery

Valvular surgery may involve closed or open heart surgery. A closed procedure does not require the use of the cardiopulmonary bypass. A valvotomy is a closed technique involving balloon dilatation of the stenotic valve. This procedure is used in some cases of mitral and tricuspid stenosis and pulmonic stenosis, especially in children. It is not recommended in cases of aortic stenosis where the heavily calcified and immobile valve causes left ventricular outflow tract obstruction.[18] Other closed procedures include annuloplasty, commissurotomy, and valvotomy. Annuloplasty involves the trimming of the valve ring with the insertion of an atrioventricular ring into the annulus or, in cases involving the tricuspid valve, with a purse-string suture. A commissurotomy involves the trimming of the valve leaflets to increase the size of the valve opening.[18]

An open valvotomy is useful in mitral stenosis.[18] The appropriate atrium is opened, the valve cusps are split, and the subvalvular papillary muscles are split or incised to give better mobility to the valve cusps and ventricular cavity. In regurgitant mitral or tricuspid disease, the atrioventricular ring can be treated with an annuloplasty, which reduces the size of the stretched annulus and improves coarctation of the valve cusps.[18]

Valve replacement, which involves the surgical removal of a diseased valve and the insertion of a prosthetic valve, requires the use of cardiopulmonary bypass. The choice of the prosthesis is determined by the design of the valve, its durability, potential for thromboemboli, and hemodynamic properties. In addition, the patient's age, size, medical history, activity level, and tolerance to anticoagulant therapy are of prime importance in the decision-making process.

Types of Prosthetic Heart Valves

There are two types of prosthetic heart valves: mechanical or prosthetic valves and tissue or bioprosthesis valves. Mechanical valves or lateral flow valves are highly durable and highly responsive to changes in chamber pressure. Biologic valves are less durable but have a lower incidence of thromboemboli. The most hemodynamically perfect tissue valve is the aortic homograft from a cadaver. It is used to replace diseased aortic and pulmonic valves. Most of the tissue valves used are derived from pig or calf pericardium. They are functionally as good as the mechanical valves but degenerate in time. Approximately 70% to 80%

last 10 years. Refer to Tables 20–2 and 20–3 for more information about artificial heart valves.

Complications of Valve Replacement

General complications of valve replacement include thromboembolism, prosthetic malfunction, paravalvular leaks, hemolysis, hemolytic anemia, prosthetic valve endocarditis, and calcification of porcine and pericardial bioprostheses. The mortality rate of prosthetic valve replacement is 5% to 10%, depending upon the patient's overall condition.

Nursing Care in Valve Replacement

The preoperative and postoperative care of the patient with a valve replacement is similar to that for the patient with CABG surgery, with two major differences.[19] First, the patient having valve replacement surgery is placed on anticoagulant therapy prophylactically to prevent embolization. Postoperatively, the patient's prothrombin time and partial thromboplastin time are closely monitored. Vigilant nursing care is essential in assessing for signs of bleeding or increased clotting time, as reflected by the appearance of petechiae, ecchymosis, oozing at puncture sites, bleeding gums, increased mediastinal tube drainage, or frank bleeding.

Second, as is the case with CABG surgery, the patient with a valve replacement is placed on intravenous antibiotic therapy, but for a longer period. Antibiotics should be started in the perioperative phase and levels maintained throughout surgery.[20] Postoperatively, it is essential that the patient receive the appropriate dosages at the proper time intervals and for the prescribed duration. This is to assure that optimal therapeutic serum levels are maintained in order to prevent not only basic postoperative infection but also prosthetic valve endocarditis (PVE). Research has demonstrated that the causative organism of PVE is a coagulase-negative staphylococcus, which is probably acquired at the time of surgery.[20]

Discharge planning specific for the patient with a valve replacement begins early on in the recuperative period. It entails patient and family education regarding the signs and symptoms of valve dysfunction. This includes sudden chest pain, fatigue, and dyspnea. The patient and family must understand the immediate need to seek medical attention when such symptoms occur. The patient must also know the importance of informing healthcare providers, especially dentists, of the valve replacement because of the higher risk of infective endocarditis. Prior to an invasive procedure, a course of prophylactic antibiotic therapy is essential.

Depending upon the type of valvular prosthesis and the presence of atrial fibrillation (or the risk of its occurrence), the patient and family need to be taught the signs and symptoms of overmedication with anticoagulants. Bleeding is the most significant side effect of anticoagulant therapy. Signs to watch for are ecchymosis, hematuria, heavier than normal menses, melena, hematoma, gingival bleeding, hemoptysis, and hematemesis. The importance of notifying the physician immediately should be emphasized.

It is important for the patient and family to understand that initially upon discharge there may be some physical restrictions, for example, no lifting objects over 10 lb, driving a car, vacuuming, and so on. Such usually temporary restrictions are necessary to allow for the sternal bone and musculature to heal properly. Within a few weeks after discharge the patient can usually resume most of his or her daily activities and should be encouraged to participate in a controlled exercise program.

VENTRICULAR ANEURYSMS

Ventricular aneurysms are defined as a systolic expansion of an ischemic, noncontractile portion of the ventricle.[21] During systole, when the ventricle contracts, the aneurysm portion bulges outward, thereby causing a decrease in the ejection fraction. Signs and symptoms are dependent on the size of the aneurysm. Ventricular aneurysms may range from 2 to 16 cm in diameter. Myocardial ischemia related to coronary artery disease is the cause of 85% to 95% of ventricular aneurysms. When occlusion of a coronary artery occurs, it promptly impedes contraction of the ischemic myocardial segment, thereby causing a relative systolic bulging or physiologic aneurysm. As the ischemia progresses, the myocardium undergoes necrosis, followed by leukocyte infiltration and replacement of the myocardium by fibrous scar tissue. Aneurysms result from the stretching of the myocardial cells so that there is a decrease in the number of cells in the transverse section. Hypertension and excessive cardiac activity during the healing phase of an MI tend to produce greater stress on the soft necrotic tissue and, therefore, promote aneurysm formation.[21] Other causes include trauma, hematomas forming in the ventricular wall, congenital defects in the myocardial attachment to the mitral or aortic valve ring, congenital diverticula, bacterial endocarditis with a mural abscess, rheumatic fever, syphilis, Chagas disease, and cardiac sarcoid granulomas.[21]

Preliminary diagnosis may be made on a chest x-ray, two-dimensional echocardiogram, and radionuclide studies. The ECG may show characteristic findings of large Q waves acorss the precordium and elevated ST segments with symmetrical inverted T waves that resemble an acute anteroseptal infarct. These changes persist after the normal healing time. Definition diagnosis is made with a cardiac catheterization, particularly a ventriculography to determine the aneurysm's size, shape, position, and degree of expansion, as well as the condition of the remaining myocardium and of the mitral and tricuspid valves.

Since ventricular aneurysms are nonfunctional seg-

TABLE 20–2
Artificial Valves Presently Used in the United States

Type	Name	Action	Special Information	Advantages	Disadvantages
Bioprosthesis					
Porcine	Hancock standard Carpentier-Edwards standard (stentless) Hancock modified orifice	Blood flows almost unobstructed through a central opening.	Aortic valve of a pig is harvested intact. Tissue is preserved with glutaraldehyde and high pressures. Mounted on a sew ring.	Biocompatible	Prone to tissue degeneration and calcification Requires short-term anticoagulant therapy
Pericardial	Carpentier-Edwards	Blood flows unobstructed through a central opening.	Most commonly used tissue valve. Calf pericardium is preserved in glutaraldehyde. Mounted on a Dacron frame.	Biocompatible Nonthrombogenic	Prone to tissue degeneration and calcification Space is restricted
Homograft		Blood flows unobstructed through the valve.	Aortic valve of a human cadaver.	Excellent hemodynamics Nonthrombogenic No need for anticoagulants	Not readily available

Mechanical

Type	Model	Description	Advantages	Disadvantages
Caged ball valve	Starr-Edwards	Blood flows through the cage and around the ball/poppet.	Durable Infrequent valve malfunction Use on children and adolescents	High incidence of thromboemboli Requires long-term anticoagulation therapy Not used for women anticipating childbearing May cause left ventricular outflow obstruction
Monoleaflet	Medtronic-Hall	Disc has wide open angle, occludes at the equator, providing maximal oriface opening. Valve is coated with pyrolytic carbon.	Very durable Biocompatible Hemodynamic performance Low incidence of valve-related complications	Susceptible to fracture, if heavily scarred or scratched during insertion Requires long-term anticoagulant therapy
Bileaflet	St. Jude Medical	Disk or leaflets open perpendicularly. Minimum obstruction to blood flow.	Used in patients with small orifices, especially children	Thromboembolism Requires long-term anticoagulant therapy

333

TABLE 20–3
Additional Valves Used Outside the United States

Type	Name
Bioprosthesis	
Porcine	Hancock II
	Carpentier-Edward supra-annular
	Medtronic intact
	St. Jude bioplant
Pericardial	Metroflow
Mechanical	
Monoleaflet	Bjork-Shiley monostrut
Bileaflet	Baxter Duramedics
	Carbomedics
	Sorin

ments of myocardium, the remaining part of the myocardium works harder, and aneurysms eventually aggravate or cause heart failure. Ventricular size and shape will be affected as well as surrounding structures such as the papillary muscles and valve supports.

Prognosis varies according to the patient's underlying health, the size of the aneurysm, its location, the type of aneurysm (refer to Figure 20–5), and the cause of the aneurysm. Embolization is a threat, due to the presence of clots in aneurysms. Recurring ventricular arrhythmias arising in the scar tissue about the edge of the aneurysm are ominous and directly proportional to the size of the aneurysm. That is, as the size of the aneurysm increases, so does the incidence of ventricular arrhythmias.

Treatment consists of surgical removal of the aneurysm if heart failure cannot be controlled with medications. If the patient is undergoing myocardial revascularization, then the aneurysm should be repaired at the same time.[21] It is easier and safer to excise the aneurysm after extensive fibrosis of its edges has occurred because the dense connective tissue permits closure of the resulting ventricular margins with less risk of the sutures tearing through. Removal of the aneurysm causes distortion in the contour of the ventricle and ventricular irritability, so that the patient is susceptible to ventricular arrhythmias.

A new procedure, ventricular endoaneurysmorrha-phy (Fig. 20–6), was developed in the late 1980s.[22] In this procedure, an oval Dacron patch, approximately 2 to 3 in by 0.5 in, is inserted through a small incision and sutured into place. The patch can be shaped and molded to the normal configuration of the left ventricle. This patch helps stabilize the ventricle, while increasing the injection fraction, and causes less irritability. This procedure can be performed in patients who would normally do poorly in the early postoperative phase with fewer complications.[22]

ARTIFICIAL HEARTS AND VENTRICULAR ASSIST DEVICES

Artificial hearts, left ventricular assist devices, and heart transplantation are usually last resorts for the failing, irreparable heart. These approaches to therapy have provoked many ethical questions and entail high risks, many complications, and a course of complex long-term care. The cost for hospitalization, surgery, and postsurgical rehabilitation can be prohibitive.

There are a number of artificial hearts that have been developed over the past decades. Probably the most famous is the Jarvik 7 artificial heart. In general, the artificial heart is made up of mechanical ventricles that are sewn to the patient's pulmonary artery and atria, and placed within the mediastinum. The mechanical heart is powered by compressed air, which activates the internal valves and diaphragm, thereby simulating the pumping action of the heart.[23]

New advances in technology have led to more compact artificial hearts as well as a decreased incidence of thromboembolic complications and device failure. Due to these advances, clinical use of the artificial heart has expanded.

Ventricular assist devices (VADs) are used to support the failing heart and reduce the work of the heart by diverting the blood from the natural ventricle to an artificial pump that maintains circulation.[24] VADs also maintain adequate systemic perfusion during episodes of ventricular fibrillation or asystole. There are two main indications for the use of a VAD[24] (Table 20–4).

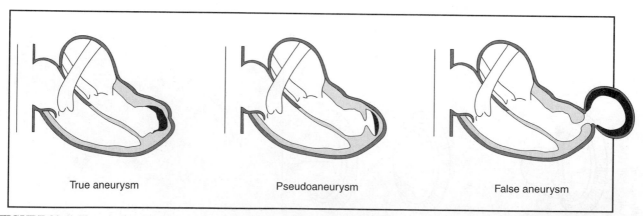

True aneurysm   Pseudoaneurysm   False aneurysm

FIGURE 20–5. Ventricular aneurysms. (Adapted from Rowe, GG: Ventricular aneurysm. Curr Conc Hosp Med 21:28, 1985.)

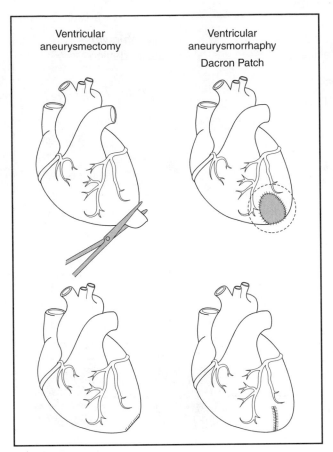

Ventricular aneurysmectomy

Ventricular aneurysmorrhaphy
Dacron Patch

FIGURE 20–6. Ventricular aneurysm repair.

First, VADs are used for patients in cardiac failure who have the potential of regaining normal heart function. Examples of this would be the patient who cannot be weaned from the bypass machine after cardiopulmonary bypass and the patient in cardiogenic shock after MI. The second situation where a VAD would be used is for the patient awaiting to receive a new heart . . . a "bridge to transport." VADs are considered only after optimal fluid therapy, pharmacologic support, and the IABP (where applicable) have been instituted. Abnormalities in electrolytes, acid-base balance, arrhythmias, hypothermia, and severe bleeding should be corrected as much as possible before the initiation of a VAD.

There are three types of VADs[23] (Fig. 20–7 and Table 20–5). The first is the right ventricular assist device. Here the right atrium is cannulated; the blood flows through the device to the cannulated main pul-

TABLE 20–4
Ventricular Assist Device: Patient Selection Criteria

1. Cardiac index <21 min^{-1} m^{-2}
2. Systolic blood pressure <90 mmHg
3. Left or right atrial pressure >20 mmHg
4. Urinary output <20 mL/h
5. Systemic vascular resistance >2100 dynes sec cm^{-5}
6. Blood lactate level >30 mg/dL

monary artery, where the blood returns back to the body. The second type is the left ventricular assist device. Here, cannulation is at the left atrium, if transplantation is going to be performed, or at the left ventricular apical area, if transplantation is expected. Blood flows to the device and re-enters the body through the cannulated ascending aorta. The third type is the biventricular assist device, where there are two devices and both ventricles are cannulated.

Nursing care is the same as that for any critically ill cardiac surgical patient, with a few additions.[23,25] Ongoing assessments are essential, but the nurse now needs to collaborate with the perfusionist to assure device functioning. Inotropic drugs and vasodilators will be administered to maintain the patient's cardiac output. This requires that arterial pressures, pulmonary artery pressures, and left atrial pressures be monitored hourly until stable. Mediastinal chest tube drainage will be monitored hourly. Drainage of >75 mL/h will require replacement blood products. Autotransfusion during the initial postoperative period is an option. Neurologic assessments, especially pupil size and response to light, will be done hourly to assess for cerebral emboli, since the formation of thromboemboli is a complication of the device. Mental alertness, strength of grip, and the ability to follow commands will probably be ineffective or inappropriate indicators since the VAD patient is frequently chemically paralyzed to prevent dislodgement of the tubes. The nurse needs to remember that the VAD patient is a surgical patient and probably in pain, so analgesics should be administered with the paralytic agent.

Infection is a very serious complication for the VAD patient. Strict sterile techniques must be followed when caring for the incision, tubes, and device. The patient's WBC count should be assessed daily and the patient's temperature should be monitored every 2 to 4 hours. Antibiotics will be ordered at any sign of infection. The chest dressings are changed daily with strict isolation and sterile technique. The wound and cannulae are generally scrubbed with povidone-iodine. Only very light pressure should be applied when scrubbing the chest. The chest is covered with a dry sterile dressing or transparent occlusive dressing. (Refer to Table 20–6 for complications of VADs.) The head of the bed may be elevated, but there cannot be any kinks in the tubing. The patient cannot be turned, only be tilted to 20 degrees. Specialized beds, that is, kinetic therapy beds, and air or water mattresses may be useful. Passive range of motion should be performed to augment circulation and maintain muscle tone. Nutrition via enteral feedings should be started within 48 hours of surgery, after bowel sounds are present. Psychological support should be intense and ongoing. See Table 20–7 for guidelines for weaning a patient from a VAD.

HEART TRANSPLANTATION

Heart transplantation involves the replacement of the patient's heart with a donor heart procured from

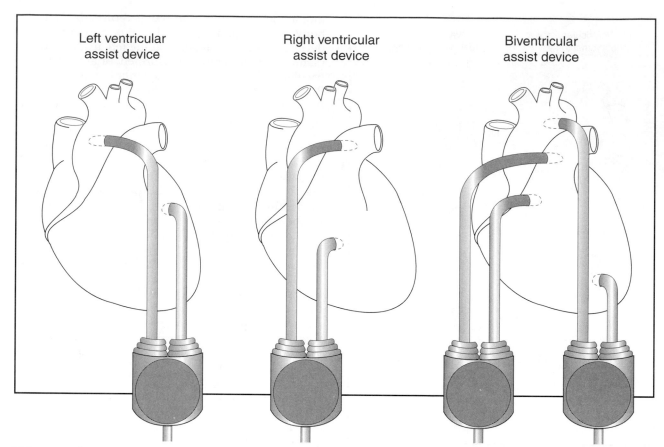

Left ventricular
assist device

Right ventricular
assist device

Biventricular
assist device

FIGURE 20–7. Types of ventricular assist devices. (Adapted from Quaal, SJ: VADs: Beyond intra-aortic balloon pumping. CV Nurse: Trends in Cardiovascular Care 5:5, and Vaska, PL: Biventricular assist devices. Crit Care Nurs 11:54.)

a brain-dead patient, the majority of whom have sustained head injuries.[26] In 1988, for the United States alone, the United Network of Organ Sharing computer listed 400 patients awaiting new hearts. Gill[26] notes that the problem is not that there is an inadequate number of potential donors but that use of the donor pool is suboptimal. Donors are either not identified, not declared brain-dead, or families are not given the option to donate. Legislation has been passed establishing a national organ procurement and transplantation network (OPTN) to establish criteria for the acquisition and distribution of organs through the regional organ procurement facilities.[26] "Required request" legislation makes healthcare facilities responsible for offering the option of organ donation to families and for notifying organ procurement agencies of potential donors. The Omnibus Budget Reconciliation Act requires (1) that all hospitals funded by Medicare have policies and procedures relating to donation and notification of designated organ procurement agencies to ensure that the families of potential donors are made aware of the option to donate and (2) that the potential donor hospital must notify a federally certified organ procurement agency (OPA). Another measure was the establishment of the National Task Force on Organ Transplantation, which

recommended that massive education efforts be directed to increasing the public and professional awareness of the need for organ donors.[26]

As of 1986, the 1-year survival rate for heart transplant patients was 85%. Of these patients, approximately 90% returned to normal activity levels. As of March 1988, the 5- to 10-year actual survival rate was 73%.[23] The best survival rate was among the elderly group (55 to 68 years old). The retransplantation 1-year survival rate for this group was 57%, and the 5-year survival rate was 53%.[27] The majority of transplants are done for end-stage cardiomyopathy and/or ischemic heart disease. Congenital anomalies, end-stage valvular disease, and cardiac tumors are less frequent conditions requiring heart transplantation.[28]

Criteria for Heart Transplant Candidacy

There are certain criteria that the potential heart transplant candidate must meet to be considered for transplant surgery. While variations may exist from center to center, these criteria usually include those listed in Table 20–8. Fulfillment of these criteria helps to insure a more successful outcome following transplantation. Medical evaluation prior to acceptance

TABLE 20–5
Ventricular Assist Device: Types of Pumps

Type	Characteristics
Centrifugal	Centrifical force propels the blood through the device. Nonocclusive. High negative inflow pressure cannot develop minimizing kinks or air entrapment.
External pulsatile	Restricted use in the United States. Two compartments separated by a diaphragm or flexible sac. Unidirectional valves direct the blood to the device from inflow cannula during the filling phase. Pressurized air causes the diaphragm or sac to move so that the blood is forced through the outflow cannula during the ejection phase.
Implantable (Heartmate)	Pneumatically driven with external console. Used to bridge patients to transplantation. Electrically driven pulsatile pump is implanted in the upper abdominal quadrant. Patients can be mobile.
Resuscitative system	Support cardiac and/or pulmonary function during heart or lung failure. Femoral to femoral extracorporeal membrane oxygenation done by percutaneous or femoral cutdown. Rapid application performed in the ICU or cardiac catherterization lab.
Rotating pump (new)	Silicon catheter is positioned through the femoral artery into the left ventricle. Electromechanically coupled propeller within the catheter draws blood into the aorta.

includes a thorough health history, physical examination, and routine laboratory and roentgenographic studies. A complete workup to determine the status of pulmonary, renal, and hepatic function is ordered. Evaluation of pulmonary hemodynamics is especially critical. If the pulmonary vascular resistance (PVR) exceeds 600 dynes/cm^{-5} or 80 Wood units, even a healthy donor heart may be unable to significantly increase the cardiac workload sufficiently to overcome such high pulmonary vascular resistance. Such a condition predisposes the new heart to early postoperative right ventricular failure.

TABLE 20–6
Complications of Ventricular Assist Devices

Bleeding
Thrombosis
Biventricular failure
Respiratory failure
Renal failure
Liver failure
Air emboli
Infection
Return cannula obstruction

TABLE 20–7
Ventricular Assist Device Weaning Guidelines

Cardiac index >2.0 L min^{-1} m^{-2}
Systolic blood pressure >90 mmHg
Mean arterial pressure >60 mmHg
Ultrasound of the left ventricle to detect thrombi
Not done before 2nd postoperative day

Two consecutive trials of decreased blood flow through the ventricular assist device are carried out 4 hours apart. If the patient is hemodynamically stable, the device is removed in the OR.

Assessment of cardiovascular function entails cardiac catheterization to evaluate right and left heart hemodynamics. A thorough evaluation of the patient's immunologic status, including compatibility between the donor heart and the recipient, is vital. The presence of donor-specific cytotoxic antibodies is a distinct contraindication for heart transplantation. The necessary immunosuppressant therapy, postoperatively, greatly increases the likelihood of life-threatening infection during this phase.

Nursing evaluation of the transplant candidate involves an assessment of the patient's functional health pattern. It is important to establish how the patient perceives health and to identify those activities performed by the patient and family that reflect the level of health care desired. An assessment of roles and relationships may help to determine the patient's psychosocial stability and available family support systems. Identifying how the patient and family cope with stress may be of assistance during the preoperative and postoperative periods, and reinforcement of formerly effective coping mechanisms may be vital to the patient's recuperation during the postoperative and rehabilitative phases of care.

TABLE 20–8
Criteria for Heart Transplant Candidacy

1. Primary end-stage cardiac disease not responding to medical or surgical management
2. Life expectancy without a transplant less than 1 year
3. Less than 65 years of age (this is not a steadfast rule since transplants are performed on newborns as well as adults 68 years of age, the average age being 42.5 years)
4. No evidence of current pulmonary infarction
5. Pulmonary hypertension <600 dyne sec cm^{-5} or 80 Wood units, or PAP >40 mmHg
6. No active infection
7. No insulin-dependent diabetes mellitus (this way vary from institution to institution)
8. No multisystem disease, including severe kidney or hepatic dysfunction, and pulmonary failure
9. No extracerebral neoplastic disease
10. Absence of donor-specific cytotoxic antibodies
11. No major psychological dysfunction, i.e., history of alcohol or drug abuse, depression, or psychosis
12. Motivated and compliant patient
13. Strong family support system

Donor Procurement

Heart donors are individuals who have sustained a irreversible brain injury, usually involving a traumatic event. Ideally the heart donor is less than 30 years old, with a heart that is typically healthy and largely free of advanced atherosclerotic disease. Refer to Table 20–9 for donor criteria.

Once a potential donor is identified, the nurse or physician should notify the OPA or transplant center immediately. The procurement coordinator conducts the initial evaluation of the donor over the telephone.[26] Table 20–10 lists information procured during the initial evaluation. If the donor appears acceptable, the procurement coordinator makes an on-site evaluation. Until the organ is removed, the patient's physiologic status must be maintained. It is estimated that 60% of all potential donors die by the 3rd day of hospitalization, so identification and evaluation of the patient must be made as soon as possible.[26]

Surgical Approaches

In the United States there are two surgical approaches to heart transplantation currently in use. The first is the orthotopic procedure. Here the recipient's heart is removed except for the posterior right and left atrial walls and the inferior and superior vena cava. The pulmonary artery and aorta are transversed just distal to the semilunar valves. Refer to Figure

TABLE 20–9
Criteria for Heart Donor Candidacy

Classical Donor Criteria
1. Men under the age of 30; women under the age of 40.
2. No cardiac or chest trauma.
3. No history of coronary artery disease: a cardiac catheterization may be required; ECG should be within normal limits, although ST-T wave changes may be accepted; normal echocardiogram, normal or minimum creatinine-kinase-myocardial band (CPK-MB).
4. No history of severe insulin-dependent diabetes (relative).
5. No history of severe chronic hypertension.
6. Absence of systemic sepsis.
7. Absence of hepatitis.
8. Absence of extracranial malignancy.
9. Hemodynamically stable, not requiring high doses of inotropic support.
10. No episodes of prolonged cardiac resuscitation, intracardiac injections, prolonged hypotension or hypoxia, or prolonged dopamine use.
11. ABO compatability with the recipient.
12. Lymphocytic crossmatch, antibody screen (negative).
13. Body size and weight comparable to recipient; weight difference less than 20% of the recipient's weight.

Extented Donor Criteria
1. Up to 50 years of age.
2. Severe chest trauma, not include chest tubes.
3. Prolonged hospitalization.
4. Short-term high doses of inotropic medication.
5. Transient reversible hypotension for 20–180 minutes.
6. Up to 32% body weight difference from the recipient.

TABLE 20–10
Donor Information Needed for the Initial Interview by the Organ Procurement Coordinator[26]

- Potential donor's name
- Demographic information: age, sex, race
- Height and weight
- Date and time of admission
- Cause of death or the nature of accident or injury—including prehospital and emergency room care
- History since admission—including invasive and/or operative procedures, cardiac or respiratory arrests
- Past medical history—family history of heart disease, signs and symptoms of cardiac disease
- Drugs used during hospitalization
- Social history including intravenous drug use, homosexuality
- Clinical status—vital signs, ECG rhythm, urine output, hemodynamic status, vasopressor support
- Laboratory date—BUN, creatinine, electrolytes, hemoglobin and hematocrit, WBC count, cardiac enzymes, cultures, and urinalysis
- Blood type
- Declaration of brain death—if yes, date and time
- Donor status—presence of donor card and limitations
- Family information—notifying next of kin and relationship; family's understanding of brain death; what the family has been told; family's knowledge of the request for organ donation
- Status of permission—if permission has been obtained, the date and time
- Donor's case type, i.e., medical examiner's case

20–8.[27] The advantage of this procedure is that the sinoatrial (SA) node and most of the internodal pathways to the AV node are preserved in the recipient heart. This is the most common procedure used in the United States. The second approach is the heterotopic, or "piggy-back," procedure. Here the donor's heart and major blood vessels are sewn to the recipient's heart and major vessels (Fig. 20–9). The donor heart is placed in the right side of the chest, while the recipient's heart remains in the left side. The blood passes through either or both hearts.[27] The major advantage of this approach is that there is a lower incidence of pulmonary hypertension and rejection. It has been reported in some cases that the recipient's own heart recovered after being allowed to rest.[29]

Postoperative Nursing Management

Nursing care of the heart transplant patient is similar in many respects to that of the myocardial revascularization patient. Unique to the postoperative care of the heart transplant patient is that the requirement of immunosuppressant therapy poses an extreme risk of infectious complications (Table 20–11). Commonly used immunosuppressant drugs are listed in Table 20–12. In some institutions the transplant patient is provided a room with strict isolation or a special airflow system. Vigilant nursing care is essential to prevent infection or to recognize its presence early on so that timely and aggressive therapy can be instituted.

Other differences compared with myocardial revascularization include conditions inherent to the sur-

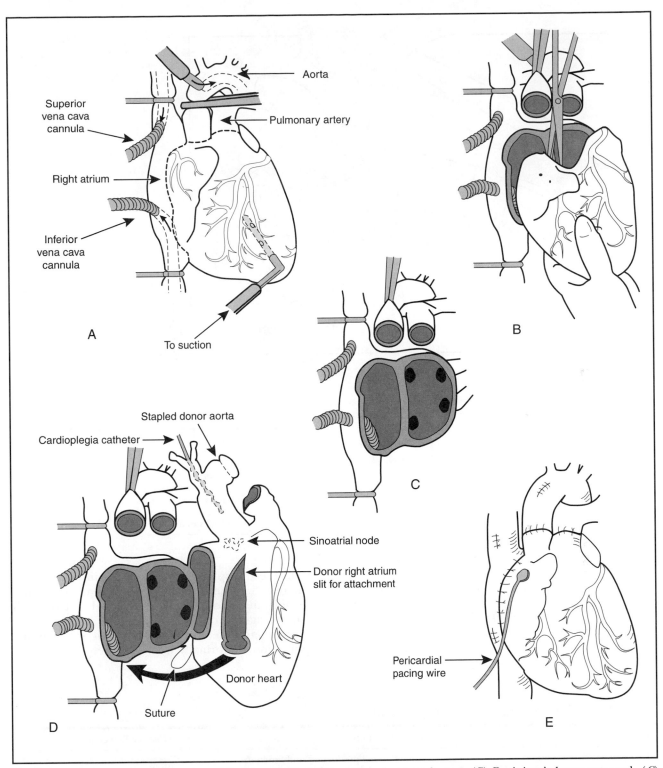

FIGURE 20–8. Heart transplantation. (*A*) Person placed on cardiopulmonary bypass. (*B*) Recipient's heart removed. (*C*) Exposed heart ready for transplantation. (*D*) Initial attachment of left atrium of donor heart. (*E*) Transplanted heart, off bypass, with epicardial pacing wire in place. (Adapted from Luckman, J and Sorensen, KC: Medical-Surgical Nursing: A Psychophysiologic Approach, ed. 3. WB Saunders, Philadelphia, 1987.)

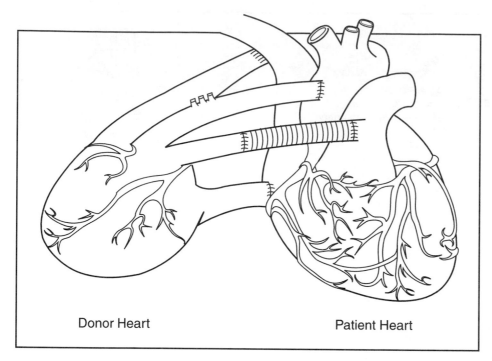

Donor Heart

Patient Heart

FIGURE 20–9. Heterotopic procedure. (Adapted from Rafalowski, M: The heterotopic heart transplant patient: Cardiac monitoring challenges. Crit Care Nurs 11:28, 1991.)

gery. First, the patient has no autonomic innervation of the heart after the procedure,[28] and the resting heart rate will be higher than normal, between 90 and 110 beats/min. Sinus rhythm is usually established, but it lacks the respiratory variations. The transplanted heart will also respond to many drugs (e.g., digoxin, verapamil) and treatment modalities (e.g., carotid sinus massage, Valsalva maneuver) in a manner that differs from that of the normal heart, so that these drugs and treatments are frequently ineffective.[28] The transplanted heart should respond appropriately to inotropic drugs. Isuprel is usually used for bradycardia instead of atropine. Caution should be used with negative inotropic drugs (i.e., calcium channel blockers and antiarrthythmics). If symptomatic supraventricular tachycardia occurs, elective cardioversion is often required. Prior to exercise these patients will require a longer warm-up period because the increase in heart

TABLE 20–11
Complications of Cardiac Transplantation

Acute cardiac failure
Low cardiac output state
Hemorrhage
Infection
Acute renal failure
Pulmonary hypertension
ECG abnormalities/arrhythmias
Cerebral vascular accident (CVA)

rate in the transplanted heart occurs in response to an increase in venous return and release of circulating catecholamines, so that the change in heart rate will be slower than normal.[28]

The second difference is the problem of orthostatic hypotension.[28] Normally when a patient sits up and

TABLE 20–12
Heart Transplantation: Immunosuppressive Drugs*

Drug	Mode of Action	Use for Rejection
Cyclosporine (Sandimmune)	Inhibits T-cell production and function	Prevention
Antithymocyte globulin (ATG, RAT6)	Suppresses T lymphocytes	Prevention and treatment
Azathioprine (Imuran)	Inhibits purine and DNA synthesis of T cells	Prevention
Corticosteroids (prednisone, methylprednisolone)	Suppress T and B lymphocytes Inhibit mobility of macrophages Inhibit leukocyte migration and vascular dilatation	Prevention and treatment
Muromonab-CD3 (Orthoclone OKT3)	Removes circulating T cells	Prevention and treatment
Methotrexate	Interferes with purine synthesis, inhibiting humoral and cellular immunity	Treatment of persistent rejection

*Can be used alone or in combination.

develops hypotension, a reflex tachycardia occurs to compensate for the drop in blood pressure. This does not occur in the transplanted heart. When getting patients out of bed, extreme caution must be taken to assure that the patient is not dizzy or hypotensive.

The next difference affects the early postoperative phase. The new heart is usually smaller. It is placed in the old pericardial sac, which is larger because the old diseased heart was enlarged. Due to the difference in size, there is room for bleeding to occur and remain unnoticed. Although the patient has a mediastinal tube in place, the nurse must promote drainage by keeping the head of the bed elevated at an angle of 30 degrees warranting patient tolerance (i.e., not hypotensive or in shock).[28]

The ECG will appear different also:
1. Usually there will be a second P wave visible. The conduction from this impulse is generated in a normal fashion from the SA node, but it never crosses the suture line.
2. If the patient is placed on cyclosporin, the voltage of the QRS complex will be decreased.
3. If a heterotopic transplant was performed, there will be two QRS complexes, one from each heart.

A final difference is that the patient will not experience any chest pain or discomfort in response to myocardial ischemia because the sensory nerves have been severed during the transplantation. Early in the postoperative course, the nurse must keep a close watch on the patient's ECG for signs of ischemia or rejection (Table 20–13). During the rehabilitative phase the patient undergoes periodic cardiac catheterization, myocardial biopsies, and exercise stress tests to detect ischemia or rejection. Once the heart transplant patient is established hemodynamically, he or she is transferred to a step-down unit. Barring complications, the patient can be discharged as early as 10 days after surgery. The patient is monitored closely for the first several weeks and then monthly for at least 3 to 6 months. After transplantation, monitoring and diagnosis of organ rejection are based on right ventricular endomyocardial biopsies, blood studies, and cardiac catheterizations, which are performed at intervals determined by the recipient's overall condition.[30] Table 20–13 lists signs of rejection.

Discharge teaching includes the conventional discharge teaching of the CABG patient, as well as patient and family education about prevention of infection, and signs and symptoms that may indicate the presence of infection and/or rejection. Patient education regarding immunosuppressant therapy and other medications, including dosage, desired actions, side effects, and precautions, is essential.

CASE STUDY: MYOCARDIAL REVASCULARIZATION

Mr. DS, who is 48 years old, was admitted for myocardial revascularization. His cardiac catheterization revealed 90% occlusion of the left main coronary artery, 85% of the left anterior descending, 90% of the circumflex, and 60% of the right coronary.

Your admission history and assessment reveal:

BP 120/70	HR 76	RR 18	T98.4°F orally
Ht 6 ft 1 in	Wt 204 lb	Heart sounds normal: no S_3 or S_4	

Peripheral pulses: +3 and equal bilaterally

Color: Normal, no cyanosis	Skin turgor: Normal
Capillary refill: <3 sec	No clubbing
ECG: Normal sinus rhythm without ectopy	ST-T waves within normal limits
Lungs clear to apex	
Chest excursion normal	No chest deformities noted

Labs: Na 140 K 4.0   Cl 101 CO_2 32   Hg 16
  ABGs: pH 7.39 PCO_2 41 Po_2 96 HCO_3- 28
         Hct 48   Ca 5.1   Mg 3.0
         SaO_2 99%
  Cholesterol 200   HDL 46 Triglycerides 156
  Blood type: A−   Platelets 280,000 PT 18
         Ptt 92   APTT 35
  Plasminogen 4.6   Bleeding time 3

Allergies: Seasonal only. Smokes 5 cigarettes a day. Drinks a glass of wine at dinner and up to 6 beers a week. Denies drug use.

Strong family history of heart disease, negative diabetes, negative COPD, negative asthma, negative peripheral vascular disease, negative seizures, negative psychiatric problems.

TABLE 20–13
Signs of Cardiac Transplant Rejection

Type	Occurrence	Cause	Diagnosis/Prevention	Treatment
Hyperacute	In the operating room	Antibodies of recipient act against donor antigens	ABO blood and lymphocyte crossmatching	Immediate retransplantation
Acute	2–12 weeks after surgery	Interstitial and perivascular mononuclear cell infiltration progresses to necrosis if not treated	Endomyocardial biopsy weekly for the first 6–8 weeks*	Immunosuppressive drugs, especially ATG or OKT3
Chronic	20–30 weeks after surgery	Immune-mediated injury to the coronary arteries, which leads to diffuse coronary artery disease	First sign is a decrease in exercise tolerance; stress tests; cardiac catheterization	Immunosuppressive drugs, retransplant

*The use of urine polyamine levels is currently under study.

DS is a policeman with 5 more years to retire. He is married, with four children ages 6, 10, 14, and 20. He is physically active, playing soccer and baseball, and working out at the gym three times a week. He coaches his children's soccer and baseball teams. He and his wife are active in the community. DS and his wife have been married for 25 years and share a strong relationship.

During the admission interview, DS says, "Why me? I do all the doctors tell me to do. I follow my diet. Why me?"

Questions

1. Based on your history and assessment findings, how would you respond to his statement?
2. DS appears to be very anxious about the surgery. What findings in your history and assessment may affect his anxiety?
3. What assessment findings need immediate attention?
4. You start preoperative teaching with DS and his wife. What aspects of preoperative teaching would you focus on initially?
5. What aspects need further input from DS and his wife?

As you continue to explain preoperative procedures to DS and his wife, he appears more relaxed and starts to ask questions concerning the surgery. Then he asks, "Am I going to die? Am I going to be an invalid? A friend of mine had this procedure and now his wife must do everything for him. What if I need blood? You know I have A− blood."

Questions

6. How would you best respond to his questions?
7. You are preparing DS for surgery the next day. For what nursing actions are you responsible other than teaching and psychological support?

DS had a triple CABG and an internal mammary graft. The surgery was uneventful. Upon arriving in the ICU, assessment findings are:

BP 140/74   HR 72   RR 26   T 93°F (core)
PAP 18   PCWP 10   MAP 80
Hg 12   Hct 36   PT 18   PTT 100
Extremities: Cold, slightly cyanotic. Pulses: +2 equal bilaterally. Capillary refill: >3 sec
ECG: Normal sinus rhythm with rare PVCs
Resp: Breathing assisted by ventilator; lungs clear
Mediastinal tubes to pleuro-vac: drainage 300 cc mark.
GU: Urine clear yellow via Foley
GI: Bowel sound absent
Neuro: Unresponsive except to pain; pupils equal and reactive

Question

8. What would your nursing actions be at this time based on these assessment findings?

First hour post-op assessment findings are:

BP 190/90   HR 120   RR 16   T 95°F (core)
PAP 27   PCWP 16   MAP 100
ECG: Sinus tachycardia with occassional PVCs
Urine output: 30 cc
Mediastinal drainage: 100 cc

Questions

9. What nursing diagnoses would you formulate at this time?
10. Based on these findings, what medications would you expect the physician to order? Why?

Second hour post-op assessment findings are:

BP 120/70   HR 88   RR 16   T 97°F (core)
PAP 21   PCWP 11   MAP 90
Color: Normal   Capillary refill: <3 sec
Urine output: 30 cc
Mediastinal drainage: 75 cc
Neuro: Responds to verbal stimuli, pupils equal and reactive

Questions

11. What potential nursing diagnoses would you formulate at this time?
12. What nursing actions would you prepare for?

Third hour post-op assessment findings are:

BP 90/50   HR 60   RR 16   T 99°F (core)
Urine output: 20 cc
Mediastinal drainage: 60 cc
Neuro: Alert, oriented, cooperative; pupils equal and reactive

Questions

13. Physiologically, what is happening?
14. What nursing actions would you expect to follow at this time?

Fifth hour post-op assessment findings are:

BP 120/68   HR 52   RR 16   T 99°F (core)
Hg 12   Hct 36
Urine output: 35 cc
Mediastinal drainage: 60 cc

Questions

15. What nursing diagnosis would you establish at this time?
16. What nursing actions would you anticipate?

Seventh hour post-op assessment findings are:

BP 100/56   HR 60   RR 20
Hg 10   Hct 30
ECG: 100% paced rhythm
Urine output: 25 cc/h for the past 2 h
Mediastinal drainage: 100 cc the 6th hour, 120 cc the 7th
Neuro: Alert, slightly confused, restless

Questions

17. What additional parameters need to be monitored?
18. What nursing actions would you anticipate?

Day 1 post-op: DS is now hemodynamically stable. You are getting ready to get him out of bed for the first time.

Questions

19. What preparations do you need to do before getting DS out of bed?
20. How would you respond to DS stating "I can't get out of bed. My chest will burst open"?

Day 2 post-op: DS's mediastinal tubes are to be discontinued. He is to be transferred to the step-down unit later this afternoon.

Questions

21. What preparations would you make prior to the mediastinal tubes being discontinued?
22. What teaching would you do to get DS prepared for transfer?
23. DS asks "What about the incisions? Aren't they too red? Who'll take care of them?" These questions are demonstrating what?
24. How would you respond to the above questions?

Day 5 post-op: DS is to be discharged tomorrow.

Question

25. In preparing DS for discharge, what aspects of care would you emphasize?

CASE STUDY: CARDIOPULMONARY BYPASS

Mr. ED is a 68-year-old man who, coming off cardiopulmonary bypass, was hemodynamically unstable and was placed on the IABP. He has been on IABP for 3 days and the surgeons are considering placing him on ventricular assist.

Questions

1. What nursing diagnoses would you formulate at this time?

2. What nursing activities would you expect that would be different from those initiated for the CABG patient?

CASE STUDY: MITRAL VALVE PROLAPSE

Mrs. AF is a 28-year-old with a history of mitral prolapse. She has been treated medically but now is in severe heart failure. A mitral valve replacement is planned for tomorrow.

Questions

1. What preoperative teaching would you expect to do?
2. What type of valve would you expect to be implanted? Why?
3. How would the postoperative teaching topics differ from those of a CABG patient?

CASE STUDY: CARDIAC TRANSPLANTATION

DJ is a 38-year-old man in end-stage cardiac failure, with approximately 3 months to live. He is awaiting heart transplantation. He is 5 ft 8 in and weighs 170 lb. He has a wife, three children, two brothers, and one sister.

BA is a 42-year-old woman with a brain tumor. She was declared brain dead 4 days ago. She is hemodynamically stable. She is 5 ft 7 in tall, weighs 120 lb.

RZ is a 16-year-old male declared brain dead 15 minutes ago. He was in an motorcycle accident and sustained head and severe chest injuries. He is 5 ft 8 in tall and weighs 220 lb.

ZA is a 40-year-old woman who was robbed and pushed down the subway stairs. She suffered severe head injuries. She is a newly diagnosed diabetic, diet controlled. She is 5 ft 5 in tall and weighs 140 lb.

Questions

1. What criteria for transplantation does DJ meet?
2. Which of the above patients would be a potential donor for DJ? Why?
3. When the transplant coordinator calls concerning the potential donor, what information should be available?
4. What lab studies will be done to confirm compatibility between donor and recipient?
5. What preoperative teaching will DJ need?
6. What postoperative teaching will DJ need?

REFERENCES

1. McHale, DJ: Interventions for acute myocardial infarction: PTCA and CABGS. Critical Care Nurse Quarterly 12(2):38–47, 1989.
2. Penchofer, SM and Holm, K: Women undergoing coronary artery bypass surgery: Physiological and psychosocial perspectives. Cardiovascular Nursing 26(3):13–18, 1990.
3. Allen, JK: Physical and psychosocial outcomes after coronary

artery bypass surgery: Review of the literature. Heart Lung 19:49–54, 1990.

4. Pollick, C: Coronary artery bypass surgery: Which patients benefit? Canadian Family Physician 39(2):318–323, 1993.

5. Kenner, CV, Guzzetts, CE, and Dossey, BM: Critical-Care Nursing: Mind-Body-Spirit, ed 2. Little Brown, Boston 1985.

6. Weeks, LC (ed): Advanced Cardiovascular Nursing. Blackwell Scientific, Boston, 1986.

7. Lewis, SM and Collier, IC: Medical-Surgical Nursing: Assessment of Clinical Problems. McGraw-Hill, New York, 1983.

8. Cisar, NS and Morphew, SF: Preoperative teaching: Aortocoronary bypass patients. Focus on Critical Care 10(1):21–25, 1983.

9. Sadler, D: Nursing for Cardiovascular Health. Appleton-Century-Crofts, Norwalk, CT, 1984.

10. Zoche, DA (ed): Mosby's Comprehensive Review of Critical Care, ed 3. CV Mosby, St. Louis, 1986.

11. Zellinger, M and Leinberger, TP: Use of the rubber dam after open heart surgery. Critical Care Nurse 11(3):24–27, 1991.

12. Marshall, J, Penckofer, S, and Llewellen, J: Structured postoperative teaching and knowledge and compliance of patients who had coronary bypass surgery. Heart Lung 15:76–82, 1986.

13. Penckofer, S and Llewellen, J: Adherence to risk-factor instructions one year following coronary artery bypass surgery. Journal of Cardiovascular Nursing 3(3):10–23, 1989.

14. Gortner, SR, Dirks, J, and Wolfe, MM: The road to recovery for elders after CABG. Am J Nurs 92:44–49, 1992.

15. Culligan, M: Preventing graft leg complications in CABG patients. Nursing 20(6):59–61, 1990.

16. Packa, DR: Quality of life of cardiac patients: A review. Journal of Cardiovascular Nursing 3(2):1–9, 1989.

17. Koroteyev, A, et al: Skeletal muscle: New technique for treating heart failure. Journal of the Association of Operating Room Nurses 53(4):1005–1020, 1991.

18. Kolvekar, S and Forsyth, A: Valvular surgery. Cardiology Update 5(32):48–49, 1991.

19. Hamilton, HK (ed): Nurse's Clinical Library: Cardiovascular Disorders. Springhouse, Springhouse, PA, 1984.

20. Akins, CW: Review of the global experience with the Medtronic-Hall valve. Eur J Cardiothorac Surg 6:568–573, 1992.

21. Rowe, GG: Ventricular aneurysm: Current concepts. Hospital Medicine 21(9):21–34, 1985.

22. Dacron patch improves outcome of ventricular aneurysm. CV Nurse: Trends in Cardiovascular Care 5(1):9, 1992.

23. Barden, C and Lee, R: Update on ventricular assist devices. AACN Clinical Issues in Critical Care Nursing 1(1):13–29, 1990.

24. Quaal, SJ: VADs: Beyond intra-aortic balloon pumping. CV Nurse: Trends in Cardiovascular Care 5(1):4–8, 1992.

25. Vaska, PL: Biventricular assist devices. Critical Care Nurse 11(6):52–60, 1991.

26. Gill, B: Cardiac transplantation: Issues of donor procurement and management. Journal of Critical Care Nursing 2(2):32–38, 1988.

27. Imperial, FA, Cordova-Manigbas, L, and Ward, CR: Cardiac transplantation. Critical Care Nursing Clinics of North America 1(2):399–415, 1989.

28. Funk, M: Heart transplantation: Postoperative care during the acute period. Critical Care Nurse 6(2):27–46, 1986.

29. Painvin, GA, et al: Cardiac transplantation: Indications, procurement, operation and management. Heart Lung 14:484–489, 1985.

30. Murdock, DK, et al: Rejection of the transplanted heart. Heart Lung 16:237–245, 1987.

SUGGESTED READINGS

Abou-Awdi, N: High-tech help for the failing heart. RN 54(5):42–44, 1991.

Akins, CW: Hypothermic fibrillatory arrest for coronary artery bypass grafting. Journal of Cardiac Surgery 7(4): 1992.

Allen, JK, Becker, DM, and Swandk, RT: Factors related to functional status after coronary artery bypass surgery. Heart Lung 19:337–342, 1990.

Artinian, NT: Family member perceptions of a cardiac surgery event. Focus on Critical Care 16(4):301–308, 1989.

Artinian, NT: Stress experience of spouses of patients having coronary artery bypass during hospitalization and 6 weeks after discharge. Heart Lung 20:52–58, 1991.

Barr, WJ: Teaching patients with life-threatening illnesses: Disease, transplantation, and organ donation. Nurs Clin North Am 24:639–644, 1989.

Ball, GB and Grap, MJ: Postoperative GI symptoms in cardiac surgery patients. Critical Care Nurse 12(1):56–62, 1992.

Bayer, AS, Nelson, RT, and Slama, TG: Current concepts in prevention of prosthetic valve endocarditis. Chest 97:1203–1207, 1990.

Bradley, KM and Williams, DM: A comparison of the preoperative concerns of open heart surgery patients and their significant others. Journal of Cardiovascular Nurse 5(1):43–53, 1990.

Brenner, ZR: Patient's learning priorities for reoperative coronary artery bypass surgery. Journal of Cardiovascular Nursing 7(2):1–12, 1992.

Buse, SM and Peiper, B: Impact of cardiac transplantation on the spouse's life. Heart Lung 19:641–647, 1990.

Carbone, S, Gheen, ML, and McKenna, BG: A patient-education path for cardiac surgery. Am J Nurs 92:24D, 1992.

Cardan, S and Clark, S: A nursing diagnosis approach to the patient awaiting cardiac transplant. Heart Lung 14:499–504, 1985.

Cifani, L and Vargo, R: Teaching strategies for the transplant recipient: A review of future directions. Focus on Critical Care 17(6): 1990.

Copel, LC and Stolarik, A: Impact of nursing care activities on $S\dot{V}O_2$ levels of postoperative cardiac surgery patients. Cardiovascular Nursing 27(1):1–5, 1991.

Cupples, SA: Effects of timing and reinforcement of preoperative education on knowledge and recovery of patients having coronary artery bypass graft surgery. Heart Lung 20:654–660, 1991.

Dargie, HJ: Late results following coronary artery bypass grafting. Eur Heart J 13:89–95, 1992.

Dault, LA, Nagy, CS, and Collins, JA: Reversing cardiac transplant rejection with Orthoclone OKT3. Am J Nurs 89:953–955, 1989.

Edwards, BS and Rodeheffer, RJ: Prognostic features in patients with congestive heart failure and selection criteria for cardiac transplantation. Mayo Clin Proc 67:485–492, 1992.

Fitzgerald, ST: Occupational outcomes after treatment for coronary heart disease: A review of the literature. Cardiovascular Nursing 25(1):1–6, 1989.

Futterman, LG: Cardiac transplantation: A comprehensive nursing perspective, I. Heart Lung 17:499–509, 1988.

Garvin, BJ, Huston, GP, and Baker, CF: Information used by nurses to prepare patients for a stressful event. Applied Nursing Research 5(4):158–163, 1992.

Gillis, CL, et al: A randomized clinical trial of nursing care for recovery from cardiac surgery. Heart Lung 22:125–133, 1993.

Gillis, CL, Neuhaus, JM, and Hauck, WW: Improving family functioning after cardiac surgery: A randomized trial. Heart Lung 19:648–653, 1990.

Grady, KL: Development of a cardiac transplantation program: Role of the clinical nurse specialist. Heart Lung 4:490–494, 1984.

Grady, KL: Evolution of a cardiac transplantation program: Role of the clinical nurse specialist. Focus on Critical Care 16(2):130, 1989.

Grady, KL, et al: Symptom distress in cardiac transplant patients. Heart Lung 21:490–494, 1992.

Halfman, M, Gabel, K, and Berg, DE: Reoperation: Cardiac surgery. AACN Clinical Issues in Critical Care Nursing 1(1):72–78 1990.

Hill, M: Teaching after CABG surgery: A family affair. Critical Care Nurse 9(4):59–72, 1989.

Hutchings, SM and Monett, ZJ: Caring for the cardiac transplant patient. Critical Care Nursing Clinics of North America 1(2):245–261, 1989.

Jameison, WR: Modern cardiac valve devices—bioprostheses and mechanical prostheses: State of the art. Journal of Cardiac Surgery 8(1):89–98, 1993.

King, KK, et al: Patient perceptions of quality of life after coronary artery surgery: Was it worth it? Res Nurs Health 5:327–334, 1992.

Knapp-Spooner, C and Yarcheski, A: Sleep patterns and stress in patients having coronary bypass. Heart Lung 21:342–439, 1992.

Kretten, CK and Bass, L: Valvular heart disease: Surgery and post-op care. RN 50(12):38–43, 1987.

Lang, SS, et al: Issues in transplantation: Infection control practices in cardiac transplant recipients. Heart Lung 21:101–105, 1992.

Leahy, NM: Neurologic complications of open heart surgery. Journal of Cardiovascular Nursing 7(2):41–51, 1993.

Lough, ME: Quality of life for heart transplant recipients. Progress in Cardiovascular Nursing 2(2):11–22, 1986.

Luquire, R and Houston, S: Ethical concerns regarding cardiac retransplantation. Nursing Economics 10(6):413–417, 1992.

Lyons, M: Immunosuppressive therapy after cardiac transplantation: Teaching pediatric patients and their families. Critical Care Nurse 13(9):39–45, 1993.

Mahon, PM: Orthoclone OK3 and cardiac transplantation: An overview. Critical Care Nurse 11(3):42–47, 1991.

Marchetta, S and Stennis, E: Ventricular assist devices: Applications for critical care. Journal of Cardiovascular Nursing 2(2):39–55, 1988.

Menkis, AH, Carley, SD, and Clough, TM: Reoperation after coronary bypass grafting. Canadian Family Physician 39(2):325–332, 1993.

Miller, KM and Perry, PA: Relaxation technique and postoperative pain in patients undergoing cardiac surgery. Heart Lung 19:136–143, 1990.

Miller, P, et al: Marital functioning after cardiac surgery. Heart Lung 19:55–61, 1990.

Muirhead, J: Heart and heart-lung transplantation. Critical Care Nursing Clinics of North America 4(1):97–109, 1992.

Nolan, MT, et al: Perceived stress and coping strategies among families of cardiac transplant candidates during organ waiting period. Heart Lung 2:540–547, 1992.

O'Mara, RJ: Dilemmas in cardiac surgery: Artificial heart and left ventricular assist device. Critical Care Nurse Quarterly 10(2):48–55, 1987.

Payne, JL: Immune modification and complications of immunosuppression. Critical Care Nursing Clinics of North America 4(1):43–57, 1992.

Pedersen, A, et al: Intramuscular administration of RATG in the heart transplant patient. Critical Care Nurse 13(1):22–31, 1993.

Pieper, B, Lepczyk, M, and Caldwell, M: Perceptions of the waiting period before coronary artery bypass grafting. Heart Lung 14:40–44, 1985.

Porter, RR, et al: Stress during the waiting period: A review of pre-transplantation fears. Critical Care Nurse Quarterly 13(4):25–31, 1991.

Rafalowski, M: The heterotopic heart transplant patient: Cardiac monitoring challenges. Critical Care Nurse 11(2):28–30, 1991.

Rice, VH, Mullin, MH, and Jarosz, P: Preadmission self-instruction effects on postadmission and postoperative indicators in CABG patients: Partial replication and extension. Research in Nursing and Health 15(4):253–259, 1992.

Schoen, FJ and Levy, RJ: Heart valve bioprostheses: Antimineralization. Eur J Cardiothorac Surg 6 Suppl 1:591–593, 1992.

Smith, A: Case example: Embolization after prosthesis implantation. Am J Nurs 91:65–66, 1991.

Smith, A: Case example: Cardiac tamponade after coronary bypass. Am J Nurs 91:69–70, 1991.

Stewart, JV, et al: Cardiomyoplasty: Treatment of the failing heart using the skeletal muscle wrap. Journal of Cardiovascular Nursing 7(2):23–31, 1993.

Valente, M, et al: Heart valve bioprosthesis durability: A challenge to the new generation of porcine valves. Eur J Cardiothorac Surg 6:582–590, 1992.

Vargo, RL: Bridging to transplant: Mechanical support for heart failure. Critical Care Nursing Clinics of North America 5(4):649–659, 1993.

Walden, JA, et al: Heart transplantation may not improve quality of life for patients with stable heart failure. Heart Lung 18:497–505, 1985.

Whitman, GR and Hicks, LE: Major nursing diagnoses following cardiac transplantation. Journal of Cardiovascular Nursing 2(2):1–10, 1988.

Weiland, AP: A review of cardiac valve prostheses and their selection. Heart Lung 12:498–504, 1983.

CARE PLAN FOR PREOPERATIVE CARE OF THE CARDIAC SURGICAL PATIENT

Nursing Diagnoses

Nursing Diagnosis #1
Anxiety, related to upcoming cardiac surgery

Desired Patient Outcomes

The patient will demonstrate decreased anxiety by indicating willingness to discuss the following:
1. Normal function of the heart
2. Disease process including:
   • Risk factors
   • Surgical procedure
   • Expected outcomes of the surgery

Nursing Interventions

• Teach the patient about the normal function of the heart; underlying disease process including risk factors; the surgical procedure; and the expected outcomes of the surgery.

• Use simple terms or explain medical terms used.

• Utilize posters, models, and handouts/pamphlets.
• Teach in short blocks if time allows.

• Observe patient's nonverbal cues.

• Allow time for questions.

Rationales

• Teaching provides a basic understanding of the problem, the solution, and what to expect, thereby decreasing the patient's anxiety. However, not all patients experience a decreased level of anxiety when bombarded with new information.
• Using simple terms for explaining medical terms enhances learning because the patient can understand the explanations. Using medical terms sometimes confuses and overwhelms the patient.
• Visualization aids learning.
• Allows assimilation of information before more is added, and thus enhances learning.
• Enables the nurse to evaluate patient's understanding and anxiety level. The nurse can determine whether to proceed, reiterate, or stop.
• Relieves anxiety, clarifies information, and prevents misconceptions.

CARE PLAN FOR PREOPERATIVE CARE OF THE CARDIAC SURGICAL PATIENT
(*Continued*)

Nursing Interventions	Rationales
• Answer questions honestly.	• Establishes a trusting relationship and attains patient cooperation.
• Maintain a calm, relaxed, nonrushed atmosphere with little or no interruptions.	• Enhances the learning experience.
• Have the patient discuss the information in his or her own words.	• Assists in evaluating what has been learned.
• Correct any misconceptions.	• Patient knows what to expect, thereby reducing some of his or her anxiety.

Nursing Diagnoses	Desired Patient Outcomes
Nursing Diagnosis #2 Knowledge deficit regarding preoperative and postoperative expectations	Patient will verbalize an understanding of the preoperative routine: 1. Tests, procedures 2. Medications 3. The night before the surgery 4. The day of the surgery 5. The immediate postoperative care Patient will demonstrate activities expected to be performed in the postoperative period: 1. Coughing and deep breathing (see Table 20–3) 2. Splinting the chest incision 3. Use of the incentive spirometer 4. Arm and leg exercises 5. Turning side to side 6. Getting out of bed the day after the surgery

Nursing Interventions	Rationales
• Provide information regarding the following: ○ Tests and procedures that will be performed before surgery:	○ This is a time when the patient needs and wants to be with family but is frequently interrupted, causing frustration and sometimes anger. Knowing about these studies ahead of time will help in coping with the interruptions.
▫ Blood studies: CBC, serum electrolytes, BUN, creatinine, cardiac enzymes, clotting time, prothrombin time, fibrinogen levels, platelets, type and crossmatch of blood, arterial blood gases	▫ To evaluate baseline values. If any abnormal values are present, treatment can be initiated so as to prevent complications intraoperatively and postoperatively. Patient is typed/crossmatched to ensure blood is available if needed.
▫ ECG	▫ Provides a baseline for comparison.
▫ Chest x-ray	▫ To examine for abnormalities; provides a baseline for comparison.
▫ Urinalysis	▫ To evaluate for signs of infection.
▫ Pulmonary function tests (PFTs)	▫ To evaluate patient's pulmonary status.
○ Changes in medication regimen and necessary preoperative medication:	○ Changes in medication regimen can cause anxiety. Understanding of what the changes will be helps decrease anxiety and enhance patient cooperation.
▫ Sedation the evening prior to surgery.	▫ Decreases anxiety, allows a good night's sleep
▫ All aspirin, anticoagulants, and anti-inflammatory drugs should be discontinued at least 2 days prior to surgery.	▫ Prevents bleeding due to altered coagulation characteristics.
▫ Digitalis is usually held 1–2 days prior to the surgery unless the patient is in uncontrolled atrial fibrillation.	▫ Digitalis toxicity is a common complication postoperatively, related to low potassium levels. If digitalis is given to control atrial fibrillation, the patient must be monitored closely for signs of toxicity postoperatively, especially in the immediate postoperative phase.
▫ Diuretics are discontinued the day of surgery.	▫ Diuretics increase the loss of fluids and potassium, which could cause adverse reactions postoperatively (i.e., hypovolemia, acidemia, hyponatremia, digoxin toxicity).

CARE PLAN FOR PREOPERATIVE CARE OF THE CARDIAC SURGICAL PATIENT
(*Continued*)

Nursing Interventions

□ Nitroglycerin is given at c/o cp at the bedside and can be taken for chest pain or discomfort (as per protocol).
□ Long-acting insulin is changed to regular insulin and patient is placed on a sliding-scale coverage the day of surgery.

□ Potassium supplements may be given to maintain the patient's potassium level at 4.0 mEq/L.

□ Norpace may be discontinued 24 h prior to the surgery.
□ Antiarrhythmics are maintained to control the arrhythmias.

□ Antihypertensive medications are maintained.

□ Prophylactic antibiotics may be given prior to the surgery and continued for 2 days postoperatively.
○ Check the patient for allergies to any medications, especially antibiotics, iodine preparations, or fish.
• The night before the surgery, the patient will:
○ Receive a light dinner, then nothing to eat or drink after midnight.
○ Be shaved from the chin to the toes (CABG) or chin to shins (valve replacement).
○ Shower with an antibacterial agent (e.g., Betadine).

• The morning of the surgery, the patient will:
○ Shower again with the antibacterial agent.
○ Put on a hospital gown.
○ Receive a preoperative sedative.
○ Receive family for a brief visit (according to hospital policy).
○ Give valuables to the family to take home.

○ Be transferred to a stretcher and transported to the OR.
• Explain the immediate postoperative care and inform the patient of the ICU routine:
○ Patients remain in the ICU for 2–3 days if no complications occur.
○ The unit may be noisy and the lights left on.
○ Patients are checked frequently for vital signs and assessments.
○ Visiting hours are restricted to brief periods.
○ A tour of the unit is offered to those who want it. Patient may be able to meet the nurse who will be taking care of her or him in the ICU.

• Explain expectations of postoperative period (e.g., equipment, routines). Patient will:

○ Have an endotracheal tube connected to a ventilator that will help with breathing

Rationales

□ Relieves chest pain associated with anxiety.

□ Insulin requirements change due to the stress of the surgery and NPO status. Administration of insulin on a sliding scale provides a more precise dosage to meet the patient's needs, thereby preventing hyperglycemia or hypoglycemia.
□ To prevent intraoperative and postoperative complications (e.g., acidemia, digoxin toxicity, arrhythmias).
□ Norpace may cause heart failure in the postoperative phase.
□ To prevent further decrease in the cardiac output related to the arrhythmias; to help prevent serious or life-threatening arrhythmias.
□ To maintain the patient's blood pressure. Nitroprusside (Nipride) can be given intraoperatively.
□ To prevent infection.

○ Prevents anaphylaxis.

○ Prevents aspiration of the stomach contents.

○ Decreases the possibility of infection since skin and hair harbor bacteria.
○ Decreases the possibility of infection by decreasing the number of bacteria on the skin.

○ Decreases anxiety and helps the patient to relax.
○ Allays anxiety of patient and family.

○ There is little room in the ICU for the patient's personal effects. Family will be told what to bring in when it is needed.

• Knowing what to expect decreases the patient's anxiety and enhances cooperation.

○ The patient should understand that frequent assessments are part of usual ICU protocols. It does not mean that anything is wrong.
○ Awareness of the unit's environment will decrease the anxiety level for some patients. The patient will not become alarmed in response to the noise, frequent monitoring of vital signs, and absence of family except during brief visits.
• Knowledge regarding expectations of care enables the patient to be cooperative and participate in care (e.g., not trying to pull the tubes out, fighting procedures, afraid of moving). The patient needs to know that needs will be anticipated and a method of communication must be worked out. This serves to reduce anxiety.
○ The endotracheal tube is usually left in place for 8–24 h.

CARE PLAN FOR PREOPERATIVE CARE OF THE CARDIAC SURGICAL PATIENT
(*Continued*)

Nursing Interventions

- ○ Be unable to talk

- ○ Experience breathlessness when suctioned

- The patient will:
  - ○ Have a Foley catheter postoperatively
  - ○ Have peripheral, jugular, and subclavian IVs

  - ○ Have an arterial line for approximately 1 day

  - ○ Be connected to a cardiac monitor
  - ○ Have mediastinal tubes in place for approximately 2 days

- Explain the various suture lines.

  - ○ Advise the patient that Ace bandages or elastic stockings are applied postoperatively.

- Demonstrate and have the patient demonstrate activities to be performed postoperatively:

  - ○ Pain medication will be given prior to the exercises (as indicated).
  - ○ Coughing and deep breathing: take 4–5 deep breaths, then cough.

  - ○ Splinting the chest incision.
  - ○ Arm exercises–range of motion and walking up the wall.
  - ○ Leg exercises–ankle range of motion, "ankle pump," and dorsiflexion.
  - ○ Turning side to side every 2 h.
  - ○ Getting out of bed—splint chest.
  - ○ Inch legs over the side of the bed. Sit up straight on the edge of the bed, then ease the feet down to the floor. Nurses will be present for support and guidance of tubings.

Rationales

- ○ An alternate means of communication should be set up (e.g., mouthing words, finger writing, sign language).
- ○ The patient should know that the feeling of breathlessness, should it occur, will last only a few seconds.
- ○ The patient should be encouraged to breathe with the ventilator and not to "fight" the ventilator.

- ○ Allows for accurate measurement of urine output.
- ○ Access for emergency medications, fluids, blood and blood products, and plasma expanders as needed. Once the patient is stabilized postoperatively, all but one will be discontinued while in the ICU.
- ○ Access for arterial blood gases and other blood specimens. Allows for continuous monitoring of arterial blood pressure.
- ○ To monitor heart rhythm and rate.
- ○ Allows evaluation of bleeding in the chest, which may indicate improper closure of a graft, cardiac tamponade, or coagulation abnormality.
- ○ The drainage will be bloody initially and then gradually become serous.

- Patient will have a midline chest incision (medial sternotomy) that will be dressed initially. The dressing is usually removed 24 h postoperatively. Patient may have some chest discomfort related to the sternum being opened; this pain differs from the chest pain experienced previously. Pain medication will be available.
- Patient will have an incision in one or both legs. It may extend from the thigh to the knee, the thigh to the ankle, or the knee to the ankle, depending on the amount of graft needed, the surgeon's preference, and the condition of the vein.
- Note: When a mammary artery is used as bypass graft, incisions in lower extremities are unlikely.
  - ○ Ace bandages/elastic stockings aid in the venous return from the legs; they are also used to prevent thrombi.
- Enhances cooperation in the postoperative activities needed to prevent complications. Ensures that the patient knows what must be done, why, and how it is to be done.
  - ○ Decreases the amount of pain so the exercises can be done effectively.
  - ○ Prevent atelectasis and pneumonia.
  - ○ Deep breaths loosen the secretions so they can be mobilized.
  - ○ Decreases the amount of pain.
  - ○ Prevent frozen shoulder.

  - ○ Increase circulation in the lower extremities and prevent stasis and thrombosis. Range of motion also prevents foot drop.

  - ○ Early ambulation helps prevent many complications, especially pneumonia and thrombosis. It is not as simple a task postoperatively as patients may believe.

CARE PLAN FOR EARLY POSTOPERATIVE CARE OF THE CARDIAC SURGICAL PATIENT

Nursing Diagnoses

Nursing Diagnosis #1

Cardiac Output, decreased, related to:
1. Cardiopulmonary bypass
2. Low cardiac output syndrome

Desired Patient Outcomes

Patient will demonstrate stabilization of body function as supported by monitoring and life-support systems:
1. Arterial blood pressure within 10 mmHg of patient's baseline
2. Stable pulmonary artery pressures:
   - PAP <25 mmHg
   - PCWP 8–12 mmHg
   - CVP 0–8 mmHg
3. Cardiac output ~ 5 L/min
   - Heart rate between 60 and 100 beats/min
4. Urine output >30 mL/h
5. Alert mental status: oriented to person, place, time
6. Electrolyte balance
7. Acid-base balance:
   - pH 7.35–7.45
   - Pao_2 >80 mmHg
   - $Paco_2$ 35–45 mmHg
8. Stable hematology profile:*
   - Hct: Male, 45%–52%
     Female, 37%–48%
   - Hgb: Male, 13–18 g/100 mL
     Female, 12–16 g/100 mL
   - Platelet count: 150,000–450,000/mm³

Nursing Interventions

- Monitor vital signs (BP, heart rate, respiratory rate, and temperature) q5 min while rewarming, then q15 min until stable, then q1h×12.
- Assess the patient q1h until stable, including heart sounds; ECG changes; cardiac rhythm; neck veins; lung sounds; peripheral pulses; capillary refill; skin turgor, color, and temperature; movement and sensation.

- Monitor hemodynamic parameters: Mean arterial pressure (MAP), pulmonary artery pressure (PAP), pulmonary capillary wedge pressure (PCWP), central venous pressure (CVP) or right atrial pressure (RAP), and left atrial pressure (LA).
- Assess the pacemaker concerning type (fixed or demand), the rate it is set at, the milliamperes (mA), and whether it is functioning properly.

   ○ Keep exposed wires wrapped in gauze and place in a plastic covering.
- Report any abnormalities in vital parameters to physician immediately:
   ○ BP: Systolic <80 mmHg, >180 mmHg
        Diastolic >100 mmHg
   ○ MAP: <60 mmHg, >100 mmHg
   ○ CVP: <5 cmH₂O, >15 cmH₂O

   ○ Heart rate: <60 beats/min, >100 beats/min

Rationales

- Frequent monitoring of the vital signs allows early detection of abnormalities, and treatment can be initiated to prevent complications.
- Changes may indicate hemodynamic decompensation or complications. Signs of low cardiac output syndrome include a decrease in arterial pressure, urine output below 30 mL/h, signs of vasoconstriction (cool, pale, or cyanotic skin and mucous membranes), tachycardia, arrhythmias, tachypnea, narrow pulse pressure, weak peripheral pulses, decrease in level of consciousness, restlessness.
- Parameters will reflect left ventricular function, fluid status, and arterial perfusion.

- Need to be familiar with equipment in order to use it properly, identify if it is functioning properly, and how to troubleshoot problems. Pacemaker is usually kept on standby to keep the patient's heart rate above 60 beats/min and to treat other arrhythmias. (Cardiac pacing is discussed in detail in Chapter 17.)
   ○ Prevents the possibility of electric shock or short circuit.
- Immediate intervention can be ordered to prevent further deterioration/complications.
   ○ Pressures below 80 mmHg could cause graft closure or indicate shock; pressures above 180 mmHg could cause the graft to "blow," or could cause a CVA.
   ○ CVP readings below 5 cmH₂O indicate inadequate intravascular fluid; readings above 15 cmH₂O indicate fluid overload.
   ○ Heart rates below 60 beats/min could cause graft closure; rates above 100 beats/min will decrease the oxygenation to the myocardium and increase the workload of the heart.

CARE PLAN FOR EARLY POSTOPERATIVE CARE OF THE CARDIAC SURGICAL PATIENT
(*Continued*)

Nursing Interventions	Rationales
° Temperature: remains hypothermic or rises above 101°F.	° Hypothermia prolongs vasoconstriction, adding to low cardiac output syndrome. Temperatures above 101°F may indicate infection.
° Monitor the patient for shivering. Use methods to enhance body warming and prevent shivering, e.g., warm blood products, heart shields, warming blankets or lamps. Administer morphine sulfate or meperidine to decrease shivering.	° Shivering is the body's natural response to cooling. It is triggered in the postanesthesia period by return of the central nervous system's thermoregulatory functions. Shivering increases the body's metabolic rate, oxygen consumption, carbon dioxide production, and myocardial workload. It depresses myocardial contractility and heart rate. It also increases BP.
° Excessive or bloody chest tube drainage >100 mL/h	° Excessive and/or bloody drainage suggests bleeding at surgical site.
° Urine output <30 mL/h	° Reduced urine output warns of prerenal failure.
° Extremities: cool, moist, mottled, with sluggish capillary refill and poor or absent peripheral pulses	° Signs of decreased peripheral perfusion related to emboli or decreased cardiac output. If accompanied by pain, arterial occlusion of the extremity may have occurred.
° A decrease in movement or sensation	° May indicate possible neurologic involvement or may be due to the effect of the anesthesia.
° Presence of anginal pain or ECG changes: ST segment elevation or depression; T wave peaked/inverted	° Indicative of myocardial ischemia.
□ Administer nitroglycerine drip as ordered.	□ Nitroglycerin will cause vasodilation and increase O_2 supply to the myocardium, thereby decreasing angina. Nitroglycerin drips are also used in patients who have had an internal mammary graft to decrease the risk of spasm.

Nursing Diagnoses	Desired Patient Outcomes

Nursing Diagnosis #2
Breathing Pattern, ineffective, related to:
1. General anesthesia
2. Incisional pain with splinting
	The patient will maintain:
	1. A patent airway.
	2. Respiratory rate <25–30/minute; eupneic rhythm.
	3. ABGs within normal range:
	  • pH 7.35–7.45
	  • Pao_2 >80 mmHg
	  • $Paco_2$ 35–45 mmHg
	  • HCO_3 22–26 mEq/L

Nursing Interventions	Rationales
• Assess respiratory function: rate, rhythm, pattern, chest excursion, use of accessory muscles; breath sounds; presence of adventitious sounds.	• It is essential to establish baseline function with which to compare subsequent findings: assists in following trends.
• Maintain patient on ventilator at prescribed settings.	• Maintains patient's respirations when the respiratory center is depressed due to the anesthesia and narcotics. Provides adequate oxygenation. Decreases the workload of the heart.
° Check the endotracheal cuff for adequate inflation.	° Improper cuff inflation reduces tidal volume and may compromise ventilation.
• Administer pain medications to decrease pain and prevent "fighting" the ventilator.	• Pain and "fighting" the ventilator can lead to hyperventilation, which may predispose to respiratory alkalosis. Acid-base imbalances can cause arrhythmias.
	° Tachycardia related to pain can increase workload of the heart.
• Suction prn. Sigh the patient before and after suctioning. (Sigh is a deeper than normal breath with 100% oxygen.)	• Remove secretions for adequate oxygenation and gas exchange. Sighing the patient before and after expands the alveoli, mobilizes the secretions, and prevents drastic drops in the patient's oxygen levels.
° Use hand resuscitator bag to ventilate and preoxygenate prior to and following each suction pass (some mechanical ventilators have "sigh" capability.)	

CARE PLAN FOR EARLY POSTOPERATIVE CARE OF THE CARDIAC SURGICAL PATIENT
(*Continued*)

Nursing Interventions

- Monitor ABGs q1–4 h as the patient's condition warrants; or continuously monitor mixed venous gases ($S\bar{v}O_2$) as prescribed. (*Note:* $S\bar{v}O_2$ is discussed in Chapter 16)
- Wean patient off the ventilator as prescribed, when alert, breathing spontaneously, and demonstrating adequate ABGs and appropriate ventilatory parameters (e.g., inspiratory pressure, expiratory pressure, tidal volume, minute volume, and vital capacity).
- Administer oxygen through a heated humidified face mask or tent after weaning.

- Encourage patient to cough and deep breathe hourly; administer chest percussion; encourage the use of the incentive spirometer q1–2 h while awake.
  - Have respiratory therapist administer intermittent positive pressure breathing and nebulizer treatments as ordered.
- Assess breath sounds q2 h and/or when indicated.

- Notify the physician of any significant abnormalities in respiratory parameters.

Rationales

- Respiratory and metabolic alterations are reflected in the ABGs. Adjustment in the ventilator settings or pharmacologic interventions can be initiated to prevent severe imbalances.
- The patient must be able to breathe spontaneously with adequate respiratory excursion, tidal volume, minute ventilation, and peak inspiratory pressure.

- Provides oxygenation with humidification to assist in thinning the secretions and thereby facilitating deep breathing and coughing.
- Loosens and mobilizes the secretions, thereby preventing atelectasis and pneumonia. Incentive spirometer provides patients with a visual feedback as to how well they are breathing.

- Decreased breath sounds may indicate atelectasis, pneumonia, or poor breathing technique due to splinting. Absence of breath sounds on one side suggests atelectasis or malpositioning of the endotracheal tube. Endotracheal tube may have slipped down into right bronchus. Pneumothorax, if present, is usually accompanied by unequal chest excursion and shifting of trachea to opposite side.
- Interventions may be taken expeditiously to prevent complications.

Nursing Diagnoses

Nursing Diagnosis #3
Fluid Volume deficit, actual and risk for related to:
1. Surgery-related blood loss or hemorrhage
2. NPO status
3. Peripheral vasodilation associated with rewarming (disproportion between size of vascular bed and intravascular blood volume)

Desired Patient Outcomes

Patient will:
1. Maintain stable hemodynamic parameters:
   - BP, pulses, CVP, PAP, PCWP (See Nursing Diagnosis #1, above.)
2. Demonstrate adequate peripheral perfusion; peripheral pulses 2+ bilaterally; brisk capillary refill; skin warm, no cyanosis of nailbeds or mucous membranes
3. Be alert and oriented
4. Maintain urinary output above 30 mL/h with no hematuria
5. Show no sign of hemorrhage (stable vital signs)
6. Maintain a hematocrit above 30%

Nursing Interventions

- Monitor vital signs q15 min while the patient is rewarming.

- Administer fluids as ordered. (Usually less than 100 mL/h total volume unless the patient is hypovolemic).

- Monitor the patient's intake and output carefully. Weigh daily.

Rationales

- The vascular bed increases during rewarming, causing a disproportion in the vascular volume and the vascular bed size. If the disproportion is great enough, the patient will become hypotensive, predisposing to shock. Under these circumstances, there is a risk that the grafts may close off. In response to the hypotension, the patient may develop myocardial ischemia with arrhythmias, prerenal failure, or DIC.
- Adequate fluids are necessary to prevent hypovolemia; overhydration can cause the patient to develop pulmonary edema.
- Patient may be retaining fluid if fluid intake is greater than output plus the insensible losses. Daily weighing is a reliable indicator of hydration status (2.2 lb is equal to 1 L of fluid).

CARE PLAN FOR EARLY POSTOPERATIVE CARE OF THE CARDIAC SURGICAL PATIENT
(*Continued*)

Nursing Interventions	Rationales
• Monitor urine output q1 h; specific gravity q2 h.	• Urine output less than 30 mL/h may indicate decreased cardiac output, hypovolemia, or renal failure. A decrease in specific gravity indicates hypovolemia.
• Monitor BUN and creatinine.	• The BUN is an indicator of renal function and fluid status; the creatinine is an indicator of renal function. The physician should be notified of an increase in either, or of any change in BUN/creatinine ratio.
• Assess skin turgor and mucous membranes for hydration status.	• Tenting of the skin when pinched indicates dehydration. Edema indicates fluid excess or decreased cardiac output. Dry mucous membranes indicate dehydration; moist mucous membranes indicate adequate hydration.
• Monitor hemodynamic parameters, especially when rehydrating the patient.	• PAP, LAP, and CVP will be decreased in volume depletion. As fluids are administered the pressures also will increase. Pressures will be elevated in fluid overload.
• Monitor serum electrolytes and hemoglobin and hematocrit (Hgb and Hct). Administer potassium to maintain level at 4.0 mEq/L.	• Low Hgb and Hct are indicative of blood loss or hemodilution; an elevated Hct is indicative of hemoconcentration. • Elevation of potassium may be related to renal failure, cardiopulmonary bypass, or acid-base imbalance. Abnormal potassium levels can cause arrhythmias.
• Monitor amount and color of chest tube drainage.	• Chest tube drainage greater than 100 mL/h for the first 4 h is indicative of abnormal bleeding, which could be related to platelet destruction, inadequate reversal of the heparin, inadequate suturing of arteries during the surgery, or diffuse intrathoracic ooze.
○ Observe the dressings and bedding for signs of hemorrhage.	○ Bleeding may occur at the suture line. Excessive bleeding may ooze down the patient's side and pool under him or her.
• Monitor coagulation studies.	• Abnormal coagulation caused by anticoagulants or DIC can cause hemorrhage related to oozing at injection sites, suture lines, insertion sites of IVs.
• Administer blood, plasma expanders, and clotting factors as prescribed.	• Blood and plasma expanders are given to maintain the intravascular volume. Fresh-frozen plasma and cryoprecipitate may be administered to bolster concentration of clotting factors to ensure appropriate blood coagulation and prevent hemorrhaging.
○ Autotransfusions may be considered during early post-operative phase.	○ Giving back the patient his or her own blood decreases the possibility of infection by hepatitis or HIV. It also decreases the possibility of transfusion reactions, especially if the patient has a rare blood type or antibodies.

Nursing Diagnoses	Desired Patient Outcomes
Nursing Diagnosis #4 Tissue Perfusion, altered peripheral, related to low cardiac output syndrome	Patient will: 1. Demonstrate normotension (MAP within 10 mmHg of patient's baseline) 2. Demonstrate normothermia (98.6° F, 37.0°C) 3. Maintain palpable peripheral pulses and brisk capillary refill 4. Exhibit warm, dry skin, pink in color with good turgor 5. Maintain heart rate >60 beats/min <100 beats/min 6. Maintain urine output >30 mL/h

Nursing Interventions	Rationales
• Assess peripheral pulses. Compare right with left. Note characteristics: rate, rhythm, quality (bounding, weak, and thready), and equality. ○ Mark sites of pulses if difficult to palpate.	• Peripheral pulses are indicators of the arterial flow through the extremity. An absence or decrease in the pulse may indicate occlusion of the vessel due to emboli. ○ Marking the sites makes it easier to find the pulse, especially if the pulse is weak.
• Assess the skin for temperature, color, capillary refill, breakdown, and sensation.	• Indicators of peripheral perfusion. A decrease may be indicative of poor perfusion.

CARE PLAN FOR EARLY POSTOPERATIVE CARE OF THE CARDIAC SURGICAL PATIENT
(*Continued*)

Nursing Interventions	Rationales
• Have patient perform leg and arm exercises as taught in the preoperative phase.	• Exercises increase circulation.
• Apply elastic stockings or Ace bandages to lower extremities as prescribed. ○ Check size of elastic stockings and apply properly; check pulses q4h, administer skin care. Remove stockings once each shift.	• Properly applied elastic stockings and Ace bandages assist in venous return, reducing risk of venous stasis.
• Assess the patient for calf tenderness, swelling, and a positive Homan's sign.	• Signs of thrombophlebitis.
• Measure girth of calves and thighs bilaterally.	• A deep venous thrombosis can often be detected by monitoring the circumference.
• Do not use a Gatch bed or use pillows under the knee. Discourage the patient from crossing knees and/or ankles.	• Applies pressure under the knee, thereby decreasing circulation to the lower leg.

Nursing Diagnoses	Desired Patient Outcomes
Nursing Diagnosis #5 Tissue perfusion, alteration in cerebral, related to: 1. Anesthesia 2. Cardiopulmonary bypass 3. Narcotics 4. Postcardiotomy delirium (PCD)	Patient will: 1. Demonstrate an intact, direct, and consensual pupillary light reflex bilaterally 2. Demonstrate an intact gag reflex 3. Be alert and oriented to person, place, and time 4. Follow commands and behave appropriately 5. Speak clearly and understandably 6. Demonstrate movement in all extremities equal to preoperative state

Nursing Interventions	Rationales
• Assess neurologic status at least every 2–4 h, or when indicated: pupils—size and equality, reaction to light; level of consciousness; orientation; speech; response to directions; movement of all extremities.	• Abnormal neurologic findings may be indicative of permanent or temporary alterations related to the anesthesia, intraoperative stroke, cardiopulmonary bypass machine, hypothermia, decreased cardiac output. Abnormal findings may occur in the immediate postoperative phase, but they should gradually return to baseline within the initial 4–8 h postoperatively.
• Assess the patient's behavior every shift. Orient to person, place, and time. Provide frequent explanations. Allow family to visit. Reinforce normality of the disorientation (if no other signs of neurologic deficit are present).	• Confusion and disorientation may be indicative of postcardiotomy delirium (PCD). Frequent explanations, reorientation, and visits from family help the patient cope with PCD. Postcardiotomy delirium is associated with cardiopulmonary bypass and is manifested in some patients after bypass by changes in behavior, confusion, and frank psychosis.

Nursing Diagnoses	Desired Patient Outcomes
Nursing Diagnosis #6 Infection, risk for, related to: 1. Interruption in integrity of skin barrier (surgical incision) 2. Invasive monitoring 3. Chest tubes, Foley catheter	The patient will remain infection free: 1. Temperature at baseline (98.6°F) 2. WBC at baseline 3. Incisional area clean, dry, and healing

Nursing Interventions	Rationales
• Assess incision, IV sites, intravascular lines for signs of infection (warmth, redness, swelling).	• The skin is the first line of defense against infection. Any break in the skin's integrity is prone to infection.
• Change IV lines and hemodynamic lines per hospital protocol. Maintain sterility of the lines.	• These are access sites through which bacteria enter.
• Change dressings daily or according to hospital protocol.	• Dressing changes permit visualization of the surgical site. Redness, warmth, and swelling suggest infection.
• Culture any draining wound.	• Detection of the causative organism is necessary so that appropriate antibiotic therapy can be prescribed.
• Administer antibiotics as prescribed.	• Timely and accurate administration of antibiotics helps to maintain therapeutic blood levels.

CARE PLAN FOR EARLY POSTOPERATIVE CARE OF THE CARDIAC SURGICAL PATIENT
(*Continued*)

Nursing Interventions

- Assess breath sounds and appearance of sputum.

- Maintain the Foley catheter as a closed system. Discontinue as soon as possible.
- Assess the patient for signs of systemic infection (sepsis): change in behavior, hyperthermia/hypothermia, chills, diaphoresis.
- Practice good handwashing technique.

Rationales

- Presence of adventitious sounds and sputum production can signal possible onset of pneumonia.
- Foley catheters are a common source of infection and can lead to gram-negative sepsis.
- The first sign of sepsis is a change in behavior. Timely and aggressive intervention is necessary to prevent septic shock and multisystem organ dysfunction.
- Good handwashing technique is the main way to prevent inspection or its spread.

Nursing Diagnoses

Nursing Diagnosis #7
Anxiety, related to:
1. Outcome of surgery
2. Recuperative period
3. Lack of sleep/rest
4. Noisy ICU environment

Desired Patient Outcomes

Patient will verbalize:
1. Feeling less anxious
2. Ability to rest and to sleep
3. Progess made in recuperation
4. Willingness to cooperate in care
5. Desire to make decisions concerning care

Nursing Interventions

- Familiarize patient with ICU environment: equipment, procedures, and protocols.
- Explain condition and treatments. Stress the patient's progress.
- Administer pain medication as needed. Withhold medication if the patient is hypotensive, is being weaned off the ventilator, or has neurologic changes.

- Provide rest periods. Administer sedatives/pain medication to enhance sleep at night.
- Allow the patient to take an active part in care; allow patient to make decisions concerning care.

- Allow the family to visit as much as possible according to unit/hospital policy.

Rationales

- Appropriate explanation decreases anxiety.

- Reassures the patient. Gives positive reinforcement.

- Decreasing the pain will decrease the patient's anxiety by breaking the pain-fear-anxiety triangle. Narcotics are not given if they will interfere with assessment or stabilization of the patient.
- Sleep and rest deprivation causes irritability, which increases anxiety.
- Decision-making and active participation in care give positive feedback to the patient that he or she is making progress, as well as giving the patient a sense of self-worth.
- The family is a support system that the patient depends on. Family interaction helps prevent social isolation and gives the patient a sense of being needed.

*Some hemodilution is expected with bypass and fluid retention; thus, lower hematocrits may be acceptable.

C H A P T E R   21

Nursing Management of the Patient in Shock

Cathy J. Thompson

CHAPTER OUTLINE

LEARNING OBJECTIVES

After completing this chapter, you should be able to:

1. Define shock and its classifications.
2. Describe the pathophysiology underlying the effect of shock on body organ systems.
3. Identify major compensatory mechanisms triggered in response to shock, including neural, hormonal, and chemical influences.
4. Identify key factors to be assessed in the early recognition and treatment of shock.
5. Describe hypovolemic shock, its etiology, pathophysiology, diagnosis, treatment, and management.
6. Discuss the role of the nurse regarding the patient with shock.
7. Delineate the nursing process in the care of the patient with hypovolemic shock, including assessment, diagnosis, and planning of desired patient outcomes and nursing interventions.

Shock is a complex clinical syndrome that may result from, and complicate, many disease processes. The nurse has a critical role in the identification and management of the patient in shock. This chapter will present a review of the basic pathophysiologic mechanisms underlying the shock state, briefly discuss cardiogenic and distributive forms of shock, and detail the management of the patient with hypovolemic shock. Current research regarding the treatment and management of the shock patient is included where applicable.

Shock is a state of impaired cellular metabolism that occurs as a consequence of inadequate tissue perfusion. It is a syndrome characterized by a disturbance in circulation that results in impaired nutrient transport and an imbalance between oxygen supply and demand.[1] Impaired tissue oxygenation occurs when there is an absolute or relative decrease in circulating blood volume and/or an ineffective cardiac pump. Oxygen deprivation is the end result of inadequate tissue perfusion.

Shock is a complex process that begins as a compensatory response to some insult or trauma and may rapidly progress to multiorgan dysfunction. The cyclic, self-perpetuating nature of the shock state presents a significant challenge to the critical care nurse and medical team. Without early and aggressive intervention based on clinical observations and patient response, shock can be life-threatening.

BASIC PATHOPHYSIOLOGY OF SHOCK STATES

Shock begins at the cellular level. It may evolve rapidly if not recognized and treated early. Timely and definitive intervention is the key to preventing widespread cellular injury and progression of the shock state.

Disruption of Cellular Function

The effects of shock at the cellular level are significant (Table 21–1). Blood carries oxygen and energy substrates to the cells and the tissues. The ability of the cells to use these nutrients is influenced by the amount of substrate available. When oxygen transport decreases, oxygen delivery to the tissues is compromised.

Oxygen is the necessary ingredient for cell metabolism to produce energy in the form of adenosine triphosphate (ATP). Aerobic respiration is an efficient means of energy production needed for normal cell functioning producing 38 moles of ATP per 1 mole of glucose. As the shock state persists, cellular metabolism becomes progressively disturbed. The sluggish microcirculation diminishes the availability of oxygen to the tissues, and cell respiration shifts from aerobic to anaerobic. Anaerobic respiration produces only 2 moles of ATP per 1 mole of glucose. In addition, anaerobic glycolysis produces large amounts of lactic acid, which accumulate in the tissues. This predisposes the patient to metabolic acidosis and other metabolic derangements.

Cellular reactions are reduced as stores of ATP are used up. Active transport of sodium and potassium through the cell membrane is greatly diminished. As a result, sodium and water accumulate within the cell, while there is a potassium efflux from the cell. Cells may begin to swell. Cellular responsiveness to catecholamines and calcium regulation, both of which play vital roles in the production of an action potential and the ability of the heart and muscles to respond to nervous stimulation, is also reduced.

As shock progresses, further deterioration in cellular function occurs and chemical mediators are released. These substances cause local damage to adjacent tissues and capillaries by altering blood flow and activating the immune process and coagulation cascade. Lysosomal disruption causes the release of hydrolytic enzymes within the cell, thereby initiating the self-destruction or self-digestion of the cell by enzymes from within the cell itself (cell autolysis). The end result is cellular death and tissue damage.[2]

Stages of Shock

The body's response to the effects of shock are described as occurring in four stages. Keep in mind that all patients will not necessarily experience every stage. Indeed, the primary goal of care is directed at recognizing the signs and symptoms of shock early to prevent progression to the next stage. The *initial* shock stage begins at the cellular level. The shift from aerobic to anaerobic respiration occurs, and cardiac output and tissue perfusion begin to decrease. Generally, this stage does not present with any obvious clinical signs of deterioration.[2]

The second stage of shock is one of *compensation* (Table 21–2). The body attempts to maintain adequate functioning, in terms of an adequate cardiac output and arterial pressure, through mediation of nervous, hormonal, and chemical mechanisms (Figs. 21–1, 21–2, and 21–3). The effects of these mechanisms on the body are responsible for the clinical signs and symptoms typically associated with the shock state (Table 21–3). It should be noted that conditions such as diabetes, renal failure, normal aging, and drug therapy (e.g., β-blockers or vasodilators) can "mask" the expected compensatory responses of tachycardia and vasoconstriction,[3] so that the nurse needs to be knowledgeable about the patient's medical history and drug therapies when assessing for shock. As cellular function deteriorates, signs of tissue and organ impairment

TABLE 21–1
Disruption of Cellular Function

Decreased tissue perfusion
Oxygen deficit
Decreased energy production
Deterioration of cellular function
Excess production of lactic acid
Eruption of the intracellular membrane
Cell death
Local tissue damage

Source: Adapted from Rice, V: Shock, a clinical syndrome: An update, I. Critical Care Nurse 11(4):27, 1991, with permission.

TABLE 21–2
Compensatory Mechanisms Initiated in Shock

Central Nervous System/Endocrine
Mediation of homeostatic mechanisms (sympathetic, hormonal, and chemical)
Anterior pituitary secretes corticotropin → stimulates adrenal cortex
Posterior pituitary secretes ADH
Vasoconstriction of cerebral blood vessels

Cardiovascular
↑ Heart rate, ↑ contractility → ↑ CO
↑ Cardiac work → ↑ MVO_2
↑ Vascular resistance (arterial and venous)
Shunting of blood to heart and brain

Respiratory
↑ Respiratory rate and depth
Bronchial smooth muscle dilation

Renal/Endocrine
Renin-angiotensin-aldosterone-ADH secretion → conservation of water and sodium
Adrenal medulla → catecholamine secretion (epinephrine, norepinephrine)
Adrenal cortex → glucocorticoids produced → elevated glucose levels

Splanchnic Organs/Skin
↓ Blood flow → vasoconstriction

ADH = antidiuretic hormone; CO = cardiac output; MVO_2 = myocardial oxygen consumption.

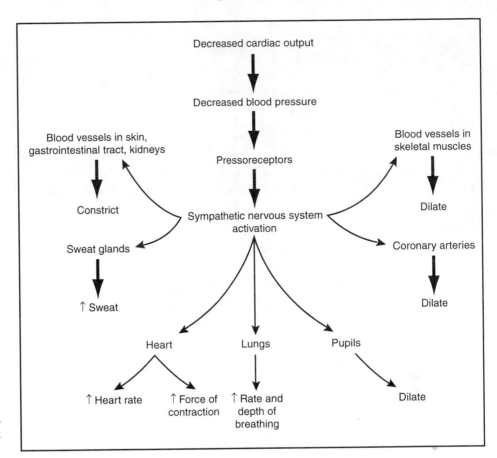

FIGURE 21–1. Neural compensation in shock. (Adapted from Rice,[2] p 76.)

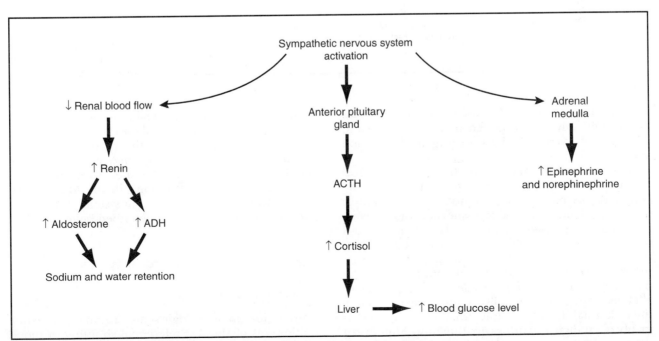

FIGURE 21–2. Hormonal compensation in shock. (Adapted from Rice,[2] p 78.)

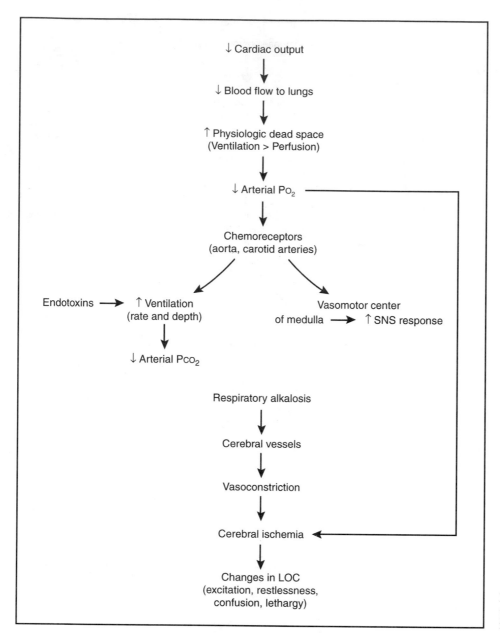

FIGURE 21–3. Chemical compensation in shock. (Adapted from Rice,[2] p 80.)

become more marked. Compensatory mechanisms are only effective for a limited time before demand exceeds capacity and signs of organ dysfunction appear.

Decompensation marks the third stage and is referred to as the *progressive* stage. In this stage, the compensatory mechanisms are not able to effectively maintain adequate levels of tissue perfusion. Hypoperfusion of all organ systems leads to ischemia and necrosis. The loss of autoregulatory control and increased capillary membrane permeability contribute to the reduction in cardiac output and coronary perfusion.[2] The decline in cardiac output causes a parallel decrease in oxygen delivery and oxygen demand: the cells are not able to extract what oxygen is present in great enough quantities to function. Multiorgan dysfunction syndrome (MODS) and organ failure follow.

Should the shock state remain unresolved, the progressive deterioration of circulatory and cellular function leads to a state where the body is unable to respond to treatment. The *refractory* stage is the final and irreversible stage in the shock syndrome and leads, ultimately, to the patient's death. At all stages, shock affects virtually every organ system of the body. Specific effects of shock are described below.

Impact on the Body's Organ Systems

Neurologic System

Alterations in neurologic status are typically the first subtle signs of shock. Preferential shunting of blood to the heart and the brain preserves neurologic functioning to a certain extent. As long as the mean arterial

TABLE 21–3
**Clinical Signs and Symptoms Associated with
Compensatory and Progressive Stages of Shock**

	Compensatory Stage	Progressive Stage
Neurologic	↑ Level of consciousness Restlessness Agitation Lethargy Confusion	Unresponsive
Cardio-vascular	Adequate BP ↑ HR 101–150 beats/min Weak, thready pulse Cool, clammy, pale	SBP <80 mmHg ↑↑ HR >150 beats/min May be absent Cold, cyanotic, mottled
Respiratory	RR > 20/min, deep ↓ PaCO₂ Respiratory alkalosis ↑ pH Hypoxemia	Rapid rate, ↑ PaCO₂ Shallow Rales, rhonchi Metabolic and respiratory acidosis ↓ pH Hypoxemia
Urine	<30 mL/h ↑ specific gravity	< 20 mL/h ↑ BUN/CR ↓ specific gravity
Pupils	Dilated (6–8 mm) Brisk	Dilated Sluggish
GI	Hypoactive bowel sounds Mild abdominal distension	Absent
Lab Values	↑ Glucose ↑ Sodium ↑ Lactate	↑ Liver enzymes ↑ Pancreatic enzymes ↑ BUN/CR ↓ NaHCO₃

pressure is approximately 60 mmHg, cerebral blood flow is usually maintained at essentially normal levels. Metabolic derangements such as electrolyte abnormalities and changes in acid-base status, decreased perfusion, and resulting hypoxemia influence cerebral blood flow and therefore affect mental functioning.[4] Compensatory responses of the nervous system, in response to shock, occur within seconds and are influenced by negative feedback control mechanisms.

Cardiovascular System

Initial compensatory mechanisms activated in response to shock significantly affect the cardiovascular system. A decrease in circulating blood volume causes a drop in mean arterial pressure and consequently the degree of stretch of the vessel walls. Baroreceptors, located in the aortic arch and carotid sinus, sense this pressure change and send impulses to the vasomotor center in the cerebral medulla. An immediate sympathetic response occurs, with the release of norepinephrine at adrenergic nerve endings. The adrenal medulla is also stimulated to secrete epinephrine and, to a lesser extent, norepinephrine.

Physiologically, the body's overall response to increased sympathetic activity involves an increase in heart rate (chronotropic effect); an increase in the force of myocardial contraction (inotropic effect); and vasoconstriction of resistance vessels (arterioles and precapillary) and capacitance vessels (venules and veins). The net result of these activities provides an increase in venous return and hence an increase in cardiac output (via increased heart rate and stroke volume) and an increase in total systemic vascular resistance (SVR). The increased cardiac output (CO) and SVR result in a return of the mean arterial blood pressure to within the physiologic norm.

Stimulation of β-adrenergic receptors, by direct sympathetic drive and catecholamine release, contribute to the chronotropic and inotropic effect on the heart, as well as to the slight vasodilation of the coronary circulation and that of skeletal muscle. α-Adrenergic stimulation to the skin, splanchnic circulation, and kidneys causes these vessels to vasoconstrict, thereby shunting blood to the priority organs, the heart and the brain. Sympathetic stimulation does not cause significant vasoconstriction of the cerebral vasculature, as blood flow through the cerebral circulation is, to a large extent, intrinsically regulated via the phenomenon of autoregulation.

The body's ability to compensate for a significant reduction in arterial blood pressure has its limitations. As shock progresses, these compensatory mechanisms fail and circulatory and cellular deterioration begin. As stores of energy used to maintain the vasoconstrictive state become depleted, the heart itself becomes weakened and fails to pump effectively. The result is a reduction in cardiac output that decreases coronary artery perfusion and leads to myocardial ischemia, serious arrhythmias, and heart failure; the consequent reduction in blood flow to the tissues and end-organs predisposes to hypoxia and organ failure.

Impaired tissue perfusion reduces oxygen delivery. In the presence of an oxygen deficit, cells must produce the energy needed for normal cell functioning via anaerobic glycolysis. A major end-product of this series of reactions is lactic acid, which is responsible for the metabolic acidosis associated with the shock state. Lactic acidosis depresses the myocardium and decreases the peripheral vascular responsiveness to catecholamines (e.g., epinephrine, norepinephrine, and dopamine). The accumulation of lactate in the bloodstream is an important marker of the degree of anaerobic metabolism and oxygen supply and demand.[3] Lactate levels greater than 4 mmol/L indicate severe acidemia, with a poor prognosis for recovery.[5]

Tissue hypoxia also triggers the release of chemical mediators, which potentiate the severity of the shock state. Two of these mediators, bradykinin and histamine, are especially potent vasodilators that contribute to the pooling of blood in the vascular bed and in the microcirculation. Disruption of the capillary membranes, as well as relaxation of precapillary sphincters, leads to the shifting of fluid from the capillaries into the interstitium. This not only adds to the pooling of blood, but, more importantly, further reduces blood volume and venous return to the heart.

Microvascular injury has been shown to lead to the trapping of platelets in affected organs.[6] The accumulation of cellular elements of blood, platelet microaggregates, and other particulate matter leads to the sludging of blood in the microcirculation. Such sludging precipitates thrombosis and intravascular coagulation abnormalities (see Chapter 53).

Respiratory System

Hyperventilation is generally observed in the early stages of shock. Changes in the pH of the cerebrospinal fluid and the presence of hypercarbia stimulate the brain to increase the rate and depth of respiration. Although the tidal volume may be reduced, the respiratory rate increases by two- or three-fold, resulting in a minute ventilation that is often one and a half to two times normal.[7] As shock progresses, the increased work of breathing and decreasing energy stores lead to a decline in ventilatory effort: respiratory rate remains rapid, but shallow. Mechanical ventilation is often indicated to support the patient. Underlying the respiratory dysfunction is a disruption in pulmonary capillary dynamics that predisposes to pulmonary edema (see Fig. 34–1). In patients with cardiogenic shock, pulmonary edema is a result of hydrostatic pressure changes. In contrast to cardiogenic pulmonary edema, *noncardiogenic* pulmonary edema is associated with an increase in permeability of the alveolar capillary membrane, often as a result of trauma or injury. Noncardiogenic pulmonary edema is also termed adult respiratory distress syndrome (see Chapter 25).

Chemically Activated Compensatory Mechanisms. Closely associated with pulmonary function are compensatory mechanisms that respond to chemical stimuli, especially those directly related to serum concentrations of oxygen, carbon dioxide, and hydrogen ions (Fig. 21–3). When cardiac output is reduced, blood flow to the lungs is also reduced. This contributes to an imbalance in the ratio of ventilation to perfusion, the consequence of which is a decrease in oxygen tension of arterial blood (PaO_2) leaving the lungs.

Chemoreceptors located in the aortic arch and carotid bodies sense this reduced PaO_2 and send impulses to the vital centers in the medulla. The physiologic response is to increase the rate and depth of respirations. Chemoreceptors also respond to the rise of carbon dioxide and hydrogen ion concentrations of circulating blood, and elicit a response similar to that described for oxygen. The increase in alveolar ventilation acts to "blow off" the excess carbon dioxide (CO_2), thereby reducing the arterial carbon dioxide tension ($PaCO_2$) and the hydrogen ion concentration, while increasing the PaO_2 to within an acceptable physiologic range. This reaction also results in a rise in pH.

Renal and Endocrine Systems

In response to shock, the kidneys function to restore tissue perfusion by conserving sodium and water through the interaction of central nervous and hormonal mechanisms. Juxtaglomerular cells in the kidney are sensitive to decreases in cardiac output and mean arterial pressure and are thus stimulated to secrete renin. Renin, a proteolytic enzyme, triggers the conversion of angiotensin I to angiotensin II. Angiotensin II exerts a potent vasoconstrictor effect on both arteries and veins. The resulting increase in systemic vascular resistance raises blood pressure and increases venous return to the heart.

Angiotensin II also stimulates the secretion of aldosterone by the adrenal cortex. Aldosterone, in turn, acts on the distal renal tubule to increase reabsorption of sodium, which is accompanied by the reabsorption of water. In this way, the body's compensatory mechanisms attempt to overcome the effects of the shock state.

Reabsorption of water is facilitated by the action of antidiuretic hormone (ADH; vasopressin), which is released from the posterior pituitary gland in response to a sensed increase in blood osmolality. This hormone acts on the distal kidney tubules and collecting ducts to increase the permeability of these cells to water, thus facilitating the passive reabsorption of water in conjunction with enhanced sodium reabsorption. ADH also exerts the body's most potent vasoconstrictor effect on the systemic vasculature.

In addition, the increase in sympathetic activity in response to shock stimulates the anterior pituitary gland to release corticotropin (ACTH). This hormone acts directly on the adrenal cortex to promote the release of glucocorticoids. Glucocorticoids act to elevate the serum glucose concentration to provide a ready source of energy for cellular metabolism; increased serum glucose concentration also contributes to the osmolality of the circulating blood.

Gastrointestinal System

The research literature has indicated that the gastrointestinal (GI) mucosa is particularly vulnerable to the effects of shock.[8] The splanchnic organs are among the first to suffer from the effects of hypoperfusion as the body preferentially shunts blood away from these organs to the vital organs (heart and brain) during the early compensatory stage of shock. Through the use of a gastric tonometer, researchers have correlated the gastrointestinal intramucosal pH (pHi) with the degree of anaerobic respiration: a low pHi indicates an increased anaerobic rate in the gastric mucosa (and therefore a decreased oxygen supply to the mucosa)[8,9] (see Research Application Box).

Decreased perfusion to the GI tract during shock, and reperfusion injury following treatment, has been implicated in the development of pathogenic bacterial movement (translocation) into the systemic circulation, with consequent infection.[6,10–12] In fact, the GI tract has been pinpointed as the initial reservoir of the endotoxin responsible for the development of gram-negative sepsis.[10]

Significant gastrointestinal bleeding may also occur from erosions and ulcerations in the mucosal lining. In the stomach, these alterations are associated with an impairment of the gastric mucosal barrier. Normally, gastric cells are protected from the destructive effects of hydrochloric acid secretion by the thick secretions (mucus) of the goblet cells. Maldistribution of blood flow to the mucosal lining inhibits this protective effect.[11] The back-diffusion of hydrogen ions across the friable mucosa causes an autodigestion of the lining and development of ulcerated areas.

Hepatic complications may also develop in response to preferential shunting of blood away from the liver. Ischemic injury of the liver is associated with fatty infiltrates and centrilobar necrosis, impaired synthesis of vital proteins and clotting factors, and alterations in immune function.[4] Prolonged impairment of hepatic blood flow in shock can increase the tendency for severe acute failure of other organ systems. The liver plays a key role in the removal of potentially toxic substances absorbed from the GI tract and splanchnic tissues during shock. Many of these substances cause further impairment of cardiovascular function, and a vicious downward cycle of progressive end-organ failure is perpetuated.

Microcirculation

Tissue hypoxia in the microcirculation is potentiated by the effects of mediator responses and coagulation abnormalities. Sluggish blood flow in the microcirculation is a result of the accumulation of tissue fragments, platelet aggregation,[6] abnormalities in red blood cells, and fibrin deposits.[4] Alterations in capillary membrane permeability foster the movement of fluid into the tissues and thereby interfere with the diffusion of oxygen and carbon dioxide.[4] The abnormal activation of the coagulation cascade precipitates the development of disseminated intravascular coagulation (DIC).

CLASSIFICATION AND ETIOLOGY

Shock can be classified according to three major pathophysiologic mechanisms: (1) a dysfunction in the pumping effectiveness of the heart (cardiogenic shock), (2) an abnormal distribution of vascular volume (distributive or vasogenic shock), and (3) a reduction in intravascular volume (hypovolemic shock). The end result of each type of shock is a reduction in cardiac output that compromises oxygen delivery to the tissues.

Cardiogenic Shock

Cardiogenic shock is caused by the inability of the heart to function effectively as a pump. Dysfunction of either the right or left ventricle can precipitate cardiogenic shock, though it occurs most often as a result of primary left ventricular pathology. The most common pathology responsible for the development of cardiogenic shock is in the setting of an acute myocardial infarction (MI) in patients with severe coronary artery disease. Development of cardiogenic shock carries a high mortality rate (75% to 95%) and occurs in approximately 15% of MI patients.[2] The *cumulative* amount of infarcted muscle is directly related to the risk of developing shock. Patients suffering from anterior infarctions or those who have sustained previous muscle damage (i.e., "old" MIs) are at greatest risk. Any condition that affects the ability of the heart to contract can cause cardiogenic shock (Table 21–4).

Damage to 40% or more of the left ventricular muscle mass severely jeopardizes the ability of the heart to eject its volume (pump) into the systemic circulation. Forward flow of blood is impaired, and the reduction in stroke volume leads to decreases in tissue perfusion. Blood that is not ejected collects in the ventricles, and the volume increases with each filling period. With progressive heart failure, this extra volume increases ventricular filling pressures (increases left ventricular end-diastolic pressure [LVEDP]) and is transmitted backwards into the pulmonary system, which is consequently disposed to pulmonary edema. High pressures in the pulmonary circuit increase right ventricular afterload and cause impaired ejection of blood volume from this chamber as well. This further decreases the volume (preload) delivered to the left ventricle and therefore cardiac output.

Hemodynamically, patients with cardiogenic shock experience a fall in mean arterial pressure, which is associated with an inadequate cardiac output and reduced stroke volume (SV). Tachycardia occurs as an immediate compensatory measure to boost cardiac output (CO = HR × SV). With the increase in heart rate (HR), there is a consequent decrease in ventricular diastolic filling time and coronary artery perfusion. Attempts by the body to maintain blood pressure are demonstrated as an increase in systemic vascular resistance (MAP = CO × SVR). Reflex sympathetic

TABLE 21–4
Causes of Cardiogenic Shock

Coronary Causes
Atherosclerotic coronary artery disease
  (acute myocardial infarction)

Noncoronary Causes
Septal rupture
Papillary muscle rupture
Valvular heart disease
Cardiomyopathy
Myocarditis
Arrhythmias
Massive pulmonary embolism
Cardiac tamponade
Tension pneumothorax
Hypothermia

activity is also detrimental because an increase in heart rate and contractility increases myocardial oxygen consumption and potentiates myocardial ischemia.

The increase in afterload associated with systemic vasoconstriction similarly increases the work of the heart. As the pulmonary artery wedge pressure rises (PAWP > 18 to 20 mmHg) and the cardiac index falls (CI < 2.2 L/min), cardiogenic shock becomes definitive. The effect of decreases in end-organ perfusion and oxygen delivery present as the clinical signs and symptoms of cardiogenic shock (see Table 19–11).

Treatment of cardiogenic shock involves manipulation of oxygen transport variables and the determinants of cardiac output: preload, afterload, and contractility. Maintenance of an adequate circulating blood volume through careful volume administration and vigilant monitoring of hemodynamic parameters is very important. Inotropic and vasodilating drugs optimize contractility and vascular resistance. In cases of severe cardiogenic shock, mechanical assistance via the intra-aortic balloon pump, Hemopump, or other ventricular assist devices may be employed for patient recovery. (For a detailed discussion and care plan for the patient with heart failure, see Chapter 19.)

Distributive (Vasogenic) Shock

Distributive, or vasogenic, shock is a broad category that includes several types of shock, all of which are characterized by peripheral vasodilation with a disproportion between the usual circulating blood volume and the size of the vascular bed. This alteration in blood vessel radius leads to a decrease in systemic vascular resistance and an increase in vascular capacity. The pooling of blood in the periphery causes a "relative hypovolemia." The resulting decrease in venous return (decreases in preload) reduces cardiac output and therefore tissue perfusion and oxygen transport. Subclassifications of distributive shock include (1) anaphylactic, (2) neurogenic, and (3) septic shock.

Anaphylactic Shock

Anaphylactic shock is a dramatic clinical event associated with a type I hypersensitivity reaction. It involves an immediate systemic response that occurs when an individual who has been sensitized to an antigen from a previous exposure (i.e., an individual who has preformed antibody) is again exposed to the antigen in question. The consequent interaction between the antigen and preformed antibody causes mast cells to release their chemical mediators (e.g., histamine, serotonin, and slow-reacting substance of anaphylaxis [SRS-A]). When released, these chemical mediators cause vasodilation, an increase in vascular permeability, and bronchial hyperactivity. The consequent fluid shifts and vasodilation result in a relative hypovolemia predisposing to a significant, symptomatic hypotensive state. Bronchial edema and bronchospasm lead to alveolar hypoventilation and acute respiratory distress.

Therapeutic management consists of immediate recognition of the signs and symptoms, maintenance of a patent airway, removal of allergen and/or prevention of allergen spread, administration of drugs (antihistamines, antipruritics, bronchodilators), and general measures to treat shock. (For a detailed discussion and care plan for the patient with anaphylactic shock, see Chapter 57.)

Neurogenic Shock

Neurogenic shock, also called vasomotor shock, is characterized by an abnormal distribution of blood volume caused by massive vasodilation of the systemic vasculature as a result of an *interruption or loss of sympathetic innervation*. It is a temporary condition that is associated with injury or disease of the brainstem or of the upper spinal cord (above T-4 to T-6). It may also occur following administration of general anesthesia or spinal anesthesia that extends upward in the spinal cord, drugs that block sympathetic activity, or significant pain or emotional stress.[13]

Loss of sympathetic vasoconstrictor tone below the level of injury, in arterioles, precapillaries, and venules results in a significant decrease in peripheral vascular resistance and venous pooling. Consequently, there is a reduction in venous return to the heart, a decrease in stroke volume, and symptomatic hypotension. Bradycardia is also characteristic of neurogenic shock, due to the loss of sympathetic tone on the heart. Vasodilatation and loss of the sweat response below the level of injury produces warm, dry skin. Treatment consists of inotropic and vasopressor support, regulation of body temperature, and careful monitoring of fluid status.[14] (See Chapter 33 for further discussion of neurogenic shock.)

Spinal Shock. Spinal shock should *not* be confused with neurogenic shock. It differs from neurogenic shock in that the patient suffers from a *loss of control of reflex activity* below the level of injury. Spinal shock and neurogenic shock are frequently seen together. This type of shock is a temporary condition which develops within 30 to 60 minutes of acute spinal cord trauma.[14,15] Paralytic ileus and bladder atonicity are clinical manifestations of spinal shock. Treatment of paralytic ileus consists of nasogastric tube placement, prohibition of food and drink, administration of IV fluids and/or total parenteral nutrition (TPN), and assessment of bowel sounds for return of peristalsis. Bladder atonicity is treated by placement of a Foley catheter for initial monitoring of urine output, followed by an intermittent catheterization protocol.[15]

Septic Shock

Sepsis is a systemic inflammatory response to an infectious process.[16] More than 40% of hospitalized patients who develop sepsis will progress to septic shock; mortality ranges from 40% to 90%.[13] Septic shock is characterized by an abnormal distribution of intravascular blood volume due to massive vasodilation associated with an overwhelming infection or septicemia. Both exotoxin, released from gram-positive organisms, and endotoxin, released from gram-negative organisms, can cause septic shock. Gram-negative organisms are the most common cause of septic shock in the ICU setting.[16] The endotoxin released by the causative microorganism acts to trigger a variety of biochemical reactions that adversely affect the body and predispose to the shock state. Included among these reactions is activation of the complement, clotting, and kinin systems. In addition, endotoxin triggers the release of vasoactive mediators from the damaged tissues. Clinically, septic shock is seen to progress through the stages of hyperdynamic shock, hypodynamic shock, and multisystem organ dysfunction.

The hyperdynamic stage is characterized by profound peripheral vasodilation, which is depicted hemodynamically as a decreased systemic vascular resistance. The consequent reduction in afterload eases the workload of the heart and promotes an increase in cardiac output. However, the patient becomes hypotensive despite the increased output because of the disproportion between the blood volume and the size of the vascular bed. Clinically, the septic patient in this stage does not "look" like a patient in shock. Typical signs and symptoms will include: a high cardiac output, a low SVR, tachycardia, hyperthermia (from the pyrogens released from the endotoxin), warm, flushed skin (vasodilation and fever), normotension or hypotension, with a high mixed venous oxygen saturation ($S\bar{v}O_2 > 80\%$) because the tissues are unable to extract and utilize the oxygen delivered by the circulation.

The signs and symptoms of the hypodynamic stage are more typical of a classic shock pattern. In this stage, the hypermetabolism of the first stage is reversed and compensatory mechanisms are stimulated. Systemic vascular resistance is increased as vasoconstriction occurs. The increased afterload (increase in SVR) and decreased preload (decreased SV) contribute to a reduction in cardiac output, to hypotension, and to decreased tissue perfusion. In addition, the patient presents with cool, clammy skin, tachycardia, hypothermia, and a decreased $S\bar{v}O_2$. Without timely and aggressive intervention, the patient rapidly

decompensates and progresses to multisystem organ dysfunction and organ failure.

Current treatment of septic shock includes identification and antibiotic treatment of the causative organism, good handwashing and aseptic technique, monitoring and support of the cardiovascular system (optimize preload, contractility, and vascular resistance), and maximizing oxygen delivery/demand ratio. Multiple new therapies, such as the use of mediator-specific monoclonal antibodies, are being investigated for the treatment of sepsis and septic shock.[16] (For a detailed discussion and care plan for the patient with septic shock, see Chapter 56.)

Hypovolemic Shock

Hypovolemic shock is characterized by a significant reduction in effective circulating intravascular volume in relation to the vascular space.[7] Cardiac output is jeopardized due to the reduction in preload and, in the scenario of hemorrhagic shock, a decrease in the oxygen-carrying capacity of the blood. Volume loss can be divided into four classes (Table 21–5). An acute blood volume loss of 35% can be life-threatening.[3] (The remainder of this chapter will include an in-depth discussion of hypovolemic shock, its etiology, diagnosis, treatment, and nursing care.)

Etiology

Hypovolemic shock reflects a depletion of extracellular fluid caused either through external losses from the body (absolute hypovolemia) or an internal maldistribution of blood between the intravascular and the extravascular compartments (relative hypovolemia). A variety of conditions can cause hypovolemic shock, including one or more of the following: (1) an actual decrease in blood volume (i.e., hemorrhagic shock) associated with bleeding related to trauma, surgery, childbirth, coagulation defects, or gastrointestinal bleeding; (2) a decrease in intravascular fluid volume associated with fever or profuse diaphoresis, gastrointestinal dysfunction, including a reduction in fluid intake, severe vomiting or continuing nasogastric

TABLE 21–5
Classes and Clinical Signs of Hemorrhagic Shock

	Class I	Class II	Class III	Class IV
Blood loss (mL)	Up to 750	750 to 1500	1500 to 2000	2000 or more
% Blood volume	Up to 15%	15% to 30%	30% to 40%	40% or more
Heart rate (beats/min)	<100	100 to 120	120 to 140	>140
Blood pressure	Normal	Normal	Decreased	Severe hypotension
Pulse pressure	Normal or increased	Decreased	Decreased	Decreased
Respirations (per min)	14 to 20	20 to 30	30 to 40	>35 (shallow)
Urine output (mL)	>30	20 to 30	5 to 15	<5
Capillary blanch	Normal	Slight delay	Defined delay	No filling noted
Skin	Pink, cool	Cold, pale	Cold, moist	Cold, cyanotic, mottled

Source: Adapted from Sommers, MS: Fluid resuscitation following multiple trauma. Critical Care Nurse 10(10):74–81, 1990.

suctioning, diarrhea, or fistula or wound drainage; (3) renal dysfunction (e.g., tubular damage with sodium and protein depletion, or overzealous use of diuretics); (4) endocrine dysfunction (e.g., diabetes insipidus); (5) arterial or venous pooling (i.e., vaso-dilation secondary to drugs or associated with vaso-genic shock); and (6) third-spacing (i.e., a shifting of fluid into intracellular spaces as occurs with hypopro-teinemia [severe burns, ascites]; capillary leakage causing pleural effusion; or intestinal obstruction with mobilization of fluid within the proximal in-testinal lumen), which depletes the intravascular volume.

Pathophysiology

The stages of shock for hypovolemic shock are the same as previously described in the general presenta-tion of the stages of shock. Compensatory mechanisms are activated in hypovolemic states, with progressive deterioration of essential body functions unless aggressive interventions are instituted. Hemorrhage is the most common cause of hypovolemic shock.[4,13,17] Hemorrhagic shock can be classified by severity based on the amount of blood volume lost (i.e., from trauma, surgery, childbirth) or displaced (from other causes of hypovolemia). These classes correlate with the presentation of clinical signs and symptoms cor-responding to the four stages of shock (see Table 21–5).

In class I hemorrhagic shock there is a decrease in venous return to the heart and therefore a reduced stroke volume and cardiac output. This is a direct con-sequence of a reduction in circulating blood volume of 750 mL or less (up to 15% of total blood volume). This is analogous to the *initial* stage of shock. While subtle changes are occurring at the cellular level, there may be no clearly evident clinical manifestations to suggest the presence of an underlying pathophysio-logic process, outside of a slight increase in heart rate. A *resting* tachycardia, in any patient, should alert the nurse to the possibility of a fluid deficit.

Class II shock signifies a volume loss of 15% to 30% and marks the onset of the *compensatory* stage. The body responds to the fluid volume deficit by the acti-vation of neural, hormonal, and chemical mechanisms (Figs. 21–1, to 21–3) in an attempt to restore cardiac output, mean arterial pressure, and tissue perfusion. The typical signs and symptoms of shock are exhibited during this stage (Table 21–3). Recognition of this early stage of shock and prompt treatment are essen-tial to the successful outcome of the patient.

Class III shock coincides with a 30% to 40% loss in volume, at which point the body's ability to compen-sate is overwhelmed. The signs and symptoms are sim-ilar to the *progressive* stage. The condition of the micro-circulation continues to deteriorate, resulting in stasis of blood and third-spacing of fluid. Intravascular vol-ume is further reduced.

With a fluid or volume loss greater than or equal to 40%, class IV hemorrhagic shock is equivalent to shock in its *final* stage: the body's response is charac-terized by severe acidemia/acidosis associated with impaired cellular function. Failure of the major organ systems (cardiovascular, pulmonary, renal, and hepatic) develops as a result of inadequate tissue per-fusion, with consequent cellular ischemia and tissue necrosis. Disseminated intravascular coagulation fre-quently occurs as a bleeding diathesis manifested by the depletion of clotting factors and thrombosis of the microcirculation. Death eventually ensues as a result of vasomotor failure and severely compromised cere-bral perfusion.

Diagnosis and Clinical Assessment

The diagnosis of hypovolemic shock must be made swiftly and precisely so that appropriate and aggressive treatment may be initiated. The diagnosis is based on analysis of the patient's medical history, physical find-ings, and clinical indices of tissue perfusion (Table 21–6), laboratory data, assessment of fluid loss, and serial hemodynamic measurements. Efforts in this regard are undertaken after the patient's condition is suffi-ciently stabilized so that there is no imminent danger of ventilatory and/or circulatory compromise. Essen-tial information to be elicited during the early phase of treatment includes the time and circumstances sur-rounding the triggering event, the patient's status dur-ing the interval since the onset, and the patient's cur-rent physiologic, psychological, and emotional state.

It is important to remember that body fluids account for 60% of lean body weight.[3] Extracellular

TABLE 21–6
Clinical Indices of Inadequate Tissue Perfusion Due to Hypovolemia

Neurologic
Decreased level of consciousness
Restlessness
Anxiety

Cardiovascular
↑ Heart rate
↓ Systolic blood pressure
↑ Diastolic blood pressure (↑ afterload)
↓ CVP/PAWP (↓ preload)
Flat jugular veins
Decreased pulse quality
Delayed capillary refill

Respiratory
↑ Respiratory rate and depth
Respiratory alkalosis → acidosis

Renal
↓ Urine output
(<0.5–1.0 mL/kg)
↑ BUN and CR

Integumentary
Skin cool, clammy, mottled
Pale, ashen
Cyanotic

CR = creatinine; CVP = central venous presure; PAWP = pul-monary artery wedge pressure.

fluid comprises 27.5% of the total body water (TBW). The extracellular fluid is separated into the interstitial fluid (20% TBW) and the intravascular fluid (7.5% TBW). The normal blood volume in the average adult amounts to about 6 L, of which red blood cells constitute 45% and plasma 55%. This translates to about 13% of the TBW. A fluid loss of greater than 25% from the extracellular space is a significant loss of TBW. In the early stages of shock the fluid deficit is in the interstitial space as interstitial fluid moves to refill the vascular space.[3] This is called *transcapillary refill* and leads to dehydration of tissue and dilution of the blood.[17]

Initial estimates of fluid loss usually guide resuscitation therapy. In hemorrhage, estimation of acute blood loss can be accomplished by matching the clinical signs with which the patient presents to the class of severity (see Table 21–5). Dehydration or water overload from alterations in salt and water balance can be estimated from clinical signs such as thirst, lethargy, and fainting.[17] The parameters most commonly assessed in the diagnosis of shock include vital signs, hemodynamic parameters, urine output, acid-base status, and the degree of tissue perfusion.[2]

Blood Pressure. In all cases of shock there is a decrease in mean arterial blood pressure. The pattern reflected by changes in the three components of arterial blood pressure (i.e., pulse pressure, systolic pressure, and diastolic pressure) varies, based on the underlying cause of the shock state. These pressure findings, which may be subtle in the early stages, serve as an early indication of underlying hemodynamic changes.

The *pulse pressure* is the difference between the systolic and diastolic pressures and primarily reflects stroke volume and the compliance of the aorta and larger arteries. Pulse pressure is generally about 40 mmHg. During shock, the pulse pressure is considered a more accurate indicator of changes in cardiac output than is systolic pressure and changes in pulse pressure occur before systolic pressure begins to fall.[7] In hypovolemic shock, changes in stroke volume can be detected by the narrowing or widening of the pulse pressure. Major reductions in stroke volume are reflected in a narrowing pulse pressure and decreased peripheral pulses. For example, a blood pressure that changes from 120/80 mmHg to 120/100 mmHg shows a narrowing pulse pressure and thus a decrease in stroke volume.

The *diastolic* blood pressure (DBP) largely reflects the degree of arteriolar constriction and gives the nurse a noninvasive way to estimate SVR, or afterload. In the compensatory stage, diastolic pressure may increase as a response to sympathetic activity. Thus, in the previous example, the increase in diastolic blood pressure from 80 mmHg to 100 mmHg indicates vasoconstriction and an increase in afterload (increased SVR). The *systolic* blood pressure (SBP) is determined by ventricular ejection and arterial compliance. Systolic pressure may be normal to high, due to sympathetic stimulation in early shock. As the shock state progresses and the compensatory mechanisms fail,

both the systolic and diastolic pressures fall and the pulse pressure remains steady. Consequently, low SBP is a *late* sign of shock. *Mean arterial pressure* (MAP) is the average "driving force" propelling the volume of blood downstream. The average arterial blood volume and resistance in the arterial system determine the MAP.[18]

When assessing blood pressure it is important that the nurse be aware of *the patient's* normal blood pressure values. While shock has been traditionally defined as an SBP of less than 90 mmHg, not all people with a systolic pressure below 90 mmHg are in shock! Hypertensive patients may be assessed as having a "normal" blood pressure and being in profound shock. In shock patients, initial blood pressure readings may be normal or high due to compensatory effects.

Keep in mind that obtaining blood pressure by cuff may not produce an accurate central reading.[4,18] Vasoconstriction, the body's attempt to increase venous return (and therefore stroke volume), results in a weak blood flow that may not produce audible Korotkoff sounds.[7,18] In this case, arterial blood pressure, in the critically ill, may be actually higher, by 10 to 60 mmHg, than the cuff BP reading.[18] Use of a Doppler apparatus may aid the nurse in hearing Korotkoff sounds.

Direct arterial measurement is preferred in shock patients because this technique is not readily affected by vasoconstriction, enables continuous monitoring of arterial blood pressure, and provides an easy access to the arterial circulation for the frequent lab samples (i.e., blood gases, hematologic, and chemistry studies) that are needed. Monitoring of the waveform for catheter whip (fling) and dampened waveforms is a nursing responsibility associated with direct hemodynamic monitoring (see Table 16–2).

Palpation of the pulse points is a method that may be used to estimate systolic blood pressure when Korotkoff sounds cannot be heard. The presence of a palpable radial pulse gives an estimate of the systolic blood pressure at 80 mmHg; a palpable femoral pulse correlates with an SBP of 70 mmHg, and a palpable carotid pulse with 60 mmHg.[19]

Peripheral Pulses. The adequacy of peripheral blood flow and stroke volume can be measured by evaluating arterial pulses. All major peripheral pulses should be assessed for rate, rhythm, quality, and character. Carotid, radial, femoral, popliteal, dorsalis pedis, and posterior tibial pulses are typically weak and thready in shock. The pulse rate is expected to be greater then 100 beats/min. Arrhythmias will alter the pulse regularity.

Respiration. Increases in respiratory rate and depth are provoked by changes in the chemical composition of the blood: PaO_2 decreases and $PaCO_2$ increases due to the imbalance in oxygen supply. Efforts to increase oxygen supply and eliminate the accumulated CO_2 occur when the cerebral medulla stimulates the patient to breathe more deeply and rapidly. Respiratory rates greater than 20 breaths/min and large tidal volumes (double the norm) are common findings in the shock patient. In the later stages of shock, this increased work of breathing eventually takes its toll and the patient suffers from respiratory muscle fatigue. The respiratory rate remains fast, but shallow. Since CO_2 cannot be eliminated, the CO_2 levels rise, the pH of the arterial blood declines, and a respiratory acidosis ensues.

Temperature. Temperature alterations vary with the mechanism of the shock state. Early septic shock usually presents with an elevated temperature due to the hypermetabolic state and the immune response toward the presence of pyrogen in the bloodstream; fever with anaphylactic shock is also a result of an immune reaction with the antigen. In cardiogenic shock, temperature is usually associated with an inflammatory response to the myocardial damage.

Hypovolemic shock can present with a variable temperature, depending on the basal metabolic rate. Core temperature monitoring (i.e., pulmonary artery temperature) produces the most accurate and least variable values. *Great toe temperature* monitoring is not used regularly in adults, but may provide an indication of reductions in cardiac output via reductions in perfusion.[20] Toe temperatures around 22°C signal vasoconstriction. The normal toe temperature range is 28°C.[5]

Hemodynamic Parameters. Hemodynamic parameters are measures of circulatory effectiveness. Early recognition and treatment of shock require a clinical assessment of the determinants of cardiac output. Assessment of these parameters aids in delineating the etiology of the shock state and provides baseline data that aid in determining initial therapy and evaluating the patient's response to therapy (Table 21–7).

A pulmonary artery (PA) catheter is commonly used to measure cardiac output, right and left heart pressures, and pulmonary artery pressures (PAP). Elevations of pulmonary artery pressures are seen with hypoxia, as the vessels constrict to shunt blood from underventilated alveolar units, and with vasoconstriction stimulated by sympathetic activity. For an in-depth discussion of hemodynamic monitoring, please refer to Chapter 16. See Appendix F for hemodynamic formulas.

Cardiac Output and Cardiac Index. Data from the pulmonary artery catheter enable cardiac output and cardiac index to be calculated. These measures quantify the adequacy of systemic perfusion. Cardiac output is the product of heart rate and stroke volume; stroke volume is determined by preload, afterload, and contractility (see Chapter 12 for detailed descriptions of cardiac output determinants). Cardiac index, which is the cardiac output indexed for body size, is a more accurate indicator of individual ventricular performance, as it gives a better idea of the adequacy of cardiac output for the patient's size. For example, a cardiac output of 4 L/min may adequately perfuse a 5 ft 2 in, 100 lb person, but may be dangerously low for a 6 ft 3 in, 250 lb person. The cardiac index value would take the body size into account and result in a truer measure of cardiac efficiency. A new technique used to measure cardiac output noninvasively is called thoracic electrical bioimpedance (TEB). Trends in cardiac output values seem to be accurately monitored with this technique.[7]

Heart Rate. In patients with hypovolemic shock, a sinus tachycardia (commonly greater than 120 beats/min) is present and reflects the body's attempt to compensate for the decrease in cardiac output. It is important to appreciate that as heart rate increases, stroke volume declines, due to decreases in the time available for left ventricular filling and thus for coronary artery perfusion. This further compromises systemic and coronary blood flow. Any increase in *resting* heart rate (without provocation) of 10 beats/min in the elderly to 20 beats/min in the younger patient[5] should signal the bedside clinician to assess the patient and intervene accordingly.

In addition to changes in heart rate, patients with hypovolemic shock may experience arrhythmias (especially premature ventricular contractions). This is especially true in patients with underlying coronary artery disease. Decreased coronary artery perfusion causes ischemia, which irritates the myocardium and predisposes to arrhythmia formation. Arrhythmias may also be precipitated by severe metabolic derangements associated with acid-base imbalance and tissue hypoxia.

TABLE 21–7
Hemodynamic Patterns in Shock

	CO/CI	MAP	CVP	PAP	PAWP	SVR	SⱽO₂
Cardiogenic	↓ ↔	↓ ↔	↓ ↔	↑	↑	↑	↓
Hypovolemic	↓	↓	↓	↓	↓	↑	↓
Neurogenic	↓	↓	↓	↓	↓	↓	↓
Anaphylactic	↓	↓	↓	↓	↓	↓	↓
Septic							
Early	↑	↔	↔	↓	↓	↓	↑
Late	↓	↓	↓	↑	↓	↑	↓

↑ = increased, ↓ = decreased, ↔ = no change. CO = cardiac output, CI = cardiac index, MAP = mean arterial blood pressure, CVP = central venous pressure, PAP = pulmonary artery pressure, PAWP = pulmonary artery wedge pressure, SVR = systemic vascular resistance, $S\bar{v}O_2$ = mixed venous oxygen saturation.

Preload. The pressure exerted upon the walls of the myocardium from the volume of blood in the ventricles at end-diastole is defined as *preload.* Filling pressures are determined by the amount of venous return, ventricular compliance, and the adequacy of systolic function.[4] Preload can be accurately determined by monitoring direct hemodynamic parameters, including central venous pressure (CVP) or right atrial pressure (RAP) in the right heart and pulmonary artery wedge pressure (PAWP) or left atrial pressure (LAP) in the left. The PAWP most closely reflects left ventricular end-diastolic pressure in the presence of a functioning mitral valve.[21] Since LVEDP reflects the preload of the left heart, monitoring the PAWP helps to assess how well the left heart is managing the volume presented to it. The pulmonary artery diastolic (PAD) pressure can estimate PAWP in the event of the inability to wedge the PA catheter, providing that valve disease is not a problem. During open heart surgery, a left atrial catheter may be placed to measure left heart pressures directly. In the patient with hypovolemic shock, all of these parameters are generally decreased, largely as a result of the decreased intravascular blood volume. Preload can be estimated noninvasively by assessing the appearance of the jugular veins (see Fig. 13–2). The patient in hypovolemic shock should present with flat jugular veins (no jugular venous distention).

Afterload. Afterload is the degree of systemic (SVR) and peripheral vascular resistance.[4] It is reflected in the diastolic arterial blood pressure, and it may be normal to high in the patient with hypovolemic shock, due to extensive vasoconstriction. Pulmonary vascular resistance (PVR) reflects the afterload of the right heart. Both parameters can be calculated to fine-tune therapy (see Appendix F). Note that a high CVP/RAP does not always signify a high *volume load* in the right ventricle. High resistance in the pulmonary circuit (increased PVR) will cause a *pressure overload,* which is then reflected back into the right heart and causes CVP/RAP to rise.

Contractility. Contractility is more difficult to assess directly, but palpation of the heart at its point of maximal impulse (PMI) may provide some appreciation as to the heart's thrust. *Ejection fraction* is a measurement of contractility obtained by angiography, echocardiography, or right ventricular catheters,[7] or by radionuclide studies.[4] Contractility is evaluated at the bedside by calculating the right and left ventricle's stroke work indexed for body size (RVSWI/LVSWI). Data from the PA catheter are needed to calculate these formulas (see Appendix F). The Frank-Starling principle describes the force of ventricular contraction as directly related to the filling volume, up to a physiologic limit, in the form of a *ventricular function curve* (Fig. 21–4). Ventricular function curves provide the most reliable reflection of the state of contractility and can help to differentiate the problems of insufficient volume (decreased preload) from impaired contractility.[4] Stroke work is plotted against measures of volume to determine the optimal wedge pressure for the particular patient and thereby individualize interventions.

Urine Output and Composition. In the scenario of shock, the renal system is not viewed as a vital organ. Consequently, regardless of its underlying cause, the presence of a shock state will cause blood to be shunted away from the kidneys to the heart and brain, resulting in *renal hypoperfusion.* As compensatory mechanisms are initiated, this decrease in renal blood flow is reflected clinically by a reduction in urine output. Since renal perfusion depends on the cardiac output,

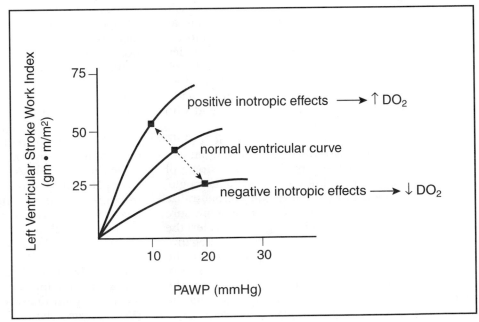

FIGURE 21–4. Left ventricular function curve: Relationship between PAWP and LVSWI. *LVSWI* is left ventricular stroke work indexed for body size. *PAWP* is the pulmonary artery wedge pressure. *DO$_2$* is oxygen delivery. (Adapted from Epstein and Henning,[23] p 335.)

any alteration in this parameter will greatly influence urine output. Thus, if cardiac output falls abruptly, the consequent decrease in renal perfusion will be reflected by a corresponding fall in urine output. Urine outputs of less than 30 mL/h for periods of 2 hours or more should be reported to the physician.

With a gradual fall in cardiac output and renal perfusion, the *composition* of the urine may change *prior* to changes in urine output. Glomerular filtration decreases as a result of reduced renal blood flow and vasoconstriction. Increased absorption of sodium and water causes a fall in urine sodium concentration, coupled with a rise in urine osmolality. These changes may be noted before there is any reduction in the urine output.[7] In the differential diagnosis of reduced renal perfusion, low urine sodium concentrations and high urine osmolality point to hypovolemia as the probable cause. Urine specific gravity will also be elevated in hypovolemic states.

Acid-Base Changes. In the early stages of hypovolemic shock, the patient may present with a respiratory alkalemia associated with tachypnea and a noticeable increase in the work of breathing. Normally, efforts to breathe are not obvious. Failure of the shock patient to hyperventilate is a sign of ventilatory deterioration and a warning of the potential need for mechanical intervention.[7] As shock progresses, the lactic acid produced from anaerobic metabolism accumulates and metabolic acidosis results. In late shock the eventual development of a combined metabolic and respiratory acidosis carries a poor prognosis.[7]

Serum Lactate Levels. Lactate levels should be periodically evaluated in all shock patients. Lactate is the end product of anaerobic metabolism and is formed when pyruvate cannot be converted to acetyl CoA because of an oxygen deficit. The evaluation of serum lactate provides the nurse with an estimation of the degree of oxygen balance (oxygen demand versus supply) and consequently tissue perfusion. An increase in demand coupled with a decreased supply leads to an accumulation of lactic acid, which contributes to the development of metabolic acidosis. Serum lactate levels normally range from 0.6 to 1.8 mmol/L. Levels greater than 2 mmol/L suggest a moderate acidosis and greater than 4 mmol/L indicate a severe acidemia.[7] High lactate levels are directly correlated with decreased chance of survival[4] (Fig. 21–5).

Base Excess and Anion Gap. The improvement of tissue perfusion, in the early shock stages, can often correct the acid-base abnormality. The body's stores of buffering agents (e.g., sodium bicarbonate, hemoglobin, proteins, phosphates) are designed to neutralize acids in the blood and plasma.[7] *Base excess,* a measure usually reported with arterial blood gases, can alert the nurse to changes in the buffer base stores. A negative base excess (base deficit) refers to a decrease in the buffer base stores or an increase in acid stores. Another indicator of the accumulation of acids is the *anion gap.* The anion gap is calculated by adding the serum chloride and serum carbon dioxide levels (bicarbonate) together and subtracting this total from

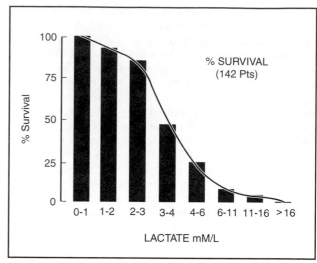

FIGURE 21–5. Relationship between arterial lactate levels and survival from circulatory shock. (Adapted from Weil, MH, and Afifi, AA: Experimental and clinical studies on lactate and pyruvate as indicators of the severity of acute circulatory failure (shock). Circulation 41:989–1001, 1970, with permission.)

the measured sodium level. The normal anion gap is about 12 mEq/L. An increase in the calculated anion gap points to an increase in acid production.

Tissue Perfusion. Perfusion of the tissues and organs is the goal of the cardiovascular system. All shock states result in decreases in tissue perfusion and may lead to organ failure. Clinical parameters of tissue perfusion are vitally important for the nurse to evaluate the adequacy of systemic perfusion.

Tissue perfusion can be evaluated noninvasively by assessing the following clinical parameters: mentation, skin and mucous membranes, vital signs, capillary refill, pulse pressure, and pulse quality. Clinical assessment is essential but when subjective in nature may not provide a reliable comparison of data from nurse to nurse. For example, the assessment of pulse quality as "weak and thready" is based on fairly subjective descriptors. Oxygen transport variables and intramucosal pH, mixed venous oxygen saturation, cardiac output, urine output, and serum lactate levels provide objective, quantitative data regarding tissue perfusion but require invasive monitoring techniques.

Objective measures of oxygen transport, intramucosal pH, and venous carbon dioxide levels are being recognized as the earliest indicators of shock.[1,20,22] Mixed venous oxygen saturation and transcutaneous monitoring techniques also provide important information to the bedside clinician regarding oxygen balance.

Oxygen Transport. In all forms of shock, the delivery of oxygen is compromised. Oxygen transport variables include oxygen delivery (DO_2), oxygen consumption ($\dot{V}O_2$), oxygen demand, and oxygen extraction ratio (OER)[23] (see definitions in Tables 21–8 and 21–9).

TABLE 21–8
Definitions of Oxygen Transport Variables

Oxygen delivery (DO$_2$) is the volume of oxygen delivered to the tissues by the left ventricle each minute. DO$_2$ is the product of cardiac output and arterial blood oxygen content. When indexed to body surface area, normal DO$_2$ is approximately 600 millimeters per minute per meter squared (mL min^{-1} m^{-2})

Oxygen consumption (V̇O$_2$) is the volume of oxygen consumed by the tissues each minute. V̇O$_2$ is the product of cardiac output times the arterial minus the venous blood oxygen content difference. Normal V̇O$_2$ is approximately 250 mL/min. When indexed to for body surface area, the normal V̇O$_2$ is approximately 120 to 140 mL min^{-1} m^{-2}

Oxygen demand is the amount of oxygen needed by cells for aerobic metabolism. Oxygen demand is determined by the metabolic need for oxygen in peripheral tissues. Although difficult to quantify clinically, oxygen demand may be roughly estimated in patients by measurements of V̇O$_2$.

Oxygen extraction ratio (OER) is the ratio of oxygen consumption to oxygen delivery (V̇O$_2$/DO$_2$). The OER provides an estimate of the balance between oxygen demand (consumption) and oxygen supply (delivery).

Source: From Epstein, CD and Henning, RJ: Oxygen transport variables in the identification and treatment of tissue hypoxia. Heart Lung 22:328–345, 1993, with permission.

Serial measurements of oxygen transport parameters are an objective way of evaluating the patient's response to the interventions designed to increase oxygen supply and decrease demand; the therapies can then be revised, if needed, to produce positive patient outcomes.

Oxygen delivery reflects the ability of the circulatory system to supply oxygen to the tissues.[1] The variables that influence oxygen delivery are the cardiac output, hemoglobin (Hgb), and arterial oxygen saturation

TABLE 21–9
Definitions of the Oxygen Parameters of the Blood

Oxygen content of blood is the total amount of oxygen transported in the blood, including oxygen combined with hemoglobin and oxygen dissolved in plasma. CaO$_2$ refers to the oxygen content of arterial blood, and CvO$_2$ refers to the oxygen content of mixed venous blood.

Oxyhemoglobin (HbO$_2$) refers to oxygen combined with hemoglobin.

Oxygen capacity is the maximum amount of oxygen that can be bound to hemoglobin. One gram of hemoglobin when fully saturated with oxygen reversibly binds 1.39 mL of oxygen. In a patient with a hemoglobin concentration of 15 grams per deciliter (g/dL) and an oxygen saturation of 100%, the oxygen capacity of hemoglobin is 21 milliliters of oxygen per deciliter (mL/dL) of arterial blood.

Oxygen saturation is the percent of oxyhemoglobin divided by the total amount of saturated and unsaturated hemoglobin (HbO$_2$/Hb + HbO$_2$). That is, oxygen saturation is the oxygen content of the blood divided by the oxygen capacity. The oxygen saturation of arterial blood (SaO$_2$) is approximately 98%, while the oxygen saturation of mixed venous blood (Sv̄O$_2$) is about 75%.

Source: From Epstein, CD and Henning, RJ: Oxygen transport variables in the identification and treatment of tissue hypoxia. Heart Lung 22:328–345, 1993, with permission.

(SaO$_2$). The body normally delivers three to four times more oxygen than is needed for normal usage.[23] The additional amount returns to the lungs and is used as an *oxygen reserve*.[24] Normal values for DO$_2$ are 1000 mL/min, and the calculation of DO$_2$ is found in Appendix F. *Oxygen consumption* represents the body's demand for oxygen and thus the general state of tissue metabolism.[1] However, V̇O$_2$ is not always equal to the amount of oxygen needed. The tissues may be unable to extract all of the oxygen needed from the blood, even if oxygen is available (e.g., in early sepsis). A measure of V̇O$_2$ reduction is common in all shock states and the degree of V̇O$_2$ deficit has been directly correlated with mortality.[1,22,23,25] Normal values for V̇O$_2$ are 250 mL/min. Both these values can be individualized by indexing for body size (divide value by body surface area). The *oxygen extraction ratio* provides an indication of the ability of the tissues to actually use the oxygen delivered. Normal values for OER range from 22% to 32%. High values indicate an increased peripheral tissue demand and low values signify decreased demand or utilization ability.[23]

In the critically ill patient, oxygen needs, to support the patient through stressors such as hospitalization, therapy, and wound healing are greatly increased. It is understandable, then, that acutely stressed patients would try to extract more oxygen in order to meet this increased demand: V̇O$_2$ does increase in critically ill patients. However, hypermetabolic demands for oxygen soon outstrip the supply, V̇O$_2$ falls, and an *oxygen debt* builds. Supranormal levels of DO$_2$ and V̇O$_2$, in vulnerable patients, are vital to assure oxygen diffusion and uptake to the cells to prevent or reverse oxygen debt during shock. These parameters need to be maintained at higher levels after the patient has been stabilized to "repay" the oxygen debt.[7] Recent research studies have shown that supranormal levels of oxygen transport variables significantly decreased the mortality rate in critically ill patients.[16,23,26]

Treatment measures are primarily focused on methods to increase cardiac output, which is the major determinant of DO$_2$. Many researchers contend that oxygen transport variables should be both the therapeutic starting points and end points for the titration of pharmacologic interventions (Table 21–10).[1,16,23,26,27]

Intramucosal pH. Recent research focuses on gastric intramucosal pH (pHi) readings as one of the earliest indicators of tissue hypoxia.[8,9] The gastrointestinal tract, kidneys, and liver are among the first organs to be affected by low-flow states as blood is shunted away from these organs to the "priority" organs (the heart and brain). Therefore, it makes sense that as the gut switches to an anaerobic pathway for energy production and lactic acid accumulates, the pH of the gastric mucosa will fall. Tonometry (the measurement of the partial pressure of a gas) is used to obtain a PCO$_2$ reading of the gastric mucosa, which is correlated with the arterial bicarbonate value; pHi is then calculated using the Henderson-Hasselbalch equation (Fig. 21–6). Gastric tonometry provides a useful, relatively noninvasive

TABLE 21–10
Therapeutic End Points in the Treatment of Shock

HR	<100 bpm
CVP	15 mmHg (ref 3)
PAWP	10–12 mmHg or 18–20 mmHg* (ref 3)
Serum lactate	<2 mmol/L[3]
Vo_2I	≥170 mL min^{-1} m^{-2} (ref 23)
Do_2I	>800 mL min^{-1} m^{-2} or 300–400 mL min^{-1} m$^{-2†}$ (ref 23)
CI	>4.5 L/min/m^2 (ref 23)
OER	<31% (ref 23)

HR = heart rate, CVP = central venous pressure, PAWP = pulmonary artery wedge pressure, Vo_2I = oxygen consumption index, Do_2I = oxygen delivery index, CI = cardiac index, OER = oxygen extraction ratio.

*Suggested for patients with hypertension or left heart failure.
†Suggested for patients with cardiogenic shock. Values are indexed (I) to body size.

method to detect early changes in perfusion and tissue hypoxia.[9]

Venous Hypercarbia. The difference between rising venous carbon dioxide levels ($Pvco_2$) and decreasing arterial carbon dioxide levels ($Paco_2$) can also be evaluated as early signs of lactic acidosis and decreased tissue perfusion.[20,28] The principle is based on the fact that typically CO_2 is rapidly cleared when circulation is unimpaired; thus the presence of venous hypercarbia signifies impaired perfusion. The re-establishment of effective circulation clears accumulated CO_2 within 2 minutes; blood lactate is cleared in about 4 hours.[28] Therefore, venous CO_2 levels are very sensitive markers of decreases in perfusion and resulting lactic acidosis. Buildup of CO_2 in the tissues and venous blood is correlated with decreases in cardiac output and organ ischemia.[28]

The end-tidal CO_2 ($EtCO_2$) monitor, placed in line with the endotracheal tube, is a noninvasive method that has been suggested as a useful adjunct in evaluating early acidosis and systemic perfusion. As cardiac output is reduced, blood flow to the pulmonary circuit is reduced and CO_2 elimination is reduced. This is evidenced as a low $EtCO_2$ reading.[20,29]

Mixed Venous Oxygen Saturation. Trends in cardiac output and tissue perfusion can also be evaluated by monitoring mixed venous oxygen saturation ($S\bar{v}o_2$) as obtained via a fiberoptic PA catheter. The oxygen saturation of mixed venous blood in the pulmonary artery is an average of total body saturation that reflects the match of oxygen delivery to oxygen demand.[24] The $S\bar{v}o_2$ reading averages 75%, with a normal range of 60% to 80%. $S\bar{v}o_2$ decreases as oxygen delivery variables (CO, Hgb, Sao_2) decrease, or as oxygen demands increase; $S\bar{v}o_2$ is increased as oxygen demands decrease, or in conditions where the oxygen

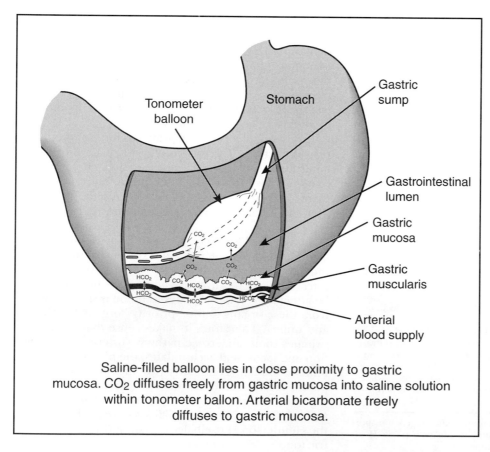

Saline-filled balloon lies in close proximity to gastric mucosa. CO_2 diffuses freely from gastric mucosa into saline solution within tonometer ballon. Arterial bicarbonate freely diffuses to gastric mucosa.

FIGURE 21–6. Principles of Pco_2 and HCO_3^- diffusion in gastric tonometry. (Adapted from Clark and Gutierrez,[9] p. 55.)

RESEARCH APPLICATION: COMPARISON OF GASTRIC INTRAMUCOSAL pH WITH MEASURES OF OXYGEN TRANSPORT AND CONSUMPTION IN CRITICALLY ILL PATIENTS
Gutierrez, G, et al. Crit Care Med 20:451–457.

Purpose: The purpose of this article was to compare assessment of decreases in gastric mucosal tissue perfusion by a noninvasive method with oxygen transport variables in critically ill patients. Changes in intramucosal pH and oxygenation variables were correlated with mortality.

Methods: This was a prospective, nonintervention study set in the medical and surgical ICUs of a large metropolitan university teaching hospital. The sample consisted of 22 critically ill patients requiring pulmonary artery monitoring and nasogastric tubes. The ages ranged from 26 to 82 years (52.1 ± 3.6) and illness severity, using the APACHE II scoring system, ranged from 12 to 32 (20.3 ± 1.4). Sixteen of the 22 patients were diagnosed with sepsis, ARDS, or both.

Gastric intramucosal pH measurements were obtained using a TRIP™ gastric tonometer, which is a nasogastric (NG) tube that has been adapted with a gas-permeable silicone balloon. After ensuring correct positioning of the NG tube, the silicone balloon is infused with 2.5 mL of normal saline and allowed to remain undisturbed in the stomach for about 1 hour. The saline is then withdrawn and the P_{CO_2} level is analyzed and reported. This reading is correlated with the arterial bicarbonate level from a blood sample drawn at the same time gastric sampling occurs. The intramucosal pH (pHi) is then calculated using the Henderson-Hasselbalch equation. Hemodynamic and serum lactate measurements were also obtained at the time of gastric and arterial sampling. Calculations of systemic oxygenation (DO_2I, $\dot{V}O_2I$, OER, PvO_2, and mixed venous pH) were then calculated.

Results: The nonsurvivors group was found to have definitive signs of decreased tissue perfusion and resultant acidosis. Oxygen consumption and extraction needs ($\dot{V}O_2I$ and OER) were higher in nonsurvivors than survivors, as were serum lactate levels; DO_2I, mixed venous pH and PO_2, arterial pH and gastric intramucosal pH were found to be lower in nonsurvivors. These researchers found pHi readings of <7.32 to be very sensitive and specific indicators of early mortality.

Practice Implications: The gastrointestinal tract is among the first organs to be denied an adequate blood flow in the evolution of the shock state: blood is shunted to priority organs as a compensatory measure. The cells shift to the anaerobic form of energy production as oxygen delivery decreases with decreases in perfusion. Lactic acid accumulates in the cell and eventually causes cell death and local tissue destruction. Low pHi readings are associated with the degree of anaerobic activity. Early detection of mucosal acidosis enables the clinician and medical team to implement aggressive treatment in hope of preventing the progression of shock to the deadlier stages.

Care of the patient with a gastric tonometer is no different from routine nasogastric tube care. Attention must be given to maintaining the patency of the NG tube, and the integrity of the patient's skin and airway. The technical aspects of the use of this tonometer may preclude its use in everyday monitoring. The nurses must be familiar with the rationale for use; receive technical training regarding the proper priming, sampling, and documentation procedures; and be able to act upon the pHi results.[9] The use of gastric tonometry in the critically ill promises to provide early information of systemic acidosis. Early diagnosis and intervention in systemic hypoxia and circulatory shock states should help to decrease mortality and morbidity.

---

supply is increased, such as those where the ability of the cell to use oxygen is impaired (as in early septic shock).

Research studies have demonstrated that changes in $S\bar{v}O_2$ readings occurred *before* obvious changes in vital signs or preload indicators.[24] Therefore, changes in $S\bar{v}O_2$ readings provide the bedside clinician with an early warning system of deteriorating cardiopulmonary function and an objective indicator of the patient's tolerance to pathologic conditions and response to therapeutic interventions (Table 21–11). Typical nursing care activities such as dressing changes, baths, and obtaining weights on a sling scale can increase the patient's $\dot{V}O_2$ by 10%, 23%, and 36%,

respectively.[24] $S\bar{v}O_2$ will decrease in the acutely ill patient. A decrease of 5% to 10% from baseline should alert the nurse to possible alterations in cardiopulmonary function; an $S\bar{v}O_2$ reading of less than 60% suggests compromised tissue perfusion or increased oxygen extraction/consumption by the tissues and requires immediate action by the clinician.

Transcutaneous Oxygen Monitoring. Other noninvasive measures of detecting impaired tissue perfusion include the use of pulse oximetry (SpO_2) and transcutaneous gas measurements (Ptc). *Pulse oximetry* estimates oxygen saturation of hemoglobin via a reflectance meter. SpO_2 values greater than or equal to 92% are generally desired. Actual oxygen saturation read-

TABLE 21–11
Increases in Resting S$\overline{\text{v}}$O$_2$ Associated with Pathologic Conditions and Common Nursing Care Activities

Pathologic Conditions	(%)	Nursing Care Activities	(%)
Fever (each 1°C)	10	Dressing change	10
Fractures (each)	10	Electrocardiogram	16
Agitation	18	Physical exam	20
Chest trauma	25	Visitors	22
Work of breathing	40	Bath	23
Critically ill in emergency room	60	Chest x-ray	25
Severe infection	60	Endotracheal suctioning	27
Shivering	50–100	Nasal intubation	25–40
Sepsis	50–100	Turn to side	31
Head injury, sedated	89	Chest physiotherapy	35
Head injury, not sedated	138	Weight on sling scale	36
Burns	100		

Source: Adapted from White, KM: Using continuous S$\overline{\text{V}}$O$_2$ to assess oxygen supply/demand balance in the critically ill patient. AACN Clinical Issues in Critical Care 4(1): 134–147, 1993.

ings (acquired during arterial blood gas [ABG] analysis) are normally less than SpO$_2$ by 2% to 5%.[29] A major limitation to the use of pulse oximetry in shock patients is the need for pulsatile flow to accurately measure oxygen levels. The oximetry probe that is located in areas of decreased blood flow will therefore not provide valuable data. *Transcutaneous oxygen* (PtcO$_2$) and carbon dioxide gas measurements are not yet widely used in the clinical setting but have been encouraged for use as measurements of regional tissue perfusion. Decreases in peripheral blood flow result in a decrease in the amount of oxygen that diffuses from the vessels.[29] Placement of the PtcO$_2$ probe on specific sites will reflect the local reduction in blood flow.

Mentation. Changes in level of consciousness are often the subtle, first signs of shock. The effectiveness of cerebral perfusion is reflected by the patient's demeanor and general cerebral functioning (e.g., mental status; orientation to person, time, and place). Reduced cerebral perfusion is exhibited by an altered level of consciousness, restlessness, anxiety, apathy, lethargy, and confusion. As the shock state deepens and coma ensues, the patient's response to pain may progress from flexion, to extension, to no response. Severe cerebral ischemia leads to depression of the vasomotor center and sympathetic activity. The loss of sympathetic tone causes the systemic vasculature to dilate, resulting in the pooling of blood in the periphery. This further reduces venous return to the heart and cardiac output.

Skin and Mucous Membranes. Widespread peripheral vasoconstriction in response to intense sympathetic stimulation causes the skin to appear pale and mottled, and to feel cool to the touch. Increased sweat gland activity causes the skin to feel clammy and moist. Assessment of mucous membranes will reveal pale, dry mucosa. These findings become apparent once the shock state is well established. Cyanosis is a *late* sign in shock. In patients with hemorrhagic shock, a severe loss of blood may preclude this finding.[19,30]

These typical findings are not observed in shock complicated by sepsis or spinal trauma. These patients may present with signs of vasodilatation rather than vasoconstriction: the skin is warm and dry, and may be flushed. In the early stage of septic shock, the release of vasoactive substances in response to the endotoxin(s) underlies the vasodilatation and SVR is decreased (see Chapter 56). In the patient with neurogenic shock, the loss of autonomic tone is responsible for the difference.

Capillary Refill. Assessment of capillary refill is a quick way to determine the adequacy of the peripheral circulation. Tissues that blanch for longer than 2 seconds indicate poor perfusion of the capillary bed. However, keep in mind that the patient in the early stages of shock may still demonstrate capillary blanching of less than 2 seconds.[30]

Diagnostic Tests/Studies

In the scenario of shock or trauma, the principal diagnostic tests include radiographic and laboratory studies. A simple chest x-ray provides immediate information about intrathoracic injury. Pneumothorax, hemothorax, mediastinal or diaphragmatic injury, and rib fractures can usually be determined in chest x-ray. The chest x-ray is also helpful in determining underlying pulmonary congestion as exhibited by pulmonary infiltrates and lymphatic enlargement. Depending on the underlying condition, and a high index of suspicion, other visualization studies may be requested, including computed tomography (CT scan) and magnetic resonance imaging (MRI). Contrast imaging studies such as intravenous pyelography and angiography may also be requested.

Implementation of hemodynamic monitoring is invaluable, both in determining the patient's hemodynamic status and in managing the shock state. As discussed previously, use of a PA catheter facilitates assessment of left heart function and mixed venous oxygen saturation; central venous pressure measurements reflect venous return and right heart function.

Arterial pressure monitoring enables ongoing assessment of mean arterial pressure; evaluation of the arterial pressure waveform; and, very importantly, blood sampling for arterial blood gases, a hematology profile, serum electrolytes, glucose, blood urea nitrogen (BUN) and creatinine, plasma proteins, serum lactate, and a coagulation profile. Urine studies, as described earlier, are also assessed.

Treatment and Management

The overall goal in therapeutic management of the patient with hypovolemic shock is to restore the effective circulating blood volume and tissue perfusion. Basic resuscitative measures that may have to be implemented prior to determining the underlying problem include establishing and/or maintaining an airway to ensure adequate ventilation and oxygenation; treatment of obvious fluid volume deficit with rapid infusion of crystalloids, colloids, and blood and/or blood products; correction of electrolyte abnormalities (e.g., hyperkalemia) and acidosis; and initiation of pharmacologic therapy, titrated to maintain blood pressure at the desired level. In the scenario of acute blood loss, regardless of the underlying cause, treatment is based on the magnitude of the loss based on the patient's initial clinical presentation (Table 21-5).

Once the underlying diagnosis is established, outcomes of therapy are directed toward the following: (1) reduction in anaerobic cellular respiration with correction of consequent acidosis; (2) reduction in intrapulmonary shunting and improved gas exchange as reflected by an increase in arterial oxygenation ($PaO_2 > 80$ mmHg); (3) improvement in tissue perfusion with increased cerebral blood flow, as determined by improvement in mental status and state of consciousness; increased renal perfusion, as reflected by an increased in hourly urine outputs; increased peripheral perfusion, as reflected by well-perfused, warm, dry skin and moist mucous membranes; and (4) treatment of the underlying cause (e.g., gastrointestinal bleeding associated with peptic ulcer disease; thoracic, abdominal, or long-bone trauma).

Ventilation/Oxygenation

Oxygen deprivation of the tissues is the major endpoint in the pathophysiology of the shock state. The inability to maintain tissue perfusion and oxygenation leads to metabolic acidosis and tissue hypoxia. Therefore, establishing and maintaining a patent airway with the necessary ventilation and oxygenation are of prime importance.

Patients in early shock can be observed to be hyperventilating and tachypneic, with a minute volume twice the normal and a $PaCO_2$ that usually ranges between 25 and 35 mmHg. These are anticipated compensatory responses to enhanced chemoreceptor stimulation in the presence of a lowered PaO_2, a raised $PaCO_2$, and a decreasing pH. The shock patient who

TABLE 21-12
Criteria for Mechanical Ventilatory Assistance for Patients in Shock

1. Minute ventilation less than 9–12 L/min (or greater than 18 L/min)
2. Tidal volume less than 4–5 mL/kg
3. Vital capacity less than 10–12 mL/kg
4. $PaCO_2$ greater than 45 mmHg if a metabolic acidosis is present or $PaCO_2$ greater than 50–55 mmHg with normal bicarbonate
5. PaO_2 less than 60 mmHg on 40% O_2 or PaO_2 less than 200 mmHg on 100% O_2
6. Respiratory rate greater than 30–35 per minute
7. Excessive ventilatory effort

Source: From Wilson, RF: Critical Care Manual: Applied Physiology and Principles of Therapy, ed 2. FA Davis, Philadelphia, 1992, with permission.

is not hyperventilating should be assessed for the presence of a serious problem with ventilation and aggressive ventilatory support should be considered.[7] Indications for endotracheal intubation and implementation of ventilatory assistance in patients with shock are listed in Table 21-12. In all patients in shock, including those in whom spontaneous ventilation is adequate, oxygen therapy should be administered during the initial 4 to 6 hours of the resuscitative period, to maintain a PaO_2 greater than 80 mmHg.[7]

Resuscitation Strategies

The main goal of therapy in the hypovolemic patient, regardless of the etiology, is to restore circulation to a level where oxygen is available for tissue metabolism. Oxygen utilization is affected by the adequacy of blood flow (cardiac output) and the oxygen content in the blood (Hgb and SaO_2). Cells have the ability to adjust the amount of oxygen being extracted (used) according to changes in oxygen delivery; however, this mechanism can be impaired in the critically ill patient[23] and this impairment necessitates therapeutic intervention.

Fluid Volume Replacement. Aggressive fluid administration is the most efficient treatment for the patient with hypovolemic shock.[4,7,15,17,19,31] The first goal is to support the circulation. Fluid volume replacement helps to re-establish an effective circulating blood volume essential for adequate tissue perfusion. After the blood volume has been reestablished, the second goal is to improve tissue oxygenation. In the anemic patient, the administration of blood and/or blood products is necessary to assist in restoring and maintaining the oxygen-carrying capacity of the intravascular volume.

The choice of the *initial* fluid therapy is related to the ability of the product to increase blood flow.[3] Common fluids used in resuscitation are isotonic crystalloids such as lactated Ringer's solution, normal (0.9%) saline, and colloids such as albumin, hetastarch, and dextran (Table 21-13). Controversy continues to exist over the efficacy of crystalloids ver-

TABLE 21–13
Types of Replacement Fluids

Type	Description	Uses	Complications
Colloids			
1. Normal human serum albumin (5% or 25%)	Blood plasma derivative approximately 96% albumin, a simple protein; rapidly expands intravascular volume	Increases plasma colloidal oncotic pressure (PCOP)	Volume overload; circulatory failure Rare: transmission of hepatitis; urticaria; febrile reactions; clotting abnormalities
2. Plasma protein fraction	Albumin and other proteins in NSS	Same as albumin	Same as albumin; paradoxical hypotension; hypersensitivity
3. Dextran	Nonprotein glucose polymer with molecules larger than albumin in either NSS or dextrose solution	Rapid expansion of plasma volume	Interference with blood typing; allergic reactions; anaphylaxis; clotting abnormalities; increased blood viscosity
4. Hetastarch	Synthetic colloid made from heterogeneous group of starch molecules in NSS	Expand plasma volume	Clotting abnormalities; circulatory overload; increased amylase; decreased PCOP
Crystalloids			
1. Lactated Ringer's injection	0.9% NaCl in water with added potassium, calcium, and sodium lactate buffers	Replace body fluid; to provide bicarbonate to buffer body fluids	Large volumes may increase lactic acidosis in shock (due to lactate); fluid retention; circulatory overload
2. Normal saline solution	0.9% NaCl in water	Raise plasma volume when red blood cell mass is adequate; replace body fluids	Fluid retention; circulatory overload

NSS = normal saline solution.
Source: Adapted from Sommers, MS: Fluid resuscitation following multiple trauma. Critical Care Nurse 10(10):74–81, 1990.

sus colloids in resuscitation of the hypovolemic patient. Colloids have demonstrated the ability to increase intravascular fluid volume and cardiac output more rapidly and with a greater effect on cardiac output than crystalloids.[3]

Crystalloids. Crystalloids include solutions of dextrose dissolved in water or electrolytes dissolved in water. If the goal is fluid volume expansion of both the intravascular and interstitial compartments, crystalloid solutions may be indicated. It is important to note, however, that only 20% of the crystalloid volume infused remains in the intravascular space; the remainder moves into the interstitial space.[3,7] Therefore, if the goal is predominantly to expand the intravascular fluid volume, then these agents are not the solutions of choice. The main ingredient in crystalloid solutions is sodium. Since sodium is the major extracellular ion, infused sodium (via crystalloids) moves into the interstitial space and thus restores the interstitial fluid volume deficit that exists in hypovolemia.[3] However, movement of the fluid into the interstitial compartment may also predispose to systemic and pulmonary edema.[7,32] Crystalloid infusion is reported to be favored by some as the primary fluid of choice for acute volume loss, despite the large volume usually required for adequate resuscitation.[31–33] Advantages of crystalloids in general include the following: they are cost effective, readily available, nonallergenic, and have a long shelf life.[7]

Administration of *0.9% normal saline*, an isotonic solution, is well tolerated in the hypovolemic patient. It is necessary to cautiously monitor serum electrolytes during therapy because large amounts of normal saline can disrupt serum electrolyte balance and predispose to hyperchloremia, hypernatremia, hypokalemia, and metabolic acidosis.

Administration of *lactated Ringer's (LR)* solution is also used in the treatment of hypovolemic shock. In addition to volume replacement, this agent helps to buffer the acidosis since the lactate contained therein is converted to bicarbonate in the liver. Metabolic alkalosis is a potential complication of infusion of large amounts of LR, especially in the presence of renal or liver failure.[7,32] In the presence of cardiac disease, half normal saline (0.45%) may be indicated because of its lower sodium content.

Dextrose in water (D_5W) is administered in hypovolemic shock and in states of severe dehydration because this solution is evenly distributed throughout the body. D_5W should always be given in conjunction with other fluids for resuscitation.[19] As is the case with all replacement fluid, serum electrolytes need to be closely monitored because replacement solutions tend to dilute serum concentrations of electrolytes. Keep in mind that the hematocrit will also drop when fluids are used to increase the plasma volume: this is due to a dilution in the proportion of red cells to plasma and *not* due to acute blood loss.[3]

The latest research has focused on the use of *hypertonic saline solutions (HSS)* in trauma and hypovolemic shock.[7,32–34] HSS (3%, 5%, 7%) exerts an osmotic effect that draws fluid into the vascular space, much like colloidal solutions. One advantage of HSS, therefore, is that less total volume is required for resuscitation than with isotonic saline; thus the potential for complications is decreased.[32–34] Other advantages may include a beneficial inotropic effect on the myocardium and vasodilator properties.[7,32] The main disadvantages are listed as the risk of hypernatremia, hyperosmolality, and hyperchloremia.[34] Serum sodium levels of greater than 160 mEq/L are indications for discontinuing any HSS infusion.[7]

Colloids. Colloids are solutions that contain large proteins or starches, which exert an oncotic force that causes fluids to be retained in the vascular space. In contrast to crystalloids, the colloids generally cannot traverse the capillary endothelium. Thus, these agents play a pivotal role in maintaining the osmotic pressure within the vascular space and are ideal for rapid intravascular fluid volume expansion in patients with hypovolemic shock. One-third less volume is required to increase cardiac output with colloid solutions than with crystalloids.[31] Studies have shown that colloids are more effective in rapidly expanding blood volume than blood or crystalloids in acute hypovolemic states, and therefore are the fluids of choice for expanding the intravascular volume.[1,3,31] Colloid solutions that are frequently used include albumin, hetastarch, and dextran.

Albumin is a human protein available in 5% and 25% concentrations with oncotic pressures of 20 mmHg (normal body value) and 70 mmHg (hyperoncotic), respectively.[3] Albumin is the most common protein found in plasma and is responsible for the colloid osmotic force in the intravascular space.[7,32] Albumin's advantages include the ability to retain fluid in the intravascular space for long periods of time, protection against edema formation by maintaining colloid oncotic pressure, and improving immune function.[34] Disadvantages include the prohibitive cost (up to 30 times more expensive than crystalloid solutions[7]) and potential deficits in coagulation function.[32]

Hetastarch (Hespan) is the colloid of choice in patients who have a religious objection to the administration of human blood products. Hetastarch is a synthetic starch similar to albumin in its plasma volume expansion capability, and its effect can last up to 36 hours. *Dextran* preparations are frequently used for rapid volume expansion. Use of these two agents has been associated with coagulation and bleeding complications because they reduce platelet adhesiveness. Prothrombin time, partial thromboplastin time, and platelet count should be monitored.

Blood and/or Blood Products. After the immediate need to replenish the intravascular volume has been met, replacement of blood and blood products may be indicated in cases of hypovolemic shock related to hemorrhage. Available products include fresh whole blood, stored whole blood, packed red cells, fresh-frozen red cells, platelet concentrate, fresh-frozen plasma, Plasmanate, and cryoprecipitate. Packed red blood cells are the most common type of blood product used.

The ability to store blood makes it readily available, but blood decreases in quality with long storage times. Stored blood has a higher concentration of potassium and citrate levels, and lower concentrations of 2,3-diphosphoglyceric acid (2,3 DPG), ATP, and platelets. Citrate, an anticoagulant blood preservative, binds calcium and magnesium and may affect normal functions of conduction and contraction as a result. Patients requiring great quantities of blood should have their calcium and magnesium levels checked, since the electrolytes may require replacement.

The ultimate goal of blood replacement therapy in the critically ill is to keep the hematocrit levels at 30% to 35%. Increased hematocrit levels have been associated with decreased mortality.[7] Autotransfusion, pharmacologic stimulation of erythropoiesis, and the development of synthetic red blood cell products provide additional strategies for blood replacement.

Autotransfusion. Autotransfusion is the reinfusion of the patient's shed blood. It is accomplished through (1) planned preoperative donation and designation of the patient's own blood, (2) collection of blood in the immediate preoperative period, and (3) intra- and postoperative autotransfusion.[33] Autologous blood infusion benefits include the elimination of blood-borne pathogen risks and allergic reactions, cost-effectiveness, and less stress on blood bank stores. Disadvantages include the potential for reinfusion of shed blood affected by heparin therapy (as in cardiac surgery patients), reduced clotting factors (increasing bleeding tendencies), and a predisposition to DIC.[7] Autotransfusion benefits the patient with planned blood loss (as in surgery) and may aid in preventing hypovolemic shock.

Erythropoietin Stimulation. The ability to stimulate red cell growth factors in the bone marrow has been a recent advance in blood replacement therapy. Recombinant human erythropoietin (rHuEPO) has been shown to stimulate the bone marrow to produce red blood cells and thus hasten recovery after acute blood loss. Though administered in the acute period, this treatment does not have an immediate effect on blood volume; clinical effects are not evident until about 1 week into therapy.[33]

Artificial Blood. Two types of artificial blood currently being investigated include stroma-free hemoglobin (SFH) and fluorocarbons. Both products are colloids with the ability to carry and release oxygen.[34] SFH is hemoglobin that has been separated from the red blood cell membrane;[33] because it is a hemoglobin it has a very high affinity for oxygen and therefore does not easily release oxygen for use by the tissues. Poly SFH-P is a newer SFH product that has physiologic properties similar to those of stored red blood cells, and early studies have shown promising results.[33] Fluosol-DA 20% (Flusol) has been used in emergency situations to treat patients who refused blood therapy for religious reasons,[7] but it has not been found to be particularly beneficial as a substitute blood product because its oxygen-carrying capacity is limited.[33] Complications of fever, leukocytosis, diffuse pulmonary infiltrates, and hypoxemia have been encountered in

TABLE 21–14
Drugs That Boost Cardiac Output

Drug; Use	Usual IV Dose	Onset/Duration	Heart Rate/Contractility	Afterload	Preload	Cautions
Nitroglycerin (Nitro-Bid IV, Nitrostat, Tridil) To relieve angina, congestive heart failure (CHF) associated with acute MI, and perioperative hypertension	*Initial:* 5 μg/min *Titrate:* at 5–10 μg/min q 5 min to response or max dose of 400 μg/min	*Onset:* 5 min *Duration:* 15 min	↑ 2° to ↓ BP/↑	Small ↓ with high doses	→	• Side effects: hypotension, headache, tolerance • 40%–80% absorbed by plastic and PVC tubing; mix in glass bottle, administer through non-PVC, nitroglycerin tubing
Nitroprusside (Nipride) To lower pressure in hypertensive crisis, to lower afterload and preload in CHF	*Initial:* 0.5–1.0 μg kg^{-1} min^{-1} *Titrate:* to response up to 10 μg kg^{-1} min^{-1}; stop if no response to this dose within 10 min	*Onset:* immediate *Duration:* 1–10 min	May ↑ /No effect	→	→	• Side effects: hypotension, cyanide toxicity • Dilute only with D$_5$W • Photosensitive when diluted; protect solution from light
Dobutamine (Dobutrex) To boost cardiac output during decompensation 2° to CHF or cardiac surgery	*Initial:* 2–10 μg kg^{-1} min^{-1} *Titrate:* to response or max 20 μg kg^{-1} min^{-1}	*Onset:* 1–2 min *Duration:* 10 min	No effect/↑		→	• Side effects are dose-related: atrial or ventricular ectopic beats (though risk of arrhythmias slightly less than with dopamine); occasional tachycardia, though usually no rise in heart rate • Do not add dobutamine to bicarbonate or other strongly alkaline solution • Solution with dobutamine may turn pink due to slight oxidation of drug, but does not affect potency
Dopamine (Intropin) To boost cardiac output during shock not induced by fluid loss, during cardiac decompensation in CHF, and after open heart surgery. Simulation of dopaminergic receptors produces vasodilation; of β-adrenergic receptors, faster heart rate; of α-adrenergic receptors, faster heart rate, and vasoconstriction	*Initial:* 1–5 μg kg^{-1} min^{-1} for dopaminergic response; 5–10 μg kg^{-1} min^{-1} for β-adrenergic response; > 10 μg kg^{-1} min^{-1} for α-adrenergic response *Titrate:* to response or max 50 μg kg^{-1} min^{-1}	*Onset:* within 5 min *Duration:* less than 10 min	↑ /↑	↓ at low (1–5 μg kg^{-1} min^{-1}) doses ↑ at high (5–50 μg kg^{-1} min^{-1}) doses	Same as effect on afterload	• Side effects: hypertension at high doses, may lower circulation in arms and legs • Extravasation can lead to necrosis; antidote is to infiltrate area with 5–10 mg phentolamine (Regitine) diluted in 10–15 mL NaCl

Drug / Indication	Dose	Onset / Duration				Side effects
Amrinone (Inocor) To raise cardiac output in CHF after digitalis, diuretics, and vasodilators have failed	*Initial:* 0.75–3 µg/kg infused slowly over 2–3 min *Maintenance:* 5–10 µg kg⁻¹ min⁻¹ to response	*Onset:* within 5 min *Duration:* 0.5–2 h	No effect/↑	↓	↓	• Side effects: thrombocytopenia, hepatotoxicity, hypotension, arrhythmias in CHF
Norepinephrine (Levophed) To raise pressure in acute hypotension	*Initial:* 0.05 µg kg⁻¹ min⁻¹ or 8–12 µg/min *Titrate:* to patient response	*Onset:* immediate *Duration:* 1–2 min	May ↓ from vagal stimulation or ↑ from β stimulation/↑	↑	↑	• Side effects: ischemia due to potent vasoconstriction causing tissue hypoxia, bradycardia associated with hypertension, headache, dyspnea • Constriction can produce some leakage of drug out of the vein and blanching along the infused vein • Extravasation results in necrosis; see dopamine for antidote
Epinephrine (Adrenalin) To raise cardiac output in shock not related to fluid loss and to relieve respiratory distress 2° to bronchospasm	*Initial:* 0.5–1 mg bolus *Titrate:* at 0.05 mg kg⁻¹ min⁻¹ to response	*Onset:* immediate *Duration:* 5 min	↑/↑	↓ at low doses ↑ at high doses	Same effect as afterload	• Side effects: tachycardia, hypertension, ventricular arrhythmias • Extravasation results in necrosis; see dopamine for antidote
Phenylephrine (Neo-Synephrine) To raise pressure in acute hypotension	*Initial:* 0.2 mg bolus *Repeat dose:* 0.1–0.5 mg no more frequently than q 10–15 min *Titrate:* 40–180 µg kg⁻¹ min⁻¹ to response	*Onset:* 1–2 min *Duration:* 15 min	↓ 2° to vagal effect/no effect	↑	↑	• Side effects: severe peripheral and visceral vasoconstriction, hypertension with reflex bradycardia, decline in cardiac output from vagal stimulation • Extravasation results in necrosis; see dopamine for antidote

Source: From Murphy, TG, et al: Drugs that boost cardiac output. Am J Nurs 92:38–39, 1992, with permission.

its use.[7] While current use of artificial blood products is still largely investigational, there is a promise of conventional use of these products in the future.

Gravity and Mechanical Resuscitation. *Gravity Methods.* The goal of redirecting pooled blood from the periphery back into the central circulation is also a type of autotransfusion. Two temporary measures that are used frequently in a shock setting are placing the patient in the Trendelenburg position or elevating the lower extremities. These methods are intended to "pour" blood into the central circulation; however, because the venous system absorbs rather than transmits pressure, the expected pressure gradient does not develop.[3] The Trendelenburg position has been studied in animal models and has demonstrated a decrease in cerebral blood flow. In patients, this could cause an increase in intracranial pressure. Therefore, gravity measures to increase central blood flow have not demonstrated efficacy and may be unsafe in certain patient populations.[3]

Military Antishock Trouser (MAST). The MAST is an external counterpressure device consisting of an inflatable unit with three chambers—an abdominal chamber and two leg chambers—each chamber inflating separately from the others. The MAST—also called the pneumatic antishock garment (PASG)—is a form of circulatory assistance that has been used in trauma situations, particularly scenarios of severe hemorrhage and hypovolemic shock. The theory behind the device is that it assists in increasing arterial pressure by compression of vascular beds by the inflatable layers to increase SVR; compression also redistributes blood flow from the peripheral circulation, thus increasing venous return and making it available for the perfusion of vital organs. However, despite its accepted use in emergency situations, clinical studies have *not* shown the application of MAST to significantly improve survival in the shock patient.[35] MAST garments have been used beneficially as a tamponade device to stop bleeding and as a splint for fractures of the pelvis or long bones of the lower extremities.[30]

Nursing Care Considerations. Key nursing considerations for the patient receiving treatment with the MAST device include careful monitoring of the patient's arterial blood pressure and respiratory function, and vigilant maintenance of the equipment to ensure optimal effect while minimizing complications. A baseline cardiopulmonary assessment should be performed prior to inflation of the device. Prior to inflation, it is useful to pad all bony prominences and pressure points. This helps to prevent an impairment in skin integrity. When applying the garment, it is important to avoid positioning it over the lower costal margins, so as not to interfere with respiratory excursion. Sudden deflation must be avoided to prevent an abrupt fall in blood pressure. If the garment is to be used for a prolonged period, it is useful to insert a nasogastric tube. Pressure on the abdominal viscera may cause vomiting, as well as defecation and urination. A Foley catheter is also indicated.

While the MAST device is in use, the patient should be assessed for compartment syndrome, as reflected by pain, redness, swelling, and tenderness. Loss of peripheral pulses is an ominous sign. During the course of therapy the patient should also be monitored for signs that counterpressure can be discontinued. This may be indicated by an adequate volume replacement or control of bleeding. When the therapy is to be discontinued, it must be done gradually, with sequential release of pressure in each compartment, beginning with the abdomen. Blood pressure should be monitored closely and volume replacement instituted immediately if the blood pressure drops by 5 mmHg. Subsequent deflation should proceed only if the patient remains hemodynamically stable.

Pharmacologic Support

The mainstay of treatment for the patient with hypovolemic shock is fluid volume replacement. The combination of fluids used (crystalloids, colloids, and/or blood and blood products) depends on the nature of the fluid loss. Use of vasopressors is usually contraindicated because of the intense vasoconstriction of the microcirculation associated with shock-induced enhanced sympathoadrenal activity.

- Epinephrine and norepinephrine may be used if vasopressor support is indicated. If fluid volume replacement therapy and the inherent sympathetic response are inadequate in maintaining blood pressure, a drug whose effects are dose-dependent, such as dopamine, may be prescribed. At low doses (less than 5 μg kg^{-1} min^{-1}), dopamine acts selectively to stimulate dopaminergic and mesenteric receptors to improve blood flow, especially to the kidneys (*dopaminergic* effect). Its inotropic effect increases cardiac contractility and improves cardiac output at doses from 5 to 10 μg kg^{-1} min^{-1} (*beta effect*), with α-receptors being stimulated above 10 μg kg^{-1} min^{-1} (*alpha effect*). Dobutamine affects contractility without significantly increasing heart rate and provides some systemic vasodilation as well. Refer to Table 21–14 for a review of drugs commonly used to increase cardiac output.
- Glucose-insulin-potassium (GIK) polarizing solution is an infusion therapy used to increase myocardial energy substrate and thus improve myocardial function.[7]
- Furosemide or mannitol may be indicated if urine output does not increase with fluid volume replacement therapy.
- Vasodilators are used with caution to combat severe vasoconstrictive states. The patient must have sufficient fluid volume or the increase in vascular capacity will cause a precipitous drop in blood pressure. Fluid status monitoring is extremely important.
- Patients who receive transfusions of stored whole blood may require calcium therapy because a reduction in ionized serum calcium may occur.

- Steroids may be administered, but their use remains controversial.[7]
- Antibiotics are given as appropriate.
- Antiarrhythmic agents may be prescribed for patients experiencing arrhythmias.

Sodium Bicarbonate Administration. In severe acid-base disturbances (pH < 7.10), sodium bicarbonate may be prescribed to increase the pH to the range 7.20 to 7.25, but studies have demonstrated mixed results regarding the efficacy of sodium bicarbonate administration in the patient with acidemia.[25] Generally, both clinical and laboratory studies have shown no benefits from bicarbonate administration in the treatment of acidosis; in fact, some studies reveal detrimental consequences, especially in relation to oxygen delivery.[25] If sodium bicarbonate is ordered, it is important to administer it carefully so as not to overcorrect the acidosis and to avoid precipitating an alkalotic state.

Nutritional Support

The important role that nutritional status plays in the shock patient is beginning to be appreciated. Alteration in the barrier mechanisms of the GI tract have been associated with bacterial translocation, which leads to sepsis and multisystem organ failure.[10-12,36-38] Critical illness influences gut integrity by altering gut mucosal permeability. Changes in mucosal permeability are a result of systemic insults such as shock or cancer, direct mucosal injury, impaired host defenses, intestinal atrophy, and an increase in intestinal bacteria (Fig. 21–7).[38] Adequate nutritional support of the shock patient preserves mucosal integrity, enhances immune function, promotes wound healing, and decreases the incidence of septic complications.[11]

The GI tract contains the largest reservoir of immunologic tissue in the body. Gut-associated lymph tissue (GALT) functions to control local immune response to bacterial pathogens. Secretory IgA is the primary protective immunoglobin in the intestine that suppresses bacterial migration. It is secreted in response to oral or enteral feedings. Mucus production is increased in the presence of endotoxin to protect the stomach from mucosal damage and bacterial colonization.

The shock patient suffers from deterioration of these gut immune defenses, partly as a result of commonly used treatment modalities.[11] Treatment of the shock patient may include the use of antibiotics, H_2 (histamine) blockers, antacids, narcotics, and steroids, all of which override normal mucosal defense mechanisms and encourage bacterial growth. "Bowel rest" protocols[11,38] and the provision of total parenteral nutrition[11,39] decrease stimulation of the gastric mucosa and predispose the patient to mucosal atrophy.[11,38]

"If the gut works, use it" is a valuable maxim for therapy. The implementation of early enteral nutrition (within 8 to 12 hours after surgery or trauma) is supported in the literature as an inhibitor of intestinal atrophy and subsequent bacterial translocation.[11,38] Typically, the decision of when to restart enteral feedings was based on the presence of bowel sounds: par-

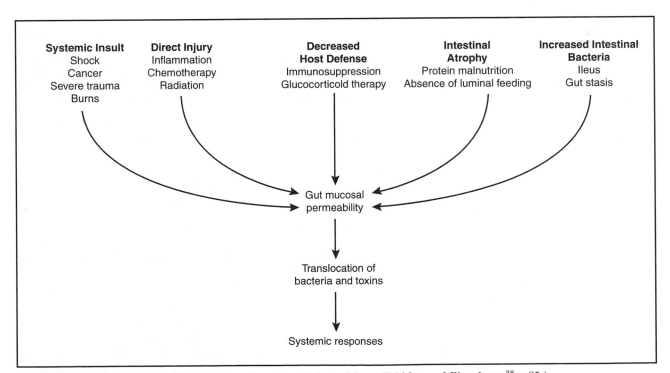

FIGURE 21–7. Mechanisms of bacterial translocation. (Adapted from Keithley and Eisenberg,[38] p 25.)

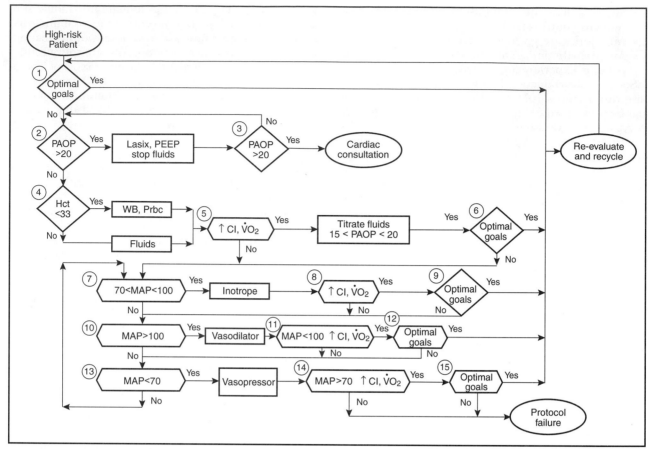

FIGURE 21–8. Decision-making algorithm to evaluate the adequacy of tissue perfusion in response to therapy. (Adapted from Shoemaker et al,[27] p 686.)

Step 1. Determine if the patient has reached the optimal goals. Measure cardiac index, $\dot{D}O_2$, and $\dot{V}O_2$. If cardiac index >4.5 L/min·m², $\dot{D}O_2$ >800 mL/min·m², $\dot{V}O_2$ >170 mL/min·m², the goals are reached, and the first objective of the algorithm has been achieved. Reevaluate and recycle at intervals to maintain these goals. If any of the preceding optimal values were not reached, proceed to step 2.

Step 2. Take pulmonary artery occlusion pressure (PAOP). If PAOP >20 mmHg, proceed to step 3; if PAOP <20 mmHg, proceed to step 4.

Step 3. If PAOP >20 mmHg, and there is clinical or radiographic evidence of salt and water overload or clinical findings of pulmonary congestion, give furosemide IV at increasing doses to produce diuresis and lower PAOP. If not, consider vasodilators, nitroprusside or nitroglycerin if MAP >80 mmHg and systolic arterial pressure (SAP) >100 mmHg; titrate the dose needed to maintain 15 <PAOP <20 mmHg and MAP >80 mmHg. If unsuccessful, obtain cardiology consult and place on cardiac protocol.

Step 4. If hematocrit (Hct) <33%, give 1 U of whole blood or 2 U of packed RBC. If hematocrit >33%, give a fluid load (volume challenge) consisting of one of the following (depending on clinical indications of plasma volume deficit or hydration): 5% plasma protein factor, 500 mL; 5% albumin, 500 mL; 25% albumin (25 g), 100 mL; 6% hydroxyethyl starch 500 mL; 6% dextran-60, 500 mL; lactated Ringer's solution, 1000 mL.

Step 5. If the blood or fluid load improves cardiac index (CI), $\dot{D}O_2$, or $\dot{V}O_2$, continue to give appropriate fluids to increase these variables; if these are improved with adequate volume, proceed to step 8. Continue to infuse fluids until 15 < PAOP <20 mmHg; if PAOP reaches 20 mmHg before optimal goals are reached, proceed to step 8.

Step 6. If optimal goals are reached, recycle; if not, proceed to step 8.

Step 7. If MAP >70 mmHg and <100 mmHg, give dobutamine by constant IV infusion to optimize cardiac index, $\dot{D}O_2$, and $\dot{V}O_2$.

Step 8. Titrate dobutamine beginning with 2 μg/min·kg and gradually increasing to 20 μg/min·kg, provided there is improvement in cardiac index (CI), $\dot{D}O_2$, or $\dot{V}O_2$ without further lowering of BP until goals are met.

Step 9. If goals are reached, reevaluate and recycle. If goals are not reached or it becomes evident that higher drug doses are not more effective or that they produce hypotension, tachycardia, or dysrthythmia, continue dobutamine at its most effective dose range and proceed to step 10.

Step 10. If MAP >10 mmHg, give vasodilator, such as nitroprusside, nitroglycerine, labetalol, prostaglandin E_1, and so on.

Step 11. Titrate vasodilators to decrease MAP and increase cardiac index (CI), $\dot{D}O_2$, or $\dot{V}O_2$. If there is no improvement in cardiac index, $\dot{D}O_2$, $\dot{V}O_2$, with the vasodilator, and if hypotension (MAP <80 mmHg, SAP <110 mmHg) occurs, reduce or discontinue the vasodilator. If there is improvement in cardiac index, $\dot{D}O_2$, or $\dot{V}O_2$, titrate vasodilator to its maximum cardiac index, $\dot{D}O_2$, or $\dot{V}O_2$ effects consistent with satisfactory pressures.

alytic ileus and gut stasis are common in the postoperative and/or postinjury period. The small bowel is functional within hours after acute traumatic injury or surgery, however, thus allowing the implementation of jejunal feeds.[11,38] Early nutritional support preserves the normal immune and defense functions of the GI tract and prevents the movement of bacteria and endotoxin across the mucosal barrier and into the systemic circulation.

Therapeutic End Points

A number of measures can be used to judge the effectiveness of resuscitation strategies in shock (see Table 21–10). Heart rate should decrease as cardiac output increases. Hemodynamic parameters (CI, LVSWI, PAWP, and CVP) are used to gauge and thus optimize preload in the shock patient. The oxygen transport variable end points (Do_2, $\dot{V}o_2$, OER) are manipulated so as to provide supranormal levels of oxygen delivery to meet the increased oxygen demand of the critically stressed patient and to normalize oxygen extraction. A treatment algorithm for determining if optimal patient hemodynamic and oxygen delivery goals are met is demonstrated in Figure 21–8. The provision of supranormal levels of oxygen delivery during the early critical phases of shock has been shown to improve patient survival.[1] Tissue ischemia can be monitored by serial measurements of serum lactate levels[3] and gastric tonometry.[8,9]

NURSING CARE OF THE PATIENT WITH HYPOVOLEMIC SHOCK

The immediate goal in the treatment of the patient with hypovolemic shock is to restore effective circulating fluid volume, control bleeding (if present), and stabilize hemodynamic function. It is critical to restore an adequate intravascular volume so that tissue perfusion can be maintained and the metabolic needs of the cells fulfilled. In the patient with hypovolemic shock this is achieved by timely and aggressive fluid and/or blood replacement therapy.

It is essential to establish baseline assessment data when caring for the patient with hypovolemic shock. Such data are used to assess the patient's subsequent response to treatment and to determine the effectiveness of that therapy in meeting the patient's desired outcomes. Identifying trends, or a series of patient responses over time, is of greater clinical significance than any isolated reading.

TABLE 21–15
The Nurse's Role in Shock

Recognize/identify early signs and symptoms
Communicate and collaborate with the medical team
Implement interventions promptly
Evaluate the patient's response to therapy (patient outcomes)
Collaborate and revise the plan according to patient outcomes
Document

The Nurse's Role

The nurse's role in the care and management of the shock patient is a crucial one (Table 21–15). The nurse must first *recognize* the early signs and symptoms signaling the onset of the shock state. The nurse who is aware of a patient's high risk for the development of shock may detect subtle changes in the patient's condition before the shock state progresses far. For example, the coronary care nurse should be aware that patients at particularly high risk of developing cardiogenic shock are those who have suffered anterior myocardial infarctions or those patients with a history of previous MIs. The total cumulative amount of ventricular damage is significant in this diagnosis. Likewise, the patient with spinal cord trauma is at high risk for neurogenic shock, and so on.

Early communication and collaboration with the medical team and prompt implementation of the treatment plan are vital to a successful patient outcome. Evaluation of the patient's response to the interventions and revision of the plan, as needed, help to assure positive patient outcomes. Documentation of all steps is critical to providing a complete record of care.

Therapeutic Goals

Implementation of the nursing process in the care of the patient with hypovolemic shock involves consideration of the following therapeutic goals:

1. Restoring and/or maintaining hemodynamic stability via fluid and blood replacement therapy to improve tissue perfusion and oxygenation
2. Maintaining adequate ventilation and oxygenation
3. Restoring and/or maintaining fluid and electrolyte balance

---

Step 12. If optimal goals are reached, reevaluate and recycle at intervals to maintain optimal goals.
Step 13. If these goals are not reached and MAP <80 mmHg, SAP <110 mmHg, give dopamine or other vasopressor.
Step 14. Titrate doses of vasopressor (dopamine) in the lowest dose that maintains MAP >70 mmHg, SAP >110 mmHg, and increases cardiac index, $\dot{D}o_2$, and $\dot{V}o_2$ to their optimal values. If pressures cannot be maintained or optimal goals reached, the patient is considered to be a protocol failure; consider reevaluation and recycling.
Step 15. If optimal goals are reached, reevaluate and recycle.

4. Maintaining therapeutic milieu with optimal rest and comfort to minimize bleeding or rebleeding
5. Reducing anxiety and apprehension
6. Providing hydration and nutritional support to maintain ideal weight, facilitate the healing process, and prevent bacterial translocation
7. Preventing and/or monitoring for complications of shock, including adult respiratory distress syndrome (ARDS), acute renal failure, and DIC
8. Preventing infection
9. Providing emotional and psychological support to patient and family
10. Initiating activities to assist the patient in health management

Nursing Diagnoses, Desired Patient Outcomes, and Nursing Interventions

Pertinent nursing diagnoses, desired patient outcomes, nursing interventions, and their rationales are presented in the care plan for the patient with hypovolemic shock at the end of this chapter. In addition, see the care plan for the patient with acute upper gastrointestinal bleeding in Chapter 44..

It is to be emphasized that the following plans are guidelines for nursing care. The expected outcomes should always be individualized for each specific patient to provide the most effective and appropriate care.

CASE STUDY: PATIENT IN SHOCK

JS, a 45-year-old accountant, is brought into the emergency room complaining of abdominal pain, nausea, vomiting of frank blood, and black, tarry stools. His wife states that he had vomited "small" amounts of blood over the last 8 hours but he would not go to the hospital. Mrs. S states that she finally convinced her husband to come to the emergency room after he "threw up about a cup of blood" about an hour ago.

Physical assessment reveals an anxious man, oriented × 3, in increasing distress. Mr. S is tachycardic and hypotensive, with a thready pulse. He is complaining of nausea and dizzyiness when he sits up. Respirations are shallow and 26. Mucous membranes are pale, the skin is cool. Hemoglobin is 10.5 and hematocrit is 29%. Mrs. S states that her husband has been under an increased amount of stress lately. Mr. S's past history includes treatment for a peptic ulcer.

A nasogastric tube is placed and iced saline lavage is initiated. Oxygen is administered via nasal cannula at 4 L/min and two 14-gauge peripheral IV lines are started. Lactated ringer's solution is infused at 150 mL/h and two units of packed red blood cells are ordered for immediate infusion. Mr. S asks the nurse if blood transfusions are "really necessary."

REFERENCES

1. Shoemaker, WC: Relation of oxygen transport patterns to the pathophysiology and therapy of shock states. Intensive Care Med 13:230–243, 1987.
2. Rice, V: Shock, a clinical syndrome: An update, Part 2. Crit Care Nurse 11(5):74–83, 1991.
3. Marino, PL: The ICU Book. Lea & Febiger, Philadelphia, 1991.
4. Astiz, ME, Rackow, EC, and Weil, MH: Pathophysiology and treatment of circulatory shock. Crit Care Clinics 9:183–203, 1993.
5. Houston, MC: Pathophysiology of shock. Critical Care Nursing Clinics of North America 2:143–149, 1990.
6. Sigurdsson, GH, Christenson, JT, El-Rakshy, MB, and Sadek, S: Intestinal platelet trapping after traumatic and septic shock. An early sign of sepsis and multiorgan failure in critically ill patients? Crit Care Med 20:458–467, 1992.
7. Wilson, RF: Critical Care Manual: Applied Physiology and Principles of Therapy, ed 2. FA Davis, Philadelphia, 1992.
8. Gutierrez, G, Bismar, H, Dantzker, DR, and Silva, N: Comparison of gastric intramucosal pH with measures of oxygen transport and consumption in critically ill patients. Crit Care Med 20:451–457, 1992.
9. Clark, CH and Gutierrez, G: Gastric intramucosal pH: A noninvasive method for the indirect measurement of tissue oxygenation. American Journal of Critical Care 1(2):53–60, 1992.
10. Marshall, JC, et al: The microbiology of multiple organ failure: The proximal GI tract as an occult reservoir of pathogens. Arch Surg 123:309–315, 1988.
11. Phillips, MC and Olson, LR: The immunologic role of the gastrointestinal tract. Critical Care Nursing Clinics of North America 5(1):107–120, 1993.
12. Deitch, EA, Berg, R, and Specian, R: Endotoxin promotes the translocation of bacteria from the gut. Arch Surg 122:185–190, 1987.
13. Rice, V: Shock, a clinical syndrome: An update, I. Critical Care Nurse 11(4):20–27, 1991.
14. Laskowski-Jones, L: Acute SCI: How to minimize the damage. Am J Nurs 93:23–32, 1993.
15. Hickey, JV: The Clinical Practice of Neurological and Neurosurgical Nursing, ed 3. JB Lippincott, Philadelphia, 1992.
16. Bone, RC: Toward an epidemiology and natural history of SIRS (systemic inflammatory response syndrome). JAMA 268:3452–3455, 1992.
17. Meyers, KA and Hickey, MK: Nursing management of hypovolemic shock. Critical Care Nursing Quarterly 11(1):57–67, 1988.
18. Gorney, DA: Arterial blood pressure measurement technique. AACN Clinical Issues in Critical Care 4(1):66–80, 1993.
19. Sommers, MS: Fluid resuscitation following multiple trauma. Critical Care Nurse 10(10):74–81, 1990.
20. Astiz, ME and Rackow, EC: Assessing perfusion failure during circulatory shock. Crit Care Clin 9:299–311, 1993.
21. Daily, EK and Schroeder, JS: Techniques in Bedside Hemodynamic Monitoring, ed 4. CV Mosby, St. Louis, MO, 1989.
22. Shoemaker, WC: Tissue perfusion and oxygenation: A primary problem in acute circulatory failure and shock states. Crit Care Med 19:595–596, 1991.
23. Epstein, CD and Henning, RJ: Oxygen transport variables in the identification and treatment of tissue hypoxia. Heart Lung 22:328–345, 1993.
24. White, KM: Using continuous $S\dot{V}O_2$ to assess oxygen supply/demand balance in the critically ill patient. AACN Clinical Issues in Critical Care 4(1):134–147, 1993.
25. Mathieu, D, Neviere, R, Billard, V, Fleyfel, M, and Wattel, F: Effects of bicarbonate therapy on hemodynamics and tissue oxygenation in patients with lactic acidosis: A prospective, controlled clinical study. Crit Care Med 19:1352–1356, 1991.
26. Yu, M, Levy, MM, Smith, P, Takiguchi, SA, Miyasaki, A, and Myers, SA: Effect of maximizing oxygen delivery on morbidity and mortality rates in critically ill patients: A prospective, randomized, controlled study. Crit Care Med 21:830–838, 1993.
27. Shoemaker, WC, Appel, PL, and Kram, HB: Oxygen transport measurements to evaluate tissue perfusion and titrate therapy: Dobutamine and dopamine effects. Crit Care Med 19:672–688, 1991.

28. Johnson, BA and Weil, MH: Redefining ischemia due to circulatory failure as dual defects of oxygen deficits and of carbon dioxide excesses. Crit Care Med 19:1432–1438, 1991.
29. Ahrens, T: Respiratory monitoring in critical care. AACN Clinical Issues in Crit Care 4(1):56–65, 1993.
30. Campbell, JE (ed): Basic Trauma Life Support: Advanced Prehospital Care. Prentice-Hall, Englewood Cliffs, NJ, 1988.
31. Rackow, EC, et al: Fluid resuscitation in circulatory shock: A comparison of the cardiorespiratory effects of albumin, hetastarch and saline solutions in patients with hypovolemic and septic shock. Crit Care Med 11:839–850, 1983.
32. Haupt, MT: The use of crystalloidal and colloidal solutions for volume replacement in hypovolemic shock. Crit Rev Clin Lab Sci 27:1–26, 1989.
33. Gould, SA, et al: Hypovolemic shock. Crit Care Clin 9:239–259, 1993.
34. Imm, A and Carlson, RW: Fluid resuscitation in circulatory shock. Crit Care Clin 9:313–333, 1993.
35. Pepe, PE, Bass, RR, and Mattox, KL: Clinical trials of the pneumatic antishock garment in the urban prehospital setting. Ann Emerg Med 15:1407–1410, 1986.
36. Saadia, R, et al: Gut barrier function and the surgeon. Br J Surg 77:487–492, 1990.
37. Border, JR, et al: The gut-origin of septic states in blunt multiple trauma in the ICU. Ann Surg 206:427–448, 1987.
38. Keithley, JK and Eisenberg, P: The significance of enteral nutrition in the intensive care unit patient. Critical Care Nursing Clinics of North America 5(1):23–29, 1993.
39. Alverdy, JC, Aoys, E, and Moss, GS: Total parenteral nutrition promotes bacterial translocation. Surgery 104:185–190, 1988.

SUGGESTED READINGS

Murphy, TG and Bennett, EJ: Low-tech, high-touch perfusion assessment. Am J Nurs 92:36–47, 1992.
Rackow, EC, Astix, ME, and Weil, MH: Cellular oxygen metabolism during sepsis and shock. JAMA 259:1989–1993, 1988.
Rice, V: Shock, a clinical syndrome: An update, III. Critical Care Nurse 11(6):34–39, 1991.
Rice, V: Shock, a clinical syndrome: An update, IV. Critical Care Nurse 11(7):28–41, 1991.

CARE PLAN FOR THE PATIENT WITH HYPOVOLEMIC SHOCK

Nursing Diagnoses

Nursing Diagnosis #1

Tissue Perfusion, alterated, cardiovascular GI, renal, and peripheral, related to:
1. Reduced circulating blood volume
2. Fluid volume deficit

Desired Patient Outcomes

Patient will maintain adequate tissue perfusion AEB:
1. Arterial blood pressure within 10 mmHg of baseline.
2. Heart rate <100 beats/minute.
3. Mental status: Alert; oriented to person, time, and place.
4. Skin warm, dry to touch; usual color, good turgor, capillary refill <2 seconds.
5. Palpable pulses 2+/4+
6. Lungs clear; respiratory rate 12–20/min unlabored, regular
7. Urinary output ≥ 30 mL/hr.
8. Arterial blood gases within normal range:
   - PaO_2 > 80 mmHg
   - $PaCO_2$ 35–45 mmHg
   - HCO_3 22–26 mEq/L
   - pH 7.35–7.45
9. $S\bar{v}O_2$ 60%–80%

Nursing Interventions

- Assess for signs/symptoms of hypovolemic shock:

  - Assess cardiovascular function:
    - Blood pressure (orthostatic)

    - Heart rate, rhythm

    - Resting peripheral pulses
    - Check capillary refill

    - Skin color, moisture, temperature, and turgor

  - Assess neurologic function:
    - Mental status
    - Orientation

Rationales

- A baseline assessment is necessary to establish stage of shock and to determine emergent measures indicated; serves as a measure of the patient's response to therapy.

  - A drop in blood pressure of 10–15 mmHg from supine to sitting/standing position suggests blood loss of about 1 L.
  - Reflects compensatory effect of decreased intravascular volume on cardiac function.
  - Peripheral pulses, if palpable, may be weak and thready due to decrease in stroke volume and peripheral vasoconstriction.
  - When tissue perfusion is decreased, skin becomes cool and clammy to the touch and pale in color; cyanosis may occur if reduced hemoglobin concentration exceeds 5 g/100 mL. If blood loss is significant, cyanosis may not be present.
  - Appropriateness of patient's behavior and responses reflects adequacy of cerebral tissue perfusion.

CARE PLAN FOR THE PATIENT WITH HYPOVOLEMIC SHOCK (*Continued*)

- ○ Assess renal function:
  - □ Urine output
  - □ Intake and output
  - □ Urine specific gravity
  - □ Daily weight
- ○ Assess gastrointestinal function:
  - □ Bowel sounds, abdominal distention, pain
  - □ Obtain serial pHi measurements (if gastric tonometer in place).

- Establish/maintain 1 or more large-gauge intravenous access sites.

- Initiate timely and aggressive fluid replacement therapy and monitor response to therapy:
  - ○ Administer crystalloids, colloids.
  - ○ Transfuse blood/blood products.
- Assess oxygenation status:
  - ○ Lung auscultation
  - ○ Respiratory rate, depth, character

  - ○ Arterial blood gases
  - ○ Mixed venous oxygen saturation ($S\bar{v}O_2$)
  - ○ Calculate oxygen transport variables (DO_2, VO_2, OER) if PA catheter in place
  - ○ Administer oxygen; monitor vent settings.
- Initiate hemodynamic monitoring: Arterial, pulmonary artery, and pulmonary capillary wedge pressures.

  - ○ Initiate monitoring of mixed venous blood ($S\bar{v}O_2$).
- Monitor hydration status during fluid replacement therapy:
  - ○ Assess respiratory function:
    - □ Respiratory rate, rhythm, chest excursion, breath sounds, use of accessory muscles; status of neck veins
  - ○ Record daily weight.
  - ○ Document intake and output.
- Insert Foley catheter to measure hourly urine output.

- Insert nasogastric tube.

- Monitor hematology profile:
  - ○ Hematocrit, hemoglobin, RBCs, platelets

- ○ Reduced circulating blood volume and hypotensive state compromise renal perfusion. Urine output is a reliable indicator of renal perfusion. Urine specific gravity >1.025 reflects fluid volume depletion.

- ○ Decrease in blood flow to splanchnic area depresses bowel motility and peristalsis.
- ○ Decreased perfusion to the GI tract increases lactic acid production and local tissue damage. pHi readings aid in evaluation for early intervention.
- Rapid administration of fluids and fluid volume expanders and blood and blood products may be necessary to restore circulating blood volume.
- See above rationale

- ○ Decreases in perfusion to the lungs will be demonstrated as adventitious breath sounds and the development of acute respiratory distress.
- ○ Assessment of arterial and venous blood gases provides data regarding the patient's response to therapy.
- ○ Oxygen transport variables can help to dictate and evaluate therapeutic interventions.

- Insertion of systemic arterial and pulmonary artery catheters in the setting of massive hemorrhage and/or fluid loss with massive fluid volume replacement is essential to accurately follow trends and evaluate patient's response to therapy.
  - ○ Status of mixed venous blood reflects adequacy of peripheral tissue perfusion and oxygen extraction.

- ○ Detection of adventitious breath sounds (crackles, rhonchi) in previously clear lungs suggests overhydration.
- ○ Most accurate measure of hydration status.

- Hourly urine outputs reflect status of renal perfusion and underlying hemodynamic status.
- Decompresses stomach to facilitate respiratory excursion and prevent aspiration of stomach contents, and affords means to monitor for gastrointestinal bleeding.
- Reflects hemoglobin oxygen-carrying capacity; decrease in hemoglobin levels compromises oxygen delivery to tissues.

Nursing Diagnoses
Nursing Diagnosis #2
Fluid Volume, deficit in, related to:
1. Hemorrhage
2. Fluid shifts associated with loss of plasma proteins (hypoproteinemia, hypoalbuminemia)

Nursing Interventions
- Maintain fluid and electrolyte balance
  - ○ Administer prescribed fluid volume.

Desired Patient Outcomes

Patient will:
1. Maintain body weight within 5% of baseline
2. Balance fluid intake and output
3. Exhibit good skin turgor, absence of peripheral edema, absence of jugular venous distention, absence of adventitious breath sounds
4. Maintain serum electrolytes within normal limits

Rationales
- Fluid therapy is the mainstay of treatment of hypovolemic shock to restore/maintain tissue perfusion.

CARE PLAN FOR THE PATIENT WITH HYPOVOLEMIC SHOCK (*Continued*)

○ Document intake and output, urine specific gravity.
○ Record daily weight
○ Monitor serum electrolytes.

• Implement nursing measures to improve and/or maintain cardiac output
  ○ Assist patient into positions of comfort that facilitate breathing.
    □ Elevate head of bed to 20-30 degrees.
    □ Administer inotropic drugs.

  ○ Monitor hemodynamic parameters:
    □ Arterial blood pressure
    □ Pulmonary artery pressure parameters
    □ Central venous pressure
    □ Cardiac output
• Assess skin, capillary refill, turgor, peripheral edema
  ○ Provide special care to back and to skin over joints and pressure points.
  ○ Assist with passive range-of-motion exercises.

  ○ Maximize patient activities in accordance with the acuity and limitations of the illness.
• Auscultate lungs.
• Assess for jugular venous distention.

○ Close monitoring of urine output helps to evaluate renal perfusion and assess overall hemodynamics.
○ Rapid and massive fluid volume replacement therapy can dilute electrolytes and precipitate electrolyte imbalance.

○ Placing patient with hypovolemic shock into Trendelenburg's position (i.e., the legs higher than the head) may be of little value to hemodynamics or to improvement of cardiac output. Optimal ventilation/perfusion matching occurs in dependent areas of lungs.
○ These measures best reflect the patient's status and response to therapy. Rapid administration of crystalloids and colloids may precipitate fluid shift between extracellular and intracellular compartments.

○ Compromised circulation in a patient with reduced tissue perfusion increases the risk of tissue ischemia and stasis of blood predisposing to venous thrombosis, and reduces venous return and cardiac output.

○ Nursing interventions are implemented to maximize circulation, prevent pooling or stasis of blood, ensure adequate venous return, and promote comfort.

Nursing Diagnoses

Nursing Diagnosis #3
Anxiety, related to:
1. Hemorrhage
2. Transfusion therapy
3. Inherent sympathoadrenal activity (enhanced)
4. ICU setting

Nursing Interventions

• Assess signs/symptoms of anxiety:
  ○ Restlessness, agitation, diaphoresis; tachypnea, tachycardia, palpitations; uncooperative or noncompliant behavior; verbalization of fears and concerns.
• Examine circumstances underlying anxiety and validate with the patient.
  ○ Manipulate ICU environment to provide calm, restful periods.

• Assess patient coping behaviors and their effectiveness in dealing with current stressors.
  ○ Provide positive reinforcement when desired outcome is achieved.
• Initiate interventions to reduce anxiety:
  ○ Relieve pain or other discomfort:
    □ Medication for pain; monitor response
    □ Comfort measures
  ○ Monitor effectiveness of ventilation and oxygenation.
  ○ Serial arterial blood gases.

  ○ Listen attentively, encourage verbalization, provide a caring touch.

Desired Patient Outcomes

Patient will
1. Verbalize feeling less anxious
2. Demonstrate relaxed demeanor
3. Perform relaxation techniques with assistance
4. Verbalize familiarity with ICU setting

Rationales

• Thorough assessment assists in discerning underlying cause of anxiety and provides a basis for therapy. Patients with hypovolemic shock may experience anxiety associated with massive sympathoadrenal output.

• Removal of precipitating cause may reduce anxiety.

  ○ Reduction in stimuli is essential to assist patient to relax. This is especially important in the patient at risk of bleeding or rebleeding.
• Experiencing a bleeding episode can be very distressing.

  ○ Positive feedback and reassurance nurture self-confidence and confidence in health team.

  ○ Pain precipitates and/or aggravates anxiety.

  ○ Inadequate gas exchange, "air hunger," hypoxemia, and/or hypercapnia may cause the patient to experience a "sense of impending doom."
  ○ These nursing activities reassure the patient that he/she is not alone.

CARE PLAN FOR THE PATIENT WITH HYPOVOLEMIC SHOCK (*Continued*)

- ○ Let the patient know it's okay to feel anxious and afraid.
- ○ Remain with patient during periods of acute stress.
- • Assess readiness to learn and implement the following when appropriate:
  - ○ Orient patient to environment, ICU equipment and routines, and staff.
    - □ Explain all procedures and activities involving patient.
  - ○ Involve patient in decision making regarding care when possible and appropriate.
  - ○ Assist in establishing short-term goals and desired patient outcomes.
  - ○ Instruct patient in relaxation techniques when it is prudent to do so.

- ○ Reassurance helps patient to focus on feelings and to work them through.

- • Readiness to learn facilitates meaningful learning and a sense of accomplishment.
  - ○ Knowing what to expect helps to reduce anxiety.

- ○ Helps patient to maintain some degree of control of health management.
- ○ Builds and reinforces self-confidence.

- ○ Use of energy-release techniques allows an outlet for pent-up feelings; enables patient to have some control over anxiety.

UNIT THREE

Respiratory System

UNIT OUTLINE

C H A P T E R   2 2

Anatomy and Physiology of the Respiratory System

Betty S. Henderson

CHAPTER OUTLINE

LEARNING OBJECTIVES

After completing this chapter, you should be able to:

1. Describe the functional anatomy of the respiratory system and its role in the process of respiration.
2. Identify the major features of the respiratory alveolar-pulmonary capillary membrane that facilitate its role in gas exchange.
3. Examine the unique features of the bronchopulmonary vasculature in terms of its responses to ventilation and oxygenation.
4. Describe the essential aspects of the mechanics of breathing.
5. Define compliance and its impact on the ``work'' of breathing.
6. Outline strategic pulmonary defense mechanisms.
7. Describe the underlying mechanisms of pulmonary ventilation.
8. Discuss the clinical significance of maximal expiratory flow studies.
9. Describe the mechanisms underlying diffusion of gases between the alveoli and pulmonary capillaries and between the circulating blood and body tissues.
10. Examine ventilation-perfusion relationships and their clinical significance.
11. Discuss mechanisms of oxygen and carbon dioxide transport in body fluids.
12. Review the clinical significance of the oxyhemoglobin dissociation curve.
13. Describe the intricate mechanisms in the control of respiratory function.

The process of respiration involves the following physiologic activities: (1) the mechanics of pulmonary ventilation (i.e., the movement of air into and out of the lungs; (2) the exchange of oxygen and carbon dioxide between the alveoli and the blood by diffusion; (3) the transport of oxygen and carbon dioxide throughout the circulatory system; (4) the exchange of oxygen and carbon dioxide between the circulating blood and the cells by diffusion; and (5) the regulation of the activities involved in respirations. Each of these activities is examined in this chapter. The discussion begins with a review of the overall organization of the respiratory system.

ORGANIZATION OF THE RESPIRATORY SYSTEM

Upper and Lower Airways of the Respiratory Tract

The entire pathway for the flow of air between the external environment and the lungs extends from the mouth or nose down to the alveolar sacs. Inhaled gas is conducted through the *upper* airways, which include the nose, nasal cavity, paranasal sinuses, mouth, oropharynx and nasopharynx, and the larynx, down through the *lower* airways, which include the tracheobronchial tree, terminal bronchioles, respiratory bronchioles, and ending in tiny blind sacs, the alveoli.

Throughout this system, a progressive dichotomous branching of bronchi and bronchioles occurs. The trachea divides at the carina into right and left mainstem bronchi (Fig. 22–1), which, in turn, branch into lobar bronchi (three on the right, two on the left), segmental and subsegmental bronchi, smaller bronchi, and bronchioles. In all, these conducting airways divide about 15 to 17 times down to the level of terminal bronchioles, which are the smallest units that do not participate in gas exchange (Fig. 22–2).

Larynx

The larynx and pharyngeal musculature provide clinically significant protective functions essential for maintenance of normal lung physiology. The critical dividing point in separating solids and liquids from air occurs within the laryngopharynx. Here, the passageway bifurcates into the larynx and esophagus, and the pharyngeal muscles function to close the glottis while initiating the *swallowing reflex*. In this way, the lungs are protected from aspiration.

Cough Reflex. The cough reflex is a major physiologic mechanism for clearing and protecting the airways. It protects against aspiration of food or other foreign material into the airway and assists in clearing the tracheobronchial secretions produced within the tracheobronchial tree. The cough reflex is usually initiated by stimulation of irritant receptors found primarily in the larynx, trachea, and major bronchi, and especially at points of bifurcation of the air passages.

Trachea

The trachea is about 11 to 13 cm in length and extends from the cricoid cartilage in the neck into the thorax, where it branches into the right and left mainstem bronchi at a point called the *carina* (Fig. 22–1).

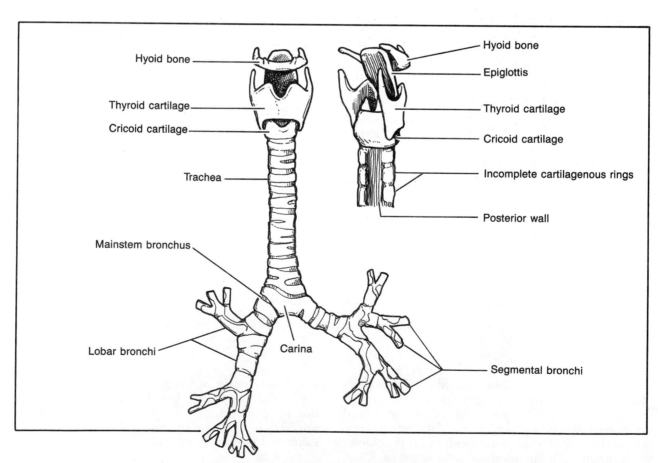

FIGURE 22–1. Structure of cartilaginous airways, including the trachea and major bronchi.

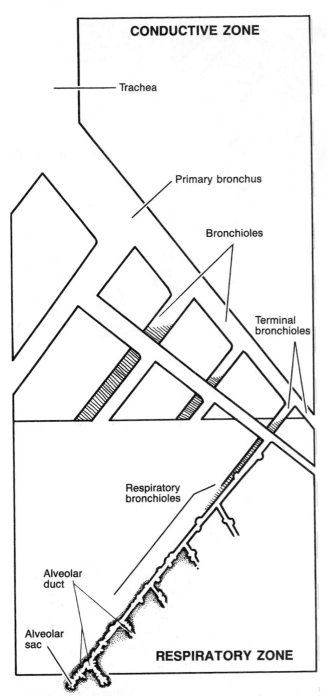

CONDUCTIVE ZONE

Trachea

Primary bronchus

Bronchioles

Terminal bronchioles

Respiratory bronchioles

Alveolar duct

Alveolar sac

RESPIRATORY ZONE

FIGURE 22–2. Functional zones of the respiratory tract. The area from the trachea to the terminal bronchioles is called the "conductive zone" because these airways transport (conduct) inhaled gas to and from the respiratory zone. Gas exchange takes place increasingly in the respiratory bronchioles, alveolar ducts, and alveolar sacs. Collectively, these areas constitute the "respiratory zone."

The carina is highly innervated and can produce severe bronchospasm and coughing when stimulated (as frequently occurs in endotracheal suctioning). The carina also serves as a strategic landmark when evaluating the placement of an endotracheal tube on a chest x-ray.

Bronchi

The right and left mainstem bronchi are anatomically asymmetrical (Fig. 22–1). The right bronchus is shorter and wider than the left bronchus and continues from the trachea in a more nearly vertical course. The left mainstem bronchus is longer and narrower and continues from the trachea at a more acute angle.

The clinical implications of these anatomic characteristics are noteworthy. When an endotracheal tube is passed too far, it will enter the right mainstem bronchus. If this occurs and the cuff is inflated, the left lung cannot be ventilated, a situation that can rapidly lead to atelectasis of the left lung with hypoxemia. It is essential to observe for bilateral equal chest expansion and to auscultate both anterior upper lung fields immediately upon intubation. A chest x-ray may confirm proper positioning of the endotracheal tube.

Respiratory Epithelium

The airways that extend from the nose down to and including the terminal bronchioles function primarily to prepare and condition the inhaled gas by filtering, warming, and humidifying it and by facilitating its flow throughout the respiratory tract to the alveoli. These airways are especially well suited for these critical functions. The nose, nasal cavity, turbinates, and paranasal sinuses provide an extensive, highly vascularized surface to which inhaled gas is exposed as it flows through the respiratory tract. The luminal surface layer or mucosa of both upper and lower airways is lined with a specialized *respiratory epithelium,* or pseudostratified ciliated columnar epithelium with goblet cells (Fig. 22–3). The cilia function to protect the deeper airways by propelling tracheobronchial secretions toward the pharynx where they can be coughed up, swallowed, or expectorated.

The epithelial surface is covered by a "mucous blanket," which is secreted largely by submucosal mucous glands and, to a lesser extent, the goblet cells. Fine particles within the inhaled gas are trapped in the mucous blanket, which is continuously propelled by the cilia toward the pharynx by a process termed *mucociliary transport* or *mucociliary clearance.*

Bacteria inhaled on dust particles are similarly trapped in the mucous blanket. In this way, the mucociliary clearance mechanism contributes to the body's total defense against bacterial infection. A reduction in ciliary activity, as occurs with cigarette smoking, combined with an increase in mucus secretion, also induced by noxious agents such as cigarette smoke, predisposes the airway to congestion and obstruction by stationary mucus.

A rich underlying vascular network warms the gas as it flows toward the distal or peripheral areas of the tracheobronchial tree. It is largely by the "conditioning activities" of the respiratory epithelium on inhaled gas that the gas reaching the alveoli is dust-free, at body temperature, and 100% humidified.

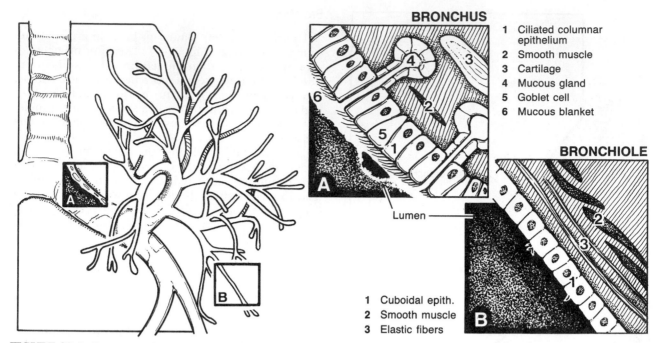

BRONCHUS

1 Ciliated columnar epithelium
2 Smooth muscle
3 Cartilage
4 Mucous gland
5 Goblet cell
6 Mucous blanket

Lumen

BRONCHIOLE

1 Cuboidal epith.
2 Smooth muscle
3 Elastic fibers

FIGURE 22–3. Structure of respiratory epithelium that lines the respiratory passages and the tracheobronchial tree. Note differences in structure of the epithelium that lines a larger bronchus as compared with that which lines a bronchiole. Such differences reflect underlying function, including the air-conditioning and conducting activities of the upper and lower airways, respectively.

Functional Zones of the Respiratory Tract

The lower respiratory tract subdivides into "generations" of airways, with each generation containing progressively narrower, shorter, and more numerous branches (Fig. 22–3). The conductive airways include the bronchi and bronchioles, which transport inhaled gas to and from the alveoli. These airways take no part in gas exchange and constitute the *anatomical dead space*. Anatomical dead space contains about 2 mL/kg of body weight, or about 150 mL, of inhaled gas that does not participate in gas exchange.

The respiratory bronchioles participate in gas exchange because their walls contain alveoli. Gas exchange primarily occurs, however, in the alveolar ducts and alveoli (Fig. 22–2).

Airway Structure

Definitive structural changes occur as the airways progress distally in the tracheobronchial tree. These structural changes involve the respiratory epithelium, the smooth muscle layer, the elastic layer, and the cartilaginous structure of the airways.

There is a progressive thinning of the *respiratory epithelium* as it changes from the ciliated columnar cells of the bronchi to the cuboidal, sparsely ciliated cells of the terminal bronchioles. Goblet cells, which are numerous throughout the upper airways and proximal lower airways, decrease in number until they actually disappear at the level of the respiratory bronchioles (Fig. 22–4).

Significant changes in the *smooth, muscle layer* of the airways occur at different levels of the tracheobronchial tree. In the trachea and large bronchi, the smooth muscle layer occurs as bands or a spiral network; in the small bronchi and bronchioles, the smooth muscle layer completely surrounds the airway wall. With the progressive diminution in airway size distally, the smooth muscle layer increasingly occupies the greater portions of the total wall thickness, becoming maximal at the level of the respiratory bronchioles.

Elastic tissue, although present in the larger airways, makes up a significant part of the walls of smaller airways and alveoli. In emphysema, the elastic tissue in the respiratory bronchioles and alveoli is destroyed.

The *cartilaginous structure* of the airways also changes in configuration. In the trachea, cartilage occurs as incomplete rings, whereas in the larger bronchi, it occurs as sheets or plates of cartilage. These cartilaginous sheets become progressively smaller and less numerous, until they disappear completely at the level of the bronchioles.

Site of Gas Exchange: The Acinus

The respiratory bronchioles, alveolar ducts, and alveolar sacs (alveoli) collectively constitute the pulmonary functional unit, or acinus (Fig. 22–5).

Alveoli. The enormous surface area within the alveoli provides for a most efficient mechanism for the exchange of oxygen and carbon dioxide between the alveolar spaces and pulmonary capillary blood. The adult human lung has about 300 million alveoli, a total

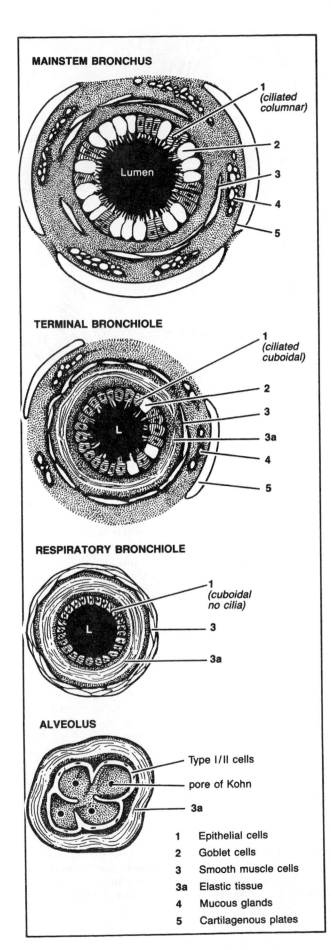

MAINSTEM BRONCHUS

Lumen

1 (ciliated columnar)
2
3
4
5

TERMINAL BRONCHIOLE

L

1 (ciliated cuboidal)
2
3
3a
4
5

RESPIRATORY BRONCHIOLE

L

1 (cuboidal no cilia)
3
3a

ALVEOLUS

Type I/II cells
pore of Kohn
3a

1   Epithelial cells
2   Goblet cells
3   Smooth muscle cells
3a   Elastic tissue
4   Mucous glands
5   Cartilagenous plates

surface area approximately the size of a tennis court. Extensive networks of capillaries weave their way back and forth through the interstitium of the interalveolar septum creating a communication meshwork that facilitates exchange of gases.

Cell Types. Two different types of epithelial cells, or *pneumocytes,* line the luminal surface of the alveolar wall; these include type I and type II cells. *Type I* cells are much smaller and more numerous than type II cells; they are relatively flat cells with characteristically long cytoplasmic extensions that line about 90% of the alveolar luminal surface (Fig. 22–5). It is through the flattened extension of these cells that gas exchange predominantly occurs. Type I cells also function as a barrier to prevent free movement of fluid from the alveolar wall into the alveolar lumen.

In contrast, *type II* cells are larger than type I cells and account for less than 5% of the alveolar surface. Their major function is to produce *surfactant,* a substance that reduces surface tension within the lungs and is a major contributing factor to total lung compliance.

A third type of cell identified within the alveoli is the pulmonary alveolar *macrophage.* By the process of *phagocytosis* (engulfment/digestion of foreign material), macrophages function as a major defense against inhaled substances that have escaped the defense mechanisms of the upper and lower airways. Through their ability to process antigenic material, macrophages also play a vital role in the body's immunologic defense system.

Pores of Kohn. The *pores of Kohn* are alveolar-septal pores, or openings, within the alveolar wall that facilitate alveolar-alveolar communication and *collateral ventilation.*[1] These pores allow movement of gases between alveoli, reducing the incidence of atelectasis. They also facilitate movement of macrophages between alveoli.

PULMONARY VASCULATURE

Bronchial and Pulmonary Circulations

All portions of the airways and the alveoli receive a rich supply of blood. The pulmonary vasculature encompasses a dual blood supply by the bronchial and pulmonary vessels. The *bronchial* circulation, which is actually part of the systemic circulation, provides nutrient blood flow to the bronchi and larger bronchioles. Distal to the terminal bronchioles including all the acini, blood in the pulmonary capillaries provides the necessary blood supply. Communication between the bronchial and pulmonary circulations

FIGURE 22–4. Microanatomy of airways in cross-section, at various points within the tracheobronchial tree, including the mainstem bronchus proximally, down to the alveolus, distally. Refer to Figure 22–2 to appreciate the relationship between structure and function of these various airways.

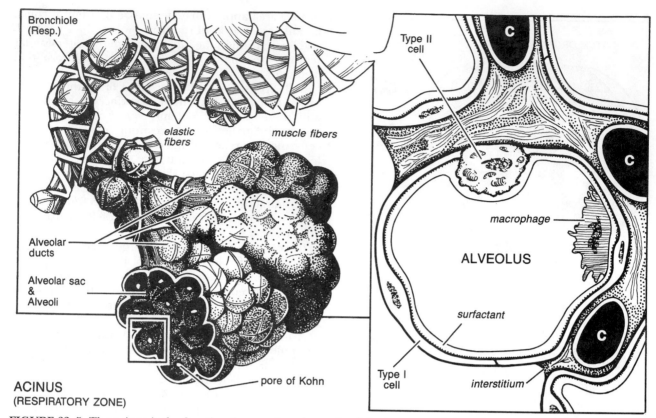

FIGURE 22–5. The acinus is the functional gas-exchanging unit of the lungs, consisting of respiratory bronchiole, alveolar ducts and sacs, and alveoli. The pores of Kohn play a unique role in alveolar: alveolar communication and collateral ventilation. *Inset,* ultrastructure of a pulmonary alveolus and capillaries (C).

occurs at the level of the terminal bronchioles, and the blood originating in the bronchial arteries returns to the heart by way of the pulmonary veins. In this instance, venous blood is returned to vessels transporting oxygenated blood to the left heart.

The *pulmonary* circulation is responsible for transporting deoxygenated blood from the right ventricle to the lungs by the pulmonary artery and returning oxygenated blood to the left atrium by the pulmonary veins. Although the pulmonary circulation handles about the same cardiac output from the right ventricle as does the systemic circulation from the left ventricle at a resting cardiac output (about 5 L/min), blood supply to the lungs is uniquely different in several respects.

The pulmonary vasculature is characterized by its great distensibility, attributed largely to its thin-walled blood vessels with minimal smooth muscle. Thus, these blood vessels offer a low resistance to right ventricular ejection, reducing the work of the right ventricle.

During exercise or under conditions of increased cardiac output, the pulmonary circulation is actually able to *decrease* its resistance so that overall, only a minimal increase in pulmonary artery pressure occurs. Mechanisms underlying this response include

(1) recruitment of blood vessels, which, under normal resting conditions, essentially receive no blood, and (2) distensibility of thin-walled pulmonary vessels, which can enlarge their diameter under increased pressure to accommodate additional blood flow (Fig. 22–6). The ability to increase the total cross-sectional area of the pulmonary vasculature on demand enables the pulmonary circulation to lower its resistance when the need for increased blood flow arises.

There is an uneven distribution of pulmonary blood flow that is strongly influenced by the low-pressure hemodynamics and the effects of gravity. In the upright position, blood flowing to the apex of each lung must flow against gravity. Under normal conditons, a mean pulmonary artery pressure of 15 mmHg is usually just sufficient to achieve adequate flow to this region.

In contrast, blood flow to the base of each lung is assisted by gravity; thus, there is a substantially greater blood flow to this region than to the apices. Gravity also becomes a factor with respect to blood flow to dependent areas associated with position (i.e., the supine or prone positions; Fig. 22–7). The distribution of blood flow to the lungs has major implications for the matching of ventilation with perfusion, and local mechanisms within the lungs function to ensure opti-

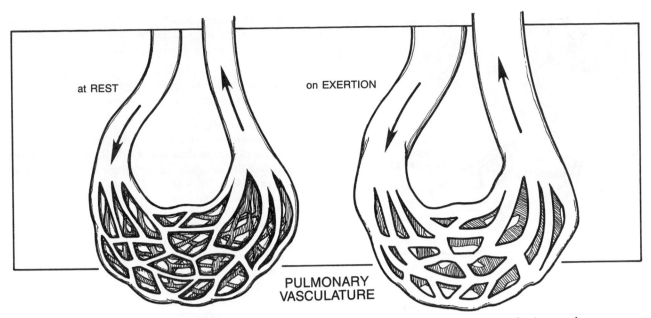

FIGURE 22–6. Effects of increases in pulmonary arterial blood pressure and blood flow (on exertion) on pulmonary vasculature resistance. Recruitment and distention of pulmonary vessels actually result in a decrease in pulmonary vascular resistance in the face of increases in pulmonary blood flow, assuming that lung volumes and left atrial pressure remain constant.

mal matching of ventilation and perfusion to individual alveoli.

One mechanism functions to adjust ventilation to perfusion by reflex changes in bronchiolar smooth muscle tone in response to local carbon dioxide concentrations. If an alveolus is well ventilated but its blood supply is reduced, there is a consequent decrease in the alveolar carbon dioxide concentration (P_{ACO_2}). This reduction in P_{ACO_2} in turn causes a reflex constriction of bronchioles in the underperfused area. The end-result is a decrease in ventilation to the area to more closely match ventilation with the available blood supply.

A second mechanism functions to adjust perfusion to ventilation by reflex changes in the smooth muscle tone of pulmonary blood vessels in response to local oxygen concentrations. A decrease in alveolar oxygen concentration (i.e., the P_{AO_2}) causes nearby pulmonary blood vessels to vasoconstrict, thereby shunting blood away from alveoli with reduced ventilation. Thus, unlike blood vessels in the systemic circulation that dilate in the presence of hypoxemia, the pulmonary vasculature constricts. Pulmonary vasoconstriction in response to alveolar hypoxia is a protective mechanism designed to reduce blood flow to poorly ventilated alveoli, thereby minimizing ventilation/perfusion ($\dot{V}/\dot{Q}$) mismatch.

Although these two mechanisms are effective in matching ventilation with perfusion, even in healthy persons some $\dot{V}/\dot{Q}$ mismatching exists. This largely accounts for the fact that arterial gas pressures are not exactly the same as alveolar gas pressures; that is, a gradient exists between oxygen tension in alveolar air and in arterial blood. (See Alveolar-Arterial Oxygen Difference [A-a Gradient] later in this chapter.)

A reduction in arterial pH is also known to cause pulmonary vasoconstriction and, together with hypoxemia, may have a synergistic effect on increasing pulmonary vascular resistance. (See Control of Respiration later in this chapter.)

The pulmonary circulation also plays an important role in the metabolism of some biologically active substances, for exampe, 5-hydroxytryptamine (serotonin), bradykinin, and prostaglandins. Converting enzyme, synthesized by pulmonary vascular endothelial cells, is responsible for the proteolysis of angiotensin I to angiotensin II. Angiotensin II is a major stimulator of aldosterone synthesis and secretion by the adrenal glands. It is also a powerful vasopressor.

Pulmonary Lymphatic Network

An extensive network of lymphatic channels occurs within the lungs in close proximity to small pulmonary blood vessels and airways. The lymphatic system functions to return to the systemic circulation fluid and solutes (e.g., albumin) that diffused into the interstitium from pulmonary capillaries and were not reabsorbed. In this way, the pulmonary lumphatic system helps to prevent pulmonary congestion and pulmonary edema, while helping to maintain intravascular blood volume and, very important, serum albumin levels.

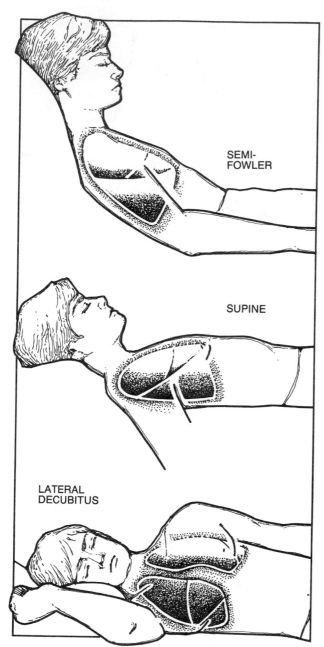

SEMI-
FOWLER

SUPINE

LATERAL
DECUBITUS

FIGURE 22–7. The effect of various position changes on the ratio of ventilation ($\dot{V}$) to perfusion ($\dot{Q}$) throughout regions of the lungs. In the uppermost lung regions, the $\dot{V}/\dot{Q}$ ratio is greater than that in dependent lung regions. In general, ventilation and perfusion are more closely matched in dependent lung areas, a factor that may be of significance when turning and positioning patients.

PULMONARY VENTILATION

Mechanics of Pulmonary Ventilation

Air, like blood or water, flows from a region of higher pressure to one of lower pressure. Inspiration occurs when alveolar pressure is less than atmospheric pressure; expiration occurs when alveolar pressure is greater than atmospheric pressure. The changes in alveolar pressure are caused by changes in the dimensions of the lungs.

Functional Elastic Properties of Pulmonary Structures and Intrapleural Pressure

The lungs are highly elastic organs, open at one end to the atmosphere and enclosed within the thoracic cavity. The pleura, a thin sheet of collagen and elastic tissue, lines the thoracic cavity (parietal) and encases the lungs (visceral). A thin film of pleural fluid is in the intrapleural space, which allows the two pleural surfaces to glide over each other during respiration, but prevents their separation from one another. This relationship between the thoracic wall and the lungs is analogous to two glass slides that are stuck together with water. The slides easily glide over one another, but they cannot easily be pulled apart.

Although both the lungs and the thoracic wall have highly elastic properties, they act in *opposition*. The recoil tendency of the lungs, attributed to its elastic structure, functions to collapse the lung and pull it away from the chest wall; the elastic properties of the chest wall, in turn, function to expand the thoracic cavity. The consequence of these opposing recoil tendencies is the creation of a net *subatmospheric* (negative) pressure within the intrapleural space relative to atmospheric (external) pressure (Fig. 22–8). The point in the respiratory cycle at which these opposing forces are balanced, that is, when pressure across the lungs and chest wall is zero, is the normal *resting end-expiratory phase,* or functional residual capacity.

Mechanics of Inspiration

At the end-expiratory position in the respiratory cycle, the intrapleural pressure is subatmospheric, the alveolar pressure is atmospheric, the respiratory muscles are relaxed, and there is no air flow. *Inspiration* is initiated by contraction of the diaphragm (predominantly) and the inspiratory musculature (external intercostals and the accessory muscles—sternocleidomastoid, scalene), which causes an increase in the size of the thoracic cavity. As the thoracic cage expands it pulls ever so slightly away from the lung surface, causing the intrapleural pressure to become more negative. Because of the changes in intrapleural pressure, the lungs are also forced to expand. This increases the size of the alveoli, causing the pressure within them to become subatmospheric (negative). The consequent difference between atmospheric and intra-alveolar pressures causes the bulk flow of air into the lungs (Fig. 22–8).

Mechanics of Expiration

A reversal of the inspiratory process occurs on expiration when the inspiratory muscles relax and the lungs recoil. The elastic recoil of the lungs causes gas

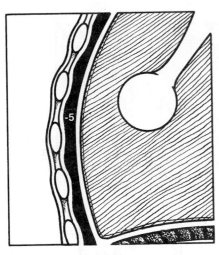
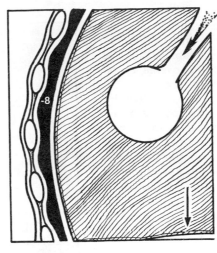
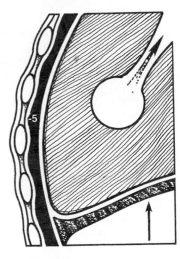

| End-expiratory phase | Inspiratory | Expiratory |

FIGURE 22–8. Pulmonary forces during quiet breathing. A schematic depiction of changes in intrapleural and intra-alveolar pressures at end-expiratory, inspiratory, and expiratory phases. A representative alveolus is depicted within the lung: lung expansion occurs as the chest cage expands and diaphragm descends (*down arrow*); lung recoil occurs as diaphragm relaxes (*up arrow*); numerical values represent change in intrapleural pressures during each phase. *End-expiratory phase:* At end-expiration, the tendency of the lungs to recoil is balanced by the opposing recoil tendency of the chest wall to bow out, resulting in a subatmospheric intrapleural pressure (−5 mmHg). The pressure in the alveolus is atmospheric, and there is no air flow. *Inspiratory phase:* On inspiration, contraction of inspiratory muscles (predominantly diaphragm) increases the size of the thoracic cavity, causing the intrapleural pressure to become increasingly subatmospheric (−8 mmHg) with consequent expansion of the lung. Intra-alveolar pressure becomes subatmospheric and air flows into the lung. *Expiratory phase:* On expiration, the respiratory muscles relax and the size of the thoracic cavity decreases, reducing the intrapleural pressure (−5 mmHg); the consequent recoil of the lung compresses the alveolus so that intra-alveolar pressure momentarily exceeds atmospheric pressure, and air flows out of the lung.

within the alveoli to become temporarily compressed. The consequent increase in intra-alveolar pressure momentarily exceeds atmospheric pressure, and air flows out of the lungs (see Fig. 22–8). In contrast to inspiration, expiration is largely a passive process.

Compliance

Compliance refers to the distensibility of the lungs and thorax and reflects the ease with which lungs can be inflated. The normal compliance of both lungs in the average adult is about 200 mL/cm of water pressure, the expression of unit change in lung volume per unit change in respiratory pressure.[2] When lung compliance is diminished, the work of breathing is increased and a greater amount of energy is expended for a given amount of chest expansion.

Work of Breathing

The work or energy required to expand the lungs and thorax is generated by the contraction of the inspiratory musculature, that is, the diaphragm (predominantly), intercostal muscles, and accessory muscles (if necessary). The actual work of breathing can be divided into three components: (1) *compliance* work reflects the work required to expand the lungs against the elastic forces; (2) *tissue resistance* work is the work expenditure required to overcome the viscosity of the

lungs and chest wall; and (3) *airway resistance* work reflects the work required to overcome resistance to air flow through the bronchi and respiratory bronchioles.[3]

Clinically, the different types of work of breathing may be increased in pulmonary disease. Compliance work and tissue resistance work are frequently increased in pneumonia, pulmonary edema, adult respiratory distress syndrome (ARDS), and pulmonary fibrosis, among others. Airway resistance work is especially increased by diseases causing airway obstruction such as asthma and chronic bronchitis. A more detailed discussion of some of these pathologic conditions can be found in subsequent chapters within this unit.

Airway Resistance

The volume of gas that flows in or out of the alveoli per unit time is directly proportional to the pressure difference between the atmosphere and the alveoli and inversely proportional to the airway resistance to gas flow.

Resistance to gas flow into the alveoli is directly proportional to the degree of interaction between the flowing gas molecules and airway length and inversely proportional to airway radius or diameter. The radius or diameter of airways is the predominant factor determining overall airway resistance. Specifically, the medium-to-large airways rather than the more numerous small airway provide greater resistance to air flow. The reason for this is that, despite their small diameter, the enormous number of these smaller airways makes up the greater portion of the overall cross-sectional area of the tracheobronchial tree.

Total airway resistance in the average healthy individual is so small that at rest only a pressure of about 1 mmHg needs to be generated with each breath to move a volume of 500 mL of gas into the lungs. Airway resistance becomes a significant factor in the presence of pulmonary disease. For example, bronchospasm and the hypersecretion of bronchial mucous glands associated with asthma cause an increase in airway resistance, which can seriously compromise ventilation.

Pulmonary Volumes and Capacities

Volume changes that occur with breathing do so within the boundaries of the maximum excursion of the respiratory apparatus. Four pulmonary lung volumes have been defined, which, when summed up, equal the maximum volume to which the lungs can be expanded. These four volumes include the tidal volume (V_T), inspiratory reserve volume, expiratory reserve volume, and residual volume (Fig. 22–9).

Tidal volume (V_T) is the volume of air inspired or expired with each normal breath. Under resting conditions in the average adult, it is about 500 mL.

Inspiratory reserve volume (IRV) is the extra volume of air that can be inspired over and above the resting tidal volume. It amounts to about 3000 mL.

Expiratory reserve volume (ERV) is the amount of air that can still be expired by forceful contraction of the expiratory musculature after the end of a normal tidal volume expiration. It amounts to about 1100 mL.

Residual volume (RV) is the volume of air still remaining in the lungs after the most forceful expiration. It amounts to about 1200 mL.

When describing events in the respiratory cycle, two or more volumes can be combined, called *pulmonary capacities*. They include the inspiratory capacity, functional residual capacity, vital capacity, and the total lung capacity (see Fig. 22–9).

Inspiratory capacity (IC) is equal to the sum of the tidal volume plus the inspiratory reserve volume. It amounts to about 3500 mL.

Functional residual capacity (FRC) is equal to the sum of the expiratory reserve volume plus the residual volume. It amounts to about 2300 mL. The functional residual capacity is significant in that the volume of gas remains in the lungs at end-expiration during quiet breathing, available to ensure that the gas exchange process continues uninterrupted.

Vital capacity (VC) is equal to the sum of the inspiratory reserve volume plus the tidal volume plus the expiratory reserve volume. It amounts to about 4600 mL.

Total lung capacity (TLC) is equal to the sum of the

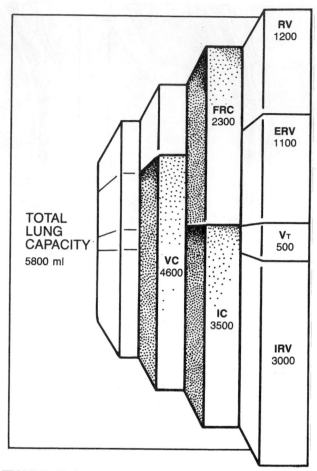

FIGURE 22–9. Lung volumes and capacities: total lung capacity, a total of 5800 mL (as seen at left), and its breakdown into its component lung volumes and capacities, all of which total 5800 mL (as seen at right).

vital capacity plus the residual volume. It amounts to about 5800 mL. In this instance, the forceful contraction of the inspiratory muscles causes maximal expansion of the chest wall. Further outward expansion of the chest wall is limited by the inward elastic recoil of the lungs. At the opposite extreme is the residual volume, wherein further forceful contraction of the expiratory muscles is unable to decrease the lung volume any more because of the outward recoil of the chest wall and airway closure.

Alveolar Ventilation

To maintain arterial blood gas parameters within the normal physiologic range to ensure adequate gas exchange to the tissues, a volume of gas must be presented to the lungs that is sufficient for the necessary oxygen uptake and carbon dioxide elimination.

The average person under resting conditions breathes about 12 to 20 times per minute and exchanges about 500 mL gas with each breath (V_T).

The total volume of gas inspired each minute (i.e., respiratory rate times the V_T amounts to 6 to 8 L/min and is called the *minute ventilation* (V_E). Thus,

$$V_E = f \times V_T$$

where f represents the respiratory rate or frequency of breaths per minute.

Not all the gas inspired with each breath is used for gas exchange. Rather, the portion of the total minute ventilation that occupies the space within the upper airways and tracheobronchial tree, that is, the *conducting* zone, does not participate in gas exchange and constitutes the *anatomical dead space* (see Fig. 22–2). This "wasted" volume of gas amounts to about 1 mL per pound of body weight or, on the average, about 150 mL.

The portion of the V_T that reaches the gas exchanging zones of the lungs (i.e., *respiratory* zone) is called the *alveolar volume* and usually amounts to about 350 mL per single normal breath. *Alveolar minute ventilation* (V_A) is equal to the number of breaths per minute (i.e., the frequency) times the V_T minus the anatomical dead space volume (V_D); thus,

$$V_A = f \times (V_T - V_D)$$

Total (Physiologic) Dead Space

The anatomical dead space is not the only type of dead space. For example, areas of the lung that normally participate in gas exchange and are fully ventilated but do not receive adequate blood flow, contribute additional dead space volume. This volume of air is called the *alveolar* dead space. Thus, *physiologic* dead space is equal to the *anatomical* dead space plus the *alveolar* dead space.

The relationship between dead space volume and the depth and rate of breathing is clinically significant. Rapid, shallow respirations with a V_T of 150 mL and a respiratory rate of more than 40 can seriously compromise alveolar ventilation because the patient is essentially moving only dead space gas and the alveoli are not being ventilated. On the other hand, any

increase in V_T and reduction in the rate of breathing will enhance alveolar ventilation.

DIFFUSION

Behavior of Gases in Air and Body Fluids

The underlying process responsible for the net movement of oxygen and carbon dioxide between the alveoli and the blood and between the blood and the cells of the body is diffusion. *Diffusion is the random movement of molecules from an area of greater concentration to one of lesser concentration.* The energy that fuels this process is derived from the kinetic motion of the molecules themselves. The constant impact of these molecules against a surface exerts a force or pressure, and this pressure, which is a function of the amount of the gas present, is called the partial pressure (P) of the particular gas (e.g., P_{O_2}, P_{CO_2}).

Atmospheric air at sea level is composed of about 79% nitrogen and 21% oxygen and exerts a total pressure of 760 mmHg (Fig. 22–10). Each of these gases contributes to the total pressure in direct proportion to their relative concentrations or partial pressure. Nitrogen contributes 79% of the 760 mmHg or a partial pressure of 600 mmHg; oxygen contributes 21% or a partial pressure of 159 mmHg.

Vapor Pressure

When gas is inhaled into the respiratory tract, it is immediately conditioned by the specialized epithelium lining the respiratory passageways. This means that the inspired gas is filtered, warmed, and humidified. Humidification of gas occurs because, like other dissolved gas molecules, water molecules are continually escaping from the fluid into the gaseous state. The pressure exerted by water molecules as they escape from the water surface is called *vapor pressure*. At normal body temperature (98.6°F), the vapor pressure is 47 mmHg.

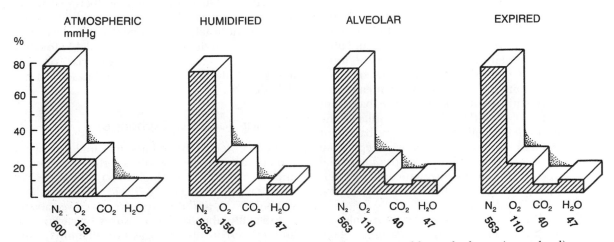

FIGURE 22–10. Partial pressures of respiratory gases as they enter and leave the lungs (at sea level).

Solubility of Gases

Gases dissolved in body fluids similarly exert a partial pressure because dissolved molecules move randomly and generate kinetic energy as do molecules in the gaseous state. Factors that determine the concentration of a gas in solution include the pressure exerted by the relative concentration of the gas and by its *solubility coefficient*. The *solubility coefficient* refers to the extent that molecules of a gas are physically or chemically attracted to water molecules. The greater the attraction, the greater the number of molecules that become dissolved. This is an important factor in determining the rate at which a gas can diffuse through the tissue. A point to remember is that carbon dioxide is 20 times more soluble than oxygen in body fluids.

Composition of Alveolar Gas

The composition of *alveolar* gas is different from that of atmospheric air (Fig. 22–10). This difference is attributed largely to the following: (1) oxygen is constantly being absorbed from the alveoli into pulmonary capillary blood, and (2) carbon dioxide is constantly diffusing from the pulmonary blood into the alveoli. Thus, the partial pressure of oxygen in alveolar air is about 14% or about 110 mmHg compared with its concentration or partial pressure in atmospheric air, which is about 21% or about 159 mmHg, respectively. The partial pressure of carbon dioxide in alveolar air is 40 mmHg.

Diffusion of Gases Through the Alveolar-Capillary Membrane

Gas exchange between the alveoli and the blood in the pulmonary capillaries occurs at the alveolar-capillary membrane. The structural layers of this membrane allow for alveolar gases to be in close proximity to the blood within the capillaries, thus facilitating the exchange of these gases.

Structurally, the layers of the respiratory membrane through which gases are exchanged include the following (Fig. 22–11): (1) a fluid layer lining the alveolar lumen and containing surfactant; (2) the long, narrow cytoplasmic extensions of type I alveolar epithelial cells; (3) epithelial cell basement membrane; (4) narrow interstitial space between the basement membrane of alveolar epithelial cells and that of the pulmonary endothelial cells; (5) capillary basement membrane, which commonly fuses with epithelial basement membrane, thus obliterating the interstitial space in a large portion of the alveolar-capillary interface; and (6) the capillary endothelial cell and the red blood cell (RBC; Fig. 22–11).

The overall thickness of the respiratory membrane varies from 0.2 μm (micrometers) to an average of 0.6 μm; its total surface area approaches about 50 to 100

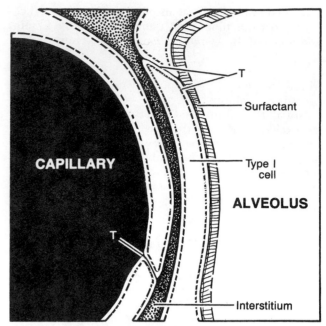

FIGURE 22–11. Ultrastructure of the alveolar-capillary membrane shown in cross-section: pathway of diffusion. Diffusion of gases occurs through the various structural layers of the membrane, including the fluid surfactant layer that lines the alveolus, alveolar epithelial type I cell, epithelial basement membrane, interstitial space, capillary basement membrane, capillary endothelial cell, and the red blood cell (not depicted). Tight junctions (T) are also depicted.

m² in the normal adult. The average diameter of the pulmonary capillary is 7 to 9 μm. Because the diameter of an RBC is about 7.0 μm, one can appreciate the close intimate interface that occurs between the RBC and the alveolar lumen as blood flows through the pulmonary circulation.

The usual transit time for an RBC traveling through the pulmonary capillaries is about 0.75 second. The diffusion of respiratory gases through the alveolar-capillary membrane is so rapid that full equilibration of partial pressures of these gases between the alveoli and pulmonary capillaries occurs within the initial one third of the total transit time, or 0.25 second. Thus, there is a pulmonary "reserve" available for diffusion if transit time decreases, as in exercise, or if disease alters the alveolar-capillary membrane and impairs diffusion.

Alveolar-Blood Gas Exchange

Blood entering the pulmonary capillaries by the pulmonary arterial circulation is systemic *venous* blood, and as such contains a high $P\bar{v}CO_2$ (46 mmHg) and a low $P\bar{v}O_2$ (40 mmHg) (Fig. 22–12). (The small $\bar{v}$ in the symbols $P\bar{v}CO_2$ and $P\bar{v}O_2$ reflects mixed venous blood.)

Normally, the partial pressures of carbon dioxide and oxygen in alveolar gas are 40 mmHg and 110 mmHg, respectively (Fig. 22–10). The net gradient

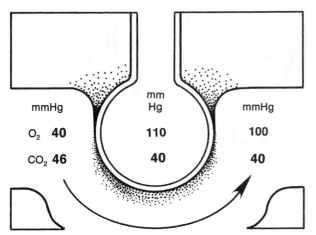

	mmHg		mm Hg		mmHg
O_2	40		110		100
CO_2	46		40		40

FIGURE 22–12. Transfer of oxygen and carbon dioxide between alveolus and capillary blood. The net gradients between the partial pressure of oxygen and carbon dioxide on the two sides of the alveolar-capillary membrane provide the driving force that underlies gas exchange within the lungs. These pressure differences facilitate carbon dioxide release and oxygen uptake as blood flows through the pulmonary circulation. Following gas exchange, the partial pressures of these gases in arterial blood leaving the pulmonary circulation are 95 and 40 mmHg, respectively. The difference between the alveolar oxygen tension (110 mmHg) and that of arterial blood (100 mmHg) is largely attributed to "physiologic" dead space (i.e., the sum of anatomical and alveolar dead space). This difference is referred to as the A-a gradient.

between the partial pressures of carbon dioxide and oxygen on the two sides of the alveolar-capillary membrane result in a net diffusion of carbon dioxide into the alveoli and of oxygen into the blood.

In summation, diffusion of carbon dioxide and oxygen is influenced by the integrity of the alveolar-capillary membrane, the surface area available for gas exchange, the solubility coefficient of each gas, the net pressure gradients between the alveolar and pulmonary capillary gas pressures, the total RBC count, and the amount of hemoglobin.

VENTILATION/PERFUSION RELATIONSHIPS

The extensive network of the pulmonary capillary bed interfacing with alveolar walls provides for an enormous surface area of intricate contact between RBCs and alveolar gas. For gas exchange to be most efficient, the appropriate amount of alveolar gas and capillary blood should be available to each gas-exchanging unit.

Ventilation/Perfusion ($\dot{V}/\dot{Q}$) Ratio

Ideally, optimal efficiency for gas exchange would be provided by an even distribution of ventilation and perfusion throughout the lung so that ventilation and

perfusion are always matched. Clinically, this is not the case even in healthy individuals. *Overall, alveolar ventilation is normally about 4 L/min, and pulmonary capillary blood flow is about 5 L/min, making the average ratio of ventilation to blood flow 4:5, or about 0.8. This relationship is called the $\dot{V}/\dot{Q}$ ratio.*

Although the overall $\dot{V}/\dot{Q}$ ratio is about 0.8, the ratio varies remarkably throughout the lung. The dependent areas of each lung receive a disproportionately larger share of the perfusion, whereas areas in the apices of the lungs are relatively underperfused. In the normal person in the upright position, the alveoli in the apices of the lungs receive a moderate amount of ventilation but little blood flow. As a result, the $\dot{V}/\dot{Q}$ ratio in the upper regions of the lungs is greater than 0.8.

Gradations of ventilation occur throughout each lung, with a greater portion going to dependent lung areas. However, ventilation and perfusion are not matched in the dependent areas because the gradient is more marked for perfusion than for ventilation. As a result, the $\dot{V}/\dot{Q}$ ratio is lower than 0.8 in the lower lung regions. Thus, gas exchange throughout the lung is not uniform but varies according to the ratio of ventilation to perfusion in each region. Clinically, the position assumed (e.g., supine, prone, side-lying) is an important factor to be considered in terms of ventilation and perfusion to dependent areas as patients are turned and positioned (Fig. 22–7).

Dead Space Versus Shunt Units

To better understand the effects of alterations in the $\dot{V}/\dot{Q}$ ratio on gas exchange, it is useful to consider the dynamics of a single alveolar-capillary unit. In such a unit, a continuum of possible $\dot{V}/\dot{Q}$ relationships exists (Fig. 22–13). As discussed, in the normal situation the ventilation and perfusion are well matched and the $\dot{V}/\dot{Q}$ ratio is ideally 0.8 (or rounded off to 1/1, for this discussion). At one extreme of the continuum, ventilation is maintained, but perfusion approaches zero. The $\dot{V}/\dot{Q}$ ratio in this instance approaches infinity (1/0). Insofar as gas exchange is concerned, because the alveolus is not perfused, the ventilation is "wasted" and the alveolus becomes part of the "dead space" ventilation.

At the opposite extreme of the continuum, ventilation approaches zero, whereas perfusion is preserved. The $\dot{V}/\dot{Q}$ ratio in this instance approaches zero (0/1). When there is no ventilation (V = 0), a shunt exists, and oxygenation does not take place during the transit of the blood through the pulmonary circulation.

Clinically, $\dot{V}/\dot{Q}$ ratios within specific alveolar-capillary units can fall anywhere along the continuum from a ratio of 1/0 (i.e., dead space) to a ratio of 0/1 (i.e., shunt). Pulmonary dead space and shunt units may occur simultaneously in the ill person; such $\dot{V}/\dot{Q}$ ratio inequality is responsible for some compromise in gas exchange.

In the healthy lung, regional differences in $\dot{V}/\dot{Q}$ matching affect oxygen and carbon dioxide tensions

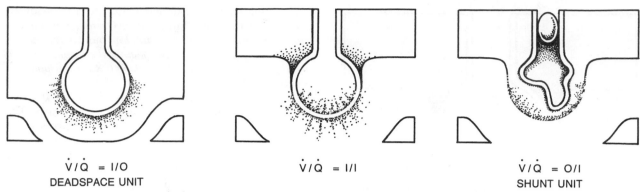

$$\dot{V}/\dot{Q} = 1/0$$
DEADSPACE UNIT

$$\dot{V}/\dot{Q} = 1/1$$

$$\dot{V}/\dot{Q} = 0/1$$
SHUNT UNIT

FIGURE 22–13. Continuum of $\dot{V}/\dot{Q}$ relationships reflecting the extremes of ventilation-perfusion matching. From the dead space unit, $\dot{V}/\dot{Q} = 1/0$ (i.e., ventilation but no perfusion), to the ideal unit, $\dot{V}/\dot{Q} = 1/1$ (i.e., ventilation and perfusion optimally matched). Two examples of respiratory disorders and their effect on the $\dot{V}/\dot{Q}$ ratio include pulmonary embolism, which causes an increase in dead space ventilation, and adult respiratory distress syndrome, in which the predominant $\dot{V}/\dot{Q}$ pattern is the shunt.[5]

in blood coming from specific regions, as well as the overall gas tensions in the resulting arterial blood returning to the left ventricle. For example, at the apex of each lung where the $\dot{V}/\dot{Q}$ ratio approaches 3.3, the PaO_2 is about 132 mmHg and the $PaCO_2$ is about 28 mmHg. At the bases, where the $\dot{V}/\dot{Q}$ ratio approaches 0.63, the PaO_2 is about 89 mmHg and the $PaCO_2$ is about 42 mmHg. The net PaO_2 and $PaCO_2$ of the combined blood returning from the apices, the bases, and areas in between is a function of the relative amounts of blood from each of these areas and the gas tensions of each.[4]

In respiratory disease, the $\dot{V}/\dot{Q}$ ratio is always altered, resulting in clinically significant gas exchange abnormalities. For example, in disorders that reduce alveolar ventilation, the affected lung areas receive little to no ventilation in relation to blood flow, causing the $\dot{V}/\dot{Q}$ ratio to decrease. Consequently, blood coming from these areas has a low oxygen content and saturation, which cannot be compensated for by blood from relatively preserved regions of the lung. Respiratory disorders that decrease the $\dot{V}/\dot{Q}$ ratio include hypoventilation from any cause, obstructive lung disease (e.g., asthma, emphysema, and chronic bronchitis) and restrictive lung disease (e.g., pneumonia, ARDS).

In respiratory disorders that reduce pulmonary perfusion, the affected lung area receives little to no blood flow in relation to ventilation, causing the $\dot{V}/\dot{Q}$ ratio to increase. Consequently, a larger portion of the alveolar ventilation will constitute dead space ventilation. When the $\dot{V}/\dot{Q}$ ratio increases, the PaO_2 also increases and the $PaCO_2$ decreases. Respiratory disorders that increase the $\dot{V}/\dot{Q}$ ratio include pulmonary embolism with partial or complete occlusion of the pulmonary artery or one of its branches; altered pulmonary vascular dynamics associated with pneumothorax or hydrothorax and tumors; and actual destruction of pulmonary blood vessels as occurs, in emphysema.

Alveolar-Arterial Oxygen Difference (A-a Gradient)

Theoretically, under normal physiologic conditions the PaO_2 in blood leaving the pulmonary capillary bed should be in equilibrium with the PAO_2. Physiologically, this is not the case because the PAO_2 (alveolar oxygen tension) is greater than PaO_2 (arterial oxygen tension) in the healthy person, or about 110 mmHg and 100 mmHg, respectively. The difference between the *alveolar* and *arterial* oxygen tensions is called the *alveolar-arterial oxygen difference,* or the A-a gradient.

The existence of this gradient is attributed to the presence of normal physiologic shunt. This includes the exiting of blood from lung regions with low $\dot{V}/\dot{Q}$ ratios (i.e., alveoli that are underventilated in proportion to the pulmonary blood flow); drainage of venous blood from the bronchial circulation into the pulmonary veins; and drainage of coronary venous blood directly into the left atrium by the thebesian veins.

Normally, the A-a gradient is less than 15 mmHg. An A-a gradient greater than 15 mmHg reflects an underlying pathologic process. There are several reasons for an elevated A-a gradient in disease: intracardiac shunts such as atrial or ventricular septal defects, pulmonary arteriovenous malformations, pulmonary disease wherein the alveoli are filled with fluid or exudate (e.g., pulmonary edema, ARDS, or complete alveolar collapse (e.g., pneumothorax).

$\dot{V}/\dot{Q}$ mismatch may also cause the A-a gradient to be elevated. Even when total ventilation and perfusion to both lungs are normal, if some areas receive less ventilation and more perfusion (low $\dot{V}/\dot{Q}$ ratio) whereas others receive more ventilation with less perfusion (high $\dot{V}/\dot{Q}$ ratio), the end-result can be an increase in the A-a gradient with hypoxemia.

The physiologic mechanism underlying this phenomenon is that areas with a low $\dot{V}/\dot{Q}$ ratio provide relatively desaturated blood with a low oxygen content; blood coming from regions of high $\dot{V}/\dot{Q}$ ratio cannot compensate for the alteration because the hemoglobin is already fully saturated and cannot increase its oxygen content further by increased ventilation.

Calculation of Arterial/Alveolar Ratio (a/A Ratio) and Alveolar-Arterial Gradient (A-a Gradient)

The calculation of the (a/A ratio) and the A-a gradient can be extremely helpful in the clinical setting, particularly when one is trying to determine the reason why a patient is hypoxemic. Both these calculations are relatively simple to determine and require only two parameters to do so: the arterial oxygen pressure (PaO_2) value obtained from an arterial blood sample and the alveolar oxygen pressure (PAO_2), which can be determined using the alveolar gas equation[6,7]:

$$PAO_2 = FIO_2(PB - PH_2O) - \frac{PaCO_2}{RQ}$$

where FIO_2 is the fraction of inspired oxygen; PB is the barometric pressure (assumed to be 760 mmHg at sea level); PH_2O is the vapor pressure of water in the alveoli (assumed to be 47 mmHg); $PaCO_2$ is the partial pressure of carbon dioxide in arterial blood as determined on blood gas analysis; and RQ is the respiratory quotient, which reflects carbon dioxide production divided by oxygen consumption, usually a factor of about 0.8. Accordingly, the *a/A ratio* can be calculated as follows:

$$a/A\ ratio = \frac{PaO_2}{PAO_2}$$

The A-a gradient can be calculated as follows:

$$A\text{-}a\ gradient = PAO_2 - PaO_2$$

Venous Admixture (Intrapulmonary Shunting)

Limitations in the use of the a/A ratio and A-a gradient calculations occur in the scenario of venous admixture (i.e., the mixing of shunted unoxygenated blood with oxygenated blood distal to the alveoli). Venous admixture commonly occurs with many respiratory disorders, such as when the alveoli are filled with edema fluid (pulmonary edema) or inflammatory cells (pneumonia). To determine the degree of shunting, the *classic shunt equation* is used.

$$\frac{Qs}{QT} = \frac{CcO_2 - CaO_2}{CcO_2 - CvO_2}$$

where Qs is cardiac output that is shunted, QT is total cardiac output, CcO_2 is oxygen content of capillary blood, CaO_2 is oxygen content of arterial blood, and CvO_2 is oxygen content of mixed venous blood.

To obtain the data necessary to calculate the degree of pulmonary shunting, the following information must be obtained: PB (barometric pressure); PaO_2 (partial pressure of arterial oxygen); Hb (hemoglobin concentration); PAO_2 (partial pressure of alveolar oxygen); FIO_2 (fraction of inspired oxygen); and PvO_2 (partial pressure of mixed venous oxygen).[7,8]

TRANSPORT OF OXYGEN

Oxygen is transported in the blood in two distinct ways: by being dissolved in blood and by being bound to hemoglobin within the RBCs. Under normal physiologic conditions, about 97% of oxygen is transported from the lungs to the tissues in chemical combination with hemoglobin. The remainder is dissolved in blood, the amount dissolved being directly proportional to its partial pressure (PaO_2). Because oxygen is relatively insoluble in plasma, only about 3% of total oxygen is transported in this manner.

Hemoglobin consists of four polypeptide chains, each containing a heme group. Oxygen specifically binds to the iron atom found within each of the four heme groups. Thus, each hemoglobin molecule can combine with four molecules of oxygen. When all four iron atoms (i.e., binding sites for oxygen) in each molecule of hemoglobin are bound with oxygen, the hemoglobin molecule is said to be fully saturated. *Saturation* is defined as the degree to which binding sites are occupied by a particular molecule—in this case, oxygen. Hemoglobin bound with oxygen is called *oxyhemoglobin*; when not in combination with oxygen, the hemoglobin is called *reduced hemoglobin*.

Oxyhemoglobin Dissociation Curve

The amount of oxygen bound to hemoglobin is a function of the partial pressure of oxygen. The quantitative relationship between oxygen bound and the partial pressure of the gas is characterized by the *oxyhemoglobin dissociation curve*. (Fig. 22–14). This curve is S-shaped with a steep slope below a PO_2 of 60 mmHg and a plateau portion between a PO_2 of 60 to 100 mmHg. The cooperative binding that occurs between the heme groups in a given hemoglobin molecule accounts for its sequential increase in oxygen affinity as reflected by the sigmoidal-shaped curve. As oxygen binds to one heme group, this facilitates the rapid binding of oxygen with the remaining heme groups within the same hemoglobin molecule. Thus, at the lower PO_2, the extent to which hemoglobin combines with oxygen increases very rapidly from 10 to 60 mmHg, so that *at a PO_2 of 60 mmHg, 90% of the total hemoglobin is bound to oxygen.*

At higher PO_2 levels, the oxyhemoglobin dissociation curve reaches a plateau, which reflects that *hemoglobin can only bind to so much oxygen before the binding sites become fully saturated.* In general, as the PO_2 increases, there is a progressive increase in the percentage of hemoglobin bound with oxygen. This is

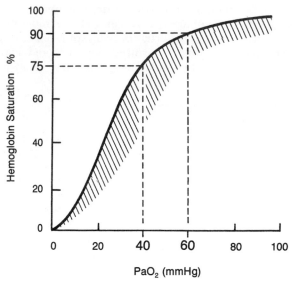

FIGURE 22–14. Oxyhemoglobin dissociation curve, relating the percent of hemoglobin saturation and the partial pressure of oxygen (PO_2). The unique structure of the hemoglobin molecule accounts for the unusual affinity this molecule has for oxygen. When the PO_2 is high as in the lungs (*plateau portion*), oxygen readily binds with hemoglobin; when the PO_2 is low as in the tissue (*steep portion*), oxygen is readily released. Note that at a PaO_2 of 60, approximately 90% of the hemoglobin is saturated. Thus, clinically, oxygen therapy is often instituted to maintain a PaO_2 of 60 minimally, in the patient with compromised pulmonary function. Oxygen unloading at the cellular level is enhanced when the oxyhemoglobin dissociation curve is shifted to the right (*striped area*). The presence of acidemia (i.e., an increase in hydrogen-ion concentration), an increase in body temperature, and increased levels of 2,3-DPG all function to shift the curve to the right. Alkalemia, hypothermia, and reduced levels of 2,3-DPG function to shift the curve in the opposite direction, thereby reducing the release of oxygen at the cellular level.

called the *percent saturation of hemoglobin* (SO_2). The usual saturation of arterial blood (SaO_2) is about 97% at sea level; in venous blood, the $P\bar{v}O_2$ is about 40 mmHg with saturation of hemoglobin ($S\bar{v}O_2$) about 75%.

Factors Affecting Hemoglobin Saturation

Several factors can cause the oxyhemoglobin dissociation curve to shift, resulting in a greater or lesser affinity of hemoglobin for oxygen. A shift of the curve to the right means that, at a given PO_2, hemoglobin has a decreased affinity for oxygen. By contrast, a shift of the curve to the left means that at any given PO_2, hemoglobin has an increased affinity for oxygen.

Hydrogen-Ion Concentration

Acidemia (i.e., an increase in hydrogen-ion concentration of the blood [pH less than 7.35]) can cause a shift of the entire oxyhemoglobin dissociation curve

to the *right*. Clinically, the more metabolically active a tissue is (e.g., heart, nerves, or an exercising muscle), the greater is its production of hydrogen ions and carbon dioxide. The high concentrations of hydrogen ions and carbon dioxide enhance oxygen unloading. As the blood concentrations of these substances increase, a shift of the oxyhemoglobin dissociation curve to the right occurs. In contrast, hypocapnia and alkalemia may cause a shift of the curve to the left.

Effect of Temperature

The effect of an increase in body temperature resembles that of increased acidity (i.e., the oxyhemoglobin curve shifts to the right). Clinically, this suggests that an actively metabolizing tissue (e.g., an exercising muscle) has a consequent elevation in temperature, which facilitates the release of oxygen from hemoglobin as blood flows through the tissue capillaries. Hypothermia, however, causes a shift of the curve to the left.

Effect of 2,3-Diphosphoglycerate

2,3-Diphosphoglycerate (DPG) is produced by RBCs during glycolysis. This molecule binds reversibly with hemoglobin and causes it to have a reduced affinity for oxygen. Thus, as with increased hydrogen-ion concentration and temperature elevation, *DPG likewise shifts the oxyhemoglobin dissociation curve to the right*.

Clinically, tissues experiencing ischemia or anaerobic glycolysis generate an increased supply of DPG. This increase in turn causes the enhanced unloading of oxygen as blood passes through the tissue capillaries. In this way, additional oxygen is made available to the tissues.

Factors Determining Tissue Oxygen Delivery

The percent saturation of hemoglobin is predominantly a function of the PO_2. Additional factors concerned with oxygen delivery to the tissues include the hemoglobin level and the cardiac output.

Reductions in the hemoglobin level can seriously compromise oxygen delivery to the tissues. In anemia, for example, with the reduction in hemoglobin levels there is a concomitant reduction in the number of oxygen binding sites, with a consequent decrease in the total oxygen content of the blood delivered to the tissues. In this circumstance, oxygen tissue delivery capability may be reduced, even though PaO_2 remains within acceptable physiologic range (higher than 60 mmHg). Because oxygen delivery to the tissues depends on blood flow, any alteration in cardiac output can compromise oxygenation at the tissue level.

TRANSPORT OF CARBON DIOXIDE

Carbon dioxide is transported in the circulation in three different forms: (1) as bicarbonate ion (HCO_3),

(2) as dissolved carbon dioxide, and (3) bound to hemoglobin (*carbamino*hemoglobin). Bicarbonate is quantitatively the largest fraction and results from the combination of CO_2 and H_2O in a reaction catalyzed by the enzyme, *carbonic anhydrase:*

$$\text{Carbonic anhydrase}$$
$$\downarrow$$
$$CO_2 + H_2O \leftrightarrow H_2CO_3 \leftrightarrow H^+ + HCO_3$$

This reaction takes place within the RBC. HCO_3 then diffuses into the plasma in exchange for chloride (Cl^-) called *chloride shift*).

CONTROL OF RESPIRATION

Central Neuronal Control

Alveolar ventilation requires a rhythmic, coordinated sequence of events involving the activity of the respiratory muscles (respiratory pump) under the control of the central nervous system (CNS). No single "respiratory center" controls breathing. Rather, several neuronal networks are involved in coordinating the respiratory efforts. Breathing depends on the cyclic innervation of the inspiratory musculature (diaphragm and intercostal muscles) by neurons from these networks.

Major neuronal networks that have been identified include[9] (1) dorsal and ventral respiratory neuronal networks located within the medulla, (2) the *pneumotaxic* center located in the superior pons, and (3) a less well-defined *apneustic* center located in the lower pons (Fig. 22–15).

The basic rhythm of breathing is generated within the medullary groups of neurons. Innervation of the inspiratory musculature occurs characteristically by alternating cycles of neuronal firing and quiescence. At the end of expiration, there is some degree of muscle tone involving the diaphragm and intercostal muscles, but not of sufficient magnitude to move the chest wall.

Inspiration is initiated by an increased firing of impulses to the motor units, which begin to contract more forcefully. The inspiratory force increases as it proceeds, until there is an abrupt cessation of impulse firing and the inspiratory muscles relax. At this point, expiration begins. Expiration is largely a passive process, and all that is required for expiration to occur is a cessation of inspiratory neuronal activity.

The pneumotaxic center in the pons functions primarily to limit inspiration. Because limiting the inspiratory phase also shortens the entire period of the respiratory cycle, there is a secondary effect on the respiratory rate.

The apneustic center in the pons may signal the dorsal medullary network so as to prevent a "switch-off" of inspiratory effort. The function of the apneustic center may be to provide extra drive to inspiration, but this effect is overridden by impulses from the pneumotaxic center.

Control of respiration by the major neuronal networks in the medulla and pons requires an intricate feedback system to "fine-tune" the neural output of the CNS to the pulmonary musculature. In this way, the CNS is able to respond to the varied needs of the individual by appropriately increasing ventilation as during exercise or strenuous activity, while maintaining arterial blood gases within the acceptable physiologic range.

Autonomic Nervous System Control

Regulation of respiratory function is largely under autonomic nervous system control including parasympathetic and sympathetic innervation. Specific effects of autonomic innervation on respiratory physiology include the following:

	Parasympathetic	*Sympathetic*
Bronchiolar smooth muscle	Contraction	Relaxation
Pulmonary vasculature smooth muscle	Vasodilatation	Vasoconstriction
Mucous/serous glandular secretion	Stimulation	Inhibition

Chemical Control of Respiration

The major neuronal networks are concerned with the mechanisms that generate spontaneity and rhythmicity of breathing. These networks in turn receive afferent inputs from a variety of sources.

The most important of these inputs concerned with the involuntary control of ventilatory volume include *peripheral chemoreceptors*, which monitor PaO_2, $PaCO_2$,

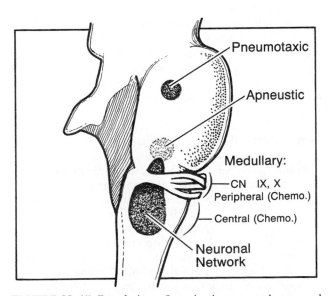

FIGURE 22–15. Regulation of respiration: central neuronal networks.

and hydrogen-ion concentrations; and *central chemoreceptors,* which monitor the hydrogen-ion concentration of the brain's interstitial fluid. Respiratory control is designed to maintain arterial blood gas parameters within the acceptable physiologic range: PaO_2 greater than 60 mmHg; $PaCO_2$, 35 to 45 mmHg, and a pH, 7.35 to 7.45.

Control of Ventilation by Oxygen Concentration

Large decreases in PaO_2 (e.g., less than 60 mmHg) act as a stimulus to reflexly increase ventilation. Because the oxygen content of arterial blood is not really compromised at a PaO_2 above 60 mmHg (e.g., percent oxygen saturation of hemoglobin is 90), it is usually when the PaO_2 falls below 60 mmHg that a significant increase in ventilation occurs.

Peripheral chemoreceptors that respond to changes in the PaO_2 include the *carotid* and *aortic bodies.* The chemoreceptors sense the PaO_2 and respond specifically to dissolved oxygen and not to oxyhemoglobin. Afferent nerve fibers arising from these chemoreceptors pass to the medulla by way of the vagus and glossopharyngeal nerves, and stimulate the medullary inspiratory neuronal network. A compensatory increase in ventilation occurs to return the PaO_2 toward normal.

Control of Ventilation by Carbon Dioxide and Hydrogen-Ion Concentration

A decrease in alveolar ventilation raises the $PaCO_2$, and accordingly an elevation in $PaCO_2$ occurs. Unlike the PaO_2 wherein a large decrease in PaO_2 (less than 60 mmHg) must occur before the chemoreceptors respond, *an increase in $PaCO_2$ of but 2 to 5 mmHg can cause a 100% increase in ventilation.*[10] The slightest change in $PaCO_2$ is associated with a significant reflex change in rate and depth of ventilation. The increased ventilatory effort promotes elimination of carbon dioxide by the lungs, thus returning the $PaCO_2$ toward normal.

Conversely, a decrease in $PaCO_2$ below normal reflexly reduces the ventilatory stimulus, enabling metabolically produced carbon dioxide to accumulate. In this way, the $PaCO_2$ is returned toward normal (i.e., above 35 mmHg).

There are no definitive receptors for carbon dioxide per se. Rather, the impact of changes in $PaCO_2$ on the ventilatory effort are mainly due to the consequent increase in hydrogen-ion concentration that occurs with an increase in carbon dioxide concentration. According to the law of mass action, an increase in $PaCO_2$ drives this reaction to the right, thereby increasing the hydrogen-ion concentration.

Hydrogen-ion receptors include the peripheral chemoreceptors, the carotid bodies. Thus, these receptors are triggered by either a low PaO_2 or a high hydrogen-ion concentration in arterial blood. The major hydrogen-ion reflex involves the *central* chemorecep-

tors located in the medulla. Carbon dioxide diffuses rapidly across the blood-brain barrier. Thus, any increase in $PaCO_2$ causes a rapid, similar increase in the PCO_2 of the brain's interstitial fluid. Accordingly, by the law of mass action (see previous equation), there is a consequent increase in the hydrogen-ion concentration of the brain's interstitial fluid.

The increase in hydrogen-ion concentration stimulates the central chemoreceptors in the medulla, which in turn stimulate the inspiratory neuronal networks to enhance the ventilatory effort. The end-result is a closely regulated hydrogen-ion concentration within the normal range. The normal pH of cerebrospinal fluid ranges beween 7.32 and 7.35.

In addition to carbon dioxide–induced changes in hydrogen-ion concentrations, peripheral chemoreceptors are also responsive to changes in hydrogen-ion concentration associated with conditions other than an elevated $PaCO_2$. For example, metabolically induced increases in hydrogen-ion concentration associated with increased lactic acid production can precipitate hyperventilation. *Kussmaul's* breathing (i.e., rapid, deep breathing) associated with diabetic ketoacidosis is an example of how an increase in hydrogen-ion concentration can alter the ventilatory response.

In these instances, central chemoreceptors do not respond to increases in hydrogen-ion concentrations because, unlike carbon dioxide, the charged hydrogen ion does not easily penetrate the blood-brain barrier. Therefore, the hydrogen concentration of the brain's interstitial fluid is not appreciably increased, at least not initially.

Clinically, reflex hyperventilation associated with an increase in hydrogen-ion concentration functions effectively to restore arterial pH toward normal. (i.e., 7.35 to 7.45). Hyperventilation decreases the carbon dioxide concentration, which, by the law of mass action (see previous equation), lowers the hydrogen-ion concentration.

Although the stimulatory effects of carbon dioxide on ventilation have been discussed, it is essential to appreciate that very high levels of carbon dioxide may have just the opposite effect, that is, a *depressant* effect on the CNS, including the various neuronal networks concerned with respiration.

Other Controls of Ventilation

Pulmonary stretch receptors, which lie in the airway smooth muscle layer, are activated by expansion of the lung on inspiration and may provide an important "cut-off" signal for inspiration. These receptors are activated when very large tidal volumes (more than 1 L) are exchanged, as during exercise.

Irritant reflexes are elicited by stimulation of irritant receptors located within the luminal lining of the airways. Cough, bronchospasm, and tachypnea may occur in response to a noxious stimulus such as inhaled dust, chemicals, or cigarette smoke. Tachypnea may also occur in response to stimulation of *juxtacapillary* or *j receptors,* found within the pulmonary interstitium in response to an inflammatory process, or the presence of fluid and congestion in the interstitial compartment. These receptors are thought to be the source of dyspnea that occurs with pulmonary edema.

REFERENCES

1. Des Jardins, TR: Cardiopulmonary Anatomy & Physiology: Essentials for Respiratory Care. Delmar Publishers, New York, 1988, p 28.
2. Porth, C: Pathophysiology: Concepts of Altered Health States, ed 4. JB Lippincott, Philadelphia, 1994, p 507.
3. Guyton, AC: Textbook of Medical Physiology, ed 8. WB Saunders, Philadelphia, 1991, p 406.
4. Weinberger, SE: Principles of Pulmonary Medicine. WB Saunders, Philadelphia, 1986, p 16.
5. King, G: Respiratory failure in the critically ill. In Sibbald, WJ (ed): Synopsis of Critical Care, ed 3. Williams & Wilkins, Baltimore, 1988, p 55.
6. Ahrens, T and Rutherford, K: The new pulmonary math applying the a/A ratio. Am J Nurs 87 (3):337, 1987.
7. Goodnough-Hanneman, SK: Ventilatory management. In Boggs, RL and King, MW (eds): AACN Procedure Manual for Critical Care, ed 3. WB Saunders, Philadelphia, 1993, pp 96–164.
8. Des Jardins, TR: Cardiopulmonary Anatomy & Physiology: Essentials for Respiratory Care. Delmar Publishers, New York, 1988, p 177.
9. Guyton, AC: Textbook of Medical Physiology, ed 8. WB Saunders, Philadelphia, 1991, p 444.
10. Vander, A, Sherman, J, and Luciano, D: Human Physiology: The Mechanisms of Body Function, ed 4. McGraw-Hill, New York, 1985, p 412.

CHAPTER 23

Acid-Base Physiology and Pathophysiology

Sandra K. Hanneman

CHAPTER OUTLINE

LEARNING OBJECTIVES

After completing this chapter, you should be able to:

1. Define acidemia and alkalemia.
2. Describe the compensatory mechanisms, including the major buffering systems, and their critical role in the maintenance of acid-base balance.
3. Describe the respiratory response to changes in hydrogen-ion concentration.
4. Identify key factors in the renal regulation of hydrogen-ion concentration.
5. Define the clinical significance of blood acid-base parameters (pH, $Paco_2$, HCO_3^-, and base excess); list normal values.
6. Contrast respiratory acidemia with respiratory alkalemia.
7. Contrast metabolic acidemia with metabolic alkalemia.
8. Describe the procedure for analyzing arterial blood gases.
9. Describe procedures for obtaining an arterial blood gas sample.

The optimal physiologic range for acid-base balance is a pH between 7.35 and 7.45. Deviations from this range can disrupt intracellular chemical reactions and vital electrochemical processes critical to nerve conduction.

Maintaining the physiologic pH takes on added significance when one considers that the waste products of metabolism are primarily acidic. Carbon dioxide combines with water to form carbonic acid, the most ubiquitous body acid. Fat and protein metabolism contribute other acid by-products. Mechanisms within the body function to resist changes in the pH, which would otherwise occur in the presence of large quantities of acid by-products. Such mechanisms facilitate the excretion of these substances at a rate that matches their generation.

DEFINITION OF TERMS

pH

The *pH* of a solution is a measure of its hydrogen-ion concentration. Specifically, pH reflects the *negative logarithm* of the hydrogen-ion concentration. For example, water, which consists of hydrogen ions (H^+) and hydroxyl ions (OH^-) has a pH of 7. Numerically, the expression pH of 7 reflects the actual concentration of hydrogen ions in water, which is 0.0000001, or the negative logarithm of 10^{-7}.

Thus, the pH and hydrogen-ion concentration are *inversely* related. As the hydrogen-ion concentration rises, the pH falls; as the hydrogen-ion concentration decreases, the pH rises. A low pH indicates the solution is more *acidic*; a high pH indicates the solution is more *alkaline*. The normal pH range is 1 to 14, where 7 is about neutral (i.e., the concentrations of acid and base in the solution are about equal). In water, which has a neutral pH of 7, the concentrations of hydrogen ions and hydroxyl ions are about the same.

Acids

An *acid* is a substance that can donate hydrogen ions, or protons, to a solution (i.e., proton donor). A distinction is made between strong and weak acids. *Strong* acids have a strong tendency to discharge hydrogen ions into solution and thus become completely dissociated or ionized in solution.

Weak acids also donate hydrogen ions to solution, but they do so far less vigorously than do strong acids. Weak acids are only partially dissociated in acidic solutions.

Bases

A *base* is a substance that can accept or combine with hydrogen ions to remove these ions from solution (i.e., proton acceptor). A distinction similar to that for acids is made between strong and weak bases. *Strong* bases remove hydrogen ions from solution and remain dissociated. *Weak* bases also combine with hydrogen ions in solution, but they do so much less vigorously than do strong bases. Weak bases are only partially dissociated in alkaline solutions.

In the body, weak acids and weak bases regulate acid-base balance to prevent sudden and precipitous changes in the pH of body fluids. For example, if hydrochloric acid, a strong acid, is added to water (pH 7), the pH drops precipitously to 1. If however, sodium bicarbonate, a weak base, is added to the solution, it functions to neutralize the strong acid (i.e., the hydrochloric acid) and, in turn, produces the weak acid, carbonic acid. The weak base thus minimizes the change in pH by converting a strong acid into a weak acid solution.

The following equation expresses this reaction:

$$\underset{\substack{\text{(Weak} \\ \text{base)}}}{NaHCO_3} + \underset{\substack{\text{(Strong} \\ \text{acid)}}}{HCl} \rightarrow \underset{\substack{\text{(Weak} \\ \text{acid)}}}{H_2CO_3} + \underset{\substack{\text{(Salt} \\ \text{[sodium} \\ \text{chloride])}}}{NaCl} \quad (1)$$

Similarly, a weak acid, carbonic acid, functions to neutralize a strong base, sodium hydroxide. When sodium hydroxide is added to water (pH 7), the pH rises precipitously, approaching 14. The addition of carbonic acid to this solution produces the weak base, sodium bicarbonate, thus minimizing the change in pH. The following equation expresses this reaction:

$$\underset{\substack{\text{(Weak} \\ \text{acid)}}}{H_2CO_3} + \underset{\substack{\text{(Strong} \\ \text{base)}}}{NaOH} \rightarrow \underset{\substack{\text{(Weak} \\ \text{base)}}}{NaHCO_3} + \underset{\text{(Water)}}{H_2O}$$

$$(2)$$

In each of these reactions, a strong acid (base) is converted to a weak acid (base), thus minimizing the consequent change in pH. In other words, the strong acid (base) has been buffered by the addition of a weak acid (base).

COMPENSATORY MECHANISMS IN ACID-BASE BALANCE

Maintenance of acid-base balance in the extracellular and intracellular fluids is accomplished by the precise regulation of the free hydrogen-ion concentration. These control mechanisms are so effective that the pH is normally stabilized at 7.4 for arterial blood and 7.35 for venous blood. The lower pH of venous blood is due to an increased concentration of acid by-products of cellular metabolism. The major control mechanisms responsible for the regulation of hydrogen-ion concentration include chemical buffers, lungs, and kidneys.

CHEMICAL BUFFERS

A chemical buffer is a combination of a weak acid and its conjugate base (e.g., carbonic acid and bicarbonate), which together minimize a change in pH when either acid or base is added to the buffered solution.

Equations 1 and 2 in the above section demonstrate the buffering reactions. The buffer in Equation 1 is the weak base, sodium bicarbonate; in Equation 2, the buffer is the weak acid, carbonic acid.

There are four major chemical buffers in body fluids: the carbonic acid/bicarbonate system, the hemoglobin/oxyhemoglobin system in red blood cells (RBCs), the phosphate system, and the protein buffers. The significance of chemical buffers is that they react *immediately* to prevent any major, consequential changes in hydrogen-ion concentration. Combined with the dilutional effect of circulating blood, they constitute the first line of defense in preventing immediate shifts in pH. Eventually, excess hydrogen ions are eliminated by way of the lungs (carbon dioxide) and kidneys.

Carbonic Acid/Bicarbonate System

Roughly 50% of the extra acid load or base load is buffered in minutes within the extracellular fluid. The other 50% is buffered in the intracellular fluid in 2 to 6 hours. Carbon dioxide and water, the end-products of energy metabolism, react to form carbonic acid; carbonic acid dissociates to form hydrogen and bicarbonate ions:

$$CO_2 + H_2O = H_2CO_3$$
$$= H^+ + HCO_3^- \quad (3)$$

The Henderson-Hasselbalch equation describes the dissociation of carbonic acid and expresses the relationship between pH and the ratio of bicarbonate to carbonic acid:

$$pH = pK + \log \frac{HCO_3^-}{H_2CO_3} \frac{Base}{Acid} \quad (4)$$

The pK is a constant that reflects the pH of an acid at which it is half-dissociated (i.e., when half of the solution occurs as carbonic acid, and the other half is ionized as hydrogen and bicarbonate ions). The pK for carbonic acid is 6.1.

In 1 liter of extracellular fluid, there are 24 to 28 mEq/L of bicarbonate ions and 1.2 to 1.4 mEq/L of carbonic acid. Thus, the base-to-acid ratio is 20:1. Because carbonic acid exists in the body predominantly as carbon dioxide gas, the value of PCO_2 (i.e., the partial pressure of carbon dioxide) is substituted in the denominator as follows:

$$pH = pK\ (6.1) + \log \frac{HCO_3^-}{PCO_2} = \frac{20}{1}\ Ratio \quad (5)$$

Calculate the pH, where the pK for carbonic acid is 6.1, and the log of 20 is 1.3:

$$pH = 6.1 + 1.3 \quad (6)$$
$$pH = 7.4\ (arterial\ blood)$$

Hemoglobin/Oxyhemoglobin System

Hemoglobin is an effective body buffer. The reaction between hemoglobin and free hydrogen ions occurs within the RBCs, which are readily permeable to bicarbonate ions. For every free hydrogen ion bound by hemoglobin, a corresponding bicarbonate ion diffuses out of the RBC into the plasma. To maintain electrical neutrality across the RBC membrane, bicarbonate ions are exchanged for chloride ions (Cl^-). As venous blood leaves the tissues, this exchange of bicarbonate ions for chloride ions is designated the *chloride shift* and accounts for the greater chloride content of venous blood, which, in contrast to arterial blood, has a greater carbon dioxide tension (PCO_2).

Protein and Phosphate Buffers

In addition to hemoglobin, other proteins act as buffers both intracellularly and extracellularly. Phosphate ions exert their buffer effects primarily in the intracellular fluid.

Lungs

Because carbon dioxide gas is the predominant state of carbonic acid in the body, any increase in the concentration of carbon dioxide gas in body fluids decreases the pH; any decrease in the concentration of carbon dioxide gas causes the pH to rise.

The major factor regulating the carbon dioxide gas concentrations in body fluids is alveolar ventilation ($\dot{V}A$). An increase in alveolar ventilation (*hyper*ventilation) causes carbon dioxide gas to be blown off by way of the lungs, thus decreasing the concentration of carbon dioxide in body fluids, with a consequent increase in the pH; conversely, a decrease in alveolar ventilation (*hypo*ventilation) allows body fluid concentrations of carbon dioxide to increase, with a consequent decrease in the pH. See Helpful Hint #1.

The slightest change in carbon dioxide is associated with significant reflex changes in the rate and depth of breathing.

Peripheral chemoreceptors (e.g., carotid and aortic bodies) respond to changes in carbon dioxide in the arterial blood ($PaCO_2$) by reflexly stimulating medullary inspiratory neuronal networks and an increase in alveolar ventilation occurs. This response is designed to promote elimination of carbon dioxide by way of the lungs, thus reducing the $PaCO_2$ and returning the hydrogen-ion concentration of circulating blood toward normal.

A decrease in $PaCO_2$ reflexly decreases alveolar ventilation to some extent.

Central chemoreceptors located in the medulla consist of a major reflex mechanism whereby the hydrogen-ion concentrations of circulating cerebral blood and the brain's interstitial fluids regulate the rate and depth of alveolar ventilation. An increase in the hydrogen-ion concentration and the corresponding drop in pH can increase the rate of alveolar ventilation several times normal, depending on the magnitude of the change; conversely, a reduction in hydrogen-ion concentration and corresponding increase in pH can decrease the rate of alveolar ventilation to a fraction of normal.

Thus, the respiratory system acts as a *feedback* regulatory system for controlling hydrogen-ion concentration. When hydrogen-ion concentrations become high (i.e., low pH), alveolar ventilation increases. Any increase in alveolar ventilation wherein carbon dioxide is eliminated by way of the lungs causes the reaction to be driven to the *right* (see Equation 3 earlier in chapter). The end-result is a decrease in the hydrogen-ion concentration.

Conversely, when hydrogen-ion concentrations

become low (i.e., high pH), alveolar ventilation becomes depressed, carbon dioxide accumulates, and the hydrogen-ion concentration rises. Any decrease in alveolar ventilation reduces the elimination of carbon dioxide by the lungs, causing the reaction to be driven to the *left* (see Equation 3). The concentration of hydrogen ions increases accordingly.

Respiratory control of the hydrogen-ion concentration is rapid and occurs within minutes to several hours. However, it is limited in that such control cannot return the hydrogen-ion concentration to its normal value reflected by a pH of 7.4. The reason for this is that, as the pH approaches normal, the stimulus for the increase or decrease in alveolar ventilation is removed.

Kidneys

The renal response to changes in hydrogen-ion concentration occurs much more slowly than does the respiratory response, usually over several days. The renal system functions to maintain physiologic pH by regulating the bicarbonate-ion concentration in extracellular fluid and by ridding the body of acid by-products of metabolism that cannot be eliminated by the lungs (i.e., fixed acids).

Bicarbonate is freely filtered at the glomerulus. Key events involved in its reabsorption include hydrogen-ion secretion, combination of hydrogen ions with bicarbonate ions in the renal tubules, and the reabsorption of sodium in exchange for hydrogen ions (Fig. 23–1).

The net result of these events is that, for each hydrogen ion secreted into the tubular lumen, a bicarbonate ion is absorbed into the extracellular fluid and peritubular capillaries.

The greater the concentration of carbon dioxide in body fluids, the greater the rate of hydrogen-ion secretion. Thus, any factor that increases carbon dioxide

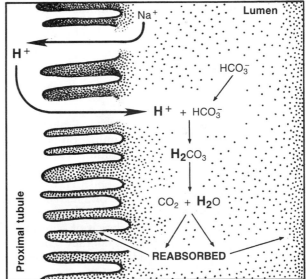

BICARBONATE BUFFER

FIGURE 23–1. Bicarbonate "reabsorption" from the proximal tubular epithelial cell. Within the tubular cell, carbon dioxide is hydrated to form carbonic acid, a reaction catalyzed by the enzyme, carbonic anhydrase, and followed by the almost immediate dissociation of the acid into hydrogen ions and bicarbonate ions. The bicarbonate ion thus generated is "reabsorbed" by diffusing into the peritubular interstitium. The hydrogen ion formed in this reaction (as depicted) is pumped out of the cell into the tubular lumen (in exchange for sodium), where it is available to combine with filtered bicarbonate to form carbonic acid. This, in turn, is converted to carbon dioxide and water. The carbon dioxide enters the tubular cell, where the entire process is again replicated. Note that the bicarbonate ion reabsorbed is not the same one filtered; note also that the hydrogen ion is not excreted but is available to be used for bicarbonate "reabsorption."

tensions in body fluids (e.g., reduced alveolar ventilation, increased metabolic rate) also increases the rate of hydrogen-ion secretion. Conversely, any factor that decreases carbon dioxide tensions (e.g., hyperventilation, or decreased metabolic rate) decreases the rate of hydrogen-ion secretion.

These events of hydrogen-ion secretion and bicarbonate absorption occur throughout the renal tubular system, except for the descending loop of Henle. The proximal tubule absorbs 80% to 90% of the total bicarbonate filtered. The conversion of such large quantities of intraluminal carbonic acid to carbon dioxide and water in the proximal tubule is catalyzed by the enzyme, carbonic anhydrase, which resides in the microvilli of the proximal tubular epithelial cells.

Fixed acid by-products of metabolism are excreted in the urine with the assistance of the phosphate and ammonia buffer systems. These urinary buffer systems function in a similar fashion to the bicarbonate buffer system. Differences include that the respective end-products of monosodium dihydrogen phosphate and ammonium ion are excreted in the urine, taking the dissociated hydrogen ion with them, and that these reactions occur largely in the distal tubules. Thus, with the phosphate and ammonia buffers, for each bicarbonate ion absorbed, a hydrogen ion is excreted. This represents a net gain of base in conjunction with the renal excretion of fixed acids.

ACID-BASE BALANCE

The normal ranges of values for blood acid-base parameters are shown in Table 23–1. Evaluation of acid-base balance depends on examination of arterial or mixed venous blood gases in conjunction with the patient's history and physical examination. *Acidemia* is definitively diagnosed by a low blood pH, that is an arterial pH (pHa) of less than 7.35 or a mixed venous pH (pHv̄) of less than 7.30. This condition reflects an excess of acid or, conversely, a deficit of base in the blood. Thus, the base excess generally correlates directly with the pH. If the pH is low, the base excess is usually negative.

Alkalemia is a condition in which the hydrogen-ion concentration of the blood is reduced. Alkalemia is definitively diagnosed by blood pH, with a pHa of more than 7.45 or a pHv̄ of more than 7.40. This condition reflects a deficit of acid or, conversely, an excess of base in the blood. As with acidemia, the base excess generally correlates directly with the pH. If the pH is high, the base excess is usually positive.

Acidosis is the process that causes acidemia; *alkalosis* is the process that causes alkalemia. The two categories of processes are respiratory and metabolic. The respiratory process is reflected by carbon dioxide tension (PCO_2); the metabolic process is reflected in the bicarbonate level.

Carbon Dioxide (PCO_2): Respiratory Parameter

Carbon dioxide (CO_2) gas is considered an *acid* substance because, when it combines with water, carbonic acid is formed; this weak acid dissociates into hydrogen and bicarbonate ions (see Equation 3). Carbon dioxide is a major by-product of aerobic metabolism. The body eliminates carbon dioxide by way of the lungs.

A direct relationship exists between alveolar ventilation and the concentration of carbon dioxide in arterial blood ($PaCO_2$). Any alteration in the respiratory elimination of carbon dioxide out of proportion to its metabolic production can result in abnormalities of arterial PCO_2 and pH.

A general rule (see Helpful Hint #2) regarding the expected change in pH resulting from changes that occur in $PaCO_2$ is:

pH will rise or fall 0.08 in the appropriate direction for every 10-mmHg change in $PaCO_2$.

Any factor that decreases the rate of alveolar ventilation (i.e., *hypo*ventilation) increases the concentration of dissolved carbon dioxide in the extracellular fluid ($PaCO_2$ greater than 45 mmHg); conversely, any factor that increases the rate of alveolar ventilation (i.e., *hyper*ventilation) decreases the concentration of dissolved carbon dioxide in body fluids ($PaCO_2$ less than 35 mmHg).

TABLE 23–1
Parameters of Blood Acid-Base Balance*

Parameter[†]	Arterial Blood	Mixed Venous Blood	>Normal	<Normal
pH	7.35–7.45	7.31–7.41	Alkalemia	Acidemia
PCO_2	35–45	41–51	Acidosis	Alkalosis
HCO_3^-	22–26	22–26	Alkalosis	Acidosis
Base excess	−2 to +2	−2 to +2	Alkalosis	Acidosis

*Values are normal ranges at sea level.
[†]Note that vegetarians may have a higher normal range of bicarbonate.
pH = concentration of free hydrogen ions in solution; PCO_2 = partial pressure of carbon dioxide; HCO_3^- = bicarbonate ion concentration in blood.

Acute changes in Pa_{CO_2} from 20 to 60 mmHg
will cause an *approximately* reciprocal change in
hundredths of pH units.

Pa_{CO_2}	=	20	40	60
pH	=	7.60	7.40	7.20

Clinical Abnormalities

Two pathophysiologic conditions are associated
with an alteration in the ventilatory effort: respiratory
acidosis and respiratory alkalosis.

Respiratory Acidosis

Respiratory acidosis is characterized by an increase in
Pa_{CO_2} (more than 45 mmHg). As the concentration
of carbon dioxide in the extracellular fluid increases,
the reaction depicted in Equation 3 is driven to the
left (i.e., there is an increase in the formation of carbonic
acid, with a consequent increase in hydrogen-ion
and bicarbonate-ion formation). Acidosis results
from the increase in hydrogen-ion concentration.

As shown in the Henderson-Hasselbalch equation
(Equation 5), as the carbon dioxide component
(denominator) increases, the pH decreases. Thus, respiratory
acidosis is reflected clinically by a Pa_{CO_2}
greater than 45 mmHg and a pH less than 7.35.

Respiratory Alkalosis

Respiratory alkalosis is characterized by a decrease in
Pa_{CO_2} (less than 35 mmHg), associated with hyperventilation.
What occurs is a reversal of the process
described for respiratory acidosis. As carbon dioxide
is blown off and its concentration in extracellular fluid
decreases, the reaction depicted in Equation 3 is
driven to the *right* (i.e., there is a reduction in the
hydrogen-ion concentration resulting in alkalemia).
Referring again to the Henderson-Hasselbalch equation,
as the denominator decreases, the pH increases.
Thus, respiratory alkalosis is reflected clinically by a
Pa_{CO_2} less than 35 mmHg, and a pH greater than 7.45.

For information related to the pathophysiology, etiology,
clinical presentation, and treatment of respiratory
acidosis and respiratory alkalosis, see Table 23-2.

Bicarbonate-Ion (HCO_3^-) and Base Excess: Metabolic Parameters

Metabolic acid-base abnormalities include all acid-base
disturbances other than those caused by excess
or insufficient carbon dioxide in extracellular fluid

(i.e., respiratory parameter). Two pathophysiologic
conditions are associated with alteration in the metabolic
parameters of acid-base balance: metabolic acidosis
and metabolic alkalosis.

Metabolic Acidosis

Metabolic acidosis is associated with the accumulation
of fixed acid or with a loss of bicarbonate from extracellular
fluid. A distinction is made between *fixed* acid
and the *respiratory* acid, carbonic acid. By convention,
carbonic acid, which results from dissolved carbon
dioxide, is considered part of the *respiratory* parameter.
All other acids, whether metabolically produced or
ingested, constitute the *metabolic* parameter.

Clinically, metabolic acidosis is characterized by a
decrease in bicarbonate-ion concentration in extracellular
fluid (<22 mEq/L), by a base deficit, and by
a pHa < 7.35 (Table 23-1). The reduction in bicarbonate-ion
concentration is associated with an
increase in fixed acid. For example, with hyperkalemia,
potassium ions move into the cells and displace
hydrogen ions into the extracellular fluid. The consequent
increase in hydrogen-ion concentration necessarily
uses up bicarbonate and other anions (see following
text) as part of the body's buffering response
to neutralize the high acid load, preventing the pH
from falling too low.

Anions and the Anion Gap. Metabolic acidosis is
commonly divided into those causes in which there is
an increase in unmeasured anions and those in which
bicarbonate is lost without an increase in unmeasured
anions. An *anion* is a substance with a net negative
charge.

The ionic composition of the major fluid compartments
is such that, overall, body fluids are essentially
electroneutral, that is, the number of cations (positively
charged ions) match the number of anions (negatively
charged ions).

Sodium accounts for 90% of the cations in extracellular
fluid. The positively charged sodium ions are
matched rather well by the sum of chloride and bicarbonate
anions and to a much lesser extent by minor
anions such as sulfates, phosphates, and organic acids.
Laboratory measurements of plasma concentrations
of sodium, chloride, and bicarbonate ions can readily
be made. Other anions (e.g., sulfates, phosphates, and
organic acids) are difficult to assess and are referred
to as the *unmeasured anions*, or more conveniently, as
the *anion gap*.

The normal range of the anion gap is 10 to
14 mM/L. The anion gap is calculated as follows:

$$\text{Anion gap} = Na^+ - (Cl^- + HCO_3^-)$$
$$= 140 - (102 + 26)$$
$$= 140 - 128$$
$$\text{Anion gap} = 12 \text{ mM/L}$$

which shows the plasma sodium concentration
minus the sum of plasma chloride and bicarbonate.

TABLE 23–2
Respiratory Acid-Base Abnormalities

	Respiratory Acidosis	Respiratory Alkalosis
Definition	Respiratory acidosis is caused by a process that raises the $Paco_2$, with pHa < 7.35. Primary abnormality: $Paco_2 > 45$ mmHg	Respiratory alkalosis is caused by a process that reduces $Paco_2$, with pHa > 7.45. Primary abnormality: $Paco_2 < 35$ mmHg
Pathophysiology	Underlying process: Alveolar *hypo*ventilation. When the lungs fail to eliminate metabolically produced carbon dioxide, for whatever reason, $Paco_2$ rises, resulting in an increase in hydrogen-ion concentration with pHa < 7.35, termed *hypercapnia*.	Underlying process: Alveolar *hyper*ventilation Hyperventilation (i.e., blowing off CO_2) causes a decrease in hydrogen-ion concentration, with pHa > 7.45, termed *hypocapnia*.
Etiology	CNS depression of respiratory centers in pons and medulla: Drug overdose Respiratory depressants Neuromuscular conditions: Guillain-Barré syndrome Myasthenia gravis Thoracic restrictions: Kyphoscoliosis Massive obesity (pickwickian syndrome) Airway patency: Chronic obstructive pulmonary disease Parenchymal disorders: Adult respiratory distress syndrome Pneumonia Pulmonary edema Pain (thoracic and upper abdominal incisions)	CNS dysfunction of respiratory centers in pons and medulla: Fever Head trauma Cerebrovascular accident Anxiety Brain tumor Salicylates Alterations in pulmonary function related to: Pneumonia Pulmonary embolism Congestive heart failure Interstitial lung disease Asthma Mechanical ventilation Hypoxemia Gram-negative septicemia Pain
Clinical presentation	Hypercapnia is usually associated with hypoxemia, which dominates the clinical presentation: 1. Altered neurologic function: restlessness, irritability, headache (related to increase in cerebral blood flow due to vasodilatory response of cerebral vasculature to hypercapnia), drowsiness, confusion, coma 2. Cardiac arrhythmias 3. Neuromuscular status: weakness, tremors, asterixis 4. Altered pulmonary function: tachypnea, dyspnea, respiratory distress	Hypocapnia is manifested by the following: 1. Altered neurologic function: changes in level of consciousness (hypocapnia causes cerebral vasoconstriction); coma, lightheadedness, giddiness, seizures, hyperactive deep tendon reflexes, convulsions 2. Cardiac arrhythmias 3. Neuromuscular status: paresthesias, weakness, muscle cramps, tetany 4. Altered pulmonary function: tachypnea, hyperpnea
Laboratory values	pHa < 7.35 $Paco_2 > 45$ mmHg Serum electrolytes—Renal compensation may produce hypochloremia.	pHa > 7.45 $Paco_2 < 35$ mmHg Serum electrolytes—Occasionally associated with hypokalemia and hypocalcemia
Physiologic responses	Buffering: The increase in hydrogen-ion concentration is immediately buffered by noncarbonate buffers including hemoglobin and other proteins in extracellular fluid, and phosphates, proteins, and lactate in intracellular fluid.	The decrease in hydrogen-ion concentration within the extracellular fluids prompts an immediate release of hydrogen ions from the intracellular compartment, usually in exchange for potassium. Cellular metabolism contributes to restoring the level by increasing production of lactate and other metabolic acids.
Renal compensation	The kidneys increase hydrogen-ion secretion while reabsorbing HCO_3^-; the increased $Paco_2$ directly stimulates an increase in hydrogen-ion secretion, which is associated with an increased reabsorption of sodium (to maintain appropriate electrochemical balance). In acute respiratory acidosis, more sodium is reabsorbed in exchange for hydrogen ions, resulting in an increased chloride secretion. Renal compensation also includes an increased excretion of ammonium ion (NH_4^+) and an increase in chloride secretion. The net result is an increase in HCO_3^- concentration in extracellular fluid.	The kidneys reduce net excretion of hydrogen; there is a decreased reabsorption of HCO_3^- in the renal tubules. Because it is necessary for HCO_3^- to react with hydrogen ions to be "reabsorbed," all excess bicarbonate ions are excreted in the urine, usually with sodium. Net renal response: sodium bicarbonate is removed from extracellular fluid, and the pH decreases toward normal.

continued

TABLE 23–2
Respiratory Acid-Base Abnormalities (*Continued*)

	Respiratory Acidosis	Respiratory Alkalosis
Correction of primary problem (pulmonary in origin)	Restoration of effective alveolar ventilation (In patients with chronic hypercapnia associated with irreversible lung disease, only a partially corrected acid-base balance may be possible.)	Restoration of effective alveolar ventilation. It is necessary to alleviate hyperventilation. Hyperventilation associated with mechanical ventilation can be easily corrected; a reduction of stimulation of respiratory centers in the pons and medulla may be more difficult to achieve; if due to an irreversible pathologic process, correction may not be possible.
Treatment	Treatment goal: To restore and maintain effective alveolar ventilation. Specific therapy may entail vigorous pulmonary toilet or mechanical ventilation. Oxygenation as indicated by PaO_2, patient history, and physical examination. Close monitoring of cardiopulmonary and neurologic function and fluid and electrolyte status is essential in acid-base imbalances.	Treatment goal: To correct or ameliorate the underlying disorder causing the hyperventilation. Oxygenation to treat hypoxemia. Patients on mechanical ventilation who manifest neuromuscular irritability, twitching or seizures, or cardiac arrhythmias, may benefit from decreasing the minute ventilation and/or increasing dead space ventilation. Occasionally, treatment with an inhaled gas mixture containing 3% carbon dioxide may be helpful when used for short periods of time. Close monitoring—same as in respiratory acidosis.
Nursing diagnoses	Breathing pattern, ineffective: hypoventilation. Airway clearance, ineffective with potential for: Sensory-perceptual alteration—altered level of consciousness Alteration in thought processes Potential for injury: cardiac arrhythmias Potential for electrolyte imbalance	Breathing pattern, ineffective: hyperventilation. Anxiety. Sensory-perceptual alteration: altered level of consciousness. Potential for injury: seizure activity, tetany, cardiac arrhythmias. Potential for electrolyte imbalance.

$PaCO_2$ = arterial carbon dioxide tension; pHa = pH of the arterial blood; HCO_3^- = bicarbonate blood level; PaO_2 = arterial oxygen tension.

Anion Gap Greater Than 15 mM/L. An increase in unmeasured anions (i.e., the anion gap) is always present when metabolic acidosis is caused by the *addition* of acid from an endogenous or exogenous source. For example, accumulations of lactic acid (anaerobic metabolism), ketoacids (diabetic ketoacidosis), or sulfates, phosphates, creatinates, and proteinates (renal failure) are *endogenous* sources of unmeasured anions. *Exogenous* sources include drug overdose or poisoning attributed, for example, to salicylates, ethylene glycol, or methyl alcohol or to ingestion of other acidic substances. In each of these examples, there is an increase in the hydrogen-ion concentration of the extracellular fluids, which consumes bicarbonate ions in the buffering process, eventually replacing the bicarbonate with an increased concentration of unmeasured anions.

Normal Anion Gap (10 to 14 mM/L). Not all episodes of metabolic acidosis are attributed to an increase in unmeasured anions. The anion gap remains normal in acidosis associated with loss of bicarbonate ion, as occurs with diarrhea and lower gastrointestinal dysfunction (e.g., fistulas, drainage of

pancreatic juices, ureterosigmoidostomy) among others. Such conditions are usually associated with *hyperchloremia*. The loss of bicarbonate ion in excess of a concomitant loss of chloride ions will reduce the bicarbonate-ion level of extracellular fluid, while the chloride-ion concentration rises. See Table 23–3 for other details related to metabolic acidosis.

The pathophysiology, etiology, clinical presentation, and treatment of metabolic acidosis are summarized in Table 23–2. A general rule (see Helpful Hint #3) for the administration of sodium bicarbonate to treat metabolic acidosis is to give 50% of the calculated dose of $NaHCO_3$ and monitor pHa and HCO_3^- concentration.

Metabolic Alkalosis

Metabolic alkalosis may be associated with a net *loss* of hydrogen ions or a net *gain* of bicarbonate ions in extracellular fluids or with a loss of chloride ions in excess of bicarbonate ions. Hydrogen-ion depletion of extracellular fluid may occur by way of the gastrointestinal tract and kidneys. Gastric losses due to vomit-

---

**RESEARCH APPLICATION: BRAIN pH EFFECTS OF NaHCO$_3$ AND CARBICARB®
IN LACTIC ACIDOSIS**

Kucera, RR, et al. Critical Care Medicine 17(12):1320–1323, 1989.

Purpose: The purpose of this study was to compare the effects of sodium bicarbonate (NaHCO$_3$), the standard buffer; Carbicarb, an experimental buffer; and normal saline, a control buffer, on arterial and intracellular brain pH.

Methods: An experiment was conducted with 11 rats that were instrumented for infusion of buffer, monitoring of mean arterial pressure, and sampling for blood gas and lactate. The animals were mechanically ventilated, sedated, and placed in a nuclear magnetic resonance (NMR) magnet. A combined metabolic and respiratory acidosis was induced to mimic conditions of human cardiopulmonary arrest. Intravenous NaHCO$_3$, Carbicarb, or saline was infused, and arterial blood gases and lactate were sampled at 2-, 10-, and 15-minute periods afterward. NMR spectroscopy was used to measure intracellular brain pH (pHi) from the chemical shifts observed in cerebral metabolites. The investigators were blinded to the identity of the buffers. Analysis of variance techniques were used to compare the buffer effects.

Results: All three buffers had similar effects on mean arterial pressure and lactate levels. Saline had no effect on arterial pH (pHa) or pHi. NaHCO$_3$ transiently raised pHa, but this effect was not sustained at the 10-minute measurement period; NaHCO$_3$ had no effect on pHi. Carbicarb, on the other hand, improved both arterial and intracellular brain pH over the 15-minute measurement period, with the peak effect occurring at 2 minutes after infusion. The different alkalinization effects of NaHCO$_3$ and Carbicarb may be related to carbon dioxide. NaHCO$_3$ generates carbon dioxide, and the arterial carbon dioxide tensions (PaCO$_2$) were significantly elevated after NaHCO$_3$ infusion. Carbicarb infusion did not affect PaCO$_2$.

Practice Implications: Intravenous NaHCO$_3$ is the primary treatment used to combat lactic acidosis during cardiopulmonary arrest. The minimal and transient increase in pHa and the decrease in brain pHi found in this study with sodium bicarbonate administration raises concerns about the efficacy of this buffer as a treatment for acidosis. Although Carbicarb corrected both pHa and pHi acidosis in this animal model, further research is needed before alternative buffers will become standard therapy in the clinical setting. First, the physiologic significance of the study findings, particularly with respect to patient outcomes, is uncertain. Second, further studies in clinical populations are needed.

---

ing or continuous nasogastric suctioning can cause a considerable loss of hydrogen ions as well as chloride ions. Serum bicarbonate levels rise if hydrogen-ion loss is greater than that gained by the diet or body metabolism.

Clinically, metabolic alkalosis is characterized by an increase in bicarbonate-ion concentration in extracellular fluid (more than 26 mEq/L), by a base excess, and by a pHa greater than 7.45 (Table 23–1).

Hypochloremic, Hypokalemic Metabolic Alkalosis. A reciprocal relationship exists between bicarbonate (HCO$_3^-$) and chloride (Cl$^-$) concentrations: When plasma bicarbonate concentration rises, there is a concomitant fall in the plasma chloride concentration. Chloride is the only anion, other than bicarbonate, which occurs in significant concentrations in extracellular fluid; it is readily reabsorbed by the kidneys in conjunction with the reabsorption of sodium. Thus, any reduction in chloride levels seriously compromises bicarbonate excretion and actually favors its reabsorption.

Hypochloremia contributes to the maintenance of metabolic alkalosis in another way. Normally, reabsorption of sodium (cation) is largely accompanied by the reabsorption of chloride (anion) to preserve electrochemical gradients along the renal tubular system.

Sodium is also reabsorbed by way of an exchange mechanism wherein it is reabsorbed, whereas another cation (e.g., potassium or hydrogen ion) is secreted. When the latter mechanism becomes predominant (as in hypochloremia), the additional loss of hydrogen ions that results contributes further to the alkalemic state.

In addition, because there is a limited concentration of potassium ions available for exchange with sodium, hypokalemia may rapidly ensue. Thus, the patient with metabolic alkalosis may ultimately experience a *hypochloremic, hypokalemic metabolic alkalosis.* See Table 23–3 for other details related to metabolic alkalosis.

Extracellular Fluid Volume Depletion: Impact on Metabolic Alkalemia

Extracellular fluid volume depletion is also instrumental in maintaining metabolic alkalemia. The kidney preserves the extracellular volume by its reabsorption of sodium, which, in turn, facilitates the reabsorption of water along osmotic gradients and in the presence of antidiuretic hormone (ADH). Volume depletion is known to increase sodium reabsorption,

TABLE 23–3
Metabolic Acid-Base Abnormalities

	Metabolic Acidosis	Metabolic Alkalosis
Definition	Metabolic acidosis is caused by a process that increases hydrogen-ion (H^+) concentration in conjunction with a decrease in bicarbonate ions (HCO_3^-), resulting in a decrease in pHa < 7.35.	Metabolic alkalosis is caused by a process that increases bicarbonate-ion concentration (or decreases hydrogen-ion concentration), with consequent increase in pHa > 7.45.
Pathophysiology	The HCO_3^- concentration can be reduced in the following ways[1]: 1. Buffering activity—buffering of a strong, highly dissociated acid with HCO_3^- 2. Loss of HCO_3^- from body fluids especially by way of gastrointestinal tract and kidneys 3. Rapid hemodilution of fluid in extracellular space with a noncarbonate-containing fluid (e.g., isotonic saline)	The HCO_3^- concentration can be elevated in the following ways[1]: 1. A net loss of hydrogen ions from extracellular fluid 2. A net addition of HCO_3^- to the extracellular fluid 3. Chloride loss from extracellular fluid in excess of HCO_3^-

Etiology	Causes of metabolic acidosis[1-5]:
	1. Increase in unmeasured anions (anion gap >15 mM/L)
	  • Diabetic ketoacidosis
	  • Starvation ketoacidosis
	  • Alcoholic ketoacidosis
	  • Poisonings: salicylate, ethylene glycol, methyl alcohol
	  • Lactic acidosis
	  • Shock; cardiac arrest; left ventricular failure
	  • Renal failure
	2. Normal anion gap (hyperchloremia)
	  • Diarrhea
	  • Drainage of pancreatic juice
	  • Ureterosigmoidostomy
	  • Obstructed ileal loop
	  • Ammonium chloride therapy
	  • Renal tubular acidosis
	  • Dilutional acidosis
	  • Hyperalimentation
	  • Acetazolamide therapy*
		Causes of metabolic alkalosis[1-5]:
		1. Fluid loss from upper gastrointestinal tract:
		  • Vomiting
		  • Nasogastric suctioning
		2. Rapid correction of chronic hypercapnia
		3. Diuretic therapy
		4. Corticosteroid therapy
		5. Severe hypocalemia
		6. Alkali administration ($NaHCO_3$, antacids)

Clinical presentation	Severe metabolic acidosis may cause the following:
	1. Alterations in neurologic function:
	  • Headache, change in level of consciousness, drowsiness, confusion, coma
	2. Alteration in cardioavascular function:
	  • Depressed cardiac function, cardiac arrhythmias
	  • Decreased peripheral vascular resistance, with hypotension, shock, tissue hypoxia
	3. Alteration of pulmonary function:
	  • Deep, rapid respirations (Kussmaul's breathing), which is especially evident when bicarbonate levels are <15 mEq/L
	4. Alterations in gastrointestinal function:
	  • Nausea, vomiting, anorexia
		A high index of suspicion is necessary in examining the patient with metabolic alkalemia because there are no specific signs and symptoms unique to this disorder.
		A history of vomiting, diuretic usage, and complaints of weakness may provide important clues.
		Specific considerations:
		1. Alteration in neuromuscular function:
		  • Irritability, muscle cramps, hyperactive deep tendon reflexes, tetany (hypocalcemia is frequently an associated problem because levels of ionized calcium decrease as pH increases).
		  • Muscle weakness
		2. Alteration in cardiovascular function:
		  • Cardiac arrhythmias

Laboratory values	pHa < 7.35
	Pa_{CO_2} normal; or decreased with compensation
	HCO_3^- < 20 mEq/L
	Anion gap: normal or increased, depending on the underlying cause
	Serum electrolytes:
	  • Potassium ions—Normal or increased. (In the presence of excess hydrogen ions, these ions shift into cells in exchange with potassium ions.)
		pHa > 7.45
		Pa_{CO_2} normal; or increased with compensation
		HCO_3^- > 26–30 mEq/L
		Serum electrolytes:
		  • Potassium ions decreased
		
		  • Chloride ions decreased

continued

TABLE 23–3
Metabolic Acid-Base Abnormalities (*Continued*)

	Metabolic Acidosis	Metabolic Alkalosis
Physiologic responses	1. Buffering: Intracellular buffers such as hemoglobin and phosphates actively participate in the buffering process, as bicarbonate ions are used up buffering the excess hydrogen-ion concentration. 2. Respiratory compensation: As the pH decreases, a concomitant fall in Pa_{CO_2} is essential to reestablish the 20:1 ratio (Henderson-Hasselbalch equation) and return the pH to within the normal range: 7.35–7.45. • The respiratory system compensates for acidemia by increasing alveolar ventilation. As the lungs "blow off" carbon dioxide, a reduction in the hydrogen-ion concentration occurs. • The stimulus for the increased ventilatory effort is an increase in hydrogen-ion concentration of cerebral fluids. • The respiratory response occurs quickly (within minutes) but may be limited by inadequacy of the respiratory center or ventilatory mechanics. 3. Renal compensation: The kidney is responsible for excreting the acid load; reabsorbing and generating bicarbonate ions. • A lag time of up to 24 hours occurs before the kidneys begin to impact the acidemic state; up to 4 or 5 days may be required for maximal excretion of the acid load. • The major renal mechanism for excreting excess hydrogen ions is by the urinary buffers: Ammonia/ammonium ion buffer Phosphate buffer system	1. Buffering: Excess bicarbonate ions are buffered primarily by hydrogen ions derived from intracellular phosphates and proteins, which shift to the extracellular fluid compartment. 2. Respiratory compensation: As the pH increases, a concomitant increase in Pa_{CO_2} is essential to reestablish the 20:1 ratio (Henderson-Hasselbalch equation), which is necessary to achieve a pH within the normal range: 7.35–7.45. • Alveolar hypoventilation occurs to retain carbon dioxide and increase the Pa_{CO_2}. The degree of compensation is limited by the requirement to maintain Pa_{O_2} at acceptable level ($Pa_{O_2} > 60$ mmHg). • Upper limits of Pa_{CO_2} compensation in patients without pulmonary disease is usually about 55 mmHg, but may be higher. 3. Renal compensation: The kidney has the ability to rapidly excrete HCO_3^- and restore normal levels of bicarbonate in extracellular fluid. • Hypochloremia can seriously compromise renal excretion of bicarbonate, because one method of sodium reabsorption requires the concomitant reabsorption of a negatively charged ion (e.g., chloride or bicarbonate ions). In the presence of chloride-ion depletion, reabsorption of bicarbonate ion can actually be enhanced. • Reabsorption of sodium in exchange for hydrogen or potassium ions further depletes hydrogen ions.
Treatment	Therapeutic goal: To treat the underlying disease process responsible for the depletion of body buffers. 1. Major therapeutic considerations: • Severe metabolic acidosis (pH < 7.0) may require intravenous sodium bicarbonate to raise pH to >7.20, and bicarbonate levels to >15 mM/L • Very rapid and total (See Helpful Hint #3) correction of acidemia should be avoided. 2. Specific therapeutic considerations when administering sodium bicarbonate: • Cerebrospinal fluid acidosis may worsen initially, causing changes in the level of consciousness (see Research Application in this chapter). • Hemoglobin delivery of oxygen to the tissues may be retarded. • Continuous infusion with sodium bicarbonate may compromise cardiac function; the additional sodium intake can predispose to congestive heart failure and pulmonary edema in the compromised renal or cardiac patient. • Close monitoring of cardiopulmonary function and fluid and electrolyte balance is essential. • Close monitoring of neurologic and neuromuscular status is necessary.	Therapeutic goal: To treat the underlying disease process responsible for the alkalemia, and correct factors maintaining it. Specific therapeutic considerations: • Correct volume depletion. • Replace chloride so that kidney has the option of reabsorbing or secreting HCO_3^-. • Sodium and potassium replacement therapy will correct volume depletion and hypokalemia. • Administration of ammonium chloride may be used in compromised cardiac or renal status. • Intravenous acetazolamide may be useful because it will increase renal excretion of bicarbonate. • Close monitoring of cardiopulmonary function and fluid and electrolyte balance is essential. • Close monitoring of neurologic and neuromuscular status is necessary.

continued

TABLE 23–3
Metabolic Acid-Base Abnormalities (*Continued*)

	Metabolic Acidosis	Metabolic Alkalosis

Nursing diagnoses	Thought processes, alteration in
	Sensory-perceptual alteration:
	    Altered level of consciousness
	Electrolyte imbalance, potential for
	Potential for injury:
	    Altered level of consciousness
	    Cardiac arrhythmias
		Sensory-perceptual alteration
		Electrolyte imbalance, potential for:
		    Hypochloremia
		    Hypokalemia
		    Hypocalcemia
		Potential for injury:
		    Altered level of consciousness
		    Cardiac arrhythmias
		    Neuromuscular irritability
		    Seizure activity, tetany

*Acetazolamide inhibits intracellular and luminal (tubular) carbon anhydrase. It delays the hydrolysis of carbonic acid to carbon dioxide and water, allowing hydrogen ions to increase in the lumen, creating a gradient against hydrogen-ion secretion by tubular epithelial cells. Intracellularly, acetazolamide inhibits hydration of carbon dioxide to carbonic acid, thus reducing the subsequent production of hydrogen and bicarbonate ions.

HELPFUL HINT #3 FOR ACID-BASE IMBALANCE TREATMENT Formula for NaHCO$_3$ Administration During Metabolic Acidosis

$$HCO_3^- = \text{needed}$$
(24 mEq/L – HCO$_3^-$)
normal   observed
value   value
$\times$
(0.3 $\times$ body weight in kg)

To avoid giving too much HCO$_3^-$, NaHCO$_3^-$ (sodium bicarbonate) is administered as half the dose calculated with the above formula. A partial dose only is given because overcorrection will result from the additive effects of endogenous buffer systems. The arterial pH and HCO$_3^-$ concentration are monitored closely to avoid the iatrogenic creation of metabolic alkalosis.

---

as well as bicarbonate reabsorption in the proximal tubule. Increased hydrogen-ion secretion is associated with the generation of bicarbonate (Fig. 23–1).

SUMMARY OF ACID-BASE RELATIONSHIPS: IMPACT ON pH

Referring again to the Henderson-Hasselbalch equation, the following generalities can be made:

$$pH = pK + \text{Log} \frac{HCO_3^- \ (\text{Base})}{P_{CO_2} \ (\text{Acid})} = \qquad (5)$$

Acid-base parameters
$\frac{20}{1}$ Ratio $\frac{\text{Metabolic (kidneys)}}{\text{Respiratory (lungs)}}$

- Any increase in the numerator (HCO$_3^-$, other anions) without a corresponding increase in the denominator (P$_{CO_2}$) to maintain the 20:1 ratio will increase pH. A pH change due primarily to alterations in bicarbonate and other anions (the numerator) is attributed to *metabolic* (nonrespiratory) causes.
- Any increase in the denominator (P$_{CO_2}$) without a corresponding increase in the numerator (HCO$_3^-$, other anions) to maintain a 20:1 ratio will decrease the pH. A pH change due primarily to alterations in P$_{CO_2}$ (the denominator) is attributed to *respiratory* causes.
- Any change in both the HCO$_3^-$ (numerator) and P$_{CO_2}$ (denominator) that preserves the 20:1 ratio will result in a pH within the normal physiologic range (7.35 to 7.45).
- Causes of acidemia and alkalemia:

Acidemia   Respiratory $\uparrow$ P$_{CO_2}$
pH < 7.35
            Metabolic $\downarrow$ HCO$_3^-$
Alkalemia   Respiratory $\downarrow$ P$_{CO_2}$
pH > 7.45
            Metabolic $\uparrow$ HCO$_3^-$

ACID-BASE ABNORMALITIES

Acute Uncompensated

Acute or uncompensated acid-base abnormality is characterized by an abnormal pH and a change in *one* blood parameter, either the respiratory parameter (P$_{CO_2}$) or the metabolic parameters (HCO$_3^-$ and base excess).[2]

Compensated

Compensated acid-base abnormality is characterized by a change in pH, an abnormal parameter associated with the primary disorder (respiratory or metabolic), and a change in the other parameter, to maintain a bicarbonate to carbonic acid (HCO_3^-) ratio of about 20:1.

Fully Compensated

In fully compensated acid-base abnormality, the pH is normal. Both HCO_3^- and $PaCO_2$ parameters may still be abnormal, but the ratio between them remains 20:1.

Partially Compensated

The pH in partially compensated acid-base abnormality may have improved toward the normal range but is still slightly abnormal. In this situation, all three values—pH, PCO_2, and HCO_3^-—are abnormal.

Compensation occurs much more slowly than the initial, immediate buffering processes, but it is much more effective in returning the pH to within the normal physiologic range. The respiratory system ($PaCO_2$) compensates for an underlying metabolic disorder; the renal system (HCO_3^-) compensates for an underlying respiratory disorder.

Corrected

Corrected acid-base abnormality is characterized by all acid-base parameters (pH, PCO_2, and HCO_3^-) returning to normal. The primary disorder is rectified: the lungs remedy the respiratory parameter while the kidneys correct the metabolic parameter.

PROCEDURE FOR ANALYZING ARTERIAL BLOOD GASES TO DETERMINE ACID-BASE ABNORMALITIES[3,4]

1. Establish pH using 7.40 as a guide to acidemia or alkalemia.
2. Examine respiratory parameter, $PaCO_2$. Does it explain the change in pH?

3. Examine metabolic parameters, HCO_3^- and base excess. Do these factors explain the change in pH?

ANALYSIS AND INTERPRETATION OF ARTERIAL BLOOD GASES: CASE STUDIES

1. An 18-year-old woman was admitted to the hospital after taking an overdose of phenobarbital.

Data	Analysis
pH 7.18	(a) pH < 7.4; therefore, underlying condition is *acidemia*.
$PaCO_2$ 60 mmHg	(b) Respiratory parameter is elevated—*primary* cause of the acidemia.
HCO_3^- 26 mEq/L	(c) Metabolic parameters are within normal physiologic range.
Base excess +1	

Diagnosis. Acute uncompensated respiratory acidemia caused by severe hypoventilation

2. A 17-year-old semicomatose man is seen in the emergency department. His breath has a fruity odor; he has insulin-dependent diabetes.

Data	Analysis
pH 7.20	(a) pH < 7.4; therefore, underlying condition is *acidemia*.
$PaCO_2$ 40 mmHg	(b) Respiratory parameter is within normal physiologic range.
HCO_3^- 13 mEq/L	(c) Metabolic parameters are significantly reduced—*primary* cause of the acidemia.
Base excess −4	

TABLE 23–4
Drawing Arterial Blood Sample from Indwelling Line

Procedure	Rationale/Precautions
1. Place unheparinized syringe in 3-way stopcock nearest the patient and withdraw flush solution until blood fills the line; discard syringe and flush solution.	Maintain sterile technique throughout procedure to decrease risk of infection. Flush solution is withdrawn so as not to dilute the sample.
2. With a heparinized syringe, withdraw about 2 mL blood; maneuver stopcock to closed position and remove the syringe.	Stopcock should be adjusted so that it is closed to the syringe port prior to removing syringe.
3. Immediately expel any air from the syringe, cap the syringe with rubber stopper or cork, immerse in ice, and deliver for analysis.	To avoid inaccuracy in results, it is essential to prevent any air from getting into the syringe. Immersion in ice slows oxygen consumption and carbon dioxide production in the sample.[4]
4. Flush the stopcock used to obtain the sample, and flush the arterial line.	
5. Return stopcock to original position so that it is off to air and the flush solution is opened to the patient.	Assess line to make sure that no air bubbles were introduced into the system.

TABLE 23–5
Drawing Arterial Blood Sample by Percutaneous Puncture

Procedure	Rationale/Precautions
1. Select site to be used for percutaneous stick. Arterial blood can be obtained from radial, brachial, or femoral artery. Radial and brachial arteries are preferred sites.	Maintain sterile technique throughout procedure to decrease risk of infection. Radial and brachial arteries have readily palpable pulses and are easily accessible.
2. If radial artery is selected, collateral circulation to the hand via the ulnar artery should be determined with the Allen's test. *To perform Allen's test*[7]:	Femoral artery usually used as a last resort because of higher incidence of hematoma or infection. The Allen's test is performed to determine collateral circulation to the hand.
a. Occlude both radial and ulnar arteries while patient clenches hand.	
b. Ask patient to unclench and relax hand, and observe blanched palm of the hand.	
c. Release pressure on ulnar artery while maintaining pressure on the radial artery.	
d. If the hand quickly becomes pink, collateral circulation is good and the radial site is usable.	
3. Assemble necessary equipment. Arterial blood gas sampling kit may be available. Specific equipment:	
• 3- or 5-mL syringe	
• Rubber or cork cap	
• 1-mL ampule heparin (1000 U/mL)	
• Povidone-iodine or alcohol swabs	
• 2 needles: 22 gauge, 1½ inch and 25 gauge, ⅝ inch	
• Gauze pads/dressing	
• Appropriate laboratory request slip with necessary information	Information on laboratory slip should include: patient's temperature, fraction of inspired oxygen (FIO_2), method of oxygen delivery, ventilator settings if applicable, and patient's position.
4. Prepare heparinized syringe by drawing up heparin from the ampule using the 22-gauge needle. Switch to 25-gauge needle and, after rinsing syringe barrel with heparin, discard excess heparin and air from the syringe while holding the syringe with needle pointing upward.	Care should be taken to remove excess heparin and air, since these may cause inaccurate results.
5. Explain to the patient what is to be done and what to expect.	An arterial stick is uncomfortable and may cause a burning sensation. An informed patient may be a cooperative one.
6. Position the patient's wrist in mild hyperextension by placing a small rolled towel under it, with the palmar surface of the hand facing upward.	Proper positioning makes the artery more accessible, and it is easier to determine point of maximal impulse.
7. Wash hands thoroughly and use gloves.	Diligent hand-washing helps to decrease risk of infection. Gloves are used for universal precautions.
8. Carefully palpate pulse, determining the approximate point for the puncture.	
9. Cleanse site with povidone-iodine or alcohol swab. Start at the puncture site and move outward, using circular motion. Always prep from the center outward.	Cleansing minimizes contamination of puncture site.
10. Hold the syringe and needle (bevel up) directly over insertion site while stabilizing artery with fingers of other hand.	
11. Pierce the skin at about a 60-degree angle. As soon as the artery is punctured, blood will forcefully enter the syringe.	After the skin is penetrated, the high blood pressure within the artery forces blood into the syringe.
12. Collect about 2 mL blood and withdraw needle and syringe.	
13. Apply firm pressure immediately with one hand. With other hand, hold syringe with needle upright to expel any air, and promptly cork or apply a rubber stopper. Place in ice and have specimen transported for analysis without delay.	Firm, *continuous*, pressure needs to be applied for at least 5 minutes to prevent bleeding and hematoma formation. Remember that the high pressure within the artery can easily cause bleeding at puncture site.
14. After applying continuous, firm pressure to puncture site for 5 minutes, assess site for bleeding and apply pressure dressing.	
15. Leave pressure dressing in place for about 30 minutes, assessing the site periodically.	

Diagnosis. Acute uncompensated metabolic acidemia. The anion gap in this situation would be expected to be elevated due to excess ketoacids associated with diabetic ketoacidosis.

3. A 62-year-old woman presents with a history of severe vomiting over the past 48 hours; she complains of severe weakness and muscle cramps.

Data	Analysis
pH 7.56	(a) pH > 7.40; therefore, underlying condition is *alkalemia*.
$PaCO_2$ 44 mmHg	(b) Respiratory parameter is within normal physiologic limits.
HCO_3^- 33 mEq/L	(c) Metabolic parameters are elevated—*primary* cause of the alkalemia.

Base excess +7

Diagnosis. Acute uncompensated metabolic alkalemia, probably associated with hypochloremia (vomiting) and hypokalemia (weakness). Muscle cramps may be related to the effect of the alkalemic state. Alkalemia increases the protein-bound calcium with a resultant decrease in free, ionized calcium. This patient is at risk for developing tetany. (Note: Vomiting causes loss of hydrogen ions as well as chloride.)

4. A 62-year-old man with long-standing chronic obstructive pulmonary disease (COPD) is admitted to the hospital with possible gastrointestinal bleeding.

Data	Analysis
pH 7.34	(a) pH borderline *acidemia*
$PaCO_2$ 60 mmHg	(b) Respiratory parameter significantly elevated
HCO_3^- 32 mEq/L	(c) Metabolic parameters elevated

Base excess +5
PaO_2 75 mmHg
O_2 Saturation 80%

Diagnosis. Fully compensated respiratory acidemia. Long-standing COPD suggests respiratory acidosis as the primary cause of the acidemia. The elevated base reflects renal compensation, and the nearly normal pH suggests that compensation is largely complete.

5. A 54-year-old woman with long-standing pulmonary disease is admitted to the emergency department with severe dehydration and prostration. Her family reports that she has had the flu for the past week.

Data	Analysis
pH 7.24	(a) pH < 7.35; therefore, underlying mechanism is *acidemia*.
$PaCO_2$ 55 mmHg	(b) Respiratory parameter is elevated.
HCO_3^- 20 mEq/L	(c) Metabolic parameters are reduced.

Base excess −6

Diagnosis. Combined respiratory and metabolic acidemia. The elevated $PaCO_2$ and history suggests that the primary disorder is respiratory acidemia. The metabolic parameters also suggest acidemia because these values are considerably reduced. In the setting of long-standing chronic respiratory acidemia, the expectation would be for HCO_3^- and base excess to be elevated (renal compensation) with a pH reflective of partial to full compensation. This is not the case here because the pH is 7.24.

ARTERIAL BLOOD GASES: DRAWING THE SAMPLE

Arterial blood for blood gas analysis needs to be obtained using an appropriate technique to ensure the integrity of the sample and to prevent complications of bleeding and infection. For specific details related to obtaining the sample, care of the puncture site, and appropriate disposition of the sample, see Tables 23–4 and 23–5.

SUMMARY

An understanding of the principles underlying acid-base physiology is essential to the care of the critically ill patient. Acid-base imbalances are constantly encountered in the critical care setting, and they make an impact on total body function. Together with clues derived from the patient's ongoing history, physical examination, and other laboratory tests and studies, information garnered from arterial blood gas analysis and interpretation assists in assessing the patient's status and overall response to therapy. It is important to develop a systematic approach to analyzing and evaluating such data in terms of total body function.

REFERENCES

1. Schrier, N: Renal and Electrolyte Disorders, ed 3. Little, Brown & Co, Boston, 1986.
2. Goodnough, SK: Advanced Pulmonary Critical Care Course Syllabus, vol 1. Hermann Hospital, Houston, 1983, pp 59–102.
3. Martin, L: All You Really Need to Know to Interpret Arterial Blood Gases. Lea & Febiger, Philadelphia, pp. 6–45; 101–186, 1992.
4. Shapiro, BA, et al: Clinical Application of Blood Gases, ed 4. Mosby–Year Book, Chicago, 1989.
5. Malley, WJ: Clinical Blood Gases: Application and Non-invasive Alternatives. WB Saunders, Philadelphia, 1990.
6. Kucera, RR, et al: Brain pH effects of $NaHCO_3$ and Carbicarb® in lactic acidosis. Crit Care Med 17(12):1320, 1989.
7. Respiratory Support. Springhouse Corporation, Springhouse, PA, 1991, pp 40–44.

CHAPTER 24

Respiratory Assessment: Clinical History and Physical Examination

Terry L. Jones

CHAPTER OUTLINE

Clinical History
- Cardinal Respiratory Signs and Symptoms
- Extrapulmonary Findings
- Past Medical History

Physical Examination
- Thoracic Landmarks—Location of Underlying Lung Lobes
- Techniques of Physical Examination

Radiographic Examination
- Techniques for Obtaining Quality Chest Films
- Basic Principles of Chest X-Ray Interpretation

References

LEARNING OBJECTIVES

After completing this chapter, you should be able to:

1. Outline essential aspects of the clinical history as they pertain to respiratory function and dysfunction.
2. List the cardinal signs and symptoms and extrapulmonary findings of respiratory disease.
3. Locate and describe specific anatomic landmarks and imaginary lines of the anterior, posterior, and lateral thorax.
4. List the four techniques used in the physical examination of the lungs and thorax, and the order in which they are performed.
5. Describe essential information to be obtained on inspection of the lungs and thorax.
6. Describe the key aspects of the palpatory examination of the lungs and thorax.
7. Discuss the significance of percussion in assessing for underlying pathophysiology of the lungs and thorax.
8. Describe normal breath sounds and locate the area of the chest wall where they are normally heard.
9. Define adventitious breath sounds and discuss the possible underlying pathophysiology that they may reflect.
10. Discuss techniques to improve the quality of portable chest x-ray films.
11. Discuss radiographic findings associated with common chest disorders.
12. Discuss radiographic findings used in the verification of invasive monitoring and therapeutic devices.

The major components of the patient's assessment are significant clinical history, physical examination, arterial blood gas studies, pulmonary function tests, x-rays, and other studies. In this chapter, emphasis is placed on the clinical history and the physical examination of the lungs and thorax. Basic principles of chest x-ray interpretation are also discussed.

The most important factor in appraising clinical status is a carefully elicited and comprehensive history. The history provides data for developing a differential diagnosis; it establishes a baseline with which to evaluate the patient's clinical course and responsiveness to therapy.

So much of a productive, long-standing relationship among patient, family, and healthcare providers depends on establishing a rapport with open communication for joint caring, sharing, and learning. A thorough, ongoing history offers the information and clues on which to develop a working relationship—one that assists each participant to more fully realize his or her potential.

CLINICAL HISTORY

In initiating the respiratory assessment, it is essential to determine the patient's immediate status to ascertain whether the patient is experiencing respiratory or other distress. The extent and thoroughness of the initial history and examination should be modified accordingly. In the presence of moderate to severe distress, as is frequently encountered in the critical care setting, eliciting a detailed and comprehensive history from the patient is contraindicated. Rather, the focus is on prompt identification and evaluation of the signs and symptoms reflective of the most life-threatening problems.

In assessing the symptomatology, including the cardinal signs and symptoms of respiratory disease, it is important to establish the onset, progression, and current status of the illness. This is followed by a careful examination of the severity, frequency, and duration of symptoms, as well as their precipitating, aggravating, and alleviating factors (see SLIDT tool, Table 35–1).

Cardinal Respiratory Signs and Symptoms

Four commonly occurring respiratory-related complaints are dyspnea, cough, hemoptysis, and chest pain. Such symptoms may reflect serious underlying chest disease and consequently warrant thorough investigation.

Dyspnea

Dyspnea reflects an uncomfortable awareness of one's own sensation of breathlessness or difficulty breathing. The exact mechanism responsible for the perception of dyspnea remains unclear. It may reflect the intensity of stimulation generated by activation of various receptors associated with the act of breathing.

The patient may complain of "shortness of breath" or "difficulty catching my breath." By definition, the perception of dyspnea is highly subjective and difficult to quantify. When evaluating reports of dyspnea, it is important to remember that the degree of severity perceived by the patient does not consistently correlate with objective indicators of respiratory distress such as respiratory rate and arterial oxygen and carbon dioxide tension.[1] Consequently, all reports of dyspnea warrant careful exploration, regardless of initial objective findings.

When assessing dyspnea, it is important to elicit information pertaining to time of onset, pattern, precipitating events, and associated signs and symptoms.

RESEARCH APPLICATION:
PSYCHOPHYSIOLOGIC ASPECTS OF DYSPNEA IN CHRONIC OBSTRUCTIVE PULMONARY DISEASE: A PILOT STUDY
Gift, AG and Cahill, CA. Heart Lung 19(3), 252–257, 1990.

Purpose: The purpose of this study was to explore the relationships among selected psychological and physiologic variables known to be related to dyspnea and to compare them during times of high and low levels of dyspnea.

Methods: Six male patients with chronic obstructive pulmonary disease (COPD) were assessed for clinical signs believed to be associated with dyspnea. The clinical signs included respiratory rate and depth, use of accessory muscles, paradoxical breathing and sighing. Somatization and depression were measured using the Brief Symptom Inventory (BSI), and anxiety was measured using the Spielberger State Anxiety Inventory (SAI). Plasma cortisol levels and $PaCO_2$ and PaO_2 were also recorded.

Following the assessment, patients were asked to rate their feelings of breathlessness on a vertical analog dyspnea scale (VADS). Measurements were taken at the same time each morning until they reported a change in dyspnea greater than 20 cm (1 SD) on the VADS.

Results: Degrees of anxiety and depression were significantly higher during times of more severe dyspnea when compared with times of less severe dyspnea, as were plasma cortisol and $PaCO_2$ and use of accessory muscles. No significant differences were found for somatization, PaO_2, respiratory rate and depth, sighing, or paradoxical breathing during periods of high and low levels of dyspnea. The use of accessory muscles was the single best indicator of the level of dyspnea perceived.

Practice Implications: The perception of dyspnea is associated with both physiologic and psychological factors. Evaluation of dyspnea in the clinical setting should consequently include assessment of both physiologic and psychological parameters. More specifically, use of accessory muscles and a rise in $PaCO_2$ may indicate worsening dyspnea for the patient. The absence of a decrease in PaO_2, however, does not exclude progression of perceived dyspnea. The identification and exploration of clinical indicators of perceived dyspnea will result in more effective treatment for patients experiencing dyspnea.

Progression from dyspnea on exertion (DOE) to dyspnea at rest suggests progression of disease. Several tools have been developed to aid in the quantification of dyspnea.[2] A gradual onset of dyspnea over the course of months or years is usually associated with chronic lung disease or malignancy, whereas a sudden onset of dyspnea is usually associated with more life-threatening disorders requiring immediate intervention (e.g., pulmonary embolism, pneumothorax, and acute pulmonary edema).[3] Two well-defined patterns of onset have been identified and, because of their association with specific physiologic alterations, warrant further discussion.

Orthopnea. Orthopnea is described as shortness of breath on reclining. It is often quantified by the number of pillows the patient requires to sleep comfortably (e.g., three-pillow orthopnea). Orthopnea generally reflects significant pulmonary or cardiovascular disease. The increase in venous return to the heart in the recumbent position results in left heart decompensation for the patient with congestive heart failure. The pooling of secretions and increase in viscous resistance associated with the recumbent position serve to reduce lung volumes and increase the work of breathing in the patient with chronic lung disease.

Paroxysmal Nocturnal Dyspnea (PND). Paroxysmal nocturnal dyspnea occurs at some point after the patient has been sleeping in the recumbent position. The sudden onset of shortness of breath typically occurs 1 to 2 hours after the patient has fallen asleep, causing him or her to awaken gasping for breath. Following such an episode of PND, patients may sleep undisturbed for the remainder of the night. PND is a classic symptom of left ventricular heart failure but occurs less frequently in patients with pulmonary disease.[2,3]

Virtually all disorders that affect pulmonary function may manifest as shortness of breath. Differential diagnosis of dyspnea includes obstructive airway disease (e.g., asthma, chronic obstructive pulmonary disease [COPD], malignancy); parenchymal lung disease (e.g., pneumonia, interstitial or fibrotic processes, adult respiratory distress syndrome); disorders of the pleura (e.g., pleural effusion, pneumothorax), and pulmonary vascular disorders (e.g., pulmonary embolus, pulmonary hypertension). Cardiovascular disorders commonly associated with dyspnea are left heart failure with a consequent increase in pulmonary pressures (as in pulmonary edema) and severe anemia. Dyspnea may also be anxiety-related.

Cough

The cough reflex is an inherent protective reflex against food or other substances entering the respiratory tract. In conjunction with the intrinsic mucociliary clearance mechanism of the respiratory epithelium, coughing functions to clear secretions produced within the tracheobronchial tree. The cough reflex results from stimulation of extrathoracic cough receptors (found in the nose, oropharynx, larynx, and upper trachea) or intrathoracic, rapidly adapting, irritant receptors (found in the epithelium of the lower trachea and large bronchi).[4]

When evaluating the clinical significance of a cough, the following features should be addressed: Was the onset of the cough acute or chronic? Is it productive? What is the character of the cough? Does the frequency vary in a pattern? What is the character of the sputum?

An acute cough is associated with an infectious process or inhalation of noxious or allergenic substances, whereas a chronic cough is more likely the result of chronic bronchitis, bronchogenic carcinoma, or bronchiectasis. A productive cough is associated with an inflammatory process that may or may not be infectious. Mechanical, thermal, or chemical stimulation of cough receptors (e.g., neoplasms, temperature changes, and pharmacologic agents) may produce a nonproductive cough.

A dry hacking cough may reflect airway irritation from cardiac disease, mechanical obstruction, fibrotic lung disease, or atypical pneumonia. A barking cough is associated with upper airway obstruction or croup, whereas a loose cough is suggestive of the presence of excess secretions, and a congested cough implies an upper respiratory infection or bronchitis.

A cough that occurs primarily in the morning is frequently associated with COPD and results from pooling of secretions throughout the night. Smokers also frequently report increased coughing in the morning. A cough that occurs mainly at night can result from chronic postnasal drip, sinusitis, or congestive heart failure.

Yellow-green sputum reflects the presence of anti-inflammatory cells associated with bacterial infection; a tenacious mucoid purulent sputum, laden with neutrophils and eosinophils, is seen in acute asthma; blood-tinged or rust-colored sputum may be associated with trauma caused by coughing as well as underlying pathology (e.g., pulmonary infarction, pneumococcal pneumonia); and pink, frothy sputum may be encountered in advanced pulmonary edema. Anaerobic infections may yield foul-smelling sputum, especially when accompanied by a lung abscess or necrotizing pneumonia. The presence of *Pseudomonas* infection frequently yields a bluish-green sputum.

Hemoptysis

Hemoptysis is defined as coughing up blood originating within the airways or the lung parenchyma itself. Hemoptysis is frequently associated with significant disease and warrants thorough evaluation. The origin of the bleeding is not always apparent and must be distinguished from that originating in the nasopharynx (e.g., common nosebleed), mouth (e.g., lip or tongue biting), or upper gastrointestinal tract (e.g., esophagus, stomach, or duodenum). It may be confused with hematemesis or associated with aspiration.

In the differential diagnosis, hematemesis is acidic—usually dark red or the color of coffee grounds—often contains food particles, and is accompanied by reports of nausea. Hemoptysis is usually frothy and alkaline and is frequently accompanied by expectoration of sputum.

Airway disease is the most common cause of hemoptysis. Bronchitis/bronchiectasis and bronchogenic carcinoma are the leading causes in the critical care unit. Pulmonary embolism associated with pulmonary infarction and congestive heart failure may also be accompanied by some degree of hemoptysis. Intubated patients may exhibit blood-tinged secretions as a result of the trauma imposed by the act of intubation or frequent endotracheal suctioning.

Assessing and recording the amount of hemoptysis contributes significantly to the differential diagnosis. Massive hemoptysis is said to occur if more than 200 to 600 mL of blood are expectorated within 24 hours and is most frequently the result of acute pulmonary tuberculosis or bronchiectasis. Ordinary hemoptysis involves expectoration of less than 200 mL in 24 hours and is most frequently the result of bronchiectasis or pulmonary neoplasm.[4]

Chest Pain

Chest pain usually originates in the cardiovascular, pulmonary, or gastrointestinal system.[5] Because the severity of the pain or discomfort described does not correlate with clinical significance and because potential morbidity is associated with delayed treatment of chest pain, all reports of chest pain should be taken seriously and warrant thorough evaluation. Chest pain reflective of pulmonary disease does not originate in the lung itself, because this organ is free of sensory (afferent) pain fibers, as is the visceral pleura. However, there are pain receptors so close to the parietal pleura that it is considered to be sensitive to pain. Pleural pain then stems from intercostal muscles, ribs, and overlying skin, the diaphragm, parietal pleura, or mediastinum, each of which is highly innervated by sensory nerve fibers specific for pain.

Chest pain of pulmonary origin has some distinctive features that contribute significantly to the differential diagnosis. Parietal pleural pain is usually well localized over the involved site, sharp in nature, and worsened on inspiration or with coughing or sneezing. Any movement of the upper torso can increase pleural pain. Consequently, patients experiencing pleuritic pain have a tendency to restrict their movement and exhibit splinting of the involved site.[3,4] When the diaphragm is involved, the pain is referred to the ipsilateral shoulder (reflective of phrenic nerve distribution). A sudden onset of pleuritic pain may reflect a pulmonary embolism or pneumothorax, whereas a slightly slower onset (over a few hours) may reflect pneumonia, especially when accompanied by a fever and chills.

Extrapulmonary Findings

Clubbing

Clubbing is a change in the shape and configuration of the nails and distal phalanx of fingers and toes. These changes are characterized by a loss of the normal angle between the nails and skin with an increase in the curvature of the nail, an increased sponginess of the tissue beneath the proximal part of the nail, and a bulbous appearance of the fingertip with flaring or widening of the terminal phalanx (Fig. 24–1).

Clubbing is observed most commonly in long-standing respiratory disease including, especially, bronchogenic carcinoma, chronic lung infection (bronchiectasis and lung abscess), and interstitial lung disease. Carcinoma of the lung parenchyma or pleura is the single most common cause of clubbing. Nonpulmonary causes of clubbing include cardiovascular disease (subacute bacterial endocarditis or congenital intracardiac disease with right-to-left shunting), and chronic diseases of the gastrointestinal system (chronic liver disease or inflammatory bowel disease). The pathophysiologic mechanism underlying clubbing remains undefined.

Cyanosis

Cyanosis is a bluish discoloration of skin, nailbeds, lips, and mucous membranes. It is associated with an increased level of deoxygenated or reduced hemoglobin. Central or generalized cyanosis is linked to a low partial pressure of arterial oxygen (PaO_2), resulting in insufficient oxygenation of hemoglobin in the lungs. A decreased PaO_2 may also occur when systemic blood flow is reduced, with a subsequent extraction of oxygen from the blood by peripheral tissues. Peripheral or localized cyanosis is attributed to the latter mechanism. A reduction in venous oxygen saturation accounts for the bluish discoloration. More specifically, central cyanosis is exhibited when there are at least 5 g of reduced hemoglobin per 100 mL of capillary blood present.[6] Patients with normal or elevated levels of hemoglobin exhibit central cyanosis more

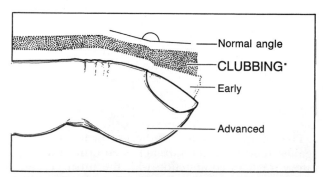

FIGURE 24–1. There is progressive loss of the angle formed at the juncture of the nails and skin of the distal phalanx. The result is an increased curvature of the nail and widening of the terminal phalanx.

readily than patients with lower hemoglobin concentrations given the same change in arterial oxygen saturation (SaO_2). Consequently, the presence of central cyanosis is an unreliable indicator of hypoxemia.

Past Medical History

The patient's past medical history may provide valuable information regarding the underlying etiology and pathophysiology of respiratory disease. It is important for the critical care nurse to elicit information regarding the presence of chronic lung disease (e.g., COPD, asthma, and pulmonary fibrosis). Such disorders significantly affect the patient's response to acute interventions and must be considered when establishing realistic predicted outcomes.

Clinical history related to cardiovascular function should be ascertained because of the close relationship between cardiovascular and pulmonary function. Evidence of hypertension, myocardial infarction, congestive heart failure, anemia, and hypoproteinemia should be carefully documented. Recent chest or lung-related surgery or other procedures (bronchoscopy, thoracentesis) should likewise be noted.

PHYSICAL EXAMINATION

Thoracic Landmarks—Location of Underlying Lung Lobes

To localize and describe findings on examination of the lungs and thorax, it is important to be familiar with the anatomic surface landmarks and imaginary lines drawn on the anterior and posterior thorax.

Sternal Angle (Angle of Louis)

The ability to number the ribs accurately on the anterior chest, the sternal angle, or the angle of Louis provides the best guide.[3,4] The sternal angle is the horizontal bony ridge that joins the manubrium to the body of the sternum (Fig. 24–2). Lateral to this ridge is the 2nd rib and costal cartilage. The intercostal space immediately below is the 2nd intercostal space. Beneath this intercostal space is the 3rd rib, counting downward along the anterior chest. Always start from the sternal angle and 2nd rib when locating ribs or interspaces in the anterior thorax.

Imaginary Lines of the Anterior Thorax

When inspecting the anterior thorax, there are three imaginary lines with which one needs to be familiar: the midsternal line, midclavicular line (a vertical line from the midpoint of the clavicle), and the anterior axillary line (a vertical line from the anterior axillary fold; see Fig. 24–2).

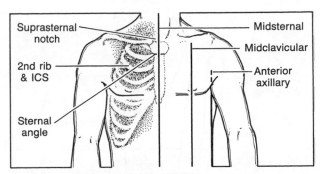

FIGURE 24–2. The sternal angle is located adjacent to the 2nd rib and costal cartilage, making it an ideal anatomical landmark to guide the identification of the intercostal spaces on the anterior thorax. The midsternal, midclavicular, and anterior axillary lines are used to describe the location of underlying structures and assessment findings in the thoracic cavity.

Anatomic Landmarks of the Posterior Thorax

When inspecting the posterior thorax, the scapulae provide an anatomic landmark in that the inferior angle (pole of each scapula lies about at the level of the 7th rib or intercostal space; Fig. 24–3).

Findings may also be localized according to their relationship to the spinous processes. When the head is flexed on the chest, the most prominent spinous process is usually that of the cervical C-7 or thoracic T-1 vertebra. The spinous processes below this level can often be felt and numbered, especially when the spine is flexed. The spinous processes of the thoracic vertebrae T-4 through T-12 angle obliquely downward so that each overlies the body of the vertebra below it. For example, the spinous process of the thoracic T-6 vertebra overlies the thoracic T-7 vertebra and is adjacent to the 7th rib.

Imaginary Lines of the Posterior Thorax

The posterior thorax has two imaginary lines: the vertebral line, which occurs along the spinous pro-

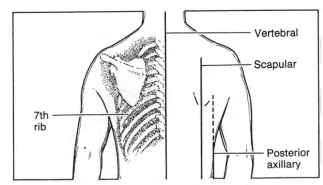

FIGURE 24–3. The inferior angle of the scapula can be used to locate the 7th rib on the posterior thorax. The vertebral, scapular, and posterior axillary lines are used to describe the location of assessment findings from the posterior thorax.

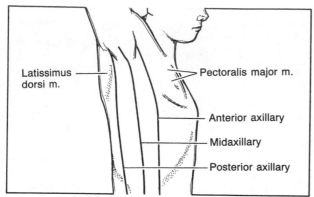

FIGURE 24–4. The posterior axillary, midaxillary, and anterior axillary lines are used to describe the location of the assessment findings on the lateral thorax.

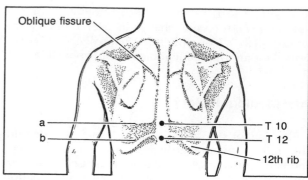

FIGURE 24–6. On the posterior thorax, the inferior border of each lung extends to the level of the thoracic T-10 vertebra. During full inspiration the inferior level of the lungs may descend to the level of the thoracic T-12 vertebra.

cesses, and the scapular line, which is vertical from the inferior angle of the scapula (Fig. 24–3).

Imaginary Lines of the Lateral Thorax

The imaginary lines in the lateral view are the anterior axillary line, midaxillary line (a vertical line from the apex of the axilla), and the posterior axillary line (a vertical line from the posterior axillary fold; Fig. 24–4).

Lung Borders

When examining the lungs and thorax, it is important to consider the location of the underlying lungs and their lobes with respect to anterior landmarks and imaginary lines. In the anterior view (Fig. 24–5), the apex of each lung rises above the medial aspect of each clavicle; the inferior border of each lung crosses the sixth rib at the midclavicular line and the eighth rib at the midaxillary line. Posteriorly, the lower border of each lung occurs at the level of the thoracic T-10 vertebra and may descend to the T-12 process with full inspiration (Fig. 24–6).

Lung Fissures

An oblique fissure divides each lung into upper (anterior) and lower (posterior) lobes (Fig. 24–7). The apex of each lung is actually the superior projection of the upper lobes. The lower lobes project anteriorly and laterally. The right lung is further divided by a horizontal fissure, which delineates the right middle lobe (Fig. 24–5).

The anatomic position of each lobe of the lungs within the thorax has implications for the actual examination of the lungs. A complete examination of the apex of each lung, for example, requires both anterior and posterior examination. Anteriorly, palpation, percussion, and auscultation of the supraclavicular space are required; posteriorly, the examination should begin across the top of each shoulder.

To examine the right middle lobe (RML) appropriately, visualize its position in the right chest in the area circumscribed by the 4th rib superiorly, the 6th rib inferiorly, and laterally to the midclavicular line (Figs. 24–5 and 24–7). This is especially important because the RML is implicated frequently in aspiration

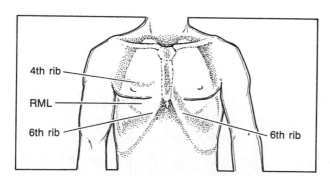

FIGURE 24–5. The inferior border of each lung lies at the level of the 6th rib at the midclavicular line. The right middle lobe is evaluated from the anterior thorax in the area extending from the 4th to the 6th rib between the midsternal and midclavicular lines.

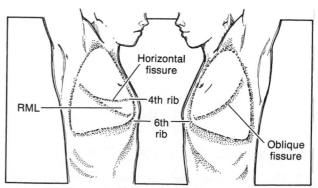

FIGURE 24–7. On the lateral aspect of the thoracic wall, the lungs descend to the 8th rib. The oblique fissure divides the lungs into upper and lower lobes at the level of the 6th rib. Note that the lower lobes primarily project posteriorly and laterally.

pneumonia. The more vertical course of the right mainstem bronchus from the bifurcation of the trachea makes the RML more vulnerable to aspiration. Last, appreciate the anterior and lateral projections of the lower lobe of each lung, which descend to the 6th and 8th ribs, respectively (Fig. 24–7).

Techniques of Physical Examination

Four methods are used in the physical examination of the lungs and thorax. These are inspection, palpation, percussion, and auscultation, in that order. The examination should be organized and systematic. The extent of the initial examination depends on the patient's condition. It is important to compare one side with the other whenever symmetry of structure allows. This comparison allows the patient to serve as his or her own control. Throughout the examination, try to visualize underlying tissues, including the location of lobes of the lungs to surface landmarks.

Inspection

General observation of the patient entails a determination of airway patency, level of consciousness, pain, restlessness, agitation, fear, acute distress, evidence of debilitation, malnutrition, and chronic illness. The respiratory rate, pattern, symmetry of chest wall excursion, work of breathing (use of accessory muscles), body position assumed, and nasal flaring are ascertained, and baseline function is established. Inspect color of skin and mucous membranes for signs of cyanosis, and look for the presence of clubbing. Observe the ease with which the patient speaks and eats. A patient experiencing dyspnea frequently exhibits a disconnected speech pattern and tense facial, neck, and shoulder muscles and may lean forward in the sitting position. A severe or prolonged increase in the work of breathing may lead to decompensation.

The shape and contour of the thoracic cage should be observed for deformities. A "barrel chest" may suggest advanced COPD. Respiratory motion should be observed during quiet breathing and then during deep inspiration whenever possible. Oxygen delivery devices should be observed and evaluated for proper fit and appropriate oxygen delivery. Monitoring devices such as pulse oximeters should be observed and evaluated for accuracy of measurement and intact alarm systems. Chest drainage systems also warrant close inspection to ensure the integrity and proper functioning of the system.

The presence of "paradoxical respirations" (a reversal of normal respiratory mechanisms wherein the thoracic rib cage is observed to passively collapse on inspiration while the diaphragm descends and to expand on expiration as the diaphragm ascends) may reflect disruption of intrapleural pressures, as occurs with thoracic trauma (e.g., multiple rib fractures, flail chest, and disruption of the costosternal cartilaginous

joints) or paralysis of respiratory muscles associated with cervical spinal cord injury. Asymmetry of respiratory motion may also be observed with a large pneumothorax. In these instances, tracheal deviation to the unaffected side may be observed as well. Patients observed splinting one side of the chest when breathing or coughing may be experiencing pleuritic chest pain.

Frequently in the critical care unit, patients are endotracheally intubated while receiving mechanical ventilation. Inspection of such patients should include the entire patient-ventilator unit. Ventilator circuit connections should be observed for looseness or disconnections, and endotracheal tubes should be observed for the presence of secretions. The critical care nurse must observe the patient's respiratory pattern, giving special attention to the extent to which the patient assists the ventilator. Asynchronous breathing patterns should be noted and evaluated for etiology. Visible diaphragmatic contraction reflects spontaneous respiratory effort, which is of great significance in patients requiring pharmacologic paralysis for effective ventilator management.

Palpation

The chest is palpated to identify moisture (e.g., diaphoresis), elasticity, and texture of the skin and to determine the presence of any painful area, enlarged or tender lymph nodes, or crepitus. Muscle tone, extent of respiratory excursion, asymmetry, and intercostal retraction also need to be assessed. Assess for tracheal deviation (deviation away from defect—large pneumothorax, thyroid enlargement, neck mass, pleural effusion, or expiratory phase of flail chest; deviation toward defect—atelectasis or inspiratory phase of flail chest); neck vein distention; and tactile fremitus (diminished fremitus—pleural effusion, pneumothorax with lung collapse, obstruction of mainstem bronchus, or emphysema; increased fremitus—pneumonia with consolidation, lung tumors, or pulmonary infarction).

Fremitus refers to the palpable vibrations transmitted through the tracheobronchial tree to the chest wall when the patient speaks. Usually, the palmar surface of each hand is placed flat on the posterior chest, and the patient is asked to say "99." Liquid and solid materials transmit vibrations better than air-filled spaces.

It is also important to assess for the presence of subcutaneous emphysema, which occurs when the air leaks into the subcutaneous tissue. Assessment for the presence of subcutaneous air involves gently pressing down on the skin during palpation. A "crunching" or "crackling" is felt as the subcutaneous air is displaced; this is often referred to as *crepitus*. It is especially important to assess for subcutaneous air in patients with new tracheostomies, chest tubes, thoracotomy incisions, chest trauma, barotrauma, or neck surgery. Patients receiving positive pressure mechanical ventilation, especially in conjunction with high levels of positive end-expiratory pressure (PEEP), have an even greater risk of developing subcutaneous emphysema. Occasionally, the development of gas gangrene may also result in subcutaneous emphysema as the gas produced by the bacteria leaks into the subcutaneous tissue.

Percussion

In percussing, the examiner notes the quality of sound elicited by tapping the middle finger of one hand against the middle finger of the opposite hand, which is applied to the chest wall. The underlying principle is similar to that of tapping a surface and judging whether what is underneath is solid or hollow. Normally, percussion of the chest wall overlying air-containing lung produces a resonant sound; in contrast, percussion over a solid organ, such as the liver, produces a dull sound. This contrast in sounds allows the examiner to detect areas with something other than air-containing lung beneath the chest wall. For example, the sound elicited over fluid in the pleural space (pleural effusion) or airless (consolidated) lung in both cases is dull to percussion. At the other extreme, air in the pleural space (pneumothorax) or a hyperinflated lung (emphysema) may produce a hyperresonant or more hollow sound, approaching what one hears when percussing over a hollow viscus such as the stomach (tympany; Table 24–1).

Auscultation

Goals of auscultation are twofold: to assess the quality of breath sounds and to detect the presence of abnormal or adventitious sounds. When the examiner places the diaphragm of the stethoscope firmly on the chest wall, the sound of airflow can be heard when the patient takes a breath that is a little deeper than normal, with the mouth open. Exactly what is heard depends on where the stethoscope is placed. Sounds heard over the trachea tend to be loud, harsh, and high-pitched, with the expiratory phase being slightly longer than the inspiratory phase. In contrast, when the stethoscope is placed over peripheral lung fields, sound is heard almost exclusively during the inspiratory phase, and the quality of the sound is much softer. When interpreting the quality of breath sounds, it is important to be cognizant of two facts[8]: (1) Normal transmission of sound depends on airway patency; and (2) the presence of air or fluid in the pleural space acts as a barrier to sound.

Normal Breath Sounds. Normal breath sounds are described as vesicular, bronchial, and bronchovesicular.

Vesicular Sounds. Vesicular sounds are soft, quiet, and low-pitched. They consist of a fine rustle or swishing sounds and are heard primarily during the inspiratory phase and early expiratory phase. The inspiratory phase is about three times longer than the expiratory phase.

The actual sounds produced are thought to be due to distention and separation of alveoli during the inspiratory maneuver. These sounds are the predominant breath sounds, and they are heard over most lung areas. Vesicular sounds are produced in the alveoli and fine terminal and respiratory bronchioles, which make up the lung parenchyma.

Bronchial Sounds. Bronchial sounds are normally heard over the trachea and sternum. They are described as loud "tubular" sounds resembling wind blowing through a long tube. These sounds are both low-pitched and high-pitched with an expiratory phase that is longer than the inspiratory phase. There is a

TABLE 24–1
Respiratory Pathophysiology—Physical Findings[7]

Condition	Tactile Fremitus	Percussion	Breath Sounds	Adventitious Sounds
Normal	Normal	Resonant	Vesicular over peripheral lung fields; bronchovesicular over large bronchi; bronchial over trachea and sternum	Usually none; transient rales (crackles) after sleep or recumbency
Atelectasis (collapsed air sacs)	Decreased to absent	Dull	Decreased vesicular to absent	None
Bronchitis (partial airway obstruction)	Normal	Resonant	Normal to prolonged expiratory phase	Rales (crackles); wheezes; rhonchi
Emphysema (hyperinflated lung)	Decreased	Hyperresonant	Decreased vesicular, frequently with prolonged expiratory phase	None unless bronchitis is also present
Pleural effusion or pleural thickening	Decreased to absent	Dull to flat	Decreased or absent	None unless underlying airway or lung parenchymal disease
Pneumothorax (air in pleural space)	Decreased to absent	Hyperresonant	Decreased to absent	None
Pneumonia (pulmonary consolidation)	Increased	Dull	Bronchial	Rales (crackles)
Pulmonary edema (left ventricular failure)	Normal	Resonant	May be prolonged on expiration	Rales (crackles) at lung bases; wheezes may be detected

momentary pause between these phases during which no noise or breath sound is heard. When bronchial breath sounds are heard other than over the trachea and sternum, they may be associated with a pathologic process (e.g., pneumonia, pleural effusion, or major atelectasis).

Bronchovesicular Sounds. Bronchovesicular sounds reflect a mixture of both bronchial and vesicular breath sounds. They are heard best where normal lung overlies the large mainstem bronchi at the first and second intercostal space at the left and right sternal borders, below the clavicles anteriorly, and between the scapulae posteriorly. Bronchovesicular sounds are heard about equally through the inspiratory and expiratory phases. Vesicular, bronchial, and bronchovesicular sounds all are normal breath sounds when heard in the appropriate area of the thorax.

In general, sound generated by airflow is transmitted better through consolidated than air-containing lung. Thus, a bronchial-type sound might be detected over lung tissue that is consolidated because of pneumonia. Furthermore, a difference exists not only in the quality of sound, but in its relative duration of inspiration and expiration.

Diminished Breath Sounds.[3,4] A decrease in intensity of breath sounds may occur throughout the lung fields or in localized areas. The decrease in intensity may reflect shallow respirations or hypoventilation states involving small volumes of air movement. Disorders commonly associated with diminished breath sounds in localized areas include pleural effusion, pneumothorax, pneumonia, malpositioned endotracheal tube, atelectasis, and neoplasm.

Adventitious Breath Sounds.[3,4,9] The second goal of auscultation is to detect adventitious or abnormal breath sounds. The major types of adventitious sounds are rales or crackles, wheezes, rhonchi, friction rubs, and stridor.

Rales (Crackles). Rales are described as a series of popping or clicking noises heard over an involved area of lung. The quality of these sounds may range from rubbing two hairs together, to the sound of soda fizzing, to the sound generated by opening a Velcro fastener or crumpling a sheet of cellophane. The sounds are often referred to as "opening" sounds, reflective of the opening of small airways and alveoli that may have been atelectatic or poorly ventilated or that may be partially filled with fluid or inflammatory exudate. These sounds are heard throughout or at the latter part of the inspiratory phase. Rales are most commonly associated with pulmonary edema, atelectasis, pneumonia, and interstitial lung disease (idiopathic pulmonary fibrosis, fibrosis associated with collagen diseases—systemic lupus erythematosus, scleroderma, sarcoidosis, and others). Rales often develop in dependent areas. Consequently, it is important to listen to the lung bases with the patient positioned upright and to the posterior lung regions with the patient positioned supine.

Wheezes. Wheezes are high-pitched sounds, often of a "whistling" quality that are produced by airflow through narrowed airways. Airway narrowing may be caused by bronchiole smooth muscle contraction, edema, excessive secretions, or airway collapse due to inadequate support. Under normal physiologic circumstances, the diameter of the airways is decreased during expiration; consequently, wheezing is more pronounced during the expiratory phase. During expiration, there is some loss of the "tethering" effect by virtue of the elastic recoil of the lung parenchymal tissue. This may account, in part, for the narrowing of airways during expiration.

It is important to note that for wheezing to occur, there must be a certain minimal amount of airflow. If airway narrowing becomes sufficiently severe and ventilation is seriously compromised, wheezing may no longer be heard and the patient's condition may rapidly decompensate leading to respiratory failure (Table 24–1).

Rhonchi. Rhonchi is a term that describes sound generated by secretions within the airways. It usually reflects breath sounds that are lower-pitched and somewhat coarser in quality than wheezes.

When rales or rhonchi are heard, ask the patient to cough. If these sounds do not disappear or if they become accentuated with coughing, they are usually clinically significant, reflective of fluid and secretions in the tiny airways, alveolar ducts, and alveolar sacs.

Friction Rub. A friction rub is the term used to describe the sounds caused by the rubbing together of inflamed or roughened pleural surfaces. These sounds are raspy in quality and mimic the rubbing together of two pieces of leather. They occur continuously throughout the respiratory cycle. Pleuritic pain and splinting may accompany friction rub. Clinically, a friction rub may be associated with a primary acute inflammatory disease of the pleura, or it may be caused by lung parenchymal pathologic processes that penetrate the pleural surface (e.g., pneumonia, pulmonary infarction, and others).

Stridor. Stridor is a high-pitched noisy respiration like the blowing of the wind. Its presence usually reflects some type of respiratory obstruction, particularly in the trachea or larynx (the upper airways). In the acute setting, the larynx is probably the major area subject to obstruction. Infection (e.g., with *Haemophilus influenzae*), thermal injury and consequently laryngeal edema from smoke inhalation, foreign body aspiration, laryngeal edema associated with allergic reaction (anaphylaxis), and premature extubation all have been implicated as causes of stridor.

The critical care nurse should remember that the presence of mechanical ventilation may alter normal breath sounds. As a result of high flow rates and turbulent flow through the endotracheal tube, breath sounds are frequently louder and less "breezy" in patients receiving mechanical ventilation. Patients receiving PEEP may exhibit a decrease in the intensity of breath sounds. Auscultation of patients with stiff noncompliant lungs (as with adult respiratory distress syndrome) may reveal localized areas throughout the lung fields that sound less breezy for reasons not clearly understood.[3]

A gurgling sound may also be heard because of the condensation of water having accumulated in the ventilator circuit tubing. To prevent such extraneous sounds from drowning out potentially clinically significant adventitious sounds, the circuit tubing should be emptied and the patient suctioned prior to auscultation of breath sounds. Auscultation of patients with a chest tube may also reveal unusual sounds. Frequently "squeaks" or "crunches" are heard, which may be the result of chest tube movement with respirations. Bubbling or wheezelike sounds may also be transmitted from the suction apparatus of chest drainage systems or nasogastric tubes.

RADIOGRAPHIC EXAMINATION

Chest x-rays are frequently ordered for critically ill patients for diagnosing and monitoring chest disorders and for verifying placement of a host of invasive monitoring and therapeutic devices (e.g., endotracheal tubes, tracheostomy tubes, central venous catheters, pulmonary artery catheters, intra-aortic balloons, pacemakers, dialysis catheters, and nasogastric tubes). The most common view ordered in the critical care unit is the anteroposterior (AP) frontal view with the patient sitting upright or lying supine. In this view, the x-ray beam is delivered from the machine toward the patient's anterior chest with the film cassette positioned behind the patient adjacent to the posterior thorax. Although the posteroanterior (PA) view generally produces a higher-quality film, it is contraindicated in most critically ill patients because it must be done in the radiology department with the patient standing.

Techniques for Obtaining Quality Chest Films

The critical care nurse should provide appropriate assistance to the x-ray technician to help ensure optimum quality of the film. When positioning a patient for a portable AP film, the sitting position is preferred over the supine position because the supine position may result in the appearance of elevated hemidiaphragms, redistribution of pulmonary blood flow, and a larger heart and mediastinum in the absence of pathology.[3,10] Fluid levels of pleural effusions may not be clearly visible in the supine position. The patient's back should be flat against the x-ray cassette and the head of the bed elevated so that the x-ray beam can be delivered at a perpendicular angle. Even a slight rotation of the patient's body may result in asymmetry or distortion of structures on the film, making accurate interpretation difficult.

Objects in contact with the patient's chest should be removed or repositioned above the shoulder, away from areas of suspected pathology whenever possible (e.g., jewelry, snaps on gowns, ECG electrodes, binders, external portion of central venous and pulmonary artery catheters, and pacemaker wires). It is important to communicate the patient's diagnosis and purpose of the chest x-ray to the x-ray technician so that appropriate adjustments can be made on the equipment to provide optimum visualization of the areas of interest to the diagnostician.

Basic Principles of Chest X-Ray Interpretation

The Normal Chest X-Ray

Chest x-ray interpretation involves a systematic approach to the visualization of the following structures: soft tissues, trachea, bony thorax, intercostal spaces, diaphragm, pleural surfaces, mediastinum, hila, and lung fields. The normal or nonpathologic chest x-ray is symmetric in appearance, with the tra-

TABLE 24–2
Radiographic Findings Associated with Common Chest Pathology[3,4,9,11]

Disorder	Findings
Pneumothorax	Tracheal deviation away from affected side, widened intercostal spaces, diaphragmatic elevation, fissure displacement; mediastinal shift, hilar displacement, increased density of collapsed lung
Pleural effusion	Widened intercostal spaces, blunted posterior costophrenic angle, horizontal or meniscus fluid level, increased thickness of involved fissures, area of increased density
Pulmonary congestion/edema	Hilar clouding, increased vascular markings, changes in the distinctiveness of vessel borders
Pneumonia	Dulled posterior costophrenic angle, hilar displacement, well-defined area of increased density, air bronchogram sign
Obstructive lung disease	Widened intercostal spaces, diaphragmatic depression or flattening
Atelectasis	Narrowed intercostal spaces, dulled posterior costophrenic angle, fissure displacement; well-defined area of increased density, shift of cardio-mediastinal silhouette to ipsilateral side, overexpansion of contralateral lung
Adult respiratory distress syndrome	Irregular, patchy distribution of areas of increased density; "whited out"

TABLE 24–3

Radiographic Findings Reflecting Proper Placement of Common Invasive Monitoring and Therapeutic Devices[3,9,11,12]

Device	Placement Verification
Endotracheal tube	Tip should lie about 5 cm above the carina when the head is in the neutral position.
Central venous catheter or dialysis catheters	Tip should lie just below the junction of the left or right bracheo-cephalic veins or just above the junction of the superior vena cava and right atrium.
Pulmonary artery catheter	Tip should lie in the right or left main pulmonary artery.
Intra-aortic balloon catheter	The proximal end should lie in the descending thoracic aorta 1–2 cm below the origin of the left subclavian artery. The distal end of the balloon should lie above the origin of the renal arteries.
Transvenous pacemaker	Tip should lie in the apex of the right ventricle.
Nasogastric tube	A thin radiopaque line should descend down the center of the chest into the stomach.
Tracheostomy tube	Tip should lie one half to two thirds of the distance between the tracheal stoma and the carina. The lumen should be two thirds of the diameter of the trachea.

chea in the midline position and consistency of intercostal space width. The hemidiaphragms are dome-shaped, the right side typically 1 to 3 cm above the left side. The pleura, when visible, is of consistent thickness and adjacent to the chest wall, and the interlobar fissures are in the correct anatomic location in relation to the ribs (Fig. 24–7).

The mediastinal profile consists of distinct curves with a cardiothoracic (CT) ratio of less than 1:2. The hilar area contains shadows of the pulmonary arteries and upper lobe veins. The left hilum may be slightly higher than the right, and the left pulmonary artery is often visible projecting outward from the hilar profile, unlike the right pulmonary artery, which remains

in the pericardial sac until the point of bifurcation. The costophrenic angles should be well defined. The largest structures on the chest film are the lung fields. Bronchovascular markings branch out from the hilar area, taper toward the periphery, and disappear in the outer third of the lung fields. The degree of density should be symmetric with increasing blackness toward the periphery.

Common Diagnostic Radiographic Findings

Radiographic findings associated with disorders frequently encountered in the critical care unit are summarized in Table 24–2. Radiographic findings associated with placement of invasive monitoring and therapeutic devices are summarized in Table 24–3.

REFERENCES

1. Gift, AG and Cahill, CA: Psychophysiologic aspects of dyspnea in chronic obstructive pulmonary disease: A pilot study. Heart Lung 19:252, 1990.
2. McCord, M and Cronin-Stubbs, D: Operationalizing dyspnea: Focus on measurement. Heart Lung 21:167, 1992.
3. Kirsten, LD: Comprehensive Respiratory Nursing. WB Saunders, Philadelphia, 1989.
4. Murray, JF: Diagnostic evaluation: History and physical examination. In Murray, JF and Nadal, JA (eds): Textbook of Respiratory Medicine. WB Saunders, Philadelphia, 1988, p 431.
5. Forshee, T: Systemic origins of chest pain. Nursing '87 17:30, 1987.
6. Mortin, L and Khahil, H: How much reduced hemoglobin is necessary to generate central cyanosis? Chest 97:182, 1990.
7. Bates, B: A Guide to Physical Examination, ed 6. JB Lippincott, Philadelphia, 1995.
8. Weinberger, S: Principles of Pulmonary Medicine. WB Saunders, Philadelphia, 1986, p 33.
9. Ahrens, T: Pulmonary data acquisition. In Kinney, MR, Packa, DR, and Dunbar, SB (eds): AACN's Clinical Reference for Critical Care Nursing. CV Mosby, St. Louis, 1993, p 689.
10. Greenspan, RH and Mann, H: Radiographic techniques. In Murray, JF and Nadal, JA (eds): Textbook of Respiratory Medicine. WB Saunders, Philadelphia, 1988, p 478.
11. Turner, AF: Interpretation of the conventional chest x-ray in the critically ill and injured. In Shoemaker, WC, et al (eds): Textbook of Critical Care Medicine, ed 2. WB Saunders, Philadelphia, 1989, p 230.
12. Hartnett, TM and Gaffney, T: Intra-aortic balloon size selection. In Quail, SJ: Comprehensive Intraaortic Balloon Counterpulsation, ed 2. CV Mosby, St. Louis, 1993, 207.

C H A P T E R   25

Nursing Management of the Patient with Acute Respiratory Failure

Dorothy M. Kite-Powell

CHAPTER OUTLINE

Respiratory Failure
- Classification of Acute Respiratory Failure
- Gas Exchange Abnormalities

Acute Respiratory Failure
- Clinical Presentation
- Treatment and Management

Adult Respiratory Distress Syndrome
- Pathogenesis
- Pathophysiology
- Clinical Presentation
- Treatment

- Nursing Care of the Patient with ARDS
- Research and ARDS

Therapeutic Modalities in the Treatment of Acute Respiratory Failure
- Oxygen Therapy
- Chest Physiotherapy–Bronchial Hygiene
- Airway Management
- Mechanical Ventilation

References
Suggested Readings

LEARNING OBJECTIVES

After completing this chapter, you should be able to:
1. Describe the four pathophysiologic mechanisms that can impair gas exchange and cause hypoxemia:
   a. Alveolar hypoventilation
   b. Ventilation/perfusion ($\dot{V}/\dot{Q}$) mismatch
   c. Intrapulmonary (right-to-left) shunt
   d. Impaired diffusion
2. Examine the etiology and pathophysiology of the two types of respiratory failure:
   a. Hypoxemic
   b. Hypercapnic/hypoxemic
3. Describe the clinical presentation of acute respiratory failure (ARF).
4. Outline medical and nursing management of ARF.
5. List the disorders commonly associated with the development of adult respiratory distress syndrome (ARDS).
6. Compare and contrast the noncardiogenic pulmonary edema of ARDS and cardiogenic pulmonary edema.
7. Identify the role of mechanical ventilation and positive end-expiration pressure (PEEP) therapy in the treatment of ARDS.
8. Describe the nursing care of the patient with ARDS based on the nursing process.
9. State the primary goal and indications for use of oxygen therapy.
10. List the complications of oxygen therapy.
11. Describe types of artificial airways in current use and discuss implications for nursing care.
12. Identify the primary goals and indications for mechanical ventilation therapy.
13. Describe the types of ventilators in current use, modes of ventilatory assistance, and ventilator controls.
14. List the complications of mechanical ventilation therapy.
15. Outline nursing considerations for the patient receiving mechanical ventilation therapy.
16. Describe indications for and basic approaches to the weaning process.

The normal function of the respiratory system is to facilitate gas exchange. Without an adequate exchange of oxygen and carbon dioxide, the metabolic demands of the tissues would not be met and body systems would rapidly fail. Many different types of respiratory diseases are capable of disrupting the lung's normal function. Some of these diseases cause a mild impairment of gas exchange with little or no consequences; other dysfunctions lead to a life-threatening event.

When respiratory function is compromised to the degree that arterial blood gases (ABGs) cannot be maintained within an acceptable range, the patient is said to be in respiratory failure. Acute respiratory failure (ARF) requires early recognition and prompt treatment to improve the patient's chances of survival. Respiratory failure can develop acutely in the patient with or without preexisting respiratory disease. The primary cause of the failure may be respiratory in origin, or it may evolve from an acute illness involving another organ system, which is complicated by respiratory problems.

RESPIRATORY FAILURE

Respiratory failure has been defined as the inability of the respiratory system to adequately oxygenate the blood with or without an impairment of carbon dioxide elimination. Respiratory failure is present when the partial pressure of arterial oxygen (PaO_2) is less than or equal to 50 mmHg or when the partial pressure of arterial carbon dioxide ($PaCO_2$) is greater than or equal to 50 mmHg of breathing ambient air composed of 21% oxygen. Other clinical criteria are a decreasing pH of less than 7.35 and a decreasing percent saturation of hemoglobin (SaO_2) of less than 90%. Respiratory failure is considered acute if the lungs are unable to maintain adequate oxygenation in a previously healthy person, with or without an impairment of carbon dioxide elimination.

Classification of Acute Respiratory Failure

Hypoxemia, defined as subnormal oxygenation of arterial blood with a PaO_2 of less than 60 mmHg and an SaO_2 of 90% or less, develops when there is a significant alteration in the physiologic status of one or more of these factors. Hypoxemia is a feature of virtually all patients with ARF. Respiratory failure is broadly categorized into two types, based on the pattern of blood gas abnormalities.

Type I is hypoxemic respiratory failure, in which the PaO_2 is less than 50 mmHg and the $PaCO_2$ is normal to low. The major pathophysiologic mechanisms causing hypoxemic respiratory failure usually involve a combination of ventilation/perfusion ($\dot{V}/\dot{Q}$) mismatching and right-to-left shunting.

Type II is hypercapnic/hypoxemic respiratory failure, in which the $PaCO_2$ is greater than 45 mmHg, accompanied by a lower-than-normal PaO_2, pathologically caused by alveolar hypoventilation. The pathophysiology underlying hypercapnic/hypoxemic respiratory failure is the inability of the patient to maintain alveolar ventilation at a level sufficient to eliminate carbon dioxide while keeping the PaO_2 within an acceptable range (PaO_2 higher than 60 mmHg). See Table 25–1 for a comparison of hypercapnic/hypoxemic and hypoxemic respiratory failure.[1]

Gas Exchange Abnormalities

Four pathophysiologic mechanisms can impair gas exchange, lead to hypoxemia, and contribute to respiratory insufficiency and failure: alveolar hypoventi-

TABLE 25–1
Comparison: Hypercapnic/Hypoxemic and Hypoxemic Respiratory Failure

	Hypercapnic/Hypoxemic	Hypoxemic
Incidence	Relatively common	Common
Clinical history	Usually long-standing antecedent chronic obstructive pulmonary disease (COPD)	Usually normal lung function prior to acute pulmonary insult
	Evidence of neurologic, neuromuscular disorders; chest cage defect; impaired airway patency	
Underlying pathophysiologic mechanism	Alveolar hypoventilation	$\dot{V}/\dot{Q}$ mismatching
Typical arterial blood gas values	Some $\dot{V}/\dot{Q}$ mismatching	Right-to-left intrapulmonary shunting
Resting lung volume	↓ PaO_2; ↑ $PaCO_2$	↓ PaO_2; $PaCO_2$ normal or ↓
Lung compliance	May be high (e.g., emphysema)	Low
Alveolar ventilation	Increased	Decreased
	Decreased	Increased
Assisted ventilation	COPD: Avoid, if titrated oxygen therapy and airway therapy effective	Early institution
	Others: Observe criteria for intubation and mechanical ventilatory assistance	

TABLE 25–2
Alveolar Hypoventilation

Hypoxemia is always accompanied by hypercapnia (↑ $PaCO_2$). For causes refer to Figure 25–1.

1. Hypoventilation with normal lungs
   a. Damage to or depression of the pons and medullary centers in the brain
      (1) CNS depressant drugs
      (2) CVAs
      (3) Trauma
   b. Defects in the neuromuscular connections
      (1) Guillain-Barré syndrome
      (2) Amyotropic lateral sclerosis
      (3) Muscular dystrophy
   c. Defects in the chest bellows
      (1) Kyphoscoliosis, pleuritis, spinal cord injury
2. Hypoventilation with abnormal lungs
   a. Obstructive airway disease
      (1) Chronic obstructive pulmonary disease (COPD)
      (2) Asthma
      (3) Cystic fibrosis
   b. Alveolar disease
      (1) ARDS
      (2) Pneumonia
      (3) Atelectasis
      (4) Pulmonary embolism

Goals of therapy are to improve ventilation. Specific therapy is related to the specific cause.

lation, $\dot{V}/\dot{Q}$ mismatch, intrapulmonary (right-to-left) shunt, and diffusion impairment.

Alveolar Hypoventilation

Alveolar ventilation (Table 25–2) is the prime determinant of $PaCO_2$, and an elevation in $PaCO_2$ signals inadequate alveolar ventilation, or alveolar hypoventilation (Table 25–2). Indeed, hypoventilation may be defined as an elevated PaO_2. Alveolar hypoventilation is characterized by ABG values that reflect an increase in $PaCO_2$, a decrease in $PaCO_2$, and a decrease in SaO_2, or hypercapnic/hypoxemic respiratory failure. Physiologically, effective alveolar ventilation requires an intact series of interconnected anatomic-physiologic "links" (Fig. 25–1). It is essential to review these links because a disturbance of more than one link in this cycle contributes largely to alveolar hypoventilation and hypercapnic/hypoxemic respiratory failure. These links include (1) the pons and medullary center; (2) the neuromuscular connections from the respiratory center to the chest cage; (3) the chest bellows or chest cage itself, and the respiratory musculature; (4) patent airways; and (5) intact alveoli. Patients with alveolar hypoventilation are usually treated with supplemental oxygen, specific therapy related to the eti-

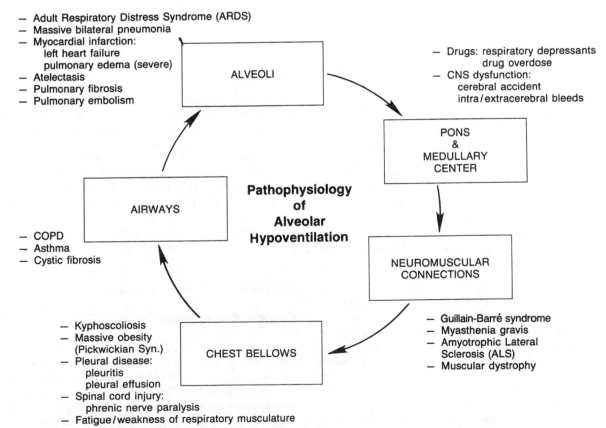

FIGURE 25–1. A cycle depicting the interconnected anatomic-physiologic links essential for effective alveolar ventilation; and the possible disease entities that can disrupt the integrity of these links, individually and/or collectively, predisposing to alveolar hypoventiliation.

TABLE 25–3
Hypoxemia Due to V̇/Q̇ Mismatching

1. Pathophysiology
   a. Low V̇/Q̇ units, with perfusion in excess of ventilation, result in hypoxemia because the blood traversing these units is not fully oxygenated.
   b. Low V̇/Q̇ units may result from partial obstruction of airways by foreign bodies, secretions, edema, inflammation, bronchospasm, or other conditions.
2. Etiology
   a. Obstructive airway disease: chronic bronchitis, emphysema, asthma
   b. Restrictive airway disease: obesity, kyphoscoliosis, interstitial lung disease
   c. Pulmonary vascular disease
3. Diagnosis
   a. History: clues to the above diagnoses
   b. Physical exam: abnormal chest wall motion, abnormal distribution of breath sounds, bronchospasm
   c. Laboratory data: ABGs with hypoxemia and a widened alveolar-arterial gradient; characteristic change on chest x-ray, pulmonary function tests, V̇/Q̇ scan
4. Treatment
   a. Supplemental oxygen
   b. Identification of underlying cause
   c. Specific therapy variable depending on specific cause

Source: From Ahrens, T and Nelson, G: Pulmonary anatomy and physiology. In Kinney, M, Packa, D, and Dunbar, S (eds): AACN's Clinical Reference for Critical Care Nursing, ed 3. CV Mosby, St Louis, p 685, with permission.

TABLE 25–4
Hypoxemia Due to Shunting (R → L)

1. Pathophysiology
   a. Hypoxemia results from venous admixture when deoxygenated; mixed venous blood bypasses functional alveolar-capillary units and mixes with normally oxygenated blood in the systemic circulation.
   b. Shunts may be either anatomic or physiologic.
2. Etiology
   a. Anatomic shunts—blood bypasses the alveolar-capillary unit.
      (1) Normal anatomic shunts: bronchial, pleural, thebesian veins
      (2) Intrapulmonary shunts: pulmonary atrioventricular fistulas
      (3) Intracardiac shunts: tetralogy of Fallot, Eisenmenger's syndrome
      (4) Other pathologic shunts: shunts associated with neoplasms
   b. Physiologic shunts—blood is shunted through nonfunctional alveolar-capillary units.
      (1) Alveolar collapse: atelectasis, pneumothorax, hemothorax, pleural effusion
      (2) Alveoli filled with foreign material: pulmonary edema, pneumonia, ARDS
3. Diagnosis
   a. Hypoxemia with a normal or decreased $PaCO_2$ and a widened alveolar-arterial difference
   b. 100% oxygen test: widened alveolar-arterial difference persists; shunt may be estimated
4. Treatment
   a. Oxygen—little effect
   b. Depends on specific etiology

Source: From Ahrens, T and Nelson, G: Pulmonary anatomy and physiology. In Kinney, M, Packa, D, and Dunbar, S (eds): AACN's Clinical Reference for Critical Care Nursing, ed 3. CV Mosby, St Louis, p 687, with permission.

ology, and, in acute cases, intervention with mechanical ventilation.

Ventilation/Perfusion (V̇/Q̇) Mismatch

Effective gas exchange depends largely on the degree to which ventilation is matched with perfusion throughout the lung. Clinically, there is an uneven distribution of ventilation and perfusion in the normal lung, because not all alveoli are completely ventilated and perfused. Normally, these individual areas of the lungs balance out to maintain an overall PaO_2 within normal physiologic range. If, however, there is a greater-than-normal variability in these V̇/Q̇ match-ups, the overall ratio of ventilation to perfusion is disturbed and hypoxemia develops. V̇/Q̇ mismatch is the most common cause of hypoxemia (Table 25–3).

Shunt

A pulmonary shunt occurs when unoxygenated blood returns to the left heart and to the systemic circulation after passing through nonventilated alveoli (Table 25–4). The result is a decrease in PaO_2 that is commonly accompanied by a normal or decreased PaO_2, or hypoxemic respiratory failure. Administration of 100% oxygen may not improve the shunting problem or relieve the associated hypoxemia, because the shunted blood has no opportunity to come into contact with gas exchange tissue.

Diffusion Impairment

Gas exchange between the alveoli and the pulmonary capillaries occurs across the alveolar-capillary membranes, which are normally thin structures, freely permeable to carbon dioxide and oxygen (see Figs. 22–10 and 22–11; Table 25–5). Because diffusion of these gases occurs so rapidly, an impairment in this process alone rarely becomes significant enough to alter oxygenation. The combination of a diffusion abnormality with V̇/Q̇ mismatching or hypoventilation could lead to hypoxemia in the critically ill patient.

ACUTE RESPIRATORY FAILURE

Clinical Presentation

When patients develop ARF, their symptom complex usually includes the manifestations of hypoxemia or hypercapnia or both and the specific symptomatology associated with the underlying precipitating disorder. The signs and symptoms of hypoxemia, hypercapnia, and acidemia are widespread, involving all major body systems. It is essential for the critical care nurse to appreciate the underlying etiology, pathophysiology, and clinical presentation of ARF. Patients

TABLE 25–5
Hypoxemia Due to Diffusion Abnormalities

1. Pathophysiology
   a. Increased diffusion pathway—prevents equilibrium between alveolar oxygen and pulmonary capillary blood, so that blood exiting the capillary is hypoxemic
   b. Decreased diffusion area—destruction of membrane surface area available for diffusion and loss of pulmonary capillary bed
2. Etiology:
   a. Increased diffusion pathway
      (1) Accumulation of fluid: congestive heart failure and pulmonary edema
      (2) Accumulation of collagen in the pulmonary interstitium: idiopathic pulmonary fibrosis, sarcoidosis, and collagen-vascular disease
   b. Decreased diffusion area
      (1) Pulmonary resection
      (2) Destructive lung diseases: emphysema and obliterative pulmonary vascular diseases
3. Diagnosis
   a. History and physical findings compatible with the primary diagnosis
   b. Laboratory
      (1) Pulmonary function tests reveal decreased diffusing capacity for carbon monoxide, exercise ABG measurements reveal arterial desaturation
      (2) Chest x-ray compatible with interstitial fibrosis, emphysema, and so on
4. Treatment
   a. Oxygen administration
   b. Evaluation of need for home oxygen therapy

Source: From Ahrens, T and Nelson, G: Pulmonary anatomy and physiology. In Kinney, M, Packa, D, and Dunbar, S (eds): AACN's Clinical Reference for Critical Care Nursing, ed 3. CV Mosby, St Louis, p 685, with permission.

who have a high risk of developing ARF can be identified, and the early, often subtle, signs and symptoms can be recognized, possibly preventing actual respiratory arrest. It is *anticipatory* nursing care that makes a significant impact on the successful management of the patient with or at risk of developing ARF. Clinical signs and symptoms of hypoxemia with hypercapnia are presented in Table 25–6.

Treatment and Management

Acute respiratory failure reflects the inability of patients to maintain adequate gas exchange. In some patients, impairment of gas exchange is mild and patients are responsive to "conservative" therapeutic techniques, whereas in others, it may be life-threatening and require emergency intervention. The survival of these patients depends on their ability to maintain adequate gas exchange over the course of the respiratory failure with the aid of timely, aggressive, and supportive forms of therapy. By supporting gas exchange for as long a period as necessary, the patient can be maintained while the underlying pathophysiologic process causing the failure is treated or allowed to resolve spontaneously. The overall goal of treatment and management of ARF is to "normalize" the

disturbed gas exchange and maintain the PaO_2 and pH. Normal gas exchange involves the adequate uptake of oxygen by the blood, transport of oxygen to the tissues, and the elimination of carbon dioxide. To achieve optimal oxygen transport to the tissues, it is essential to maintain PaO_2 of more than 60 mmHg; an SaO_2 of more than 90 mmHg; an acceptable hemoglobin level (hemoglobin, 12 g/100 ml; hematocrit 37% to 42%); and an adequate cardiac output (5 L/min).[2]

Carbon dioxide elimination by way of the lungs is essential for maintaining acid-base balance. In managing patients with ARF who have impaired elimination of carbon dioxide, the primary goal is to achieve a pH within the acceptable physiologic range (7.35 to 7.45) and not necessarily a "normal" $PaCO_2$. This distinction is particularly important in patients with a hypercapnic/hypoxemic form of ARF who have a prior history of chronic respiratory disease with chronic hypercapnia. An abrupt restoration of the $PaCO_2$ to normal ($PaCO_2$ of 35 to 45 mmHg) in these patients can result in alkalemia and serious complications (e.g., cardiac arrhythmias and seizures).

In ARF involving hypoxemia without hypercapnia, aggressive treatment with high fraction of inspired oxygen (FIO_2) is needed because severe hypoxemia is rapidly fatal. Interventions are aimed at increasing the SaO_2 to 90%. The initiation of mechanical ventilation in hypoxemic patients is considered when hypoxemia is refractory to increasing FIO_2 or when retention of carbon dioxide occurs leading to mental confusion or increased fatigue. Respiratory failure associated with hypoventilation and hypercapnia requires interventions that improve ventilation. Examples include the use of a narcotic antagonist to treat opiate overdose or mechanical ventilation if the disorder results from neuromuscular disease or neurologic trauma. For patients with acute, decompensating respiratory failure in whom gas exchange is seriously compromised (PaO_2 less than 50 mmHg; $PaCO_2$ greater than 50 mmHg), treatment and management involve timely and aggressive respiratory support therapy. This

TABLE 25–6
Hypoxemia and Hypercapnia: Physiologic Responses

Body System	Physiologic Responses
Neurologic	Restless, anxious, confused, disoriented, eventual lapse into coma
Cardiovascular	*Early:* tachycardia, increased contractility, peripheral vasoconstriction *Late:* depression of cardiac function due to increased acidemia; arrhythmias, decreased cardiac contractility
Respiratory	Increased respiratory rate and depth; dyspnea due to the increased work of breathing; ABGs: ↑ PCO_2, ↓ O_2
Metabolic	↓ pH, which continues to worsen over time
Renal	Decreased urine; acute tubular necrosis may develop
Gastrointestinal	↓ Bowel sounds; could progress to ischemic bowel

TABLE 25–7
Nursing Care Guidelines for the Patient with ARF

1. Continue to assess and monitor the patient's overall condition.
2. Establish and maintain a patent airway.
3. Provide appropriate ventilatory support and oxygenation.
4. Provide necessary cardiovascular support to maintain cardiac output and reduce occurrence of tissue hypoxia.
5. Treat the underlying primary disease.
6. Administer prescribed drug therapy and monitor the patient's response to therapy.
7. Maintain hydration and nutrition.
8. Correct or maintain fluid and electrolyte balance.
9. Prevent complications related to mechanical ventilation and artificial airway management.
10. Prevent infection.
11. Provide emotional and psychological support to patient and family.
12. Assist the patient in maintaining optimal physical function and performance of activities of daily living.

TABLE 25–8
Disorders Associated with ARDS

ARDS may result from a direct insult to the lung or from a systemic insult.

Lung Injury
Pneumonia: viral, bacterial, or fungal; *Pneumocystis carinii* infection
Embolism: fat, air
Lung contusion
Tuberculosis
Aspiration: gastric contents; fresh/salt water (near-drowning)
Inhaled toxins: oxygen toxicity, smoke, ammonia
Direct lung injury secondary to trauma

Systemic Causes
Shock of any type
Sepsis, especially gram-negative infections
Severe pancreatitis
Uremia
Drug overdose: narcotics (heroin, methadone); sedatives (barbiturates)
Neurogenic: head injury, intracranial trauma
Severe trauma of any type (massive motor vehicle accident)
Hematologic disorders: disseminated intravascular coagulation (DIC), massive transfusions, transfusion reactions

TABLE 25–9
Diagnostic Criteria for ARDS

Clinical presentation
  Tachypnea
  Dyspnea
  Use of accessory muscles
Medical history
  Direct lung injury or indirect systemic process (see Table 25–8)
Gas exchange
  Profound hypoxemia refractory to increased FIO_2 ($FIO_2 > 50\%$)
Pulmonary mechanics
  Increased FRC
  Decreased compliance
Chest x-ray
  Diffuse pulmonary infiltrates on exam
Hemodynamics
  PCWP within normal limits or <18 mmHg

includes oxygen therapy, chest physiotherapy, bronchial hygiene, airway management, and mechanical ventilation. The immediate therapeutic goals in the treatment and management of the patient with ARF are to relieve the hypoxemia and return the pH to within the acceptable physiologic range. See Table 25–7 for nursing care guidelines for the patient with ARF.

ADULT RESPIRATORY DISTRESS SYNDROME

Adult respiratory distress syndrome (ARDS) is characterized by a rapidly progressing and fulminating form of hypoxemic respiratory failure, which often occurs in previously healthy persons who have sustained a severe physiologic insult—pulmonary or nonpulmonary in origin. ARDS has been associated with a variety of causes or precipitating events (Table 25–8). Regardless of the underlying insult, ARDS is the final common clinical and pathologic pattern predisposing to the demise of the individual. The onset of ARDS usually occurs within hours or 3 to 4 days after the precipitating event. Despite intensive research and advances in supportive care over the past two decades, the mortality rate associated with ARDS varies from 50% to 76%.[3]

No single test is diagnostic of ARDS; rather, its identity is based on a description of its clinical presentation. See Table 25–9 for diagnostic criteria for ARDS.

Pathogenesis

The pathology underlying ARDS involves an increase in the permeability of the alveolar-capillary membrane leading to pulmonary interstitial and alveolar edema, or, as it is frequently termed, "noncardiogenic pulmonary edema." It is important to distinguish between the noncardiogenic pulmonary edema of ARDS and the cardiogenic pulmonary edema associated with left heart failure. See Table 25–10 for a comparison of cardiogenic and noncardiogenic pulmonary edema.

Under normal physiologic conditions, there is always a small net movement of fluid out of the pulmonary capillaries (intravascular space) into the lung interstitium (Fig. 25–2). An accumulation of this fluid within the interstitium does not normally occur, because any excess fluid or protein is drained by the pulmonary lymphatic system and eventually returned to the blood. Pulmonary edema occurs when there is an abnormal accumulation of fluid within the interstitial and air spaces of the lungs. The mechanisms underlying the pathogenesis of pulmonary edema may involve one or more of the following: (1) an increase in the hydrostatic pressure within the pulmonary capillaries; (2) an increase in the permeability of the alveolar-capillary membrane; and (3) an alteration in pulmonary lymphatic drainage.

Cardiogenic (Hydrostatic) Pulmonary Edema

Cardiogenic pulmonary edema occurs most often in the scenario of left heart failure. Its cause is essentially an imbalance between the hydrostatic and osmotic pressures that govern fluid movement within the lungs (see Fig. 25–2). As the volume of blood in the left ventricle at the end of diastole increases, the left ventricular end-diastolic pressure (LVEDP) increases and is reflected back to the pulmonary capillary bed. This increase in pulmonary intravascular hydrostatic pressure (represented clinically by an increase in the pulmonary capillary wedge pressure (PCWP) forces fluid out of the pulmonary capillaries and into the interstitium, causing pulmonary congestion.[4] When the amount of fluid in the interstitium exceeds the drainage capacity of the pulmonary lymphatic system or lymphatic drainage is impeded (e.g., after irradiation for lymph fibrosis and neoplasms), fluid is forced into the alveoli, causing pulmonary edema. In this form of pulmonary edema, the permeability of the microvascular membrane remains intact, limiting movement of protein out of the capillaries.

Noncardiogenic Pulmonary Edema

The mechanism leading to noncardiogenic pulmonary edema, or ARDS, involves an increase in the permeability of the alveolar-capillary membrane usually in the presence of normal pulmonary capillary hydrostatic pressure. As a consequence of the increase in permeability, plasma proteins and red blood cells, in addition to fluid, move out of the intravascular space and into the pulmonary interstitium. The exact cause (or causes) of the increase in membrane permeability remains undefined, but the theory is that it is related to mediators that cause lung injury.[5]

Initial pathologic changes reflect disruption of the capillary endothelium, which leads to leakage of fluid, protein, and cellular material into the interstitial space. This is followed by involvement of alveolar epithelial cells including both type I cell sloughing and type II cell dysfunction.

Damage to alveolar epithelial cells has profound effects on lung function. Type I cells are especially vulnerable to injury with limited reparative capabilities. Damage to these cells results in at least three pathophysiologic phenomena: alveolar edema, atelectasis, and decreased lung compliance associated with the atelectasis and loss of type I cell elasticity.[6] Type II cells, in contrast, are far less susceptible to injury and have notable reparative capabilities. Injury to these cells largely accounts for the severely decreased lung compliance and alveolar atelectasis secondary to surfactant dysfunction.

The pathology involved in ARDS leads to right-to-left shunting, evidenced by hypoxemia refractory to increasing FIO_2, and $\dot{V}/\dot{Q}$ mismatching. See Table 25–10 and the following explanations for a summary of pathophysiologic events underlying noncardiogenic pulmonary edema.

Pathophysiology

Shunting and $\dot{V}/\dot{Q}$ Mismatching

The pathologic processes of ARDS previously described play a major role in altering gas exchange and disrupting the mechanical properties of the lungs. Flooding the alveoli with fluid prevents ventilation of lung units, whereas perfusion may be relatively preserved. Consequently, unoxygenated blood is shunted into the pulmonary venous circulation and on into the left heart. This right-to-left shunting is a primary cause of hypoxemia in patients with ARDS and largely accounts for the refractoriness of the hypoxemia to supplemental oxygen therapy. In addition to areas of true shunting, there are also regions of $\dot{V}/\dot{Q}$ mismatching due in part to the uneven distribution of the pathologic processes within the lungs. Changes in blood flow do not necessarily follow those related to ventilation.

Altered Lung Compliance

Alterations in the mechanical properties of the lungs include a decrease in pulmonary compliance and a decrease in functional residual capacity (FRC). The presence of increased pulmonary interstitial fluid, together with alveolar collapse, contributes to a "stiffening" of the lung parenchyma. As a result, a progressively greater effort is expended to expand the lungs and maintain adequate alveolar ventilation. The increased work of breathing is associated with decreased tidal volume (V_T) and an increase in respiratory rate, which increases the relative dead space ventilation (V_{DS}/V_T).

Reduction in Lung Volumes

As a consequence of the increase in fluid occupying air spaces and widespread atelectasis, the volume of gas within the lungs is significantly reduced. Specifically, the FRC is significantly decreased (i.e., the volume of gas remaining within the lungs at end-expiration). Thus, not only is the work of breathing increased, but the volume of gas moved with each breath is also reduced. This rapid, shallow pattern of breathing, which necessitates increased energy expenditure, contributes significantly to the dyspnea so characteristic of patients with ARDS.

Clinical Presentation

After the initial physiologic insult, several hours to 1 day or more may elapse before consequences of the underlying pathologic processes of ARDS become evident clinically. Dyspnea and tachypnea are usually the

TABLE 25–10
Cardiogenic and Noncardiogenic Pulmonary Edema

	Noncardiogenic Pulmonary Edema (NCPE)	Cardiogenic Pulmonary Edema (CPE)
Etiology	See Table 25–8.	Occurs in the setting of left heart failure. Mitral stenosis/regurgitation can cause CPE with normal LVEDP.
Pathogenesis	Noncardiogenic pulmonary edema involves an increase in the permeability of the alveolar-capillary membrane, permitting the movement of fluid and protein out of the pulmonary capillary (intravascular) space into the pulmonary interstitium and alveolar air spaces.	An increase in LVEDP is reflected back to the pulmonary capillary bed increasing pulmonary intravascular hydrostatic pressure (PCWP).
Pulmonary capillary wedge pressure (PCWP)	Pulmonary hydrostatic pressures (PCWP) usually remain within normal limits, 8–12 mmHg.	An increase in PCWP forces fluid out of pulmonary capillaries into the lung interstitium, causing pulmonary congestion. When the fluid in the interstitium exceeds the reabsorptive capacity of the pulmonary lymphatic system, fluid is forced into the alveoli, causing pulmonary edema.
Pathology	Alteration in permeability of the alveolar-capillary membrane permitting a net egress of fluid and *protein* from the pulmonary intravascular into interstitial and alveolar spaces. Initial pathologic changes reflect disruption of the capillary endothelium followed by injury to types I and II pneumocytes. Resulting pathology includes: 1. Alveolar edema, atelectasis 2. Loss of type I cell elasticity 3. Altered surfactant activity Underlying initiating factors predisposing to acute lung injury:[1] 1. Increased accumulation of polymorphonuclear neutrophilic leukocytes (PMNs) in the patient with ARDS; release of potentially toxic mediators by these cells may account for injury to, and increased permeability of, the alveolar-capillary membrane. 2. Activated *complement* (C5a) promotes adherence of circulating granulocytes to pulmonary capillary endothelium (*leukotaxis*); it may induce release of chemotactic factor from alveolar macrophages. 3. Alveolar macrophages elaborate proteases, which perpetuate the inflammatory process. 4. Platelets release mediators (e.g., serotonin), which cause pulmonary arterial vasoconstriction. 5. Mast cells trigger release of vasoactive substances. The above factors may contribute to the self-destructive inflammatory response that occurs in the setting of ARDS.	In left heart failure, as cardiac output decreases, there is a "back-up" of blood, which accumulates in the pulmonary capillary bed, raising pulmonary capillary hydrostatic pressure. When capillary hydrostatic pressure exceeds pulmonary capillary oncotic pressure (see Fig. 25–2), fluid leaks into the pulmonary interstitium; when the reabsorptive capacity of the pulmonary lymphatic system is exceeded, fluid fills the alveoli causing pulmonary edema. CPE involves the increased infiltration of a *protein-poor* fluid across the microvascular membrane. This is contrary to noncardiogenic pulmonary edema wherein the defect in endothelial permeability involves the movement of both fluid and protein. Summary of pathophysiologic stages in cardiogenic pulmonary edema: 1. *Interstitial* stage—Lung interstitium swells with fluid as lymphatics are unable to reabsorb excess fluid. Patient may become restless and anxious. 2. *Alveolar* stage—Alveolar flooding with significant decrease in PaO_2, $PaCO_2$, and a rising pH. Tachypnea increases venous return and increases the volume of blood within the pulmonary capillary bed. 3. *Bronchial stages*—Infiltration of fluid within air spaces alters surfactant activity with atelectasis. Frothy, tenacious, often blood-tinged sputum may become evident; there is the appearance of rales (crackles). 4. *Final* stage—Tissue hypoxia occurs as the patient tires; hypoventilation ensues with consequent respiratory/acidemia (pH falls <7.35).
Pathophysiology Arterial blood gases	$\downarrow\downarrow$ PaO_2 (severe hypoxemia) $\downarrow$ To normal $PaCO_2$ (hypocapnia) Respiratory alkalemia	$\downarrow$ PaO_2 $\downarrow$ $PaCO_2$ early stage with respiratory alkalemia
Ventilation	$\uparrow$ Minute alveolar ventilation ($\dot{V}A$) (>20 L/min) $\uparrow$ Respiratory rate $\uparrow$ Dead-space ventilation (VDS) Reduced residual volume Reduced functional residual capacity (FRC)	Hyperventilation initially Advanced stage: $\uparrow$ $PaCO_2$ associated with patient exhaustion and compromised ventilatory effort $\uparrow$ Respiratory rate

TABLE 25–10
Cardiogenic and Noncardiogenic Pulmonary Edema (*Continued*)

	Noncardiogenic Pulmonary Edema (NCPE)	Cardiogenic Pulmonary Edema (CPE)
Pulmonary mechanics	↓ In lung compliance—stiffening of lung parenchyma ↓ FRC ↑ Work of breathing and increased respiratory rate resulting in decreased tidal volume	↓ In lung compliance especially with alveolar flooding; loss of surfactant activity to reduce surface tension ↑ Work of breathing ↓ FRC
Pulmonary pressures	Significantly widened alveolar-arterial oxygen tension ($P_{AO_2} - Pa_{O_2}$) Significant right-to-left shunting, which causes hypoxemia to be refractory to supplemental oxygen therapy even with an $F_{IO_2} > 60\%$ $\dot{V}/\dot{Q}$ mismatching Gas exchange compromised by alteration in surfactant activity Increase in pulmonary vascular resistance Pulmonary pressures: PCWP within 8–12 mmHg Pulmonary capillary permeability: increased Protein content of edema fluid: high	Widened $P_{AO_2} - Pa_{O_2}$ gradient $\dot{V}/\dot{Q}$ mismatching Right-to-left shunting (minimal) Hypoventilation in later stages Same as for noncardiogenic pulmonary edema during bronchial and final stages Pulmonary pressures: PCWP > 18 mmHg Transudation of fluid from intravascular to interstitium and alveoli; alveolar-capillary membrane intact Protein content of edema fluid: low
Clinical presentation	Hallmarks: 1. Marked respiratory distress with dyspnea and tachypnea; use of accessory muscles; increased work of breathing 2. Profound hypoxemia 3. Decrease in functional residual capacity and residual volume 4. Decreased lung compliance 5. Appearance of diffuse pulmonary infiltrates on chest x-ray 6. Physical findings: skin warm; full bounding pulses with increase in cardiac output; breath sounds reveal coarse rales: no jugular venous distention	Left-sided heart failure: 1. *Initial* stage: anxiety, restlessness, tachypnea, dyspnea, orthopnea, paroxysmal nocturnal dyspnea (PND), insomnia 2. *Advanced* stage: Tachycardia; palpitation; hypotension, diaphoresis Reduced lung compliance = ↑ work of breathing Cough productive of frothy, often blood-tinged sputum; pallor or cyanosis; cool mottled periphery Basilar rales; bronchial wheezing Increased jugular venous distention Gallop rhythm (S_3, S_4) Chest x-ray: initial interstitial pattern followed later by a pattern of diffuse airway disease 3. *Acute* stage: decreased level of consciousness with compromised cerebral perfusion; severely deranged gas exchange causes tissue hypoxia with shock and ventricular arrhythmias
Diagnostic criteria	1. Precipitating factor(s) or catastrophic physiologic insult (see Table 25–8) 2. Physiologic parameters: $Pa_{O_2} < 60$ mmHg with an $F_{IO_2} > 50\%$. Respiratory compliance decreased. 3. Chest x-ray with diffuse bilateral infiltrates 4. PCWP ~ 12 mmHg (8–12 mmHg)	In the early stages, it may be difficult to distinguish whether the pulmonary edema is cardiogenic or noncardiogenic in origin. Differential diagnosis: 1. Presence of precipitating event 2. Clinical presentation 3. Chest x-ray findings
Clinical history	Commonly, the patient is essentially healthy prior to precipitating event.	Frequently the patient presents with a history of chronic congestive heart failure or acute event preceding episode of pulmonary edema (e.g., myocardial infarction, pulmonary embolism).
Physical examination	Physical findings reflect high cardiac output (see clinical presentation) Lack of cardiomegaly Absence of extra heart sounds	Physical findings reflect low cardiac output; see clinical presentation above. Cardiomegaly is a frequent finding. S_3, S_4 frequently present.
ECG findings	ECG usually normal	ECG possibly reflective of signs of ischemia, injury, or infarction and previous pathology
Chest x-ray	Diffuse pulmonary infiltrates	Butterfly distribution of pulmonary infiltrates
Intrapulmonary shunt	Large increase characteristic of ARDS	Small increase
Hemodynamic parameters	Central venous pressure ~ 10 cm H_2O PCWP 8–12 mmHg	Central venous pressure > 20 cm H_2O PCWP > 18 mmHg
Other		Cardiac enzyme studies may point to cardiogenic pulmonary edema in early stages.

Continued

TABLE 25–10
Cardiogenic and Noncardiogenic Pulmonary Edema (*Continued*)

	Noncardiogenic Pulmonary Edema (NCPE)	Cardiogenic Pulmonary Edema (CPE)
Treatment (overall)	Initial treatment: 1. Establish or maintain patent airway. 2. Oxygen therapy to maintain $Pao_2 > 60$ mmHg. 3. Provide ventilation therapy to maintain $Paco_2$ 35–45 mmHg. 4. Correct acid-base abnormalities. 5. Correct electrolyte abnormalities.	
Goals of treatment	1. Treat precipitating event/disorder. 2. Stabilize permeability defect in alveolar-capillary membrane. 3. Support gas exchange until adequate pulmonary function is restored. 4. Prompt recognition with early institution of supportive therapy. 5. Prevent or decrease risk for additional insults that further deteriorate patient's clinical status.	1. Therapy in left ventricular failure: a. Reduce PCWP. b. Reduce venous return (preload). c. Reduce circulating blood volume. d. Reduce systemic blood pressure (afterload). e. Increase cardiac contractility.

Specific therapeutic modalities	Mainstay of treatment:
	Intubation with mechanical ventilation, PEEP, and oxygenation
	1. PEEP therapy
	  a. Indications for PEEP therapy[1]
	    • $Pao_2 < 60$ mmHg with $Fio_2 > 50\%$
	    • Diffuse lung disease bilaterally
	    • Prophylactic use at high risk of developing ARDS
	  b. Contraindications for PEEP therapy:
	    • Reduced extracellular fluid volume
	    • Patchy, necrotizing pulmonary process
	    • Unilateral lung disease
	  c. Desired effect: recruits and maintains open lung units that are otherwise collapsed
	    • Increases FRC
	    • Increases V_T and helps to prevent atelectasis
	    • Allows for better arterial oxygenation with lower Fio_2
	  d. Administration of PEEP early in disease course (dose)
	    • Early 5–15 cm H_2O
	    • Late 20–30 cm H_2O PEEP level sought: Progressive increments of 3–5 cm H_2O that allow maintenance of a hemoglobin-saturating Pao_2 with minimal compromise of cardiac output and oxygen transport
	  e. Assessment of response to PEEP therapy:
	    • Arterial blood gases
	    • Alveolar-arterial oxygen gradient
	    • PCWP and cardiac output
	    • Mixed venous oxygen tension
	    • Frequent determination of static compliance; large tidal volume plus PEEP allows for optimal lung compliance
	  f. Adverse effects of PEEP:
	    • ↓ Venous return = ↓ cardiac output
	    • ↑ Intracranial pressure by impeding cerebral venous drainage by jugular veins
		1. Venodilation therapy:
		  a. Increases size of venous capacitance vessels enabling a larger volume of blood to pool in the venous system, thus reducing venous return to the heart.
		  b. Specific drug therapy: *Morphine* is the most effective drug in emergency treatment of pulmonary edema. Its actions include vasodilatation; sedation, which relieves anxiety and fosters muscle relaxation; it reduces myocardial oxygen demand. *Diuretic therapy:* Furosemide increases venous capacitance, reducing venous return; it causes diuresis, which reduces circulatory blood volume. *Vasodilator therapy:* Nitroprusside, nitroglycerin, nitropaste, and others reduce vascular hydrostatic pressure and thus PCWP; they facilitate an increase in cardiac output by decreasing LVEDP. Use of intravenous nitroprusside and nitroglycerin decreases both preload and afterload by their vasodilating effects on systemic venous and arterial blood vessels. *Aminophylline therapy:* Used in conjunction with furosemide, may induce an enhanced diuresis; it also enhances cardiac output, increasing renal perfusion; it improves the Pao_2 by its bronchodilator effect.
		2. *Inotropic agents:* These agents improve cardiac output by increasing myocardial contractility; there is a concomitant reduction in left ventricular preload, which, in turn, reduces PCWP. Inotropic agents increase myocardial oxygen consumption and must be used with caution in the setting of myocardial infarction. Specific agents include digoxin, ouabain, dopamine, dobutamine, primacor, inocor.
		3. *Antiarrhythmia therapy* (e.g., lidocaine, quinidine, procainamide, calcium channel blockers).
		4. Intubation and mechanical ventilation with PEEP may be instituted in pulmonary edema, which is refractory to other therapeutic modalities.
		  a. Use of PEEP reduces intrapulmonary shunting; it also reduces left ventricular preload by a vasodilator effect on the venous capacitance system and by its effects on pleural pressures; PEEP decreases LVEDP, which may improve left ventricular ejection fraction and thus reduce PCWP.

TABLE 25–10
Cardiogenic and Noncardiogenic Pulmonary Edema (*Continued*)

	Noncardiogenic Pulmonary Edema (NCPE)	Cardiogenic Pulmonary Edema (CPE)

	• Barotrauma (pneumothorax, pneumomediastinum)
	• Reduced bronchial blood flow to lungs
	• Reduced renal perfusion
	• Negative inotropism of prostaglandins
	2. Supportive fluid therapy:
	  • Maintain PCWP between 8 and 12 mmHg to maintain cardiac output during positive-pressure and PEEP therapy.
	3. Treatment of underlying cause or precipitating event (e.g., use of antibiotics to treat infection)
	  • Avoid prophylactic use of antibiotics.
	4. High-dose corticosteroids: Definitive benefit questionable; use in ARDS controversial
	5. Supportive therapy to reduce hypoxemia/hypoxia:
	  a. Increase oxygen delivery to tissues.
	    • Administration of packed red blood cells to maintain hemoglobin ~11 g/100 mL
	    • Treatment of respiratory alkalemia and hypophosphatemia to shift oxygen-dissociation curve to right (enhances oxygen unloading at the tissue level)
	  b. Decrease in oxygen demand/consumption
	    • Hypothermia: decreases in cardiac output = ↓ shunt fraction; decreases oxygen demand
	    • Cautious use of sedatives (diazepam) in restless patient to keep patent airway secure
	  Mental status evaluation is essential to evaluate response to therapy. Use of sedation must be minimized.
	    • Muscle paralysis may be necessary in the extremely restless, hypoxic patient in whom a decrease in oxygen demand is necessary
	    • Pancuronium bromide (Pavulon) is the drug of choice, administered with diazepam to reduce anxiety associated with muscle paralysis
	6. Ancillary supportive measures:
	  a. Rigorous chest physiotherapy (bronchial) hygiene
	  b. Use of aminophylline for wheezing
	  c. Intravenous or enteral nutrition or both	

Complications	Outcome depends on nature and extent of pulmonary insult.
	Mortality: ~50%
	After illness sequelae: mild restrictive disease
	Mild impairment of gas exchange: ↓ PaO_2 especially during exercise
	Airflow obstruction of smaller airways
		Progressive deterioration of cardiopulmonary function:
		Serious cardiac arrhythmias
		Complications of treatment:
		  Digitalis toxicity
		  Fluid/electrolyte imbalance
		  Oxygen toxicity
		Cardiogenic shock

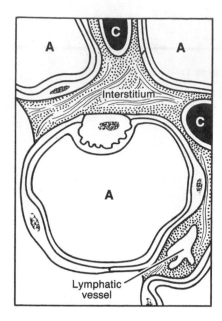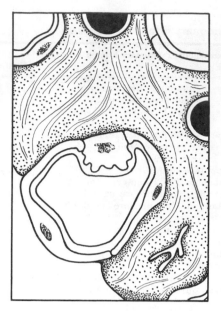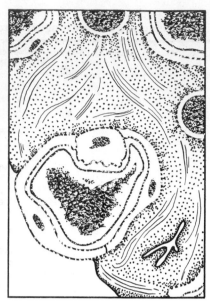

PULMONARY EDEMA

	NORMAL (mmHg)	CARDIOGENIC (mmHg)	NONCARDIOGENIC (mmHg)
Capillary hydrostatic pressure 8-12		> 12	~ 8-12
Capillary oncotic (osmotic) pressure 23-25		~ 23-25	Decreased (early) <23
Interstitial hydrostatic pressure −3		Increased	Increased
Interstitial oncotic (osmotic) pressure 16-19		~ 16-19	Increased > 19
Alveolar-capillary membrane permeability		Intact	Increased
Pulmonary lymphatic drainage		Intact (early)	Intact (early)

FIGURE 25–2. Underlying pathophysiology differentiating cardiogenic from noncardiogenic pulmonary edema. In cardiogenic edema, the alveolar-capillary membrane remains intact, but the capillary hydrostatic pressure is increased (>12 mmHg), thereby increasing movement (transudation) of fluid from the pulmonary capillary (C) (i.e., the intravascular space) into the interstitium. In noncardiogenic pulmonary edema, the capillary hydrostatic pressure remains within normal limits (~8–12 mmHg), but there is a significant drop in capillary osmotic pressure (<23 mmHg) and an increase in interstitial osmotic pressure (>19 mmHg) attributed to disruption in permeability of the alveolar—capillary membrane. This allows movement of proteins, fluid, and cells from the intravascular space (i.e., the capillary) into the interstitium and, thence, into the alveolus (A), with the consequent pressure changes.

initial symptoms experienced by the patient. ABGs usually reflect a disturbance in oxygenation (a decrease in PaO₂); PaCO₂ may be reduced because the patient is able to maintain adequate alveolar ventilation in the early period. An increase in the alveolar-arterial oxygen gradient (PAO₂ − PaO₂) may also become evident. Chest x-rays at this stage may be unremarkable.

With disease progression and continued leakage of fluid, protein, and blood cells from the intravascular space into interstitial and alveolar spaces, clinical findings become more definitive. The patient may become extremely dyspneic and tachypneic; breath sounds may reveal crackles; hypoxemia worsens with significantly widened PAO₂ − PaO₂; and chest x-rays become grossly abnormal, revealing significant infiltrates reflective of the fluid and protein within air spaces.

The progression of ARDS is variable from patient to patient, but affected patients generally become gravely ill as reflected by a mortality rate of 50%. Prior to the initial insult, many of these patients have normal pulmonary function. Yet within a matter of a few days, they may progress to life-threatening respiratory failure. Those fortunate enough to recover may have surprisingly few sequelae with pulmonary function returning essentially to premorbid status.

Treatment

Effective treatment of patients with ARDS requires a continuous effort to diagnose and treat the underlying precipitating event (Table 25–8). Goals of treatment are aimed at maintaining tissue oxygenation and reducing pulmonary edema. Effective treatment of the precipitating disorder, control of the permeability defect responsible for the leakage of fluid and protein, and support of gas exchange until adequate pulmonary function is reestablished are major goals in the treatment and management of patients with ARDS.[7] Prompt recognition of the syndrome with early institution of supportive measures remains a fundamental goal of therapy.

Intubation and mechanical ventilation are key treatments for ARDS, since fatigue and ventilatory failure occur. With hypoxemia that becomes refractory to increasing FIO_2, addition of positive end-expiratory pressure (PEEP) is generally necessary. PEEP, discussed in detail later in this chapter, reestablishes and maintains the patency of airways and alveoli and reduces the amount of right-to-left shunting. This, in turn, allows reduction of the FIO_2 necessary to relieve hypoxemia and reduces the potential for the development of oxygen toxicity associated with administration of high oxygen concentrations (FIO_2 greater than 50%).

Patients with an early form of noncardiogenic pulmonary edema may show significant improvement in gas exchange with a PEEP of 5 to 15 cm H_2O; those with severe ARDS may require as much as 15 to 30 cm H_2O of PEEP. Subsequent increments in PEEP are based on ABG analysis (PaO_2), mixed venous oxygen tension (PvO_2), lung compliance, and status of hemodynamic parameters (e.g., PCWP and cardiac output). The goal is to achieve a PEEP level that allows maintenance of a hemoglobin-saturating PaO_2 without significant compromise of cardiac output and oxygen transport.

Fluid and Electrolyte Management

Fluid management is a major consideration in the treatment of patients with ARDS. Overly vigorous administration of fluids may increase hydrostatic pressure within the pulmonary capillary bed and increase fluid content within the lung interstitium and air spaces. The consequence may be a larger shunt fraction contributing to hypoxemia. The goal of fluid therapy is to maintain cardiac output and blood flow to major organs while avoiding elevations in PCWP. Maintaining this delicate fluid balance requires continuous monitoring of pulmonary artery pressure and PCWP, together with appropriate pharmacologic manipulation.

Supportive Measures

Additional measures to be considered to achieve an increase in tissue perfusion include correction of respiratory alkalemia and hypophosphatemia. These conditions cause a shift of the oxygen dissociation curve to the right, reducing the amount of oxygen released to the tissues (see Fig. 22–14). Methods for decreasing oxygen demand and consumption may also be instituted. Careful use of sedatives (e.g., diazepam) or a muscle-paralyzing agent (e.g., pancuronium) reduces oxygen consumption by decreasing muscle tone and activity. Hypothermia also reduces oxygen demand. Use of the various modalities may allow FIO_2 to be reduced to less than 50%, thus minimizing the danger of oxygen toxicity while effectively treating the hypoxemia.

Positioning the patient with ARDS to maximize oxygenation is an important independent nursing function. In a review of research, Schmitz[8] concluded that patients with basilar or diffuse bilateral disease such as ARDS should be tried in the prone position. This position may improve $\dot{V}/\dot{Q}$ mismatching and alveolar ventilation.

Successful treatment and management of ARDS depend to a large extent on the nurse's awareness of the patient's entire clinical status in addition to the mechanical ventilatory and pharmaceutical support. Meticulous attention to the patient's responses to therapeutic modalities as well as knowledge of the adverse effects of these modalities are important considerations in the ongoing monitoring and care of the patient with ARDS.

Nursing Care of the Patient with ARDS

The critical care nurse plays a crucial role in the assessment, diagnosis, and management of the patient with ARDS who develops hypoxemic respiratory failure. The immediate therapeutic goal in the nursing care of these critically ill patients is to act in a timely and purposeful manner to relieve life-threatening hypoxemia and to assist in reestablishing adequate gas exchange. To effectively meet the challenge presented by ARDS, it is essential that critical care nurses have a thorough grasp of underlying cardiopulmonary physiology and an in-depth understanding of this syndrome—the setting in which it occurs, its pathophysiology, clinical manifestations, and necessary therapeutic interventions.

What makes ARDS particularly challenging to diagnose and treat is that no clinically valid diagnostic tests or procedures have been developed to assist in its early diagnosis. This is regrettable because therapeutic intervention instituted early in the course of ARDS can often mean the difference between the patient's complete recovery and his or her ultimate demise. This fact serves to punctuate the necessity for thorough ongoing assessment and monitoring of patients who are at risk of developing ARDS.

Goals of Nursing Care

The overall therapeutic goal in the management of the patient in hypoxemic respiratory failure associated with ARDS is to maintain adequate gas exchange through timely, aggressive, and supportive interventions. Meticulous supportive nursing care is necessary to maximize the therapeutic effects and prevent complications. Nursing functions to maintain the essential bodily processes within the patient until effective spontaneous physiologic functions are restored. Through ongoing assessment and timely, appropriate interventions, the astute critical care nurse provides the quality of care necessary not only to maintain these patients over the critical course of the illness, but also to make a positive impact on the patient's ultimate prognosis. Implementation of nursing process in the care of the patient with ARDS and hypoxemic respiratory failure revolves around the therapeutic goals listed in Table 25–7. Pertinent nursing diagnoses, desired patient outcomes, nursing interventions, and their rationales are presented in the care plan for the patient with ARDS at the end of this chapter.

Research and ARDS

Experimental treatments for ARDS include extracorporeal carbon dioxide removal, a concept that actually allows mechanical ventilation of these patients with lower airway pressures.[9] Because the high pressures that are required to ventilate ARDS patients can actually damage the lungs, this device offers hope for the future. Extracorporeal carbon dioxide removal is still experimental. Other experimental treatments include the use of surfactant replacement, which has shown success in neonates, but has been used on a limited basis with ARDS.[10] Surfactant replacement to improve lung compliance and increase alveolar surface area for oxygen exchange in ARDS shows promise and will continue to be investigated. The use of inhaled nitric oxide to reduce pulmonary vascular resistance in ARDS is a controversial treatment still under investigation.[11]

Other research has demonstrated the potential benefits of using nonsteroidal anti-inflammatory drugs (NSAIDs) such as indomethacin and ibuprofen because of their ability to diminish platelet and neutrophil aggregation and the generation of oxygen radicals.[10] Human studies have demonstrated a benefit in

using NSAIDs with sepsis, but further investigations are needed to demonstrate benefits with acute lung injury.

Medical interventions such as oxygenation, mechanical ventilation, and cardiovascular stabilization ensure tissue oxygenation and remain the backbone of treatment of ARDS. New therapies that attempt to prevent or interrupt the destructive effects of the mediators that cause lung injury, replace surfactant, and extracorporeally extract carbon dioxide continue to be investigated so that more positive patient outcomes can be achieved.

THERAPEUTIC MODALITIES IN THE TREATMENT OF ACUTE RESPIRATORY FAILURE

A continuous supply of oxygen to the tissues is essential to sustain cellular metabolism, prevent tissue hypoxia, and maintain life processes. Regardless of its underlying cause, treatment of patients with hypoxemia may require timely and aggressive respiratory support therapy, such as oxygen therapy, airway management, chest physiotherapy, and mechanical ventilation. These therapeutic modalities, together with implications for nursing care, are examined more closely in the discussion that follows.

Oxygen Therapy

Therapeutic Goals

The purpose of oxygen therapy is to relieve hypoxemia and prevent tissue hypoxia. Although the basic treatment of hypoxemia is the treatment of its cause, the immediate potentially life-threatening problem may be tissue hypoxia as a consequence of severely lowered PaO_2. Tissue hypoxia is assumed to be present at a PaO_2 of less than 60 mmHg and a lowered SaO_2 of less than 90%. Thus, regardless of the underlying cause of hypoxemia, oxygen is the initial and perhaps most important drug in its treatment.

Dosage and Methods of Oxygen Administration

Low-Flow Oxygen Systems. Low-flow oxygen systems do not provide sufficient gas to supply the entire inspired volume.[12] The term "low-flow" implies that the concentration of oxygen delivered relies on a mixture of ambient air and oxygen. The overall oxygen concentration will be altered by VT and ventilatory pattern.

Nasal cannulas and catheters are the most commonly used devices for administering low-flow oxygen and can provide from 24% to 50% oxygen at flow rates up to 6 L/min. Nasal catheters are not used very often because of the need to move the catheter every day to the alternate nare to minimize pharyngeal damage. Nasal cannulas are the most commonly used device for oxygen administration and are usually well tolerated by patients. Care must be taken not to use greater than 6 L/min flow for the nasal cannula to prevent drying and irritation of the nasal mucosa.

Simple oxygen masks deliver about 35% to 60% oxygen with flow rates of 5 L/min or more. Masks with reservoir (rebreathing or nonrebreathing) are capable of delivering a high FIO_2 of greater than 50%. A more recent method of oxygen delivery for patients requiring continuous oxygen therapy is the transtracheal oxygen delivery system, a small tracheal catheter that replaces the nasal cannula for low-flow oxygen delivery.[13] This device may decrease the oxygen flow rate needed to support the same oxygenation as nasal oxygen and can potentially improve oxygentation in some patients.

High-Flow Oxygen Systems. High-flow oxygen systems can provide flow rates that completely satisfy the patient's inspiratory demand, either by entrainment of ambient air or by a high flow of gas. These systems can provide either high or low FIO_2.

Venturi masks are designed to deliver 24%, 28%, 35%, and 40% oxygen. The recommended flow rates are 6 L/min, 6 L/min, 10 L/min, and 10 L/min, respectively. Venturi masks can be used with patients who have chronic obstructive lung disease, because they deliver a precise concentration of oxygen. Reservoir nebulizers and humidifiers with aerosol masks, face tents, continuous positive airway pressure (CPAP) masks, T tubes, or tracheostomy collars provide both supplemental oxygen and increased water vapor mist.

Complications of Oxygen Therapy

It is essential for the critical care nurse to be familiar with the adverse effects of oxygen therapy. Some of these are oxygen toxicity, absorption atelectasis, oxygen-induced hypoventilation, drying of respiratory mucosa, and psychological dependence.

Oxygen Toxicity. Oxygen toxicity is associated with long-term exposure to high inspired oxygen concentrations (FIO_2 greater than 60% for more than 2 to 3 days). Topical damage to alveolar tissue may lead to the development of a thickened alveolar-capillary membrane with consequent diffusion impairment. The earliest signs and symptoms include substernal chest pain and cough with tracheal irritation. Late symptoms are inspiratory pain and dyspnea. The pathophysiologic changes that occur with oxygen toxicity are similar to those which occur with ARDS: (1) interstitial noncardiogenic pulmonary edema, (2) alveolar hemorrhage with destruction of the surfactant-producing cells, and (3) consolidation and fibrosis of the lungs.

Intermittent exposure to oxygen appears to be .he strongest factor that may impede the onset of oxygen toxicity. Because most critically ill patients become hypoxemic at some point, oxygen administration is the drug of choice. The potential for oxygen toxicity may be avoided by limiting prolonged exposure to high concentrations of oxygen. The use of other modes of treatment such as CPAP and PEEP may be beneficial in allowing reductions of oxygen concentrations. However, patients should not suffer from tissue hypoxia to limit the potential for oxygen toxicity. The best approach is careful administration of oxygen to limit hypoxemia without overtreatment.

Absorption Atelectasis. Breathing high concentrations of oxygen increases tension PAO_2, while decreasing the level of nitrogen. Nitrogen does not diffuse from the alveolus into the pulmonary capillary as oxygen does. It remains in the alveolus and is responsible for keeping the alveolus open. For a patient on high concentrations of oxygen, the nitrogen that is normally in the alveolus is "washed out" and replaced by the oxygen, eventually leading to alveolar collapse.

Oxygen-Induced Hypoventilation. This complication is seen in patients who develop ARF superimposed on chronic lung disease. The increased carbon dioxide tension associated with chronic alveolar hypoventilation causes the patient's respiratory centers to become insensitive to normal fluctuations in $PACO_2$. As a consequence, the patient's respiratory stimulus becomes a low arterial oxygen tension or hypoxic drive. Administration of oxygen in concentrations sufficient to obliterate this hypoxic drive may cause apnea, which is the underlying reason for administering supplemental oxygen at controlled low concentrations in patients with hypercapnic/hypoxemic respiratory failure.

Drying of Respiratory Mucosa. Drying of the respiratory mucosa occurs when oxygen is administered without humidification. It results in a thickening of respiratory secretions with disruption of the integrity of the respiratory epithelium. Mucosal bleeding may occur, and the patient has an increased risk of developing retained secretions, leading to atelectasis or infection.

Principles of Oxygen Therapy

For a review of the basic principles of oxygen therapy, see Table 25–11.[14]

Chest Physiotherapy-Bronchial Hygiene

Therapeutic Goals

Retained pulmonary secretions predispose to atelectasis and infection (e.g., pneumonia) with a consequent increase in $\dot{V}/\dot{Q}$ mismatch and right-to-left shunting. The end-result is hypoxemia with tissue hypoxia.

Chest physiotherapy is a series of manipulative assistive techniques designed to be both preventive and therapeutic. Chest physiotherapy techniques, in conjunc-

TABLE 25–11
Principles of Oxygen Therapy

1. A patent airway must be maintained. Oxygen therapy is of no use without a patent airway.
2. Oxygen is a potent drug and, as such, should be administered in a prescribed dose (the FIO_2 is the dose) and evaluated for desired, as well as adverse, effects.
3. If high concentrations are necessary, duration of administration should be kept to a minimum and reduced as soon as possible.
4. The goal is to maintain PaO_2 greater than 60 mmHg to produce acceptable saturation of hemoglobin (SaO_2 >90%) without damaging lungs or causing carbon dioxide retention.
5. Response to oxygen therapy should be evaluated in terms of its effect on tissue oxygenation rather than its effect on ABG values alone.
6. Periodic ABG monitoring is a necessary assessment parameter when oxygen concentrations above 40% are administered.
7. The pathophysiology of the patient's disease is a major determinant of the effectiveness of oxygen therapy.
8. Delivered concentrations of gas from low-flow or high-flow oxygen systems are subject to the condition of the equipment, technique of application, cooperation of the patient, and the rate, depth, and pattern of the patient's ventilations. Oxygen analyzers should be used periodically to determine actual FIO_2.
9. Low-flow oxygen systems do not provide the total inspired gas (patient is breathing some ambient air) and therefore are effective only if V_T is adequate, respiratory rates are not excessive, and the ventilatory pattern is stable. Variable oxygen concentrations of 21%–90+% are provided, but the FIO_2 varies greatly with changes in V_T and breathing patterns.
10. High-flow oxygen systems provide the entire inspired gas (patient is breathing only the gas supplied by the apparatus) and are adequate only if flow rates exceed inspiratory flow rate and minute ventilation. Both high and low oxygen concentrations may be delivered by high-flow systems (FIO_2 24%–100%).
11. Concerns about "oxygen toxicity" should *never* prevent adequate oxygenation of the patient. Although the phenomenon of oxygen toxicity is very real, hypoxemia "kills."

Source: Modified from Neagley, S: The pulmonary system. In Alspach, J (ed): AACN's Core Curriculum for Critical Care Nursing, ed 4. WB Saunders, Philadelphia, p 76, 1991.

tion with bronchial hygiene (pulmonary toilet), assist in mobilizing bronchial secretions, facilitating their removal from the respiratory tract, and preventing accumulation of secretions within the tracheobronchial tree. Techniques of chest physiotherapy are postural drainage, percussion and vibration techniques, deep-breathing exercises, incentive spirometry, and intermittent positive-pressure breathing. A systematic approach to the implementation of these techniques should be used.[15]

Airway Management

Therapeutic Goals

A major goal of effective respiratory care is to establish or maintain a patent airway to ensure adequate alveolar ventilation. Airway management is concerned with maintaining the integrity of respiratory passageways to allow for proper ventilation and to facilitate removal of secretions.

Risks of Airway Management

The major risk encountered in airway management is a disruption of the normal integrity of the respiratory tract, with consequent contamination and potential infection of the respiratory system. The placement of artificial airways extending into the trachea bypasses the normal protective mechanisms of the upper airways involved in warming, filtering, and humidifying inhaled gases. Bypassing the upper airway defense mechanisms allows microorganisms and other foreign matter in the unfiltered inspired gas to enter the lower airways.

Under normal physiologic circumstances, the respiratory tract is considered to be sterile distal to the larynx. Consequently, all procedures involving artificial airways should be performed using aseptic technique. Placement of an artificial airway through the glottis interferes with or reduces the effectiveness of the coughing mechanisms, which plays a crucial role in clearing secretions from the respiratory tract.

Bypassing the humidification function of the upper airway increases the risk of dehydration of the respiratory mucosa. Consequent loss of the mucociliary transport activity of the respiratory epithelium compromises movement of secretions toward the large bronchi and trachea, where they are accessible to removal by suctioning. Accumulation and pooling of secretions within the tracheobronchial tree predispose to airway obstruction and provide a milieu conducive to colonization by microorganisms. The patient is at increased risk of developing infection (pneumonia). Humidification devices are required when artificial airways are used.

Placement of most artificial airways eliminates the ability of the patient to communicate verbally. Special adaptors for tracheostomies enable the patient to talk while mechanical ventilation is maintained. These devices are usually reserved for the stable patient who has a minimal amount of secretions. In patients with standard endotracheal tubes, it is imperative that some form of communication be established to enable the patient, family, and healthcare providers to understand each other more clearly.

If the patient is able to write, a writing pad should be provided. A chalkboard can be very helpful, if available. Picture cards can also be used to facilitate communication. A signal method, such as a shake of the head, blinking of the eyes, or movement of fingers, can be implemented.

Patients often become frightened when they realize that they cannot ask questions regarding their condition or care. Patients need frequent reassurance that their needs will be met and that someone is always nearby, anticipating needs or attending to problems and concerns as they arise.

Artificial Airways

Pharyngeal Airways. The nasopharyngeal and oro-pharyngeal airways are used for short-term airway maintenance. They function to hold the tongue away from the posterior wall of the pharynx. Pharyngeal airways are designed to allow air flow around or through them, and they easily accommodate the passage of a suction catheter into the laryngopharynx. The oro-pharyngeal tube may cause gagging, vomiting, or laryngospasm in the conscious or semiconscious patient (Fig 25–3).

Endotracheal Tubes

Endotracheal tubes are flexible, hollow cylindrical airways designed for nasal or oral insertion (Fig. 25–3). They come equipped with an inflatable balloon or cuff, which provides a seal to prevent aspiration of oral secretions and facilitates mechanical ventilation.

The endotracheal tube may be placed orally or nasally. Nasal intubation is frequently used for long-term intubation because it is easier to stabilize, has a decreased risk of extubation, and is usually better tolerated by the conscious patient. Its major drawback is that a smaller diameter tube is required, which can potentially increase airway resistance.

More frequently, endotracheal intubation is accomplished using the oral approach, especially in an emergency situation. Oral intubation requires a tube with a larger diameter, which reduces airway resistance and facilitates spontaneous or mechanical ventilation. Oral intubation may be especially indicated for the patient with thick, copious pulmonary secretions, which require a larger size suction catheter for effective secretion removal.

Preparation for Intubation. Prior to intubation, competency of the cuff is established by injecting 10 mL of air into it, or the amount indicated on the tube. Appropriate explanations are made to the patient, if possible, and the patient is then sedated if awake and alert. Medication administration allows for a more controlled intubation and reduces the possibility of trauma and laryngospasms. Prior to actual intubation, the laryngoscope blade is attached to verify that the light works. At least three people are necessary for intubation: (1) a person properly credentialed in intubation; (2) a person to manage the airway, provide supplemental oxygen, and set up respiratory modalities after intubation; and (3) a person to attend to the patient's needs, to give medications, and to assist with airway care.

Assessment for Correct Airway Placement. Upon insertion of the endotracheal tube, it is essential to assess for correct placement by following the techniques listed in Table 25–12. There is always the danger that, if the endotracheal tube is passed too far, it will enter the right mainstem bronchus, which continues from the bifurcation of the trachea in a nearly vertical course (see Fig. 22–1). If this occurs, upon cuff inflation ventilation will be exclusively to the right lung. The unventilated left lung will develop atelectasis, and respiratory insufficiency with hypoxemia and tissue hypoxia may rapidly ensue.

Ideally, the tip of the endotracheal tube should be about 3 cm above the carina. Adequate stabilization of the airway is a major nursing concern to ensure optimal ventilation. After airway placement is confirmed, the endotracheal tube should be marked at the point at which it emerges from the mouth. The tube should be taped securely because body movements may lead to accidental extubation or endobronchial intubation. If an oral endotracheal tube is inserted, an oral airway may also be inserted as a "bite block." The position of the endotracheal tube should be changed from side to side every 8 hours to relieve pressure on the lips and tongue. Frequent and aggressive oral hygiene should be provided.

Cuff Inflation and Deflation. Endotracheal tubes in current use have cuffs that are soft and pliable and of low pressure if inflated properly. This has allowed endotracheal tubes to remain in place for increased periods of time. Three weeks is now considered standard. If longer-term airway management is anticipated, a tracheostomy is usually performed.

The responsibility of the critical care nurse is to make sure that an optimal low pressure is always maintained. Cuff inflation requires only the amount of air

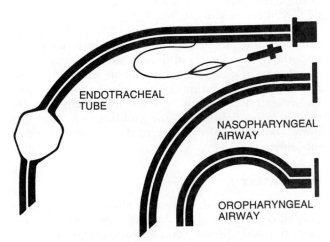

FIGURE 25–3. Artificial airways.

ENDOTRACHEAL TUBE

NASOPHARYNGEAL AIRWAY

OROPHARYNGEAL AIRWAY

TABLE 25–12

Assessment for Correct Endotracheal Tube Placement

Immediately after intubation, the cuff is inflated and the patient is ventilated and oxygenated.
Placement verification:
1. Auscultation for bilateral breath sounds
2. Feeling/listening for air flow through the tube opening
3. Observation for symmetric, bilateral chest movement
4. Immediate chest x-ray

necessary to achieve a minimal air leak. Tracheal damage occurs when the pressure extended by the inflated cuff against the tracheal walls exceeds the tracheal capillary pressure, which is about 25 mmHg. Usually the maximum pressure exerted by an inflated cuff is about 15 to 20 mmHg. The actual pressure can be determined by connecting the balloon port to a manometer. If increasing amounts of air are needed to obtain a seal, tracheal dilation or a leak in the cuff should be suspected. Regardless of cuff design or pressure characteristics, all cuff pressures should be evaluated every 4 to 8 hours.

Complications of Endotracheal Intubation. Problems encountered with use of endotracheal tubes usually occur at pressure points along the respiratory tract (Table 25–13).[16,17] Nasal endotracheal tubes, for example, may cause nosebleed, sinusitis, pressure necrosis to the cartilaginous structure of the nose, or turbinate fracture. Both nasal and oral endotracheal tubes have the potential to cause pressure-induced trauma to the glottis, the subglottic area, and the larynx.

Commonly, complications involving these areas

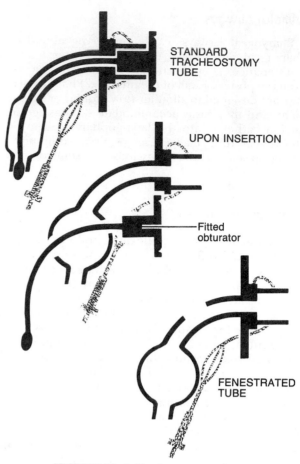

FIGURE 25–4. Tracheostomy tubes.

TABLE 25–13
Complications of Endotracheal Intubation

Complications of Laryngoscopy
Lip lacerations
Tooth avulsion
Esophageal lacerations
Aspiration

Complications During Intubation
Laryngospasm
Bronchospasm
Cardiac arrhythmias
Labile blood pressure
Misplacement of tube
  Nasal intubation:
    Nosebleed, sinusitis, otitis media
    Pressure necrosis of nose cartilage
    Turbinate fracture
  Tracheostomy:
    Bleeding, hematoma formation
    Subdermal tissue dissection with consequent inability to pass
      tube into trachea
    Subcutaneous emphysema
    Tracheostomy tube obstructed by blood, tissue, or secretions
    Aspiration
    Pneumothorax, pneumomediastinum

Complications After Intubation
Endotracheal tube kinked or obstructed
Increased airway resistance leading to increased work of breathing
  due to small diameter of tube
Aspiration
Pneumothorax, pneumomediastinum
Endotracheal tube cuff leak

Complications After Confirmation of Correct Placement
Dislodgement of tube due to patient movement (tube must be
  secured with tape)

Source: Modified from Hoffman, L, Mazzucco, L, and Roth, J: Fine tuning your chest PT. Am J Nurs 87:1566, 1987; and Boggs, R: Airway management. In Boggs, R and Wooldridge-King, M (eds): AACN Procedure Manual for Critical Care, ed 3, WB Saunders, Philadelphia, p 1–54.

become especially significant after extubation. Complications after correct endotracheal tube placement has been verified by chest x-ray and can occur with patient movement. Neck extension causes the tube to move up. With upward movement, the endotracheal tube cuff may become positioned above the vocal cords. If this occurs, an increase in cuff inflation may become necessary to maintain a seal, and the tube may be forced out of the trachea.

Whenever a leak arises around the endotracheal tube cuff, the cuff should be completely deflated, the endotracheal tube repositioned, and the cuff reinflated so as to maintain a minimal air leak. If a sealed airway is desired, a minimal occlusive volume is used. Head flexion causes the tube to move down into the mainstem bronchus, and the endotracheal tube can move about 2 cm from a neutral position with head movement.

Tracheostomy

Tracheostomy is the airway of choice for long-term assisted or controlled mechanical ventilation. It facilitates removal of thick, tenacious secretions. A tracheostomy may be established to bypass an upper airway obstruction. It may be more comfortable than other

TABLE 25–14
Tracheostomy Tube Styles

Style Name	Description
Shiley, Portex, National	A plastic tube usually composed of parts: an inner cannula—disposable or nondisposable—an obturator, and a soft cuff. (Some Portex tubes do not have inner cannulas)
Lanz	A plastic tube with a pressure-regulating valve, soft cuff, and external balloon
Fenestrated	A tube with precut openings in the outer cannula, useful in weaning patients from long-term mechanical ventilation
Kamen-Wilkinson	A foam-filled plastic tube without an inner cannula that requires minimal air for inflation
Jackson	A metal tube with an inner cannula and an obturator; uncuffed and designed for long-term usage
Kistner	Also referred to as a tracheostomy button, one-way valve attached to the outer cannula; permits airflow through the tube during inspiration and closes during expiration; permits speaking and coughing
Pitt Trach Speaking Tube	A tube that permits speaking and coarse whispers in the presence of continuous air/oxygen ventilation

Source: From Boggs, R: Airway management. In Boggs, R and Wooldridge-King, M (eds): AACN Procedure Manual for Critical Care, ed 3, WB Saunders, Philadelphia, p 56, with permission.

airways and allows the patient to eat and, with some adaptations, to speak.

The standard tracheostomy tube is designed for placement beneath the second cartilaginous ring below the cricoid cartilage (see Fig. 22–1). As a sterile procedure, it is preferable to perform a tracheostomy on an elective basis in an operating room setting. However, it may be performed at the bedside in the ICU setting, or in an emergency situation. Upon insertion of the tracheostomy tube, the cuff is inflated, and the airway is assessed immediately for patency and correct placement. Auscultation for breath sounds and examination for bilateral chest wall excursion are performed. A chest x-ray is obtained to ascertain exact tube position within the trachea.

Each tracheostomy tube is packaged with a fitted obturator, which is used only for insertion or reinsertion (Fig. 25–4). This device should be kept wrapped and in an obvious place at the patient's bedside to be available for reinsertion of the tube, if necessary. The obturator, with its rounded tip, eliminates the blunt edge of the tracheostomy tube and facilitates reinsertion. See Table 25–14 for the different types of tracheostomy tubes and their potential uses.[16]

Complications of Tracheostomy. The most immediate complication of a tracheostomy is local wound bleeding. Aspiration of blood into the tracheobronchial tree may obstruct airways with clots, leading to atelectasis. Clotted blood also serves as an excellent culture medium for bacterial colonization with consequent infection. See Table 25–15 for the major

TABLE 25–15
Complications of Tracheostomy

Laryngospasm, bronchospasm (usually observed during procedure)
Cardiac arrhythmias, labile blood pressure (usually observed during procedure)
Bleeding, hematoma formation
Subdural tissue dissection with consequent inability to pass tube into trachea
Subcutaneous emphysema
Tracheostomy tube obstructed by blood, secretions, or tissue
Aspiration
Pneumothorax, pneumomediastinum
Infection

immediate and long-term complications associated with tracheostomy.

Tracheostomy Care. Tracheostomy care is performed at least every 8 hours, or more frequently if needed, to maintain airway patency, to reduce the risk of infection, and to make the tracheostomy more aesthetically acceptable to patient, family, and significant others. See Table 25–16 for key points in tracheostomy care.[18]

Airway Suctioning. Airway suctioning with secretion removal is a major goal in airway management (Table 25–17).[16] Suctioning should be performed on an as-needed basis limiting the duration to 10 seconds or less. Although frequently performed, endotracheal suction is associated with several complications: hypoxemia, cardiac arrhythmia, hypotension, hypertension, increased intracranial pressure, atelectasis, trauma to the airway, and nosocomial infections.[19]

Techniques to prevent complications are hyperinflation and hyperoxygenation prior to suctioning. These procedures can be done through the use of a manual resuscitation bag or with the assistance of the ventilator (see the Research Application box on page 453). A newer technology used to prevent hypoxemia during suctioning is the closed tracheal suction system (CTSS). Research related to this device is controver-

TABLE 25–16
Tracheostomy Care Guidelines

Nursing care for the patient with a tracheostomy centers around two important goals: maintenance of a patent airway and prevention of complications.
Key points of tracheostomy care:
1. Assess respiratory rate, rhythm, depth, and quality at least once a shift.
2. Suction as needed.
3. Keep obturator at bedside for reinsertion of tube should it become dislodged.
4. Assess color, viscosity, and quality of secretions.
5. Monitor stomal site for redness, swelling, and odor.
6. Provide stomal care at least once a shift and as needed per hospital policy, replacing or cleaning inner cannula at this time.
7. Assess for vascular sensitivity. (If tube fluctuates with patient's pulse, suspect that it is rubbing against an artery, which could cause erosion.)

Source: Adapted from Weilitz, P and Dettenmeier, P: Test your knowledge of tracheostomy tubes. Am J Nurs 94:49, 1994.

TABLE 25–17
Procedure for Endotracheal Suctioning

Procedure	Rationale
1. Assess for signs and symptoms indicative of need for suctioning.	Unnecessary suctioning should be avoided because it is uncomfortable and may be hazardous to the patient.
2. In the conscious patient, the procedure should be clearly explained. Stress necessity and importance of procedure in maintaining airway patency.	This encourages patient's cooperation during the procedure.
3. Position patient in semi-Fowler's sitting position at about 45-degree angle.	This facilitates airway alignment; straightening of trachea ensures greater patency; it allows for full use of respiratory musculature, and improves coughing.
4. Wash hands.	
5. Assemble sterile suctioning equipment. (A 14F catheter is commonly used in adults; catheter should be less than one third the inner airway diameter.)	Catheter exceeding one third the airway diameter increases risk of suction-induced hypoxia and atelectasis.
6. Preoxygenate and hyperventilate patient with 100% oxygen using resuscitator bag, or ventilator.	This helps to minimize suctioning hypoxia and atelectasis.
7. Glove and maintain sterility of dominant hand; glove and maintain clean technique of nondominant hand. (Two-glove technique may be preferred.)	Sterility decreases the incidence of contamination and infection.
8. Using nondominant hand, remove ventilation tube or open suctioning port on swivel adapter. Place ventilator tubing end on sterile gauze pad or drape.	Sterile handling prevents contamination of ventilator tubing.
9. Using sterile gloved dominant hand, pick up catheter and connect to suction source; thumb of opposite "clean" gloved hand controls suction port.	
10. Lubricate catheter with sterile saline.	Surgical lubricant is usually unnecessary and may accumulate on inner surface of endotracheal tube.
11. Using sterile gloved hand, insert catheter into endotracheal tube as far as it will go. Do not force catheter.	Do not apply suction while advancing catheter because this will "steal" oxygen from within the airway.
12. Withdraw catheter 1 cm to free it from respiratory mucosa; apply intermittent suction by quickly opening and closing suction thumb port.	Application of continuous suction should be avoided to prevent the catheter from "grabbing" the respiratory mucosa and causing trauma.
13. Withdraw catheter using a rotating motion; entire suctioning pass should not exceed 10 sec.	Rotating motion sweeps the catheter tip against all sides of the airway as the catheter is withdrawn.
14. Hyperinflate patient's lungs with 100% oxygen using resuscitator bag.	Hyperinflation helps to re-expand sections of the lung that may have collapsed with evacuation of air; it minimizes hypoxia due to suction-induced atelectasis.
15. The above steps should be repeated each time the suction maneuver is done.	Maintain rigorous aseptic technique because impaired pulmonary defense systems place the patient at high risk of infection.
Note: If the endotracheal tube cuff is to be deflated, suction above the cuff prior to deflation.	Suctioning will prevent secretions from being deposited within the tracheobronchial tree.
	Never use the same catheter to suction oral and nasal cavities and then lower airways.
16. Reconnect patient to ventilator or close suction port of the swivel adapter.	
17. Reassess patient's airway status.	
Additional tips	
18. Minimize frequency and duration of suctioning when PEEP is required.	Small suction-induced changes may have profound effects on a high-risk, refractory, hypoxemic patient.
19. Patient's hydration status should be monitored closely, including daily weight and intake and output. Maintain humidification of inspired gas.	Hydration helps to minimize viscosity of pulmonary secretions, facilitating their removal. Humidification prevents drying of respiratory epithelium.

Source: Modified from Hoffman, L, Mazzucco, M, and Roth, J: Fine tuning your chest PT. Am J Nurs 87:1566, 1987.

sial. The benefits of CTSS have been identified as (1) the maintenance of CPAP, (2) the continuation of oxygen supply, and (3) the stability of PEEP.[19] Related potential complications with this device are excess negative pressure, airway trauma, and increased incidence of colonization without an increased incidence of nosocomial pneumonia.

The instillation of normal saline during suctioning once was routine. Normal saline was used to loosen tenacious secretions. However, past research related to use of normal saline and whether it actually increased the amount of secretions obtained has been conflicting.[20,21] Recent research describes the deleterious effects of normal saline instillation on oxygen saturation.[22] (See the Research Box on page 454.)

Extubation

Endotracheal extubation is appropriate when the underlying problem that necessitated placement of an

---

RESEARCH APPLICATION: NURSES' ABILITY TO ACHIEVE HYPERINFLATION AND HYPEROXYGENATION WITH A MANUAL RESUSCITATION BAG DURING ENDOTRACHEAL SUCTIONING
Glass, C, et al. Heart Lung 22(2):158, 1993.

Purpose: Endotracheal suctioning has been associated with detrimental side effects such as arrhythmias and respiratory decompensation. Hyperoxygenation and hyperinflation prior to suctioning can prevent or minimize these untoward effects. This study was designed to determine the nurse's ability to deliver a hyperinflated V_T volume at 100% FiO_2 with a manual resuscitator bag (MRB) during endotracheal suctioning and to identify nurse and patient characteristics associated with volume and oxygen delivery during suctioning.

Methods: The subjects were drawn from the 200 nurses employed full-time or part-time in the adult critical care units of a university-affiliated tertiary care hospital. Each nurse was asked to perform the suctioning procedure using normal routine. Using a stopwatch, the investigator measured the total time that the nurse spent ventilating the patient with the MRB. A rate of bag compressions was determined by multiplying the number of MRB compressions by 60 and dividing the total time for the episode in seconds. Exhaled volumes were measured by a spirometer as a measure of delivered V_T volume. V_E was calculated by multiplying the mean V_T delivered by the bagging rate for each hyperinflation episode. The patient's SaO_2, heart rate, and mean arterial pressure were recorded immediately before and after each episode of hyperinflation. MRB delivered oxygen concentration with each breath was recorded using an oxygen analyzer attached to the MRB. After all suctioning observations were completed, hand length, width, and grip strength were measured for each nurse.

Results: Two different methods of bag compression were observed, a one-handed method and a hand-to-forearm method. The one-handed method delivered a significantly greater amount of oxygen (74.14%) to the patient than those using the one-handed technique (66.86%), although neither method constantly delivered the standard 100%. The hand-to-forearm method produced a significantly greater volume overall (64.5%, $P = .000$).

the oxygen liter flow to the MRB was not set consistently at 15 L and alone accounted for 12% of the variance in oxygen delivery. The one-handed method produced a significantly higher rate ($P = .001$). The mean MRB volume delivered was 625.68 mL, significantly less than the standard of 1.5 times the ventilated volume (mean = 752.06).

Although most nurses did not achieve the standard hyperinflation volume with either of the two methods, nurses using the hand-to-forearm method came closer to the standard (696.3 mL) than nurses using the one-handed method (574.6 mL). The patient's dynamic lung compliance was significantly correlated with the amount of volume delivered ($r = .11$; $P = .04$), although the correlation was minimal. No significant change was noted in patient outcomes using SaO_2, heart rate, and mean arterial pressure as criteria. Hand size and strength were determined to be insignificant factors.

Practice Implications: The purpose of hyperoxygenation and hyperinflation prior to suctioning is to prevent hypoxemia. In this study, nurses were unable to adequately hyperoxygenate and hyperinflate manually. Overall, patient outcomes were unchanged. However, in individual cases SaO_2 did drop considerably. The method used to hyperoxygenate and hyperinflate can be an important factor for patients who are dependent on consistent delivery of oxygen and V_T.

This study emphasizes the need to evaluate individual practitioner technique and points to using the ventilator to hyperoxygenate and hyperventilate whenever possible. Oxygen liter flow to the MRB, which can be easily maintained, was the most important determinant of oxygen delivery. Hand-to-forearm compression was significantly better than the one-handed method in V_T delivery and may be useful for ventilating patients with large V_T requirements. Overall, identification of patients at risk for complications associated with low levels of V_T and oxygen delivery should guide nurse's decisions concerning suctioning technique.

---

artificial airway and mechanical ventilation has been resolved. In assessing the patient's readiness for extubation, the following factors need to be evaluated:

1. Level of consciousness; intact protective reflexes—cough, gag, and epiglottal closure
2. Ability of patient to effectively remove secretions from the lungs
3. Effectiveness of spontaneous respirations as reflected by respiratory parameters:
   Tidal volume (V_T) of 10 mL/kg or more

Minute volume (V_E) about 10 L
Vital capacity greater than 12 to 15 mL/kg
Peak inspiratory pressure -20 cm H_2O or more
Respiratory rate less than 28/min
ABG values: $PaCO_2$ 35 to 45 mmHg (may be more than 45 mmHg in chronic lung disease); PaO_2 greater than 60 mmHg; SaO_2 greater than 90%

4. Hemodynamic stability—vital signs (blood pressure, heart rate)
5. Cardiac status (absence of arrhythmias)

RESEARCH APPLICATION: THE EFFECT OF SALINE LAVAGE PRIOR TO SUCTIONING
Ackerman, M. Am J Crit Care 2(4):326, 1993.

Purpose: The purpose of this study was to evaluate the effect on oxygen saturation of instilling normal saline into artificial airways prior to suctioning. Artificial airway was defined as either an endotracheal tube or a tracheostomy.

Methods: A single-case, repeated-measured, counterbalanced design was used to allow subjects to serve as their own controls. The target population consisted of 40 critically ill male patients in three different ICUs requiring mechanical ventilation. Subjects were alternately suctioned with or without saline for a period of 24 hours or until the endotracheal tube or tracheostomy was removed. The length of time that either device was in place was not controlled. Protocol for the saline bolus procedure included (1) ventilator set to 100% suction mode for 1 minute, (2) 5 mL of normal saline (NS) instilled into the airway, (3) five manual V_T breaths with ventilator, and (4) patient suctioned until clear.

The other part of the procedure included suctioning in the same way, just without saline. Use or nonuse of saline was then alternated each time the subject was subsequently suctioned whenever needed, as assessed by the bedside nurse. Suctioning was performed by nine staff nurses employed in critical care units who volunteered for special training in the research protocol. Oxygen saturation was measured with a noninvasive pulse oximeter connected to a finger or ear probe immediately before and after suctioning at 1-minute intervals after suctioning for 5 minutes. Heart rate, blood pressure, and respiratory rate were also obtained.

Results: Data analysis determined that the instillation of saline had a negative effect on oxygen saturation at each time period after suctioning when compared with suctioning not using saline. These changes were significant at 2 minutes ($P = .05$), 3 minutes ($P = .05$), 4 minutes ($P = .01$), and 5 minutes ($P = .001$). The negative change caused by saline indicates that, on average, the instillation of saline prior to suctioning had a more detrimental effect on oxygenation than not using saline. The interesting findings are that the negative effect increases over time, with the greatest effect being at 5 minutes, the longest parameter used.

Practice Implications: The purpose of suctioning is to clear the airway and ultimately improve oxygenation. These results demonstrate that subjects have better oxygenation after suctioning when an NS bolus is not used. Although standard practice in many institutions is to use saline lavage to loosen thick secretions, this practice should no longer be accepted as routine. The need and appropriateness of saline lavage should be evaluated on an individual basis and used with extreme caution because of its potential detrimental effects.

In preparation for extubation, appropriate explanations are made and the patient is placed in a semi-Fowler's position. This position ensures a more open airway after the artificial airway is removed; it allows for full use of respiratory muscles; it facilitates coughing; and it minimizes risk of vomiting and consequent aspiration. See Table 25–18 for steps in extubation.[15]

After extubation, the patient is fitted with a face mask, and the prescribed concentration of humidified oxygen is administered. The patient should be observed closely for increasing hoarseness or respiratory stridor, which warns of potential laryngeal edema or spasm. Subglottic edema is the most serious complication occurring after extubation.[23] It may be distinguished from glottic edema in that it does not respond to the typical therapy after extubation such as humidification, application of α-adrenergic medications to cause vasoconstriction and reduce edema, or corticosteroid preparations for their anti-inflammatory effect. Subglottic edema should be considered a life-threatening problem, usually requiring reintubation. Equipment for reintubation should be available at the bedside. The patient's tolerance to extubation should be monitored by clinical observation, ventilatory measurements, and ABG parameters.

Mechanical Ventilation

Mechanical ventilation therapy is critical to the effective management of patients in respiratory failure or at high risk for developing ARF. Confirmation of ventilatory failure must be determined by ABG analysis, not merely by clinical observation. By supporting ventilation and thus gas exchange, mechanical ventilators can sustain a patient for as long a period as necessary until the acute process precipitating ARF is resolved.

Primary Goals of Mechanical Ventilation

Mechanical ventilation is concerned with (1) maintaining alveolar ventilation (i.e., carbon dioxide elimination); (2) delivering appropriate concentrations of oxygen more reliably; (3) administering gas under positive pressure, which functions to increase lung volumes and reduce areas of atelectasis; (4) maintaining effective PEEP to help prevent closure/collapse of small airways; and (5) reducing the work of breathing.

If the degree of carbon dioxide retention is increased sufficiently to cause a marked decrease in the patient's pH (less than 7.25) or if the patient's

Table 25–18
Techniques Used in Extubation

Always use universal precautions. After unsecuring the endotracheal tube, continue as follows:
1. Suction pharynx with tonsil-tip catheter to remove pooled secretions above the cuff.
2. Hyperoxygenate and hyperventilate the patient with three breaths to prevent oxygen desaturation.
3. Insert syringe into one-way valve in pilot balloon.
4. Insert sterile suction catheter 1 to 2 inches below distal end of tube.
5. Instruct the patient to take a deep breath. At the peak of a deep inspiration, deflate the cuff and pull out the tube while applying suction to the catheter. This assists in preventing aspiration of mucus that may be in the tube.
6. Suction the pharynx as needed; instruct the patient to deep-breathe and cough.
7. Apply supplemental humidified oxygen.
8. Monitor the patient closely for any untoward effects.

Source: From Hoffman, L, Mazzucco, M, and Roth, J: Fine tuning your chest PT. Am J Nurs 87:1566, 1987, with permission.

level of consciousness and mental status is impaired by marked hypercapnia ($PaCO_2$ greater than 50 to 60 mmHg), mechanical ventilation may be indicated. The progression from normal values to severe hypoxemia, hypercapnia, and respiratory acidemia can occur with alarming rapidity. Without early recognition and prompt intervention, patients with ARF may be observed to pass through three phases: an early

hyperventilatory phase, a crossover phase, and full-blown ARF (Fig. 25–5).

In the early stage (hyperventilatory phase), patients can be observed using increasingly greater effort to ventilate the lungs in the face of advanced airway obstruction. There is use of accessory muscles with intercostal retraction, nasal flaring, and "pursed-lip" breathing; diaphoresis may be evident, and the patient may have tachypnea and tachycardia. BG values at this stage reflect mild-to-severe hypoxemia (PaO_2 lower than 60 mmHg) and hypocapnia ($PaCO_2$ lower than 30 mmHg), predisposing to respiratory alkalemia with a variable degree of compensation (pH 7.50 or higher). Patients are able to maintain themselves in the face of serious underlying pathophysiology (increasing alveolar hypoventilation, $\dot{V}/\dot{Q}$ mismatch, and intrapulmonary shunting) by hyperventilating (i.e., "blowing off" carbon dioxide). However, they do so at the expense of considerable energy and oxygen consumption.

As these patients become increasingly fatigued to the point of exhaustion, they eventually progress to the crossover phase (Fig. 25–5). During this phase, the patient's clinical status might suggest to an unsuspecting observer that his or her condition is actually improving. The patient appears to be breathing with less difficulty and effort; breath sounds are diminished; and ABG values reflect a normalizing pH (about 7.4) and $PaCO_2$ (about 40 mmHg). Significantly, how-

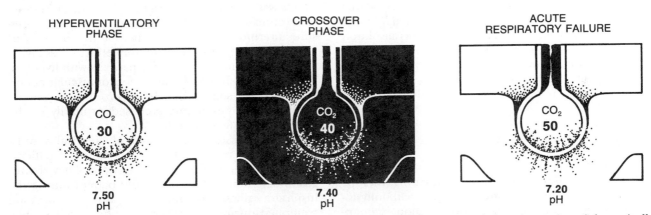

FIGURE 25–5. Blood gas and pH relationships in setting of progressive mild to severe airway obstruction. Schematically depicted are three alveoli and alveolar—capillary membranes. Numbers within the alveoli represent carbon dioxide concentrations; numbers within the capillary reflect corresponding pH.

Hyperventilatory phase: Characterized by hypocapnia ($PaCO_2$ ~30 mmHg) and respiratory alkalemia (pH 7.50). Mild airway obstruction predisposes to tissue hypoxia with clinical signs of anxiety, apprehension, and increased work of breathing with hyperventilation. Hyperventilation results in increased carbon dioxide elimination with consequent hypocapnia; hypocapnia underlies the respiratory alkalemia.

"Cross-over" phase: Characterized by seemingly "normalizing" blood gas values ($PaCO_s$ ~40 mmHg, pH ~7.40). Clinically, there are diminished breath sounds and decreased work of breathing.

Acute respiratory failure: Characterized by hypercapnia ($PaCO_2$ >50 mmHg) and respiratory acidemia (pH <7.20). With severe airway obstruction, there is increased ventilation/perfusion mismatching, and shunting. Alveolar ventilation is significantly compromised, predisposing to the hypercapnia. Hypercapnia causes respiratory acidemia, which, if untreated, can lead to acute respiratory failure.

The significance of the "cross-over" phase is that, despite a seemingly "normalizing" clinical picture, the patient is actually in need of immediate, aggressive therapy to prevent full-blown acute respiratory failure. (Not depicted here is the $PaCO_2$, which, concomitantly, progressively worsens as the patient moves from the hyperventilatory phase, to the cross-over phase, and, finally, to acute respiratory failure, if untreated.)

TABLE 25-19
Indications for Initiation of Mechanical Ventilation Therapy

Mechanical ventilation is necessary if the patient:
  Is unconscious
  Is in respiratory failure
  Has an airway obstruction
  Requires tracheal suctioning
  Is expected to require long-term ventilatory support
Mechanics
  Tidal volume (VT) <5–7 mL/kg
  Vital capacity (VC) <12–15 mL/kg
  Peak inspiratory pressure (PIP) <20 cmH_2O
  Respiratory rate (f) >30–35/min (adults)
Ventilation
  Dead space (VDS/VT) <55% of VT (normal: 25%–40%)
  PaO_2 <60 mmHg; SaO_2 <90%
  Alveolar hypoventilation: $PaCO_2$ >45 mmHg (pH <7.25)
  Alveolar hyperventilation: $PaCO_2$ <35 mmHg (pH >7.45)

Source: From King, G: Respiratory failure in the critically ill. In Sibbald, W (ed): Synopsis of Critical Care, ed 3. Williams & Wilkins, Baltimore, 1988, p 53, with permission.

ever, the hypoxemia worsens (PaO_2 of less than 50 to 60 mmHg), reflecting advancing alveolar hypoventilation, serious disturbances in $\dot{V}/\dot{Q}$ matching, and significant right-to-left shunting. Diminishing breath sounds on auscultation suggests that the patient is unable to effectively move gas into or out of the lungs.

The crossover phase is significant because it signals the need for decisive and immediate institution of timely and aggressive therapy to treat or avert full-blown ARF (pH less than 7.2; PaO_2 less than 50 to 55 mmHg; $PaCO_2$ greater than 50 mmHg). It is absolutely essential to initiate mechanical ventilation at this time to prevent further deterioration in the patient's condition. Mechanical ventilation therapy reduces the work of breathing while maintaining adequate alveolar ventilation.

Clinical Indications for Mechanical Ventilation

Indications for mechanical ventilation therapy depend largely on the degree to which pathophysiologic processes encroach upon cardiopulmonary reserves (Table 25–19). This is best assessed by the patient's clinical history and physical examination, serial measurements of spontaneous ventilatory capability, and interpretation of ABG values.

Criteria for the establishment of intubation and the initiation of mechanical ventilation are helpful in determining whether and when such therapy is indicated. This information is presented in Table 25–19.[24] These criteria may apply to any one of the following clinical situations (Fig. 25–1):

1. Central nervous system depression with apnea due to primary causes such as drugs, cerebrovascular accidents (CVAs), and increased intracranial pressure, or due to cerebral hypoxia caused by disturbances in cardiopulmonary function.

2. Increased intracranial pressure (ICP), which is very sensitive to changes in $PaCO_2$. In this situation, induced hypocapnia is used commonly to lower ICP.

3. Persistent hypoxemia (PaO_2 lower than 60 mmHg) despite maximum FIO_2 by face mask and nasal prongs.

4. In the development of acute lung disease wherein initially, hypocapnia is the rule. The onset of even mild elevation of $PaCO_2$ with a consequent decrease in pH is suggestive of disease progression to a serious potentially compromising state.

5. Deterioration of ventilatory status of patients with neurologic and neuromuscular problems such as Guillain-Barré syndrome and myasthenia gravis, respectively.

6. Flail chest if more than six ribs are broken unilaterally or four ribs are broken on each side, and there is evidence of respiratory compromise.

Types of Mechanical Ventilators

The two types of mechanical ventilators are negative-pressure ventilators and positive-pressure ventilators.[25,26]

Negative-Pressure Ventilators The first type of mechanical ventilator to be used was the negative-pressure ventilator. An example is the "iron lung," which was used for polio victims. The negative-pressure ventilator works by applying subatmospheric pressure intermittently to the trunk of the body. This assists the patient's own respiratory effort. These types of ventilators may be useful for patients with hypoventilation caused by chest wall or neuromuscular abnormalities or in some cases, by hypoxemic respiratory failure. These ventilators are used primarily in the home or chronic care setting.

Positive-Pressure Ventilators. Mechanical ventilators currently used for the management of patients with ARF are positive-pressure devices. They deliver gas under positive pressure to the patient during the inspiratory phase. In contrast, negative pressures are generated during the inspiratory phase with spontaneous ventilation.[24] With spontaneous breathing, expansion of the chest cage and lungs creates a negative pressure within the alveoli. The resulting pressure gradient between the alveoli and the atmosphere allows air to flow into the lungs.

The two types of positive-pressure ventilators are volume-cycled, in which inspiration is terminated after a preset volume has been delivered by the ventilator, with expiration allowed to occur passively; and pressure-cycled, in which inspiration is terminated when a specific airway pressure has been reached. Volume cycled ventilators are used more frequently in the critically ill adult patient because the total volume of air will be delivered despite variations in the patient's airway resistance and lung compliance. Many of the newer model ventilators can be adjusted to be volume cycled or pressure cycled.

Modes of Ventilation

The term "ventilator mode" refers to the way the machine ventilates the patient. Several different modes can be set. Each is different in determining how much work of breathing the patient has to do. See Table 25–20 for the different modes used in mechanical ventilation.

Control Mode or Controlled Mandatory Ventilation (CMV) In the control mode, ventilation is provided entirely by the ventilator at a respiratory rate, V_T, and FIO_2 prescribed by the physician. At ventilatory rates greater than 8 inspirations per minute in conjunction with a V_T of 12 to 15 mL/kg, it is reasonable to assume that full alveolar ventilatory support is adequate in most instances. The use of barbiturate coma to treat head injury is an example wherein ventilation is exclusively in the control mode. However, with the availability of the assist-control and intermittent mandatory ventilation modes, which provide full ventilatory support without the inflexibility of the control mode, this mode is used infrequently.

Assist-Control Mode. In the assist-control mode of ventilation, the ventilator is able to "sense" when the patient initiates inspiration, at which point the ventilator "assists" by delivering a specified V_T to the patient. The patient will receive a set number of breaths from the ventilator each minute. He or she may initiate a breath on his own, but it is augmented by the preset V_T from the ventilator. The total respiratory rate is determined by the number of spontaneous inspirations initiated by the patient plus the number of breaths set on the ventilator. The assist-

control mode of ventilation can result in wide swings in V_E if the patient's respiratory rate changes appreciably.

Intermittent Mandatory Ventilation (IMV). IMV allows for partial ventilatory support by delivering a present number of breaths per minute at a specified V_T and FIO_2. In between the ventilator-delivered breaths, the patient is able to breathe spontaneously through the ventilator circuit without increased resistance and at the preset FIO_2. The ventilator does not assist the spontaneous breaths, and the V_T of these breaths is determined by the patient's inspiratory effort.

Synchronized Intermittent Mandatory Ventilation (SIMV). Most ventilators in use today have the SIMV mode. This mode allows the patient to breathe spontaneously through the ventilator circuit without increased resistance, while, at predetermined intervals, the next spontaneous breath is assisted by the machine. The ventilator and self-initiated breaths do not compete as they can with the IMV mode described previously.

High-Frequency Jet Ventilation. In high-frequency jet ventilation, a high-pressure source connected to a small-bore cannula is placed in the endotracheal tube. With an interposed cycling mechanism allowing high-frequency delivery of gas, high-frequency jet ventilation delivered at 100 to 150 cycles/min can maintain adequate gas exchange for undefined periods of time. The patient is also connected to a volume ventilator. This type of ventilation provides continuous ventilation in the setting of ARF without the undesirable side effects of positive-pressure ventilation, such as high peak airway pressures, barotrauma, and cardiovascular comprise.

Adjuncts to Mechanical Ventilation

Positive End-Expiratory Pressure (PEEP). When using a positive-pressure, volume-cycled ventilator, an important option available for the intubated patient with hypoxemic ARF is PEEP. PEEP refers to the existence of an airway pressure above that of ambient air at the end of exhalation. PEEP functions to increase functional residual capacity (FRC), which appears to be the primary mechanism by which alveolar ventilation and thus gas exchange are improved when PEEP therapy is instituted. PEEP increases FRC by distending airways and increasing alveolar size by the application of positive pressure. In fact, in ventilated patients receiving PEEP, the entire respiratory cycle is maintained under positive pressure.

PEEP functions to reduce the incidence of atelectasis, particularly in the scenario of altered surfactant activity. The application of PEEP therapy has been associated with an improvement in arterial oxygenation and overall lung compliance; it reduces pulmonary vascular resistance. PEEP may be the most effective therapy in ARF where right-to-left shunting is a significant problem, because it helps to balance the

---

TABLE 25–20
Modes of Mechanical Ventilation

Control Mode (CV)
Ventilation is completely provided by the mechanical ventilator with a preset V_T, respiratory rate, and FIO_2.

Assist-Control (A/C)
Ventilator "senses" patient's inspiratory effort and delivers breath at a preset V_T and FIO_2. A back-up respirator rate is set. If the patient fails to breathe, the ventilator takes over and controls ventilation at a preset rate.

Synchronized Intermittent Mandatory Ventilation (SIMV)
SIMV delivers a preset number of positive breaths at a selected rate that is synchronized with the patient's ventilatory effort. The patient can spontaneously initiate a breath while the ventilator delivers only humidified oxygen.

Pressure Support Ventilation (PSV)
Ventilator applies a predetermined amount of positive pressure to the airways upon inspiration. PSV is used to decrease the work of breathing and can be added to other modes such as SIMV or used alone for a spontaneously breathing patient.

Continuous Positive Airway Pressure (CPAP)
A variation of PEEP, CPAP applies positive pressure at the end of expiration. It is used for a spontaneously breathing patient.

distribution of the inspired volume of gas throughout the lungs.

Continuous Positive Airway Pressure (CPAP). For patients breathing spontaneously, CPAP, a variation of PEEP, is available. Principles underlying CPAP are similar to those of PEEP except that the patient is breathing spontaneously without any breaths from the mechanical ventilator. Benefit is derived from the positive pressure maintained within the airways and alveoli at the end of expiration.

Pressure Support Ventilation (PSV). A newer mode of ventilatory support, PSV is used primarily for weaning from mechanical ventilation. It is designed to maintain a constant preset amount of positive pressure during ventilation. Augmentation of inspiration with positive pressure helps to overcome airway resistance and assists in reducing the work of breathing. PSV may be combined with other modes of ventilation such as IMV. PSV alone requires patient-generated breaths. Therefore, a safe mode of ventilation must either incorporate a backup ventilatory rate, such as IMV, or use a ventilator with an apnea mode that will convert to a programmed ventilator rate and volume if a period of apnea is detected.

Pressure-Controlled Inverse Ratio Ventilation (PC-IRV). This application of mechanical ventilation is used for hypoxemia that is refractory to increases in FIO_2 and PEEP therapy. PC-IRV reverses the normal inspiratory to expiratory time (I:E ratio). The ventilator delivers a long inspiration and a short expiration instead of a short inspiration and a long expiration. I:E ratios may be as high as 3:1 or 4:1. PC-IRV is still experimental but has been beneficial when used for patients with ARDS.[27]

Ventilator Controls. See Table 25–21 for information regarding ventilator controls.[26]

Monitoring the Ventilated Patient: Nursing Care Considerations

General monitoring of the patient on continuous ventilatory support should include (1) ongoing patient assessment, that is, the status of neurologic, respiratory, cardiovascular, renal, and gastrointestinal function; (2) monitoring of ventilatory settings; (3) monitoring of ABGs; (4) laboratory studies; (5) pulmonary function studies; and (6) radiology studies—daily chest x-ray. See Table 25–22 for mechanical ventilation guidelines for nursing.

Complications of Mechanical Ventilation Therapy

Complications of mechanical ventilation therapy may involve problems related to the treatment of ARF, as well as medical complications that may arise during the course of ARF. Intubation and mechanical ventilation therapy are not without risks or complications.

Equipment failure or mechanical malfunction is always a potential danger of mechanical ventilation therapy. A resuscitator bag and oral airway must always be available at the bedside, and the patient should be manually ventilated until the malfunction is corrected. Inappropriate or inadequate ventilatory settings related to V_T, respiratory rate, and airway pressure may predispose to hypoventilation with consequent hypercapnia and respiratory acidemia. For details regarding complications, see Table 25–23.

Weaning from Mechanical Ventilation Therapy

Weaning is the gradual process of removing the patient from mechanical ventilation therapy.[28–30] The duration of the process is affected largely by the length of time that the patient has been on the mechanical ventilator; the patient's physical condition, including the tone and strength of respiratory muscles; nutritional status; underlying disease status; and the presence or absence of psychological dependence. When patients have been maintained on mechanical ventilatory therapy, a period of gradual separation is necessary before spontaneous respiration can effectively meet ventilatory needs. Long-term mechanically ventilated patients may have their weaning complicated by infection, anemia, hemodynamic instability, nutritional and metabolic disturbances, altered elimination patterns, and sleep disturbances.

The basic guide to beginning the weaning process

TABLE 25–21
Ventilator Controls

Respiratory rate—Number of breaths the ventilator will deliver a minute. It is usually set at 10 to 16 bpm to achieve the required $PaCO_2$. Total respiratory rate equals patient rate plus ventilator rate.

Tidal volume (V_T)—Volume of gas delivered to a patient during a ventilator breath. It is normally set between 5 to 15 mL/kg.

Fraction of inspired oxygen concentration (FIO_2)—Percent of oxygen concentration that the patient is receiving. Use of the lowest FIO_2 that achieves the desired PaO_2 is recommended. The ventilator should be checked frequently with an oxygen analyzer to ensure that the desired FIO_2 is actually being delivered to the patient.

Inspiration to expiration ratio (I:E ratio)—Determined by the rate of inspiratory flow and the V_T on volume ventilators. Typical ratio is 1:2 unless inverse ratio ventilation is used.

Sensitivity—Adjusts the ventilator's response to initiation of breath by the patient. Sensitivity is usually adjusted so that minimal patient effort (i.e., about −2 cm H_2O) is required to trigger the machine.

Sighs—Allows periodic selection of a larger-than-normal V_T. Sighs substitute for the normal sighing reflex.

Pressure limits—Used to regulate the maximal pressure that the ventilator can use to deliver the V_T. Once the pressure limit is reached, the machine will spill undelivered volumes into the atmosphere to protect the patient from barotrauma.

Alarm systems—Mechanical ventilators that incorporate audible and visual alarm systems, which act as immediate warning signals to altered ventilation. Alarms can usually be set for low or high pressures and low volume to ensure delivery of the appropriate V_T to the patient. Other alarms guarantee appropriate I:E ratio, appropriate concentrations of oxygen, and fail-safe alarms, which warn of disconnection or unplugging of the ventilator.

TABLE 25–22
The Mechanically Ventilated Patient: Nursing Care Considerations

Nursing Interventions	Rationales
• Maintain a patent airway by proper endotracheal tube placement/taping.	• Because of the anatomic structure of the mainstem bronchi, the endotracheal tube may slip into the right mainstem if positioned too low, thereby obstructing air flow to the left lung.
• Inflate tracheal/endotracheal tube cuff using the minimal air leak or minimal occlusive technique.	• The cuff must be adequately inflated to provide a closed system between the patient and the ventilator. Underinflation of the endotracheal tube cuff may allow aspiration of gastric contents or saliva and loss of desired VT. Overinflation may cause tracheal tissue necrosis or may herniate the cuff over the tip of the tube causing partial or complete airway obstruction.
• Turn patient every 1–2 hours; alternate side-to-side and semi-Fowler's position.	• Both ventilation and perfusion can be preferentially delivered to the segments of the lung through positioning maneuvers that promote drainage of some segments and ventilation of others.
• Use nonverbal as well as verbal communication; provide slate/pencil; maintain IV in nonwriting arm.	• Intubated patients experience fear, helplessness, and despair, and communication is necessary.
• Evaluate respiratory status periodically noting bilateral breath sounds and symmetry of chest movement.	• Auscultation provides information regarding the flow of air through the tracheobronchial tree and the presence of fluid, mucus, or obstruction. Evaluation of symmetry with respirations provides information about air flow to lungs and may identify inadvertent right mainstem intubation.
• Suction airway as necessary.	• The endotracheal intubated patient usually has an ineffective cough reflex because of the interference of the tube with glottic closure. Suctioning should not be routine because unnecessary suctioning may produce excessive tracheal irritation and increase risk of infection.
• Hyperventilate with resuscitator bag and oxygenate before and after suctioning with 100% oxygen for 3–6 breaths.	• Hyperventilation minimizes atelectasis related to suctioning. High concentrations of oxygen provided before and after suctioning assist in preventing myocardial hypoxia and cardiac arrhythmias.
• Monitor ECG during suctioning.	• Hypoxia is a common cause of arrhythmias. Ventilated patients have $\dot{V}/\dot{Q}$ imbalances and often have hypoxia/hypoxemia.
• Maintain respiratory parameters within normal limits by frequent checks on ordered ventilatory settings: Oxygen percentage	• The lowest possible FiO$_2$ capable of promoting adequate oxygenation should be provided to the patient; lower levels (<50%) can be used for long periods of time without evidence of oxygen toxicity.
VT	• Changes may indicate leakage through the machine or cuff and will affect ventilation and oxygenation.
I/E ratio	• Usual I:E is 1 to 2 or 1 to 3. Changes in the I:E will change the ventilatory rate and affect the $\dot{V}/\dot{Q}$ ratio.
Sensitivity	• If the sensitivity is not adjusted, the patient can hyperventilate or, at the other extreme, fight for air.
Airway pressure	• Once the VT has been established, the airway pressure should remain relatively constant. An increase in the pressure reading on the manometer may reflect an increase in the amount of pressure needed to deliver a set volume of gas as occurs with increases in airway resistance or decreases in lung compliance as may occur with pneumothorax, pulmonary edema, and misplacement of the endotracheal tube.
Sigh (frequency and volume)	• Frequency and volume of sigh affect alveolar ventilation, promote cough, and help prevent atelectasis.
Humidity and temperature	• The usual warming/humidifying function of the nasopharynx has been bypassed with intubation. Humidification is necessary to maintain secretions at normal viscosity. The temperature of inspired gas should be maintained at about body temperature.
Rate	• Respirations should be counted for 1 full minute comparing the patient's respiratory rate with set ventilatory rate. Rapid respiratory rate due to the patient's triggering of the ventilator can produce abnormal blood gas values.
Alarm system	• Mechanical ventilators involve a series of audible and visual alarms to reflect abnormal ventilator changes and increase ventilator efficiency and patient safety, (e.g., low-high-pressure alarms, I:E ratio alarms, oxygen alarms.) These alarms should never be turned off even when suctioning.
• Evaluate response to mechanical ventilation: level of consciousness and responsiveness; monitor ABGs.	• Assess mental state, orientation to person, place and time; level of consciousness. Changes in arousability or behavior, or ability to follow commands, may be early indicators of hypoxia, as noted by ABG values.
• Check patient respirations related to ventilator.	• If the patient is *bucking* or *fighting* the ventilator, it may be appropriate to sedate the patient.

Continued

TABLE 25–22
The Mechanically Ventilated Patient: Nursing Care Considerations (*Continued*)

Nursing Interventions	Rationales
• Constant supervision and care are required if pancuronium is used.	• Complete paralysis makes the patient totally dependent on the ventilator for breathing and on nursing staff for general care.
• Maintain optimal PEEP; avoid routine suctioning.	• Each time the ventilator is disconnected, the PEEP is lost, and it takes time to reestablish effective alveolar pressures again.
• Recognize side effects/complications: atelectasis evidenced through auscultation/palpation.	• Localized atelectasis may occur as a result of retained secretions.
• Monitor for decreased cardiac output evidenced by decrease in blood pressure and pulse.	• The positive pressures generated increase the intrathoracic pressure, which can potentially decrease venous return, resulting in a decrease in cardiac output (especially with the use of PEEP).
• Monitor for signs of pneumothorax (barotrauma): asymmetrical chest movements; diminished/absent breath sounds on affected side; tachycardia with weak pulse; cyanosis; decreased cardiac output with hypotension; accumulation of air under skin, crackling of skin with palpation; displacement of trachea; note tracheal position.	• Pressures generated by the PEEP mode of ventilation may promote rupture of the alveolar walls, allowing air leaks into the pleural space, mediastinum, or subcutaneous spaces. The patient becomes at risk for lung collapse with compromise of cardiopulmonary function.
	• Trachea shifts away from the affected side. Depending on the size of pneumothorax or mediastinal or subcutaneous emphysema, chest tube insertion may be necessary.
• In preparation for weaning: Monitor the tests related to respiratory status.	• Monitor ABGs, VT on spontaneous breathing, VC >12 to 15 mL/ kg; ease of breathing.
Assess respirations and ventilator breaths per minute; record VT for each during use of IMV for weaning. Monitor for signs of respiratory distress.	• IMV allows the patient's own breathing pattern to be maintained with positive breaths delivered intermittently by the ventilator.
	• Early detection and treatment of respiratory difficulty minimize the possibility of return to the ventilator.

Medical Management

• Arterial line and serial ABGs	• ABG values help to assess effectiveness of ventilatory effort, gas exchange, and the weaning process
• Bronchodilators	• Use may improve ventilation compromised by bronchial edema and bronchospasms.
• Pancuronium	• Sedation or paralysis alleviates the problem of "fighting the ventilator," but makes the patient completely dependent on mechanical ventilation.
• Sedatives	• Pavulon does not affect the ability to think, and sedation is important to reduce the unpleasant feelings that accompany the use of this drug.
• Addition of PEEP to ventilator regimen	• PEEP promotes alveolar expansion and helps to prevent shunting of blood through unventilated areas of the lung, thereby increasing FRC and optimizing the oxygen gradient across the alveolar/capillary membrane.
• IMV, SIMV, or other appropriate weaning techniques	• Weaning promotes use and gradual strengthening of the respiratory muscles.

is to establish whether or not the indications for the implementation of mechanical ventilation have improved. Criteria for weaning are reflected in Table 25–24.[29] The three basic approaches to weaning are the T-piece trial, the intermittent mandatory ventilation (IMV) method, and pressure support ventilation (PSV).

T-Piece Trial. For patients in whom there is a good potential for successful weaning, a trial of breathing humidified oxygen through a T piece is indicated. During T piece weaning, periods of ventilatory support are alternated with spontaneous breathing. CPAP can be added to the T piece to increase FRC. CPAP will also improve the distribution of ventilation by opening smaller airways and maintaining alveolar stability.[30] Some patients require gradual weaning with T-piece trials, increasing the time off the ventilator with each trial. Care must be taken to avoid respiratory muscle fatigue with this process.

Intermittent Mandatory Ventilation (IMV). The second approach to weaning involves application of IMV. The number of mechanical breaths delivered to the patient per minute is decreased to allow the patient to increasingly contribute to ventilatory demand by spontaneous breathing. Singular use of the SIMV mode for weaning is controversial.[30] Some SIMV systems require the patient to generate negative pressure to open the demand valve, which would definitely increase the work of breathing. It is extremely important to assess the patient for respiratory muscle fatigue when reducing the IMV rate. The SIMV mode of weaning can be effective for some patients, perhaps better if it is used in conjunction with PSV.

Pressure Support Ventilation (PSV). PSV is a newer mode of weaning patients from mechanical ventilation. With PSV, the patient breathes spontaneously with a preset pressure assisting each spontaneous inspiration. PSV is noted for maximizing patient con-

TABLE 25–23
Complications of Mechanical Ventilation Therapy

Complication	Cause and Clinical Presentation	Management Considerations
Acid-Base Disturbances		
1. Posthypercapnic alkalemia	Too-rapid reduction in $Paco_2$ by mechanical ventilation, in a patient with chronic lung disease (long-standing hypercapnia with elevated serum bicarbonate; renal compensation to maintain pH within normal limits). Reduction in $Paco_2$ exposes underlying alkalemia. Signs/symptoms of severe alkalemia: 1. Depression of respiratory centers for ventilation 2. Reduced serum ionized calcium level 3. Increased central nervous system irritability (potential seizures); muscle weakness, ileus 4. Cardiac arrhythmias (pH > 7.55)	Provide enough mechanical ventilation to reduce $Paco_2$ only to a level that normalizes the pH. Replace chloride ion to allow kidney to excrete bicarbonate (HCO_3^-).
2. Metabolic alkalemia/alkalosis	Associated with hypokalemia and hypochloremia related to: 1. Increased renal loss of potassium by diuretics, steroids, penicillins, and other drugs 2. Shift of K^+ intracellularly in exchange with H^+ in presence of underlying alkalemia 3. Inadequate intake of potassium 4. Increased aldosterone secretion 5. Loss of gastric acid by nasogastric drainage 6. Renal retention of bicarbonate in the presence of hypercapnia Respiratory compensation for metabolic alkalemia involves alveolar hypoventilation.	Alkalemia may interfere with weaning. Acetazolamide therapy—renal response significantly enhanced with excretion of large urine volumes with increased bicarbonate. Administration of saline or potassium chloride. Alveolar hypoventilation predisposes to atelectasis.
3. Respiratory alkalemia/alkalosis	Respiratory alkalemia can be artificially produced by overventilation of the patient. Spontaneous hyperventilation may also cause respiratory alkalemia. Signs/symptoms: 1. Reduced cardiac output 2. Cardiac arrhythmias 3. Decreased lung compliance 4. Increased airway resistance 5. $\dot{V}/\dot{Q}$ mismatch 6. Increased right-to-left shunt 7. Seizures	Ventilatory therapy should be closely controlled to produce an acceptable pH, but not necessarily a normal $Paco_2$. Decrease alveolar ventilation: • Decrease V_T • Decrease respiratory rate • Add mechanical dead space Changing ventilatory mode to IMV may alleviate problem if due to patient "out of sync" with ventilator or assist-control. Diazepam, morphine, and pancuronium may be necessary to control. spontaneous hyperventilation while the patient is mechanically ventilated.
4. Hypercapnic respiratory acidemia/acidosis	Inadequate alveolar ventilation or alveolar hypoventilation Retention of carbon dioxide leads to acidemia with decreased pH (pH <7.35)	Increase (V_E) or (V_A) ventilation. • Larger V_T • Increase in respiratory rate
Pulmonary Alterations		
1. Atelectasis	Collapse of alveoli associated with airway obstruction Use of low V_Ts with mechanical ventilation therapy without a periodic "sigh" Signs/symptoms: 1. Diminished breath sounds 2. Increase in alveolar-arterial oxygen gradient 3. Reduced lung compliance	Institute use of "sigh" or large V_T Institute vigorous chest physiotherapy and pulmonary hygiene Provide increased humidification of inspired gas Provide vigorous tracheal suctioning

Continued

TABLE 25–23
Complications of Mechanical Ventilation Therapy (*Continued*)

Complication	Cause and Clinical Presentation	Management Considerations
2. Oxygen toxicity	Prolonged administration of high concentration of oxygen (FIO_2 >60%) may cause: 1. Absorption atelectasis (at FIO_2 100%) 2. Impaired surfactant activity 3. Pulmonary interstitial edema; fibrosis and thickening of alveolar-capillary membrane (may impair diffusion and gas exchange).	Frequent monitoring of ABGs with use of $FIO_2 > 40\%$ Periodic oxygen analysis to confirm that oxygen concentration reaching the patient is at the prescribed level Always use lowest possible oxygen concentration to maintain $PaO_2 > 60$ mmHg
3. Barotrauma: pneumothorax, pneumomediastinum, subcutaneous emphysema	Associated with positive-pressure ventilation; especially with PEEP Signs/symptoms: 1. Restlessness; agitation 2. Asymmetrical chest wall excursion 3. Altered breathing pattern; tachypnea 4. Diminished breath sounds on affected side; hyperresonance on percussion 5. Tachycardia; cyanosis	Patients with COPD are at high risk. The effects of excessive pressure and volume combined within the alveoli can lead to rupture of the membrane. Possibility of tension pneumothorax must always be considered. Chest x-ray.
4. Inability to wean	A major problem in patients with chronic lung disease, debilitation (as in elderly), musculoskeletal disorders, cystic fibrosis	Intubation and initiation of mechanical ventilation therapy should be done only if absolutely necessary.
5. Tracheal/laryngeal damage	Pressure necrosis 1. Tracheal stenosis 2. Tracheomalacia 3. Tracheoesophageal fistula 4. Tracheoinnominate fistula	Ongoing assessment for: 1. Proper placement of tube 2. Maintenance of cuff pressure sufficient to achieve a minimal leak/seal 3. Properly secured tube to prevent movement of the tube or accidental extubation 4. Necessary humidification of inspired gas 5. Airway patency: effectiveness of secretion removal 6. Use of aseptic technique in suctioning 7. To minimize trauma to the airway, alleviate clinical problems that result in disruption of tube placement (e.g., restlessness, agitation, "bucking vent," or seizure activity) Support tube/tubing during patient movement to reduce traction or friction on airway
6. Pulmonary embolism	Immobilization associated with mechanical ventilation therapy High incidence of thrombocytopenia in adult respiratory distress syndrome	Range-of-motion exercises Support stockings to lower extremities Careful assessment for calf tenderness; measure circumference of calf and thighs each shift Prophylactic heparin therapy

Cardiovascular Alterations
1. Cardiac arrhythmias
  a. Supraventricular
  b. Ventricular
	Hypoxemia, hypercapnia, pH changes, increased catecholamine secretion, hypokalemia, and hypocalcemia
	1. Disrupt depolarization and repolarization phases of action potential.
	2. Increase automaticity.
	3. Increase reentry phenomenon.
	Tracheal intubation and suctioning can stimulate vagal reflexes and predispose to arrhythmias.
		Treat hypoxemia/hypoxia.
		Maintain continuous ECG monitoring.
		Monitor electrolytes.

2. Decreased cardiac output
  a. Tachycardia
  b. Hypotension
  c. Tissue hypoxia
	Positive intrathoracic pressures reduce preload (venous return).
	Signs/symptoms of decreased cardiac output:
	1. Reduced blood pressure; tachycardia
	2. Decreased urine output
		Maintain intravascular volume to minimize effects of changes in intrathoracic pressures on venous return to the heart.
		Provide careful ongoing assessment of V_T, airway resistance, PEEP adjustments.

TABLE 25–23
Complications of Mechanical Ventilation Therapy (*Continued*)

Complication	Cause and Clinical Presentation	Management Considerations
Fluid and Electrolyte Disturbances		

1. Water and salt retention	Controlled mechanical ventilation causes:
	  1. Alteration in renal blood flow
	  2. Increased secretion of antidiuretic hormone (ADH) resulting in decreased urinary output
	  3. Increase in aldosterone secretion
	Hypoalbuminemia and decreased colloidal oncotic pressure predispose to pulmonary interstitial edema.
	Fluid retention results from overhydration by humidification.
		Close monitoring of intake and output
		Daily weight
		Respiratory assessment every 1–2 h for abnormal or adventitious breath sounds.
		Monitor serum electrolytes; serum proteins.
		Monitor ABGs and alveolar-arterial gradient.
		Monitor vital capacity and lung compliance.

2. Electrolyte imbalances
  a. Hypokalemia
  b. Hypochloremia
	(See acid-base disturbances earlier in table.)
	Associated with metabolic alkalemia
	  1. Sodium renal reabsorption is associated with potassium excretion in presence of reduced hydrogenion concentration.
	  2. Shift of potassium intracellularly in exchange for hydrogenion movement into blood.
	  3. Renal reabsorption of bicarbonate in response to hypercapnia is associated with chloride excretion = hypochloremia.
	Hypokalemia resulting from large renal losses of potassium in response to drugs:
	  1. Diuretics
	  2. Penicillins (carbenicillin; ticarcillin, piperacillin)
	  3. Adrenocorticosteroids: endogenous and exogenous sources
	Signs/symptoms:
	  1. Muscle weakness, which may interfere with weaning
	  2. Arrhythmias associated with or without digitalis toxicity
		Monitor as above:
		  1. Serial electrolytes, BUN, creatinine.
		  2. Drug therapy—avoid potassium-depleting medications.
		  3. Serum digitalis levels if the patient takes digoxin; assess for signs of digitalis toxicity.
		    CNS–fatigue, headache, muscle weakness, mental depression: paresthesias
		    Cardiovascular—Decreased cardiac output with hypotension; arrhythmias.
		    GI—nausea, vomiting, diarrhea
		  4. Continuous ECG.

c. Reduced ionized serum calcium	Alkalemia increases the fraction of protein-bound calcium, thus reducing available ionized calcium. 1. Serum calcium levels <8.0 mg/100 mL can precipitate neuromuscular irritability.	Correct hypercapnia and acidemia to reduce obligatory renal reabsorption of bicarbonate. Monitor serum calcium/phosphorus levels. Assess for signs of hypocalcemia.
Gastrointestinal Alterations		
1. Acute upper GI bleeding due to stress ulcer, peptic ulcer, gastritis 2. Paralytic ileus (most commonly associated with hypokalemia) 3. Gastric distention related to intubation and air swallowing 4. Pulmonary aspiration of gastric contents	Gastrointestinal complications are frequently associated with ARF. Hypoxia enhances gastric acidity; acute increases in gastric acidity play a role in the increased incidence of peptic ulcer disease associated with chronic lung disease and ARF.	Abdominal assessment: bowel sounds Antacid prophylaxis to keep gastric pH >4.5 Cimetidine or ranitidine therapy: 1. Note side effects—lethargy, confusion, depressed ventilatory drive, thrombocytopenia; cardiac arrhythmias, GI symptoms, other. Periodic testing of gastric aspirate and stools for guaiac.
Infections		
1. Pulmonary infections: pneumonias 2. Septicemia 3. Urinary tract infection	Debilitated and aged at increased risk Multiple invasive lines Malnutrition/protein catabolism; alteration in surfactant activity; alteration in respiratory epithelium (Replication invites infection and ulceration.) Use of antibiotics that alter normal flora Increased risk of aspiration Artificial airway and other respiratory adjuncts interfering with nonpulmonary defenses; increased risk of airway contamination Immunosuppression/decreased immunocompetence	Obtain baseline cultures of sputum, urine, blood. Monitor white blood cells, leukocytosis, body temperature, presence of purulent tracheobronchial secretions. Pulmonary infiltrates on chest x-ray Monitor pulmonary function. Provide vigorous chest physiotherapy (bronchial hygiene), postural drainage, percussion, regular turning/positioning. Use aseptic technique in suctioning, care of monitoring lines. Provide therapeutic bronchoscopy. Administer appropriate antibiotic therapy. Maintain nutrition.

Continued

TABLE 25–23
Complications of Mechanical Ventilation Therapy (*Continued*)

Complication	Cause and Clinical Presentation	Management Considerations
Malnutrition		
1. Critical illness and increased stress cause hypermetabolic state • Protein catabolism 2. Increased carbon dioxide production with respiratory acidosis 3. Energy demand greater than energy supply • Fatigue and weakness of respiratory muscles	Critical illness with inadequate nutritive intake = semistarvation Prolonged mechanical ventilation, resulting in atrophy of diaphragm and respiratory muscles Excess glucose alimentation resulting in increased carbon dioxide production and added demands on ventilatory system	Assess nutritional status. Provide appropriate total parenteral nutrition. Maintain alveolar ventilation.
Psychological Depression Anxiety: patient and family	Inability to communicate normally during mechanical ventilation therapy Psychological dependence on mechanical ventilation Sensory/sleep deprivation Sensory overload	Develop system of communication that is comfortable for patient. Anticipate needs. Monitor continuously. Establish rapport with family, keep patient/family informed, involve in care planning. Offer reassurance; take time to listen and answer questions. Help nurture feelings of security and human worth.

trol of inspiration, decreasing the work of breathing, and allowing a slow progression for the patient to assume the total responsibility for the work of breathing.[10] The latter is accomplished by slowly decreasing the amount of pressure over time.[31]

Monitoring During Weaning

The patient should be closely monitored during the weaning process for signs of poor tolerance and decreased oxygenation. Three types of devices used to

TABLE 25–24
Weaning Parameters

Awake and alert
PEEP $<$/=5 cm H_2O
$PaO_2 > 60$ mmHg on $FIO_2 < 50\%$
$PaCO_2$ acceptable with pH of 7.35–7.45
f $<$25 inspirations/min
VT 4–5 mL/kg
VC > 10–15 mL/kg
VE 5–10 L/min (equals f $\times$ VT)
  VE $>$ than 10 L/min is associated with respiratory muscle fatigue and increased work of breathing.
Maximum voluntary ventilation 10–20 L/min
  MVV is the maximum amount of air that can be inhaled and exhaled as rapidly as possible over 1 minute; determined by measuring 2 maximum exhaled volumes and multiplying by 4. Normal = 50–250 L/min. MMV assesses respiratory muscle endurance.
NIF > -20 cm H_2O
  NIF is measured with an inspiratory force manometer; indicates patient's ability to take a deep breath and cough.

Source: Modified from Weilitz, P: Weaning a patient from mechanical ventilation. Crit Care Nurse 13(4):34–35 1993.

monitor the patient are pulse oximetry (SaO_2), end-tidal carbon dioxide, and continuous ABG monitoring. These devices may be used not only during the weaning process, but also during the entire mechanical ventilation period.

Pulse oximetry is a noninvasive monitoring technique to measure SaO_2. Oxyhemoglobin is determined by measuring the variation in light absorbance between reduced and oxygenated hemoglobin.[31] Two wavelengths of light—red and infrared,—are transmitted through a highly vascular area. The SaO_2 is measured by analyzing the change in optical density of the transmitted light as arterial blood flows into a vascularized area. The photodetector signal is transformed into a digital display of percent saturation and pulse rate. Research has demonstrated that continued measurement of SaO_2 can be used in a safe and effective protocol for nurses to use to wean patients from toxic oxygen levels.[32] Monitor SaO_2 can decrease the incidence of hypoxemia in susceptible patients.

End-tidal carbon dioxide capnography is the measurement of the end-tidal partial pressure of carbon dioxide, also referred to as $PetCO_2$. The patient's inhaled and exhaled carbon dioxide is displayed as a waveform and as a number. Correct interpretation and application of this information include the ability to understand (1) the normal components of this waveform, (2) the normal relationship between $PaCO_2$ and $PetCO_2$ values, and (3) the physiologic relationships for disruptions of this relationship.

Intra-arterial blood gas monitoring is a newer method of monitoring oxygenation and ventilation designed to give continuous ABG readings.[33] In vitro measurement of pH, oxygen, and carbon dioxide has been

TABLE 25–25
Assessment Criteria for Termination of Weaning

Decrease level of consciousness
Diastolic blood pressure > 100 mmHg
Fall in systolic blood pressure
Heart rate > 110 bpm or a > 20 bpm increase over baseline
f > 30 inspirations/min or a > 10 inspirations/min increase over
    baseline
V_T <250–300 mL
pH < 7.35
$Paco_2$ increased by 8 mmHg
Premature ventricular contractions > 6/min or salvos
Changes in ST segment (usually elevation)
Ventricular condition changes

Source: From Weilitz, P: Weaning a patient from mechanical ventilation. Crit Care Nurse 23(4):37, 1993, with permission.

made possible by the development of highly sensitive optical fibers. The system attaches to an arterial line and gives a continuous digital readout of oxygen, carbon dioxide, pH, and temperature. Continuous ABG monitoring has the potential to allow for timely intervention during the initial stages of ARF. Early intervention may contribute to an improved outcome for these critically ill patients.

Tips for Weaning

With any successful weaning process, eventually the patient assumes complete ventilatory responsibility by spontaneous breathing.[33] Some of the factors that have to be corrected before weaning can actually begin are acid-base abnormalities, fever, infection, anemia, hyperglycemia, fluid imbalance, protein loss, electrolyte abnormalities, and sleep deprivation.[29] Successful weaning is evaluated using one or more of the monitoring devices previously described. Serial ABG values in conjunction with Sao_2 may be used as parameters for determining continued decrease in the ventilatory rate.

Explanation of the weaning process to the patient is essential for success. Keep the patient informed of his or her progress. Before weaning is initiated, all central nervous system depressant drugs should have been held for at least 4 hours. The patient should be kept in a position in which all respiratory muscles are maximally functioning. See Table 25–25 for criteria for termination of weaning.[29]

REFERENCES

1. King, G: Respiratory failure in the critically ill. In Sibbald, W (ed): Synopsis of Critical Care, ed 3. Williams & Wilkins, Baltimore, 1988, p 53.
2. Weinberger, SE: Principles of Pulmonary Medicine. WB Saunders, Philadelphia, 1986, pp 311–312.
3. Suchyta, M, et al: The adult respiratory distress syndrome: A report of survival and modifying factors. Chest 101:1074, 1992.
4. Campbell, M and Greenberg, C: Reading pulmonary artery wedge pressure at end-expiration. Focus Crit Care 15(2):60, 1988.
5. Ahrens, T: Respiratory disorders. In Kinney, M, Packa, D, and Dunbar, S (eds): AACN's Clinical Reference for Critical Care, ed 3. CV Mosby, St Louis, 1993, p 703.
6. Shapiro, BA: Noncardiogenic edema, adult respiratory distress syndrome, and PEEP therapy. In Cane, RD and Shapino, BA (eds): Case Studies in Critical Care Medicine. Year Book Medical Publishers, Chicago, 1985, p 184.
7. Bradley, R: Adult respiratory distress syndrome. Focus Crit Care 14(5):48, 1987.
8. Schmitz, T: Fact or myth? Patients with pulmonary disease should be placed in the semi-Fowler's position. Focus Crit Care 18(1):58, 1991.
9. Vaughn, P and Brooks, C: Adult respiratory distress syndrome. Crit Care Clin North Am 2:235, 1990.
10. Hall, J and Wood, L: Acute hypoxemic respiratory failure. In Hall, J, Schmidt, G, and Wood, L (eds): Principles of Critical Care. McGraw-Hill, New York, 1992, p 1646.
11. Rossaint, R, et al: Inhaled nitric oxide for the adult respiratory syndrome. N Engl J Med 326:399, 1993.
12. Fulmer, JD and Snider, GL; American College of Chest Physicians/National Heart, Lung, and Blood Institute National Conference on Oxygen Therapy. Heart Lung 13(4):550, September, 1984.
13. Pfister, S: Management of a transtracheal oxygen catheter in a mechanically ventilated patient. Crit Care Nurse 13(4):52, 1993.
14. Neagley, S: The Pulmonary System. In Alspach, J (ed): AACN's Core Curriculum for Critical Care Nurses, ed 4. WB Saunders, Philadelphia, 1991, p 76.
15. Hoffman, L, Mazzucco, M, and Roth, J: Fine tuning your chest PT. Am J Nurs 87:1566, 1987.
16. Boggs, R: Airway management. In Boggs, R and Wooldridge-King, M (eds): AACN Procedure Manual for Critical Care. WB Saunders, Philidelphia, p 1.
17. Don, H: Decision Making in Critical Care. CV Mosby, St Louis, 1985, p 106.
18. Weilitz, P and Dettenmeier, P: Test your knowledge of tracheostomy tubes. Am J Nurs 94(2):46, 1994.
19. Noll, M, Hix, C, and Scott, G: Closed tracheal suction systems: Effectiveness and implications. AACN Clin Iss in Crit Care Nurs 1(2):318, 1990.
20. Gray, J, MacIntyre, N and Kronenberger, G: The effects of normal-saline instillation in conjunction with endotracheal suctioning. Resp Care 35(8):185, 1990.
21. Hanley, M, Rudd, T, and Butler, J: What happens to intratracheal saline instillations? Am Rev Resp Dis, 117:124, 1978.
22. Ackerman, T: The effect of saline lavage prior to suctioning. Am J Crit Care 2(4):326, 1993.
23. Emanuelsen, K and Densmore, MJ: Acute Respiratory Care. Fleschner Publishing, Bethany, CT, 1981, p 155.
24. King, G: Respiratory failure in the critically ill. In Sibbald, WJ (ed): Synopsis of Critical Care, ed 3. Williams & Wilkins, Baltimore, 1988, p 53.
25. Chalikian, J and Weaver, T: Mechanical ventilation: For CE credit where it's at, where it's going. Am J Nurs 84:1372, 1984.
26. Ahrens, T: Mechanical support of ventilation. In Kinney, M, Packa, D, and Dunbar, S (eds): AACN's Clinical Reference for Critical Care, ed 3. CV Mosby, St Louis, 1993, p 741.
27. Marcy, T and Marini, J: Inverse ratio ventilation in ARDS: Rationale and implementation. Chest 100:494, 1990.
28. Norton, LC and Neureter, A: Weaning the long-term ventilator-dependent patient: Common problems and management. Crit Care Nurse 9(1):42–46, 1989.
29. Weilitz, P: Weaning a patient from mechanical ventilation. Crit Care Nurse 3(4):34–35, 1993.
30. Weilitz, P: Weaning from mechanical ventilation: Old and new strategies. Crit Care Nurs Clin North Am, 3:585, 1991.
31. O'Grady, S, Egstrom, S., and Fisher, J: Special pulmonary procedures. In Boggs, R and Wooldridge-King, M (eds): AACN Procedure Manual for Critical Care, WB Saunders, Philadelphia, p 199.
32. Rotello, L, et al: A nurse-directed protocol using pulse oximetry to wean mechanically ventilated patients from toxic oxygen concentrations. Chest 102:1833, 1992.

33. Marshall, W and Foster-Smith, R: Intra-arterial blood gas monitoring. Part 1: Optical sensor technology. Progress Notes. Spring, 1992, Puritan-Bennett p 6.
34. King, G: Respiratory failure in the critically ill. Synopsis of Critical Care, ed 3. Williams & Wilkins, Baltimore, 1988, p 60.

SUGGESTED READINGS

Ahrens, T and Rutherford, K: The new pulmonary math applying the a/A ratio. Am J Nurs 87:337, 1985.

Applefeld, JH: Acute Respiratory Care. Blackwell Scientific Publications, Boston, 1988.

Ayers, S, Schlichtig, R, and Sterling, M: Care of the Critically Ill, ed 3. Year Book Medical Publishers, Chicago, 1988.

Belshe, R: Viral respiratory disease in the intensive care unit. Heart Lung 15:222, 1986.

Bradley, R: Adult respiratory distress syndrome. Focus Crit Care 14(5):48, 1987.

Case, S and Sabo, C: Adult respiratory distress syndrome: A deadly complication of trauma. Focus Crit Care 19(2):116, 1992.

Clochesy, J, Daly, B, Montenegro, H: Weaning chronically ill adults from mechanical ventalatory support: a descriptive study. Am J Crit Care 4(2):93, 1995.

Flynn J-B and Bruce, N: Introduction to Critical Care Skills. CV Mosby, St Louis, 1993.

Holloway, N: Critical Care Care Plans. Springhouse Corporation, Springhouse, PA, 1989.

Kacmarek, R and Stoler, J: Current Respiratory Care. BC Decker, Philadelphia, 1988.

Lewis, R: Tracheostomies: Indications, timing, and complications. Clin Chest Med 13:137, 1992.

Macintyre, N: Techniques for weaning from mechanical ventilatory support. J Crit Illness 6(1):91, 1991.

Mathay, M: The adult respiratory distress syndrome. West J Med 150:187, 1989.

Pierce, L: Guide to Mechanical Ventilation and Intensive Respiratory Care. WB Saunders, Philadelphia, 19   .

Pierce, J, et al: Pressure support ventilation: Reducing the work of breathing during weaning. Dimensions in Critical Care Nursing 12(6):282, 1993.

Raymond, S: Normal saline before suction: helpful or harmful? Am J Crit Care 4(4):267, 1995.

Roberts, S and White, B: Common nursing diagnoses for pulmonary alveolar edema patients. Dimensions in Critical Care Nursing 11(1):13, 1992.

Shapiro, BA: Noncardiogenic edema, adult respiratory distress syndrome and PEEP therapy. In Cane, RD and Shapiro, BA (eds): Case Studies in Critical Care Medicine. Year Book Medical Publishers, Chicago, 1985.

Stoller, J and Kacmarek, R: Ventilatory strategies in the management of the adult respiratory distress syndrome. Clin Chest Med 11(4):755, 1990.

Vincent, E: Medical problems in the patient on a ventilator. Crit Care Q 6(2):40, 1983.

Williams, M: An algorithm for selecting a communication technique for intubated patients. Dimensions in Critical Care Nursing 11(4):222, 1992.

CARE PLAN FOR THE PATIENT WITH ADULT RESPIRATORY DISTRESS SYNDROME IN HYPOXEMIC ACUTE RESPIRATORY FAILURE

Nursing Diagnoses

Nursing Diagnosis #1
Gas exchange, impaired, related to:
1. Right-to-left shunting
2. $\dot{V}/\dot{Q}$ mismatch

Desired Patient Outcomes

Patient will:
1. Be alert and oriented to person, place, and time.
2. Demonstrate appropriate behavior.
3. Maintain effective cardiovascular function:
   - Blood pressure within 10 mmHg of baseline
   - Cardiac output ~ 5 L/min
   - Cardiac index 2.5–4 L/min
   - Without cyanosis if preexisting pulmonary function normal
   - Lab values:
     Hematocrit
       Male: 45%–52%
       Female: 37%–48%
     Hemoglobin
       Male: 13–18 g/100 mL
       Female: 12–16 g/100 mL
4. Maintain optimal arterial blood gases:
   pH 7.35–7.45
   $Pa_{O_2} > 60$ mmHg
   Pa_{CO_2} ~ 35–45 mmHg
5. Alveolar-arterial oxygen gradient ($PA_{O_2} - Pa_{O_2}$): <15 mmHg on room air.
6. $Sp_{O_2} > 90\%$
7. Capillary refill ≤ 3 sec

Nursing Interventions

- Perform neurologic assessment:
  - Mental status, level of consciousness
  - Appropriate behavior
  - Protective and deep tendon reflexes
- Monitor respiratory function:
  - Respiratory rate and pattern

Rationales

- Hypoxemia may predispose to cerebral tissue hypoxia.

CARE PLAN FOR THE PATIENT WITH ADULT RESPIRATORY DISTRESS SYNDROME IN HYPOXEMIC ACUTE RESPIRATORY FAILURE (*Continued*)

Nursing Interventions

- ○ Use of accessory muscles

- ○ Status of weakness and fatigue
- ○ Degree of chest wall excursion
- ○ Increase in fremitus

- ○ Presence of dullness on percussion

- ○ Abnormal breath sounds
- ○ Adventitious breath sounds

- • Assess cardiovascular function:
  - ○ Heart rate
  - ○ Hemodynamic parameters:
    - ▫ Systemic arterial pressure
    - ▫ PCWP
    - ▫ Cardiac output/cardiac index
  - ○ Evidence of cyanosis
  - ○ Pulse oximetry
  - ○ Capillary refill
  - ○ Cardiac arrhythmias

  - ○ ABG values: pH

- • Monitor laboratory data:
  - ○ ABG values
    pH
    PaO_2 significantly reduced < 60 mmHg
    $PaCO_2$ reduced early < 35 mmHg
           increased late >45 mmHg
  Calculate alveolar-arterial gradient.

  - ○ Hematology: hematocrit, hemoglobin

- • Administer prescribed humidified oxygen therapy.

Rationales

- ○ Increased work of breathing fatigues the patient and predisposes to alveolar hypoventilation with hypercapnia and respiratory acidemia.

- ○ Consolidated lung tissue transmits vibrations better than air-filled lung spaces.
- ○ Percussion over consolidated lung produces a "dull" sound.
- ○ Bronchial breath sounds are often heard in areas of the lung that normally would reflect vesicular sounds; rales (crackles) may also be heard.
- • Hemodynamic parameters reflect tissue perfusion.

- ○ Cyanosis is a late sign reflecting the desaturation of at least 5 g hemoglobin; evidence of $\dot{V}/\dot{Q}$ mismatch and right-to-left shunt.
- ○ Hypoxemia is commonly associated with myocardial irritability.
- ○ A metabolic acidemia is often associated with decreased tissue perfusion; the consequent anaerobic metabolism causes a rise in serum lactate levels with a progressive metabolic acidosis.
- ○ Metabolic acidosis may depress myocardial function and predispose to arrhythmias.

- ○ ABG values most closely reflect effectiveness of gas exchange.
- ○ Extensive right-to-left shunting causes the hypoxemia to be refractory to oxygen therapy.
- ○ Tachypnea and dyspnea cause carbon dioxide to be eliminated, predisposing to hypocapnia.
- ○ Alveolar-arterial gradient >250–300 mmHg with an FIO_2 of 100% is a hallmark of ARDS.
- ○ Maintenance of normal physiologic levels of hemoglobin ensures maximal oxygen transport and release of oxygen to the tissues; increased hemoglobin levels increase blood viscosity.
- • Oxygenation is the mainstay of treatment of ARDS; a large right-to-left shunt predisposes to a hypoxemia refractory to administration of even high concentrations (FIO_2 > 50%) of oxygen.
  - ○ Oxygen is administered in conjunction with mechanical ventilation and PEEP therapy.
  - ○ Precautions associated with oxygen therapy:
    - ▫ Oxygen is a potent drug necessitating cautious use.
    - ▫ Oxygen concentrations should be kept to a minimum to maintain PaO_2 > 60 mmHg.
    - ▫ Duration of oxygen therapy should be kept to a minimum.
  - ○ Prolonged administration of high oxygen concentrations predisposes to oxygen toxicity.
  - ○ Frequent monitoring of ABGs is a mandatory safety measure when an FIO_2 > 40% is used.

CARE PLAN FOR THE PATIENT WITH ADULT RESPIRATORY DISTRESS SYNDROME IN HYPOXEMIC ACUTE RESPIRATORY FAILURE (*Continued*)

Nursing Interventions

- Implement PEEP therapy in conjunction with mechanical ventilatory support.
  - Dosage: early noncardiogenic pulmonary edema; 5–15 cm H_2O pressure; severe ARDS 15–30 cm H_2O pressure.

  - Criteria used to determine effective PEEP level: ABG analysis; mixed venous oxygen tension; lung compliance; hemodynamic parameters: pulmonary artery pressure; PCWP; cardiac output.
  - PEEP—usually increased in increments 3–5 cm H_2O pressure until "best PEEP" is achieved.
  - Monitor for complications of PEEP therapy: reduction in venous return to the heart and cardiac output; reduction in cerebral perfusion—assess mental status.
  - Barotrauma.

- Monitor fluid status.

Rationales

- PEEP therapy maintains airway opening pressure at end-expiration above atmospheric pressure. This distending airway pressure increases lung volumes including FRC; it prevents airway collapse; it enhances gas exchange and oxygen transport; and it functions to reduce right-to-left shunting.
  - Use of PEEP therapy increases PaO_2 without requiring an increase in FIO_2.
  - Lung compliance is determined by dividing the peak inspiratory pressure (PIP) into the V_T.
  - "Best PEEP" is the level at which maximal benefit of PEEP is realized (i.e., $PaO_2 > 60$ mmHg on FIO_2 50%).
  - Positive intrathoracic pressure generated by PEEP is applied to the great veins within the chest, reducing venous return to the right heart.
  - Overdistention and rupture of alveoli are major complications of PEEP therapy.
- Overly vigorous administration of fluids may aggravate the pulmonary edema; the increased capillary hydrostatic pressure favors movement of fluid into lung interstitium.
  - Excessive fluid accumulation increases total lung water, causing an increase in $\dot{V}/\dot{Q}$ mismatching.

Nursing Diagnoses

Nursing Diagnosis #2
Breathing pattern, ineffective, related to tachypnea, hyperventilation

Desired Patient Outcomes

Patient will:
1. Achieve effective minute ventilation
   - $V_T > 5–7$ mL/kg
   - Respiratory rate < 30 inspriations/min
2. Achieve a vital capacity VC $> 12–15$ mL/kg.
3. Verbalize ease of breathing.
   - Breath sounds audible throughout anterior/posterior chest
   - Reduced to absent adventitious sounds

Nursing Interventions

- Assess respiratory function:
  - Rate, rhythm, depth, and pattern of breathing

  - Symmetry of chest wall and diaphragmatic excursion: use of accessory muscles; flaring of nares
    - Monitor for fatigue, exhaustion.
  - Lung compliance

  - Pulmonary lung volumes:
    - V_E
    - V_T
    - Respiratory rate (f)
    - Vital capacity (VC).

- Assist patient into position of comfort to allow for best lung expansion.
- Implement mechanical ventilation (see Table 25–22 for nursing care considerations)

Rationales

- Tachypnea is the compensatory mechanism for hypoxemia.
- Hyperventilatory effort is responsible for the hypocapnia observed during the *early* course of the illness.

- Accumulation of fluid, edema, and secretions within the lungs, with lung consolidation, reduces lung compliance.
- Maximal respiratory effort is made to facilitate optimum ventilation.
- A minimal volume of ventilation is necessary to ensure adequate alveolar ventilation; this minimal volume of gas enables gas exchange to occur during the phases of the respiratory cycle when no new gas is inspired (expiratory and end-expiratory phases).
- Expansion of lungs facilitates more even distribution of ventilation; increases $\dot{V}/\dot{Q}$ matching.

CARE PLAN FOR THE PATIENT WITH ADULT RESPIRATORY DISTRESS SYNDROME IN HYPOXEMIC ACUTE RESPIRATORY FAILURE (*Continued*)

Nursing Diagnoses

Nursing Diagnosis #3
Airway clearance, ineffective, related to increased tracheobronchial secretions

Desired Patient Outcomes

Patient will:
1. Be alert and oriented to person, place, time
2. Maintain effective alveolar ventilation:
   - Breath sounds audible throughout anterior/posterior chest
   - Reduced to absent adventitious sounds
   - ABG values stabilized as follows:
        pH 7.35–7.45
        $Pao_2 > 60$ mmHg
        $Paco_2$ 35–45 mmHg

Nursing Interventions

- Assess respiratory function with emphasis on status of pulmonary secretions and the patient's ability to handle secretions.
  - Presence of adventitious sounds
    - Rales (crackles), wheezes, bronchi
    - Suction endotracheal tube as necessary, using in-line suction device
- Assess fluid status.
  - Intake and output; daily weight

- Implement chest physiotherapy and bronchial hygiene measures.

Rationales

- Patients with ARDS often have increased secretions, which impair adequate ventilation, further compromising the hypoxemia.

- Even the slightest interruption of PEEP therapy can significantly increase hypoxemia.
- Excessive intrapulmonary accumulation of fluid reduces compliance and further aggravates underlying right-to-left shunting and $\dot{V}/\dot{Q}$ mismatching.
- Pooling of secretions within the tracheobronchial tree compromises ventilation and predisposes to infection.

Nursing Diagnoses

Nursing Diagnosis #4
Cardiac output, alteration in, decreased (diminished venous return)
Tissue perfusion, alteration in: cardiopulmonary status (related to ARDS)

Desired Patient Outcomes

Patient will:
1. Maintain stable hemodynamics:
   - Blood pressure within 10 mmHg of baseline
   - Heart rate < 100 bpm
   - Cardiac output ~5 L/min; cardiac index ≥2.4 L/min
   - Central venous pressure (CVP) 0–8 mmHg
   - PCWP 8–12 mmHg
2. Remain without:
   - Extreme weakness or fatigue
   - Peripheral (pedal) edema
   - Neck vein distention
   - Chest pain
   - Cardiac arrhythmias
3. Maintain fluid and electrolyte balance:
   - Stable body weight
   - Balanced intake and output
   - Hourly urine output >30 mL/h

Nursing Interventions

- Perform ongoing cardiovascular assessment:
  - Continuous cardiac monitoring (establish baseline rate, rhythm)
  - Continuous hemodynamic monitoring (establish baseline): CVP, PCWP

  - Heart sounds: loudness or intensity, splitting, extra heart sounds (S_3–S_4)?

  - Breath sounds: evidence of rales (crackles); altered pulmonary mechanics?
  - Fatigue, exhaustion?
  - Neck vein distention? Pedal edema?
  - Serial ABGs

Rationales

  - Cardiac tissue hypoxia may predispose to arrhythmias.

  - Hemodynamic monitoring offers significant data regarding cardiopulmonary function.
  - Positive-pressure mechanical ventilation increases pressure within the thorax, which impedes venous return to the heart; decrease in venous return (preload) reduces cardiac output.
  - Loud pulmonic sound or splitting is commonly found in cor pulmonale; it is related to pulmonary hypertension due to long-standing hypoxemic state.
  - In the patient with COPD, diminished breath sounds in a previously "noisy" chest may warn of hypoventilation with impending ARF.

CARE PLAN FOR THE PATIENT WITH ADULT RESPIRATORY DISTRESS SYNDROME IN HYPOXEMIC ACUTE RESPIRATORY FAILURE (*Continued*)

Nursing Interventions	Rationales

• Implement fluid replacement therapy as prescribed.
 	
   ◦ Monitor hydration status: daily weight, intake and output, urine specific gravity.
   ◦ Avoid fluid volume overload.
	• Adequate fluid replacement therapy is essential for maintaining blood volume and keeping pulmonary secretions moist and easily mobilized.
	   ◦ Long-standing pulmonary disease with pulmonary hypertension predisposes to right heart failure (cor pulmonale). (See Nursing Diagnosis #6)

Nursing Diagnoses	Desired Patient Outcomes
Nursing Diagnosis #5 Tissue perfusion, alteration in: cerebral status	Patient will: 1. Demonstrate appropriate behavior: • Oriented to person, place, time

Nursing Interventions	Rationales

• Assess ongoing neurologic function.
   ◦ Mental status, level of consciousness; behavior appropriate?
• Assess fluid and electrolyte status.
   ◦ Body weight
 	
   ◦ Intake and output (hourly urine output)
   ◦ Serum electrolytes, BUN, creatinine
 	
• Maintain a quiet, relaxed milieu.
   ◦ Use a calm, reassuring approach.
   ◦ Provide explanations of care.
   ◦ Provide frequent periods of rest and relaxation.
 	
• Monitor for effects of drugs on cardiopulmonary function.
• Monitor effects of sedatives and paralytics if in use.
	• Compromised hemodynamics and hypoxemia predispose to cerebral hypoxia with altered cerebral function.
	
	• Reduced blood volume will further compromise venous return and cardiac output; blood volume may need to be expanded to minimize this effect.
	   ◦ Reduced cardiac output may diminish renal perfusion, placing patient at risk of developing acute renal failure.
	• Minimize fear and anxiety, which increase oxygen consumption and demand.
	
	   ◦ The work of breathing is often taxing; it is important to conserve patient's energy.
	• Drug toxicity may further compromise cardiopulmonary function.

Nursing Diagnoses	Desired Patient Outcomes

Nursing Diagnosis #6
Fluid and electrolyte, alterations in (see Chapter 36 for specific fluid/electrolyte imbalances), related to increased permeability of the pulmonary capillary membranes and shifting of intravascular volume.
	Patient will:
	1. Maintain baseline body weight
	2. Balance fluid intake with output
	3. Have:
	   • Good skin turgor
	   • Absence of peripheral edema
	   • Absence of rales (crackles) on auscultation
	   • Stable vital signs
	4. Stabilize in terms of serum electrolyte, BUN, creatinine, total protein within acceptable physiologic range

Nursing Interventions	Rationales

• Monitor hydration status:
   ◦ Daily weight, intake and output, vital signs
 	
   ◦ Examine skin for signs of dehydration: poor skin turgor; sunken eyeballs; dry, parched mucous membranes.
Monitor mental status changes; lethargy; severe weakness; reduced urine output.
   ◦ Examine for signs of overhydration: peripheral edema; hypertension; tachycardia; neck vein distention; elevated pulmonary hemodynamics; shortness of breath, dyspnea.
• Monitor serum electrolytes, BUN, creatinine, total protein.
   ◦ Increase V_T.
   ◦ Decrease respiratory rate.
   ◦ If mechanically ventilated, increase V_{SP} space ventilation; decrease minute ventilation.
	• Patients receiving mechanical ventilation with humidified gas therapy are at limited risk for an increase in total body water.
	   ◦ Stress increases secretion of antidiuretic hormone (ADH) by posterior pituitary gland, increasing water retention.
	
	   ◦ Stress increases aldosterone secretion by adrenal cortex, which stimulates sodium reabsorption within the kidneys.
	
	   ◦ Increasing V_T and decreasing respiratory rate decrease total V_E; reduced ventilation enables the alveolar P_{CO_2} and, thus, the Pa_{CO_2} to return to an acceptable physiologic range (35–45 mmHg).

CARE PLAN FOR THE PATIENT WITH ADULT RESPIRATORY DISTRESS SYNDROME IN HYPOXEMIC ACUTE RESPIRATORY FAILURE (*Continued*)

Nursing Diagnoses

Nursing Diagnosis #7
Acid-base balance, alteration in, respiratory alkalosis (tachypnea, hyperventilation)

Desired Patient Outcomes

The patient's ABG values will stabilize as follows:
pH 7.35–7.45
$Pao_2 > 60$ mmHg
$Paco_2$ 35–45 mmHg

Nursing Interventions

- Assess for signs and symptoms of respiratory alkalemia:
  - Neurologic function: lightheadedness, weakness, muscle cramps, twitching; paresthesias; hyperactive deep tendon reflexes, seizure activity; tetany
  - Cardiovascular function: cardiac arrhythmias

  - Serum calcium levels
  - Serial ABG measurements

- Implement supportive therapy to maintain adequate ventilation and optimal gas exchange.

Rationales

- Respiratory failure in the patient with ARDS is associated with tachypnea and hyperventilation as the body tries to compensate for the severe hypoxemia. As the ARDs worsen, the hypoxia worsens and there is increased Pco_2 and decreased pH.
  - Hyperventilation reduces $Paco_2$ with a consequent rise in pH.
  - A rise in pH reduces the serum concentration of freely ionized calcium by causing an increase in the calcium that is protein-bound. The consequent hypocalcemia, if sufficiently severe, may predispose to neuromuscular alterations.

Nursing Diagnoses

Nursing Diagnosis #8
Nutrition, alteration in, related to less than body requirements. (See Chapter 9.)

Desired Patient Outcomes

Patient will:
1. Maintain body weight within 5% of baseline weight
2. Maintain total serum proteins ~6.0–8.4 g/100 mL
3. Maintain laboratory data within acceptable range: BUN, serum creatinine, electrolytes, fasting blood sugar, serum albumin, hematology profile, phosphate
4. Verbalize essentials of adequate diet

Nursing Interventions

- Arrange consultation with nutritionist and collaborate to perform nutrition assessment: general state of health; baseline body weight; nutritional history—likes, dislikes, meal preparation, eating habits, cultural, religious considerations.
  - Lifestyle influences
  - Physiologic factors: height, weight, triceps skinfold, mid/upper arm circumference
  - Laboratory studies: urinary/serum creatinine, BUN, fasting blood sugar, serum electrolytes, total protein (serum albumin), hematology profile
- Maintain adequate nutrition with prescribed enteral or parenteral feedings.
  - Note special nutritional considerations.

  - Avoid large glucose loads to meet caloric needs.

  - Avoid hypophosphatemia.

  - Avoid high amino acid loads.

- Place patient in optimal position during feedings (usually semi-Fowler's position).

Rationales

- Adequate nutritional intake is necessary to meet metabolic requirements to reverse acute respiratory failure.
  - Nutritional deficiencies (especially in elderly) are often associated with chronic disease.

- Clinical semistarvation leads to depression of the hypoxic ventilatory drive.
  - Patients receiving mechanical ventilation therapy are highly stressed and require nutritional supplements to meet hypermetabolic needs.
  - There is an obligate increase in carbon dioxide with increased glucose intake. Fat emulsions may be used to provide calories.
  - In patients who are mechanically ventilated or who have reduced respiratory reserve, the increased carbon dioxide can lead to hypercapnia and may precipitate ARF in the high-risk patient.
  - Reduced phosphate levels are associated with decreased energy levels, respiratory muscle weakness, and increased risk of infection.
  - High levels of amino acids increase oxygen consumption.
- Proper positioning and intact protective reflexes reduce risk of aspiration.

CARE PLAN FOR THE PATIENT WITH ADULT RESPIRATORY DISTRESS SYNDROME IN HYPOXEMIC ACUTE RESPIRATORY FAILURE (*Continued*)

Nursing Interventions	Rationales

• Confirm placement of nasogastric feeding tube in stomach before initiating feedings.
  ○ Assess for protective reflexes (gag, cough, swallowing).
• Provide frequent mouth care and other comfort measures.
 	
• Monitor daily weight, fluid and intake.
• Assess bowel function:
  ○ Assess bowel sounds.
  ○ Initiate bowel regimen, if indicated.
	• Proper placement of nasogastric tube helps to prevent aspiration.
	
	• Good mouth care may be aesthetically pleasing to patient/family.
	  ○ Oral hygiene keeps mucous membranes moist and intact and assists in preventing further infections.
	
	  ○ Good bowel regimen maintains gastrointestinal smooth muscle tone; prevents constipation or impaction.

Nursing Diagnoses	Desired Patient Outcomes
Nursing Diagnosis #9 Infection, potential for, related to compromised immune status secondary to ARDs.	Patient will: 1. Maintain normal body temperature ~98.6°F (37°C) 2. Maintain white blood count at acceptable baseline level 3. Remain without evidence of acute infection: redness, swelling, pain

Nursing Interventions	Rationales

• Identify patients at high risk for developing an infection: debilitated or elderly, chronic lung disease, multiple invasive lines, semistarvation state, immunosuppressed.
 	
• Obtain baseline cultures: sputum, urine, blood.
 	
• Monitor the following parameters:
  ○ Body temperature
  ○ Hematology profile: evidence of leukocytosis; eosinophilia
  ○ Sputum for changes in color, quantity, consistency, odor; and ability of patient to handle secretions
  ○ Chest x-ray for pulmonary infiltrates
• Institute vigorous chest physiotherapy and bronchial hygiene.
• Use aseptic technique for patient care: tracheobronchial suctioning, care of invasive lines.
• Administer prescribed antibiotic therapy.
  ○ Monitor culture and sensitivity studies to assess response to therapy.
• Maintain nutrition.
	• Patients with COPD are especially at high risk for infection because of:
	  ○ Alteration in surfactant activity.
	  ○ Alterations in respiratory epithelium replication.
	• Upon intubation, a baseline sputum specimen should be obtained.
	  ○ Use of artifical airway (endotracheal tube or tracheostomy) contaminates the tracheobronchial tree, which is usually considered to be sterile distal to the larynx.
	• Early diagnosis with institution of timely and vigorous therapy (antibiotic) may help to minimize the impact of the infectious process on total body function.
	
	• Secretion removal improves ventilation and reduces pooling of secretions, which may act as foci of infection.
	• Asepsis reduces risks of infection.

Nursing Diagnoses	Desired Patient Outcomes

Nursing Diagnosis #10
Pulmonary mechanics, alteration in, related to respiratory muscle atrophy (immobility, mechanical ventilation)
	Patient will:
	1. Perform deep breathing exercises
	2. Achieve maximum pulmonary function:
	  • $V_T > 7$ mL/kg
	  • Vital capacity > 15 mL/kg
	  • Maximal expiratory flow

CARE PLAN FOR THE PATIENT WITH ADULT RESPIRATORY DISTRESS SYNDROME IN HYPOXEMIC ACUTE RESPIRATORY FAILURE (*Continued*)

Nursing Interventions	Rationales
• Teach deep-breathing exercises.	• Use of positive-pressure ventilation predisposes to atrophy of the respiratory musculature, which can present problems for weaning.
○ Instruct about importance of deep-breathing exercises.	○ Improves pulmonary ventilation, mobilizes secretions, stimulates circulation.
	○ Teaching regarding pulmonary mechanics forms the foundation of patient's self-care after hospitalization.
○ Allow patient to demonstrate pulmonary exercises.	○ Patient should be allowed to learn one task before proceeding to the next. Always establish readiness to learn on the part of patient and family.
○ Combine deep-breathing therapy with other chest physiotherapy maneuvers.	
○ Involve patient/family in decision-making (e.g., scheduling of exercise activities).	○ The nature of chronic illness requires cooperation of all family members if exacerbations are to be prevented.
○ Encourage early ambulation (e.g., sitting up in chair).	○ Involvement in planning and decision-making enables patient and family to begin to assume responsibility for their own lives.
• Assess pulmonary volumes to determine effectiveness of therapy: VT, vital capacity.	

Nursing Diagnoses	Desired Patient Outcomes
Nursing Diagnosis #11	
Skin integrity, impairment of, related to immobility, and altered nutritional status	Patient's skin will remain intact.

Nursing Interventions	Rationales
• Establish routine for turning and repositioning.	• Exercise maintains muscle tone and prevents muscle atrophy.
• Assist with range-of-motion exercises to extremities.	• Exercise stimulates circulation and prevents stasis.
○ Provide support stockings to lower extremities.	○ Immobility predisposes to thrombophlebitis.
○ Assess extremities for calf tenderness.	○ Consult PT and OT when patient is hemodynamically stable.
○ Measure circumference of thighs and calves daily.	
• Provide special skin care to back and joints, and all pressure points.	• Maintains circulation to all areas; these patients frequently have a compromised body defense system and a high risk of infection.
○ Establish regimen for skin inspection, skin care, decubitus care, if necessary.	○ Good skin care is essential to prevent skin breakdown.
○ Provide egg-crate or air mattress; sheepskin; heel and ankle protectors.	○ Devices provide pressure relief.
○ Apply local skin care.	

Nursing Diagnoses	Desired Patient Outcomes
Nursing Diagnosis #12	Patient/family will:
Coping, ineffective individual/family	1. Verbalize knowledge and understanding of the illness
	2. Verbalize feelings as to what this potentially life-threatening illness means to each family member, individually and collectively
	3. Verbalize strengths and coping capabilities
	4. Identify family resources
	5. Make decisions regarding matters of importance to patient and family

CARE PLAN FOR THE PATIENT WITH ADULT RESPIRATORY DISTRESS SYNDROME IN HYPOXEMIC ACUTE RESPIRATORY FAILURE (*Continued*)

Nursing Interventions

- Assess patient/family perceptions regarding a potentially life-threatening illness.

  ○ Develop a trusting relationship with patient and family.

  ○ Establish a caring rapport: patient advocacy; accessible to patient/family.
  ○ Encourage verbalization of perceptions, concerns, and feelings.
- Assist patient/family to identify past coping capabilities:
  ○ Emphasize strengths.
  ○ Assist patient/family to define areas requiring problem-solving and decision-making.
    □ Support patient/family in this regard.
  ○ Involve in decision-making regarding care.
    □ Offer praise for accomplishments.
    □ Encourage development of new coping mechanisms.
    □ Assist patient/family to explore and identify options and the consequences of the options. Assist patient/family to implement chosen options.
- Initiate referrals to intrahospital and community resources for special needs: psychiatric social worker, family pastor, home care.

Rationales

- Knowledge of patient and family perceptions of the illness assists in identifying coping capabilities and potential coping problems.
  ○ A trusting, caring, supportive relationship facilitates verbalization of concerns and fears.
  ○ A definitive, dependable support system assists patient/family to assume responsibility for decision-making.
  ○ Unexpressed and unresolved fears and concerns may compromise ability to cope effectively.

  ○ Active participation in self-care assists the individual/family to gain a new sense of dignity, self-worth, and self-esteem.

- Additional resources may assist patient/family to gain increased awareness of self in the interactions among patient, family, healthcare providers, and environment.

CHAPTER 26

Nursing Management of the Patient with Respiratory Dysfunction: Pulmonary Embolism, Pleural Effusion, and Pneumothorax

Terry L. Jones

CHAPTER OUTLINE

LEARNING OBJECTIVES

After completing this chapter, you should be able to:

1. Identify predisposing factors associated with the pathogenesis and etiology of pulmonary embolism.
2. Describe the pathophysiology of pulmonary embolism and its impact on pulmonary and hemodynamic function.
3. Describe the clinical presentation and diagnostic evaluation of pulmonary embolism.
4. Define the therapeutic priorities in the treatment and management of pulmonay embolism.
5. Differentiate exudative from transudative pleural effusions.
6. List common causes of pneumothorax.
7. Describe the pathophysiology of pneumothorax.
8. Describe the clinical presentation of spontaneous and tension pneumothoraces.
9. List tentative nursing diagnoses related to the care of patients with pulmonary embolus, pleural effusion, and pneumothorax.
10. Identify implications for nursing care based on the nursing process for the patient with pulmonary embolus, pleural effusion, and pneumothorax.

PULMONARY EMBOLISM

Definition

Pulmonary embolism is the mechanical obstruction of pulmonary vessels with an embolus; it is defined as a mass of undissolved matter transferred to the lungs by blood or, less commonly, by lymphatic vessels.[1]

Pulmonary emboli constitute the most common cause of acute pulmonary disease in hospitalized patients. About 200,000 people die of pulmonary embolism each year in the United States. Fifty percent of these die within 2 hours of embolization, which is often undetected and therefore untreated.[2] Laboratory and radiographic findings of pulmonary embolism are nonspecific; thus, misdiagnosis is not uncommon. Yet, early recognition, prompt diagnosis, and treatment of this disorder reduce mortality rates from as high as 40% to less than 10%. In this regard, institution of prophylactic measures (i.e., low-dose heparin subcutaneously) has proved to be an effective therapeutic approach in certain high-risk patients.

Predisposing Factors

Most clinically detectable pulmonary emboli arise from sites of deep venous thrombosis. Ninety-five percent of such emboli originate in the lower extremities. Consequently, being at risk for deep venous thrombosis predisposes to the risk of pulmonary embolism. Furthermore, the risk of embolus is significantly higher if the thrombus is located in the more proximal veins (e.g., popliteal) in contrast to the calf veins, which are infrequently associated with pulmonary embolism. Three predisposing factors have been identified (Virchow's triad) in the pathogenesis of venous thrombosis. These include (1) venous stasis, (2) endothelial injury or vessel wall abnormalities, and (3) alteration in the mechanism of blood coagulation (hypercoagulable state).[3]

Etiologic Factors

Factors contributing to the pathogenesis of venous thrombosis and consequent thromboemboli include the following: immobility (bed rest), procedures requiring prolonged general anesthesia, injury or surgery to lower extremities or pelvis, thermal injuries, pregnancy and the postpartum state, underlying carcinoma, and the use of oral contraceptives.[1,2]

Less commonly, thrombus formation occurs in the heart in association with congestive heart failure, atrial fibrillation, cardioversion, endocarditis, and infarction. The incidence of thromboembolic disease increases with age and the length of illness.

Although extensive deep venous thrombosis has been highly implicated in the etiology of pulmonary embolism, it may be clinically undetectable. In fact, only about 50% of all patients with pulmonary embolism manifested prior clinical signs of venous thrombosis in the lower extremities or elsewhere. This underscores the necessity of obtaining a thorough history and of paying close attention to subtle clinical clues and details to even suspect pulmonary embolism.

Pathophysiology

Pathologically, embolic occlusion of a vessel may lead to pulmonary infarction (about 10% to 15% of all pulmonary emboli) or congestive atelectasis of the lung parenchyma characterized by hemorrhage and edema. Often, however, neither of these pathologic changes occurs, and there may be relatively little alteration of the lung parenchyma distal to the occlusion, presumably because of incomplete occlusion or sufficient oxygen from other sources. The dual circulation (pulmonary and bronchial systems) to the lungs, for example, may provide adequate collateral circulation in these instances. The pathophysiology of pulmonary embolism stems from the pulmonary and hemodynamic effects of occlusion of one or more pulmonary vessels.

Pulmonary Effects

Sudden obstruction of a pulmonary arterial branch results in alterations of both perfusion and ventilation. The degree of alteration in ventilation and perfusion depends on the site and degree of obstruction.

Increased Alveolar Dead Space. When total occlusion of a vessel and complete obstruction of blood flow through the lung region distal to the embolus occur, a region of alveolar dead space is created. Recall that alveolar dead space is a region that is ventilated but not perfused. Since such ventilation is not perfused, it is, in effect, wasted ventilation. If occlusion is partial, then one might expect that a region of high ventilation-to-perfusion ratio ($\dot{V}/\dot{Q}$ greater than 0.8) has been created. Because of other physiologic changes (discussed in the text that follows), however, this is not significant.[5]

Pneumoconstriction. Constriction and stiffening of the terminal bronchial airway and alveolar ducts occur following occlusion of a pulmonary arterial branch. The following four factors are believed to contribute to pneumoconstriction: (1) bronchoalveolar hypocapnia, (2) hypoxia, (3) humoral agents (e.g., serotonin and histamine) released from the thrombus or distal vascular endothelium, and (4) thrombin activation from the embolus itself.[2,4]

Physiologically, the effects of pneumoconstriction are increasing airway resistance, decreasing vital capacity and functional residual capacity, decreasing alveolar dead space, decreasing static effective compliance, and maldistribution of ventilation. Since the bronchoconstriction is not limited to those nonperfused lung regions, ventilation to adequately perfused alveoli is decreased as well. Consequently, a lower, or decreased $\dot{V}/\dot{Q}$ ratio is created (less than 0.8). This is referred to as a $\dot{V}/\dot{Q}$ mismatch and is a major contributor to hypoxemia associated with pulmonary embolism.

Loss of Surfactant. About 24 hours after a total occlusion, surfactant becomes depleted in those nonperfused alveolar zones. As a result, atelectasis and edema of these regions can occur. Resolution of the thrombus and reperfusion to these regions of atelectasis may consequently be accompanied by hypoxemia.

Hemodynamic Effects

Pulmonary Hypertension. As a result of the mechanical obstruction in the pulmonary arterial circulation, there is a reduction in the cross-sectional area of the pulmonary arterial bed. This reduction results in an increased pulmonary artery pressure and thus an increase in pulmonary vascular resistance (PVR). In addition to the anatomic obstruction that occurs, a degree of pulmonary arterial constriction also develops and contributes to the increased PVR. This pulmonary vasoconstriction is attributed to the release of various vasoactive and humoral substances (e.g., serotonin, histamine, and thromboxane) from the thrombus and distal endothelium. The extent of the anatomic obstruction, together with the degree of vasoconstriction that ensues, determines the severity of hemodynamic alteration.[2,3]

Right Ventricular Failure. The increase in PVR increases the resistance against which the right ventricle must pump. This then imposes a greater workload on the right ventricle, which normally pumps against a very low pressure system. If this workload becomes excessive, right ventricular failure ensues and is pronounced in the context of pre-existing cardiopulmonary compromise. In cases of massive pulmonary embolism, a profound acute right ventricular failure occurs accompanied by shock and possibly death.

Clinical Presentation

Most pulmonary emboli do not produce any significant symptoms, and the entire embolic episode may go unnoticed. When the patient becomes symptomatic, the clinical presentation may vary from mild to severe, depending on the extent and severity of the pulmonary embolism.

At physical examination, the nonspecific findings of dyspnea, tachypnea, and tachycardia are common. Dyspnea is almost universally experienced by patients suffering a pulmonary embolism and is the most common presenting complaint. Dyspnea is attributed to stimulation of the J receptors in the alveolar capillary junction. Pleuritic chest pain and hemoptysis are associated with pulmonary infarction and thus are uncommon as presenting symptoms of pulmonary embolism. The chest examination may be entirely normal, or it may reveal diminished breath sounds, localized rales (crackles), or wheezing. When atelectasis and edema

develop following loss of surfactant, a pulmonary effusion may develop accompanied by a pleural friction rub.

Hypoxemia

Some degree of hypoxemia is common in the course of a pulmonary embolism. Many novice clinicians have attributed the hypoxemia of pulmonary effusion to the increase in alveolar dead space that is created. However, since no venous admixture occurs in the context of dead space ventilation, it does not result in hypoxemia. The three factors believed to contribute to the hypoxemia of pulmonary embolism are a widening of the arteriovenous oxygen difference, decreased $\dot{V}/\dot{Q}$, and loss of surfactant. These factors are discussed in greater detail in the following text.

$\dot{V}/\dot{Q}$ Mismatch. Because of mechanisms previously discussed, areas of poorly ventilated alveoli are overperfused. As a result, this blood is not well oxygenated, and a venous admixture is said to occur. Consequently, arterial hypoxemia develops.

Widening Arteriovenous Oxygen Difference. As a result of the acute right ventricular failure resulting from the increased PVR, there is a decrease in cardiac output. Subsequently, the tissues extract more oxygen from the arterial blood, lowering the mixed venous oxygen content. This reduction in mixed venous oxygen then contributes to arterial hypoxemia as it perfuses poorly ventilated lung regions created by the pneumoconstriction previously discussed. The widening oxygen difference then magnifies the venous admixture effect created by the $\dot{V}/\dot{Q}$ mismatch and contributes significantly to arterial hypoxemia.[4]

Loss of Surfactant. After total occlusion of a vessel, there is a loss of surfactant in the nonperfused alveoli. With this loss of surfactant, atelectasis ensues. As the thrombus undergoes normal resolution, reperfusion of the previously occluded vessel occurs. Perfusion of these now-nonventilated regions creates a venous admixture effect and results in arterial hypoxemia. This "reperfusion hypoxemia" occurs 1 to 2 days after the initial embolic event.

Evidence of acute right ventricular overload (cor pulmonale) may be revealed on cardiac examination. A split S_2 or right-sided S_4 may be present, along with a murmur throughout the lung field reflecting turbulent blood flow through the partially occluded vessel. Jugular venous distention may be observed as well as cardiac arrhythmias—frequently atrial in origin—and electrocardiogram (ECG) changes reflective of right heart strain.

Diagnostic Evaluation

As previously mentioned, a diagnosis of pulmonary embolism is often difficult to make because the clinical presentation varies according to the size and location of the embolic episode. Many of the diagnostic studies do not enable a definitive diagnosis of pulmonary embolism to be made, but, rather, assist in differential diagnosis by ruling out other possibilities. To date, pulmonary angiography is the only definitive diagnostic test available. Diagnostic tests and procedures used in the diagnostic evaluation of pulmonary embolism are listed in Table 26–1.[2,6]

Treatment and Management

Therapeutic Priorities

In the setting of an acute embolic episode, the first priority may be to treat severely compromised cardiopulmonary function. Once the patient's cardiopulmonary status is stabilized, the next priority is to prevent recurrent embolization.[7]

Cardiopulmonary Support Therapy. The major considerations in initiating cardiopulmonary support in the scenario of acute pulmonary embolism is the maintenance of ventilation, oxygenation, and circulation.

Ventilatory Support. In patients with pulmonary embolism, the usual ventilatory consequence observed is hyperventilation with hypocapnia. In patients experiencing a massive pulmonary embolism associated with severe obtundation, hypoxemia and carbon dioxide retention with hypercapnia may occur, necessitating intubation and mechanical ventilation. Tidal volume and respiratory rate are adjusted to maintain the partial pressure of arterial carbon dioxide $PaCO_2$ within the range of 35 to 45 mmHg.

Oxygen Therapy. Basic principles pertaining to the management of hypoxemia require maintenance of a patent airway, with intubation and initiation of mechanical ventilation as needed to (1) prevent aspiration in the patient who is obtunded and in severe hypervolemic shock and (2) administer oxygen therapy at inspired oxygen concentrations (FIO_2) necessary to achieve a PaO_2 of more than 60 mmHg.

Circulatory Support. In obstructing the pulmonary vasculature, a pulmonary embolism reduces flow of blood to the left heart, decreasing the preload, or left ventricular end-diastolic volume (LVEDV). This in turn results in a reduction of cardiac output and systemic arterial blood pressure.

Currently, in response to the embolic episode, the pulmonary vasculature may itself reflexly trigger systemic peripheral arteriolar vasodilatation, which likewise reduces systemic arterial blood pressure. The consequence is a "relative" volume depletion or, if severe, hypovolemic shock. Treatment involves intravascular volume expansion to raise systemic blood pressure. Administration of intravenous fluids is best guided by hemodynamic pressure monitoring. Hypovolemic shock may require use of vasopressor therapy (dopamine).

Prevention of Recurrent Embolization

Anticoagulant Therapy. Concomitant with the implementation of definitive therapy to maintain cardiopulmonary function until resolution of the embolic

episode occurs, anticoagulant therapy is initiated to prevent recurrent embolization.[8] The major goal of anticoagulant therapy is to prevent further formation of intravascular clot with embolic potential.

The mainstay of anticoagulant therapy during the acute phase is heparin. The use of heparin has several advantages. Although it does not dissolve clots that have already embolized in the lungs, it does prevent formation of new thrombi or propagation of old ones.

Heparin also acts to block platelet-thrombin interactions on the embolus, which might otherwise lead to release of chemical mediators (e.g., serotonin) associated with bronchospasm and hypotension. Heparin enhances fibrinolytic activity on fresh thrombi. A major advantage of the drug is that its anticoagulant effects are promptly reversible with protamine sulfate if bleeding occurs. Heparin has an immediate onset of action.

Standard treatment for uncomplicated pulmonary embolism is anticoagulation with heparin during the acute phase, followed by Coumadin for 6 weeks to 6 months. Longer anticoagulant therapy is reserved for patients with conditions predisposing to recurrent emboli or who have a continuing predisposition to venous thrombosis. Because the action of Coumadin is mediated through altered production of vitamin K–dependent coagulation factors in the liver (factors II, VII, IX, X), the onset of action is not immediate. Hence, the initiation of Coumadin therapy should be overlapped by 2 or 3 days of heparin therapy at a slightly reduced dosage before heparin is discontinued.

Thrombolytic Therapy. Another option for treating pulmonary embolism is the use of thrombolytic agents—streptokinase or urokinase. These agents, which may actually lyse recent blood clots, must be given within the first several days of the embolic event to be effective. Patients with massive pulmonary embolus or those with hemodynamic compromise as a result of vascular occlusion are most likely to benefit from thrombolytic (fibrinolytic) therapy. Use of thrombolytic agents is generally continued for 24 to 48 hours and is followed by standard anticoagulant therapy.

Inferior Vena Cava Filter. Surgical intervention in the treatment of pulmonary embolism involves placement of a filtering device into the inferior vena cava. Also referred to as the "umbrella" device, the filter functions to trap thrombi originating in the deep veins of the pelvis or lower extremities, en route to the pulmonary circulation. These devices are indicated in situations in which anticoagulant therapy is contraindicated (e.g., in the presence of a bleeding problem) or in which the patient's pulmonary vascular reserve is so compromised that an individual embolus to the lungs could prove fatal.

Prophylactic Anticoagulation. Prophylactic anticoagulation to prevent deep venous thrombosis in high-risk patients has proved to be an effective therapeutic approach. The most common prophylaxis is heparin administered subcutaneously in low dosage, usually 5000 U every 8 to 12 hours. For nursing implications in heparin therapy (Table 26–2).[2,3,4,9]

TABLE 26–1
Diagnostic Evaluation of Pulmonary Embolism

Tests/Studies/Findings	Clinical Significance
Laboratory	
• Arterial blood gases: pH > 7.45 PaO_2 < 60 mmHg $PaCO_2$ < 35 mmHg	Hypocapnia with consequent respiratory alkalemia related to tachypnea and hyperventilation is a common finding when clinical manifestations of the embolic episode become evident. Hypoxemia in pulmonary embolism is largely due to $\dot{V}/\dot{Q}$ mismatching.
• Alveolar-arterial oxygen tension gradient = 15 mmHg (normal = <15 mmHg)	The norm for this gradient varies with age. Patients over 60 years may have an increased alveolar-arterial gradient.
• Hematology: Leukocyte count < 15,000 cells/mm³	
• Serum enzyme studies: CPK-MB SGOT LDH (lactic dehydrogenase)	These studies assist in differential diagnosis of myocardial infarction.
• Blood coagulation studies: fibrin degradation products = increased	Coagulation studies may reflect an underlying hypercoaguable state commonly associated with thromboembolic disease and pulmonary embolism.
X-ray studies	
• Chest x-ray: nonspecific, frequently normal; may indicate the following findings: Hemidiaphragmatic elevation: areas of atelectasis	Areas of elevation suggest reduced lung volumes; in the presence of an embolic episode, such findings may reflect reduced ventilation associated with tachypnea and increased airway resistance due to bronchospasm.
Pulmonary infiltrates Pleural effusion, unilateral	Pulmonary infiltrates may reflect a pulmonary infarction or congestive atelectasis and hemorrhage associated with pulmonary embolism.
Special studies	
• Perfusion lung scan (may demonstrate absence of perfusion to the region of the lung supplied by the occluded blood vessel)	Perfusion scan is a major screening test for pulmonary embolism. If perfusion scan is normal, pulmonary embolism is largely ruled out; abnormalities do not automatically indicate presence of embolic disease; false-positive scans are common because local decreases in blood flow may result from a pre-existing lung disease.
• Ventilation lung scan (involves inhalation of xenon radioisotope)	Ventilation scan assists in differential diagnosis: If regions of decreased perfusion are secondary to airway disease, a concomitant ventilation abnormality should also be present.
• Pulmonary angiography (done within 2 weeks of the suspected embolic event)	It is the most definitive diagnostic procedure for pulmonary embolism and is usually reserved to last because of the invasive nature of the procedure.
• Contrast venography • Radionuclide venography	Highly effective for detection of occlusive venous disease proximal to the knee. A sensitive test to detect the presence of small thrombi in the calves.
• Radioactive fibrinogen test • Impedance phlebography	A noninvasive method for quantitating blood volume changes in the leg: obstruction of major veins in the leg decreases rate at which blood flows out of leg; reflects capacity of venous system to accommodate additional blood volume in the presence of temporary venous outflow obstruction.
• Impedance plethysmography ¹²⁵I fibrinogen scan: screening for deep venous thrombosis (DVT)	
Electrocardiogram	
• Findings are commonly nonspecific.	
• The following may be evident: Arrhythmias Peaked P waves S wave in lead I Q wave in lead III An S_1, Q_3, T_3 together with right bundle branch block ST-segment depression T-wave inversion lead III	

TABLE 26–2
Heparin Therapy: Nursing Considerations

Actions of Heparin
Heparin is an anticoagulant agent that potentiates the inhibitory activity of antithrombin III on several clotting factors essential for normal blood coagulation. (See Chap. 51 for physiology underlying coagulation.)
- The key reactions that are blocked include:
  - Conversion of prothrombin to thrombin
  - Conversion of fibrinogen to fibrin
- Heparin inhibits the formation of new clots.
- Heparin may prevent extension and propagation of pre-existing clots but does not facilitate lysis of these clots.

Uses of Heparin
- Treatment of deep venous and arterial thrombosis, or pulmonary embolism
- Prophylaxis of thromboembolic complications associated with surgery and venostasis
- Treatment of disseminated intravascular coagulation (DIC) (rarely)

Dosage and Administration
Common approaches to heparin therapy:
- Use of loading dose: 5000–15,000 IU by IV bolus followed by continuous IV heparin therapy.
- Maintenance dose: continuous infusion of heparin 500–3000 IU hourly as determined by activated partial thromboplastin time (aPTT) and coagulation tests
- Use of continuous IV heparin infusion:
  - Facilitates administration
  - Avoids uneven anticoagulation
- Intermittent heparin therapy:
  - 10,000–15,000 IU by IV bolus: followed by
  - Maintenance dose: 5000–6000 IU every 4 h as determined by aPTT
- Prophylactic anticoagulation therapy
  - 5000 IU every 8–12 h subcutaneously

- Heparin lock flush solution to maintain patency of vascular access site.
  - Concentrations of heparin/saline flush solution typically range from 10–1000 U/mL, and volume varies from 2–3 mL to 6–8 mL/flush procedure. The volume used should be sufficient to exceed the capacity of the heparin lock catheter.
  - Flush heparin lock set with normal saline (1–2 mL) before and after a medication is administered.

Initiation of Heparin Activity
- Intravenous route: Begins within minutes with clotting time returning to baseline within 2–6 h after discontinuation
- Subcutaneous route: Begins within 20–60 min; lasts for 8–12 h, with wide variations
- Intramuscular route: unpredictable and unreliable

Duration of Heparin Therapy
- Course of heparin therapy is 8–10 days
- Coumadin therapy usually initiated during last 2–3 days of heparin therapy

Heparin Pharmacokinetics
- 95% protein-bound
- Small amount taken up by mast cells
- Metabolism: reticuloendothelial system and liver
- Elimination by urine as partially degraded heparin; some heparin possibly eliminated unchanged

Contraindications to Heparin Therapy
- Active bleeding, recent surgery, stroke
- Hypersensitivity

Precaution: Advanced renal, liver, or biliary disease

Nursing Considerations/Rationales
A loading dose is used to achieve a therapeutic blood level rapidly.

During administration of heparin therapy, periodic blood samples are obtained to determine the patient's response to heparin and dosage adjustments.

aPTT is the blood test commonly used to monitor effects of heparin therapy on blood coagulation.

Goal: To maintain aPTT 1.5–2.5 times normal baseline (usually ~65–80 s)

Prophylactic approach is commonly used in patients at risk for developing deep venous thrombosis, e.g., the immobilized patient or the patients who are about to undergo or who have recently undergone major thoracic and abdominal surgery.

Use of heparin flush in this instance is *not* intended for heparin therapeutic purposes.

Heparin is a highly acidic molecule; avoid mixing drugs with heparin to prevent potential drug interaction. Clinical relevance of the drug interaction is dubious.

Nursing Considerations/Rationales
A clot takes 8–10 days to adhere to the vessel wall.

The action of Coumadin is mediated by altered production of vitamin K–dependent clotting factors and requires several days for its action to take effect.

Altered metabolism may alter the action of heparin and its duration.

TABLE 26–2
Heparin Therapy: Nursing Considerations (*Continued*)

Adverse/Side Effects
- Spontaneous bleeding
- Sensitivity reaction at injection site
- Thrombocytopenia and platelet antibodies

Baseline platelet count should be obtained, followed by serial platelet determinations every 3 days during heparin therapy.
Increased bleeding and thrombosis have been related to heparin-induced thrombocytopenia.

Heparin Antidote[3]
Protamine sulfate (1% solution)
1. Onset of action of IV protamine is ~5 min with a duration of up to ~2 h.
2. Dosage: 1 mg of protamine neutralizes the effect of 90–110 IU of heparin.
3. Administration involves: slow injection of the drug not to exceed 50 mg in any 10-min period
   a. Loading dose may be given: 25–50 mg by slow injection followed by a continuous intravenous infusion.
4. Monitor vital signs.

The strongly basic protamine combines with the highly acidic heparin to form a stable compound and, thus, nullifies the anticoagulant effect.

Dosage is guided by blood coagulation studies; monitor aPTT and clotting time.

Nursing Interventions
- Obtain baseline studies including:
  1. Blood
     a. Coagulation studies
        (1) aPTT
        (2) Coagulation (clotting) time
     b. Hematology
        (1) Hemoglobin, hematocrit
        (2) RBC count; platelet count
- Monitor aPTT after each dosage change and daily after the maintenance dose is established.
- Identify patients at higher risk of developing spontaneous bleeding (e.g., patients receiving prophylactic heparin therapy postsurgery; the elderly; patients with renal, hepatic or biliary disease).
- Assess all organ systems prior to initiation of heparin therapy to establish baseline function.
  1. Reassess for signs/symptoms of bleeding every 2 h.
  2. Monitor the following parameters at regular intervals:
     a. Vital signs: heart rate, blood pressure; respiratory rate and rhythm; body temperature
     b. Neurologic status: mental status, level of consciousness; behavioral changes; complaints of headache, dizziness
     c. Petechiae: soft palate, conjunctiva, retina
     d. Ecchymosis
     e. Hematuria
     f. Hematemesis; red/black stools
  3. Continuous intravenous heparin therapy requires the following interventions:
     a. Addition of heparin in the prescribed strength and dose to the infusion fluid; invert 5–6 times to ensure adequate distribution of heparin.
     b. An infusion pump should be used to deliver accurate heparin dose.
     c. Examine insertion site carefully for signs of infiltration or tube kinking.
     d. Inspect all invasive sites each shift for bleeding, hematoma formation, or signs of inflammation.
  4. Subcutaneous administration of heparin therapy: Recommended guidelines/techniques.[9]
     a. Deep subcutaneous (SC) injection, preferably made to fatty layer of the abdomen or just above iliac crest.
     b. Use tuberculin syringe, 25–26 gauge, $\frac{1}{2}$–$\frac{5}{8}$ inch needle.
     c. Discard needle used to withdraw heparin from vial.
     d. Prepare site with alcohol sponge and allow to dry.
     e. Gently bunch up a defined roll of subcutaneous tissue.
     f. Insert needle into roll at 90-degree angle to skin surface.

Rationales
These tests are performed periodically throughout heparin therapy to monitor patient's response to therapy and determine appropriate dosage adjustments.
Heparin-induced thrombocytopenia may predispose to bleeding and thrombosis.

aPTT is a specific test reflecting effects of heparin therapy.

Establishing a baseline assists in assessing patient's overall response to therapy.

Changes in neurologic status may reflect intracranial bleeding.

This distribution of petechiae may reflect thrombocytopenia and warrants the determination of the platelet count.

It is necessary to read the label carefully because heparin comes in different strengths.
It is important to prevent pooling of heparin in the solution to ensure appropriate continuous dose.
Use of pump facilitates close monitoring.

Shallow SC injection should be avoided because it may be more painful, is associated with high risk of hematoma formation, and has variable duration of desired effect.
Ensures accuracy in measuring dose.

Avoid massaging the injection site to prevent injury to small blood vessels.
Avoid pinching in order to prevent injury to small blood vessels.

Continued

TABLE 26–2
Heparin Therapy: Nursing Considerations (*Continued*)

g. While maintaining support of tissue, slowly and steadily inject the drug.

Do not withdraw plunger to check for blood because of risk of tissue injury.

h. Hesitate before withdrawing needle; withdraw needle quickly in the same direction it was introduced; simultaneously, release hold of subcutaneous tissue.

Pause prevents trailing of drug through needle tract.

i. Apply gentle pressure to insertion site for about 1 min; do not massage the area.

j. Optional application of ice to puncture site may reduce incidence of hematoma or ecchymosis.

k. Keep a chart indicating rotation of injection sites.

Rotation of injection sites minimizes tissue injury and altered distribution and absorption of the drug.

- Patient/family education

Critical phase of illness: Limits educational process.

1. Instruct on preventive activities to reduce risk of deep venous thrombosis and pulmonary embolism.

Stasis or stagnation of blood, and endothelial or vessel wall injury have been implicated in the pathogenesis of venous thrombosis.

   a. Provide antiembolic stockings or support hose.

   b. Avoid positions that compromise blood flow (e.g., crossing legs, prolonged sitting in one position, or pillow under knees).

Instruction should involve ways to minimize stasis of blood or vessel injury and, thus, reduce risk of thrombus recurrence.

   c. Encourage active range-of-motion exercises hourly; initiate and maintain daily exercise schedule.

Exercise of lower extremities assists the "skeletal muscle pump" to return venous blood to the heart; such exercises minimize stasis of blood in the lower extremities. Deep venous thrombosis of lower extremities has been definitively implicated as a major etiologic factor in pulmonary embolism.

   d. Instruct patient/family regarding the following:

      (1) Avoid exposure to cold.

      (2) Stop smoking.

      (3) Maintain ideal body weight.

      (4) Maintain hydration.

Hydrated state ensures adequate blood volume; hemoconcentration associated with the dehydrated state may result in sluggish blood flow.

      (5) Avoid use of oral contraceptives.

These medications are considered to increase the risk of thrombus formation.

      (6) Avoid massaging any area of suspected deep venous thrombosis or thrombophlebitis.

Such activity may increase the risk of pulmonary embolism.

2. Instruct regarding medication therapy including:

   a. Underlying indication/rationale

   b. Dosage schedule and the importance of taking the medication as prescribed (correct dose taken at same time daily)

Following pulmonary embolism, patients are commonly maintained on long-term (6 weeks–6 months) oral anticoagulant therapy (coumarin derivative, e.g., warfarin and dicumarol).

   c. Adverse side effects

   d. Necessary regular follow-up including periodic blood studies

   e. Importance of not taking other medications including over-the-counter drugs, without first consulting with the physician

Many over-the-counter drugs contain aspirin (salicylates), which potentiates the anticoagulant effect and may cause spontaneous bleeding.

   f. Necessity of reporting to physician any unusual prolonged or excessive bleeding:

Early recognition of a bleeding problem may prevent serious complications in the patient on anticoagulant therapy.

      (1) Excessive bleeding from gums, mouth; epistaxis; excessive bruising (ecchymosis); hematuria; coffee-ground hematemesis; tarry stools; excessive menses

      (2) Other significant signs/symptoms: headaches, dizziness, behavioral/personality changes; sudden chest or shoulder pain; dyspnea or tachypnea; redness, swelling or pain in an extremity

   g. Importance of wearing Medic-Alert band identifying the patient as being on anticoagulant therapy

3. Instruct regarding precautions to be used in activities of daily living:

Knowledge and awareness of situations that can potentially precipitate bleeding assist in minimizing the risk of bleeding while the patient is on anticoagulant therapy.

   a. Use of electric rather than straight-edge razor

   b. Gentle flossing and brushing of teeth

   c. Careful trimming of nails

   d. Careful blowing of nose

   e. Avoidance of straining at stool

4. Reinforce the necessity of following prescribed care including the follow-up visits with healthcare providers.

The informed patient is more likely to exhibit compliance with prescribed treatment regimen.

   a. Provide written instructions regarding overall plan of care.

Involvement of other family members in decision-making activities and overall treatment plan may provide the patient with additional resources and support.

   b. Include names and telephone numbers of key healthcare providers involved in patient's care.

   c. Allow time for questions and clarification of information provided.

Nursing Care of the Patient with Pulmonary Embolism

The critical care nurse plays a crucial role in the prevention of pulmonary embolism in critically ill patients. Through the identification of those patients considered to be at great risk and recognition of those factors contributing to the pathogenesis of deep venous thrombosis, the critical care nurse can implement appropriate and timely interventions directed toward decreasing the risk of pulmonary embolism, preventing or eliminating those factors implicated in its pathogenesis, or, if a pulmonary embolic event occurs, preventing recurrent thrombus formation and embolization.

Therapeutic Goals

Specific nursing interventions in the care of the patient with pulmonary embolism are related to the following therapeutic goals:
1. Establish or maintain a patent airway and initiate mechanical ventilation and oxygen therapy as determined by the patient's clinical status and arterial blood gas values.
2. Provide hemodynamic support to maintain cardiac output and tissue perfusion.
3. Relieve anxiety precipitated by the acute onset of respiratory insufficiency, requiring aggressive therapy within the confines of an unfamiliar, often frightening and intimidating intensive care setting.

Nursing Diagnoses, Desired Patient Outcomes, and Nursing Interventions

Pertinent nursing diagnoses, desired patient outcomes, and nursing interventions are presented in the care plan for the patient with pulmonary embolism, in the following section.

CASE STUDY WITH SAMPLE CARE PLAN: PATIENT WITH PULMONARY EMBOLISM
(By Kathleen Daley White and Margaret Connelly)

A 62-year-old obese woman was admitted to the telemetry unit for monitoring of recent onset of atrial fibrillation with a ventricular rate of 80 to 100 bpm. Patient had history of an anterior myocardial infarction 6 years prior to this admission, with mild congestive heart failure controlled by no restricted diet, digoxin, and furosemide. The patient had had dyspnea on exertion over the past 2 weeks. When she went to her doctor, the atrial fibrillation was discovered. She denied having chest pain, syncope, dizziness, palpitations, and shortness of breath at rest.

The nurse found decreased peripheral pulses (+1) in both extremities; pedal pulses were auscultated with Doppler color flow imaging. Extremities were cool to

the touch. Patient stated that she has never had good circulation in her legs.

2/3, 3:00 AM—Patient sat up suddenly in bed complaining of dyspnea, unable to catch her breath and rang for the nurse. Nurse notified physician and respiratory therapist immediately. Vital signs: BP 120/80, heart rate 120 (atrial fibrillation), respiratory rate 36 and tachypneic. ABGs on room air: alkalosis, decreased $PaCO_2$, and decreased PaO_2.

The patient was placed on 4 L nasal oxygen and prepared for transfer to ICU with possible diagnosis of pulmonary embolus.

2/3, 4:00 AM—Patient admitted to MICU, where her condition continued to deteriorate. Dyspnea persisted, with cyanosis, diaphoresis, and fatigue. The patient was intubated at that time. The patient remained alert, awake, and oriented. Chest x-ray was within normal limits; ECG showed an old anterior wall myocardial infarction; there was no evidence of pulmonary hypertension (no right axis shift, no peaked P wave, and no ST-segment changes).

Continuous heparin therapy was started; bedside $\dot{V}/\dot{Q}$ scan was positive for pulmonary embolus. Maintenance heparin was established, PT/PTT = 19.5/52.5.

2/5—With improvement in ABGs, the patient was weaned off the ventilator using a T piece. Heparin therapy was continued for a period of 10 days.

2/15—Patient was discharged home with prescriptions for digoxin, quinidine, Coumadin, ASA daily, and follow-up visit in 1 week.

Initial Nursing Diagnoses
1. Impaired gas exchange, related to decreased pulmonary blood flow ($\dot{V}/\dot{Q}$ mismatching)
2. Potential for decreased cardiac output, related to decreased pulmonary artery blood flow, pulmonary hypertension, or right heart failure
3. Potential for physiologic injury: bleeding, related to anticoagulation therapy

PLEURAL EFFUSION

Pathophysiology

The dynamics of pleural fluid formation and its resorption from the intrapleural space are related to the difference in driving pressures at the interface of visceral and parietal pleural surfaces. While the blood supply to the parietal pleura originates from the high-pressure systemic arterial circulation (largely by way of intercostal arteries), the visceral pleura receives its blood supply from the low-pressure pulmonary arterial 4circulation.

Pleural fluid is formed since the high hydrostatic pressure at the arteriolar end of the parietal pleural capillary bed favors the movement of fluid from the capillaries into the intrapleural space. There is minimal fluid movement across the capillaries in the visceral pleura because the low hydrostatic pressure within these vessels is not sufficient to overcome the colloidal osmotic pressure exerted by plasma pro-

SAMPLE CARE PLAN FOR THE PATIENT WITH PULMONARY EMBOLISM

Nursing Diagnoses

Nursing Diagnosis #1

Impaired gas exchange, related to:
1. Altered pulmonary blood flow
2. $\dot{V}/\dot{Q}$ mismatching

Desired Patient Outcomes

Patient will maintain optimal arterial blood gas parameters:
- pH 7.35–7.45
- Pao_2 > 80 mmHg
- $Paco_2$ 35–45 mmHg
- HCO_3^- 22–26 mEq/L

Nursing Interventions

- Assess for signs/symptoms of hypoxia, anxiety, tachypnea, dyspnea, air hunger, tachycardia, hypertension, or hypotension.

- Assess level of fatigue

- Monitor arterial blood gas parameters.

- Administer prescribed humidified oxygen therapy.

  ○ Prepare for intubation.

Rationales

A classic sign of a pulmonary embolism is a subtle, mild dyspnea. In the presence of pulmonary infarction associated with an embolism, sudden and severe dyspnea may reflect an underlying total or partial obstruction of pulmonary blood flow.
- The increased work of breathing may predispose to fatigue; fatigue may result in alveolar hypoventilation with worsening hypoxemia, and it predisposes to hypercapnia.
- A metabolic acidemia is often associated with decreased tissue perfusion; the consequent anaerobic metabolism causes a rise in serum lactate levels. Arterial blood gas parameters must closely reflect effectiveness of gas exchange and pH.
- Oxygenation is effective in the treatment of $\dot{V}/\dot{Q}$ mismatch.
  ○ Compromised ventilatory effort, $\dot{V}/\dot{Q}$ mismatch, and right-to-left shunting may compromise gas exchange sufficiently to require mechanical ventilation.

Nursing Diagnoses

Nursing Diagnosis #2

Potential for decreased cardiac output related to:
1. Pulmonary hypertension
2. Right-sided heart failure
3. Decrease in LVEDP

Desired Patient Outcomes

Patient will maintain stable hemodynamics:
- Heart rate < 100 bpm
- Central venous pressure 0–8 mmHg
- Pulmonary capillary wedge pressure < 25 mmHg
- Cardiac output 4–8 L/min

Nursing Interventions

- Assess for signs/symptoms of right-sided heart failure: weight gain, imbalance in intake and output; hemodynamic changes—neck vein distention, tachycardia, extra heart sounds (S_3 and S_4); edematous lower extremities.
- Administer prescribed medication regimen to treat right heart failure:
  ○ Vasopressor therapy, cardiac glycosides, morphine, diuretics, and sedatives
- Monitor response to drug therapy.

Rationales

- Pulmonary hypertension is the major hemodynamic disturbance of pulmonary embolism. Hypoxemia, acidemia, and a reduced cross-sectional area of the pulmonary capillary bed contribute to the development of pulmonary hypertension.
- Therapies are directed toward decreasing myocardial oxygen consumption and demand.
  ○ Morphine increases systemic venous capacitance; the reduced venous return decreases the work of the heart.

Nursing Diagnoses

Nursing Diagnosis #3

Potential for physiologic injury, bleeding, related to anticoagulant therapy

Desired Patient Outcomes

Patient will experience an absence of bleeding:
- Stable hematocrit/hemoglobin (for patient)
- Stable vital signs
- Absence of petechiae, ecchymosis, hematuria, occult blood in stools, or bleeding at invasive sites

SAMPLE CARE PLAN FOR THE PATIENT WITH PULMONARY EMBOLISM (*Continued*)

Nursing Interventions

- Assess closely for signs/symptoms of bleeding.

- Teach patient to examine self for signs of bleeding: petechiae, easy bruising, changes in color of urine or stools.
- Obtain daily serum coagulation parameters (prothrombin [PT] and partial thromboplastin [PTT] times); monitor closely for desired range.
- Monitor all invasive sites every shift.
- Limit puncture sites and blood drawing to only when necessary.
  ○ Use only small-gauge needles when drawing blood.
- Teach patient to use an electric razor and to avoid vigorous toothbrushing.
- Maintain access to protamine sulfate for patients receiving heparin therapy.

Rationales

- Anticoagulant therapy is major treatment in patients with deep venous thrombosis. Major adverse effect of heparin is the risk of bleeding.
- An aware patient may afford early recognition of subtle bleeding.

- Usual PT/PTT is maintained $1\frac{1}{2}$–2 times the control.

- Puncture sites and invasive lines are not able to clot as quickly during anticoagulant therapy. Large hematomas may occur without appropriate application of pressure after injection and at puncture sites. It may be necessary to apply direct pressure to these sites for as long as 10 min, followed by application of pressure dressing.
- Protamine sulfate is the antidote for heparin and should be readily available for administration if necessary.

Nursing Diagnoses

Nursing Diagnosis #4
Anxiety, related to:
1. Sudden, acute respiratory insufficiency with disruption of lifestyle
2. Pain; hemoptysis
3. Knowledge deficit regarding illness and its prognosis
4. Intensive care setting

Desired Patient Outcomes

Patient will:
1. Verbalize feeling less anxious
2. Demonstrate a relaxed demeanor
3. Perform relaxation techniques with assistance
4. Verbalize familiarity with ICU routines and protocols

Nursing Interventions

- Assess for signs/symptoms of anxiety: restlessness, agitation, diaphoresis; tachypnea, sighing; tachycardia, palpitations; anorexia, nausea, diarrhea; presence of anxiety-related behaviors: nail biting, insomnia, finger tapping; uncooperative or noncompliant behaviors; verbalization of fears and concerns.
- Examine the circumstances underlying the anxiety.
  ○ Manipulate ICU environment to provide calm, restful periods.

- Assess patient/family coping behaviors and their effectiveness in dealing with current stressors.
  ○ Provide positive reinforcement when desired response is achieved.
- Initiate interventions to reduce anxiety:
  ○ Relieve pain or other discomfort.
    □ Medication for pain
    □ Comfort measures: turning, positioning, mouth care, skin care, and so forth
  ○ Monitor effectiveness of ventilatory support and oxygen therapy if these therapies are indicated.
    □ Serial arterial blood gas values
  ○ Listen patient attentively; encourage verbalization, provide a caring touch.

Rationales

- Thorough assessment assists in discerning underlying cause of anxiety and provides a basis for intervention. *Examples*: (1) Relief of pain with medication often alleviates its anxiety-related symptomatology. (2) Coping with the fear of dying with a listening ear and caring attitude may assist in reducing the patient's anxiety.
- Removal of precipitating factors may reduce anxiety.
  ○ Reduction in stimuli is essential to assist patient/family to relax and avoid useless dissipation of compromised energy stores.

  ○ Positive feedback nurtures self-confidence.

  ○ Pain precipitates or aggravates anxiety.

  ○ Inadequate gas exchange, hypoxemia, or hypercapnia precipitates symptomatology that contributes to the patient's "sense of doom."
  ○ These nursing activities reassure the patient that he or she is not alone.

SAMPLE CARE PLAN FOR THE PATIENT WITH PULMONARY EMBOLISM (*Continued*)

Nursing Interventions

- ○ Let patient know it's okay to feel anxious or to experience fear of dying.
- ○ Remain with patient during periods of acute stress.
- ○ Assess readiness to learn and implement the following when appropriate:
- ○ Orient to environment, ICU equipment, routines, and staff.
  - □ Explain all procedures and activities involving the patient.
- ○ Involve in decision making regarding care when possible and appropriate.

- ○ Help in establishing short-term goals that can be attained.
- • Instruct in relaxation techniques.

Rationales

- ○ Reassurance helps patient to focus on his or her feelings, work through them, and eventually accept them.
- ○ Readiness to learn facilitates meaningful learning and a sense of accomplishment.
- ○ Knowing what to expect helps to reduce anxiety.

- ○ Participation in decision making helps patient to maintain some degree of control over his or her body and healthcare.
- ○ Attainment of goals builds and reinforces self-confidence.
- ○ Energy-release techniques allow an outlet for pent-up feelings; enable the patient to have some control over anxiety.

Nursing Diagnoses

Nursing Diagnosis #5
Gas exchange, impaired, related to:
1. Right-to-left shunting
2. $\dot{V}/\dot{Q}$ mismatch

Desired Patient Outcomes

For specific patient outcomes related to these nursing diagnoses, see Chapter 25 care plan.

Nursing Diagnosis #6
Breathing pattern, ineffective, related to tachypnea, dyspnea

Nursing Interventions

Rationales

For specific nursing interventions and their rationales, see Chapter 25 care plan. For details related to the nursing care of the mechanically ventilated patient, see Chapter 25.

Nursing Diagnoses

Nursing Diagnosis #7
Cardiac output, alteration in: decreased, related to:
1. Pulmonary arterial hypertension
2. Right-sided congestive heart failure (cor pulmonale)
3. Decrease in left ventricular end-diastolic pressure (LVEDP)
4. Systemic arterial hypotension/hypovolemic shock

Desired Patient Outcomes

Patient will maintain stable hemodynamics:
- • Heart rate < 100 bpm
- • Central venous pressure (CVP) 0–8 mmHg
- • Pulmonary artery pressure < 25 mmHg
- • Pulmonary capillary wedge pressure (PCWP) 8–12 mmHg
- • Cardiac output ~5 L/min
- • Systemic arterial blood pressure within 10 mmHg of baseline

Nursing Interventions

- • Assess for signs/symptoms of right-sided congestive heart failure:
  - ○ Weight gain; fluid intake/output
  - ○ Hemodynamic changes:
    - □ Tachycardia (>100 bpm)
    - □ Jugular neck vein distention
    - □ Peripheral (dependent) edema
    - □ CVP > 8–12 mmHg
    - □ Extra heart sounds; S_3, S_4, systolic murmur
    - □ Fatigue; mottled appearance of skin, cool to touch; cyanosis of nailbeds

Rationales

- • The major hemodynamic disturbance associated with pulmonary embolism is *pulmonary arterial hypertension* (>25–30 mmHg), which may predispose to right ventricular failure.
  - ○ Hypoxemia, acidemia, and a reduced cross-sectional area of the pulmonary vascular bed all contribute to the development of pulmonary hypertension.
  - ○ Right ventricular failure causes alterations in systemic hemodynamics; left ventricular failure alters pulmonary hemodynamics. Commonly, failure in one ventricle causes failure of the other.

SAMPLE CARE PLAN FOR THE PATIENT WITH PULMONARY EMBOLISM (*Continued*)

Nursing Interventions

- ○ Breath sounds may be clear and without adventitious sounds diminished with localized rales (crackles) or wheezing. A pleural friction rub may be detected. Breathing pattern may reflect tachypnea, dyspnea.
- ○ Hepatic involvement:
  - □ Hepatomegaly, positive hepatojugular reflex; abdominal distention; ascites
- ○ Gastrointestinal: anorexia, nausea/vomiting; abdominal distention
- ○ Oliguria
- ○ Mental status changes
- • Monitor diagnostic tests/studies:
- ○ Laboratory studies: BUN, creatinine, hematocrit, serum albumin; electrolytes; arterial blood gases
- ○ ECG—may reflect signs of ischemia; arrhythmias (atrial)
- ○ Chest x-rays frequently reflect cardiomegaly, pleural effusion, and possibly, pulmonary edema (left-sided heart failure)
- • Administer prescribed medication regimen to treat cor pulmonale, a consequence of pulmonary hypertension
- ○ Vasopressor therapy (e.g., dopamine in the presence of heart failure and hypovolemic shock)
- ○ Cardiac glycosides (digoxin)
  - □ Positive inotropic agent = improved contractility
  - □ Negative chronotropic agent = reduced heart rate
  - □ End result = improved cardiac output
- ○ Morphine
  - □ Induces systemic venous vasodilatation
  - □ Reduces chest pain frequently associated with pulmonary embolism
  - □ Decreases anxiety and helps to reduce the work of breathing
  - □ Exerts a sedative effect, which assists in relaxing the patient
- ○ Diuretics (e.g., furosemide)

- ○ Vasodilator therapy may be initiated, especially in the setting of left ventricular compromise.
- ○ Administer anticoagulant therapy.
  - □ Heparin, Coumadin derivatives
  - □ Aspirin (antiplatelet agent)

Rationales

- ○ A massive pulmonary embolism with acute cor pulmonale may be characterized by dyspnea, cyanosis, and hypovolemic shock.

- • Serum sodium values reflect hydration status.
  - ○ Serum potassium needs to be carefully monitored, especially during diuretic therapy.

- • Therapies are directed toward decreasing myocardial oxygen consumption and demand.
  - ○ A pulmonary embolic episode may reflexly trigger systemic peripheral arteriolar vasodilatation with a consequent "relative" volume depletion, which, if severe, can cause hypotension or hypovolemic shock.

  - □ Increased pooling of blood in the periphery reduces venous return to the right heart, which helps to decrease the work of the right ventricle.

- ○ A reduction in total blood volume reduces venous return (preload) while also reducing systemic arterial blood pressure (afterload). The end-result is a decrease in myocardial work.
- ○ Use of diuretics requires the maintenance of fluid volume.
- ○ Vasodilators function to decrease preload and afterload and thus decrease the work of the heart.
- ○ Major focus of therapy in the patient experiencing a pulmonary embolic episode is to *prevent* recurrent embolization; anticoagulants function effectively in this capacity.

Nursing Diagnoses

Nursing Diagnosis #8
Fluid volume, alteration

Desired Patient Outcomes

Patient will:
1. Maintain body weight within 5% of baseline
2. Balance fluid intake with output
3. Have the following:
   - • Good skin turgor
   - • Absence of peripheral edema
   - • Absence of jugular vein distention
   - • Absence of rales (crackles) on auscultation

Serum electrolytes, BUN, creatinine, total protein will stabilize within acceptable physiologic range.

SAMPLE CARE PLAN FOR THE PATIENT WITH PULMONARY EMBOLISM (*Continued*)

Nursing Interventions

- Maintain fluid and electrolyte balance.
  - Administer prescribed fluid volume.

  - Document intake and output, urine specific gravity.
  - Record daily weight.
  - Monitor electrolytes.

- Monitor hemodynamic parameters.
  - Systemic arterial blood pressure, CVP, pulmonary artery pressure, PCWP, cardiac output.

- Administer oxygen therapy as prescribed and monitor arterial blood gases to evaluate patient's response to therapy.
- Implement nursing measures to improve or maintain cardiac output.
  - Manipulate environment to reduce stressors and promote rest and relaxation.
  - Plan frequent rest periods.

  - Maximize patient activities in accordance with the acuity of the illness.

  - Place in high Fowler's position.
  - Assist with frequent position changes.

  - Provide special care to back and to skin over joints and pressure points.
  - Assist with passive range-of-motion exercises.

Rationales

- Fluid therapy is directed toward reducing the work of the heart while still maintaining adequate tissue perfusion.
  - Close monitoring of urine output helps to evaluate renal perfusion/function; a reduction in cardiac output may reduce renal perfusion, which is manifested clinically by a decrease in hourly urine output.
- These measures best reflect the patient's response to therapy, and insertion of a pulmonary artery flotation catheter is commonly indicated in the setting of massive pulmonary embolism.
- Hypoxemia in pulmonary embolism is a consequence of $\dot{V}/\dot{Q}$ mismatching and right-to-left shunting.

- A quiet, calm environment decreases anxiety, and reduces sympathetic nervous system stimulation. The overall net effect is to reduce the work of the heart.

  - A reduction in cardiac workload reduces myocardial oxygen consumption and demand.
  - Nursing interventions are implemented to maximize circulation, prevent pooling or stasis of blood, maintain venous return, and promote comfort.
  - Facilitates ease of breathing as abdominal pressure on the diaphragm is reduced; less effort exerted = decrease in oxygen demand.
  - Compromised circulation predisposes to tissue ischemia; stasis or pooling of blood predisposes to venous thrombosis; reduces venous return, which decreases cardiac output.

Nursing Diagnoses

Nursing Diagnosis #9
Tissue perfusion, alteration in, related to:
1. Thromboembolic disorder
2. Deep venous thrombosis
3. Pulmonary embolism

Desired Patient Outcomes

Patient will remain without recurrent pulmonary embolism as reflected by:
- Absence of pain
- Stable vital signs (see Nursing Diagnosis #7)
- Stable arterial blood gases (within acceptable physiologic range)
  - pH 7.35–7.45
  - $Paco_2$ 35–45 mmHg
  - Pao_2 > 60 mmHg

Nursing Interventions

- Assess for signs/symptoms of venous thrombosis:

  - Tenderness, warmth, pain, and peripheral (pitting) edema of lower extremities
    - Evidence of edema is best assessed and monitored by determining the circumference of the limb at a designated point using a tape measure.
  - Skin color and temperature
    - Observe extremities in both dependent and elevated positions.

  - Bleeding/bruising tendency, petechiae, ecchymosis, hematuria, occult blood in stool

Rationales

- 95% of all pulmonary emboli arise in the deep veins of the lower extremities.
  - Edema is a characteristic manifestation when alteration in tissue perfusion is due to venous interference.

  - In the presence of altered tissue perfusion or venous obstruction, a bluish-red color of the skin may be observed.
  - Temperature of skin is assessed by use of touch; usually warm temperatures in the lower extremities are commonly associated with venous thrombosis.
  - Hypercoagulable state is often reflected by bleeding tendency.

SAMPLE CARE PLAN FOR THE PATIENT WITH PULMONARY EMBOLISM (*Continued*)

Nursing Interventions

- ○ Complaints of pain:
    - □ Pain associated with deep venous thrombosis may be described as heavy, aching, or cramping.
    - □ Pain associated with arterial insufficiency is characteristically sudden and sharp; the presence of cool skin temperature suggests decreased arterial blood flow.
- • Monitor for signs/symptoms indicative of extended or recurrent pulmonary embolism.
    - ○ Sudden occurrence of persistent or exacerbated chest or shoulder pain
    - ○ Onset of respiratory difficulties: tachypnea, dyspnea, cough with hemoptysis
    - ○ Alterations in cardiopulmonary function: tachycardia, hypotension, cyanosis
    - ○ Neurologic findings: restlessness, lethargy, confusion
- • Monitor laboratory data:
    - ○ Arterial blood gas values
    - ○ Hematologic studies: complete blood count, hematocrit, hemoglobin
    - ○ Coagulation studies: activated partial thromboplastin time; prothrombin time; clotting time
    - ○ Platelet count
- • Implement prescribed anticoagulant therapy.
- • Implement measures to reduce the risk of recurrent pulmonary embolism.
    - ○ Maintain hydrated state as prescribed.

    - ○ Apply antiembolic hose to both lower extremities; remove hose once per shift.
    - ○ Assist patient to perform active range-of-motion exercises; active/passive foot and leg exercises should be performed hourly unless otherwise contraindicated.

    - ○ Instruct patient to avoid positions that compromise blood flow in the extremities (e.g., gatch knees, pillow under knees, crossing of legs, prolonged sitting in one position).
    - ○ Encourage deep breathing hourly.
    - ○ Caution patient to avoid activities that involve a Valsalva's maneuver (e.g., straining to defecate, breath holding).

Rationales

- ○ Pain occurs with an alteration in tissue perfusion.

- • The presence of deep venous thrombosis places the patient at increased risk of pulmonary embolism.

- • See Table 26–2.

- ○ Dehydration increases blood viscosity. The consequent disturbed blood flow may predispose to endothelial injury within blood vessels, or a hypercoagulable state.

- ○ Exercise enhances "skeletal-muscular pump," which functions to prevent pooling of blood in the lower extremities (venous stasis) and maintains venous return to the heart.
- ○ If a thrombosis is suspected, the involved extremity should *not* be massaged or exercised to prevent possible dislodgement of thrombi with consequent pulmonary embolism.
- ○ Positions that compromise blood flow can cause circulatory stasis.

- ○ Expands lungs and minimizes areas of atelectasis.
- ○ Such activities increase risk of dislodging thrombi.

Nursing Diagnoses

Nursing Diagnosis #10
Comfort, alteration in: Pain associated with compromised pulmonary perfusion (see Nursing Diagnosis #4)

Desired Patient Outcomes

Patient will:
1. Verbalize pain relief
2. Exhibit relaxed demeanor:
    - • Relaxed facial expression and body posturing
    - • Ease of breathing

SAMPLE CARE PLAN FOR THE PATIENT WITH PULMONARY EMBOLISM (*Continued*)

Nursing Interventions

- Determine how patient usually copes with pain.
  - Pain tolerance
  - Willingness to discuss pain; or stoically "keeping it within" himself or herself
  - Willingness to use medication for pain
- Assess for nonverbal clues as to the presence of pain (e.g., restlessness or reluctance to move; tense facial features; clenched fists; diaphoresis; rapid, shallow breathing).
- Assess complaints of pain including severity, location/radiation; influencing factors (e.g., what precipitates, aggravates, or ameliorates the pain; and associated signs and symptoms such as diaphoresis), pain duration, and the quality of pain (e.g., sharp, dull, "knifelike").
- Implement measures to alleviate pain:
  - Assist patient into comfortable position (e.g., high Fowler's).
  - Encourage deep breathing hourly.

  - Teach/assist patient to splint chest with hands or pillow when coughing, deep breathing, or repositioning.
  - Stay with patient until pain is relieved.

  - Provide a listening ear and caring touch; encourage verbalization; explain procedures, routines, tests, and so forth.
  - Refrain from nonessential activities.

  - Provide comfort measures (e.g., position change, back care, reducing environmental stimuil).
- Administer analgesic medication therapy as prescribed.
  - Encourage to request medication when pain is first realized rather than wait until it gets unbearable.
  - Evaluate effectiveness of pain medication in relieving the patient's pain.

Rationales

- To assist in comprehensive assessment, see SLIDT Tool in Table 35–1.

  - Upright position favors better lung expansion; improves alveolar ventilation.
  - Minimizes atelectasis and improves distribution of ventilation.
  - Splinting may help to reduce discomfort.

  - Providing support can reduce anxiety and help the patient relax.
  - Keeping the patient informed may help to alleviate anxieties, which may potentiate pain.

  - Reducing patient's activities decreases oxygen consumption and demand.
  - Comfort measures and touch therapy are often sufficient to alleviate pain.

  - Pain medication administered early on may be more effective.

Nursing Diagnoses

Nursing Diagnosis #11
Knowledge deficit, related to:
1. Thromboembolic disease
2. Follow-up care
3. Prevention

Desired Patient Outcomes

Patient/family will:
1. Identify risk factors of significance in thromboembolic disease
2. Identify activities that promote venous blood flow and reduce risks of venous thrombosis.
   - Importance of individualized exercise program
3. Explain the prescribed treatment regimen and the importance of complying with it:
   - Rationale for anticoagulant therapy
   - Medication routine, dosage, and side effects
   - Signs/symptoms to report to healthcare provider
   - Measures to minimize risks of bleeding during anticoagulant therapy
   - Importance of follow-up care

Nursing Interventions

Rationales

See Table 26–2, section on patient/family education, for information essential to the patient/family's understanding of, and compliance with, the prescribed therapeutic regimen. See also nursing diagnoses #4 and #9.

teins.[10] Thus, pleural fluid is filtered from the parietal pleura into the intrapleural space and is reabsorbed by the lymphatic vessels within the pleura. As a result of these pressure gradients, it has been estimated that 5 to 10 liters of fluid pass through the intrapleural space each day.[11]

Pleural effusion is an accumulation of fluid within the intrapleural space that may reflect an increase in pleural fluid formation or a decrease in its reabsorption from the intrapleural space, or both. Two mechanisms may underlie pleural effusion: (1) an alteration of the permeability characteristics of the pleural surface or (2) an alteration in the pressure gradients (hydrostatic or colloidal osmotic pressure changes) between parietal and visceral pleural surfaces, or both.

Exudative Pleural Fluid

Exudates are characteristically associated with an increase in permeability of the pleural surfaces with a consequent movement of protein and fluid into the intrapleural space. Inflammatory and neoplastic disease are the two major pathophysiologic processes that may underlie an exudative pleural effusion. Parapneumonic effusions are exudative pleural effusions associated with bacterial pneumonia, lung abscess, or bronchiectasis, and they remain the leading cause of exudative effusions in the United States. Less frequently, complications of intra-abdominal disorders may result in exudative pleural effusions (e.g., esophageal performation, pancreatic disease, and intra-abdominal abscess).[12]

Transudative Pleural Fluid

Transudates occur as a result of changes in the pressure gradients between parietal and visceral pleura. Such changes may involve an increase in hydrostatic pressure within pleural capillaries (e.g., congestive heart failure) or a decrease in colloidal osmotic pressure (e.g., hypoproteinemia). Because the permeability of the pleural surfaces remains largely intact, a transudate characteristically has a very low protein content. Frequently, the etiology of transudative effusions lies in the dysfunction of organs other than the lungs (e.g., heart, liver, or kidneys). Congestive heart failure remains the most common cause of transudative pleural effusions. Pericarditis, hepatic cirrhosis, nephrotic syndrome, pulmonary embolism, and myxedema may also result in a transudative pleural effusion.

Clinical Presentation

Clinical features of pulmonary effusion depend on the size of the effusion and the nature of its pathophysiologic process. Some patients may not report any signs or symptoms of a pleural effusion. A sharp, pleuritic chest pain aggravated by breathing is often associated with an inflammatory process involving the pleura. Fever may accompany the pleuritic pain. Dyspnea may be observed if the effusion is large enough to compromise the underlying lung. A dry, irritating cough may also be present, possibly the result of pleural inflammation or compression of lung parenchyma.

On physical examination, it is important to appreciate that pleural fluid muffles all sounds. Thus, the region overlying the effusion is dull to percussion, and breath sounds may reflect decreased-to-absent vesicular breath sounds. A bronchial quality breath sound may be heard if fluid compresses the lung. Egophony may sometimes be heard at the upper level of the effusion, reflecting an increase in sound transmission resulting from compression or atelectasis of underlying lung. A scratchy friction rub may be heard over the affected area when an inflammatory process involves the pleural surface. Large pleural effusions resulting in significant reduction in lung volume and atelectasis may result in hypoxemia.

Diagnosis

Chest x-ray may be helpful in the diagnosis of pleural effusion, although its presence may not be apparent even with significant accumulation of pleural fluid. When a pleural effusion is suspected based on routine posteroanterior or anteroposterior chest views (i.e., blunted costophrenic angles or obscure diaphragms) lateral decubitus views should be obtained. Ultrasonography is especially useful in locating a small pleural effusion not apparent on physical examination. It is sometimes used to determine a suitable site for thoracentesis (withdrawal of fluid from pleural space by needle or catheter).

Sampling of pleural fluid obtained by thoracentesis allows for determination of chemical and cellular characteristics of the fluid. Common chemical criteria used to differentiate an exudative from a transudative effusion include the levels of protein and the enzyme lactic dehydrogenase (LDH) within the pleural fluid. In exudative fluid, the levels of these substances are low. Chemical analyses of pleural fluid may also include pH, glucose, and amylase levels.

Analyses of the cellular characteristics of pleural fluid include the absolute numbers and types of cellular constituents, the presence of microorganisms, and cytologic examination. A pleural biopsy may be performed to obtain a sample of pleural tissue for histologic examination.

Treatment and Management

The treatment of pleural effusion depends entirely on the nature of the underlying pathophysiologic process. A large accumulation of pleural fluid, which compromises respiratory function or causes respiratory distress, can be promptly relieved by thoracentesis.[13] Rapid drainage of transudative fluid may result in depletion of protein stores and rapid reaccumulation of fluid.

Pleural effusions are quantified radiographically by measuring the distance between the inner border of the chest wall and the outer border of the lung on lateral decubitus view. A distance of less than 10 mm reflects a small effusion requiring no immediate intervention. A distance of greater than 10 mm requires thoracentesis. Use of closed thoracotomy tube drainage may be indicated to treat complicated pleural effusion (e.g., empyema, loculated parapneumonic effusion, massive effusion) or hemothorax (blood in intrapleural space). A thoracotomy tube may also be used to instill therapeutic agents (e.g., antibiotics, chemotherapy) directly into the pleural space. Instillation of sclerosing agents (tetracycline) into the pleural space to prevent recurrence of effusions is called *pleurodesis.*

Nursing Care of the Patient with Pleural Effusion

Tentative nursing diagnoses for care of the patient with pleural effusion include the following:
1. Ineffective breathing pattern, related to altered respiratory mechanisms
2. Impaired gas exchange, related to atelectasis
3. Alteration in comfort related to pleuritic chest pain

See Tables 26–3 and 26–4 for nursing care considerations regarding thoracentesis and chest drainage, respectively.

PNEUMOTHORAX

Definition

A pneumothorax is created when air is introduced into the intrapleural space by a break in the surface of the pleural lining. Air can also be introduced from outside the lung (e.g., by chest trauma and invasive abdominal procedures). The subatmospheric pressure normally present within the pleural space allows air to readily enter into the space whenever communication with the surrounding atmospheric air occurs. Collection of air within the intrapleural space, if sufficiently large, may cause partial or total lung collapse, resulting in a decrease in vital capacity.

Etiology

A pneumothorax can be caused by the entry of air into the pleural cavity through the chest wall and parietal pleura. Common causes are chest trauma (e.g., knife or gunshot wounds; crushing injury) and introduction of air, either intentionally or inadvertently, by a needle or catheter inserted through the chest wall and into the pleural space.

Impairment of the integrity of the visceral pleura, thereby allowing communication of air between the airways and alveoli, and the pleural space may also create a pneumothorax. Rupture of a subpleural air pocket (e.g., bleb, cyst, or bulla) or necrosis of lung parenchyma adjacent to the visceral pleura (e.g., necrotizing pneumonia, or neoplasm) are examples of causes involving the visceral pleura.

Possible iatrogenic causes of spontaneous pneu-

RESEARCH APPLICATION: SENSATIONS DURING CHEST TUBE REMOVAL
Gift, AG, Bolgiano, CS, and Cunningham J. Sensations during chest tube removal. Heart Lung 20:131, 1991.

Purpose: The purpose of this study was to identify and quantify sensations experienced by patients during and immediately after the process of chest tube removal and to identify the information that patients would like to be told in preparation for this procedure.

Methods: Thirty-six patients undergoing chest tube removal were asked to describe the sensations experienced during the procedure. Using a visual analog scale, the patients were asked to indicate the intensity of each sensation experienced. The patients were then asked to describe and quantify the sensations experienced immediately after (within 15 minutes) chest tube removal in the same fashion. Finally, patients were asked to indicate what they would like to have been told before tube removal.

Results: Sensations experienced by patients during the removal of a chest tube are burning, pain or hurting, pulling or yanking, pressure, anxiety, friction, and queasiness. Burning was the most frequently reported sensation, followed by pain or hurting, pulling or yanking, and pressure. The mean intensity for the sensation of burning was highest, followed by pain or hurting, pulling or yanking, and pressure, respectively. Fewer sensations were reported in the period immediately following the procedure. Soreness was the most common complaint; however, it was reported by only five subjects. Most subjects indicated that being told that the tube was going to be removed was sufficient preparatory information, whereas three subjects indicated that they preferred not to be given additional information prior to the procedure.

Practice Implications: It has long been the role of the nurse to prepare patients for procedures during hospitalization, and favorable outcomes of procedures have been associated with adequate patient preparation. Adequate preparation of patients for the removal of chest tubes, a procedure commonly performed in critical care units, is contingent on the nurse's awareness of the sensations likely to be experienced by the patients, as well as on variables that may affect the intensity of such sensations. Armed with this information, the critical care nurse can better prepare patients for removal of chest tubes and thus enhance their coping mechanisms during the procedure and hopefully achieve positive outcomes.

TABLE 26–3
Thoracentesis: Nursing Considerations

Nursing Considerations	Rationales
Purpose	When air or fluid accumulates in the pleural space, the increase in intrapleural pressure compromises lung expansion; $\dot{V}/\dot{Q}$ mismatching is increased.
1. To remove fluid or air from the pleural space to relieve lung compression and consequent respiratory distress	
2. To obtain a fluid specimen for chemical, microbial (bacterial), and cytologic analysis	
Action	
1. Assess patient/family's understanding of the procedure including: its purpose, indications, expectation of patient's participation.	An informed patient/family promotes cooperation and ease of procedure implementation.
a. Reinforce explanation made by physician.	
b. Provide opportunity for questions/answers regarding procedure.	
c. Obtain a signed permission (as per unit protocol).	
2. Establish baseline assessment database.	Baseline assessment data provide a basis for evaluating the patient's subsequent responses to therapeutic measures.
a. Vital signs: blood pressure, heart rate, pulses; respiratory rate, pattern and work of breathing	
b. Physical examination of the chest	
• Palpation: tactile fremitus	
• Percussion: resonance, hyperresonance, dullness	
• Auscultation: breath sounds; adventitious sounds	
3. Assemble necessary equipment	
4. Assist patient to assume an appropriate, but well-supported position: Approach to thoracentesis needle/catheter insertion:	Placement of patient in an appropriate position assists in determining landmarks and reduces risk of complications.
a. Anterior approach—used to evacuate *air* from the pleural space	
Site: 2nd intercostal space	
Positions: sitting in bed in semi-Fowler's position; supine position with arm positioned under head	
b. Posterior approach—used to remove *fluid* from the pleural space	
Site: 8th–9th intercostal space at mid- or posterior axillary line	
Positions: dangling on side of bed with arms resting on a bedside table; straddling a chair, if possible with arms resting on back of chair or overbed table	
5. Monitor use of aseptic technique.	Every effort must be made to minimize risk of infection.
• Use of masks, sterile gowns, and gloves by persons at bedside	
6. Assist physician with procedure as indicated.	Spontaneous pneumothorax, hemorrhage with hemothorax, diaphragmatic injury, and abdominal viscera penetration are complications that may require immediate intervention.
7. Assess patient's condition continuously throughout the procedure.	
8. Encourage shallow, controlled breathing during needle insertion; ask patient to refrain from coughing or making any sudden movements.	Shallow breathing reduces risk of lung trauma.
• Inform physician of patient's complaints of pain, dyspnea, tachypnea, changes in respiratory pattern and rate, and other signs of respiratory distress; nausea, weakness, diaphoresis.	This clinical presentation is highly suggestive of pneumothorax. Within minutes a spontaneous or traumatic pneumothorax can progress to a life-threatening tension pneumothorax.
9. Assist patient to remain immobilized until thoracentesis needle is secured.	Immobilization prevents inadvertent or accidental advancement of needle with the potential risk of puncturing the lung.
10. Apply firm pressure to insertion site upon removal of thoracentesis needle.	
• Apply povidone-iodine ointment and sterile dressing.	
11. Encourage patient to rest after thoracentesis.	
• Monitor patient's vital signs and respiratory function.	
12. Record amount and appearance of pleural fluid removed.	
• Label specimens carefully and deliver to appropriate laboratories for prescribed analysis.	
13. Obtain chest x-ray after thoracentesis.	Chest x-ray can detect presence of pneumothorax; when compared with prethoracentesis chest x-ray, it assists in evaluating status of pleural effusion.

TABLE 26–4
Chest Drainage: Nursing Care Considerations[14–19]

Underwater-Seal Drainage System

Purpose:
1. To reexpand the involved lung (pneumothorax) and reestablish the physiologic integrity of the intrapleural space
2. To assess, measure, and record chest drainage
3. To promote ease of breathing and respiratory excursion
4. To facilitate more evenly matching of ventilation with perfusion

Types of drainage in use:
1. One-, two- and three-bottle drainage systems
2. Pleur-evac (disposable chest drainage unit)
   a. A special feature of the Pleur-evac unit is that it has a positive-pressure release valve, which prevents pressure buildup in the intrapleural space.
   b. This disposable chest drainage unit is used predominantly today because it is less cumbersome, simpler, and safer to use than the bottle chest drainage systems.

Components of a chest drainage system:
1. Three chambers:
   a. Collection chamber—Receives fluid draining from intrapleural space
   b. Water-seal chamber—Allows venting of air displaced from collection chamber, but prevents atmospheric air from entering the intrapleural space
   c. Suction control chamber—Controls the amount of suction exerted on the chest
2. Options of straight gravity drainage under low suction (external source) depend on which chambers are used.
   Low suction can be applied with the use of 2- and 3-bottle drainage systems or with the Pleur-evac unit.

Underlying physical principles of chest drainage systems:
1. All methods of chest drainage function to allow air and fluid to pass in one direction only (i.e., from an area of greater pressure [intrapleural space] to one of less pressure [collection chamber]).
2. The degree of negative pressure within the water-seal system (i.e., the pressure exerted by the water) is determined by the depth to which the distal end of the chest tube is submerged in the water (Fig. 26–1).

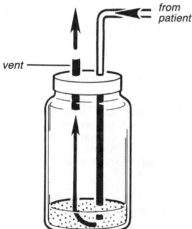

FIGURE 26–1. In the one-bottle system, the bottle acts as both a water seal and collection chamber. Air drained from the pleural space exits the system via the air vent.

   a. A depth of 2 cm is usually prescribed. If immersed under too much water, pressure accumulating within the intrapleural space cannot escape.
   b. Submersion of distal end of chest tube in water ensures "water seal," preventing retrograde flow of air or fluid into intrapleural space.
   c. Maintenance of negative pressures within the water seal system facilitates drainage of the air or fluid responsible for the disruption of normal pressures within the intrapleural space.

Setting up chest drainage:
1. One-bottle system—The bottle acts as both a water seal and collection chamber (see Fig. 26–1). An air vent in the bottle allows the air drained from the pleural space to escape, preventing pressure buildup within the system.
   a. This system is used primarily to decompress a pneumothorax; drainage of fluid along with air will cause the fluid level to rise, increasing the pressure within the system and creating a progressive resistance to drainage.
   The end-result: A greater effort must be exerted by the patient to force air or fluid, or both, into the drainage system on expiration.
2. Two-bottle system—In this system, the first bottle acts as the drainage chamber and the second bottle as the water-seal chamber (Fig. 26–2). An air vent in the second bottle allows escape of air preventing pressure buildup within the system.
   a. An advantage to this system is that the water seal is kept at a fixed level (bottle 2). This facilitates accurate assessment and recording of the amount and type of drainage.

TABLE 26–4
Chest Drainage: Nursing Care Considerations[14–19] (*Continued*)

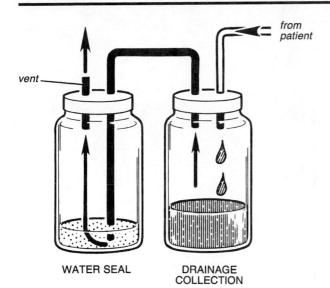

WATER SEAL   DRAINAGE
                    COLLECTION

FIGURE 26–2. In the two-bottle system, one bottle serves as a water seal with an air vent and another bottle serves as a drainage chamber.

3. Three-bottle system—In this system, there are separate bottles for each chamber: collection, water seal, and suction control (Fig. 26–3).
   a. Continuous gentle suction may be indicated if there is a considerable amount of air leaking into the intrapleural space.
   b. The amount of suction delivered by way of the chest tube is determined by the depth to which the air vent tube is submerged in the suction control chamber (bottle 3).
4. Pleur-evac (disposable chest drainage unit)—The Pleur-evac is a single molded unit with three chambers duplicating the three-bottle system (Fig. 26–3).

Nursing Considerations	Rationales
1. Assisting with chest tube insertion.	See Table 26–3 for nursing considerations in thoracentesis.
2. Additional considerations:	
a. Tape all connections securely.	Reduces risk of air leakage or inadvertent disconnection
• A Y connection may be used to connect two chest tubes to the drainage system.	Anterior chest tube (2nd intercostal space) = removal of *air*
	Posterior axillary chest tube (8th to 9th intercostal space) = removal of *fluid*
b. Maintain drainage system below level of chest tube insertion site.	Facilitates gravity drainage of air or fluid from pleural space; prevents retrograde flow of air or fluid into pleural space
c. When bottle drainage system is used, all bottles must be secured at bedside either in an appropriate holder or taped to floor.	Prevents accidental separation of tubing connections, or breakage of bottles should they be jarred
• Place calibrated tape on collection bottle to mark level of drainage.	Facilitates monitoring of quantity of drainage
d. Dressing care at chest tubing insertion site:	Reduces risk of air leak and infection
• Apply occlusive dressing using petroleum jelly gauze and dry sterile gauze pads.	
• Secure dressing with occlusive cloth tape.	
• Secure excess chest drainage tubing loosely to bottom sheet; allow sufficient tubing to enable patient to move in bed.	Prevents kinking of tubing and stress on insertion site
	Prevents accumulation of fluid in the lengths of dependent tubing, which may interfere with flow of drainage into collection chamber; or provide a milieu for bacterial growth
3. Maintenance of chest drainage:	Patency of drainage system must be maintained for therapeutic effectiveness.
a. Assess collection chamber for amount, rate, and type of drainage.	A reduction in drainage may reflect an obstruction in the system, pooling of secretions, or lung reexpansion.
(1) Mark level of drainage on calibrated tape hourly.	
(2) Notify physician if frank bleeding occurs.	
b. Place patient in semi-Fowler's position (unless contraindicated).	Semi-Fowler's position facilitates both air and fluid removal.
(1) Turn and reposition at regular intervals.	Repositioning helps to mobilize lung secretions and prevent pooling. The drainage system must remain patent; occlusion can predispose to tension pneumothorax.
c. Consider "stripping" or "milking" the tubing if fluid is not draining freely.	Use of "stripping" technique is controversial; there is some concern that such technique can generate pressures that far exceed those normally applied by gentle suction.
(1) Assess patient's status.	
(2) Consider unit protocols.	

Continued

TABLE 26–4
Chest Drainage: Nursing Care Considerations[14-19] (*Continued*)

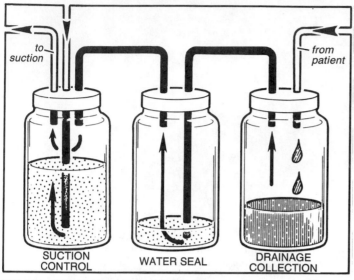

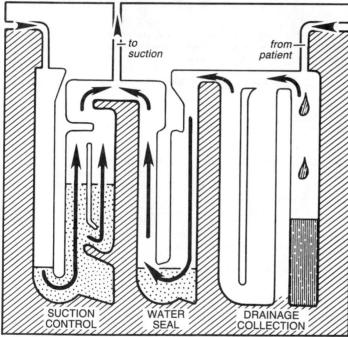

FIGURE 26–3. In the three-bottle and Pleur-evac system, there are three separate chambers, one for drainage collection, one for a water seal, and one for suction control.

Nursing Considerations	Rationales

4. Monitoring drainage system:
  a. Assess water level in water-seal chamber every 8 h.
   (1) Level usually prescribed is 2 cm.
 	
  b. Observe water-seal chamber for fluctuations:
   (1) Percuss and auscultate chest to determine if nonfluctuating water-seal chamber is due to an obstruction in the system or reexpansion of the lung.
 	
  c. Observe water-seal chamber for intermittent bubbling during expiration.
	Two little water increases risk of air entering chest; too much increases the effort necessary to generate intrapleural pressures sufficiently high to force air or fluid into the drainage system.
	Fluctuations result from changes in intrapleural pressure during respirations: With spontaneous breathing an upward movement occurs on inspiration; a downward movement on expiration. (The direction is reversed if the patient is on positive-pressure mechanical ventilation.)
	Excessive fluctuations may reflect coughing or respiratory distress; decrease in or cessation of fluctuations suggests a possible obstruction in the system, faulty suction, or lung reexpansion.
	Persistent continuous bubbling indicates an air leak within the drainage system or the patient; absence of bubbling indicates that evacuation is complete and pressure of the reexpanded lung has sealed the chest tube opening.

TABLE 26–4
Chest Drainage: Nursing Care Considerations[14–19] (*Continued*)

Nursing Considerations	Rationales

d. Observe for gentle bubbling in suction control chamber and note level of fluid.
     (1) A gentle stream of bubbling is sufficient.
   e. In bottle drainage system, check air vent patency; in Pleur-evac system, make sure the small hole in the rubber cap of the suction control chamber is not occluded.
   f. Keep two clamps at bedside to be used appropriately to:
     (1) Clamp the system briefly to locate source of air leak or to change the collection chamber.
     (2) Extra sterile bottle setup, or Pleur-evac, and thoracentesis set should be available at bedside for emergency use.
5. Implement comfort measures:
   a. Turning and positioning at regular intervals
   b. Range-of-motion exercises
   c. Splinting of chest tube insertion site during coughing or turning
6. Assisting with chest tube removal:
   a. Indications: Signs of lung reexpansion.
     (1) Cessation of bubbling in water-seal chamber
     (2) Stable clinical status
     (3) Fully aerated lungs on chest x-ray
   b. Nursing measures:
     (1) Provide appropriate explanation to patient.
 	
     (2) Premedicate as prescribed.
     (3) Monitor dressing for bleeding and reinforce if necessary.
     (4) Assess respiratory function.
	The amount of suction depends on the amount of fluid in the suction control chamber and not on setting of the external suction source.
	Occlusion increases pressure within the system and can cause tension pneumothorax. The system *must* always be vented to air.
	
	Clamping of chest tubes for more than a few seconds can lead to life-threatening tension pneumothorax.
	
	To reduce risk of pneumothorax, the able patient should be instructed to perform a Valsalva's maneuver during chest tube removal (e.g., take a deep breath and bear down).
	Chest tube removal can be painful.
	Small amount of serosanguineous drainage may occur after chest tube removal; dressing change after initial 48–72 h.

mothorax are unintentional puncture (e.g., subclavian insertion site), mechanical ventilation with positive end-expiratory pressure (PEEP) therapy, tracheostomy, and thoracentesis. It is essential for the critical care nurse to identify patients at risk and to monitor the patient closely for signs and symptoms indicative of pneumothorax.

Pathophysiology

When the normal subatmospheric intrapleural pressure is lost, there is nothing to counteract the elastic recoil tendency of the lung and the lung collapses. The degree of collapse and thus the pathophysiologic consequences of a pneumothorax depend on its size (the amount of air within the pleural space) and location. Small amounts of air may cause no symptoms and few, if any, physical signs, whereas a massive pneumothorax can result in acute cardiovascular collapse. Even relatively small decreases in vital capacity may lead to sudden and significant deterioration (e.g., respiratory insufficiency, alveolar hypoventilation, and respiratory acidosis) in patients with pre-existing respiratory compromise.[1]

Tension Pneumothorax

A tension pneumothorax occurs when air within the pleural space comes under positive pressure or "ten-

sions." This tension may be the result of a "check-valve" mechanism by which air freely enters the pleural space during inspiration but is unable to escape on expiration. Such one-way movement of air into the pleural space causes a progressive increase in intrapleural pressure with a concomitant progressive collapse of the underlying lung. When pleural pressures become sufficiently high, a shift of the mediastinum and trachea away from the side of the pneumothorax (the side with the positive intrapleural pressure) occurs. Of critical importance is that the positive pressure within the pleural space inhibits venous return by way of the superior and inferior venae cavae. This severely compromises cardiac output, and emergency treatment may be required to reverse the cardiopulmonary failure.

At high risk of developing a tension pneumothorax are patients who have sustained chest trauma and patients receiving mechanical ventilation therapy. It is important to appreciate that any pneumothorax—small or large—has the potential to become a tension pneumothorax when mechanical ventilation is initiated.

Clinical Presentation

Clinical features of pneumothorax depend largely on its size and on the presence of underlying pulmonary disease (e.g., COPD). If the pneumothorax is small and the patient is without pre-existing pulmonary disease, he or she may remain completely asymptomatic.

The most common symptoms of pneumothorax are the acute onset of chest pain or dyspnea. Physical findings reflect the presence of free pleural air on the affected side. On palpatory examination of the chest, tactile fremitus and egophony may be decreased to absent, since the air-filled pleural space muffles voice and breath sounds. A hyperresonant note may be elicited on percussion, and breath sounds may be diminished to absent on auscultation.

The patient with tension pneumothorax presents with severe respiratory distress (apprehension, agitation, dyspnea, and tachypnea) accompanied by cardiovascular collapse (tachycardia, profound hypotension, and cyanosis). The trachea and mediastinum are shifted away from the affected side; a marked elevation of jugular venous pressure is usually observed. The patient may be diaphoretic with arterial blood gases that reflect severely compromised gas exchange (e.g., hypoxemia and respiratory acidosis). In the patient who is mechanically ventilated, ventilation quickly becomes compromised, peak airway pressure rapidly increases, and gas exchange deteriorates.

Treatment and Management

Treatment of pneumothorax depends on its size and underlying cause. With a small pneumothorax causing few symptoms and no indication of expanding, no treatment other than close observation is usually necessary. Larger symptomatic pneumothoraces are best treated with chest tube insertion and decompression.[14-16]

Tension pneumothorax with hemodynamic compromise is life-threatening and requires immediate intervention. A large-bore needle placed in the 2nd intercostal space (anteriorly) usually helps to relieve the positive intrapleural pressure sufficiently to improve hemodynamics while a chest tube is being inserted. The effectiveness of decompression is reflected by an improvement in cardiac output and a rise in arterial blood pressure. Administration of 100% oxygen is indicated until stabilization of ventilatory status with tube thoracotomy.

Reexpansion Pulmonary Edema

Reexpansion pulmonary edema may occur following rapid expansion of lung after collapse from pneumothorax or pleural effusion. Although the exact physiologic mechanism for this phenomenon has yet to be precisely defined, it is believed to result from an increase in capillary permeability from the mechanical stresses of reexpansion and perhaps reperfusion injury. Reexpansion pulmonary edema is more likely to occur when the pneumothorax or effusion has been present for 3 days or when negative pressure has been applied to the pleural space (application of suction to

chest drainage systems). The clinical features of reexpansion pulmonary edema include hypoxia and at times hypotension.[20]

Tentative nursing diagnoses in the care of the patient with pleural effusion may include the following:

1. Impaired gas exchange related to $\dot{V}/\dot{Q}$ mismatch; reexpansion edema
2. Breathing pattern, ineffective, related to tachypnea, dyspnea, and altered respiratory mechanics
3. Decreased cardiac output, related to altered hemodynamics (reduced preload)
4. Alteration in comfort related to acute respiratory distress; knowledge deficit regarding illness

See Tables 26–3 and 26–4 for nursing care considerations regarding thoracentesis and chest drainage, respectively.

REFERENCES

1. Kirsten, LD: Comprehensive Respiratory Nursing. WB Saunders, Philadelphia, 1989.
2. Moser, KM: Pulmonary embolism. In Murray, JF and Nadal, JA (eds): Textbook of Respiratory Medicine. WB Saunders, Philadelphia, 1988.
3. Roberts, SL: Pulmonary tissue perfusion altered: Emboli. Heart Lung 6:128, 1987.
4. Jones, KM: Pulmonary embolus. In Mims, BC (ed): Case Studies in Critical Care. Williams & Wilkins, Baltimore, 1990.
5. Weinberger, S: Principles of Pulmonary Medicine. WB Saunders, Philadelphia, 1986.
6. Stratton, MB: Ventilation-perfusion scintigraphy in diagnosis of pulmonary thromboembolism. Heart Lung 17:287, 1990.
7. Driedger, AA and Sibbald, WJ: Acute pulmonary embolism. In Sibbald, WJ (ed): Synopsis of Critical Care, ed 3. Williams & Wilkins, Baltimore, 1988.
8. Dickinson, SP and Bury, GM: Pulmonary embolism: Anatomy of a crisis. Nursing '89, 34, 1989.
9. Mathewson, M: Pharmacotherapeutics: A Nursing Process Approach. FA Davis, Philadelphia, 1986.
10. Light, RW: Disorders of the pleura: General principles and diagnostic approach. In Murray, JF and Nadel, JA (eds): Textbook of Respiratory Medicine. WB Saunders, Philadelphia, 1988.
11. Weyrberger, SE: Principles of Pulmonary Medicine. WB Saunders, Philadelphia, 1986.
12. Light, RW: Pleural effusion. In Murray, JF and Nadel, JA (eds): Textbook of Respiratory Medicine. WB Saunders, Philadelphia, 1988.
13. Lohrman, J: Thoracentesis. In Kinkade, S and Lohrman, J (eds): Critical Care Nursing Procedures. BC Decker, Toronto, 1990.
14. Boggs, R and Woolridge, K (eds): AACN Procedure Manual for Critical Care Nursing. CV Mosby, St. Louis, 1993.
15. Carrol, P: The ins and outs of chest drainage systems. Nursing '86, 16:26, December 1986.
16. Quin, A: Thora-Drain III: Closed chest drainage made simpler and safer. Nursing '86, 16:46, September 1986.
17. Lohrman, J: Tube thoracotomy. In Kinkade, S and Lohrman, J (eds): Critical Care Nursing Procedures. BC Decker, Toronto, 1990.
18. Duncan, CR, Erickson, RS, and Wiegel, RM: Effect of chest tube management on drainage after cardiac surgery. Heart Lung 16:1, 1987.
19. Pierce, JD, Piazza, D, and Naftel, DC: Effects of two chest tube clearance protocols on drainage in patients after myocardial revascularization surgery. Heart Lung 20:125, 1991.
20. Light, RW: Pneumothorax. In Murray, JF and Nadel, JA (eds): Textbook of Respiratory Medicine. WB Saunders, Philadelphia, 1988.

UNIT FOUR

Nervous System

UNIT OUTLINE

C H A P T E R   2 7

Anatomy and Physiology of the Nervous System

Joan T. Dolan

CHAPTER OUTLINE

LEARNING OBJECTIVES

After completing this chapter, you should be able to:

1. Outline the major divisions of the nervous system
2. Describe the functional unit of the nervous system, the neuron
3. Describe the functional anatomy of the synapse and the role of neurotransmitters
4. Describe the *structural* support systems of the brain including the skull, cranial vault, and the meninges
5. Review the *functional* support systems of the brain including the ventricular system, cerebrospinal fluid, and blood circulatory systems
6. Delineate brain structures and their functions
7. Associate metabolic needs of neural tissue with autoregulation and cerebral perfusion pressure
8. Relate compensatory mechanisms to the maintenance of intracranial pressure within physiologic range
9. Describe the structure of the spinal cord including spinal nerves and plexi
10. Differentiate between ventral and dorsal spinal cord roots
11. Identify the functional components of the reflex arc
12. Trace the circuitry of primary sensory and motor pathways
13. Describe the structure and function of the autonomic nervous system

MAJOR DIVISIONS OF THE NERVOUS SYSTEM

The nervous system consists of two major divisions, the *central nervous system* and the *peripheral nervous system* (Table 27–1). The central nervous system (CNS) is composed of the brain and spinal cord; the peripheral nervous system (PNS) consists of all the nerves outside the brain and spinal cord, including 12 pairs of *cranial* nerves and 31 pairs of *spinal* nerves.

The PNS is further divided into the *afferent* and *efferent* divisions. Afferent, or sensory, nerves transmit information received from specialized *receptors* in peripheral and deep structures of the body *toward* the CNS (the brain and spinal cord); efferent, or motor,

nerves transmit information *away* from the brain and spinal cord to structures throughout the body, including skeletal muscle, cardiac muscle, and smooth muscles of visceral organs and glands. These structures are called *effectors* because it is through them that the response of the CNS is realized.

The efferent division of the PNS is further divided into the *somatic* nervous system and the *autonomic* nervous system. Nerves of the somatic nervous system are concerned with the interaction of the body with the external environment. These nerves innervate skeletal muscle cells.

The autonomic nervous system is divided into the *sympathetic* and *parasympathetic* divisions. Nerves of the autonomic nervous system are concerned primarily

501

TABLE 27–1
Divisions of the Nervous System

1. Central nervous system (CNS)
    a. Brain
    b. Spinal cord
2. Peripheral nervous system (PNS)
    a. Afferent division
    b. Efferent division
       1) Somatic nervous system
       2) Autonomic nervous system
          (a) Sympathetic division
          (b) Parasympathetic division

with visceral functions and interaction with the internal environment. These nerves innervate cardiac muscle, smooth muscle, and glands.

FUNCTIONAL MICROANATOMY OF THE NERVOUS SYSTEM

Cell Types

Neuron—The Functional Unit

The *neuron* is the functional unit of the nervous system. Neurons are among the most highly specialized cells within the human body, and although they occur in many different forms and sizes, they all have three basic fundamental properties. These include the capacity to react to stimuli, to initiate and conduct action potentials in response to stimuli, and to enable a response to occur by influencing other neurons, muscles, or glands.

Structural Components. Each neuron consists of three major structural components: the cell body, dendrites, and axon (Fig. 27–1). Dendrites and axons are collectively referred to as *nerve fibers*.

Dendrites are generally short, highly branched cytoplasmic extensions of the cell body, which receive incoming information (in the form of nerve impulses) and conduct it *toward* the cell body. The dendrite–cell body complex can be thought of as the *receptive/integrative unit* of the neuron (Fig. 27–1). Dendrites provide most of the receptor surface for incoming information from other neurons. This information is processed within the dendrite–cell body complex in such a way that the net response of the neuron reflects the integration of numerous, often conflicting bits of information received from other neurons.

The *axon* is usually a single process arising from the cell body and conducts information *away* from the cell body to the *axon terminals (synaptic knobs)* (Fig. 27–1). Some axons are covered with a lipid-protein substance called *myelin*, which insulates the axonal membrane and influences the speed of impulse conduction. Myelin is deposited along the axons in a circular manner so as to surround the axon with an outer enveloping layer called the *myelin sheath*. The myelin sheath is not a continuous layer but is segmented or interrupted at regular intervals called *nodes of Ranvier*. The presence of such nodes facilitates rapid impulse transmission.

Nerve fibers that have a myelin sheath are called *myelinated fibers* and make up the white matter of the CNS. The term "white" reflects the high lipid content in myelin. Nerve fibers without a myelin sheath are

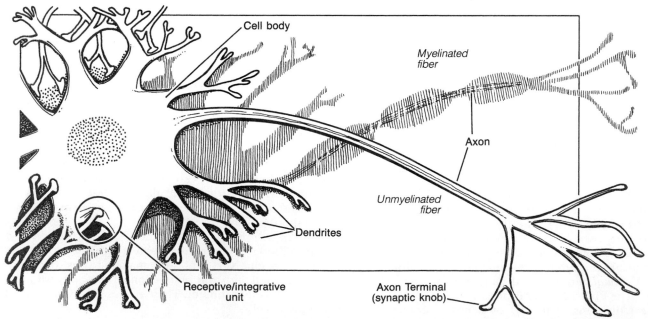

FIGURE 27–1. Neuron: functional unit of the nervous system. Major structural components include the cell body, dendrites, axon, and axon terminals (synaptic knobs). The neuron consists of receptive/intergrative units comprised of dendrite–cell body complexes. These units function by processing incoming information.

called *unmyelinated fibers* and make up the gray matter within the CNS (Fig. 27–1).

Neuroglial Cells

Neuroglial cells are specialized, non-nervous connective tissue cells within the CNS which function to sustain neurons metabolically, provide structural support, and help to regulate ionic concentrations in extracellular fluid.

Several types of neuroglial cells have been identified, including *astroglia, microglia, oligodendroglia,* and *ependymal* cells. The latter two cell types deserve special mention. *Oligodendroglia* are glial cells responsible for producing myelin within the CNS and for establishing and maintaining the myelin sheaths of myelinated axons. *Ependymal cells* are glial cells that line the ventricles and choroid plexuses and are thought to be involved in production of cerebrospinal fluid. These cells play a role in establishing and maintaining the blood-brain barrier.

Neuroglial cells are of clinical importance in that 40% to 50% of intracranial tumors are derived from glial cells *(gliomas)*. These cells, unlike neurons, can undergo mitosis. Glial scars after brain injury or surgery may result in focal seizures. The myelin sheaths, as elaborated by the oliogodendroglia, are the target of *demyelinating* diseases, such as multiple sclerosis.

Synapse

Information is communicated throughout the nervous system by both electrical and chemical processes. Transmission of impulses from one neuron to the next occurs via a synapse.

A *synapse* is a strategic, anatomically specialized junction between two neurons at which the electrical activity in one neuron influences the activity of the second neuron. At chemical synapses, this activity is communicated by a chemical "messenger" called a *neurotransmitter.*

Structurally, the synapse consists of the *synaptic knob (axon terminal)* of the *presynaptic* neuron, and the *subsynaptic membrane* of the *postsynaptic* neuron, separated by a small space called the *synaptic cleft* (Fig. 27–2). The synaptic cleft is sufficiently wide to prevent the direct propagation of electrical current from the presynaptic neuron to the postsynaptic neuron. Rather, such activity is transmitted across the synaptic cleft *chemically* by a neurotransmitter released from the synaptic knob.

In response to an action potential, which spreads over the synaptic knob depolarizing its membrane, small quantities of neurotransmitter are released into the synaptic cleft from *presynaptic vesicles*, which merge with the plasma membrane. Calcium is considered to be the link between depolarization of the presynaptic membrane by an arriving action potential and neurotransmitter release.

Once released, the neurotransmitter molecules diffuse across the cleft and bind in a transient manner and very specifically to receptor sites on the *subsynaptic plasma membrane* of the postsynaptic neuron. A neurotransmitter binding to its specific receptor causes an immediate change in the permeability characteristics of the subsynaptic membrane by opening specific ion

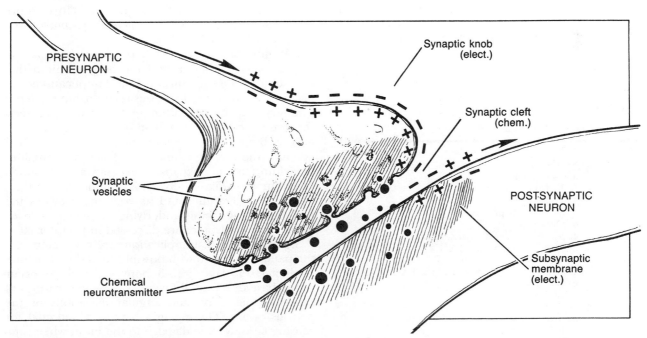

FIGURE 27–2. Diagram of synapse, a specialized junction between two neurons separated by a synaptic cleft. The presence of the synaptic cleft requires that the transfer of information between these two neurons occurs via the secretion of a chemical neurotransmitter.

channels. The type of receptor and the type of channel that the receptor controls largely determine the effects, whether excitatory or inhibitory, that the neurotransmitter has on the postsynaptic neuron.

The synaptic activity is terminated very quickly when the neurotransmitter leaves the postsynaptic receptor. Ion channels close, terminating the postsynaptic membrane potential.

It is apparent that because neurotransmitter is stored on the *pre*synaptic side of the synaptic cleft and the receptor sites occur on the *post*synaptic side, chemical synapses operate in *one* direction only. This also explains why action potentials move along multineuronal pathways in one direction.

Neurotransmitters. Neurotransmitters are the chemical messengers by which presynaptic neurons can influence postsynaptic neurons at chemical synapses. Neurotransmitters are also the vehicle by which efferent neurons influence *effector* cells (skeletal, cardiac and smooth muscles, and glands). Although there are many different neurotransmitter substances, they are highly specific, and in many instances neurons are identified by the type of neurotransmitter they release at their synapses, or at neuromuscular junctions.

In a few instances, more than one neurotransmitter may be released from the synaptic knob. Such neurotransmitters may have a *synergistic* effect on each other. More commonly, all synaptic knobs (axon terminals) on a given neuron probably release the same neurotransmitter. It is also possible for a given neurotransmitter to produce excitation at one synapse and inhibition at another. These considerations, together with the infinitesimal number of synapses within the nervous system, help to explain the degree of sophistication of integration and communication unique to the human body. Table 27–2 lists some of the more commonly known neurotransmitters.

TABLE 27–2
Classes of Neurotransmitters

1. Acetylcholine
2. Monoamines
   a. Catecholamines
      1) Dopamine
      2) Epinephrine
      3) Norepinephrine
   b. Histamine
   c. Serotonin (5-hydroxytryptamine)
3. Amino acids
   a. Aspartate
   b. Gamma-amino butyric acid (GABA)
   c. Glutamate
   d. Glycine
4. Peptides
   a. Angiotensin II
   b. Bradykinin
   c. Endorphins
   d. Enkephalins
   e. Hormones

FUNCTIONAL ANATOMY OF THE BRAIN

Structural and Functional Support Systems

Skull and Cranial Vault

The brain is enclosed within the *cranium*—that portion of the bony framework of the skull that provides a protective vault for this vital organ. The bony structure of the cranium consists of an outer and inner table of *compact bone* with a layer of *cancellous (interwoven) bone* in between. Such structure increases strength without increasing weight. A number of very small openings, or *foramina*, in the base of the skull allow for entrance and exit of blood vessels and cranial nerves. There is one large opening, the *foramen magnum*, where the brainstem connects with the spinal cord.

The floor of the cranial vault is divided into the anterior, middle, and posterior *fossae*, or compartments, which conform to and house the frontal lobe, temporal lobe, and brainstem and cerebellum, respectively (Fig. 27–3). The *anterior fossa* is formed largely by the frontal bone, except for a tiny midline section formed by the ethmoid bone. This bone contains the *cribriform plate*, which contains many openings traversed by olfactory nerve fibers.

The anterior fossa is separated from the middle fossa by the sphenoid bone. The *middle fossa* is bounded largely by the sphenoid and temporal bones. The *sella turcica*, which houses the *pituitary gland (hypophysis)*, occurs in the midline. The *optic foramina* are under the lesser wings of the sphenoid bone.

The *petrous* portion of the temporal bone provides the boundary between the middle and posterior fossae. The *posterior* fossa is the largest and is formed primarily by occipital bone. The *foramen magnum* is the most conspicuous foramen.

It is important to appreciate the structural relationship between the brain and the bony cranium that encases it because significant clinical implications may occur when the integrity of this relationship is altered by injury or pathology. Although the cranium protects the brain, it can also confine it. In the face of an insult to the brain (e.g., cerebral hemorrhage, cerebral edema), the cranium functions as a rigid container unyielding to brain expansion except via the foramen magnum (see Fig. 27–3). This unique relationship between the cranium and its contents provides the pathophysiologic basis underlying *herniation syndrome*. Herniation syndromes are discussed in Chapter 29.

Significant clinical implications are associated with the patient admitted with possible *basal* skull fracture. As depicted in Figure 27–3, bony, sharp ridges occur in the base of the skull formed by the lesser wings of the sphenoid bone and angular elevations of the petrous bones. These ridges have the potential for causing considerable damage to the brain when injurious forces applied to the head cause the brain to be thrown up against these ridges. This often results in a "shearing-type" injury to the base of the brain.

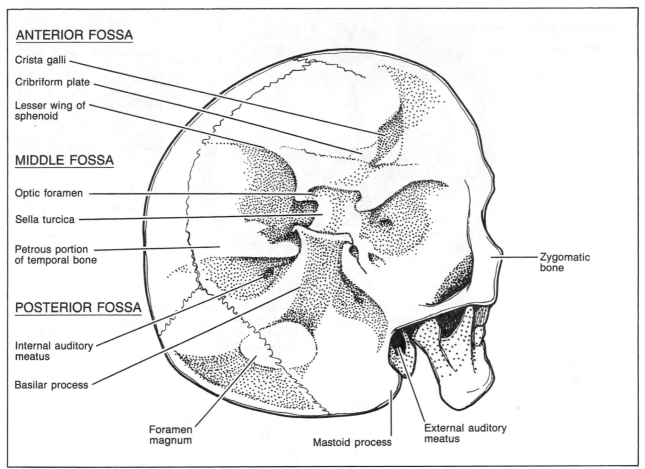

ANTERIOR FOSSA

Crista galli

Cribriform plate

Lesser wing of sphenoid

MIDDLE FOSSA

Optic foramen

Sella turcica

Petrous portion of temporal bone

POSTERIOR FOSSA

Internal auditory meatus

Basilar process

Zygomatic bone

Foramen magnum

Mastoid process

External auditory meatus

FIGURE 27–3. Intact skull and cranial vault. The floor of the cranial vault is divided into the anterior, middle, and posterior fossae (or compartments), which conform to and house the frontal lobe, temporal lobe, brainstem, and cerebellum, respectively. The intact skull has only one large opening, the foramen magnum. Expansion of the contents within the rigid skull (e.g., brain parenchyma, blood, and cerebrospinal fluid) is very limited except via the foramen magnum.

Fractures of basal skull bones and associated lacerations to brain coverings (meninges) and blood vessels may result in leakage of cerebrospinal fluid from the nose or ear, or both, and in bleeding into the cranial bones.

Meninges

The *meninges* are connective tissue membranes, which cover and surround the brain and spinal cord to support and protect these soft, delicate tissues. There are three separate and continuous layers of tissue: the dura mater, arachnoid mater, and pia mater.

The *dura mater*, the tough, fibrous outermost membrane, occurs in two layers. The outer, periosteal layer is continuous with the inner table of the bony cranium; the thick inner layer follows the contour of the skull except at sites of certain major fissures. In these locations, the dura mater is a sturdy sheath that compartmentalizes major areas of the brain. The *falx cerebri* is the sturdy midline sheath located in the *longitudinal*

fissure between the cerebral hemispheres (Fig. 27–4). The *falx cerebelli* is the dural sheath that separates the two cerebellar hemispheres. The *tentorium cerebelli* is a smaller fold of dura, which extends between the cerebral hemispheres and the cerebellum to form a "tent" over the cerebellum. A *notch,* or opening, within the tentorium accommodates the brainstem.

The *arachnoid mater,* a thin, delicate fibroelastic tissue, loosely encloses the brain but does not dip into its sulci and fissures. As this membrane skips from crest to crest over the surface of the brain, it gives rise to several large spaces called *cisterns.* The *cisterna magnum* is located between the hemispheres of the cerebellum and medulla, and the *lumbar cistern* is located in the lumbar region of the vertebral column. Both of these enlarged spaces are accessible for aspiration of cerebrospinal fluid.

The *pia mater,* a thin, delicate membrane, is attached intimately to the brain surface following every sulcus and fissure. This membrane functions to hold the brain and spinal cord substance together; it is a very vascular membrane through which pass the cerebral blood vessels that nourish the brain tissues; and it

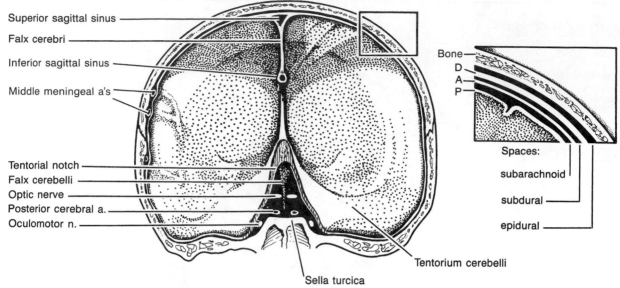

Superior sagittal sinus

Falx cerebri

Inferior sagittal sinus

Middle meningeal a's

Tentorial notch

Falx cerebelli

Optic nerve

Posterior cerebral a.

Oculomotor n.

Sella turcica

Bone

D
A
P

Spaces:

subarachnoid

subdural

epidural

Tentorium cerebelli

FIGURE 27–4. The meninges (connective tissue coverings) in a coronal section of the head with unobstructed view of the posterior wall of the cranial cavity. The meninges that surround the brain consist of three separate and continuous layers. (D = dura mater, A = arachnoid mater, P = pia mater.) Potential spaces occur between the meningeal layers. These spaces are significant clinically, in that bleeding into these spaces leads to hematoma formation.

functions as part of the *blood-brain barrier* (discussed in the following text).

The unique interrelationship of the meninges is responsible for the "spaces" within the cranial cavity. The *epidural (extradural) space* is a potential space occurring between the periosteal dura and the bone itself (Fig. 27–1). The *subdural space* is between the layers of dura and arachnoid mater. A venous vasculature traverses throughout this space. The *subarachnoid space* occurs between the arachnoid and pia mater. It contains numerous blood vessels and is the space throughout which cerebrospinal fluid circulates and is reabsorbed.

Ventricular System

The *ventricular system* includes a series of interconnected cavities within the brain, which are lined with ependymal cells and filled with cerebrospinal fluid. Two *lateral* ventricles, one in each cerebral hemisphere, communicate with the *third* ventricle via the *foramen of Monroe* (Fig. 27–5). The third ventricle communicates with the *fourth* ventricle via the *aqueduct of Sylvius*. The fourth ventricle gives rise to the *central canal* of the spinal cord and contains the *foramen of Luschka* and the *foramen of Magendie*.

Formation, Circulation, and Reabsorption of Cerebrospinal Fluid. Cerebrospinal fluid is essentially a plasma filtrate formed from the blood in the *choroid plexuses* located in portions of the lateral, third, and fourth ventricles (Fig. 27–5). Cerebrospinal fluid is a crystal clear, colorless fluid, which normally is almost completely devoid of protein but contains *glucose*. The presence of glucose helps to differentiate it from

mucous drainage from the nose in the scenario of head injury or brain surgery. Mucus contains no glucose. Other characteristics of cerebrospinal fluid are listed in Table 27–3.

In the average adult, cerebrospinal fluid is formed at the rate of about 400 to 600 mL/day. At any given moment, the volume within the cranium is about 100 to 150 mL. Because the cranium is a rigid, unyielding container, cerebrospinal fluid must be removed from the cranial cavity at about the same rate as it is formed in order to maintain intracranial pressure within normal limits. The normal pressure of cerebrospinal fluid in the lateral recumbent position is in the range of 60 to 180 mm H_2O (0 to 15 mmHg).

Cerebrospinal fluid flows from its origin in the choroid plexuses through the interconnected ventricular system into the cisterns and subarachnoid spaces occurring within and surrounding the brain and spinal cord (Fig. 27–6).

Eventually, cerebrospinal fluid is reabsorbed into the blood via the *arachnoid granulations (villi)*. These are projections of arachnoid tissue that provide for unidirectional flow of cerebrospinal fluid from the subarachnoid space into the blood.

Functions of Cerebrospinal Fluid. Cerebrospinal fluid plays a critical role in the maintenance of normal neuronal function. It provides a protective fluid "cushion" for all components of the CNS; it acts as a medium for the exchange of some nutrients and end-products of neural metabolism; it is a vital link in the regulation of the chemical environment of the CNS; it may serve as a channel for the transport of substances within the brain parenchyma; and it plays a vital compensatory role in maintaining intra-

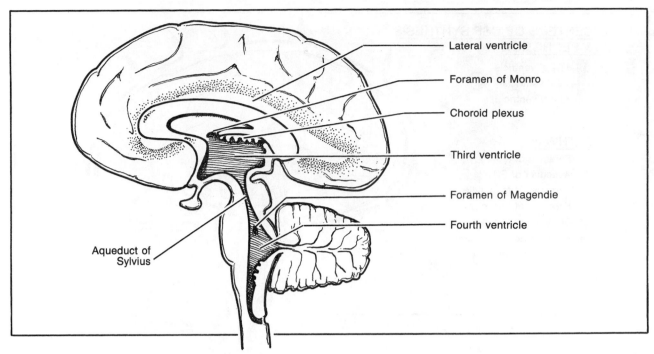

FIGURE 27–5. The ventricular system consists of a series of interconnected cavities within the brain, which contain cerebrospinal fluid.

cranial pressure within normal limits (see Chapter 29).

Cerebral Circulatory System

A constant, copious blood supply to the brain is required for normal cerebral function because the brain has little metabolic and energy reserves. Interruption of blood supply to the brain for only a few minutes may result in irreparable damage to neural tissue.

Arterial Vasculature. The major arterial blood supply to the brain is derived from two sources: the *vertebral arteries* and the *internal carotid arteries*. There is a branching anastomosing network of collateral vessels with considerable overlapping of distribution to ensure adequate blood supply to neural tissue. At the base of the cranial cavity, the *circle of Willis* connects the vertebral and internal carotid circulations (Fig. 27–7).

Vertebral Circulation. The vertebral arteries ascend from the subclavian arteries through the transverse foramina of the cervical vertebrae to enter the cranial cavity via the foramen magnum. These arteries give off branches to the spinal cord, medulla, and cerebellum before joining to form the *basilar* artery.

The basilar artery, in turn, sends branches to several regions of the brain (brainstem, cerebellum, diencephalon, internal ear) before bifurcating and terminating as the *posterior cerebral* arteries (Fig. 27–7).

The posterior cerebral arteries supply inferior and posterior portions of the cerebral hemispheres includ-

ing portions of the temporal lobes and the occipital lobe. The *primary visual cortex* within the occipital lobe is supplied by the *calcarine* artery, a branch of the posterior cerebral artery.

Internal Carotid Circulation. The *internal carotid* arteries arise from the common carotid artery and enter the cranial cavity via the *foramen lacernum*. They immediately give rise to several important arteries, including the ophthalmic, posterior communicating, anterior cerebral, and middle cerebral arteries (Figs. 27–7 and 27–18).

TABLE 27–3
Cerebrospinal Fluid: Normal Laboratory Values

Laboratory Tests	Normal Values (Adult)
Appearance	Crystal clear, colorless
Pressure (lateral recumbent)	0–15 mmHg
Protein:	
Lumbar	15–45 mg/100 mL
Ventricular	5–15 mg/100 mL
Glucose	50–75 mg/100 mL
Electrolytes:	
Sodium	~141.0 mEq/L
Potassium	~3.3 mEq/L
Chloride	120–130 mEq/L
pH	7.32–7.35
Specific gravity	1.007
Cell count:	
RBCs	None
WBCs	0–5 mm^3
Gram's stain	Negative
Culture and sensitivity	No growth of organisms

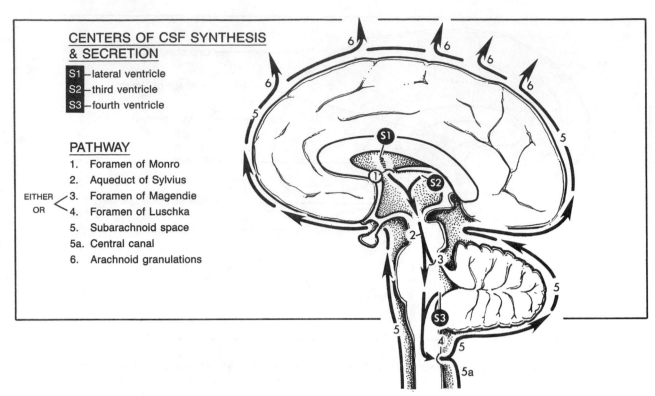

CENTERS OF CSF SYNTHESIS
& SECRETION

S1 – lateral ventricle
S2 – third ventricle
S3 – fourth ventricle

PATHWAY

1. Foramen of Monro
2. Aqueduct of Sylvius

EITHER
OR
3. Foramen of Magendie
4. Foramen of Luschka
5. Subarachnoid space
5a. Central canal
6. Arachnoid granulations

FIGURE 27–6. Formation, circulation, and reabsorption of cerebrospinal fluid. Cerebrospinal fluid is synthesized within the choroid plexus (see Fig. 27–5) and circulates via the interconnected ventricular system throughout the subarachnoid spaces occurring within and surrounding the brain and spinal cord. Eventually, cerebrospinal fluid is reabsorbed via the arachnoid granulations in the superior saggital sinus.

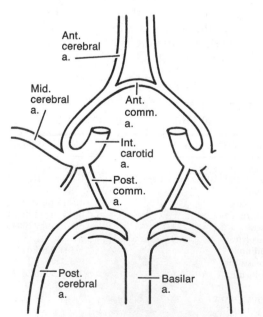

FIGURE 27–7. The circle of Willis, an anastomosing network of blood vessels at the base of the brain, which serves to connect the vertebral circulation with the internal carotid circulation.

The *anterior cerebral arteries* supply the orbital and medial aspects of the frontal lobe and the medial aspects of the parietal lobes. The *middle cerebral arteries* supply the bulk of both hemispheres including the lateral aspects of the frontal, parietal, and temporal lobes (see Fig. 27–18). The *ophthalmic arteries* can be important in common carotid or internal carotid artery occlusion because they allow collateral circulation between the *external* and *internal* carotid arteries.

Meningeal Circulation. The meninges receive an abundant blood supply via the anterior, middle, and posterior *meningeal* arteries. Branches of the *middle meningeal* artery, which arises from the external carotid artery, fan out over the lateral surfaces of dura covering the brain and are snugly nestled between the periosteal dura and inner table of compact bone (Fig. 27–4). Bleeding associated with rupture, or laceration of branches of the middle meningeal artery, results in formation of epidural hematoma.

Venous Sinuses. After flowing through the brain, blood is collected in *cerebral veins* and *venous sinuses* and ultimately leaves the cranial cavity via the *internal jugular* veins. The relatively large venous sinuses are located in the dura mater. Those of note are depicted in Figure 27–8. The *superior sagittal sinus* also drains cerebrospinal fluid. The arachnoid granulations through which cerebrospinal fluid is reabsorbed into the blood protrude into this venous sinus.

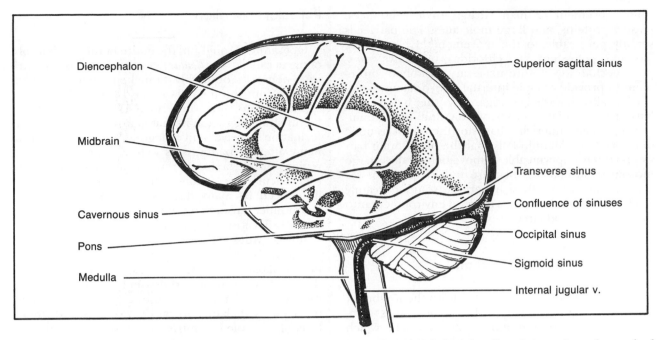

FIGURE 27–8. The venous sinuses provide a system of channels that collect blood which has flowed throughout the cerebral circulation, and they empty this blood into the internal jugular veins through which it exits from the cranial vault. The relatively large venous sinuses are located within the dura mater. The superior sagittal sinus also drains cerebrospinal fluid. The arachnoid granulations responsible for the reabsorption of cerebrospinal fluid are located within the superior sagittal sinus. (See Fig. 27–6.)

Blood-Brain Barrier

The *blood-brain barrier* is a highly selective barrier that enables the internal environment within the brain to be closely regulated. It controls both the kinds of substances that enter the extracellular space of the brain and the rate at which they enter.

The selective permeability of the blood-brain barrier is a function of its unique anatomic structure and physiologic transport systems (Fig. 27–9). It is highly permeable to water, carbon dioxide, oxygen, most lipid-soluble substances (e.g., alcohol and anesthetics), and small molecular substances. Its selectivity pre-

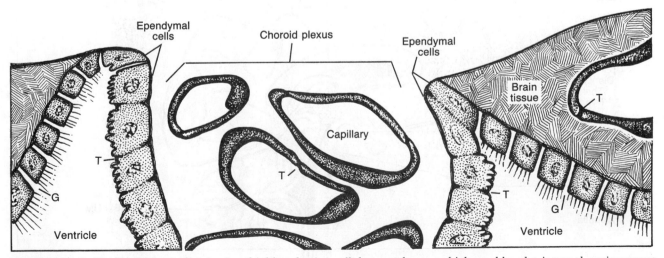

FIGURE 27–9. The blood-brain barrier is a highly selective cellular membrane, which enables the internal environment within the brain to be closely regulated. Structurally, it is characterized by the presence of specialized junctions between epithelial cells, including tight junctions (T) and gap junctions (G). Tight junctions occur when the plasma membranes of two adjacent cells are fused, as for example, between ependymal cells lining the ventricles, or between adjacent endothelial cells lining cerebral capillaries. The presence of tight junctions necessitates that substances must pass *through* these cells to gain entry into the brain's internal environment. Gap junctions, specialized channels between adjacent cells, provide a second mechanism contributing to further selectivity of substances allowed to enter the brain's internal environment via the blood-brain barrier.

vents movement of many drugs, toxic substances, plasma proteins, and large molecules. The barrier is slightly permeable to the movement of electrolytes (sodium, potassium, and chloride), but active transport mechanisms ensure necessary rapidity of movement to provide a stable internal environment.

Clinically, knowledge regarding the blood-brain barrier is essential in terms of fluid and drug administration. The underlying basis for the use of osmotic diuretics (e.g., Mannitol) is that the blood-brain barrier is largely impermeable to movement of these large molecular substances. Because water readily passes through the barrier, these hypertonic solutions readily draw water from the brain's internal environment into the systemic blood circulation.

Brain Structures and Function

The brain has three major divisions: the forebrain, brainstem, and cerebellum. The forebrain is composed of the cerebrum and upper brainstem, which includes the diencephalon. The diencephalon is, in turn, composed of the thalamus and hypothalamus. The remaining brainstem consists of the midbrain, pons, and medulla (Fig. 27–10). A review of the functional anatomy of specific brain structures is presented in Table 27–4. Primary functional areas of the cerebral cortex are depicted in Figure 27–11.

Reticular Formation

Operating throughout the entire brainstem is a core of tissue called the *reticular formation*. It consists of intricate networks of highly branched neurons, which extend from the medulla upward through the diencephalon into subcortical areas (Fig. 27–12). It is a highly strategic region in that neurons of the reticular formation receive and integrate information from many afferent pathways as well as from many other regions of the brain. As a result of such integration, the reticular formation influences and, in turn, is influenced by many different systems, somatic and autonomic, sensory and motor. Table 27–4 lists some of the effects of the reticular formation on certain bodily activities and responses.

The *reticular activating system* (RAS), an ascending neuronal pathway, conducts impulses upward through the reticular formation to the thalamus and subcortical areas. It *activates* or arouses higher cortical functions via its thalamocortical connections and, therefore, plays a role in controlling consciousness and the sleep-wakefulness cycle. A discussion regarding the physiology of consciousness is presented in Chapter 28.

Many areas of the brain operate together to produce appropriate, coordinated responses. Some of these areas are identified and described in Table 27–4.

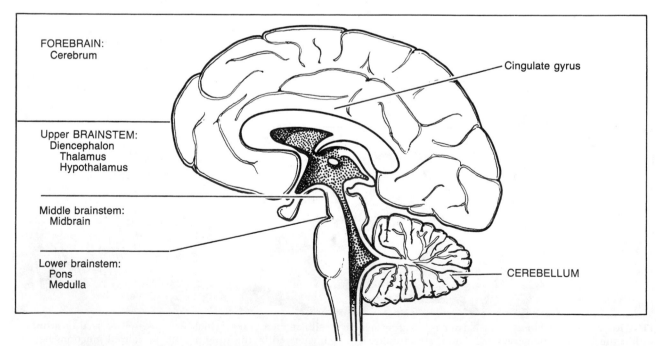

FIGURE 27–10. The gross structure of the brain is comprised of three major divisions: the forebrain, brainstem, and cerebellum. The forebrain consists of the cerebrum (center of intellectual activity and regulation of sensory and motor activity); the upper brainstem, which includes the diencephalon (the diencephalon, in turn, is composed of the thalamus [central sensory relay center] and hypothalamus [center of autonomic regulation]). The remaining brainstem consists of the midbrain and lower brainstem (central nerve tracts between cerebral hemispheres and spinal cord); the lower brainstem, in turn, is composed of the pons and medulla (center of control of vital functions, e.g., respiratory physiology, vasomotor control).

TABLE 27–4
Structures of the Brain: Functional Anatomy

Structure	Description	Function
Cerebrum (see Fig. 27–10)	Largest and most prominent component of the brain	Regulates sensory and motor activities and other activities having to do with memory, intelligence, reasoning, language, and personality • Left hemisphere largely influences symbolic language. • Right hemisphere integrates spatial (dimensional and perceptual) information.
	Divided by the *longitudinal fissure* into right and left hemispheres. The hemispheres are joined by and communicate with one another via a band of *commissural* nerve fibers called the *corpus callosum.* Each hemisphere, for the most part, innervates the contralateral (opposite) side of the body.	

Cerebral cortex	Constitutes the outer gray surface of the brain and is marked by many convolutions. The convolutions consist of *gyri* (ridges) and *sulci* (indentations), which provide for a tremendous surface area in an otherwise tight, rigid, and restrictive cranial vault. The cerebral cortex is divided into lobes:
	• *Frontal* lobe (see Fig. 27–11)
		The most complex integrating area of the nervous system
		• Operates to produce coordinated function
		
		• Operates in all cognitive and perceptive functions
		• Plays a role in reasoning, abstract thinking, creativity, memory, personality, and behavior
		  ○ Contains primary motor area concerned with voluntary muscle movement
		  ○ Plays a significant role in language; involved in the articulation of speech

	○ *Precentral gyrus*
	
	  ○ *Broca's speech area* lies adjacent to motor areas controlling muscles of face, tongue, jaw, and throat; located within left cerebral hemisphere in most individuals. Dysfunction in this area can cause an *expressive* dysphasia (aphasia) (i.e., difficulty or inability to formulate and articulate words). Patients with expressive dysphasia have great difficulty expressing their needs.
	• *Temporal lobe* (see Fig. 27–11)
	  ○ *Wernicke's area:* Connected to Broca's area by association nerve fibers. In Broca's area, the precise motor responses are programmed so that the phrase that arises in Wernicke's area can be spoken or articulated. Dysfunction in this area can result in *receptive* dysphasia (i.e., the inability to comprehend or understand language).
	• *Parietal lobe*
	  ○ *Postcentral gyrus:* All sensory information is funneled to the postcentral gyrus from the thalamus. Sensory information is received and interpreted from a variety of sensory receptors throughout the body (see Table 27–7). (See also Fig. 27–18.)
	• *Occipital lobe:* The primary visual area is composed of a number of subdivisions, each responding to a functionally distinct aspect of the visual stimulus (e.g., color of stimulus, direction of movement, contours of objects, among others). (See Fig. 27–11.)
		• Sensory receptive area for auditory stimuli
		• Involved in formulation of language, i.e., what phrase is to be said, which, in turn, is then articulated via Broca's speech center
		• Plays a major role in comprehension of spoken word and in reading and writing
		• Provides memory storage and retrieval
		
		  ○ Contains the primary sensory area enabling conscious awareness and interpretation of sensory stimuli
		
		• Contains primary visual area for integrating different aspects of visual information. This enables the conscious sensation of sight to be produced.

Subcortical areas (see Fig. 27–12)	• *Limbic system:* This is not a single area of the brain but reflects an interconnected group of structures located within portions of the frontal and temporal lobes, thalamus, and hypothalamus. Examples are the *cingulate gyrus, amygdala,* and *hippocampus.* • *Basal ganglia:* These are areas of gray matter embedded within the subcortical white matter having multiple connections throughout CNS including cerebral cortex, diencephalon, brainstem, reticular formation, and cerebellum.	• Associated with short-term memory, learning, and emotional behavior (fear, rage, sexual behavior) • Connects areas of higher brain functioning with more primitive areas and areas of autonomic and endocrine activities • Function to coordinate motor activity to ensure fine, discrete, and coordinated movements

continued

TABLE 27–4
Structures of the Brain: Functional Anatomy (*Continued*)

Structure	Description	Function
Diencephalon (upper brainstem) (see Fig. 27–10)	Uppermost portion of brainstem, which actually forms the inner core of the cerebrum. It consists of thalamus and hypothalamus.	
	• *Thalamus* ○ *Third ventricle* is located in this area.	• Functions as a major relay station and integrating center for all incoming sensory information from spinal cord and brainstem on its way to cerebral cortex • Plays a key role in refining motor responses
	○ An anatomic and functional relationship exists between the thalamus, cerebral cortex, basal ganglia, and cerebellum.	
	• *Hypothalamus:* Lies below the thalamus; contains *hypothalamic-pituitary stalk,* which directly links the nervous system to the endocrine system	• Major control area for regulating activities of the internal environment • Monitors and controls autonomic activities • Involved in regulation of body water and electrolytes, body temperature, thirst, hunger, sexual and emotional behavior
Brainstem	Literally constitutes the stalk of the brain (see Fig. 27–10).	Enables sensory input and motor output to be relayed between spinal cord and higher brain centers. • Gives rise to all cranial nerves, excluding olfactory and optic nerves • Contains afferent and efferent pathways concerned with motor coordination, and visual and auditory reflexes
	• *Midbrain:* Located between diencephalon and pons ○ *Aqueduct of Sylvius* passes through this area, connecting the third and fourth ventricles. ○ *Edinger-Westphal nucleus:* Parasympathetic nerve fibers leave midbrain via oculomotor nerve (cranial nerve III) and travel to each orbit to stimulate muscles of the iris to contract. This results in pupillary constriction. Interruption in parasympathetic innervation to the iris results in pupillary dilation.	• Contains autonomic parasympathetic reflex centers for pupillary constriction • Gives rise to cranial nerve III
	• *Pons:* The ''bridge'' that connects the cerebellum with the brainstem ○ *Pneumotaxic* and *apneustic* area ○ Contains nuclei of cranial nerves: trigeminal, abducens, facial, and acoustic	• Conductive pathway for all ascending and descending nerve tracts ○ Plays a fundamental role in respiration ○ Gives rise to cranial nerves V, VI, VII, and VIII
	• *Medulla:* Site of transition from the brainstem to spinal cord ○ Site of decussation of corticospinal motor pathways, resulting in innervation of contralateral sides of the body by each cerebral hemisphere ○ Contains nuclei of cranial nerves: glossopharyngeal, vagus, accessory, and hypoglossal	• Conductive pathway for all ascending and descending nerve tracts ○ Contains major reflex centers controlling vital activities related to cardiac, vasomotor, respiratory, sneezing, coughing, swallowing, salivating, and vomiting functions ○ Gives rise cranial nerves IX, X, XI, and XII
Reticular formation	An extensive network of fine, highly branched neurons extending throughout the core of the brainstem and ascending through the diencephalon into subcortical areas; a strategic region enabling impulses from various regions of the brain (cerebral cortex, basal ganglia, ascending and descending nerve tracts, cerebellum, nuclei of cranial nerves, and spinal cord) to converge and interact (see Fig. 27–12)	Acts to facilitate, modify, or inhibit impulse transmissions
	• *Sensory:* Linked functionally to thalamus	• Receives and integrates information from afferent pathways as they ascend through the brainstem; relays some of this information to thalamus
	○ Incredibly widespread networks of neuronal connections provide alternate pathways and mechanisms.	○ Permit qualities such as modality and localization of sensation to be discerned more clearly

continued

TABLE 27–4
Structures of the Brain: Functional Anatomy (*Continued*)

Structure	Description	Function
		○ Enhances ability to associate and discriminate sensory information ○ Maintains degree of alertness or excitability required for sensory perception ○ Actively involved in the maintenance of equilibrium, proprioception, and audition functions
	• *Motor:* A balance between excitatory and inhibitory influences; contributes to normal tone of skeletal muscles.	• Exerts both an excitatory and inhibitory effect on motor function • Provides continuous impulses to muscles to support the body against gravity; maintains posture
	• *Reticular activating systems:* An ascending neuronal pathway within the reticular formation with extensive thalamocortical connections. It is considered to be instrumental in activating or arousing higher cortical function.	• Plays a role in controlling consciousness and the sleep-wakefulness cycle • Influences attentiveness to specific tasks
Cerebellum (see Fig. 27–10)	This structure is located within the posterior fossa, where it is separated from the cerebral hemispheres by a dural fold called the *tentorium cerebelli.* It is chiefly involved with skeletal muscle function.	Functions to maintain balance Coordinates skeletal muscle activity to provide for smooth, directed movements Maintains upright posture Plays a major role in coordinating movements of speech

Cranial Nerves

The 12 pairs of cranial nerves are the *peripheral* nerves of the brain and brainstem. With the exception of cranial nerves I and II, which strictly speaking are not peripheral nerves but rather *fiber tracts* within the brain, all the other cranial nerves (III through XII) have their origin in the brainstem.

The cranial nerves occur in a *rostral* to *caudal* (head to toe) sequence, which is reflected in their numbering. Refer to Table 27–5 for details regarding the cranial nerves and their functions.

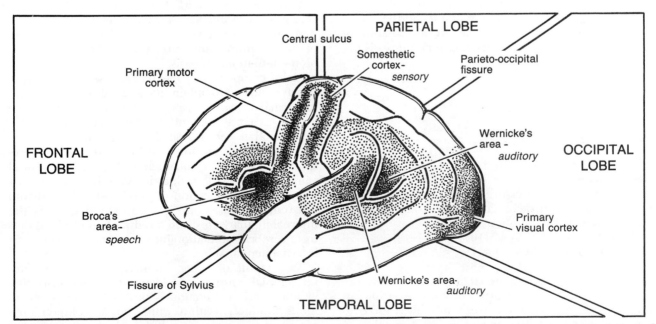

FIGURE 27–11. Primary functional areas of cerebral cortex. Frontal lobe contains Broca's speech center (articulation of language) and primary motor cortex; parietal lobe contains the primary sensory area (i.e., somesthetic cortex; see Fig. 27–18); temporal lobe contains the sensory receptive area for auditory stimuli and Wernicke's area, a more diffuse area concerned with the formulation of language; occipital lobe contains the primary visual cortex.

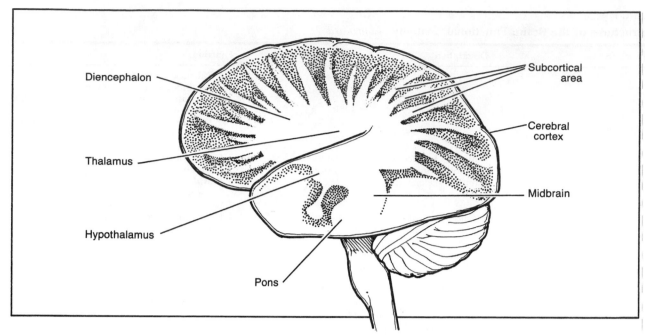

FIGURE 27–12. The reticular formation. (See text.)

The relationship of the cranial nerves to surrounding structures is of critical importance. The close approximation of the optic chiasm to the pituitary gland in the sella turcica and the relationship of cranial nerve III at the midbrain to the tentorium cerebelli (tentorial notch) are two examples wherein intracranial pathology and dysfunction may be detected by ongoing assessment of cranial nerve function. In the patient who has sustained an insult to intracranial structures, the response to therapeutic modalities can be evaluated through the assessment of cranial nerve function. Assessment of selected cranial nerves is discussed in Chapter 28.

Brain Physiology

Intracranial Pressure (ICP)

The volume of blood, cerebrospinal fluid, and brain tissue enclosed within the intracranial cavity determines intracranial pressure. The approximate percentage of total intracranial volume contributed by each of these substances is as follows:

Blood	2–10%
Cerebrospinal fluid	9–11%
Brain tissue	~88%

The volume of each of these components within the cranial vault remains nearly constant, exerting an intracranial pressure that correspondingly is also constantly maintained within narrow limits. Normal pressure within the cranial cavity (i.e., *intracranial pressure*) ranges between 0 and 15 mmHg.

Compensatory Mechanisms to Maintain Intracranial Pressure. As occupants of the mostly unyielding, inexpandable cranial vault, these three components have a *reciprocal* relationship with one another; an increase in the volume of one component must be accompanied by a *compensatory* decrease in the volume of one or both of the other two components if intracranial pressure is to remain within normal physiologic limits *(Monroe-Kellie hypothesis)*. The volumes of blood and cerebrospinal fluid both normally fluctuate over a limited range. This enables the necessary fine adjustments in intracranial pressure to be made on a moment-to-moment basis.

Major compensatory mechanisms within the brain that function to maintain intracranial pressure within its normal physiologic range include the following: the limited expansiveness of the dura mater, which can accommodate cerebrospinal fluid as it leaves the subarachnoid space; an increase in the flow of cerebrospinal fluid into the subarachnoid space and central canal of the spinal cord; a decrease in formation or increase in reabsorption of cerebrospinal fluid into the venous sinuses and systemic circulation via the internal jugular veins; and a redirection of blood flow from cerebral circulation into systemic vasculature via internal jugular veins.

As a result of these compensatory mechanisms, intracranial pressure is maintained within normal limits and cerebral function is undisturbed. There are limits, however, within which these compensatory mechanisms can function. If these limits are exceeded and the compensatory mechanisms are exhausted, intracranial pressure rises, and herniation of brain

TABLE 27–5
Cranial Nerves

Cranial Nerve	Type	Central Connection	Peripheral Connection	Function
I. Olfactory	Sensory (afferent)	Olfactory tract and bulb	Olfactory epithelium in upper nasal cavity	Smell Perception/interpretation in medial temporal lobes
II. Optic	Sensory	Optic chiasm and tract	Ganglion cells of retina	Sight Perception/interpretation in occipital lobe
III. Oculomotor	Motor (efferent)	Midbrain	Extrinsic eye muscles: superior, inferior, and medial recti, and inferior oblique, levator palpebrae muscle	Movement of eyes; elevation of upper eyelid
	Autonomic (parasympathetic)	Midbrain (Edinger-Westphal nucleus)	Intrinsic eye muscles; ciliary and pupillary muscles	Pupillary constriction; accommodation
IV. Trochlear	Motor	Midbrain	Extrinsic eye muscle: superior oblique	Movement of eyes
V. Trigeminal	Sensory	Pons	Skin and mucous membranes of face and mouth	General sensation to face via three branches: ophthalmic, maxillary, and mandibular branches; includes sensation to cornea and mucosa of nose and mouth
	Motor (mandibular division)	Pons	Muscles of mastication	Mastication; jaw clenching and lateral jaw movement
VI. Abducens	Motor	Pons	Extrinsic eye muscle: lateral rectus	Movement of eyes
VII. Facial	Sensory	Medulla	Taste buds of anterior two thirds of tongue	Taste—sweet and salty "taste center" in temporal lobe
	Motor	Caudal pons	Muscles of facial expression	Facial expression
	Autonomic (parasympathetic)	Medulla	Salivary glands (sublingual, submaxillary) and lacrimal glands	Secretion of saliva and tears
VIII. Acoustic Cochlear	Sensory	Medulla	Organ of Corti in inner ear	Hearing Perception/interpretation in temporal lobe
Vestibular	Sensory	Medulla	Receptors in semicircular canals, utricle and saccule	Equilibrium
IX. Glossopharyngeal	Sensory	Medulla	Taste buds in posterior one third of tongue; soft palate	Taste—sour and bitter "taste center" in temporal lobe
	Sensory	Medulla	Cutaneous receptors; mucous membrane pharyngeal area; carotid sinus	General sensations from external ear and surrounding area; pain and temperature. Involved in reflex control of blood pressure and respirations
	Motor	Medulla	Muscles of pharynx	Swallowing and phonation, gag reflex
	Autonomic (parasympathetic)	Medulla	Salivary gland (parotid)	Salivary secretion
X. Vagus	Sensory	Medulla	Cutaneous receptors	General sensations from skin in area surrounding ear; pain and temperature
	Sensory	Medulla	Receptors from thorax and abdomen	Sensory from visceral structures
	Motor	Medulla	Muscles of pharynx and larynx	Swallowing and control of larynx; protective reflexes: cough and gag
	Autonomic (parasympathetic)	Medulla	Smooth muscle and glands of thorax and abdomen	Regulation of smooth and cardiac muscle, and glands; carotid reflex
XI. Accessory	Motor	Medulla	Muscles of pharynx and larynx (distributed with vagus)	Swallowing and control of larynx
	Motor	Upper cervical cord segments (C-1 to C-5)	Sternocleidomastoid and trapezius muscles	Movement of head and shoulders
XII. Hypoglossal	Motor	Medulla	Extrinsic and intrinsic muscles of tongue	Movement of tongue necessary for swallowing and phonation

tissue into the tentorial notch or foramen magnum may occur.

Cerebral Perfusion Pressure

Cerebral perfusion pressure (CPP) is the driving force underlying cerebral blood flow. For cerebral blood flow to be adequate, cerebral perfusion pressure must be maintained at 60 to 90 mmHg. Determinants of cerebral perfusion pressure are the *mean arterial systemic pressure (MAP)* and the *intracranial pressure (ICP)* expressed as follows:

$$CPP = MAP - ICP$$

Any factor that *decreases* mean arterial pressure or *increases* intracranial pressure will cause a corresponding decrease in cerebral perfusion pressure. If cerebral perfusion pressure is reduced to the level of intracranial pressure, cerebral blood flow ceases.

Metabolic Needs of Neural Tissue

To maintain a state of excitability so vital to impulse initiation and propagation, neural tissue is highly active metabolically. Because energy stores within neurons are limited, there is a high and constant demand for oxygen and glucose. Any state that increases the demand of neural tissue for oxygen and glucose or decreases the blood supply of these vital substrates may alter cellular metabolism and place neural tissue at risk of developing ischemia, injury, or necrosis. Fever, for example, increases metabolic demands of neural tissue by as much as 10% for every 1°F rise in temperature. An increase in metabolic rate not only increases the demand for oxygen and glucose, but is associated concomitantly with increased levels of end-products of metabolism, including carbon dioxide and hydrogen ion concentrations.

Autoregulation

Autoregulation refers to the inherent ability of tissues to self-regulate their blood flows. Within the cerebral circulation, autoregulation functions to maintain cerebral perfusion pressure and, thus, cerebral blood flow, regardless of systemic arterial pressure. This ensures that the metabolic needs of neural tissue will be met.

Major Factors Influencing Cerebral Blood Flow

Metabolic Factors

Carbon Dioxide, Oxygen, and Hydrogen Ion Concentrations. Three metabolic factors have a potent effect on cerebral blood flow: carbon dioxide, oxygen, and hydrogen ions. Hypercapnia ($PaCO_2$ greater than 45 mmHg), hypoxia (PaO_2 less than 60 mmHg), and acidosis (increase in hydrogen ion concentration) all

result in an increase in cerebral blood flow. This is significant because the increased blood flow facilitates removal of carbon dioxide and acidic end-products of metabolism from cerebral tissues. In the normal brain, or the brain not under increased pressure, the fine moment-to-moment adjustments of cerebral vascular resistance made in response to these substances help to ensure that blood flow is adequate to meet the nutrient and oxygen needs of neural tissue.

Glucose. To meet cerebral metabolic needs adequately, serum glucose levels must be maintained at 70 to 110 mg/100 mL. A reduction in these levels below 70 mg/100 mL may predispose to an increase in cerebral blood flow.

Serum Osmolality. Serum osmolality (i.e., a measure of the number of osmotically active particles dissolved in a specific volume of fluid) must be maintained between 285 to 295 mOsm/kg. Alterations in serum osmolality are frequently associated with abnormal metabolic states (e.g., diabetic ketoacidosis; hyperosmolar hyperglycemic nonketotic coma [HHNK]; hepatic encephalopathy) and can disrupt cerebral blood flow, leading to neurologic dysfunction.

Body Temperature. Cellular metabolic activity is perhaps the most important factor influencing cerebral blood flow at the tissue level. Any increase in metabolic activity (e.g., fever) ultimately leads to an increase in cerebral blood flow. This is necessary to increase availability of oxygen and glucose to these highly active cells and to enhance removal of carbon dioxide and other metabolic end-products.

Hemodynamic Factors

Systemic Arterial Blood Pressure. Autoregulatory mechanisms within the brain function to maintain cerebral blood flow within normal physiologic limits despite wide variations in arterial blood pressure (See Table 27–6). A mean arterial pressure (MAP) of ~100 mmHg is desired to maintain adequate cerebral perfusion pressure.

Autonomic Nervous System Influence

The sympathetic and parasympathetic branches of the autonomic nervous system, as well as specialized receptors (baroreceptors and chemoreceptors) all function to maintain constant blood flow to the brain. When systemic blood pressure falls (baroreceptors) and carbon dioxide levels and hydrogen ion concentrations increase (chemoreceptors), these receptors react quickly to reflexly stimulate respiratory and vasomotor centers in the medulla (see Table 27–6).

A severe drop in systemic blood pressure evokes the *cerebral ischemic reflex*, wherein neurons in the medulla respond via increased sympathetic innervation to the heart. The response is an increase in contractility and cardiac output.

A summary of these and other major factors influencing cerebral blood flow is presented in Table 27–6.

TABLE 27–6
Summary of Major Factors Influencing Cerebral Blood Flow

Metabolic Factors	
Serum carbon dioxide levels ($PaCO_2$)	• Carbon dioxide is a potent stimulus for cerebral vasodilation. Elevated levels of carbon dioxide ($PaCO_2 > 40$–45 mmHg) cause vasodilation with an increase in cerebral blood flow.
	• Ideally, in patients at risk of developing an increase in intracranial pressure, $PaCO_2$ is maintained at $\leqq 30$ mmHg.
Serum oxygen levels (PaO_2)	• Cerebral vasodilation with an increase in cerebral blood flow occurs with lower oxygen tension ($PaO_2 < 60$ mmHg).
	• To adequately meet cerebral metabolic needs, PaO_2 should be maintained at >80 mmHg.
Hydrogen ion concentration	• An increase in hydrogen ion concentration ($\downarrow$ pH) is a potent stimulus for cerebral vasodilation with an increase in cerebral blood flow.
Serum glucose levels	• To adequately meet cerebral metabolic needs, serum glucose levels must be maintained at 70–110 mg/100 mL. Although hypoglycemia per se does not increase cerebral blood flow, it does reduce the "fuel" available for cellular activities.
Serum osmolality	• Serum osmolality must be maintained between 285–295 mOsm/kg. Alterations in serum osmolality may reflect an alteration in cellular integrity with hyperosmolality (dehydration) or hypo-osmolality (edema).
	• Hyperosmolar therapy may be prescribed to treat cerebral edema.
Body temperature	• For every degree rise in body temperature, metabolic demands of neural tissue increase by 10%.
	• Body temperature should be maintained at 98.6°F (37°C) unless hypothermia therapy is prescribed.
Seizure activity	• Seizures increase the metabolic rate of nerve cells twofold and threefold, which in turn increases need for oxygen and glucose, and removal of carbon dioxide and other metabolic end-products.
Hemodynamic Factors	
Systemic arterial blood pressure	• To ensure a cerebral perfusion pressure of >60 mmHg, mean arterial pressure should be maintained at ~ 100 mmHg.
	• Autoregulatory mechanisms maintain intracranial pressure over a wide range of mean arterial pressures (60–150 mmHg).
	• At mean systemic pressures >150 mmHg or <60 mmHg, loss of local cerebral autoregulatory capability begins to occur and cerebral blood flow becomes passively dependent on systemic blood pressure.
	• At high arterial blood pressures, cerebral vasoconstriction occurs; at lower pressures, cerebral vasodilation occurs.
Cardiac contractility	• Cardiac output must be maintained between 4 and 8 L/min to ensure a mean arterial blood pressure ~ 100 mmHg.
Blood viscosity	• An increase in blood viscosity increases resistance to blood flow, which may predispose to an increase in blood pressure.
Autonomic Nervous System Influence	
Sympathetic innervation	• Sympathetic effect causes slight vasoconstriction of cerebral blood vessels.
Parasympathetic innervation	• Parasympathetic effect causes slight vasodilation of cerebral blood vessels.
Baroreceptors	• Sense organs, especially sensitive to stretch and located in carotid sinus and aortic arch, continuously monitor and respond to changes in systemic arterial blood pressure.
Chemoreceptors	• Sense organs in carotid body and great vessels continuously monitor and respond to changes in serum levels of oxygen, carbon dioxide, and pH.
Reflexes	
Cerebral ischemic reflex	• This reflex is evoked by a severe drop in systemic arterial blood pressure. A medullary response mediated via sympathetic pathways increases cardiac contractility and cardiac output. The end-result is a rise in systemic blood pressure.
Cushing reflex	• This reflex is evoked in response to a decrease in cerebral perfusion pressure and cerebral ischemia. It functions to slow heart rate, which increases the stroke volume; it raises systolic blood pressure to levels adequate to perfuse the brain.
	• A widening pulse pressure results from the increasing systolic blood pressure and decreasing diastolic pressure.
	• Cushing's triad includes: $\uparrow$ Systolic BP with widening pulse pressure $\downarrow$ Heart rate Abnormal respiratory function

FUNCTIONAL ANATOMY OF THE SPINAL CORD

The spinal cord provides the connections between impulses coming from *re*ceptors and those going to *ef*fectors. In this way the spinal cord functions as a communication system wherein cells sensitive to changes in the environment are linked with cells responsible for carrying out the appropriate responses to minimize those changes. The spinal cord distributes responses of cerebral activities appropriately throughout the peripheral nervous system, and thus facilitates the expression of cerebral function.

Structural and Functional Support Systems

Vertebral Column and Ligaments

The vertebral column functions to support the skull and to provide protection for the spinal cord and spinal nerves. It bears the weight of the entire upper portion of the body including head, neck, trunk, and arms. *Intervertebral foramina* occurring between adjacent vertebrae accommodate the spinal nerves as they leave the spinal cord (Fig. 27–13).

There is an extensive attachment of ligaments and muscles to the vertebral processes of the uniquely structured vertebrae. This provides support to the vertebral column and, together with the *intervertebral disks*, allows for substantial stability and flexibility of the spinal column. Ligaments provide for safe, smooth movement of the head and neck and a considerable degree of movement of the entire vertebral column.

Meninges

The spinal cord is encased within the *spinal foramen (spinal canal)* of the vertebral column, which conforms to the variations in size and diameter of the spinal cord and protects and supports it. Protection is also afforded by the meningeal connective tissue sheaths, which are largely continuous with those surrounding the brain.

There occurs a distinct *epidural space* between the spinal dura and bony surface of the vertebral column. The *subarachnoid space* is continuous with that surrounding the brain. It is filled with cerebrospinal fluid, which provides a protective cushion around the spinal cord. Cerebrospinal fluid also circulates throughout the *central canal* of the spinal cord. In the event of a rise in intracranial pressure, the subarachnoid space and central canal within the cord can accommodate

an increased quantity of cerebrospinal fluid, which may help initially to *compensate* for the increase in intracranial pressure. The pia mater is closely applied to the spinal cord.

Blood Supply to Spinal Cord and Vertebral Column

There is not an extensive blood supply to the spinal cord and vertebral column. The intervertebral disks are especially limited in their blood supply. The two major arteries nourishing the spinal cord are the *anterior* and *posterior spinal* arteries, which arise from the vertebral arteries. Unlike the brain, collateral circulation to the spinal cord is not well developed. Venous drainage of the vertebral column and spinal cord follows the arterial distribution very closely.

Spinal Cord Structure and Function

The spinal cord is continuous with the medulla and extends from the foramen magnum to the upper border of the second lumbar vertebra (in adults) where it terminates as the *conus medullaris*. Spinal nerve roots descend below the conus medullaris and are known collectively as the *cauda equina*.

Thirty-one pairs of spinal nerves exit from successive levels or segments of the spinal cord via the intervertebral foramina. These include 8 pairs of cervical nerves, 12 pairs of thoracic nerves, 5 lumbar nerves, 5 sacral nerves, and 1 pair of coccygeal nerves.

Spinal Cord in Cross-Section

A significant feature in a cross-section of the spinal cord is the presence of a centrally placed area of *gray matter* occurring in the shape of an H (Fig. 27–14). These projections are known as the *dorsal* and *ventral gray horns*. They consist primarily of neuronal cell bodies, synapses, unmyelinated nerve fibers, and glial cells. Cell bodies of motor (efferent) neurons innervating skeletal muscle lie in the ventral horns. In the thoracolumbar cord, lateral projections of gray matter, the *lateral (intermediolateral) horns*, occur, which contain cell bodies of autonomic neurons innervating smooth and cardiac muscle and glands.

Surrounding the gray matter is the *white matter* of the cord, which contains bundles of longitudinal ascending or descending myelinated nerve fibers, as well as fibers entering or leaving the cord. The presence of myelin surrounding these fibers accounts for the "white" appearance.

Spinal Nerves: Dorsal and Ventral Roots

Each spinal nerve is a *mixed* nerve, formed from the union of its dorsal (sensory) root with its ventral (motor) root (see Fig. 27–14). The *dorsal root* consists

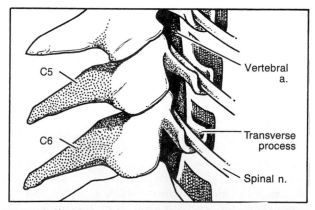

FIGURE 27–13. Intervertebral foramina occurring between adjacent cervical vertebrae. These vertebrae accommodate the spinal nerves as they leave the spinal cord via grooves within the vertebrae. The vertebral artery is depicted ascending via the transverse foramina in the transverse processes of the cervical vertebrae.

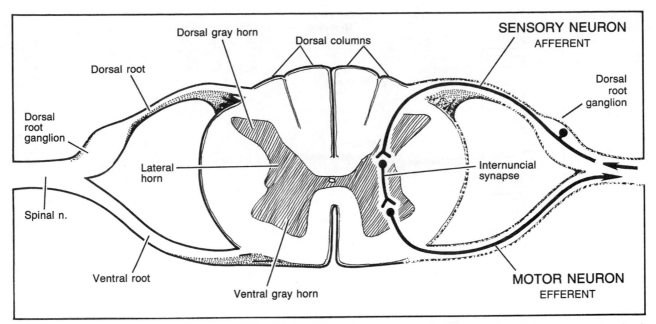

FIGURE 27–14. Spinal cord in cross-section. There is a characteristic centrally placed area of gray matter occurring in the shape of an H. The projections of gray matter are divided into the dorsal and ventral gray horns; lateral projections (i.e., lateral horn) can be observed in sections of the thoracolumbar cord. Surrounding the gray matter is a white matter of the cord composed of columns of ascending and descending nerve fibers. A spinal nerve is depicted as being composed of a dorsal root (sensory) and a ventral root (motor).

of a sensory (afferent) neuron, which transmits impulses from various sensory receptors throughout the body into the spinal cord. The cell bodies of these sensory neurons occur in the *dorsal root ganglion.* (A *ganglion* is a collection of cell bodies.) The dendritic processes extend to the periphery, while the axonal fibers enter the dorsal gray horn of the spinal cord. Thus, the dorsal root ganglion and dorsal gray horn are concerned primarily with *sensory* information.

The *ventral root* consists of a motor (efferent) neuron, which transmits impulses from the ventral gray horn within the spinal cord to the effector organs in the periphery. The ventral gray horns of the spinal cord and neurons originating therein are primarily concerned with *motor* function.

Spinal Cord Plexuses and Peripheral Nerves

Networks of spinal nerve roots join together upon leaving the spinal cord to form a *plexus*. Each plexus, in turn, gives rise to *peripheral nerves*, which provide innervation to specific areas of the body. Major plexuses include the cervical, brachial, lumbosacral, and coccygeal plexuses (Fig. 27–15).

The *cervical plexus* consists of the first four cervical spinal nerve roots and is significant in that the *phrenic nerve*, which innervates the diaphragm, arises within this plexus. The *brachial plexus*, formed by the remaining cervical nerve roots and the 1st thoracic nerve root, gives rise to the following peripheral nerves: the

median, radial, ulnar, and *musculocutaneous.* These nerves provide innervation to the upper extremities.

Spinal nerve roots from the lumbar and sacral portions of the cord overlap to form the *lumbosacral plexus.* Important peripheral nerves that arise from this plexus include the *femoral* and *saphenous nerves*, which supply in part the pelvis and hip areas and anterior portion of lower extremities. The *sciatic nerve*, which arises from the sacral portion of the lumbosacral plexus, innervates the posterior thigh muscles. The *peroneal* and *tibial nerves*, branches of the sciatic nerve, innervate most of the lower leg and foot. The *pudendal nerve*, which also arises from the lumbosacral plexus, provides innervation to the perineum.

Peripheral Nerve Distribution

The functional distribution of peripheral nerves is systematic and orderly. This is most apparent in *cutaneous* innervation wherein each segment or band of skin surface is supplied by a specific peripheral nerve derived from its specific spinal nerve roots. Such segments, known as *dermatomes*, are extremely helpful in assessing and evaluating *sensory* function. Figure 27–16 shows dermatomal distribution of sensory innervation at various cord segments. There is considerable overlap between one dermatome and the next, but generally the patterns are followed quite closely.

Distribution of motor innervation via ventral spinal roots follows a segmented pattern much like that

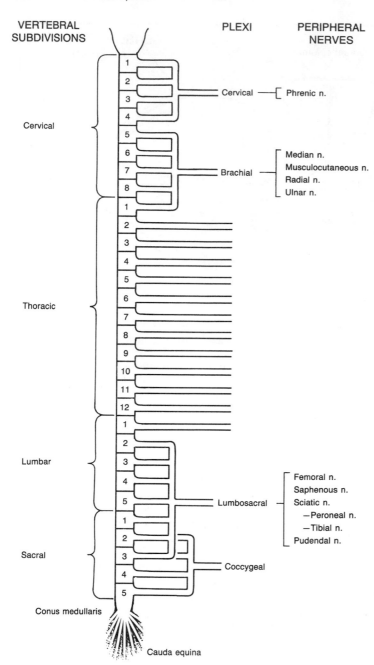

VERTEBRAL
SUBDIVISIONS
PLEXI
PERIPHERAL
NERVES

Cervical

Cervical —— [Phrenic n.

[Median n.
Musculocutaneous n.
Brachial ——— Radial n.
[Ulnar n.

Thoracic

Lumbar

[Femoral n.
Saphenous n.
Sciatic n.
Lumbosacral — —Peroneal n.
—Tibial n.
Pudendal n.

Sacral

Coccygeal

Conus medullaris

Cauda equina

FIGURE 27–15. Spinal cord plexuses and peripheral nerves. (See text.)

reflected in the dermatomes. Each peripheral nerve supplies motor innervation to several somatic or voluntary muscles (see Fig. 27–16). Familiarity with distribution of motor innervation assists in assessing and evaluating motor function including deep tendon reflexes.

Reflex and Reflex Arc

The *reflex* is the basis of nervous system function. It is a predictable and stereotyped response to a stimulus; a specific stimulus evokes the same response each time it is applied. Reflex actions underlie virtually everything we do, including the volitional functions of

skeletal muscles and the autonomic functions of cardiac and smooth muscle, and glands.

The *reflex arc* in its simplest form consists of two neurons: a *sensory neuron*, which carries impulses from receptors into the central nervous system, and a *motor neuron*, which transmits the neuronal response to the effector organ(s). This type of reflex arc involves one synapse *(monosynaptic)*. More commonly, one or more *internuncial neurons* are interposed between the sensory and motor neurons *(polysynaptic)* (see Fig. 27–14). This increases synaptic interactions not only at the entry segment of the spinal cord, but up and down the cord and into higher centers of the brain as well.

Such an arrangement is critical because it allows

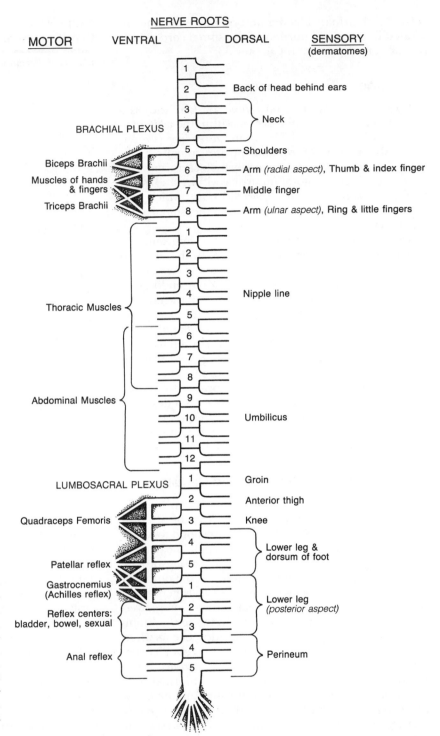

NERVE ROOTS

MOTOR   VENTRAL   DORSAL   SENSORY
(dermatomes)

BRACHIAL PLEXUS

Biceps Brachii
Muscles of hands
& fingers
Triceps Brachii

Back of head behind ears
Neck
Shoulders
Arm (radial aspect), Thumb & index finger
Middle finger
Arm (ulnar aspect), Ring & little fingers

Thoracic Muscles

Nipple line

Abdominal Muscles

Umbilicus

LUMBOSACRAL PLEXUS

Quadraceps Femoris

Patellar reflex

Gastrocnemius
(Achilles reflex)
Reflex centers:
bladder, bowel, sexual

Anal reflex

Groin
Anterior thigh
Knee
Lower leg &
dorsum of foot
Lower leg
(posterior aspect)
Perineum

FIGURE 27–16. Peripheral nerve distribution. Distribution of sensory innervation occurs via a segmented pattern wherein each segment or band of skin surface is supplied by a specific peripheral nerve derived from its specific spinal nerve roots. Such segments are referred to as dermatomes. Specific dermatomes and their dorsal roots are identified. Distribution of motor innervation, which occurs via ventral nerve roots, follows a similar segmented distribution.

reflex actions to occur within the spinal cord independent of higher brain center activity. Many responses occur automatically at this level, enabling the individual to focus attention on more sophisticated cognitive activities and functions. The multitude of internuncial connections and synaptic interactions provides for an infinite number and variety of human responses.

Major categories of reflexes include the *stretch or deep tendon reflexes, cutaneous or superficial reflexes,* and *brainstem reflexes.* A discussion of these reflexes is presented in Chapter 28. Spinal cord activities also involve *autonomic reflexes* concerned with visceral functions as, for example, control of vasomotor tone and smooth muscle tone of abdominal viscera. Reflex centers concerned with urinary bladder and rectum emptying are located in the sacral portion of the spinal cord. These reflexes are discussed in Chapter 33.

Nerve Tracts—Nomenclature

A *nerve tract* (also termed *column* or *lemniscus*) is a bundle of nerve fibers that occurs within the *white* matter of the spinal cord. There are *ascending (sensory) tracts*, which carry information up the spinal cord to the brain; *descending (motor) tracts*, which carry impulses from the brain to motor neurons within the spinal cord; and *associative (intersegmental) tracts*, which may be ascending or descending within the spinal cord segments.

Nerve tracts are named to denote origin and termination of their fibers. *Origin* refers to the location of the cell bodies of these nerve fibers; *termination* refers to the point at which the axonal endings of these nerve fibers occur. Simple analysis of tract names determines location and function. Thus, a *spinothalamic tract* has its origin in the *spinal cord* and its termination in the *thalamus*. This tract is, therefore, an ascending neuronal pathway carrying *sensory* information from the spinal cord to the brain. The *corticospinal tract* has its origin in the cerebral *cortex* and its termination in the *spinal cord*. This tract is a descending neuronal pathway carrying *motor* responses from the brain to the spinal cord. Major nerve tracts and their functions are described later in Table 27–8.

Sensory Function—Receptors and Circuitry

Receptors. All input into the CNS is provided by *sensory receptors* and/or *free nerve endings* of afferent (sensory) neurons, which detect and respond to a variety of sensory stimuli including touch, pain, heat, cold, and proprioception (position sense), among others. Each afferent fiber carries information about one such *stimulus* or *modality*. Sensory impulses thus generated may be incorporated into spinal reflexes or relayed over distinct ascending sensory pathways to the brainstem and higher cortical areas. Sensation occurs when the reticular activating system and the cerebral cortex are sufficiently aroused to process, integrate, interpret, and respond to incoming sensory information.

Sensory receptors are located throughout the body. These receptors can be classified as *mechanoreceptors*, *interoceptors*, and *special* receptors. A list of specific receptors and their functions is presented in Table 27–7.

Circuitry: Sensory Pathways. The sensation one experiences is determined by the nature of the initial stimulus, the circuitry of the specific sensory pathway or nerve tract, and the perceptive areas within the brain to which the particular pathway is directed.

The circuitry of each sensory pathway consists of a series of three neurons. Three such sensory pathways are depicted in Figure 27–17, and include the dorsal columns and the ventral and lateral spinothalamic

TABLE 27–7
Classification of Sensory Receptors

1. Mechanoreceptors	These receptors detect sensations of pressure, touch, vibration, and kinesthesia (ability to perceive direction or extent of movement)
a. Exteroceptors	Superficial or cutaneous sensations (epidermis and dermis)
Epidermis	Free nerve endings—pain, tactile, and temperature sense
	Merkel's disk—tactile
	Ruffini's end-organ—touch, pressure, position sense
Dermis	Meissner's corpuscles—tactile
Connective tissue	Pacinian's corpuscle—vibratory sense, touch, pressure
b. Proprioceptors	Endings in muscle, tendon, joints, for deep sensations
	Muscle spindle—stretch
	Golgi tendon receptors—tension
2. Interoceptors	Special receptors in visceral organs
a. Chemoreceptors	Carotid and aortic bodies—arterial carbon dioxide and oxygen levels
	Osmoreceptors in hypothalamus—osmolality of blood
b. Baroreceptors	Sensitive to stretch
	Vasomotor reflexes in carotid sinus
	Respiratory reflex (Hering-Breuer reflex) stretch receptors, which help to prevent overexpansion of lungs
c. Nociceptors	Free nerve endings in viscera—pain
d. Thermoreceptors	Cold receptors
3. Special receptors	Olfactory epithelium—small taste buds—gustatory
	Organ of Corti of inner ear—audition
	Rods and cones of retina—vision
	Hair cells in semicircular canals—equilibrium

tracts. Note that in each example, the second neuron in the series crosses over, or *decussates*, to the other side, either within the spinal cord (ventral and lateral spinothalamic tracts) or at the level of the medulla (dorsal columns). This crossing over of nerve fibers explains why the left side of the body is represented within the right cerebral hemisphere, and vice versa.

The arrangement of the ascending nerve tracts within the white matter of the spinal cord serves to provide for a certain amount of modality separation. The *dorsal columns*, for example, carry impulses concerned primarily with proprioception, touch, and movement; the *lateral spinothalamic tracts* carry impulses concerned with pain and temperature; the *ventral spinothalamic tracts* are associated with pressure and crude touch sensations. Details regarding major sensory pathways including their functions, and signs of neurologic deficits when function is disrupted, are included in Table 27–8.

Distribution of sensory innervation within the CNS can be divided into *special senses*, which include sight, hearing, taste, and smell, and *general somatic senses*, which convey information regarding pressure, touch, proprioception, temperature, and comfort. Primary receiving areas for each of these senses occur within

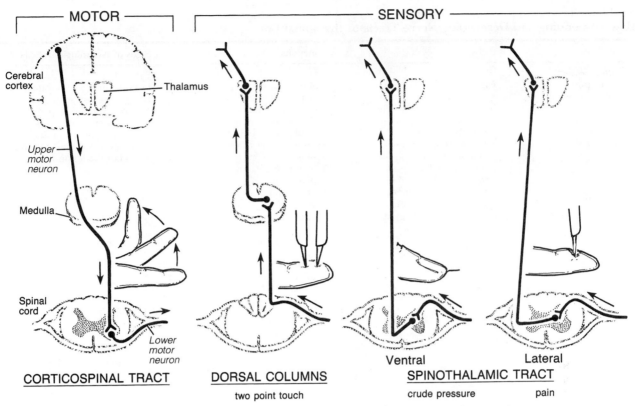

┌──────── MOTOR ────────┐ ┌──────────────────── SENSORY ────────────────────┐

Cerebral cortex — Thalamus

Upper motor neuron

Medulla

Spinal cord

Lower motor neuron

CORTICOSPINAL TRACT   DORSAL COLUMNS   Ventral SPINOTHALAMIC TRACT Lateral

two point touch   crude pressure   pain

FIGURE 27–17. Circuitry of sensory and motor tracts.

the cerebral cortex. The primary areas for the special senses are listed in Table 27–4 (see Fig. 27–11). Pathways for the general somatic senses terminate in the somatosensory area of the cerebral cortex located in the *postcentral gyrus* of the parietal lobe. This area is often called the *somesthetic cortex* because it provides a representation of senses from various segments of the body (Fig. 27–18).

Somesthetic Cortex. Regions of the body receiving a large amount of innervation receive a correspondingly larger topographic representation on the surface of the cortex. Thus, fingers (including the thumb), the lips, and tongue, having many peripheral cutaneous receptors with a high degree of sensory acuity and discrimination, receive greater cortical representation. Representation of the lower extremities, back, and lower trunk occurs over the *medial* surface of the cortex, whereas that of the hands and face is distributed over the *lateral* surface (see Fig. 27–18).

Motor Function—Circuitry and Effectors

Primary Motor Cortex. The *primary motor cortex* occurs within the frontal lobe, specifically the *precentral gyrus*, which lies just anterior to the *central sulcus* (see Fig. 27–11). It contains the cell bodies of the upper motor neurons and is concerned largely with movement of voluntary (skeletal) muscles. Representation of innervation within the motor cortex closely follows

that of the somesthetic cortex (see Fig. 27–18). Areas of the body involved in highly sophisticated and intricate function (fingers, thumbs, lips) receive a predominant portion of representation within the motor cortex.

Circuitry—Somatic Division (Skeletal Muscle)

Corticospinal Motor Pathways (Pyramidal System) The brain exerts its influence on skeletal muscle throughout the body via *descending* motor pathways. The *corticospinal pathways* are descending motor pathways that function to provide for fine, smooth, and controlled movement of the extremities. These descending pathways consist of a series of two neurons: the upper motor neuron and the lower motor neuron. (see Fig. 27–17).

Upper Motor Neuron. The upper motor neuron originates and terminates within the CNS. Its cell body occurs within the motor cortex, and it synapses directly or indirectly with the lower motor neuron within the spinal cord. About 85% of corticospinal fibers cross over to the *contralateral* (opposite) side at the level of the medulla. For details regarding these tracts, see Table 27–8.

Lower Motor Neuron. The second neuron in the descending motor pathway is the lower motor neuron, also called the *final common pathway*. This latter term reflects the fact that lower motor neurons are the *only*

TABLE 27–8
Major Ascending and Descending Nerve Tracts of the Spinal Cord

Nerve Tract	Pathway	Functions	Signs of Neurologic Deficits
Ascending–Sensory • Dorsal (posterior) columns—medial lemniscus system (see Fig. 27–17)	*First-order neuron*—enters spinal cord and ascends on the same side to the medulla *Second-order neuron*—crosses to the opposite side in the medulla and ascends to the thalamus *Third-order neuron*—fibers ascend to somesthetic cortex in the parietal lobe (postcentral gyrus)	Discriminative touch Two-point discrimination Stereognosis (perception of size, shape, and texture of objects by touch) Proprioception (position sense) Vibratory sense and weight perception Postural and "righting" sense Kinesthetic sense (awareness of position of the limbs and their movements) *Sensory receptors*—muscle spindles, Golgi tendon organs, pacinian corpuscles, and many others	Loss of touch and vibratory sense Loss of position sense Numbness, tingling, paresthesia Loss of deep tendon reflexes (The above occur on the ipsilateral side and below the level of the lesion.)
Spinothalamic tracts • Lateral spinothalamic pathway (see Fig. 27–17)	*First-order neuron*—enters cord and may ascend or descend several segments before synapsing with second-order neuron in dorsal gray horn *Second-order neuron*—crosses to contralateral side and ascends to thalamus *Third-order neuron*—relays impulse from thalamus to somesthetic cortex	Pain Temperature Nociceptive information* *Sensory receptors*—free nerve endings	Loss of pain and temperature and superficial tactile sensation on contralateral side below the level of the lesion
• Ventral (anterior) spinothalamic pathways (see Fig. 27–17)	*First-order neuron*—enters cord and synapses with the second-order neuron in the posterior horn *Second-order neuron*—crosses cord and ascends to the thalamus *Third-order neuron*—relays impulse from thalamus to somesthetic cortex	Tactile sensation Nociceptive information*	Loss of pressure and crude touch sensations on contralateral side below the level of the lesion
Spinocerebellar tracts • Dorsal (posterior) spinocerebellar pathway	*First-order neuron*—enters cord and synapses with second-order neuron in dorsal gray area of cord. *Second-order neuron*—ascends on ipsilateral side via dorsal lateral spinocerebellar tract to cerebellum. *Note:* This is a two-neuron pathway.	Unconscious proprioceptive information from lower part of body and lower extremities Fine coordination of individual muscles concerned with postural adjustments Sensations of touch and pressure *Sensory receptors*—stretch receptors including muscle spindle and Golgi tendon organs, exteroceptive receptors (touch and pressure)	There may be no abnormal signs unless there is involvement of the cerebellum. With cerebellum involvement, the following may appear: • Nystagmus • Uncoordinated movement of lower extremities • Intention tremors • Hypotonia • Decreased deep tendon reflexes

TABLE 27–8
Major Ascending and Descending Nerve Tracts of the Spinal Cord (*Continued*)

Nerve Tract	Pathway	Functions	Signs of Neurologic Deficits
• Ventral (anterior) spinocerebellar pathway	*First-order neuron*—enters cord and synapses with second-order neuron in dorsal gray area *Second-order neuron*—crosses cord immediately and ascends via the ventral spinocerebellar tract directly to cerebellum *Note:* This is a two-neuron pathway.	Conveys to the cerebellum information related to pain, tactile and pressure sensations Spinocerebellar tracts monitor ongoing activity of muscle groups and contribute to a smooth, well-coordinated performance.	
Descending—Motor *Corticospinal tracts* • Lateral corticospinal tract (see Fig. 27–17)	*Upper motor neuron* (UMN)—cell bodies of UMN occur in premotor, motor cortex of precentral gyrus, and sensorimotor cortex of postcentral gyrus. About 85–90% of these fibers cross to contralateral side at the level of the medulla. These fibers descend the cord as part of the lateral corticospinal tract.	Primarily concerned with skilled movement of muscles in the extremities Integrated movements of limbs; facilitates activity of extensor muscles while inhibiting activity of flexor muscles	Upper motor neuron paralysis • Affects groups of muscles rather than individual fibers[†] • Spasticity and hyperactivity of deep tendon reflexes • Slight muscle atrophy due to disuse • Babinski's sign • No fasciculations
• Ventral (anterior) corticospinal tract	Upper motor neuron—cell bodies of UMN in premotor, motor cortex (precentral gyrus), and sensorimotor cortex (postcentral gyrus). About 10–15% of these fibers descend the cord on the ipsilateral side and cross to the opposite side within a spinal cord segment.	Primarily concerned with voluntary muscles of the trunk	
Extrapyramidal pathways • Rubrospinal tract	Motor fibers arise from the *red nucleus* within the brainstem and function via *alpha* and *gamma* motor neurons to excite flexor muscle groups while inhibiting the activity of the extensor groups. These fibers cross immediately to the opposite side and descend the cord.	Major functions include a facilitatory or inhibitory influence on the maintenance of muscle tone, reflexes, and muscular activity concerned with posture and equilibrium, unconscious integration and coordination of muscular movement.	Muscular rigidity Involuntary tremor at rest *Athetosis*—a succession of slow, involuntary, writhing movements of hands and fingers (sometimes toes and feet) including flexion, extension, pronation, and supination
• Vestibulospinal tract	Motor fibers arise from vestibular nuclei within the brainstem.	These tracts function to maintain posture and equilibrium by influencing antigravity muscle groups. Medial pathway also influences cranial nerve nuclei (III, IV, VI) concerned with extraocular movement; coordinates head and eye movements.	

continued

TABLE 27–8
Major Ascending and Descending Nerve Tracts of the Spinal Cord (*Continued*)

Nerve Tract	Pathway	Functions	Signs of Neurologic Deficits
Medial	• Decussate and descend the cord on the opposite side		
Lateral	• Fibers remain uncrossed.		
• Reticulospinal tract	Motor fibers arise from pontine and medullary areas of brainstem and remain largely uncrossed.	These tracts function to influence muscle activities related to posture and maintenance of muscle tone.	
Medial	• Facilitates extensor reflexes while inhibiting flexors	Transmit impulses to the autonomic nervous system via spinal cord fibers, which synapse with the preganglionic fibers of sympathetic and parasympathetic branches of autonomic nervous system.	
Lateral	• Excites flexor reflex while inhibiting extensors		
• Tectospinal tract	Motor fibers arise in the midbrain, decussate and descend the cord, and terminate in the cervical cord segments.	These tracts function to influence activity of head and neck muscles in movements of the head associated with visual and auditory stimuli.	

*Note that *both* the lateral and ventral spinothalamic tracts are thought to mediate the same sensations.
†Compare with lower motor nerve paralysis.

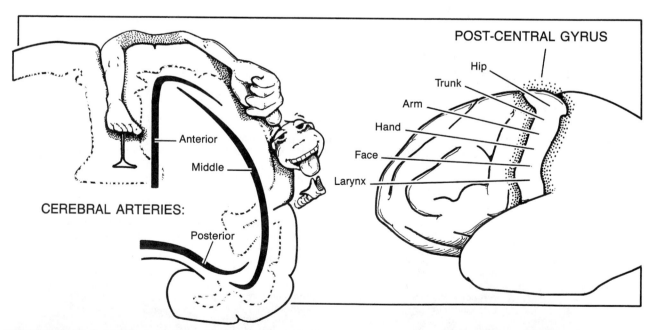

FIGURE 27–18. Somesthetic cortex refers to the topographic representation on the surface of the cortex (primary sensory cortex) of regions of the body receiving innervation. The regions of the body receiving a large amount of innervation (e.g., tongue, lips, thumb, fingers) receive a correspondingly larger topographic representation over the surface of the cortex; areas of the body receiving less innervation (e.g., lower extremities, back, and trunk) receive a correspondingly smaller representation. Note that representation of the hands and face is distributed over the lateral surface of the cortex, an area receiving its blood supply via the *middle* cerebral artery; the medial aspect of the cortex concerned with innervation to the back, trunk, and lower extremities receives its blood supply via the *anterior* cerebral artery; the visual cortex within the occipital lobe is nourished via the *posterior* cerebral artery. Knowledge of this topographic representation and blood supply is helpful in pinpointing the location of a brain lesion, based on history and physical findings.

TABLE 27–9
Responses of Effector Organs to Adrenergic* Innervation

Organ	α Receptors	β₁ Receptors	β₂ Receptors
Heart		Stimulation of these receptors increases:	
SA node		Myocardial contractility	
Atria		Conduction velocity	
AV node		Automaticity	
Ventricles		Heart rate	
		In the ventricles, an increase in the rate of idioventricular pacemakers may occur.	
Arterioles†			
Coronary	Vasoconstriction +		Vasodilation ++
Skeletal muscle	Vasoconstriction ++		Vasodilation ++
Cerebral	Vasoconstriction (slight)		
Pulmonary	Vasoconstriction +		Vasodilation
Abdominal viscera	Vasoconstriction +++		Vasodilation
Renal	Vasoconstriction +++		Vasodilation
Skin-mucosa	Vasoconstriction		
Salivary glands	Vasoconstriction		
Veins			
Systemic	Vasoconstriction ++		
Lungs			
Bronchial muscle			Relaxation (bronchodilation)
Intestinal			
Smooth muscle	Relaxation		Relaxation
Uterus	Contraction		
Ureter	Contraction		
Metabolism		β stimulation	
		Lipolysis	
		Muscle glycogenolysis	
		Insulin secretion	

*Dopaminergic receptors may be found in renal, mesenteric, splanchnic, cerebral, and coronary arteries. Vasodilation and increased blood flow to these vascular beds occurs following dopaminergic stimulation. Only *dopamine* is presently known to activate this receptor.

†Almost all arterial beds have both α- and β-receptors, and some additionally possess dopaminergic receptors. The *net* physiologic response depends almost entirely on the amount of stimulation being received by each receptor at any given time.

+Reflects degree of vasoconstriction or vasodilation, with + < ++ < +++.

neurons in the body that innervate skeletal muscle. The cell body of the lower motor neuron occurs in the ventral gray horn of the spinal cord (see Fig. 27–14), and its axonal endings terminate at the *neuromuscular junction* of individual skeletal muscle fibers.

Neuromuscular Junction. Each skeletal muscle fiber has one specialized area within its membrane called the *motor end-plate*. It is here that the lower motor neuron articulates with the individual muscle fiber. Electrical activity within the neuron is transmitted to the muscle fiber by a chemical neurotransmitter, evoking a specific motor response. This junction of nerve with skeletal muscle fiber is called the *neuromuscular junction*. The chemical neurotransmitter secreted is acetylcholine.

The ultimate message delivered to the lower motor neuron and expressed via skeletal muscle activity represents the *sum* of all excitatory and inhibitory impulses arising from many sensory and motor areas throughout the CNS.

Extrapyramidal Pathways. The extrapyramidal pathways have multiple synapses and connections with other neuronal pathways throughout the CNS. They arise from cortical and subcortical areas of the brain, basal ganglia, cerebellum, and various areas within the brainstem. These pathways do not cross over at the

medulla as do corticospinal (pyramidal) pathways, and they have been labeled *extra*pyramidal pathways.

Extrapyramidal pathways modulate the activities of the pyramidal system. Working in synchrony with the cerebellum, these pathways help to regulate and maintain activities related to muscle tone, posture, proprioception, equilibrium, and reflexes. Their excitatory and inhibitory influences are indispensable in performing fine, discrete, volitional movements. (See Table 27–8 for details regarding specific extrapyramidal pathways.)

Circuitry—Autonomic Division (Cardiac and Smooth Muscle and Glands)

The *autonomic* division of the nervous system is concerned with innervation of cardiac muscle, smooth muscle, and glands. It comprises the *sympathetic* and *parasympathetic* systems. These systems coordinate and control many vital activities including maintenance of blood pressure, heart rate, digestive processes, respiratory and excretory functions, body temperature, and emotional behavior. Many of these functions occur below the level of consciousness; most involve reflex activity. The activities of one system tend to be balanced by activities of the other.

TABLE 27–10
Autonomic Nervous System: Effect of Dual Innervation on Effector Organs

Effector Organ	Effect of Sympathetic Stimulation	Effect of Parasympathetic Stimulation
Eye		
Pupil	Dilation (mydriasis)	Contraction (miosis)
Ciliary muscle	Relaxation	Contraction
Glands		
Lacrimal	↓ Secretion	Stimulates secretion
Salivary	Scanty, viscous secretion	Profuse, watery secretion
Lungs		
Bronchioles	Bronchodilation	Bronchoconstriction
Heart	↑ Rate	↓ Rate
	↑ Conduction velocity	↓ Conduction velocity
	↑ Contractility	↓ Contractility
Gastrointestinal tract		
Lumen	↓ Peristalsis and tone	↑ Peristalsis and tone
Sphincters	↑ Tone (usually contraction)	↓ Tone (usually relaxation)
Secretions	May inhibit secretions	Stimulates secretions
Adrenal medulla	Secretion of epinephrine and norepinephrine	No significant effect
Urinary bladder		
Detrusor muscle	Relaxation (usually)	Contraction
Internal sphincter	Contraction	Relaxation
Blood vessels		
Coronary	Vasodilation	Minimal effect
Skeletal muscle	Vasodilation	Minimal effect
Splanchnic	Vasoconstriction	Minimal effect
Skin	Vasoconstriction	Minimal effect
Blood		
Glucose	Increased	
Free fatty acids	Increased	

Sympathetic and Parasympathetic Systems. The *sympathetic system* is also referred to as the *adrenergic system* because its nerve fibers release the neurotransmitter norepinephrine (or nor*adren*aline). Norepinephrine binds to two types of *adrenergic* receptors namely, α-adrenergic and β-adrenergic receptors. β-Adrenergic receptors are further classified as β_1- and β_2-receptors. *Dopamine* has been identified as another neurotransmitter within the sympathetic system, and *dopaminergic* receptors are specific for dopamine (Table 27–9).

The *parasympathetic system* is also referred to as the *cholinergic system* as its nerve fibers release the neurotransmitter, *acetylcholine*. This neurotransmitter binds specifically to *cholinergic* receptors. Most organs of the body are innervated by both the sympathetic and parasympathetic systems in what is termed *dual innervation*. Most commonly, these two systems have opposing or antagonistic effects on most organs of the body. Specific effects of this dual innervation on effector organs are listed in Table 27–10. See Table 27–2 for a partial list of other neurotransmitters that have been identified.

Activities of the autonomic nervous system are largely modulated and regulated by centers in the hypothalamus, medulla, and reticular formation. Areas within the cerebral cortex may also influence autonomic responses.

Innervation of Adrenal Medulla. The adrenal medulla functions as part of an autonomic reflex arc. The afferent or sensory limb is *neural* in nature; the efferent or motor limb is *hormonal*. Innervation of this gland occurs via sympathetic nerve fibers. The cells respond by secreting epinephrine (predominantly) and norepinephrine directly into the circulating blood, and these substances affect cells widely dispersed throughout the body. The unique structure of this autonomic reflex arc demonstrates the close interaction between the nervous and endocrine systems in regulating body functions.

CHAPTER 28

Neurologic Assessment of the Patient with an Altered Level of Consciousness

Joan T. Dolan

CHAPTER OUTLINE

Clinical History
    □ Components of Clinical History
Neurologic Examination
    □ Consciousness
    □ Cranial Nerve Function

□ Movement
Diagnostic Studies and Techniques
References
Suggested Readings

LEARNING OBJECTIVES

After completing this chapter, you should be able to:

1. Describe essential aspects of the clinical history as they pertain to neurologic function and dysfunction.
2. Elicit assessment data based on knowledge of functional health patterns.
3. Discuss the physiology of consciousness and the significance of the level of consciousness as an important indicator of neurologic function.
4. Discuss how an assessment of selected cranial nerve function assists in evaluating the level of brain function in the patient with an altered level of consciousness.
5. Review the significance of assessing movement, both somatic and autonomic, in evaluating the level of brain function in the patient with an altered level of consciousness.
6. List commonly used neurodiagnostic tests and procedures and their implications for nursing care.

Neurologic dysfunction, regardless of its cause, creates the potential for rapid deterioration in body functions and irreversible damage to fragile nerve tissue. This means that the survival of the individual and the quality of life after recovery are largely dependent upon timely diagnosis and therapeutic intervention, and upon ongoing monitoring. Serial assessments are essential to the early detection of deterioration in the patient's condition and in evaluating the patient's overall response to therapy.

The purpose of the neurologic assessment is to assist in determining (1) the presence or absence of nervous system dysfunction, including the location, type, and extent of the lesion or insult; (2) the impact of the neurologic dysfunction on the individual's self-care capabilities; and (3) the degree to which the healthy portion of the patient's nervous system can be rehabilitated. Such data provide the foundation for diagnosing and planning patient care.

To assist in diagnosing, planning, and evaluating patient care, *baseline* neurologic function must be established. This provides a measure against which to monitor changes in the neurologic status and a guide in assessing the patient's ability to adapt to environmental demands and to participate in self-care.

The major components of the patient's neurologic assessment include relevant clinical history, physical examination, and diagnostic studies and techniques. In the critical care setting, a comprehensive history may not be obtainable. Thus, the assessment should be focused on the presenting signs and symptoms, or underlying disease or insult, and the potential complications. In an emergency situation, when the patient's condition is deteriorating rapidly, or is at risk of doing so, the clinical history may be deferred or abbreviated in order to immediately establish baseline neurologic function and initiate ongoing monitoring.

CLINICAL HISTORY

The clinical history is the interview phase of the neurologic assessment. Carefully elicited from the patient and/or those familiar with the patient, the history is the initial step in the nursing process and is crucial to nursing diagnosis and patient care planning.

Because of the emergency nature of many problems presented in the intensive care setting, information about the patient is often obtained from other sources than the patient, family, or significant others. Ambulance drivers, emergency medical technicians, and police officers may prove to be valuable sources of information in establishing the patient's baseline status prior to admission. This is especially important if the patient is unconscious or unable to converse.

Components of Clinical History

Chief Complaint/History of Present Illness

The focus of the history should be to establish the patient's presenting problem, the rapidity of onset, the course since onset, and the current status. Specific details may include the location and severity of the insult, its duration, and influencing factors, including factors that may have precipitated, ameliorated (i.e., improved), or aggravated the underlying problem. The SLIDT assessment tool can be used in gathering assessment data (see Table 35–1). Examples of specific questions to be asked are included in Table 28–1. A baseline needs to be established regarding the patient's level of consciousness and mentation, along with the status of vital functions including blood pressure, breathing, and elimination.

TABLE 28–1
Eliciting Clinical History: Sample Questions

- What is the presenting symptom? When did it start? What does it feel like? Did it develop suddenly or gradually? What was the patient doing at the time? Has the condition improved or deteriorated? Does it come and go, or is it constant? Were there any precipitating factors such as infection (sinusitis, upper respiratory infection, ear or tooth infections) or trauma affecting the nervous or musculoskeletal system or both?
- What medications, prescribed or over-the-counter, does the patient take? For what reason? What is the patient's alcohol intake, type and quantity? Does the patient abuse alcohol or drugs? Has there been any recent unusual physical, mental, or emotional stress?
- If trauma to the head occurred, was the patient unconscious and, if so, for how long? Were there seizures? Was there bleeding from ear, nose, or mouth? Were there subsequent headaches, memory loss, or changes in behavior or personality? Has the patient experienced vertigo, dizziness, tinnitus, or loss of balance? Have there been problems with speaking, hearing, or seeing? Has the patient experienced alterations in sensations (e.g., numbness, tingling, pain)? Has the patient experienced muscle weakness or paresis? Does the patient have difficulty in walking or in carrying out activities of daily living? Have there been any changes in digestive, urinary, or bowel functions?

Past Medical History

Depending on the severity of the patient's underlying condition, it may be important to elicit details of the patient's past medical history to establish a relationship between past illnesses and current problems. For example, the condition of an elderly patient admitted with a seizure disorder may be related to a fall 6 months ago in which the patient sustained a Colles' fracture (fractured wrist). Other factors of importance to the neurologic assessment may include a history of transient ischemic attacks (TIAs), or stroke, hypertension, diabetes mellitus, cardiovascular disease, and pulmonary disease. Hypoxemia associated with chronic cardiopulmonary disease might underlie complaints of neurologic dysfunction (e.g., confusion, lethargy).

Functional Health Patterns[1]

As part of establishing baseline data, it is also important to begin assessing how the underlying neurologic problem affects the patient's self-care capabilities and the potential for recovery and rehabilitation. This information is especially critical to defining nursing diagnoses and to developing and implementing a plan for patient care.

Health Perception and Health Management. It is important to ascertain the patient's overall functional health status: How did the patient function prior to the illness or insult? Has there been any recent physical, mental, or emotional stress? Any significant changes in lifestyle? Have the patient's capabilities for self-care changed?

Activity and Exercise. It is important to begin exploring how the current illness might affect the patient's ability to participate in activities of daily living, and recreational and work-related activities. Potential problems for rehabilitation should be ascertained and documented, so that they may be addressed when planning care. Has the patient experienced previous difficulties in performing activities of daily living? If so, what were the nature of the difficulties and possible underlying cause? What are the current limitations involved in dressing, feeding, or bathing?

Cognitive - Perceptual. After the patient's condition has stabilized, it may be important to begin exploring some of the following concerns: Has the patient experienced previous difficulties in concentrating or problem-solving? Does the patient have difficulty recalling recent or remote experiences? Have changes occurred in the patient's sensory perception—sight, hearing, touch, taste, and smell? Have changes occurred in the patient's ability to read, speak, and understand language?

Role and Relationship. How might the patient's illness affect family dynamics and the patient's livelihood? For example, if the patient is the major "decision-maker" or "breadwinner" in the family, who will assume these responsibilities while the patient is ill?

Coping and Stress Tolerance. How do the patient and family view this illness and its impact on their lifestyle? How are they coping at present? What are the family resources, strengths, and weaknesses?

Self-Perception and Self-Concept. Often neurologic dysfunction causes changes in the patient's body image (e.g., loss of urinary and/or bowel continence, paralysis). The patient's response to these changes will need to be examined, over time, when the patient indicates a readiness to deal with the problem or concern.

NEUROLOGIC EXAMINATION

The major focus of the neurologic examination in the critical care setting is to establish a baseline as to the level of brain function, to assist in diagnosing the underlying problem more closely, and to monitor those parameters that predict whether the patient's condition is improving or deteriorating. Based upon the early *trends* in the patient's condition, as reflected by ongoing monitoring, timely therapeutic intervention can be initiated and a reversible pathophysiologic process can be prevented from becoming irreversible.

Selected aspects of the neurologic examination discussed in this chapter include an assessment of consciousness, selected cranial nerve responses, and movement. The latter includes deep tendon and cutaneous reflexes (somatic division) and brainstem function (autonomic division).

Consciousness

Consciousness is governed by the reticular activating system (RAS), a diffuse network of ascending neuronal pathways that originate in the brainstem and conduct impulses to the thalamus and subcortical areas (see Fig. 27–12). The RAS alerts the cerebral hemispheres to incoming sensory information. Because this system of anatomic and functional interrelationships is widespread, disturbances at many levels can disrupt consciousness.

The functional components of consciousness are arousal (alertness) and awareness (content). *Arousal* reflects brain activity at the level of the brainstem. Clinically, arousal is assessed by noting responses to visual, auditory, and tactile stimuli. Do the patient's eyes open spontaneously or upon being spoken to? Or do they open when a painful stimulus is applied?

Awareness reflects brain function at the level of the cerebral cortex and association fibers. Either cerebral hemisphere alone is sufficient to maintain consciousness, providing the RAS is intact. Coma ensues when the function of both hemispheres is impaired or when there is brainstem injury involving the RAS. Clinically, awareness is assessed by determining the patient's orientation to self and environment. This can be achieved by asking the questions: Who are you? Where

are you? What day is it? What is the date, month, and year?

Operational definitions of the levels of consciousness corresponding to observable verbal and tactile stimuli are commonly used. These include the following:

Alert: Awake; opens eyes spontaneously; responds appropriately to auditory, tactile, and visual stimuli; oriented to person, place, and time.

Lethargic: Sleeps often but arouses easily; may open eyes spontaneously or to stimuli; responses may be appropriate or confused.

Obtunded: Aroused by shaking or shouting; opens eyes only to stimuli; responses to verbal stimuli may be inappropriate or confused; returns to sleep.

Stuporous: Responds only to vigorous and repeated stimuli; opens eyes to painful stimuli; responses to verbal stimuli are confused or inappropriate; responds purposefully to painful stimuli.

Comatose: Does not open eyes to painful stimuli; demonstrates no spontaneous or reflex response to commands; offers no verbal response.

It should be appreciated that these terms lack precise definitions and are subject to considerable variations and inconsistencies in interpretation and usage among healthcare providers. Therefore, objective descriptions of patient responses to stimuli should be documented.

Any change in the level of consciousness is a clear indication that there is a disruption in brain function. To determine the *level* of brain dysfunction, it is necessary to assess additional parameters, including eye movements and motor function.

Glasgow Coma Scale

Using the Glasgow Coma Scale,[2] consciousness is evaluated by assessing three types of responses to stimuli: eye opening, best verbal response, and best motor response (Table 28–2). The type of stimulus required and the response obtained provide a rough measure of wakefulness or arousability. A grading scale is used to assign points based on the level of each response, and a score is obtained. A maximum score of 15 reflects a fully alert patient, who responds appropriately and follows commands; a minimum score of 3 indicates a completely unarousable, unresponsive patient. Any change of 2 points or more on the total score may reflect significant improvement or deterioration in the patient's condition.

When used in conjunction with other clinical data, for example, respiratory pattern, pupillary and motor responses, and ocular movements, the coma scale assists in judging the level of brain function and whether there is any downward progression toward brain herniation. It assists caregivers to recognize *early* the need to safeguard those functions dependent upon brainstem reflexes such as coughing, gagging, epiglottal closure, and thus, to protect the patient's airway, if necessary, by insertion of an artificial airway and nasogastric tube.

TABLE 28–2
Glasgow Coma Scale: Assessment of Arousability*

Category	Response	Score
Eyes open	Spontaneously—Eyes open spontaneously	4
	To speech—Eyes open to verbal command	3
	To pain—Eyes open to painful stimuli	2
	None—No eye opening to any stimulus	1
Best verbal response	Oriented—Converses appropriately; knows person, time, date, place	5
	Confused—Converses inappropriately; answers to questions inaccurate; uses language appropriately	4
	Inappropriate words—No sustained conversation; speech random, disorganized, and inappropriate	3
	Incomprehensible—Mumbles, moans, but does not use recognizable words	2
	None—No verbal sounds even to painful stimuli	1
Best motor response	Obeys commands—Performs simple tasks when asked to do so	6
	Localizes pain—Appropriate attempt to locate and to remove painful stimulus	5
	Flexion withdrawal—Flexes arm appropriately to withdraw from source of painful stimulus	4
	Abnormal flexion—Flexes arm at elbow, pronates, and makes a fist in response to painful stimulus; decorticate posturing (see Fig. 28–7)	3
	Abnormal extension—Extends arm at elbow and adducts with internal rotation in response to painful stimulus; decerebrate posturing (see Fig. 28–7)	2
	None—No response to painful stimulus, flaccid	1

*Maximum score 15; minimum score 3.

Some practical problems are associated with the use of the Glasgow Coma Scale in evaluating patients with an altered level of consciousness.[3] For example, eyelids may remain open after they have been drawn back, or swelling may prevent eyelid opening. Verbal response may be impaired by dysphasia or deafness; the presence of an endotracheal tube may interfere with communication.

Cranial Nerve Function

Assessment of cranial nerves provides a guide to the integrity of the brainstem. Only certain cranial nerves can be tested in critically ill patients, who may be sedated or who may have an altered level of consciousness. Testing of the cranial nerves can be accomplished by assessing brainstem reflexes. Brainstem reflexes of importance are listed later in Table 28–5. (Table 27–5 lists the central and peripheral connec-tions of cranial nerves.) Further discussion of these reflexes is presented in the sections on reflexes and on assessment of motor function: autonomic division.

Movement

The motor division of the nervous system provides the fundamental mechanism through which the activities of the nervous system are expressed and perceived. The brain and spinal cord receive sensory stimulation from a wide variety of sensory receptors throughout the body (see Table 27–7). This sensory input is sorted out, integrated, and interpreted, and the culmination of all of these activities is reflected in the motor output, or motor response. Thus, it is only in assessing motor responses that the effect of sensory stimuli on the body can be evaluated.

Assessment of Motor Function: Somatic Division

In the patient who is unable to participate in the neurologic examination, assessment of motor function is limited to those aspects of the examination that do not require the patient's cooperation. These include the testing of skeletal muscle for size, tone, and involuntary movements (Table 28–3); testing the

TABLE 28–3
Assessment of Motor Function: Somatic Division

Muscle Size
- Inspect and palpate the patient's muscles while at rest for size, consistency, and possible atrophy.
- Compare fine muscles of each hand to assess for wasting, fasciculations (twitchings), and fine tremors of a single motor unit.

Muscle Tone
- Palpate the patient's muscles at rest and note the resistance to passive movement.
- Assess for spasticity (i.e., increased resistance to passive muscle stretch), rigidity, stiffness of extremities when moved, or flaccidity (i.e., decreased resistance to passive muscle stretch).

Involuntary Movements
- Inspect for irregular, spasmodic choreiform movements (i.e., marked by involuntary muscular twitchings of the limbs and/or face), rapid myoclonic contractions, tics, or tremors. In the awake patient, a *resting* tremor is diminished by voluntary movement; an *intention* tremor is accentuated by voluntary movement.

Muscle Strength
(Requires an awake and cooperative patient)
- Ask the patient to move each of the major muscles, first without resistance, and then against resistance offered by the examiner.
- Compare corresponding muscles on each side.
- A *universal* system for recording muscle strength uses a scale rating from 0 to 5:
  - 0 = no contraction
  - 1 = trace (flicker) of contraction
  - 2 = active movements without gravity
  - 3 = active movements against gravity
  - 4 = active movements against gravity and resistance
  - 5 = usual (normal) strength

TABLE 28–4
Assessment of Motor Function: Reflexes

Deep Tendon Reflexes (DTRs)
- Elicit a reflex response by briskly striking a muscle or tendon (use a reflex hammer), which stimulates the muscle spindle stretch receptors. The expected motor response to this stretch stimulus is an action to reduce the stretch (i.e., contraction of the appropriate muscles). The presence of muscle stretch indicates that all components of the reflex arc are intact.

Reflex	Elicited by	Normal Response	Spinal Cord Segment
Biceps	Tapping biceps tendon	Flexion at elbow	C-5 and C-6
Triceps	Tapping triceps tendon	Extension at elbow	C-6, C-7, and C-8
Brachioradialis	Tapping styloid process of radius	Flexion of elbow and pronation of forearm	C-5 and C-6
Patellar (knee jerk)	Tapping patellar tendon	Extension at knee	L-2, L-3, and L-4
Achilles	Tapping Achilles tendon	Plantor flexion of foot	S-1 and S-2

Cutaneous, or Superficial, Reflexes
- Stroke skin with a moderately sharp object (not sharp enough to break the skin), and observe response of related muscles. For these reflexes the reflex arcs have sensory receptors in the skin rather than in the muscle fibers.

Reflex	Elicited by	Normal Response	Spinal Cord Segment
Epigastric	Stroking downward from nipples	Dimpling of epigastrium on the side stimulated	T-7 to T-9
Abdominal			
Upper	Stroking skin over lower costal margins toward midline	Umbilicus moves up and toward area being stroked	T-7 to T-9
Midabdominal	Stroking laterally from flanks to midline at umbilicus	Umbilicus moves toward side being stroked	T-9 to T-11
Lower	Stroking from iliac crests toward the midline	Umbilicus moves down and toward side being stroked	T-11 and T-12
Cremasteric	Stroking medial surface of upper thigh	Ipsilateral elevation of testicle	T-12 and L-1
Gluteal	Stroking skin of buttocks	Skin tenses at gluteal area	L-4 and L-5
Plantar	Scratch sole of foot on lateral surface from heel to toes	Plantar flexion of toes	L-4 and L-5
Bulbocavernous	Pinching dorsum of glans	Tensing of bulbous urethra	S-3 and S-4
Superficial anal	Pricking perineum	Tensing of external anal sphincter	S-4 and S-5, coccygeal

levels of motor responses (Table 28–2); and testing of deep tendon, and cutaneous or superficial reflexes (Table 28–4).

When assessing motor function, it is important to appreciate that smooth, coordinated somatic motor function requires that the following be structurally and functionally intact: primary motor cortex; basal ganglia; descending motor pathways, including corticospinal (pyramidal) and extrapyramidal tracts; cerebellum; lower motor neurons; neuromuscular junction; and individual skeletal muscle fibers.

It is important to remember that the majority of corticospinal fibers *cross over* to the other side at the level of the medulla. Therefore, skeletal muscle movement initiated by the motor cortex is seen on the opposite side of the body. Any weakness or absence of spontaneous movement on one side of the body usually implies disruption of motor tracts in the opposite (i.e., contralateral) cerebral hemisphere.

Levels of Motor Responses.

Levels of motor responses to specific stimuli are included as part of the Glasgow Coma Scale (Table 28–2). The patient who *obeys* a command can appreciate directions or instructions whether given verbally,

in writing, or by gesture. *Localization of pain* requires that the patient make an appropriate or purposeful attempt to remove the stimulus. *Flexion withdrawal* suggests that the patient cannot localize the stimulus but will at least flex the arm when a painful stimulus is applied (e.g., nailbed pressure). *Abnormal flexion* (decorticate) in response to a painful stimulus involves flexion at the elbow and internal rotation of the wrists. *Abnormal extension* (decerebrate) involves extension of the arm at the elbow, with adduction and internal rotation at the shoulder (see Fig. 28–7).

It should be appreciated, while observing for motor responses to the stimuli applied in this assessment, that the actual motor responses elicited also reflect how incoming sensory information is processed within the body. Eliciting a response to the stimuli applied suggests that the sensory pathways for these sensory modalities are intact. Circuitries for the sensations of crude pressure and pain are depicted in Figure 27–17; primary cortical representation of sensory innervation (somesthetic cortex) is shown in Figure 27–18.

Reflexes

Reflex activity underlies virtually everything we do. Assessment of reflexes helps to localize lesions of the

TABLE 28–5
Brainstem Reflexes

Reflexes	Elicited by	Normal Response
Pupillary		
Direct reaction	Shine bright light into eye	Pupillary constriction of ipsilateral eye
Consensual reaction	Shine bright light into eye	Pupillary constriction of contralateral eye
Note:		
Pupillary constriction—response via parasympathetic fibers of cranial nerve III		
Pupillary dilation—response via sympathetic fibers C-8, T-1, and T-2		
Corneal	Touching cornea with a wisp of cotton	Blinking of eyelids
Reflex Eye Movements		
Oculocephalic (doll's eye)	Holding both eyelids open, briskly rotate head first to one side, and then to the other	Conjugate eye deviation: if head is turned to left, eyes linger with deviation to right
Oculovestibular (caloric stimulation)	Introduction of ice water into ear canal	Nystagmus with slow component toward irrigated ear and fast component away from irrigated ear
Pharyngeal		
Gag	Stroking the pharynx	
Swallowing (pharyngeal stage)	Voluntary movement of food to posterior pharynx	

nervous system. In the patient with an altered state of consciousness, brainstem and autonomic reflexes provide critical clues as to the status of protective reflexes (ie., cough, gag, epiglottal closure) and indications of a need to safeguard the airway (see following section). Spinal reflexes that remain intact can be used as the basis for attaining autonomic control of bladder and bowel function in patients sustaining acute spinal cord injury (see Chapter 33). See Figure 27–14 for a schematic depiction of a reflex arc, which consists of a sensory neuron synapsing directly with a motor neuron. The reflex arc provides the structural basis underlying reflex activity.

Major categories of reflexes include the stretch or deep tendon reflexes (DTRs); cutaneous, or superficial, reflexes; and brainstem reflexes. When assessing deep tendon reflexes, a scale of 0 to 4 is used to quantify the degree of the reflex (0 = absent; 1 = present, but diminished; 2 = normal; 3 = increased, but not pathologic; 4 = markedly hyperactive). Table 28–4 lists some of the more important deep tendon and cutaneous, or superficial, reflexes.

Brainstem Reflexes. The brainstem reflexes are tested in the routine examination of the cranial nerves. Familiarity with the level of the cranial nerves involved is helpful in evaluting brainstem function. Table 28–5 lists some of the important brainstem reflexes, their assessment, and normal responses.

Pupillary Reactions: Direct and Consensual Light Reflex. These reflexes involve two cranial nerves: optic (II) and oculomotor (III). To assess: (1) Examine pupils, noting size, shape, and equality before testing for reactivity. Many individuals have unequal pupils. It is important to ascertain if the patient has had prior eye surgery, which may account for unequal, unusually shaped pupils. Drugs can affect pupillary size and responsiveness. A drug history may be helpful. Pupillary size may be recorded in millimeters, or as *constricted, normal,* or *dilated.* (2) Evaluate pupillary light reflexes by noting pupillary constriction in response to a light shone into each eye from the side (Fig. 28–1). Shine the light into one eye and observe the pupillary response in that eye. Next, shine the light into the same eye and observe the pupillary response in the *other* eye. When one eye is stimulated, the pupil of the other eye should also constrict (i.e., consensual light reflex). Decussation (i.e., crossing over) of optic nerve fibers at the optic chiasm provides the structural basis for the direct and consensual light reflex. To discern pupillary reactivity in extremely pinpoint pupils, darkening the room may help.

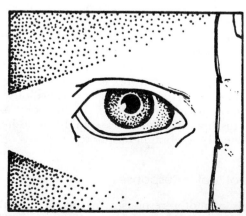

FIGURE 28–1. Evaluation of pupillary light reflexes by noting pupillary constriction in response to light shone into each eye from the sides.

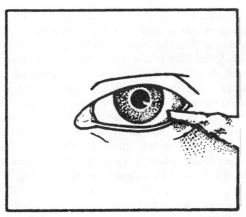

FIGURE 28–2. The corneal reflex is tested by observing whether the patient blinks in response to a light touch with a wisp of cotton on the cornea.

Corneal Reflex. The corneal reflex involves two cranial nerves: trigeminal (V) and facial (VII). To assess: Test the corneal reflex by observing whether the patient blinks in response to a light touch with a wisp of cotton on the cornea. Avoid striking only the sclera (Fig. 28–2).

Pharyngeal (Gag) Reflex. The gag reflex involves three cranial nerves: trigeminal (V), glossopharyngeal (IX), and vagus (X). To assess: Touch each side of the pharynx with a tongue depressor or Q-tip and note the gag (Fig. 28–3). The palatal reflex is tested by stroking each side of the uvula. The side touched should rise.

Swallowing. The swallowing reflex involves four cranial nerves; facial (VII), glossopharyngeal (IX), vagus (X), and hypoglossal (XII). To assess: In an awake patient, observe the ability to swallow food or liquid. If the patient swallows without difficulty, these nerves may be considered to be intact. Additional brainstem reflexes are discussed below.

Pathologic Reflexes

Babinski's Sign. To assess: Elicit reflex by briskly stroking lateral aspect of the sole and across the ball

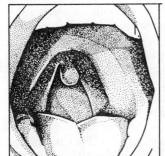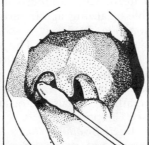

FIGURE 28–3. The pharyngeal reflex is tested by touching each side of the pharynx with a tongue depressor and noting the gag.

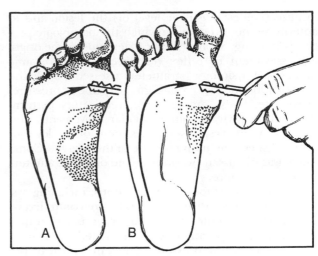

FIGURE 28–4. Plantar reflex elicited as indicated. (*A*) Normal response is the plantar flexion on the toes. (*B*) Abnormal response (i.e., Babinski's sign) is dorsiflexion of the big toe, with or without fanning of the other toes.

of the foot using a semisharp object (e.g., car key). A normal response is plantar flexion of the toes. An abnormal response (i.e., Babinski's sign) is dorsiflexion of the big toe, with or without corticospinal tract dysfunction (Fig. 28–4). Another abnormality would be the *absence* of any response.

Signs of Meningeal Irritation

1. *Nuchal rigidity:* The patient is unable to flex chin on chest. Passive flexion of the neck is limited by involuntary muscle spasm.
2. *Spinal rigidity:* Spasms of spinal muscles (erector spinae) limit movement of the spine. *Opisthotonos* is a condition of extreme spasm (tetanic contraction) producing rigid hyperextension of the entire spine; the head is forced backwards and the trunk is thrust forward.
3. *Kernig's sign:* With the patient supine, passively flex the patient's hip to 90 degrees while also flexing the patient's knee to 90 degrees. While maintaining the hip in the flexed position, attempt to extend the patient's knee. Production of pain in the hamstrings and resistance to further extension are reliable signs of meningeal irritation. This response may also occur with a herniated disk or tumors of the cauda equina.
4. *Brudzinski's sign:* With the patient supine and the limbs extended, passively flex the patient's neck. Involuntary flexion of the hip and knees is a positive sign of meningeal irritation.

Assessment of Motor Function: Autonomic Division

Patient with Altered Level of Consciousness. Evaluation as to the level of brain function in the patient with an altered state of consciousness is essential to localize (i.e., establish the level of) the lesion and to determine the direction in which the pathologic process is evolving. Such evaluation depends on the ongoing assessment of reflex responses and autonomic functions. Physiologic parameters assessed include the level of consciousness, vital signs (e.g., blood pressure, heart rate, body temperature), respiratory pattern, size and reactivity of pupils, ocular movements, and postural motor responses. Assessment of the level of consciousness, including the use of the Glasgow Coma Scale, was discussed previously. The other parameters are discussed here.

Vital Signs. Cardiovascular functions, including systemic blood pressure and heart rate, are controlled by the vasomotor center in the lower pons and upper medulla. These parameters are regulated to ensure a cerebral perfusion pressure sufficient to satisfy the metabolic needs of fragile brain tissue. Ongoing assessment of mean arterial pressure is especially important in this regard. Arrhythmias associated with structural changes (e.g., compression of brainstem) or metabolic disturbances (e.g., blood gas alterations) commonly occur, requiring close monitoring of heart rate and rhythm.

One must be cautioned about overreliance on vital signs, especially in patients at risk of developing an increase in intracranial pressure with potential brain herniation (e.g., severe head injury). An increase in systolic blood pressure, widening pulse pressure, slow bounding pulse, and alterations in respiratory pattern (Cushing reflex) signal a grave prognosis. It must be emphasized that these signs are *late* findings. They are associated with compression of vital centers in the lower brainstem and occur too late to prevent herniation and irreversible brain damage. In this clinical circumstance early initiation of intracranial pressure monitoring is essential (see Chapter 29).

Changes in body temperature significantly affect neurologic function. An increase in body temperature increases the metabolic requirements of neural tissue. *Hyperpyrexia* may reflect pathology involving the hypothalamus, or it may be indicative of infection in another part of the body. Measures should be implemented to maintain body temperature within the normal range. Hypothermia may be initiated as a therapeutic modality.

Major factors influencing cerebral blood flow (presented in Table 27–6) must be considered in the neurologic assessment.

Respiratory Patterns. Plum and Posner define breathing as a "sensorimotor act integrated by nervous influences that arise from nearly every level of the brain and upper spinal cord."[4] Regulation of breathing is an interplay of metabolic and neurogenic factors occurring at these various levels. The significance of this dual control mechanism is that pathology predisposing to the altered state of consciousness may involve structural lesions and/or metabolic disturbances, and frequently an overlapping of both.

In the patient with an altered state of consciousness, specific patterns of breathing may signify a change in the patient's status and may have localizing features reflecting the level of brain function.

Cheyne-Stokes Respiration. This is one of the most common and often earliest abnormal patterns of breathing. It reflects the presence of bilateral deep hemispheric or diencephalic lesions (upper brainstem). It is characterized by a periodic pattern of breathing in which respiratory excursion waxes and wanes, with phases of hyperpnea alternating with apnea. There is a characteristic pattern of crescendo-decrescendo breathing followed by a period of apnea (Fig. 28–5).

During the hyperpneic phase an abnormally increased ventilatory response to carbon dioxide stimulation occurs, reducing the carbon dioxide stimulus (metabolic). Apnea results and is maintained because of the abnormally decreased ventilatory stimulus (neurogenic). The stimulation to respiration does not return until there is sufficient accumulation of carbon dioxide to trigger chemoreceptors and initiate the next cycle.

Central Neurogenic Hyperventilation. This pattern reflects brainstem function at the level of the midbrain. It is characterized by a pattern of deep, rapid, and sustained hyperpnea, with consequent hypocapnia (i.e., an abnormally low tension of carbon dioxide in circulating blood) (see Fig. 28–5). The diagnosis of central neurogenic hyperventilation is made in the clinical scenario of a high respiratory rate (25 to 40/min), accompanied by arterial blood gas values indicating an elevated Pao_2 (i.e, oxygen tension in circulating blood) and a lowered $Paco_2$ (i.e., carbon dioxide tension in circulating blood), with commensurate elevated blood pH, in a patient breathing room air. The underlying pathophysiology suggests that there is an abnormally low threshold for stimulation by carbon dioxide.

Apneustic Breathing. The characteristic feature of this pattern is the long pause that occurs at full inspiration. The apneustic center occurs in the lower pons and is not very well defined.[5] Impulses generated here attempt to prevent turn-off of inspiration. Normally, these signals are overridden by those of the pneumotaxic center, which functions to limit inspiration. If impulses from the pneumotaxic center are interrupted, signals from the apneustic center are unopposed, resulting in a sustained inspiratory breathing pattern. Thus, apneustic breathing can be a very valuable localizing sign in terms of the level of brain function (Fig. 28–5).

Cluster Breathing. This pattern is associated with lesions of the pons. It is described as clusters of breaths occurring in a disorderly sequence with irregular pauses between each cluster. Onset of this type of breathing signals the occurrence of brain herniation (see Chapter 29).

Ataxic Breathing (Biot's Respirations). This breathing pattern reflects a depth and rate of breathing that are completely irregular and random, often slow with periods of apnea. Loss of the "to-and-fro" pattern of breathing suggests impairment of the reticular for-

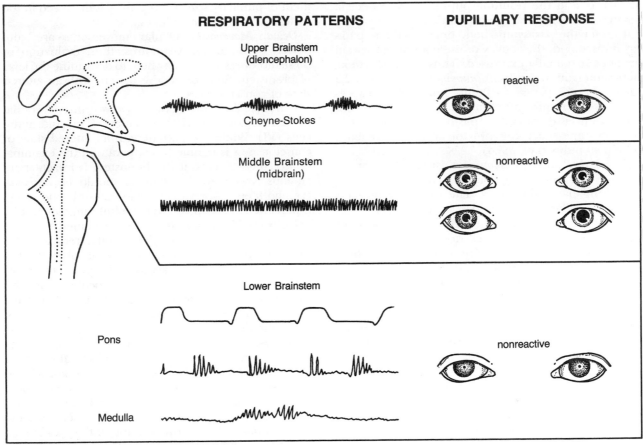

FIGURE 28–5. The presence of abnormal respiratory patterns and pupillary responses in the patient with an altered state of consciousness assists in localizing the level of brainstem function and/or signifying changes in the patient's underlying status.

mation at the level of the medulla. It differs from Cheyne-Stokes respirations in terms of its irregularity. Lesions in the posterior fossa (cerebellum), particularly rapidly expanding lesions (e.g., cerebellar or pontine hemorrhage), may precipitate this type of breathing. Complete respiratory assistance is initated as alveolar ventilation becomes compromised.

Protective Reflexes. An important component of the respiratory assessment in the patient with an altered state of consciousness is an evaluation of the status of the *protective* reflexes (e.g, cough, gag, epiglottal closure). Innervation of these reflexes occurs via neurons located in the "respiratory centers" of the pons and medulla. Loss of these reflexes presents an imminent threat to life with loss of airway patency and respiratory arrest. Immediate intubation, with initiation of mechanical ventilation, is imperative. Efforts also need to be taken to prevent aspiration of secretions. Serial arterial blood gas studies assist in assessing the effectiveness of the ventilatory effort.

Pupillary Size and Reactivity. Pupillary size and reactivity to light provide key information related to structural disturbances of the diencephalon, midbrain, and pons. Such information is significant because areas of the brainstem controlling arousal (reticular activating system) lie adjacent to those areas controlling pupillary activity. Consequently, evaluating pupillary

changes provides a guide to localizing brainstem lesions causing coma and/or determining the level of brainstem function.

Of critical importance is the circuitry of autonomic fibers to each eye. Innervation of the eye by parasympathetic and sympathetic fibers occurs over separate and distinct pathways, which assist in localizing lesions and determining the level of brain function. Parasympathetic fibers arise at the midbrain. These fibers leave the midbrain along with the oculomotor nerve (III) at a point adjacent to the *tentorial notch* (i.e, the opening in the meningeal fold, the falx tentorium, which accommodates the brainstem). From here the third nerve and parasympathetic fibers proceed directly to the orbit.

Sympathetic fibers arise in the hypothalamus and descend through the brainstem as preganglionic fibers to the lower cervical/upper thoracic spinal cord segments. Upon synapsing in the sympathetic ganglia, *post*ganglionic fibers ascend along with the internal carotid artery, eventually to reach the orbit.

Parasympathetic innervation to the eye stimulates contraction of the pupilloconstrictor muscle fibers of the iris, and the pupil becomes smaller *(miosis)*. Sympathetic innervation stimulates contraction of the pupillodilator muscle fibers of the iris, and the pupil becomes larger *(mydriasis)*. Both systems are continually active, and the resulting pupillary size reflects a balance between these two innervations.

If either the parasympathetic or sympathetic pathway is disrupted, the activity of the unopposed system becomes maximally expressed. Thus, altered sympathetic innervation results in *pinpoint* pupils (1.5 to 2.5 mm); altered parasympathetic innervation causes widely *dilated* pupils (8 to 9 mm). If innervation from both systems is disrupted, pupils become mid-sized (4 to 5 mm) and react sluggishly or become unreactive to light stimulus (i.e., fixed).

Pathologic Pupillary Responses. A variety of abnormal pupillary responses can occur depending on the underlying pathophysiology. The localizing implications of pupillary abnormalities, in terms of levels of brain function in the patient with an altered level of consciousness, have been well documented by Plum and Posner.[6] Bilateral pressure applied to the diencephalon and upper brainstem during early rostral to caudal (i.e., head-to-toe) deterioration in brain function produces symmetrically constricted pupils, but the light reflex remains intact (Fig. 28–5).

In this instance, it is also important to appreciate that metabolic disturbances can result in similar pupillary responses. Plum and Posner suggest that "because pupillary pathways are relatively resistant to metabolic insult, the presence or absence of the light reflex is the single most important physical sign potentially distinguishing structural from metabolic coma." In coma precipitated by metabolic disturbances, the pupils retain the light reflex.

Midbrain involvement is reflected in some definitive pupillary abnormalities. Midposition (4 to 5 mm) fixed (i.e., unreactive) pupils that are frequently unequal and slightly irregular in shape are caused by midbrain lesions, which interrupt both parasympathetic and sympathetic innervation of the eye (e.g., in transtentorial herniation, midbrain hemorrhages or infarctions, or tumors).

A dilated ("blown") (8 to 9 mm) pupil, which reacts sluggishly or is fixed, occurs with unilateral compression of the oculomotor nerve where it leaves the midbrain at the tentorial notch. The consequent compression of parasympathetic fibers interrupts stimulation to the eye on the same side. This results in unopposed sympathetic stimulation and, thus, the "blown" pupil (see Fig. 28–5). A unilateral fixed and dilated pupil in the patient at risk of developing an increase in intracranial pressure (e.g., acute head injury) indicates that brain herniation is occurring. This constitutes a *neurologic emergency* requiring immediate and aggressive treatment if compression of vital centers within the pons and medulla is to be averted.

Lesions of the pons may interrupt sympathetic pathways that descend through the brainstem to the spinal cord before ascending to the orbit. Pupils in this circumstance are *pinpoint* due to unopposed parasympathetic innervation, and they may be reactive.

Anoxia and ischemia (cardiac arrest) usually cause widely dilated fixed pupils. Anoxic pupillary dilation lasting longer than a few minutes yields a very grave prognosis, usually of irreversible brain damage. Assess-

ment of pupillary size and reactivity is discussed in the section on brainstem reflexes.

Ocular Movements. Ocular movements are controlled by brainstem structures; thus, evaluation of these motor responses may help to determine the level of brainstem function in the patient with an altered state of consciousness.

Extraocular movements involve three cranial nerves: oculomotor (III), trochlear (IV), and abducens (VI). While the patient with an altered state of consciousness is unable to cooperate in the examination of these nerves, if the brainstem is intact, spontaneous roving eye movements should be *conjugate* (i.e., both eyes move together so that only one image is perceived), and they cover the full range of gaze.

Reflex Eye Movements. Reflex eye movements include the oculocephalic and oculovestibular reflexes. The reflex arc for both of these reflexes involves the following cranial nerves: acoustic (vestibulocochlear; VIII) as the afferent limb and the oculomotor (III) and abducens (VI) as the efferent limb. Abnormal reflex eye movements indicate brainstem dysfunction below the midbrain.

All tests for reflex eye movements should be deferred until x-rays rule out cervical spinal injury.

1. *Oculocephalic reflex (doll's eye phenomenon).* To assess: Hold the comatose patient's eyelids open, and briskly rotate the patient's head horizontally, first to one side, and then to the other, from the midline. Observe the position of the eyes in relation to the head. The normal response is for the eyes initially to move in the direction opposite to the head turning, and then, within a few seconds, to move back to midline. If the reflex is not functioning, the eyes will move with the head as though painted on or fixed in place. Likewise, if the head is moved up and down vertically, the eyes will normally linger in the position opposite to the direction in which the head is moved. Pupils that move in the same direction as the head, as though painted on, are abnormal (Fig. 28–6).

2. *Oculovestibular reflex.* To assess: The *caloric stimulation* test is used to evaluate the oculovestibular reflex. The auditory canal is examined carefully before the test is performed to ensure that the tympanic membrane is intact. The head is raised to about 30 degrees, and up to 120 mL of ice water is slowly introduced into the auditory canal of the compromised patient. In the normal response (intact brainstem), the eyes will exhibit a horizontal nystagmus (i.e., side to side movement) with the slow conjugate component moving toward the irrigated ear and the rapid component moving away from the irrigated ear.

The oculovestibular reflex is significant in that it may be preserved somewhat longer than the oculocephalic reflex in the presence of brainstem pathology. These tests should never be performed in a patient with possible cervical spine injury. These tests are included with other brainstem reflexes in Table 28–5.

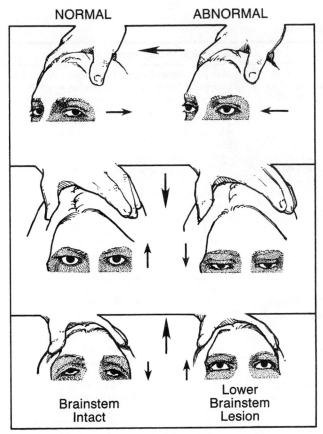

FIGURE 28–6. Oculocephalic reflex (doll's eye phenomenon).

Assessment of *horizontal* ocular movement: Normal response—with eyelids held open, the eyes should be observed initially to linger in the *opposite* direction to which the head is turned, eventually to return to the midline. Abnormal response—the eyes are observed to move in the same direction in which the head is turned. Both directions should be tested.

Assessment of *vertical* ocular movement. Head flexed (i.e., chin to chest): Normal response—the eyes will linger in the *opposite* direction in which the head is moved (i.e., looking up). Abnormal response—the eyes are observed to look downward in the *same* direction in which the head is moved.

Head hyperextended (i.e., facing the ceiling): Normal response—the eyes are observed to linger in a downward gaze in *opposite* direction to which the head is moved. Abnormal response—the eyes are observed to move in the *same* direction in which the head is moved (i.e., looking up at the ceiling).

Postural Responses. Motor function in patients with an altered level of consciousness can be assessed by applying a noxious stimulus (e.g., pressure on a nailbed) and observing the response. One of three patterns of movement may be evoked in response to such stimuli: appropriate, inappropriate, or flaccidity.

Appropriate responses include purposeful movement to push the stimulus away or the withdrawal of the limb. A facial grimace or groan may accompany the motor response. Such responses imply the presence of functioning sensory pathways and intact or partially intact descending motor pathways (corticospinal tracts).

Inappropriate motor responses include flexor spasms and extensor spasms. The pattern of these abnormal responses varies according to the site and severity of brain involvement. An abnormal *flexor* response in the arm with extension of the leg is often referred to as *decorticate* posturing or rigidity. When fully developed, this response is characterized by flexion of the arm, wrist, and fingers, with adduction in the upper extremity (Fig. 28–7) and extension, internal rotation, and vigorous plantar flexion of the lower extremity. This reflects a lesion in the cerebral hemisphere, basal ganglia, and/or diencephalon, which interrupts corticospinal pathways.

A pattern of abnormal *extensor* responses in upper and lower extremities is termed *decerebrate* posturing or rigidity. When fully developed, this response is characterized by stiffly extended, adducted, and hyperpronated arms (see Fig. 28–7); and stiffly extended legs with the feet plantar flexed. Frequently, the patient is also opisthotonic (i.e., spasm with head and heels bent backward and body thrust forward) with clenched teeth.

Flaccidity suggests an absence of motor activity and reflects dysfunction of central motor mechanisms in the pontine reticular formation or, possibly, peripheral denervation.

Clinically, the examination of motor function in the patient with an altered state of consciousness provides valuable information as to the level of the lesion and may serve as a guide to the progress of the illness. Abnormal flexor and extensor responses can shift back and forth from one combination to the other.

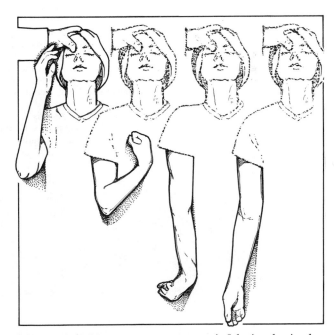

FIGURE 28–7. Motor responses to a painful stimulus in the patient with an altered state of consciousness. Appropriate response is to push the stimulus away; inappropriate responses include abnormal flexor response, abnormal extensor response, and flaccidity. These responses reflect varying degrees of responsiveness decreasing from left to right.

TABLE 28–6
Diagnostic Studies and Procedures for Neurologic Dysfunction

Test	Description/Purpose	Clinical Significance/Nursing Implications
Lumbar Puncture	Performed to 1. Measure cerebrospinal fluid (CSF) pressure (normally 50–200 cmH$_2$O). Opening CSF pressure relatively equivalent to intracranial pressure in most patients. 2. Sample CSF (normal constituents listed in Table 27–3). 3. Inject medication or contrast media. *Procedure:* A hollow needle is inserted into subarachnoid space at L3-4 or L4-5 spinal segment.	*Patient preparation:* Explain the purpose of test and procedure involved; position to be assumed (side-lying position with head and knees maximally flexed); need to avoid sudden movement or coughing; expectations about what the patient may expect to feel during and after procedure. *Postprocedure care:* Patient is advised to remain flat for 2–6 h to prevent headache; fluids are encouraged. • Clinically, presence of blood in CSF may indicate subarachnoid hemorrhage, brain laceration. • CSF glucose level approximately two thirds that of serum glucose; a blood sugar should be drawn in conjunction with lumbar puncture. • *Contraindications:* Patients with incipient brain herniation and/or posterior fossa lesions; acute head injury.
Queckenstedt's phenomenon test	Performed to detect subarachnoid obstruction (e.g., spinal tumor, vertebral compression fracture). • Performed in conjunction with lumbar puncture; involves manual compression of jugular veins for about 10 sec.	Normally a rapid rise in CSF pressure occurs during compression, with a rapid fall to normal upon release.
Radiology Studies Skull x-rays	May reveal: skull fractures or abnormalities of cranial vault; intracranial calcification; dense vascular markings; presence of tumor or congenital anomaly; possible detection of an increase in intracranial pressure.	*Patient preparation:* Explain purpose of test and procedure involved, including the need for several different radiologic views; emphasize that the procedure is painless with minimal exposure to radiation; remove all hair pins, jewelry, or other metal objects.
Spine x-rays	To identify vertebral fracture or dislocation, which may be impinging on the spinal cord or its nerve roots.	Same as above. *Note:* Any patient who has sustained a head injury should be assumed to have an associated cervical spine injury until the latter has been definitively ruled out by x-rays of the cervical spine.
Contrast Studies Cerebral angiography	An invasive procedure requiring the injection of radiopaque dye into the cerebral circulation via the carotid or vertebral arteries (also via femoral or brachial), during which time serial radiographs are taken. • Useful in the diagnosis of abnormalities of cerebral vasculature; or findings obtained by CAT scan or radionuclide studies.	*Patient preparation:* Requires thorough explanations to patient/family regarding indications and expectations of the procedure (i.e., insertion site, warm flush feeling when contrast is injected, postprocedure care). • It is essential to establish if patient has had previous allergic reaction to contrast media or if the patient is allergic to iodine-containing foods or medications; or if patient is taking anticoagulant (is so, why?). • Patient should be well hydrated to facilitate elimination of dye via kidneys. *Postprocedure care:* Monitor every 15 to 30 minutes until stable; assess for bleeding, swelling, or redness at insertion site; assess extremity distal to insertion site for signs of altered circulation caused by vessel spasm or occlusion (skin color, temperature, and peripheral pulses). • Encourage fluids to flush out contrast media. • *Complications:* Arrhythmia, allergic reaction to contrast medium, bleeding at insertion site, infection. • Clinically, confirm presence of cerebrovascular abnormalities including aneurysm, arteriovenous malformations, vessel thrombosis, stenosis, or occlusion; alteration in blood flow characteristic of arteriovenous malformation, or associated with tumor; and vascular changes associated with hematoma formation, cyst, edema, herniation, and arterial spasm.

TABLE 28–6
Diagnostic Studies and Procedures for Neurologic Dysfunction (*Continued*)

Test	Description/Purpose	Clinical Significance/Nursing Implications
Digital subtraction angiography (DSA)	An invasive procedure that produces enhanced radiographic images of extracranial vasculature, including vessel size, patency, and degree of stenosis or occlusion. • Especially indicated in studies of carotid or renal artery disease, thrombotic or embolic disease of great vessels, and in detection of aneurysms and other vascular abnormalities. • Uses a computer system in combination with a fluoroscopy apparatus capable of intensifying images. • Computer converts images into digital form and "subtracts" data compiled on plain radiography from that compiled on contrast radiographs after injection of contrast dye.	See patient preparation above. Make necessary explanations regarding procedure; patient should understand the need to remain motionless while radiographs are being taken. • Ascertain history of previous contrast studies and any reaction to contrast dye used; or allergies to foods or drugs. What other medications is the patient taking and why? Patient should be well hydrated. *Post-procedure care and complications:* See cerebral angiography, above. *Note:* Intravenous rather than intra-arterial injection of contrast medium can be used.
Myelography	An invasive procedure involving injection of contrast dye or air via puncture into spinal subarachnoid space followed by fluoroscopic or serial radiographic study.	*Procedure and preparation:* See lumbar puncture; above. *Postprocedure care:* Depending on contrast medium used, the patient may be advised to lie flat or with head slightly elevated for several hours. If a water-soluble medium is used (e.g., metrizamide), the patient's head is elevated 30 degrees for about 8 h. The head elevation prevents the contrast medium from irritating the cerebral cortex. It is absorbed into the bloodstream and eventually excreted by the kidneys. • Clinically, reveals distortions of spinal cord, spinal meninges, or intervertebral disks. Used to detect suspected spinal lesions such as tumors, cysts, herniated disks, or other lesions that may partially or totally block CSF circulation.
Computed Tomography CT scan	This study may be noninvasive or invasive (intravenous injection of contrast medium). It permits rapid, detailed screening for hematomas or other traumatic lesions, with minimum exposure to radiation. • A computerized picture is derived from the scanning of successive layers by a narrow x-ray beam. It provides a cross-sectional view of the brain, distinguishing densities. Lesions appear as variations in tissue density, differing from normal tissue.	*Patient preparation:* Explain the purpose of the test, procedure involved, and expectations of the patient. It is important for the patient to remain motionless during the procedure. Sedation should be administered if necessary. • If contrast dye is to be injected, screen for possible allergies (drug or food). • Encourage fluids if contrast dye is used. • Clinically, CT scan plays a strategic role in the *initial* diagnosis of most intracranial or spinal abnormalities, including neoplastic or vascular lesions; intracerebral hemorrhage or hematoma formation; hydrocephalus; ventricular anomalies; brain infection; or abscess. Use of contrast dye helps to define abnormalities.
Nuclear Medicine Tests Brain scan	This study employs a technique involving the intravenous administration of a radionuclide. The gamma rays emitted by the radionuclide are then detected by a scanner, which converts them into images and displays them on a screen. • The final image reflects the uptake and distribution of the radionuclide. Any alteration in the blood-brain barrier enables the radionuclide to accumulate in the affected area. • This study assists in locating areas of ischemia, infarction, hematoma, intracerebral hemorrhage, and tumors. In these areas there is an increase in radionuclide uptake. • Evidence of brain abscess or infection is indicated by a decreased uptake of the radionuclide.	*Patient preparation:* Explain purpose of the test and procedure involved. Assure patient that the amount of radionuclide administered is small and that it has a very short half-life, so there is a minimal hazard of radiation. • Determine whether patient has any allergies. • Clinically, this study is used to locate intracranial masses, vascular lesions, brain abscess, or communicating low-pressure hydrocephalus. It may also confirm the presence of a CSF leak in basal skull fractures.

continued

TABLE 28–6
Diagnostic Studies and Procedures for Neurologic Dysfunction (*Continued*)

Test	Description/Purpose	Clinical Significance/Nursing Implications
Positron emission tomography (PET)	This technique maps the brain's metabolic activity produced by the interaction of an injected radioactively tagged biochemical (e.g., glucose or oxygen) and charged electrons in the brain. The biochemical is administered intravenously or via inhalation. A scanner detects the tissue uptake of the radioactive substance, and a computer produces a color composite indicating distribution of the radioactive material corrresponding to cellular metabolism and cerebral blood flow.	*Patient preparation:* Same as for brain scan, above. • Clinically, this study provides a measure of metabolism and cerebral blood flow; it may also detect structural abnormalities (e.g., vascular disorders, tumors); or it can be used to investigate behavioral abnormalities that have a possible physiologic basis (e.g., schizophrenia). • This study is unlike x-rays and CT scans in that it shows how the organ is functioning.
Magnetic resonance imaging (MRI)	A noninvasive procedure that provides greater tissue discrimination than CT scan without the risk of ionizing radiation. • This method uses radiofrequency irradiation in a strong magnetic field rather than x-rays. The patient is placed within a high magnetic field, which aligns protons of hydrogen nuclei in body cells. Following a burst of radiofrequency energy, the protons realign, and the resulting change in the magnetic field is processed by a computer. The image that is constructed is based on the fact that different types of nervous tissue emit energy at different frequencies.	*Patient preparation:* Explain purpose of test, procedure involved, and expectations of patient. • All metal objects must be removed from the patient's body; the procedure is contraindicated in patients with previous surgery where metal hemostatic or aneurysm clips were inserted. This test is contraindicated in patients with pacemakers and metal cardiac valves. • MRI is useful in evaluating cerebral edema, hemorrhage, infarction, bone lesions, blood vessels, and spinal disk herniation. • Risk factors for this new technique have not been demonstrated. • Clinically, this test may also be helpful in detecting small lesions or in differentiating between healthy and ischemic or infarcted tissues.
Neurophysiologic Tests Electroencephalogram (EEG)	In this study, electrodes applied to the scalp produce a graphic recording of the electrical impulses generated within the cerebral cortex. • This study is used to diagnose areas of abnormal electrical activity within the cerebral cortex. • EEG monitoring is increasingly being deployed intraoperatively during various neurosurgical procedures.	*Patient preparation:* Explain purpose of tests, procedure involved, and expectations of patient. Emphasize that the patient will not experience an electrical shock. • Patient's scalp should be clean and free of hairspray or creams. • If the procedure is done at bedside, electrical devices surrounding the patient should be removed, if possible, to minimize electrical interference. • Clinically, this procedure is helpful in the diagnosis and management of seizure disorders; localization of structural abnormalities (e.g., tumors, abscesses, vascular anomalies); and investigation of metabolic alterations and sleep disturbances. • This procedure is also used in organic brain syndrome, coma, and brain death to detect characteristic patterns of electrical activity or the absence of electrical activity.
Cortical evoked potentials	These studies measure the electrical potential or activity that occurs along specific neuronal pathways in response to visual, auditory, or somatosensory (tactile) stimuli. By measuring such potentials, the integrity of visual, auditory, and somatosensory pathways can be evaluated. • This technique uses a special device, which senses cerebral cortical electrical activity via surface electrodes attached to standard sites. These potentials, evoked in response to specific stimuli, are then intensified by a computer and graphically displayed for accurate measurement.	*Patient preparation:* Tests can be performed at patient's bedside on conscious or unconscious patients. If conscious, patients need to be instructed to remain motionless as much as possible to minimize interference of musculoskeletal-derived electrical potentials. Skin or hair should be clean and free of oils, creams, or hairspray. • Depending on modality being tested, the patient can expect to receive a series of stimuli, such as flashing lights or a pattern of identifiable shapes (visual), clicking sounds delivered to the ear (auditory), or electrical stimulation of the skin (tactile-somatosensory). • The patient should be assured that no electrical shock or pain will be experienced.

TABLE 28–6
Diagnostic Studies and Procedures for Neurologic Dysfunction (*Continued*)

Test	Description/Purpose	Clinical Significance/Nursing Implications
		Clinical use: • Visual evoked potentials (responses): Assist in evaluating post-traumatic injury. • Auditory evoked potentials (responses): Assist in localizing auditory lesions and evaluating the integrity of the brainstem and the sequential auditory pathways located therein; useful in diagnosing posterior fossa lesions and multiple sclerosis; helpful in determining the reversibility of coma. • Somatosensory evoked potentials (responses): Assist in diagnosing peripheral nerve disease and lesions in the brain and spinal cord (e.g., demyelinating disease). Recordings are made via surface electrodes placed on the scalp overlying somesthetic cortical area (i.e., post-central gyrus, parietal lobe). • All methods are useful in monitoring for neurologic injury before, during, and after surgery involving nerve tissue.
Electromyography (EMG)	This study records the electrical activity of select groups of muscles at rest and during voluntary contraction. It is useful in localizing lesions and differentiating primary disease of muscle fibers or neuromuscular junction from lower motor neuron disease. • The test is not definitive as to underlying disease but assists in determining approach to more specific diagnostic workup.	*Patient preparation:* Explain purpose of test, procedure, and expectations of the patient. Emphasize that the test is similar to an electrocardiogram except a needle will be inserted into specific muscle groups. • Clinically, EMG is a useful diagnostic technique in muscular dystrophies, amyotrophic lateral sclerosis, myasthenia gravis, and peripheral denervation conditions. To differentiate muscle disorder from denervation disorders, it is necessary for results of EMG studies to be correlated with patient's history, clinical status, and other neurologic tests.
Biophyiscal Studies Ultrasound studies	Ultrasound studies use the principle that sound waves are deflected at different speeds from structures with differing densities.	Transcranial Doppler ultrasonography is a diagnostic tool used to diagnose presence of increased intracranial pressure and vasospasm.
Doppler and B-scans	The most common forms of ultrasound studies used for neurodiagnostics • In Doppler scanning, the velocity of blood flow is measured from sound waves reflecting from red blood cells. Variations in velocity are interpreted as vessel narrowing or patency. • B-scans combine Doppler estimates of velocity with images created by differing deflection of ultrasound waves from structures in the neck and pulsations within the blood vessel (e.g., carotid artery). The result is an image that reflects the patency of the vessel.	*Patient preparation:* Ultrasound studies are noninvasive. A conductive jelly is applied and a transducer is placed on the patient's neck over the carotid artery.
Continuous Monitoring Techniques SjO_2 - Jugular oxygen saturation	Continuous monitoring of jugular O_2 saturation using a fiberoptic catheter inserted into the internal jugular vein is used to detect cerebral ischemia following acute head injury. • An improvement in cerebral blood flow and, thus, cerebral oxygen delivery can be determined by monitoring the difference in O_2 saturation in the systemic circulation (i.e., SaO_2–SrO_2) and the SjO_2.	*Patient preparation:* Patient should be advised that the procedure is invasive. A catheter is placed into the internal jugular vein.

continued

TABLE 28–6
Diagnostic Studies and Procedures for Neurologic Dysfunction (*Continued*)

Test	Description/Purpose	Clinical Significance/Nursing Implications
rSo_2 - Cerebral oximetry	This technique provides clinical data regarding brain perfusion, ischemia, and hypoxia. It uses noninvasive optical spectroscopy to target the cerebral vasculature. • Infrared light sensors, capable of penetrating scalp, bone, and brain tissue to a depth of several centimeters, are used.	*Patient preparation:* Patient is advised that the procedure is noninvasive. An adhesive sensor pad is placed on the forehead. Brain oximetry values are obtained when infrared-absorbing molecules in brain hemoglobin return a nonpulsatile signal from the cerebral vasculature.
Cerebral blood flow studies	Purpose is to measure cerebral blood flow, overall or regional, by calculating the transit time of a tracer substance. • Using a radioisotope tracer, this technique calculates transit time of blood from one region of the cerebral circulation to another. • Nitrous oxide can be used as a tracer for whole-brain blood flow studies. The time it takes for a systemic arterial blood sample to appear in the internal jugular venous circulation is measured by this technique. • Clinically, cerebral blood flow techniques have been limited because of bulky equipment and difficulty interpreting results. • Regional blood flow studies have largely been limited to large clinical research programs as they require elaborate detection equipment.	*Patient preparation:* Patient should be advised that the tracer will be injected intravenously into the carotid artery, or simply inhaled as it is when nitrous oxide is used as the tracer. The relative safety of the inhalation technique has resulted in wider usage. • Extracranial probes are affixed to the scalp to detect the transit time for blood flow between areas. The tracer is eventually exhaled by the lungs. • A computer records this process and depicts the changes graphically for interpretation. • Vital signs are taken prior to the procedure and a blood specimen is drawn. • The nurse should be alert for hematoma or embolus formation if intravenous technique is used; if inhalation technique is used, any pre-existing respiratory or cardiac problems that may affect data should be noted.

Decerebrate posturing carries with it a more ominous prognosis. Its appearance during the course of rostral-caudal (head-to-toe) deterioration in brain function may herald impending brain herniation.

In terms of documentation, it is more desirable to describe abnormal motor responses as abnormal flexor, abnormal extensor, or absent (flaccid), designating the specific limbs involved, rather than to use the terms "decorticate" or "decerebrate."

DIAGNOSTIC STUDIES AND TECHNIQUES

The diagnosis of neurologic dysfunction initiated with the patient's history and neurologic examination can be verified by sophisticated diagnostic studies and techniques. Digital subtraction angiography, positron emission tomography, nuclear magnetic resonance (magnetic resonance imaging), and electrophysiology studies are major advances in neurodiagnostic testing.

Healthcare professionals must familiarize themselves with these investigative techniques: What are they? How are they performed? What patient preparation is required? What is their clinical significance? Table 28–6 briefly summarizes new as well as precedent neurodiagnostic tests and procedures most commonly performed on critically ill patients with neurologic dysfunction and includes some implications for nursing care.

REFERENCES

1. Gordon, M: Nursing Diagnosis Process and Application, ed 3. C V Mosby, St. Louis, 1994.
2. Jones, C: Glasgow Coma Scale. Am J Nurs 79:1551, 1979.
3. Brown, JD: Acute disturbances of consciousness. In Sibbald, WJ (ed): Synopsis of Critical Care, ed 3. Williams & Wilkins, Baltimore, 1988, p 163.
4. Plum, F and Posner, J: The Diagnosis of Stupor and Coma, ed 3. FA Davis, Philadelphia, 1983, p 32.
5. Guyton, A: Textbook of Medical Physiology, ed 8. WB Saunders, Philadelphia, 1991, p 445.
6. Plum, F and Posner, J: The Diagnosis of Stupor and Coma, ed 3. FA Davis, Philadelphia, 1983, p 46.
7. Caine, RM: The cutting edge in neuroscience. Supplement to Critical Care Nurse, June 1993, p 6.

SUGGESTED READINGS

Bishop, BS: Pathologic pupillary signs: Self-learning module, II. Critical Care Nurse 11(7):58, 1991.
Boss, J: Cognitive systems: Nursing assessment and management in the critical care environment. AACN Clinical Issues in Critical Care Nursing 2(4):685, 1991.
Mason, PJ: Cognitive assessment parameters and tools for the critically injured adult. Critical Care Nursing Clinics of North America 1(1):45, 1989.
Mason, PJ: Neurodiagnostic testing in critically injured adults. Critical Care Nurse 12(6):64, 1992.
Stewart-Amidei, C: Assessing the comatose patient in the intensive care unit. AACN Clinical Issues in Critical Care Nursing 2(4):613, 1991.

CHAPTER 29

Clinical Management of Patients with Intracranial Pressure Monitoring: Intracranial Hypertension and Brain Herniation Syndromes

Joan T. Dolan

CHAPTER OUTLINE

Intracranial Pressure Monitoring
- Purpose and Clinical Significance
- Intracranial Volume-Pressure Relationships
- Uses of Intracranial Pressure Monitoring
- Indications for Intracranial Pressure Monitoring
- Signs and Symptoms of Increased Intracranial Pressure (Intracranial Hypertension)
- Methods for Measuring Intracranial Pressure
- Intracranial Pressure Monitoring Waveforms: Analysis and Interpretation

Consequences of Increased Intracranial Pressure: Brain Herniation
- Pathophysiology

- Brain Herniation: Supratentorial and Infratentorial

Herniation Syndromes and Brain Dysfunction
- Central Syndrome of Rostral-to-Caudal Deterioration in Brainstem Function
- Syndrome of Uncal Herniation—Lateral Brainstem Compression

Nursing Management of the Patient with Increased Intracranial Pressure
- Intracranial Pressure Monitoring: Maintaining the Integrity of the System
- Nursing Diagnoses, Desired Patient Outcomes, and Nursing Interventions/Rationales

References
Selected Readings

LEARNING OBJECTIVES

After completing this chapter, you should be able to:

1. State the purpose of intracranial pressure monitoring and indications for use.
2. Examine intracranial volume-pressure relationships and their clinical significance.
3. List clinical signs and symptoms of increased intracranial pressure.
4. Describe methods for measuring intracranial pressure.
5. Analyze and interpret intracranial pressure waveforms in terms of intracranial volume-pressure dynamics.
6. Describe pathophysiologic mechanisms underlying the phenomenon of brain herniation.
7. Distinguish supratentorial and infratentorial herniations.
8. Contrast brain dysfunction in central herniation syndrome with that in uncal herniation syndrome.
9. Incorporate underlying physiologic principles into the nursing management of the patient with increased intracranial pressure.
10. Delineate the nursing process in the management of the patient with an increase in intracranial pressure, including assessment, nursing diagnosis, and planning, with reference to desired patient outcomes and nursing interventions.

INTRACRANIAL PRESSURE MONITORING

Purpose and Clinical Significance

Intracranial pressure (ICP) is defined as the pressure within the intracranial cavity, which is exerted by the volumes of blood, cerebrospinal fluid (CSF), and brain tissue contained therein. It is significant because it affects cerebral perfusion pressure (CPP), the driving force underlying cerebral blood flow. As ICP rises, CPP falls, and cerebral blood flow is reduced. Through intracranial pressure monitoring (ICPM) changes in the status of intracranial pressure dynamics can be detected *early*, before such changes become otherwise clinically evident. Timely therapeutic interventions can be implemented and the patient's responses monitored, thereby preventing any rapid deterioration in the patient's neurologic condition.

Intracranial Volume-Pressure Relationships

To effectively monitor and manage the patient with, or at risk of developing, an increase in intracranial pressure (i.e., intracranial hypertension), one must appreciate the intracranial volume-pressure relationships that exist between the rigid, nearly inexpandable cranium (see Fig. 27–3) and the three fluid compartments contained therein, namely, brain tissue, cere-

brospinal fluid, and blood. As explained by the Monro-Kellie hypothesis, an increase in the volume of any one of these three substances requires a reciprocal adjustment in the volumes of one or both of the other two substances in order to maintain ICP within the normal range (0 to 15 mmHg).

The ability of the brain to tolerate increases in intracranial volume without an increase in pressure is referred to as *compliance.* When brain compliance is high, large volume changes can occur without a corresponding change in ICP. When brain compliance is low, even minute changes in volume may precipitate a dramatic rise in ICP (Fig. 29–1).

Several compensatory mechanisms contribute to effective brain compliance. These include an increase in CSF reabsorption via the arachnoid granulations (see Fig. 27–6) and displacement of CSF from the cranium into the subarachnoid space and central canal of the spinal cord. The consequent reduction in the intracranial volume of CSF in turn reduces ICP. A decrease in the production of CSF may also occur, although this may not be significant unless cerebral blood flow is compromised.[1]

Autoregulatory mechanisms involving metabolic factors contribute to brain compliance by redirecting blood flow from the cerebral circulation into the systemic vasculature (see Table 27–6). This occurs when vasoconstriction associated with hypocapnia, alkalemia, and arterial PaO_2 levels over 80 mmHg reduces intracerebral blood volume, resulting in a concomi-

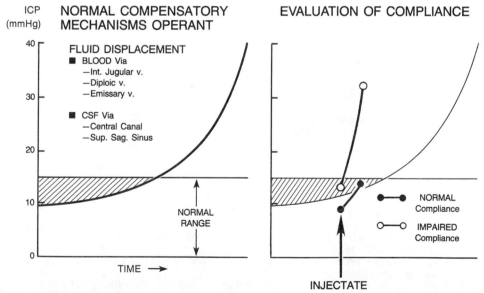

FIGURE 29–1. Intracranial volume-pressure curve. This curve relates changes in volume and pressure and reflects the degree of brain compressibility, or compliance. *(Left panel)* The normal intracranial volume-pressure curve reflects the presence of intact or operant compensatory mechanisms, thus maintaining intracranial pressure within the normal physiologic range (0 to 15 mmHg) in the face of changes in intracranial volume. *(Right panel)* Evaluation of brain compliance. When baseline intracranial pressure is within the normal range, a rise in intracranial pressure of 2 mmHg or less in response to the injectate (●—●) indicates compensatory mechanisms are operant (i.e., normal compliance); when the intracranial pressure baseline is initially high (○—○), a relatively small increase in volume (injectate) can cause potentially dangerous increases in intracranial pressure (i.e., impaired compliance). In this circumstance, compensatory mechanisms are impaired or no longer operant.

tant decrease in ICP. Vasoconstriction in response to hypocapnia is the rationale underlying use of hyperventilation therapy in the treatment of intracranial hypertension (see Chapter 30).

Hemodynamic factors also influence brain compliance and cerebral blood flow. To ensure a CPP of more than 60 mmHg, mean arterial blood pressure should be maintained at approximately 100 mmHg. Autoregulatory mechanisms maintain ICP over a wide range of mean arterial pressures (60 to 150 mmHg). At high systemic arterial blood pressures, cerebral vasoconstriction occurs and reduces cerebral blood flow; at lower pressures, cerebral vasodilation occurs to enhance cerebral blood flow. When mean arterial pressures are greater than 150 mmHg or less than 60 mmHg, loss of these autoregulatory mechanisms begins to occur.

Intracranial pressure remains nearly constant as long as the volume of CSF and/or blood displaced from the cranium vault is nearly equal to the volume of tissue or fluid added to the intracranial compartment. Eventually, if the volume added to the intracranial compartment exceeds the volume of fluid that can be displaced, ICP rises.

Volume-Pressure Curve

The volume-pressure curve relates changes in volume and pressure (see Fig. 29–1). As the intracranial volume increases (in the initial stage), intracranial pressure remains within the normal physiologic limits (i.e., 0 to 15 mmHg) because normal compensatory mechanisms (i.e., displacement of cerebrospinal fluid and blood) are operant, that is, intact and functioning (gradual slope of curve). The brain, however, has only a small capacity for compensation. When a rapidly expanding volume within the cranial vault (e.g., cerebral hemorrhage) becomes greater than that volume displaced from the vault, the compensatory mechanisms normally operant are exceeded and intracranial pressure rises (steep slope of curve). If intracranial pressure is already elevated and compensatory mechanisms are compromised, a relatively minor increase in intracranial volume can precipitate a major rise in intracranial pressure (see Fig. 29–1).

Knowledge of intracranial volume-pressure relationships and compliance is crucial to patient management. The ultimate concern is to maintain CPP within a range that ensures adequate cerebral blood flow. CPP is determined from the difference between the mean arterial pressure (MAP) and the ICP: CPP = MAP − ICP. For cerebral blood flow to be adequate, the acceptable range for CPP is 60 to 90 mmHg.

In the damaged brain, the cerebral perfusion pressure at which cerebral circulation is impaired is not so easily determined. Furthermore, depending on the underlying pathology, variations in cerebral perfusion pressure may occur from one region of the brain to the next. Techniques for evaluating the effects and treatment of ICP on cerebral blood flow are currently being investigated.[2,3] These include bedside cerebral blood flow studies, cerebral oximetry, and use of transcranial Doppler ultrasonography (see section on biophysical studies in Table 28–6).

Uses of Intracranial Pressure Monitoring

Continuous ICPM is used to facilitate (1) early diagnosis via the assessment of intracranial pressure dynamics and (2) treatment, including timely initiation of pressure-reducing measures and evaluation of the patient's response to these therapeutic measures. Timely intervention afforded by ICPM may improve prognosis as reflected by retained and potential function and reduced residual sequelae.

ICPM serves as a guide for nursing care so that sudden rises in ICP can be prevented. Various procedures (e.g., suctioning, bathing, and so forth) can be scheduled at different times so the patient is not harmed by their cumulative effects. ICPM provides the only reliable means to determine, early in the course, the presence and degree of ICP. When used in conjunction with the clinical assessment and results from noninvasive and invasive diagnostic techniques (see Table 28–6), ICPM is invaluable.

Indications for Intracranial Pressure Monitoring

Intracranial pressure monitoring is indicated for the patient who has, or is at risk of developing, an increase in ICP. Whenever a change is anticipated in intracranial volume, be it brain mass (e.g., cerebral edema or space-occupying lesions), blood (e.g., bleeding with associated head trauma, cerebral hemorrhage), or CSF (e.g., overproduction or decreased reabsorption), ICPM is indicated. Of paramount importance is the ability of ICPM to help prevent or avert the occurrence of catastrophic secondary effects (e.g., ischemia, injury, infarction, or development of cerebral edema) in what, at the onset, appeared to be an innocuous, benign, primary insult.

Brain Hyperemia

Brain hyperemia, that is, an excess of blood in the cerebral vasculature, occurs as a result of a disruption in autoregulatory mechanisms (see Table 27–6). Normally, autoregulatory mechanisms maintain ICP over a wide range of mean arterial pressures (60 to 150 mmHg). For example, as systemic pressure decreases, cerebral vasodilation occurs to enhance cerebral blood flow; at high systemic pressures, cerebral vasoconstriction occurs to prevent an increase in cerebral perfusion. When these mechanisms are disrupted, the ability of cerebral blood vessels to adjust to variable systemic blood pressures is lost, and cerebral blood flow becomes passively dependent on systemic blood pressures. Under these circumstances, high systemic blood pressures cause an increase in cerebral blood flow and intravascular blood volume, exceeding the amount required for metabolism. This results in a rise in ICP. Brain hyperemia occurs in the initial hours after acute head injury or after craniotomy surgery involving manipulation of cerebral blood vessels.

Cerebral Edema

Cerebral edema is one of the major causes of increased ICP. It represents a net increase in the water content of brain tissue, either within the cells (intracellular) or surrounding the cells (extracellular). Cerebral edema results from direct traumatic or penetrating injury to the brain tissue, or from massive tissue damage, such as might occur in cerebral infarction. Secondarily, cerebral edema may be precipitated by underlying pathophysiologic processes including ischemia, anoxia, and hypercapnia. Three types of cerebral edema have been described: vasogenic, cytotoxic, and interstitial.

Vasogenic Edema. Vasogenic edema is the most common. It is essentially an *extra*cellular edema, which results from disruption of the blood-brain barrier. Normally, the highly selective blood-brain barrier enables the internal environment within the brain to be closely regulated (see Fig. 27–9). It is readily permeable to water, small molecules, and lipid-soluble substances but prevents larger molecules, including plasma proteins, from entering into the brain's interstitial spaces. When the blood-brain barrier is disrupted, these proteins and other molecules are allowed access to the brain's interstitium and are followed by an influx of water. The end result is an increase in the water content within the brain tissue. Vasogenic edema may be caused by trauma, ischemia, tumor, infection, or brain abscess.

Cytotoxic Edema. Cytotoxic edema is *intra*cellular, with fluid accumulating within cells. The underlying pathophysiologic mechanism is thought to involve alterations in ionic transport mechanisms within cellular membranes. Inhibition of the sodium-potassium-ATPase (Na^+-K^+) pump may be involved, so that potassium leaves the cell, while sodium, chloride, and water enter it and cause the cell to swell. Failure of the Na^+-K^+ pump is a primary consideration in the presence of hypoxia and ischemia. Conditions that cause brain hypoxia and/or ischemia (e.g., trauma, cerebral hemorrhage), as well as hypo-osmolar states, may predispose to cytotoxic edema.

Interstitial (Hydrocephalic) Edema. Interstitial or hydrocephalic edema is a long-term consequence of obstructive hydrocephalus (i.e., a condition marked by excessive accumulation of fluid within the brain). An obstruction to the flow of CSF within the ventricular system causes a buildup of CSF pressure, resulting in transudation of CSF through the ependymal layer into the periventricular white matter. The location of the edema fluid is *extra*cellular. Infection, cerebral aneu-

rysm rupture, and brain tumor, among others, may predispose to interstitial edema.

The pathophysiologic effects of cerebral edema result primarily from an increase in ICP. The clinical presentation of cerebral edema may be profound (i.e., reflects significant disruption of intracranial pressure dynamics) and depends on the rapidity of formation and the extent to which brain tissues are involved.

Signs and Symptoms of Increased Intracranial Pressure (Intracranial Hypertension)

An increase in ICP may have adverse effects on cerebral structures and function. These include the mechanical deformation or shift of cerebral contents within the confines of the cranial vault and an alteration in cerebral blood flow. The end result may be a decrease in CPP leading to ischemia and an alteration in cellular metabolism. Clinically, these changes are demonstrated by the appearance of a wide range of neurologic deficits, as well as by systemic changes within the body as a whole.

Generalized signs and symptoms of increased ICP may include changes in the level of consciousness, memory loss, or alterations in thought processes. Nonspecific changes may include headache, nausea, vomiting, and diplopia (i.e., double vision). The patient may experience sensory loss and paresthesias; alterations in motor function may be exhibited by the presence of paresis or paralysis. Changes in pupillary size and reactivity, alterations in body temperature, and seizures may also become evident. In some cases, papilledema (i.e., edema of the optic disk) may be the only neurologic sign of underlying pathophysiology until ICP rises high enough to impair cerebral blood flow.

When signs and symptoms occur, they usually do so only after pathologic changes. Their appearance does not definitively reflect the magnitude of the pressure elevation. In a patient at risk for intracranial hypertension, the only reliable means to determine whether it is present is to measure ICP continuously.

In addition to its effect on brain metabolism and function, intracranial hypertension has been implicated in the dysfunction of other major organ systems. Gastrointestinal bleeding in conjunction with intracranial pathology is common. Ulcerations may result from an increase in hydrochloric acid secretion and/or disruption in the integrity of the gastric mucosal barrier.

Changes in cardiopulmonary function associated with intracranial hypertension may include a variety of electrocardiographic abnormalities (e.g., T-wave changes, ST-segment elevation or depression, or the appearance of Q waves), as well as the appearance of cardiac arrhythmias (e.g., bradycardia, atrial fibrillation). These changes have been associated with metabolic disturbances (e.g., hypercapnia, hypoxemia, hypokalemia) and with altered autonomic function (i.e., sympathetic and parasympathetic function). Specific vasomotor reactions occurring in response to severely elevated ICP have been identified. The classic Cushing triad consists of elevated systolic blood pressure with widening pulse pressure (i.e., the difference between systolic and diastolic pressures), bradycardia, and altered respiratory rate and rhythm. These are late signs, which usually reflect the presence of irreversible brain pathology, and their appearance signals a grave prognosis.

Methods for Measuring Intracranial Pressure

In ICPM, the mechanical pressure waves or pulsations of freely circulating CSF are converted into electrical impulses via a sensor or transducer. These electrical impulses, in turn, are converted into visual waveforms and digital read-outs by an oscilloscope or chart recorder.

Theoretically, because pressure exerted by fluids is distributed equally in all directions, measurement of cerebrospinal fluid is considered to be an acceptable indicator of overall intracranial pressure. It should be appreciated, however, that pressure gradients may exist between intracranial compartments, and in these cases, the pressure of cerebrospinal fluid may not accurately reflect overall intracranial pressure. ICPM can only be employed effectively if CSF is circulating freely from one intracranial compartment to the next.

Four techniques are employed for measuring ICP: (1) intraventricular, (2) subarachnoid, (3) epidural, and (4) intracerebral (intraparenchymal) (Fig. 29–2). Strict aseptic technique is mandatory during insertion and maintenance of all forms of ICPM. A continuous fluid flush device is not used for ICPM because the addition of even a small amount of fluid into the system can cause potentially dangerous increases in ICP, especially when brain compliance is decreased. The duration of ICP monitoring is approximately 3 to 5 days. Refer to Table 29–1 for a summary of the methods used in intracranial pressure monitoring, including advantages, disadvantages, and nursing considerations.

Intraventricular Method

The intraventricular method of ICPM uses a catheter, which is introduced via a burr hole in the skull and placed within the anterior (most commonly) or occipital horn of the lateral ventricle in the nondominant hemisphere (see Fig. 29–2A). The catheter is connected to the transducer via stopcocks and pressure tubing. Sterile normal saline without preservative or lactated Ringer's solution is used as the fluid column between CSF and the diaphragm of the transducer dome. Alternatively, a disposable fiberoptic transducer-tipped catheter may be placed in the ventricle. This eliminates the need for the fluid column required with external transducers. A key advantage of the intraventricular approach is that it affords direct access to CSF for purposes of diagnostic tests, administration of medication, and drainage of CSF.

The venting port of the standard-size transducer is positioned at the level of the foramen of Monro (see Figs. 27–5 and 27–6). External landmarks used to ensure correct positioning are the edge of the eyebrow and tragus of the ear (i.e., the cartilaginous projection just anterior to the external meatus of the ear). Proper positioning is critical. For every 1 inch of discrepancy between the level of the transducer and the pressure source, there is an error of about 2 mmHg.

Subarachnoid Method

The subarachnoid method uses a subarachnoid screw, which is inserted via a twist-drill or burr hole and placed so that the tip rests in the subarachnoid space (Fig. 29–2B). The cerebrum is not penetrated, and pressures are measured directly from the cerebrospinal fluid. The transducer may be attached directly to the stopcock on the screw or connected via pressure tubing. Subarachnoid pressures usually correlate well with intraventricular pressures.

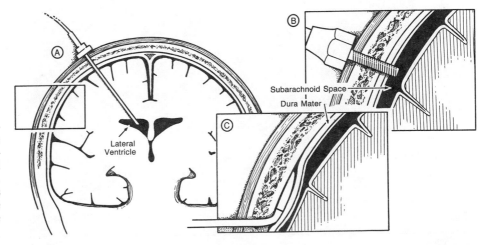

FIGURE 29–2. Methods employed in intracranial pressure monitoring. (*A*) Intraventricular method. (*B*) Subarachnoid method. (*C*) Epidural method. The intraventricular method is the most invasive and has the highest infection rate of all three approaches.

TABLE 29–1
Summary of Methods Used in Intracranial Pressure Monitoring

Method	Advantages	Disadvantages	Nursing Considerations

Ventricular
Catheter in anterior or occipital horns of lateral ventricle (anterior horn most commonly used).
	1. Direct ICP measurement
	2. Most accurate method
	3. Direct access to CSF to:
	  a. Obtain sample of CSF for analysis
	  b. Drain off CSF to reduce ICP
	4. Access to determine volume-pressure response (compliance)
	5. Access for instillation of drugs
		1. Complexity of insertion if ventricles are:
		  a. Small in size
		  b. Shifted or compressed
		2. Risk of infection
		3. Leakage of CSF
		4. Hemorrhage as catheter is placed through brain tissue
			1. Use baseline position for level of transducer to obtain consistent data.
			  a. Venting port of transducer positioned at level of foramen of Monro.
			    1) External landmarks include edge of eyebrow or tragus of ear.
			  b. All stopcocks must be in accurate position to avoid excessive drainage of CSF and sudden drop in ICP.
			    1) For each inch of discrepancy between level of transducer and pressure source, there is an error of 2 mmHg in ICP reading.
			  c. Recalibrate the transducer and monitoring equipment as indicated.
			  d. Assess catheter patency frequently. A dampened waveform may be produced if there is compression of the catheter tip by the ventricular walls or blood in the CSF. If catheter becomes obstructed, notify physician (as per hospital protocol).
			  e. Observe for any sudden changes in ICP.
			2. Correlate ICP data with total assessment of patient. Remember ICPM is another assessment technique. It is only significant when evaluated in terms of the status of the whole patient.
			3. Monitor closely for infection with this most invasive ICPM approach.
			4. Expect catheter placement to be difficult if brain is shifted or the ventricles are small or compressed. ICPM must be done in conjunction with CAT scanning.
			5. Avoid taking pressure measurements when the patient is moving, coughing, using abdominal muscle to

TABLE 29–1

Summary of Methods Used in Intracranial Pressure Monitoring (*Continued*)

Method	Advantages	Disadvantages	Nursing Considerations
			breath, or has his/her head turned to one side. These activities may cause ICP to increase.
Subarachnoid Screw is placed in subarachnoid space through burr hole in skull. Transducer may be attached directly to the screw or connected via pressure tubing in the manner described for the venticular method.	1. Direct ICP measurement 2. Access to evaluate volume-pressure response (compliance) 3. Ease and speed of insertion. 4. Lower risk of infection than in ventricular monitoring	1. Risk of infection 2. Inaccurate measurements if screw becomes occluded with brain tissue, meninges, or bone fragments from drilled burr hole 3. Unable to instill contrast medium 4. Intact skull required (no fractures) 5. Leakage of CSF	1. If waveform wanders from baseline, assess patency of screw. If screw becomes occluded, notify physician. 2. Recalibrate transducer/ monitor as indicated. 3. Monitor for signs of infection and signs of meningeal irritation (see Chap. 28).
Epidural 1. Epidural placement of a tiny balloon with radioisotopes or radiotransmitters in the epidural space via burr hole in the skull. 2. Epidural fiberoptic sensing device directly connected to bedside monitor. 3. Completely implantable epidural transducer— potential for telemetric monitoring.	1. Easily and quickly inserted into epidural space 2. Less invasive; dura is not penetrated 3. No uncontrolled loss of CSF 4. No alterations of pressure monitoring due to plugging or obstruction of sensing device 5. No insertion difficulties related to ventricular size, compression, and displacement 6. Allows greater mobility: transporting patients is easier 7. Allows for long-term use (10 to 14 days) or as long as the dura remains intact	1. Accuracy of epidural pressure monitoring questioned 2. No access for sampling or drainage of CSF 3. Cannot be recalibrated if environmental factors change 4. Inaccurate pressure readings if the dura is compressed, is thickened, or has an increased surface tension	1. Check to ensure connecting tube is inserted properly into bedside monitor. 2. Calibrate prior to insertion; discard sensor or transducer if read-outs are inaccurate.
Intracerebral (Intraparenchymal) Disposable fiberoptic transducer-tipped catheter is inserted through a subarachnoid bolt and advanced several centimeters into the white matter of the brain.	1. Accurate; correlates well with ventricular pressures 2. Easily inserted 3. Eliminates need for leveling or maintaining a fluid connection 4. Reduces risk of infection 5. Minimizes artifact, leaks, drifts 6. Requires no calibration	1. No route for CSF sampling or drainage 2. Unable to zero or calibrate after insertion 3. Catheter fragility; easily broken with bending or manipulation 4. Separate monitoring system required	1. This method provides a means of obtaining ICP recordings in patients with compressed or dislocated ventricles. 2. Mean ICP is continuously displayed on portable monitor that interfaces with a standard monitoring system for oscilloscopic display and printout of ICP waveforms and readings. 3. When a fiberoptic system is being used, it is important to prevent kinking or bending of the fiberoptic catheter.

Epidural Method

The epidural method of ICPM involves placement of an epidural device, such as a balloon with radioisotopes, a radio transmitter, or a fiberoptic transducer, between the skull and the dura (Fig. 29–2C). Unlike intraventricular and subarachnoid pressures, which correlate well with each other, there have been inconsistent correlations between cerebrospinal pressure and pressure measurements using various epidural methods.

Intracerebral (Intraparenchymal) Method

The intracerebral (intraparenchymal) approach uses a disposable fiberoptic transducer-tipped catheter, which is inserted through a small subarachnoid bolt and advanced several centimeters into the white substance of the brain. The intraparenchymal method provides a means of obtaining ICP measurements in patients whose ventricles may be compressed or dislocated. Pressures within brain tissue have been found to correlate well with ventricular pressures.

Intracranial Pressure Monitoring Waveforms: Analysis and Interpretation

ICPM reflects the status of intracranial pressure dynamics, which fluctuate continuously. ICP is routinely monitored as *mean* pressure, although systolic and diastolic pressures should be noted. Normal ICP ranges from 0 to 15 mmHg, with less than 10 mmHg being ideal and 15 mmHg reflecting the upper limit. Activities involving coughing and straining (e.g., Valsalva's maneuver) may increase ICP momentarily to as high as MAP, that is, approximately 100 mmHg. In a person with intact compensatory mechanisms, such fluctuations in pressure are well tolerated. In the acutely ill patient, symptoms may appear at pressures of 20 to 25 mmHg. This is in sharp contrast to the clinical circumstance with certain brain tumors, in which increases in ICP, occurring gradually over time, are better tolerated.

Intracranial Pressure Waveforms

The ICP waveform provides an index of intracranial pressure dynamics. The characteristics of the ICP waveforms vary depending on the method of ICPM employed and on the pathophysiology underlying the patient's condition. Because of the close proximity of circulating CSF to arterial pulsations in the cerebral vasculature, hemodynamic oscillations can be observed in ICP monitoring traces to varying degrees. At times, the waveforms resemble an arterial pressure waveform; at other times, they may resemble a central venous pressure waveform.

Abnormal Intracranial Pressure Waveforms

A waves, also called *plateau* waves because of their distinctive pattern (Fig. 29–3), are the most clinically significant waveforms. They are associated with cerebral ischemia and indicate a decreased brain compliance. The appearance of plateau waves may be sudden, paroxysmal, and transient; they usually occur in patients whose baseline ICP is elevated (>15 to 20 mmHg). *A* waves may reflect pressures between 50 and 100 mmHg, occurring at varying intervals. These increases in pressure last from 5 to 20 minutes.

The appearance of *A* waves is usually accompanied by an increase in neurologic deficits, which may resolve when ICP returns to the patient's baseline. These include alterations in the level of consciousness and in respiratory rate and pattern; headache, nausea, and vomiting (projectile); altered pupillary responses; altered motor responses (e.g., paresis, decorticate and decerebrate posturing), and changes in vital signs (i.e., blood pressure and heart rate), although these latter signs are not always a consistent finding.

A waves have been well correlated physiologically

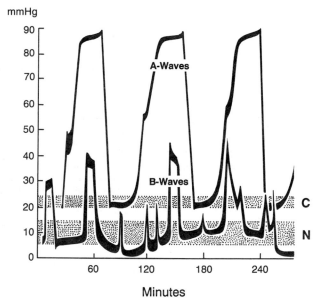

FIGURE 29–3. Intracranial pressure waveforms. Waveforms reflect pressure in mmHg and time in minutes. Two abnormal waveforms are depicted, including *A* waves and *B* waves. *A* waves reflect intracranial pressure in the range of 50 to 100 mmHg. They have a duration of 5 to 20 minutes or longer. Their waveforms have a distinctive plateau and they are referred to as "plateau" waves. *B* waves occur as sharp, peaked (sawtooth pattern), rhythmic oscillations, which may reach a peak pressure of 50 mmHg. They have a duration of ½ to 2 minutes. N refers to "normal" intracranial pressure waveforms and reflects a pressure within the range of 0 to 15 mmHg. C refers to the pressure waveform for *C* waves. *C* waves are usually rapid, rhythmic waves with an amplitude of about 20 mmHg. They occur every 4 to 8 minutes.

with the later stages of prolonged intracranial hypertension, which predisposes to cerebral ischemia, cellular hypoxia, and possibly infarction accompanied by necrosis of selected tissues. Their appearance signals that compensatory and autoregulatory mechanisms are no longer successful in controlling ICP. This loss of brain compliance resulting in elevated, sustained plateau waves is an ominous sign, and aggressive therapy needs to be provided on an emergency basis.

B waves occur as sharp, peaked (sawtooth pattern), rhythmic oscillations, which reach an amplitude of as much as 50 mmHg and may occur as frequently as every 30 seconds to 2 minutes (see Fig. 29–3). The elevated pressures are not sustained, and the rhythmic fluctuations appear to reflect respiratory and cardiovascular dynamics. A decreased arousal or wakefulness state appears to be associated with the occurrence of *B* waves. Clinically, their appearance suggests a decrease in intracranial compliance and may signal that the patient's condition is deteriorating.

C waves, also known as Traube-Hering waves, are rapid, rhythmic waves with pressures of up to 20 mmHg, occurring every 4 to 8 minutes. These waveforms reflect respiratory and cardiovascular dynamics. Their appearance may indicate severe intracranial compression.

CONSEQUENCES OF INCREASED INTRACRANIAL PRESSURE: BRAIN HERNIATION

Brain herniation refers to the shifting of intracranial structures from a compartment of high pressure to one of lower pressure. It is most commonly associated with craniocerebral trauma and usually requires emergency treatment to avert an increase in ICP and consequent decrease in CPP and cerebral blood flow.

Pathophysiology

Pathophysiologic mechanisms underlying the evolution of brain herniation are described as occurring at three stages: primary, secondary, and tertiary. The primary stage involves the actual mechanical injury or insult to brain tissue and/or its connective support systems. The secondary stage reflects pathology to brain tissue occurring as an indirect result of the primary insult and commonly involves intracerebral hemorrhage, hematoma formation, and cerebral edema. The tertiary stage involves the loss of autoregulatory and compensatory mechanisms and brain compliance, resulting in an increase in ICP.

As ICP rises, the cerebral vasculature becomes compressed, impairing blood flow. This predisposes to cerebral ischemia, cellular hypoxia, and cerebral edema, and a vicious cycle leading to herniation with infarction and necrosis of brain tissue is perpetuated (Fig. 29–4). If timely and aggressive pressure-reducing measures are not initiated, the patient will die.

Brain Herniation: Supratentorial and Infratentorial

Structurally, the cranial vault can be divided into two compartments separated by the dural fold, the tentorium (see Fig. 29–6). The supratentorial compartment is located above the tentorium. It consists of the anterior and middle fossae (see Fig. 27–3), which house the cerebral hemispheres, basal ganglia, and diencephalon (see Fig. 27–10). In the infratentorial compartment below the tentorium lies the posterior fossa, which contains the cerebellum and remaining brainstem (see Fig. 27–3 and Fig. 27–10). These two compartments are continuous with one another at the tentorial notch, or opening in the tentorium, which accommodates the brainstem.

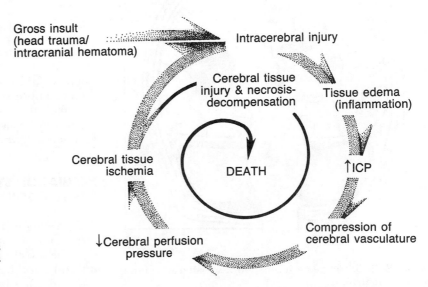

FIGURE 29–4. Pathophysiologic events leading to cerebral tissue necrosis, decompensation, and death.

Supratentorial Herniations

There are three patterns of supratentorial herniation: cingulate, central or transtentorial, and uncal. In each case, the significance of supratentorial shifts and displacements is that they compress blood vessels and brain parenchyma, causing cerebral ischemia and edema. This, in turn, further increases ICP.

Cingulate Herniation. Cingulate herniation describes an expanding hemispheric lesion that shifts medially across the midline, forcing the cingulate gyrus under the falx cerebri (Fig. 29–5). Shifting of the falx can cause compression and displacement of the great vein and branches of the ipsilateral (i.e., same side) anterior cerebral artery. This results in disruption of cerebral blood flow to the medial aspects of the cerebral hemisphere.

Central, or Transtentorial, Herniation. Central, or transtentorial, herniation is characterized by a rostral-to-caudal (i.e., head-to-toe) progression of events wherein a downward displacement of the cerebral hemispheres and basal ganglia compresses the diencephalon and eventually displaces the upper brainstem and midbrain through the tentorial notch (Fig. 29–6).

In the course of these events, other structures at the tentorial notch may be compromised. These include the oculomotor nerve (III), the posterior cerebral artery, the aqueduct of Sylvius, and subarachnoid space. Compression of these structures can, respectively, disrupt pupillary size and reactivity, cause ischemia and infarction of the occipital lobe, and interfere with the circulation and absorption of CSF. Such pathophysiologic changes underlie clinical clues as to the level of brainstem function. For example, compression of the oculomotor nerve (III) at the midbrain

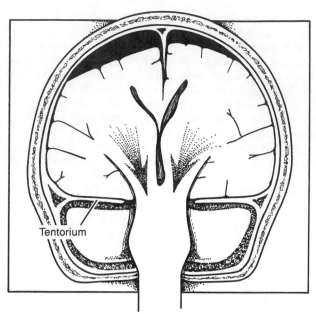

FIGURE 29–6. Central, or transtentorial, herniation associated with a subdural hematoma.

is manifested by a disruption of pupillary light reflexes. This is so because the oculomotor nerve carries parasympathetic innervation to the orbits. In this way a continuing increase in ICP reflects the brain's compromised compensatory mechanisms and reduced compliance.

Uncal Herniation. Uncal herniation is most commonly associated with an expanding lesion of the lateral middle fossa, which causes the basal medial edge, or uncus, of the temporal lobe to be forced down into the tentorial notch (Fig. 29–7). As the swollen uncus protrudes into the notch, it impinges on the oculomotor nerve and posterior cerebral artery. Lateral displacement of the diencephalon and midbrain to the side opposite that of the uncal herniation may also occur.

Infratentorial Herniations

Lesions occurring below the tentorium in the posterior fossa involve the cerebellum and lower brainstem. Underlying pathologic mechanisms include direct compression of the lower brainstem (pons and medulla), upward transtentorial herniation with midbrain compression, and downward herniation into the foramen magnum.

HERNIATION SYNDROMES AND BRAIN DYSFUNCTION

To distinguish the course of one type of supratentorial mass lesion from another, Plum and Posner[4] describe two clinically distinct syndromes, namely, *central* and *uncal* herniation syndromes. Although these two syndromes may be clinically distinct early in their

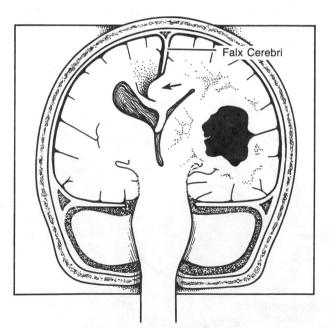

FIGURE 29–5. Cingulate herniation associated with intracerebral hematoma.

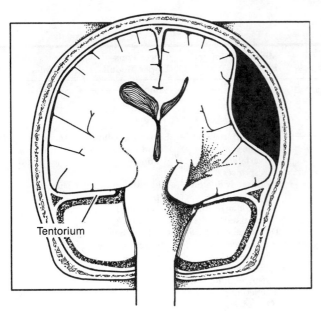

FIGURE 29–7. Uncal herniation associated with an epidural hematoma.

pathologic progression, once there is involvement of the midbrain–upper pons, their clinical pictures merge (i.e., the clinical signs of progressive uncal herniation become indistinguishable from those of central herniation syndrome).

The clinical manifestations of brain dysfunction are reflected by changes in the following parameters: level of consciousness and mentation, respiratory rate and pattern, pupillary size and reactivity, ocular movements, oculocephalic and oculovestibular reflexes, and sensorimotor responses. In the scenario of increased ICP and brain herniation, each of these parameters is described as occurring in four stages: early diencephalic, late diencephalic, midbrain–upper pons, and lower pons–upper medulla.

Central Syndrome of Rostral-to-Caudal Deterioration in Brainstem Function

The *earliest* clinical sign of the central syndrome of rostral-to-caudal deterioration in brainstem function is an *alteration in the level of consciousness*. This occurs during the early diencephalic stage (Table 29–2). As the level of brainstem function deteriorates to the late diencephalic stage, the patient becomes stuporous and eventually slips into a coma at the midbrain stage.

Referring to Table 29–2, the respiratory pattern can be seen to be eupneic during the early diencephalic stage, with perhaps an occasional deep sigh or yawn. A Cheyne-Stokes pattern of respirations may be seen at the late diencephalic stage, progressing to central neurogenic hyperventilation characteristic of the midbrain–upper pons stage (see Fig. 28–5).

Pupils initially are pinpoint but reactive during the

diencephalic stages. When the deterioration of brainstem function reaches the midbrain, pupils become moderately dilated, irregularly shaped, and unreactive (fixed) (see Fig. 28–5).

Roving ocular movements may vary from conjugate (movement of both eyes together) to dysconjugate (movement of eyes separately in different directions) during the late diencephalic stage. Oculocephalic and oculovestibular reflexes usually remain intact until the midbrain–upper pons stage. At this level the oculocephalic reflexes (doll's eye maneuver) may be abnormal or absent. (See the section on ocular movements in Chapter 28.) Oculocephalic reflexes, which reflect brainstem function, are commonly used in determining brain death. Oculovestibular reflexes are preserved somewhat longer than the oculocephalic reflexes (see Fig. 28–6).

Assessment of motor responses initially may reveal contralateral hemiparesis or hemiplegia during the diencephalic stage. This may progress to abnormal flexor (decorticate) and abnormal extensor (decerebrate) responses with progressive downward deterioration in brainstem function. Eventually, no motor response is elicited, and the extremities remain flaccid.

Syndrome of Uncal Herniation— Lateral Brainstem Compression

The syndrome of uncal herniation characterized by lateral brainstem compression (see Fig. 29–7) has an initial presentation different from that of the central syndrome (Table 29–3). The earliest sign of brain dysfunction involves changes in the level of consciousness. Associated with changes in the level of consciousness, characteristically, is the presence of a *unilateral dilated*, or *"blown," pupil* (see Fig. 28–5). Function of the diencephalon may be spared, at least initially, and it is possible that some patients may present with a "blown" pupil and still remain arousable and aware. Other than an altered state of consciousness, the dilated, sluggishly reactive pupil may be the only sign that pathology exists at the level of the midbrain in the progression of uncal herniation. Respirations may be eupneic, ocular reflexes may remain intact, and motor responses are usually appropriate.

The major concern regarding uncal herniation is that once the pupil "blows," the course of brainstem compression proceeds rapidly, and function deteriorates precipitously. The patient may progress from a state of consciousness to one of deep coma within minutes to several hours. The respiratory pattern may progress to sustained regular hyperventilation. Oculocephalic and oculovestibular reflexes become sluggish and impaired, and eventually disappear. Motor function progresses from purposeful movement to ipsilateral hemiplegia, eventually to assume abnormal flexor and abnormal extensor responses, described in central herniation syndrome. It is at this point that the clinical signs of central and uncal herniation syn-

TABLE 29–2

The Central Syndrome of Rostral-to-Caudal Deterioration

Clinical Signs	Early Diencephalon	Late Diencephalon	Midbrain–Upper Pons	Lower Pons–Upper Medulla	Medulla
Level of consciousness	Difficulty in concentration, loss of memory of recent events; agitation; drowsiness	Stupor → Coma →	Deep coma ——→	Same ——→	Same
Respiratory pattern	Eupneic, deep sighs, yawns →	Cheyne-Stokes ——→	Sustained, regular hyperventilation (variable responses) →	Eupneic, shallow,→ and rapid (>20/ min)	Ataxic (irregular in rate and amplitude)
Pupillary size and reactivity	Bilateral small and reactive → (requires close scrutiny with bright light); pupil size 1 to 3 mm	Same ——→	Moderately dilated (3 to 5 mm); irregular in shape and fixed	Mid-position, pin-point (<3 mm), and fixed	Dilated and fixed
Oculocephalic/ oculovestibular responses	Conjugate or slightly divergent roving eye movements	→ Same, with impairment of upper conjugate gaze	Doll's eye maneuver impaired (eyes move in the direction the head is turned; may be dysconjugate)	Oculocephalic → reflexes, no response	Absent
	Doll's eye manuever Full conjugate lateral gaze *opposite* to direction of turning	→ Same, but easier to obtain	(Oculovestibular reflexes are preserved somewhat longer than oculocephalic reflexes.)		
Motor responses	Bilateral signs of corticospinal and extrapyramidal dysfunction				
	Contralateral hemiparesis → or hemiplegia	Same, with addition of ipsilateral rigidity (paratonic resistance)	Usually motionless; extension of both arms and legs, particularly on side opposite to primary lesion	No purposeful movement; or possible flexor response in lower extremity to noxious stimuli	Flaccid
	Purposeful response to → noxious stimuli	Legs extended, arms rigidly flexed			Terminal stage
Babinski's sign	Absent	Bilateral	Bilateral extensor plantar responses		

dromes become indistinguishable. Often, signs of both syndromes are reflected in the same patient.

Familiarity with the clinical manifestations reflective of underlying brainstem pathology is essential to: (1) evaluate the level of brainstem function and potential threat to vital respiratory and vasomotor centers, (2) determine the direction in which the pathologic process is progressing, and (3) assess the patient's response to therapeutic interventions.

NURSING MANAGEMENT OF THE PATIENT WITH INCREASED INTRACRANIAL PRESSURE

The primary goal of medical and nursing management of the patient with, or at risk of developing, intracranial hypertension is to intervene at the primary stage to treat and/or prevent secondary and tertiary events from occurring. A potentially *reversible* insult or process must *not* be allowed to become irreversible and catastrophic.

Primary nursing responsibilities include: (1) moni-

toring for and identifying early signs of increasing ICP, (2) maintaining the integrity of the ICP monitoring system, (3) implementing measures to prevent and/ or reduce ICP, and (4) assessing the impact of the neurologic dysfunction, if present, on the individual's self-care capabilities.

It is important to appreciate that while ICPM is invaluable in the *early* diagnosis and monitoring of an increase in ICP, it is only one important parameter of the patient's total assessment. The nurse must be able to analyze and interpret data obtained via ICPM, and to evaluate the significance of those data in terms of the patient's total body function. The nurse must obtain accurate pressure measurements and be consistent in taking pressure readings. The head, for example, should always be at the same level in relation to the transducer (i.e., external landmarks: edge of eyebrow or in front of external meatus of ear). The nurse must be able to analyze pressure recordings and identify *trends*. Isolated readings are less meaningful than repeated or serial readings.

Patient activities (e.g., coughing, moving, postur-

TABLE 29–3
Syndrome of Uncal Herniation—Lateral Brainstem Compression

Clinical Signs	Early-Focal Neurologic Deficits	Diencephalon-Midbrain	Midbrain–Upper Pons	Lower Pons–Upper Medulla	Medulla
Level of consciousness	May be arousable → Perhaps some restlessness	Rapid deterioration → (once signs of herniation appear) (stupor to coma)	Deep coma ————	Same ————————→	Same
Respiratory pattern	Eupneic	Sustained, regular → hyperventilation	Same ————————→	Eupneic, shallow, and → rapid (>20/min)	Ataxic (irregular in rate and amplitude)
Pupillary size and reactivity	Unilateral dilated → pupil; sluggishly reactive	Unilateral dilated pupil, constricts sluggishly	Ipsilateral pupil widely dilated and fixed	Pupil opposite the one originally dilated may: (1) dilate widely and fix; (2) enlarge to fix in mid-position	Dilated and fixed
Oculocephalic/oculovestibular responses	Intact	Once pupil dilates, external oculomotor ophthalmoplegia appears.	Impairment of oculomotor function persists, rapidly becomes sluggish, and disappears.	No response ————→	Absent
Motor responses	Appropriate → response to noxious stimuli	Purposeful movement to noxious stimuli; contralateral paratonic resistance or rigidity	Hemiplegia develops ipsilateral to the expanding supratentorial lesion.	Extensor posturing	Flaccid Terminal stage
Babinski's sign		Contralateral extensor plantar reflex	Bilateral extensor plantar responses		

ing) may produce momentary elevations in ICP readings, and such readings may reflect normal compensatory volume-pressure responses and normal brain compliance. Changes in ICP fluctuate with cardiovascular dynamics and with changes in intrathoracic and intra-abdominal pressures reflected via the vena cavae and internal jugular veins. An appreciation of these interrelationships can help the nurse analyze and interpret data and plan patient care.

It is essential to be able to identify specific patient care activities that cause elevations in ICP. Significant study has been given to the effects of such activities in patients with actual or potential intracranial hypertension. For example, research indicates that safe and effective suctioning of patients with actually or potentially increased ICP is best performed by preoxygenating (i.e., prior to suctioning) and hyperventilating with 100% oxygen, and limiting suction passes to two, each of 15-second duration or less.[5] Neck rotation (i.e., turning the head side to side), neck flexion (i.e., touching chin to chest), and hip flexion (i.e., flexing hip at right angle to abdomen) are associated with an increase in ICP and are to be avoided.[6]

Head elevation (of about 30 degrees) has long been thought to lower ICP by improving CSF and venous outflow from the cranium. However, in patients with sustained intracranial hypertension and significantly reduced brain compliance, compensatory mechanisms may no longer be functional.[7] In these patients, head elevation may actually compromise CPP. A flat, supine position may be indicated to improve cerebral blood flow. It is essential to evaluate each patient's individual responses to head and body positions.

ICPM provides an additional assessment tool for use in planning and evaluating patient care activities. Such activities can be spaced to prevent any significant momentary increases in ICP. Planned rest periods should be incorporated into daily care, and the environment should remain as quiet as possible. The responsive patient should be taught to avoid excessive coughing, Valsalva's maneuver, isometric exercises, or pushing or pulling against siderails. The patient should be assessed for bladder distention, paralytic ileus, and constipation.

A sustained increase in intracranial pressure (>25 to 50 mmHg) for an extended period of time (15 to 20 minutes) suggests a loss of compensation and brain compliance. Under these circumstances, the nurse must recognize the clinical significance of the intracranial hypertension and act in a timely and aggressive manner to initiate prescribed treatments and nursing measures designed to reduce the intracranial pressure. (Specific therapeutic pressure-reducing measures and their nursing implications are discussed in Chapter 30.)

Intracranial Pressure Monitoring: Maintaining the Integrity of the System

A major responsibility assumed by critical care nurses caring for the neurologically compromised

TABLE 29–4
Intracranial Pressure Monitoring: Troubleshooting the System

Problem	Cause	Intervention
Absent, dampened, or drifting waveform	• Transducer stopcock turned off to patient. • Transducer connected incorrectly; loose connections. • Air between transducer diaphragm and pressure source. • Occlusion of intracranial measurement device (sensor) with blood or brain tissue; or by catheter tip pushing against ventricular wall. • Compression of monitor cable, kinking or compression of catheter tubing, or patient movement (artifact). • Incorrect gain setting for pressure, or patient having plateau waves (*A* waves). • Trace turned off.	• Turn stopcock to appropriate position. • Check all connections; be sure appropriate connector for amplifier is in use. • Eliminate air bubbles with sterile normal saline or lactated Ringer's solution; tighten all connections. • Flush intracranial device as per prescribed protocol; 0.25 mL sterile normal saline is frequently used. Note: nurses do *not* routinely inject fluid into the ICPM system. • Avoid kinking of catheter tubing as patient is moved or positioned in bed. • Adjust gain setting for higher pressure setting. • Turn power on to trace: monitor and transducer should have ample time to warm up prior to use.
False high pressure	• Transducer below level of pressure source. • Transducer incorrectly balanced.	• Place venting port of transducer at level of foramen of Monro. For every inch the transducer is below the pressure source, there is an error of approximately 2 mmHg. • Correctly position transducer and rebalance. Transducer should be balanced every 8 h, and repositioned as necessary to ensure reliable measurements. • Avoid initiating treatment for increased ICP unless read-outs are reliably accurate.
False low pressure readings	• Monitoring system incorrectly calibrated. • Air in system. Air may attenuate or amplify pressure signal. • Complete occlusion of catheter or screw device. • Air bubbles between transducer and pressure source, loose connections. • Transducer above the level of the pressure source. • Zero and/or calibration incorrect.	• Repeat calibration procedure. • Remove air from monitoring line. • Flush monitoring device. • Eliminate air bubbles with sterile normal saline or lactated Ringer's solution. Tighten all connections. • Place venting port of transducer at level of foramen of Monro. For every inch the transducer is above the level of the pressure source there will be an error of approximately 2 mmHg. • Re-zero and calibrate monitoring system.

Note: Troubleshooting and assessment of the entire monitoring system should be done frequently; the pressure waveform and digital read-outs need to be evaluated in terms of other assessment data reflective of the patient's overall status.

patient is to prevent infection. Scrupulous aseptic technique is absolutely essential when working with an ICPM system. A leak or breakdown in the integrity of the system requires immediate intervention to stop and/or control the leak, and to re-establish and maintain sterility of the system.

The ICPM system requires frequent checks to ensure that all stopcocks are in their appropriate positions. Inadvertent introduction of even small amounts of fluid may have profound, deleterious effects on the patient in whom ICP is already elevated. Leaks in the system resulting in inadvertent drainage of CSF may result in a significant lowering of ICP, causing brain tissue to be sucked up against the catheter or screw. The ventricles may collapse, precipitating a shift in intracranial contents.

The nurse must be vigilant for potential problems that may occur with the use of invasive pressure monitoring. Treatment of increases in ICP and an evalua-

tion of the patient's response to that treatment must be based on clearly established and accurate pressure measurements.

Nursing Diagnoses, Desired Patient Outcomes, and Nursing Interventions/ Rationales

Specific nursing diagnoses, desired patient outcomes, and nursing interventions concerned with the management of the patient with, or at risk of developing, an increase ICP are presented in the care plan at the end of this chapter. Additional nursing diagnoses are presented in the care plans in Chapters 30, 31, and 32. Physiologic principles underlying nursing interventions are incorporated into the rationales for decision making. Guidelines for troubleshooting the invasive ICPM system are included in Table 29–4.

REFERENCES

1. Ward, J, et al: Cerebral homeostasis and protection. In Wirth, I and Ratcheson, R (eds): Neurosurgical Critical Care. Williams & Wilkins, Baltimore, 1987, pp 207–220.
2. Dickman, CA, Carter, P, and Baldwin, HZ: Continuous regional cerebral blood flow monitoring in acute craniocerebral trauma. Neurosurgery 28:467–472, 1991.
3. Meyerson, BA, et al: Bedside monitoring of regional cortical blood flow in comatose patients using laser Doppler flowmetry. Neurosurgery 29:750–755, 1991.
4. Plum, F and Posner, J: The Diagnosis of Stupor and Coma, ed 3. FA Davis, Philadelphia, 1980, pp 153–160.
5. Rudy, EB, et al: Endotracheal suctioning in adults with head injury. Heart Lung 20:667–674, 1992.
6. Williams, A and Coyne, SM: Effects of neck rotation on intracranial pressure. American Journal of Critical Care, 2:68–71, 1993.
7. Feldman, Z, et al: Effect of head elevation on intracranial pressure, cerebral perfusion pressure and cerebral blood flow in head-injured patients. J Neurosurg 76:207–211, 1992.

SELECTED READINGS

Gilliam, EE: Intracranial hypertension: Advances in intracranial pressure monitoring. Critical Care Nursing Clinics of North America, 2(1):21, 1990.
McQuillan, KA: Intracranial pressure monitoring: Technical operatives. AACN Clinical Issues in Critical Care Nursing 2(4):623, 1991.
Richmond, TS: Intracranial pressure monitoring. AACN Clinical Issues in Critical Care Nursing 4(1):148–160, 1993.
Walleck, CA: Preventing secondary brain injury. AACN Clinical Issues in Critical Care Nursing 3(1):19, 1992.
Winkelman, C: Advances in managing intracranial pressure: A decade of selected research. AACN Clinical Issues in Critical Care Nursing 5(1):9–14, 1994.

CARE PLAN FOR THE PATIENT WITH INCREASED INTRACRANIAL PRESSURE

Nursing Diagnoses

Nursing Diagnosis #1
Tissue perfusion, altered, cerebral; related to increased ICP associated with cranial and/or cerebral insult (head injury, hematoma formation, cerebral hemorrhage, cerebral edema)

Desired Patient Outcomes

Patient will:
1. Maintain CPP >60 mmHg
   - ICP <15 mmHg
   - MAP ~80 to 100 mmHg or baseline (for patient)
2. Exhibit intact level of consciousness and mentation
3. Demonstrate eupneic breathing pattern
4. Demonstrate pupils equal in size with brisk reactivity to light stimulus
5. Demonstrate conjugate gaze
6. Follow instructions
7. Differentiate pinprick from crude pressure

Nursing Interventions

- Monitor continuously for signs and symptoms of increasing ICP.

  - Determine arousability and assess for changes in level of consciousness and mentation: restlessness, agitation, irritability; disorientation, inattentiveness; disturbed thought processes, loss of memory; inability to answer questions or follow instructions.

  - Assess for sensory function:
    - *Special senses:* visual acuity and visual fields; hearing.
    - *Somatic senses:* touch, pressure, pain, temperature, proprioception, vibration.
  - Assess for motor function (somatic): appropriate or inappropriate responses (decorticate or decerebrate posturing, flaccidity); muscle strength, tone, deep tendon reflexes.
  - Assess for motor function (autonomic): respiratory rate and pattern; pupillary size and reactivity; ocular movements: dysconjugate gaze, nystagmus; oculocephalic and oculovestibular reflexes (doll's eyes phenomenon and caloric tests).
  - Asses cranial nerves and status of protective reflexes.

  - Assess for headache, nausea, vomiting, papilledema, diplopia, blurred vision, seizures.

Rationales

- Continuous monitoring is necessary as patient responses related to ICP can change rapidly from moment to moment.
  - Arousability reflects functioning of reticular activating system within brainstem.
  - Level of consciousness provides earliest clinical evidence of a change in intracranial volume-pressure dynamics. It reflects the status of cerebral hemispheres and diencephalon.
  - Assessment of sensory function affords an evaluation of sensory pathways and functioning of primary sensory center (postcentral gyrus, parietal lobe).

  - Appropriate motor responses and deep tendon reflexes reflect intact sensory pathways and total or partial intact motor pathways and neuromuscular junctions.
  - Pupillary responses reflect status of midbrain and pons. In the patient with an altered state of consciousness who has fixed, moderately dilated pupils, ocular reflexes may provide the only clinical data reflective of the level of brainstem function.
  - Increasing ICP causes pressure on brainstem, disrupting cranial nerve function (IX and X) and compromising protective reflexes (gag, cough, epiglottal closure). This places airway in great danger.
  - Many signs/symptoms of early rise in ICP tend to be nonspecific.

CARE PLAN FOR THE PATIENT WITH INCREASED INTRACRANIAL PRESSURE (*Continued*)

Nursing Interventions

- ○ Assess vital signs: mean arterial blood pressure, pulse pressure, heart rate.

- • Implement measures to prevent rise in and/or reduce ICP.
  - ○ Maintain proper positioning: elevate head of bed 15 to 30 degrees; avoid using pillows.

  - ○ Maintain body alignment in midline, and avoid neck flexion or head rotation.
  - ○ Avoid hip flexion.
  - ○ Maintain head-neck alignment when turning.
  - ○ Prevent increase in cerebral blood flow.

  - ○ Initiate controlled hyperventilation:
    - □ Maintain $PaCO_2$ 28 to 32 mmHg, PaO_2 >80 mmHg.
    - □ Monitor arterial blood gas.

  - ○ Minimize cellular metabolism:
    - □ Relieve pain and anxiety.

- • Plan nursing care activities so as to avoid a *cumulative* increase in ICP.
  - ○ Identify activities that cause a change in ICP (e.g., coughing, suctioning, positioning).
  - ○ Incorporate planned rest periods into daily nursing care spaced between those procedures known to increase ICP.
  - ○ Administer prescribed sedatives or analgesics prior to procedures that may cause an increase in ICP.
  - ○ Avoid discussing patient's condition at the bedside or within earshot of the patient.
  - ○ Teach the responsive patient to avoid excessive coughing. Valsalva's maneuver (straining), isometric exercises, or pushing against bedrails; avoid use of footboard or restraints.
  - ○ Assess for bladder distention, paralytic ileus, constipation.
  - ○ Maintain quite environment with a minimum of stimuli; gently stroke the patient and speak with a soothing tone of voice.

Rationales

- ○ A rise in blood pressure, widening pulse pressure, and slow, bounding heart rate are classic, *late*-occurring signs of increasing ICP.

  - ○ Allows for optimal venous drainage from cranium via gravity; prevents compromise of cerebral blood flow. Response to head elevation requires close monitoring. Patients with sustained intracranial hypertension in whom compensatory mechanisms are compromised may experience a decrease in CPP and cerebral blood flow upon head elevation. Maintaining a flat, supine position may be indicated.
  - ○ Prevents compression or obstruction of jugular veins.

  - ○ May increase intra-abdominal pressure and impede cerebral drainage via jugular veins and vena cavae.
  - ○ Increase in cerebral blood volume may compromise compensation and compliance in the patient with increased ICP.
  - ○ Reduced $PaCO_2$ (*hypocapnia*) causes cerebral *vasoconstriction* and thus lowers cerebral blood volume. A reduction in cerebral blood volume augments compensatory mechanisms or compliance.
  - ○ Reduction in cellular metabolism decreases need for metabolic substrates (e.g., oxygen and glucose), while reducing the amount of metabolic waste products (e.g., carbon dioxide and hydrogen ions). The end-result is a decrease in cerebral blood flow and ICP.

- • A potential increase in ICP can occur when nursing care activities are implemented in close succession.
  - ○ Provides a guide for planning nursing care.

  - ○ These measures may prevent an inordinate increase in ICP.
  - ○ Such conversations, if overheard, could be upsetting to the patient and may predispose to an increase in ICP.
  - ○ These activities increase intrathoracic and intra-abdominal pressures, which can impede outflow of blood from cranium.

  - ○ These conditions may cause abdominal distention, thus increasing intra-abdominal pressures and limiting diaphragmatic excursion.

Nursing Diagnoses

Nursing Diagnosis #2
Potential for fluid and electrolyte imbalance, related to:
1. Osmotic diuretic therapy
2. Diabetes insipidus

Desired Patient Outcomes

Patient will:
1. Maintain baseline body weight
2. Balance fluid intake with output
3. Maintain baseline laboratory values
   - Serum electrolytes, blood urea nitrogen, creatinine, serum protein, serum osmolality
   - Urine specific gravity—0.010 to 0.025.

CARE PLAN FOR THE PATIENT WITH INCREASED INTRACRANIAL PRESSURE (*Continued*)

Nursing Interventions
- Limit or decrease cerebral edema:
  - Administer diuretic (furosemide) and hyperosmolar agents (mannitol, urea) as prescribed.

  - Administer prescribed corticosteroid therapy (dexamethasone or methylprednisolone)

  - Restrict fluid intake (usually 1200 to 1500 mL/day).

  - Meticulously record intake and output (hourly).
    - Weigh patient daily if not contraindicated.
  - Monitor urine specific gravity.
  - Monitor serum electrolytes and replace as prescribed.
  - Monitor serum osmolality and maintain at 305 to 315 mOsm/kg.

Rationales
- Fluid restriction coupled with pharmacologic therapy helps to decrease extracellular fluid volume that may contribute to cerebral edema formation. A mild dehydrated state is usually maintained.
  - Corticosteroids are thought to ameliorate cerebral edema, which occurs secondary to the primary craniocerebral insult.
  - Intake/output includes intravenous medications (IV piggybacks) and CSF.
  - Physician should be notified if urine output is <30 or >200 mL/h for 2 consecutive hours.
  - Craniocerebral insults frequently predispose to diabetes insipidus.
  - Increased serum osmolality helps to draw fluid from brain interstitium and reduce cerebral edema.

Therapeutic Modalities in the Treatment of the Patient with Intracranial Hypertension

Joan T. Dolan

CHAPTER OUTLINE

LEARNING OBJECTIVES

After completing this chapter, you should be able to:

1. Discuss why an intact blood-brain barrier is necessary for the optimal benefit of hyperosmolar therapy.
2. List important nursing considerations associated with corticosteroid therapy in the patient with intracranial hypertension.
3. Explain why sedation therapy should always be administered in conjunction with muscle relaxant therapy.
4. Discuss the physiologic, psychological, and psychosocial considerations underlying the nursing management of the patient and family in barbiturate coma therapy.
5. State the physiologic principles underlying the maintenance of optimal ventilatory function in the patient with a craniocerebral insult.
6. Analyze the hemodynamic mechanisms at work in patients with compromised autoregulatory mechanisms and reduced brain compliance.
7. Describe the physiologic basis for the clinical management of patients with actual or potential intracranial hypertension, including the following:
   a. Maintenance of a slightly dehydrated state
   b. Maintenance of appropriate body positioning and alignment
   c. Prevention of Valsalva-type maneuvers
   d. Maintenance of normothermia
8. Discuss indications and contraindications for use of cerebrospinal fluid drainage as a therapeutic intervention in some patients with neurologic dysfunction.
9. Implement the nursing process in the management of the patient with craniocerebral surgery through assessment, diagnosis, and planning with regard to desired patient outcomes and nursing interventions.

MANAGEMENT OF THE PATIENT WITH INCREASED INTRACRANIAL PRESSURE (INTRACRANIAL HYPERTENSION)

The major goals in the nursing management of the patient with increased intracranial pressure (i.e., intra-cranial hypertension) are: (1) to reduce and/or maintain intracranial pressure (ICP) within normal physiologic limits (0 to 15 mmHg); (2) to maintain cerebral perfusion pressure (CPP) above 60 mmHg; and (3) to protect the patient from any further episodes of increased ICP, which can precipitate secondary pathophysiologic changes such as cerebral ischemia, cellular hypoxia, and cerebral edema. Without timely, appropriate, and aggressive intervention, these secondary changes can lead, ultimately, to the death of the individual (see Fig. 29–4).

There is no single treatment for intracranial hypertension, except perhaps in the case of a mass lesion such as a tumor or hematoma. In these instances, surgical therapy is indicated. Overall, prognosis appears to be related to the *control* of ICP. Patients experiencing an increase in ICP (>30 mmHg) on a consistent basis or for extended periods of time (20 to 30 minutes) rarely do well. A reasonable approach in the care of these patients is to initiate treatment to maintain a *baseline* ICP of less than 20 to 25 mmHg and a CPP greater than 60 mmHg. Ideally, ICP should be maintained at less than 10 mmHg, with 15 mmHg as the upper limit, and CPP should be approximately 80 to 90 mmHg.

The current therapeutic modalities available to treat intracranial hypertension can be classified as pharmacologic, supportive, and surgical. The critical care nurse is largely responsible for implementing the plan of care and for continuously monitoring the patient to evaluate the patient's response to therapeutic measures. Emphasis is placed on monitoring the status of all major organ systems because increased ICP and therapies used to treat it have multisystem effects.

Pharmacologic Therapy in the Treatment of Intracranial Hypertension

Drug therapy can be used as a primary mode of treatment in the patient with increased ICP (e.g., in cerebral edema), or as a temporary measure to reduce intracranial volume until surgery can be performed (e.g., with an expanding space-occupying lesion). Major categories of drugs used are listed in Table 30–1.

Diuretic Therapy

Hyperosmolar Agents (Osmotherapy). Hyperosmolar agents are also called *osmotic* agents, of which *mannitol* is the most common. Their therapeutic effect is to draw fluid out of brain tissue by establishing an osmotic gradient across an intact blood-brain barrier (see Fig. 27–9). By increasing the osmolality of circulating blood, these agents cause fluid to move from the brain interstitial compartment into its intravascular compartment. Mannitol's effectiveness as an osmotic diuretic is attributed directly to the size of its molecule, which is for the most part too large to easily diffuse across an intact blood-brain barrier. A disrupted blood-brain barrier allows entry of the drug into the brain interstitium, eliminating the osmotic gradient.

Over time, with repeated use of mannitol or in the presence of an impaired or leaky blood-brain barrier

---

TABLE 30–1

Pharmacologic Therapy in the Management of Intracranial Hypertension

The following is a list of drugs commonly used in the treatment of increased intracranial pressure (intracranial hypertension):

Diuretics
Osmotic diuretic—mannitol
Loop diuretic—furosemide (Lasix)

Corticosteroids
Dexamethasone (Decadron)
Methylprednisolone (Solu-Medrol)

Sedatives
Morphine sulfate
Pentobarbital
Diazepam (Valium)

Muscle Relaxant
Pancuronium bromide (Pavulon)

Anticonvulsants
Diazepam (Valium)
Phenytoin (Dilantin)
Phenobarbital

H_2 antagonist
Ranitidine

Antihypertensives
Calcium channel blockers—verapamil, nifedipine
β-blockers—propranolol, labetalol

Antipyretic
Acetaminophen (Tylenol)

(e.g., in cerebral edema), enough mannitol molecules can move into the brain interstitium to compromise the effectiveness of the osmotic gradient. Eventually, water is drawn back into the brain interstitium from the intravascular space, thus accounting for this "rebound" effect. Careful monitoring of serum electrolytes, serum osmolality, and urinary output is essential. Seizures, fluid and electrolyte imbalance, and renal failure have been associated with repeated use of mannitol. The usual dose of mannitol is 0.5 to 1.0 g/kg, given as a bolus. Serum osmolality is maintained below 310 mOsm/kg. (Specific nursing implications regarding the administration of mannitol are listed in Table 30–2.)

Loop Diuretic. *Furosemide* (*Lasix*) acts to dehydrate the entire body. When used with mannitol, it potentiates the duration of the effect of mannitol. To an increasing extent, its effectiveness in reducing cerebral edema is making it the drug of first choice in the treatment of patients with head injury. The site of action of furosemide is the kidney tubules, where it inhibits the reabsorption of chloride and sodium. A direct reduction of sodium transport into brain tissue is also attributed to the action of furosemide.

Nursing implications related to the use of furosemide involve the potency of its diuretic effect, which can lead to a profound depletion of water and electrolytes. The peak diuretic effect occurs within 30 minutes of intravenous administration and is gone within 8 hours. The patient's vital signs, intake and output, serum electrolytes, blood urea nitrogen (BUN), and creatinine must be regularly evaluated. Serum potas-

TABLE 30–2
Administration of Mannitol: Nursing Implications

Important nursing implications related to the administration of mannitol (osmotic diuretic):

1. Mannitol needs to be warmed prior to administration if crystals are present; otherwise, use filter as prescribed.
2. An intravenous filter should be used for administration of the drug.
3. Rapid infusion of large doses of mannitol may expand the blood volume over and above the capacity of the kidneys to clear the additional fluid. The consequent circulatory overload increases cerebral blood flow, predisposing to an increase in intracranial pressure.
   a. The patient should be closely monitored for signs of increasing ICP and circulatory overload. Cardiac arrhythmias associated with circulatory overload may occur.
   b. Renal function should be closely monitored, including hourly fluid intake and output, daily weight (unless contraindicated), and laboratory data (serum BUN and creatinine).
4. Loss of electrolytes in conjunction with the diuresis may cause an electrolyte imbalance.
   a. Serum electrolytes and serum osmolality must be monitored closely.
   b. Serum potassium should be monitored regularly, particularly in patients receiving digitalis preparations. A potassium supplement may be required.
5. When using mannitol, it is necessary to monitor ICP very carefully because initially the vasodilating effect of the drug on cerebral blood vessels may aggravate an already elevated ICP, prior to the onset of its diuretic effect.
6. "Rebound" effect, an increase in ICP, can occur as much as 12 hours after the administration of mannitol. Normally, mannitol does not traverse the blood-brain barrier easily. Over time and/or in the presence of impaired or leaky cellular membranes, mannitol molecules move into the brain interstitium and eventually establish an osmotic concentration gradient. This draws fluid from the intravascular space back into the brain interstitium. The resultant increase in cerebral edema is opposite of the desired effect.

sium should be particularly closely monitored if the patient is also receiving digitalis preparations. Continuous cardiac monitoring is essential. Intravenous doses of furosemide should be administered *slowly* to minimize the risk of complications.

Corticosteroid Therapy

Corticosteroids commonly used to control intracranial pressure include dexamethasone (Decadron) and methylprednisolone (Solu-Medrol). While corticosteroid therapy has not been shown to be successful in the treatment of cerebral edema associated with head injury, it continues to be used widely, particularly in patients with tumor-related cerebral edema. The precise mechanism of action remains unknown. It has been suggested that the anti-inflammatory effects of corticosteroids may help to relieve cerebral edema through their capacity to stabilize cell membranes, thereby preventing the activation of noxious lysosomal enzymes. Steroids may also help to re-establish and maintain the integrity of the blood-brain barrier.

Nursing implications of steroid therapy include the need for close monitoring of fluid and electrolytes, because steroids, in general, promote fluid and sodium retention, and hypokalemia. Serum glucose must also be monitored closely because the hyperglycemia induced by corticosteroid therapy may be difficult to control. When administered intravenously, corticosteroids should be given slowly over at least 1 minute. High doses given for over 5 days suppress the hypothalamic-pituitary axis. Doses are tapered slowly to prevent addisonian crisis (i.e., acute adrenal insufficiency). Although the ulcer-producing properties of corticosteroids continue to make their use controversial, prophylactic therapy in this regard is usually initiated [see section on H_2 (histamine) antagonist therapy, below]. Vigilant nursing care is required, especially with patients having invasive procedures, because corticosteroids depress the immune response and may mask signs of infection, including fever.

Sedation Therapy

Sedating agents such as morphine and benzodiazepines help to stabilize ICP by reducing the patient's responsiveness to environmental stimuli. This is especially important in the presence of pain and the discomforts associated with mechanical ventilation, hemodynamic monitoring, nasogastric decompression, and related nursing interventions, including pulmonary toileting, drawing arterial blood samples, turning and positioning, maintaining protective restraints, and many other routine nursing care measures.

Morphine should be used judiciously because it depresses the level of consciousness and respirations, and it alters pupillary size and reactivity. Benzodiazepines have a dose-related depressant effect on the central nervous system and cause drowsiness and respiratory depression. Ongoing neurologic assessment requires a consideration of drug effects, which may mask underlying signs and symptoms.

Muscle Relaxation Therapy

The use of muscle-paralyzing agents is intended to reduce motor responses that have been associated with an increase in ICP. These include sustained muscle contractions such as decorticate and decerebrate posturing, as well as muscle activity involved in moving, turning, and positioning. Pancuronium bromide (Pavulon) is commonly used because of its relatively short duration of action and the ease with which its effects can be reversed. Administration of anticholinesterase agents (e.g., endrophonium and neostigmine) can be used to reverse the action of Pavulon.

Pavulon causes skeletal muscle paralysis, and its use requires the institution of continuous mechanical ventilation. Respiratory muscle paralysis occurs within 2 to 3 minutes of an intravenous dose. The effects of the drug begin to subside within 35 to 45 minutes. It is important to appreciate that this drug is not a central nervous system depressant. While motor function is lost, patients can still experience pain, and may be completely aware of what is happening around them. Consequently, such muscle relaxants should always be administered in conjunction with a sedating agent (commonly morphine or diazepam). Responsive and alert patients receiving muscle relaxant therapy require teaching and reassurance that their needs will be anticipated and met. Loss of motor control may cause anxiety and apprehension, which can themselves cause an increase in ICP.

Because muscle-paralyzing agents paralyze all skeletal muscles, patients are unable to blink or close their eyes. Consequently, it may be necessary to administer artificial tears and to keep the eyes taped shut. In addition to assessing pupillary responses, hourly examination of the eyes should also include checking for the presence of corneal moisture and any abnormal discharge.

Anticonvulsant Therapy

While the incidence of post-traumatic seizures in head-injured patients has been estimated to be only about 5%, it is nevertheless common practice for anticonvulsant therapy to be prescribed prophylactically, since seizures increase the metabolic requirements of brain tissue. The consequent increase in cerebral blood flow and blood volume places the patient at risk for an increase in ICP. Drugs commonly used for the treatment and/or prevention of seizures include diazepam, phenytoin (Dilantin), and phenobarbital. (For additional nursing implications refer to the section on seizures in Chapter 31 and Table 31–3.)

In patients receiving diazepam, intravenous doses should be administered at a rate not to exceed 5 mg/ min. The patient should be assessed for signs of respiratory depression. The anticonvulsant activity of diazepam diminishes within 15 to 30 minutes of an intravenous dose. Intravenous doses of phenytoin should be administered at a rate that achieves a therapeutic blood level of 10 to 20 μg/mL. Vital signs and cardiac rhythm should be monitored continuously. The drug must be administered with normal saline solution at a rate not to exceed 50 mg/min. Many drug interactions and adverse reactions have been associated with phenytoin.

Phenobarbital depresses all levels of CNS function. It limits seizure activity by inhibiting transmission of impulses within the nervous system and by raising the seizure threshold. Intravenous administration of the drug requires continuous monitoring of the level of consciousness and of vital signs—including respiratory status, pulse, and blood pressure. The administration rate should not exceed 60 mg/min, and the dose should be slowly titrated, based on the patient's response. Directions regarding reconstitution of the drug should be followed carefully. Solutions whose appearance does not clear within 5 minutes of reconstitution, or that contain a precipitate, should not be used. Doses may require 15 to 30 minutes to reach peak levels in the brain; therefore, it is important to administer a minimal dose and to wait to evaluate its effectiveness before administering a second dose to prevent cumulative barbiturate-induced CNS depression.

It is known that phenobarbital interacts with many other drugs. Notably, it may cause additive CNS depression when administered along with other CNS depressants (e.g., narcotics, other sedatives/hypnotics). Intravenous administration requires close monitoring because extravasation can result in tissue necrosis.

Barbiturate Coma Therapy

Barbiturate coma therapy is sometimes instituted to reduce uncontrolled intracranial hypertension that is refractory to conventional therapeutic modalities. The mechanism of action in head-injured patients is unclear, but several physiologic effects of barbiturates may account for their efficacy in reducing intracranial hypertension. These drugs cause cerebral vasoconstriction, reducing the blood volume within the cerebral vasculature. A decrease in systemic blood pressure is reflected as a lowered hydrostatic pressure within the cerebral circulation. Through these actions barbiturates may help to decrease cerebral edema.

Barbiturates also help to decrease the brain's metabolic demands for oxygen and glucose by reducing the patient's responsiveness to stimuli. Suppression of seizures also reduces the cellular demand for these metabolic substrates.

Barbiturate coma therapy requires complete, supportive care of an essentially anesthetized patient. Because of respiratory depression the patient is unable to breathe spontaneously and requires intubation and continuous, controlled mechanical ventilation. The adequacy of ventilation is evaluated by regular arterial blood gas studies. The loss of protective reflexes (cough, gag, epiglottal closure) necessitates timely suctioning of nasopharyngeal and tracheobronchial secretions to ensure a patent airway and to safeguard against aspiration. Continuous intracranial pressure monitoring is absolutely essential because the dosage of barbiturate is titrated according to ICP measurements. The usual neurologic assessment parameters (e.g., level of consciousness, respiratory pattern, pupillary and motor responses) are obliterated once coma is established, and ICP monitoring is the only reliable way to evaluate the patient's response to therapy.

Continuous hemodynamic pressure monitoring is essential to monitor CPP and to evaluate hemodynamic function. High doses of barbiturates (usually pentobarbital) can cause significant systemic hypotension, which can compromise CPP. Vasopressors (e.g., dopamine) may be required to keep the systolic blood pressure above 90 mmHg. Systemic hypotension may also be related to drug-induced myocardial depression, which can precipitate left ventricular insufficiency with a reduced cardiac output and elevated pulmonary capillary wedge pressures.

Nasogastric decompression is essential to prevent vomiting and aspiration, and to avoid compromise of diaphragmatic excursion. The abdomen should be assessed for distention in the presence of paralytic ileus and for possible fecal impaction. Gastric secretions should be monitored for pH and assessed for occult blood.

Restriction of fluid intake, use of diuretics, and continuous gastric decompression may potentially alter fluid and electrolyte balance. Thus, hourly monitoring of intake and output is essential. Serial monitoring of laboratory data, including serum electrolytes, BUN and creatinine, hematology profile, and serum osmolality, is necessary.

Nursing measures should be implemented to safeguard against infection, especially since invasive monitoring techniques, pulmonary toileting, immobility, and inadequate nutrition all place the patient at increased risk of infection.

Barbiturate Coma Therapy: Psychological and Psychosocial Impact. A major aspect of patient care involves an assessment of the emotional needs of the patient's family and/or significant others. Frequent updates regarding the patient's status and the response to therapy should be provided. Explanations may need to be repeated and clarified because stress may alter the family members' ability to comprehend. Time should be provided for the family to ask questions. The nurse should remain accessible, provide a "listening ear," and help family members and friends to identify coping mechanisms and strengths to assist them in this time of crisis. Referral of family members to a psychiatric liaison nurse, social worker, and/or chaplain may be helpful.

H₂ (Histamine) Antagonist Therapy

While there is no firm evidence that H_2 antagonists have prophylactic properties, such therapy is usually initiated in patients who have sustained a major craniocerebral insult and for whom corticosteroid therapy has been prescribed. The action of H_2 antagonists is localized to H_2 receptors within the gastric mucosa, where these drugs act to reduce acid secretion, increase gastric pH, and reduce the activity of the enzyme pepsin. In patients with a nasogastric tube, gastric pH should be monitored closely to maintain a gastric pH greater than 4.5. Nasogastric drainage and stools should also be monitored for occult blood.

Supportive Therapy

(Table 30–3)

TABLE 30–3
Clinical Management of Increased ICP: Supportive Therapy

1. Maintenance of ventilatory function: hyperventilation therapy
   a. Ensuring a patent airway through timely and appropriate suctioning
   b. Use of positive end-expiratory pressure (PEEP): acute neurogenic pulmonary edema
2. Maintenance of cerebral perfusion pressure and cerebral blood flow
   a. Hemodynamic considerations
   b. Fluid management
   c. Maintenance of optimal patient positioning
   d. Avoidance of Valsalva-type maneuvers
3. Maintenance of normothermia
4. Cerebrospinal fluid drainage

Maintenance of Ventilatory Function: Hyperventilation Therapy

Assisted mechanical ventilation with hyperventilation therapy is commonly used to control ICP. The usual goal is to maintain $PaCO_2$ at 28 to 32 mmHg and PaO_2 at greater than 80 mmHg. Both hypercapnia ($PaCO_2 > 45$ mmHg) and hypoxemia ($PaO_2 < 60$ mmHg) have a potent *vasodilatory* effect on cerebral vessels. Vasodilation increases the volume of blood within the cerebral vasculature, which, in the absence of autoregulatory and compensatory control, precipitates a rise in ICP.

On the other hand, hypocapnia ($PaCO_2 < 30$ to 35 mmHg) is a potent stimulus for cerebral *vasoconstriction.* There results a consequent reduction in cerebral intravascular blood volume which helps to reduce and/or maintain ICP at baseline. A $PaCO_2$ of less than 20 to 25 mmHg, however, may cause excessive cerebral vasoconstriction, which may lead to a reduction in cerebral blood flow and cerebral ischemia.

A major nursing responsibility is to ensure that the patient has a patent airway so that hypercapnia and hypoxemia can be prevented. A thorough assessment of respiratory parameters is necessary to determine patency of the airway. Serial arterial blood gas measurements reflect the patient's response to controlled hyperventilation therapy and indicate whether the arterial carbon dioxide and oxygen values are within the desired range. Serial assessments of tidal volume and vital capacity assist in assessing ventilatory capacity.

Timely and appropriate suctioning of the intubated patient helps to maintain a patent airway and reduces the risk of pulmonary complications (e.g., pneumonia). In the patient with unstable ICP, suctioning is especially critical to avert the reduction in alveolar ventilation that is associated with secretion buildup and to avoid consequent hypercapnia and hypoxemia.

Because suctioning can reduce the fraction of inspired oxygen (FiO_2) and thus predispose to hypoxemia, it strongly influences ICP. Therefore, this procedure should be performed when the patient is at rest and ICP is at baseline. Preoxygenating and hyperventilating the patient with 100% oxygen before and after suctioning passes, and limiting suction passes to two, each with a duration of 15 seconds or less, is considered to be a safe approach in patients with actual or potential intracranial hypertension.[1] By using continuous intracranial pressure monitoring (ICPM) as a guide for planning care, necessary procedures such as suctioning can be spaced to avoid a cumulative impact on ICP.

Suctioning may also influence ICP through its impact on the autonomic nervous system function. Suctioning enhances sympathetic output as manifested clinically by an increase in blood pressure and heart rate. The increase in intracranial blood volume afforded by an increase in CPP and cerebral blood flow may, in turn, increase ICP. Parasympathetic stimulation (e.g., vagal response) may also be triggered by suctioning. The increase in intrathoracic pressures associated with Valsalva's maneuver may contribute to an increase in ICP by impeding normal venous drainage from the cranial vault via the jugular veins.

In the absence of autoregulatory and compensatory controls, all of these responses triggered by suctioning can induce a considerable increase in ICP, which may persist after the procedure is completed.

Use of Positive End-Expiratory Pressure: Acute Neurogenic Pulmonary Edema. Acute neurogenic pulmonary edema (i.e., adult respiratory distress syndrome of neurogenic origin, for example, acute head injury, subarachnoid hemorrhage) is a critical complication of neurologic dysfunction.[2,3] It may result from an extremely rapid outpouring of nerve impulses from the injured brain, which disrupts vascular permeability and precipitates pulmonary edema.

Positive end-expiratory pressure (PEEP) is often used in the treatment of adult respiratory distress syndrome of neurogenic origin. The extra positive pressure delivered by PEEP to the lungs and thorax helps to control hypoxemia by preventing atelectasis (i.e., collapse of alveoli) and by decreasing movement of fluid and protein from the intravascular space into the pulmonary interstitium and the alveoli.

Use of PEEP presents special problems for the patient with unstable ICP. Increased intrathoracic pressures impede venous return from the intracranial venous sinuses via the internal jugular veins. This interruption of venous outflow from the brain causes intracranial fluid volume to increase and creates the potential for an increase in ICP. Increased intrathoracic pressures also restrict venous return to the heart from the systemic circulation. This causes a consequent decrease in cardiac output and systemic arterial blood pressure, which, in turn, may reduce CPP. Patients with unstable ICP should have intracranial and hemodynamic pressure monitoring so that the interaction of these physiologic phenomena can be assessed on a continuous basis.

Maintenance of Cerebral Perfusion Pressure and Cerebral Blood Flow

Hemodynamic Considerations. Cerebral perfusion pressure depends largely on: (1) mean systemic arterial blood pressure, (2) level of intracranial pressure, and (3) intact autoregulatory mechanisms within the brain that serve to maintain CPP in the face of wide fluctuations in systemic arterial blood pressure (60 to 150 mmHg).

When ICP increases beyond the autoregulatory capabilities of the brain, intracranial blood volume and cerebral blood flow become *passively* controlled by the systemic arterial blood pressure. Thus, a rise in systemic blood pressure (>150 mmHg) increases intracranial blood volume and cerebral blood flow, causing ICP to rise; a fall in systemic blood pressure (<60 mmHg) reduces cerebral blood volume and cerebral blood flow so that there is the potential for a reduction in CPP and resulting cerebral ischemia. The reduction in brain compliance associated with intracranial hypertension further complicates the patient's status because very small increases in the intracranial volume precipitate large increases in ICP (see Fig. 29–1).

To reduce and/or maintain ICP within acceptable physiologic limits (<20 to 25 mmHg) in patients with compromised autoregulatory and compensatory mechanisms, it is necessary to: (1) maintain the *mean* arterial pressure (MAP) between 80 and 100 mmHg, (2) minimize fluctuations in systemic arterial blood pressure, and (3) promote cerebral venous outflow via the jugular veins.

Patients experiencing an insult to the brain often become *hyper*tensive as the autoregulatory/compensatory mechanisms attempt to preserve CPP. High, sustained systemic arterial blood pressures (>150 mmHg) in the presence of a labile or elevated ICP requires aggressive treatment. Sedation, fluid restriction, and use of diuretic therapy are indicated. Antihypertensive drug therapy may also be indicated. It should be appreciated, however, that antihypertensive drugs may themselves increase ICP, and their administration requires close scrutiny of the patient's status.

Many antihypertensive agents (e.g., nitroprusside, nitroglycerin) exert their effect via vasodilation of peripheral blood vessels, including those within the cerebral vasculature. Consequently, care must be taken to administer drugs that have a minimal vasodilatory effect. Calcium channel blockers (e.g., verapamil) and β-blockers (e.g., propranolol and labetalol) have been prescribed with some positive results.

The presence of systemic *hypo*tension needs to be assessed carefully, especially in the trauma patient, to determine its underlying cause. Insults to the head rarely precipitate a hypotensive state unless there is a severe laceration of the scalp or damage to vital vasomotor centers in the brain. The cause of the hypotension must be diagnosed and aggressively treated because any decrease in mean systemic arterial blood

---

RESEARCH APPLICATION: EFFECTS OF NECK POSITION ON INTRACRANIAL PRESSURE
Williams, A and Coyne, SM. American Journal of Critical Care, 2(1):68–71, 1993.

Purpose: The purpose of this study was to explore the effect of non-neutral neck positions on intracranial pressure. Four neck positions were evaluated: rotation to the right, rotation to the left, flexion, and extension.

Methods: The investigators used an alternating treatment design, which included counterbalancing, and a neutral recovery period between positioning treatments. The study used a convenience sample of 10 patients (9 women and 1 man), with ages ranging from 35 to 71 years, who were currently undergoing ICP monitoring and were without contraindications to head and neck manipulation. The method of ICP monitoring was an intraventricular catheter for 9 of the subjects and subarachnoid bolt for 1 subject. Subjects served as their own controls.

Each subject experienced a unique order of experimental neck positions, which were assigned as the subjects entered the study. The head of the bed was maintained at 30 degrees throughout the investigation. Positioning began with a 5-minute baseline neutral position and was followed by each of the four experimental positions, which were maintained for a full 5 minutes. A 5-minute neutral-position recovery period was included between each experimental position. ICPs were recorded at 1-minute intervals throughout the investigation.

Results: Each subject's mean ICP was calculated for each of the experimental and neutral neck posi-

tions. The highest ICPs for the group resulted from rotation of the head to the right, to the left, and with neck flexion; these three neck positions resulted in significantly higher ICPs as compared to the baseline-neutral position ($P = .004$). ICP was highest with rotation of the head to the right, but not significantly different from rotation of the head to the left or from head flexion. Neck extension also elevated ICP from the baseline mean, but when compared to the other three experimental positions, it produced a significantly lower ICP ($P = .016$).

Practice Implications: Positioning of the head and neck in the patient with actual or potential ICP elevations is an important nursing consideration. Jugular venous return is known to decrease on the side ipsilateral to the direction of head and neck rotation. Higher ICPs associated with rotation of the head to the right may be related to the larger diameter and improved flow dynamics of the right internal jugular vein.

The authors stress that this study was conducted on subjects with compliant brains, able to effectively compensate for changes in volume. In patients with reduced intracranial vascular-autoregulatory responses, compensation may be limited. Positioning of such patients takes on paramount importance as a measure to ensure adequate vascular drainage and ICP control.

Revised by Anne W. Wojner, MSN, RN, CCRN.

---

pressure for an extended period of time can lead, eventually, to a decrease in CPP, brain ischemia, and intracranial hypertension.

Fluid Management. Careful management of fluid intake is necessary to maintain intravascular volume while also allowing the patient to be *slightly* dehydrated. The premise here is that limiting fluid intake will help to decrease extracellular fluid in *all* tissues, including the brain. This may help to minimize or prevent cerebral edema formation. The approach to fluid management in patients with actual or potential intracranial hypertension is to *restrict* fluid intake, usually to 1200 to 1500 mL/day.

Maintenance of Optimal Patient Positioning. The position a patient assumes, or is passively placed in, is a significant factor in the prevention and treatment of intracranial hypertension. Ideally, positions should be maintained that facilitate drainage of blood and cerebrospinal fluid (CSF) from the cranial vault via gravity. Unobstructed flow of blood and CSF enables the autoregulatory and compensatory mechanisms to adjust intracranial volume and pressure on a moment-to-moment basis. When such controls are impaired, maintaining free flow of CSF and blood from the brain

may help to minimize changes in intracranial volume and corresponding ICP.

Proper body alignment, with the head and neck elevated to about 30 degrees, is recommended. In addition to facilitating drainage of blood and CSF from the cranial vault via gravity, this position also allows maximum unimpeded chest excursion and lung expansion, thus facilitating ventilation and oxygenation, and reducing the risk of atelectasis.

More recently, research indicates that in patients with sustained intracranial hypertension, in whom compensatory and autoregulatory mechanisms are compromised, elevating the head of the bed may *compromise* CPP.[4] Maintaining a flat position may be more beneficial for these patients as it would improve blood flow to the cranial vault.

Neck flexion and head rotation should be avoided.[5] Hip flexion and flexion of the knees are also contraindicated because these positions may increase intraabdominal and intrathoracic pressures, which may impede free flow of blood from the cranial vault. The prone position is also contraindicated for this reason.

The patient should be turned with great care so that proper body alignment is maintained during the turning and positioning procedure. Moving the patient in this manner is essential to mobilize pulmonary secretions and to prevent pooling. Use of the kinetic bed is especially helpful in this regard. Turning and positioning also help to maximize tissue perfusion, thus promoting and maintaining skin integrity during the acute phase.

Avoidance of Valsalva-Type Maneuvers. The responsive patient at risk of developing intracranial hypertension presents a special kind of problem—how to assist the patient to avoid Valsalva-type activities, which can precipitate a rise in ICP. Valsalva's maneuver involves a forced exhalation against a closed glottis. It increases central venous and intrathoracic pressures, which impede outflow of venous return from the brain, resulting in an increase in ICP. Patient teaching is critical if Valsalva-type maneuvers are to be avoided.

The patient must be instructed to allow him- or herself to be moved passively in bed. Nurses should *lift* the patient rather than pull or tug, nor should the patient be requested to do so to avoid any potential increase in ICP that might be triggered by such maneuvers. The patient should be taught to exhale or to blow out through the mouth when moving, turning, or defecating. Exhaling requires an open glottis and thus prevents initiation of Valsalva's maneuver. Isometric exercises, such as bracing oneself to sit up or pushing against the bed frame or siderails, need to be discouraged. Use of footboards should be avoided entirely.

Coughing and sneezing increase intrathoracic and intra-abdominal pressures, which, in turn, are transmitted through blood vessels and the subarachnoid space of the spinal cord to the brain. The end-result can be an increase in ICP, and therefore these activities must be discouraged.

Maintenance of Normothermia

Temperature control is an important aspect of the management of the neurologic patient. Currently, the goal is to achieve normothermia via use of conservative methods and antipyretic therapy. Elevated temperatures increase cerebral metabolism; and the metabolic end-products, carbon dioxide and lactic acid, are both potent vasodilators of the cerebral vasculature. The consequent increases in cerebral blood volume and cerebral blood flow, in turn, increase ICP.

In the neurologic patient, an elevated temperature may be associated with infection, seizure activity, or hypothalamic dysfunction. Hyperthermia, that is, a body temperature greater than 105°F, may result from pathophysiology involving the temperature-regulating center in the hypothalamus. When the anterior portion of the hypothalamus is involved, the fever may be accompanied by profuse diaphoresis and vasodilation of blood vessels in the skin; involvement of the lateral portion of the hypothalamus is associated frequently with shivering and vasoconstriction.[6]

Therapeutic modalities used to control body temperatures and achieve normothermia (i.e., 97.7 to 100.4°F) include antipyretic medication (e.g., acetaminophen); conservative measures such as keeping the patient's environment cool and using a minimum of bed coverings; medications to prevent and/or control potential shivering; and cooling devices. Patients with hyperthermia associated with hypothalamic involvement may not respond well to antipyretic therapy. If antipyretic therapy and conservative measures to reduce body temperature are unsuccessful, or if the body temperature becomes greater than 105°F, use of the hypothermia blanket may be indicated.

*Hypo*thermia therapy, the intentional reduction of body temperature to between 86 and 89.6°F for the purpose of controlling ICP by reducing cerebral metabolic oxygen demand, is not widely accepted. Full cardiopulmonary support is necessary, and shivering, which greatly increases the body's overall metabolic requirements and lactate levels, must be prevented. Sedatives, neuromuscular blocking agents, or phenothiazines may be used for this purpose. Problems that include hemodynamic instability, acid-base imbalance, and the occurrence of cerebral edema associated with the rewarming phase contravene the wide use of this therapeutic modality.

Cerebrospinal Fluid Drainage

Cerebrospinal fluid is sometimes drained to reduce intracranial fluid volume and to relieve ICP elevations. Continuous or intermittent drainage of CSF is particularly indicated when the cause of the intracranial hypertension is increased production or obstructed circulation of CSF. Its use in the treatment of brain hyperemia or cerebral edema is usually contraindicated because, in such cases, drainage of CSF may predispose to collapse of the ventricle.

One approach to CSF removal is a ventriculostomy (i.e., the insertion of a catheter into the lateral ventricle). This procedure is performed on the nondominant hemisphere. Use of the ventricular approach allows monitoring of ICP as well as drainage (see Table 29–1). Drainage of CSF is usually performed against positive pressure to prevent rapid removal of CSF with inadvertant collapse of the ventricle. This can cause brain tissue to pull away from the supportive dura, thereby disrupting bridging veins and precipitating a subdural hematoma.

Cerebrospinal fluid shunting procedures (e.g., ventriculo-peritoneal) may also be surgically performed to establish long-term shunting of CSF from the cranial vault. Such procedures are performed to relieve obstructive hydrocephalus. A major complication of CSF drainage is infection. Strict aseptic technique must be used at all times.

Neurosurgical Techniques

Recent advances in neurosurgical techniques employ interventional radiologic and neurovascular techniques for the treatment of complicated cerebro-vascular disorders such as intracerebral aneurysm, carotid cavernous sinus fistulas, and vasospasm. These techniques utilize percutaneous balloons, which are threaded through the cerebral macrocirculation for diagnostic and therapeutic purposes. Some measures include high-resolution digital subtraction angiography with road mapping, embolization of vascular malformations, injection of a permanent solidifying substance (e.g., polymers, glues) into an arteriovenous malformation or fistula, direct injection of a thrombolytic agent (e.g., tissue plasminogen activator) to lyse emboli, as well as the use of cerebral angioplasty to dilate blood vessels. (For additional information on neurosurgical techniques, refer to the Selected Readings at the end of this chapter.)

Surgical Decompression

In the patient who has sustained an acute craniocerebral insult, immediate surgical decompression via craniotomy or burr holes may be the definitive treatment to evacuate a rapidly expanding intracranial mass lesion (e.g., epidural hematoma) and to relieve the consequent intracranial hypertension. Surgical intervention alleviates and/or prevents a precipitous rise in ICP, which might otherwise predispose to *brain herniation* with irreversible brain damage and death (see Chapter 29). Intracranial volume and pressure may be reduced surgically by arresting hemorrhaging, removing clots (e.g., hematomas), and elevating depressed skull fractures. (Acute head injury is discussed in Chapter 31).

Biophysical Techniques

Additional options in the treatment of head injury are currently being investigated. These include developing new bedside techniques both to measure cerebral blood flow and to determine whether the intracranial hypertension experienced by a patient is hyperemic in origin or secondary to ongoing cerebral ischemia and edema.[7] Investigations are ongoing as to the molecular basis of brain injury and edema attributed to intracranial hypertension, and these may offer strategies on how such injury can be treated.

NURSING DIAGNOSES, PATIENT OUTCOMES, AND NURSING INTERVENTIONS/RATIONALES IN THE CARE OF THE PATIENT WITH CRANIOCEREBRAL SURGERY

The postoperative management of the patient who has had craniocerebral surgery is especially challenging because a wide spectrum of complications is possible. Some selected postoperative complications include an altered state of consciousness, cerebral edema, intracranial bleeding, cerebral ischemia and infarction, hydrocephalus, tension pneumocephalus, and intracranial hypertension. The care plan at the end of this chapter presents specific nursing diagnoses, patient outcomes, and nursing interventions concerned with the postoperative care of the craniocerebral surgery patient. Refer also to the care plan for Chapter 29.

REFERENCES

1. Rudy, EB, et al: Endotracheal suctioning in adults with head injury. Heart Lung 20:667–674, 1992.
2. Littleton, M: Complications of multiple trauma. Critical Care Nursing Clinics of North America 1(1):75, 1989.
3. Muwaswes, M: Increased intracranial pressure and its systemic effects. J Neurosci Nurs 17:242, 1985.
4. Rosner, MJ and Daughton, S: Cerebral perfusion pressure management in head injury. J Trauma 30:933–941, 1990.
5. Williams, A and Coyne, SM: Effects of neck rotation on intracranial pressure. American Journal of Critical Care 2:68–71, 1993.
6. Snyder, M: A Guide to Neurological and Neurosurgical Nursing, ed 2. John Wiley & Sons, New York, 1991.
7. Caron, MJ, Hvoda, DA, and Becker, DP: Changes in the treatment of head injury. Neurosurgical Clinics of North America 2:483–491, 1991.

SUGGESTED READINGS

Ames, A, et al: New discoveries in neuroprotective drug therapies. Headlines January/February 1993, pp. 10–11.
Cook, H: Cerebral angioplasty: A new treatment for vasospasm secondary to subarachnoid hemorrhage. J Neurosci Nurs 22:319–321, 1990.
Doherty, MH: Benzodiazepine sedation in critically ill patients. AACN Clinical Issues in Critical Care Nursing 2(4):748, 1991.
Dupuis, RE and Miranda-Massari, J: Anticonvulsants: Pharmacotherapeutic issues in the critically ill patient. AACN Clinical Issues in Critical Care Nursing 2(4):639, 1991.
Wild, LR: Neuromuscular blocking agents in the critically ill patient: Neither sedating nor pain relieving. AACN Clinical Issues in Critical Care Nursing 2(4):778, 1991.
Wilkins, R: Neurological surgery. JAMA 268:379–380, 1992.

CARE PLAN FOR POSTOPERATIVE PATIENT WITH CRANIOCEREBRAL SURGERY

Nursing Diagnoses

Nursing Diagnosis #1
Breathing Pattern ineffective, related to:
1. Brainstem compression associated with cerebral edema (especially following *infra*tentorial craniotomy)
2. Respiratory depression associated with anesthesia, analgesia, and muscle relaxants

Desired Patient Outcomes

Patient will demonstrate effective breathing pattern:
1. Respiratory rate <25/min
2. Rhythm and depth eupneic
   - Tidal volume >7–10 mL/kg
   - Vital capacity >12–15 mL/kg
3. Adequate alveolar ventilation and gas exchange:
   - $PaCO_2$ <30–35 mmHg
   - PaO_2 >80 mmHg
   - pH 7.35 to 7.45

Nursing Interventions
- Assess respiratory function.
  - Assess spontaneous respiratory effort: rate, depth, rhythm; use of accessory muscles; dyspnea, tachypnea; hyper- or hypoventilation.
  - Assess tidal volume and vital capacity.
  - Monitor arterial blood gases.
- Implement measures to improve breathing pattern.
  - Maintain patient in semi-Fowler's position.

  - Maintain nasogastric decompression as indicated.

  - Maintain mechanical ventilation and oxygenation.

Rationales
- Adequate ventilation and oxygenation are imperative because hypercapnia and hypoxia cause cerebral vasodilation. In the patient with reduced intracranial compliance, an increase in cerebral blood flow may precipitate a significant rise in ICP.
  - Reflect adequacy of ventilation and oxygenation.

  - Permits maximal chest excursion and facilitates drainage of blood and CSF from cranial vault via gravity.
  - Prevents abdominal distention, which can compromise diaphragmatic excursion; minimizes danger of aspiration.

Nursing Diagnoses

Nursing Diagnosis #2
Airway Clearance ineffective, related to:
1. Compromised cough
2. Thick, tenacious secretions

Desired Patient Outcomes

Patient will:
1. Maintain patent airway
   - Normal breath sounds on auscultation
   - Absence of adventitious sounds (crackles, rhonchi, wheezes)
2. Demonstrate secretion-clearing cough (unless contraindicated by intracranial hypertension)

Nursing Interventions
- Assess respiratory function.
  - Assess airway patency; status of protective reflexes: cough, gag, epiglottal closure.
  - Auscultate breath sounds bilaterally.
  - Assess characteristics of sputum (e.g., color, tenaciousness, amount).

- Implement measures to maintain airway patency:
  - Humidify inspired air.
  - Initiate suctioning of tracheobronchial secretions *only* when indicated; assess effect of suctioning on patient's ICP.
  - Follow appropriate suctioning technique; minimize suctioning time; preoxygenate and hyperventilate with 100% oxygen prior to and after suctioning; limit each suction pass to 15 seconds or less.
  - Monitor hydration status.

Rationales
- Hypercapnia and hypoxia increase cerebral blood flow.
  - Compromised protective reflexes place patient at risk of aspirating tracheobronchial secretions.
  - Presence of rales (crackles), wheezes, or rhonchi suggests increased pulmonary secretions (e.g., pulmonary edema, infection) or inability to mobilize or clear secretions. Patient is at increased risk of developing a pneumonia.

  - Suctioning stimulates cough reflex and Valsalva's maneuver; these responses are associated with an increase in ICP.
  - Reduces risk of developing hypercapnia and hypoxemia; minimizes risk of increasing ICP.

Nursing Diagnoses

Nursing Diagnosis #3
Pain (headache) related to:
1. Meningeal irritation
2. Surgical scalp incision
3. Anxiety

Desired Patient Outcomes

Patient will:
1. Verbalize and/or indicate comfort
2. Demonstrate relaxed facial expression and demeanor

CARE PLAN FOR POSTOPERATIVE PATIENT WITH CRANIOCEREBRAL SURGERY
(*Continued*)

Nursing Interventions

- Assess patient for signs of pain and discomfort.
  - Symptoms may include restlessness, agitation; clenched fist, tense facial expression; photophobia.
  - Signs of discomfort may be reflected by increase in ICP, heart rate, blood pressure, and respiratory rate.
- Implement measures to reduce discomfort.
  - Administer analgesic or sedative as prescribed. Evaluate patient's response to medication.
  - Position patient to relieve muscle tension and pressure on bony prominences.
  - Make sure dressing is not too tight and constricting.
  - Provide quiet environment. Minimize environmental stimuli: dim lights, reduce noise level, restrict visitors if necessary.
  - Provide periods for uninterrupted sleep.
  - Provide touch therapy; speak softly in a soothing voice.
    - Reassure patient you are there to anticipate and fulfill his/her needs.
    - Provide appropriate explanations.
  - Employ diversional and comfort measures (e.g., soft music, mouth care, back rub).

Rationales

- The patient must be as comfortable as possible to prevent any increase in ICP. Pain, fear, anxiety, and muscle tenseness or rigidity can precipitate a rise in ICP and must be avoided.

- Nursing activities that limit sensory overload, prevent sleep deprivation, and provide reassurance help to minimize changes in the patient's ICP status; such care minimizes cellular metabolic activities, reducing demand for oxygen and glucose, and thus the need for increase in cerebral blood flow.
  - Brain tissue itself is without free pain endings; pain experienced by patients is usually related to meningeal irritation and/or injury to scalp, where free nerve endings are numerous.

Nursing Diagnoses

Nursing Diagnosis #4
Alteration in fluid and electrolyte balance
1. Fluid volume excess related to:
   - Cerebral edema
   - SIADH
2. Fluid volume deficit related to:
   - Diuretic therapy
   - Diabetes insipidus
3. Altered electrolytes related to:
   - Diuretic therapy
   - Corticosteroid therapy
   - Acid-base imbalance

Desired Patient Outcomes

Patient will:
1. Maintain hemodynamic function
   - Mean systemic blood pressure ~80 to 100 mmHg
2. Maintain balanced intake and output
   - Stable baseline daily weight (unless contraindicated)
   - Urine output >30 mL/h and <200 mL/h
   - Urine specific gravity 1.010 to 1.025
3. Demonstrate good skin turgor and moist mucous membranes
4. Maintain laboratory parameters within acceptable range

Nursing Interventions

- Monitor for signs and symptoms of diabetes insipidus: polyuria, polydipsia, and urine specific gravity <1.005; monitor fluid intake and output, weight; serum electrolytes and osmolality.
  - Monitor for signs and symptoms of dehydration.
- Implement measures to:
  - Maintain adequate fluid intake to prevent dehydration.
  - Administer prescribed medications: vasopressin replacement therapy; agents that enhance ADH secretion (e.g., chlorpropamide, carbamazepine); and monitor response to therapy.

Rationales

- Diabetes insipidus may occur secondary to craniocerebral trauma, and/or infection (e.g., meningitis), or pituitary tumors.
  - Cerebral edema related to trauma or surgery may impair synthesis and release of antidiuretic hormone (ADH) temporarily, resulting in polyuria within 24 to 48 h. As cerebral edema subsides, symptoms also regress and diminish.

Nursing Diagnoses

Nursing Diagnosis #5
Injury, risk for; related to cerebral ischemia and injury associated with surgical manipulation

Desired Patient Outcomes

Patient will be free of seizures.

CARE PLAN FOR POSTOPERATIVE PATIENT WITH CRANIOCEREBRAL SURGERY
(*Continued*)

Nursing Interventions

- Assess characteristics of seizure activity (see Table 31–1).
  - Specific signs: onset (what triggers the seizure, type, locality, presence of aura, duration of seizure); type of movement: tonic, clonic, flaccid; associated changes in level of consciousness; respiratory rate and rhythm; pupillary size and reactivity; extraocular movements; associated vomiting or incontinence (urinary, fecal).
- During seizure activity:
  - Maintain safe environment.
  - Remain with patient but do not restrain; provide reassurance.
  - Do not force airway or other objects between clenched teeth.
  - Keep resuscitative equipment at bedside.
- Implement measures to prevent seizure activity.
  - Avoid problems that cause an increase in ICP (e.g., headache, anxiety, hypoxia, urinary retention, fecal impaction, hyperpyrexia).
  - Monitor for signs of meningeal irritation (see Nursing Diagnosis #6).
  - Initiate and maintain seizure precautions: oral airway; padded siderails and headboard; keep siderails in up position.
  - Administer prescribed anticonvulsant therapy.

  - Evaluate patient's response to anticonvulsant therapy.
    - Obtain serum levels of phenytoin.
    - Be familiar with effect of phenytoin on cardiovascular hemodynamics and adverse drug reactions.

Rationales

- Seizure activity can precipitate a significant increase in ICP; it increases cellular metabolism and the demand for metabolic substrates—oxygen and glucose; it raises body temperature.
  - Postoperative seizure activity may be precipitated by hypoxia, hyperpyrexia, meningeal irritation, and bladder distention.

- A rise in ICP may precipitate seizure activity associated with cerebral ischemia.

  - See Table 31–3, Seizure Precautions.

  - Diazepam, phenytoin, and barbiturates are commonly used to prevent and/or treat seizures.

For specific information related to dose, route of administration, adverse reactions, and nursing implications for each of these drugs, see Table 31–2.

Nursing Diagnoses

Nursing Diagnosis #6
Infection, risk for meningitis related to:
1. Craniocerebral trauma
2. Surgical disruption of integrity of the meninges
3. Invasive procedures

Desired Patient Outcomes

Patient will:
1. Maintain body temperature ~98.6°F
2. Remain free of signs of meningeal irritation (nuchal rigidity, headache, photophobia, positive Kernig's and Brudzinski's signs)
3. Demonstrate normal cerebrospinal fluid analysis (white blood cell [WBC] and protein levels); serum WBC within normal range

Nursing Interventions

- Monitor for signs and symptoms of infection.
  - Assess for meningeal irritation: hyperpyrexia, chills, nuchal rigidity, photophobia, persistent headache, positive Kernig's sign (i.e., inability to extend lower leg when hip is flexed), positive Brudzinski's sign (i.e., flexion of hips and knees when head is flexed on chest).
  - Assess for otorrhea and rhinorrhea.
    - Use Dextrostix to test for presence of glucose in ear or nasal discharge.
    - Observe for clear halo around serosanguineous drainage from ear, nose, or dressing.
    - Observe for excessive swallowing or complaints of postnasal drip.
  - Assist with lumbar puncture.
    - Observe color of CSF.
    - Record cerebrospinal pressure.

Rationales

  - Meningeal tears often accompany basal skull fractures.
    - Presence of glucose in nonbloody drainage from nose or ear suggests CSF leak. Nasopharyngeal secretions do not contain glucose.

  - Presence of elevated levels of WBCs and protein in cerebrospinal fluid strongly suggests meningitis.

CARE PLAN FOR POSTOPERATIVE PATIENT WITH CRANIOCEREBRAL SURGERY
(*Continued*)

Nursing Interventions

- Implement measures to prevent infection.
  - Specific nursing actions include: strict handwashing, sterile technique in managing all invasive procedures (e.g., ICPM, ventricular shunts), sterile technique employed for all dressing changes (as per unit protocols).
  - If rhinorrhea or otorrhea are present:
    □ Caution patient not to cough, sneeze, blow the nose, or perform a Valsalva's maneuver (e.g., straining at stool).
    □ Instruct patient not to put fingers into ears or nose, and to lie quietly.
    □ Allow free flow of drainage directly onto sterile pad; change pad as soon as it becomes damp.
    □ Have patient assume a position that facilitates free drainage (e.g., semi-Fowler's position) in the presence of rhinorrhea.
    □ Provide quiet environment; minimize stimuli.
- Administer prescribed course of antibiotics.
  - Evaluate response to therapy:
    □ Monitor temperature, WBC profile.
    □ Monitor neurologic function and signs of meningeal irritation.
    □ Monitor intracranial pressure.

Rationales

- Disciplined aseptic technique is essential to prevent meningitis.

  □ These activities increase ICP and can place further stress on the dural tear.

  □ Free flow of drainage prevents pooling, which might otherwise provide a medium for bacterial colonization.
  □ Reduces risk of aggravating underlying dural tear.
- Administration of corticosteroids to reduce cerebral edema may compromise the immune response, placing patient at greater risk of developing an infection. Ongoing assessment for signs of infection must be diligent; aseptic technique must be impeccable.

Nursing Diagnoses

Nursing Diagnosis #7
Body temperature, altered, risk for, related to:
1. Cerebral edema with altered hypothalamic function
2. Infection

Desired Patient Outcomes

Patient will maintain optimal body temperature ~98.6°F

Nursing Interventions

- Monitor body temperature every 1 to 2 h if unstable.
  - Assess for signs and symptoms of hyperpyrexia (e.g., hot, dry skin; parched tongue; cool extremities; delirium).
- Obtain specimens of body fluid (e.g., blood, urine, sputum, wound drainage) for culture and sensitivity.
- Inspect all invasive sites and wounds for signs of infection (e.g., redness, warmth, swelling, pain; amount and characteristics of wound drainage).
- Implement measures to reduce body temperature.
  - Administer prescribed antibiotic and antipyretic therapy.
    □ Evaluate patient's response to therapy by monitoring body temperature and WBC profile.
  - Provide comfort measures.
    □ Remove excess clothing and blankets.
    □ Maintain room temperature at 68°F.
- Provide diligent wound care using aseptic technique.
- Implement hypothermia therapy as prescribed.

Rationales

- Hyperpyrexia increases cerebral metabolism and cerebral blood flow; an increase in ICP may result from the consequent increase in intracranial blood volume.
- In the scenario of a spiking body temperature (102.2°F–105.8°F), obtain culture of body fluids prior to initiating prescribed antibiotic therapy.

- When inducing an increase or decrease in body temperature, the change in temperature should not exceed 1°F per 15 to 20 min.

Nursing Diagnoses

Nursing Diagnosis #8
Alteration in self-concept, related to:
1. Changes in body image associated with physical appearance (e.g., shaved head) or neurologic deficits (e.g., loss of sensorimotor function)
2. Loss of self-esteem (e.g., dependence on others to achieve activities of daily living)
3. Alterations in role and personal identity

Desired Patient Outcomes

Patient will:
1. Verbalize positive feelings about self
2. Maintain interpersonal relationships with family members and significant others
3. Participate in decision-making process regarding care
4. Initiate activities related to self-care

CARE PLAN FOR POSTOPERATIVE PATIENT WITH CRANIOCEREBRAL SURGERY
(*Continued*)

Nursing Interventions

- Encourage verbalization regarding patient's perceptions of changes in appearance and body function.
  - Observe nonverbal behavior reflective of underlying feelings and concerns.
  - Listen to patient's concerns.
  - Provide information and explanations regarding patient's status and prognosis. Clarify misconceptions.
  - Ascertain patient/family expectations and understanding regarding impact of illness on family lifestyle.
  - Facilitate communication between patient, family, and significant others.
- Assist patient/family to identify coping patterns/ strengths and weaknesses.
- Assess patient/family's readiness to participate in decision-making process regarding care.
- Involve patient in making choices and decisions regarding self-care.
  - Readily identify and praise patient's accomplishments. Identify improvements in bodily functions as they occur.
- Assist patient/family in initial goal setting.

  - Refer to social worker.
    - Identify community resources.
    - Encourage use of community support groups (e.g., head injury support groups).

Rationales

- Assists patient to increase self-awareness and to recognize and vent feelings of fear, anger, or frustrations.
  - Often what the patient does not say is reflected in the body language.

- Assists patient in maintaining a sense of control over his/ her life.
  - Positive reinforcement nurtures self-motivation.

- Depending on underlying problem, a craniocerebral insult or injury can be catastrophic in terms of health-care costs, productivity, and quality of life for all concerned.
  - Early referral to social worker and community agencies should be initiated.

C H A P T E R   3 1

Clinical Management of the Patient with an Acute Brain Disorder

Joan T. Dolan

CHAPTER OUTLINE

Acute Head Injury
- Classification of Head Injury
- Mechanisms of Head Injury
- Skull Fractures: Implications for Nursing Care
- Primary Head Injury
- Secondary Head Injury

Clinical Management of the Patient with Acute Head Injury
- Nursing Management

Case Study with Sample Care Plan: Patient with Acute Head Injury
- Initial Nursing Diagnoses

Meningitis
- Pathogenesis

- Pathophysiology
- Clinical Presentation
- Clinical Management of the Patient with Meningitis

Seizures
- Pathophysiology
- Types of Seizures and Clinical Presentation
- Status Epilepticus
- Seizures: Assessment Considerations
- Clinical Management of Seizures/Status Epilepticus

Suggested Readings

LEARNING OBJECTIVES

After completing this chapter, you should be able to:

1. Describe the classification of head injury.
2. Describe mechanisms of craniocerebral injury.
3. Discuss types of skull fractures and implications for nursing care.
4. Differentiate specific types of primary head injuries, potential for neurologic dysfunction, and clinical management.
5. Discuss types of secondary head injury, potential for neurologic dysfunction, and implications for clinical management.
6. Develop a plan of care for the patient with acute head injury.
7. Discuss the significance of meningitis as an infectious disease of the central nervous system in terms of its underlying pathogenesis, clinical presentation, and clinical management.
8. List tentative nursing diagnoses that provide the basis for managing the patient with meningitis.
9. Define seizure and its underlying pathophysiology.
10. Describe types of seizures and their clinical presentation.
11. Discuss the clinical management of seizures/status epilepticus.
12. List tentative nursing diagnoses that provide the basis for managing the patient with status epilepticus.

The focus of this chapter is to examine the pathophysiology and clinical management of three disorders involving the brain that are frequently seen in the critical care setting: acute head injury, meningitis, and seizures. Initial discussion is concerned with acute head injury, followed by an examination of meningitis and seizures. A case study and sample care plan concerned with a head-injured patient are also presented.

ACUTE HEAD INJURY

Classification of Head Injury

Head injury can be classified as primary or secondary. *Primary* head injury encompasses the actual brain damage resulting from the initial force or impact of the injury; *secondary* injury reflects the pathophysiologic consequences of the initial damage as the body responds to the injury. The type of injury sustained can also be classified as open or closed. An *open* injury, sometimes referred to as penetrating, disrupts the integrity of the skull and dura, and exposes the intracranial contents to the external environment; *closed* injuries, also referred to as nonpenetrating, do not disrupt the integrity of the skull, and the skull and its contents remain intact.

Mechanisms of Head Injury

When the head strikes an object, or vice versa, kinetic energy is absorbed by the scalp, skull, and meninges. The remaining energy becomes dissipated within the contents of the cranial vault. Usually, most of this energy is absorbed effectively by the protective structural layers of hair, scalp, bony skull, and the meninges. Very often the scalp enables an energy force to glance off the head rather than causing the head to absorb the full energy of impact directly. With especially violent trauma, however, these protective layers may not be able to absorb all of the forces of impact, and the remaining energy is transmitted to the brain causing damage and disruption of these delicate tissues.

The degree of structural and/or functional disruption of neuronal activity that occurs relates most directly to the magnitude of the force applied and the time span over which it is applied. Basically, the greater the force applied and the shorter the time of impact, the greater the likelihood of neurologic damage. The protection afforded by the scalp and skull should not be underestimated. The very fact that a skull fracture occurs may be a protective mechanism that dissipates the energy of impact before it affects the fragile brain tissues.

Acceleration-deceleration forces cause injuries classified as *coup* and *contrecoup*. Coup injuries occur directly beneath the site of impact; contrecoup injuries occur opposite the site of impact. Take, for example, a passenger riding in a car that suddenly comes to a complete stop. As the forehead of the passenger hits the dashboard, a coup injury to the underlying tissues of the frontal lobe is sustained; as the brain rebounds within the skull, a contrecoup injury involving brain tissues opposite to the site of impact occurs, which in this instance is the occipital lobe.

Because of their different inertias, the skull and brain move at different velocities. In the presence of the protective cerebrospinal fluid cushion, such differences account for the acceleration, deceleration, and rotational shearing motions that can occur with head injury. The consequent intracranial stress precipitated by such forces may cause fragile brain tissue and blood vessels to be compressed, pulled, or torn apart. Shearing-type injuries to the brain can also occur when, upon impact, the base of the brain is thrown against the sharpened edges of the basal bones at the base of the cranial vault (see Fig. 27–3).

Skull Fractures: Implications for Nursing Care

The type of skull fracture sustained in head injury depends on the velocity and mass of the object, its direction, and its force of impact. Skull fractures are usually classified as linear (simple), comminuted (fragmentation of bone into pieces), depressed (interruption of contour of skull by inward displacement of bony fragments), and compound (perforated fracture that usually involves a scalp laceration creating an external pathway or openings; the dura may or may not be involved).

Of the bones comprising the cranial vault, the squamous portion of the temporal bone is the thinnest, and, thus, vulnerable to injury. The clinical significance of a fracture of this bone is discussed in the section entitled "Epidural Hematoma" (below).

Basilar Skull Fractures

Basilar fracture involves disruption of bones in the base of the cranial vault, especially in the area of the anterior and middle fossae (see Fig. 27–3). The petrous process of the temporal bone is commonly involved, as are the fragile bones comprising the paranasal sinuses (frontal, maxillary, ethmoid). Of additional consequence is the intimate attachment of the dura to these bones.

Disruption of the dura, which often accompanies a basilar fracture, accounts for leakage of cerebrospinal fluid (CSF) via the nose or ear. *Rhinorrhea* signifies drainage of CSF and blood via the nose; *otorrhea* signifies similar drainage from the ear. The importance of these signs is that dural tears or disruptions become pathways for infection (e.g., meningitis). The *halo* sign is occasionally noticed on dressing or linen. It consists of dark or bloody drainage encircled by a yellow halolike stain. It is highly suggestive of a CSF leak. Testing the drainage with a Dextrostix is more definitive. If the stick is positive, the drainage contains glucose and consists of CSF; CSF contains glucose whereas mucus is glucose-free.

Basilar skull fractures may cause injury to the cavernous sinus at the base of the brain (see Fig. 27–8); fracture of the petrous bone may cause damage to the transverse sinus, which runs in a groove adjacent to the petrous bone. Disruption of these sinuses predisposes to the spread of infection via the orbit or the ear, respectively.

Additional signs of possible basilar skull fracture reflect bleeding into bone. Ecchymosis over the mastoid process of the temporal bone (Battle's sign) becomes evident approximately 30 hours after injury; bilateral ecchymosis of medial or circumscribed orbital areas is termed "raccoon eyes."

Any patient sustaining a skull fracture should be suspected of having an associated injury to the cervical spine. Complete caution must be used in supporting the patient until fracture or dislocation of the cervical spine has been ruled out. Any patient sustaining a skull fracture should be suspected of having underlying trauma to brain tissue. Therefore, management of such fractures requires ongoing neurologic assessment with early recognition of clues suggestive of secondary injury.

In patients with possible basilar skull fracture, assessment of vital parameters is important because of the proximity of vital centers along the brainstem to the base of the skull. Patients with possible basilar skull fracture should never be suctioned, unless intubated; alert, responsive patients should be cautioned *not* to blow their noses. A nasogastric tube should not be passed in patients suspected of having a dural tear and leaking CSF. In both of these instances the concern is the introduction of infection. The patient with a basilar skull fracture is usually kept flat on complete bed rest to decrease the amount of CSF that is draining. This position may facilitate spontaneous closure of the dural tear.

Primary Head Injury

Primary head injury usually results in an alteration in the level of consciousness. In minor head injuries the loss of consciousness may be momentary to less than 20 minutes in duration, and the score on the Glasgow Coma Scale (see Table 28–2) ranges between 13 and 15. Loss of consciousness for longer than 20 minutes, and a score on the Glasgow Coma Scale of 9 to 12, implies a moderate head injury. Loss of consciousness for an extended period of time, with a score on the Glasgow Coma Scale of less than 8, defines severe head injury. Primary head injuries may occur in a focal area of the brain or be diffuse in nature. Included among these injuries are concussion, cerebral contusion, cerebral laceration, and intracranial hemorrhage with hematoma formation.

Concussion

A concussion is a mild form of diffuse brain injury characterized by a transient period of neurologic dysfunction. Loss of consciousness may or may not occur, but when present, resolves, usually in a matter of seconds to minutes. Additional transient findings seen after trauma may include headache, dizziness, confusion, inability to concentrate, drowsiness, irritability, visual changes, loss of reflexes, vital sign changes, and residual memory loss, or amnesia. Treatment involves close monitoring for up to 24 hours to detect any signs of focal or progressive neurologic changes. Recovery is usually prompt (within 48 hours), although patients sustaining a more severe concussion may experience amnesia for several weeks or up to several months.

Contusion

A cerebral contusion is an actual bruising of the brain with edema formation and capillary hemorrhages in the affected area(s) of the brain. Focal injury may result at the site of the impact (*coup* injury), and/or the side opposite to the site of impact (*contrecoup* injury). It may also result from "shearing forces" applied to the base of the brain as it is thrown against the bony ridges in the floor of the skull (see Fig. 27–3).

Clinically, the patient's behavior may range from an altered state of consciousness (e.g., confusion, restlessness, agitation, or combativeness) to a state of coma in which the patient is unresponsive to stimuli. The loss of consciousness caused by a contusion can last for hours, days, and even weeks. Additional signs and symptoms, if present, may reflect the location and extent of the contusion, and any secondary injury caused by cerebral edema and/or bleeding. Treatment is guided by serial neurologic assessments and intracranial pressure (ICP) monitoring, if indicated.

Cerebral Laceration

A cerebral laceration is an actual tear in brain tissue associated with shearing forces, which cause the brain to strike irregular, rigid bony surfaces, particularly at the base of the skull. A break in the integrity of the meningeal layers usually occurs. A laceration is a severe head injury with more extensive neurologic dysfunction than that associated with concussion.

Intracranial Hemorrhage: Hematoma Formation

A major complication of acute head injury is intracranial hemorrhage. Regardless of the severity of trauma sustained to the head, the possibility of intracranial bleeding is a major consideration and warrants ongoing neurologic assessment so that should bleeding occur, it will be diagnosed *early* in its development and treated accordingly.

Because of the structural arrangement of the meningeal layers surrounding, supporting, and protecting the brain (see Fig. 27–4), intracranial bleeding may be limited to the spaces between these membranes. Such bleeding, which is relatively or completely confined to such spaces, is referred to as a *hematoma*. Thus, bleeding into the potential space between the periosteal dural sheath and the skull is called epidural (extradural) hematoma; bleeding within the subdural space between the dural and arachnoid membranes is called a subdural hematoma; and bleeding into the parenchyma of the brain itself is called an intracerebral hematoma.

Epidural Hematoma. An epidural hematoma is a collection of blood within the potential space between the periosteal dura and the skull (see Fig. 29–7). Distinguishing features of an epidural hematoma include temporal bone fracture, rapid deterioration in the level of consciousness, and signs of uncal herniation. An epidural hematoma is a rare but extreme surgical emergency.

The squamous portion of the temporal bone is the thinnest bone of the skull, and blows to the head frequently result in a linear fracture of this bone. Such a fracture can result in a laceration of the middle meningeal artery or one of its many branches, which occupy grooves within the inner table of the bone. The consequent hemorrhage is *arterial* in origin and rapidly expands due to the high pressure in the arterial system. The increased pressure strips the periosteal dura from the inner table of the skull creating a space within which a rapidly expanding mass develops.

The classic clinical history of an epidural hematoma is a blow to the head in the temporal-parietal area following which the patient becomes momentarily unconscious. This is followed by a wakeful, lucid period lasting for an hour to several hours. But as the hematoma expands, the patient's condition deteriorates. There may be complaints of headache and noticeable changes in the level of consciousness. The rapidity of deterioration depends on how quickly the mass expands. Once clouding of consciousness develops, abnormal pupillary signs and hemiparesis rapidly ensue, accompanied by a deepening coma. An epidural hematoma occurs as a unilateral expanding lesion and eventually develops into a supratentorial herniation syndrome, most commonly that of *uncal herniation* with lateral brainstem compression. (For a discussion of uncal herniation, see Chapter 29.)

Diagnosis of epidural hematoma is based on: (1) the patient's clinical history regarding the mechanism of head injury and the events following the injury, (2) clinical manifestations, and (3) computed tomography (CT) scan. Treatment is surgical evacuation of the hematoma, which, if performed early enough, may allow for full recovery.

Subdural Hematoma. A subdural hematoma evolves from bleeding within the space between the dura and arachnoid membrane (see Fig. 29–6). It is one of the more common complications of head injury and largely results from disruption of small veins that bridge the subdural space. Contusion or laceration of the brain may also cause subdural hemorrhage.

Subdural hematomas have been classified as acute, subacute, and chronic. This classification is based largely on the clinical manifestations exhibited by the patient and the time interval between the occurrence of the head injury and the onset of symptoms.

Acute Subdural Hematoma. Acute subdural hematoma is associated with severe head injury (as determined by the magnitude of the force applied and the time span over which it is applied), with the onset of symptoms within the first 24 to 48 hours. The skull may remain intact; rather, pathology is related to contusion and/or laceration of underlying brain tissue. Signs and symptoms may initially present as headache with progression to an altered state of consciousness. Rapid deterioration of consciousness may be accompanied by abnormal changes in respiratory rate and rhythm, pupillary dysfunction, dysconjugate eye movements, and abnormal motor responses.

The subdural hematoma usually involves the accumulation of blood throughout the entire frontotemporoparietal area, which acts as a generalized expanding supratentorial lesion. In contrast to the epidural hematoma, the downward rostral to caudal (head to toe) deterioration of an acute subdural hematoma may occur without substantial associated focal signs of a hemispheric mass lesion. Rather, its pathologic course more closely reflects that of the *central syndrome* of rostral to caudal brain herniation (see Chapter 29). An acute subdural hematoma requires early diagnosis and surgical evacuation of the clot to prevent secondary injury and permanent sequelae.

Subacute Subdural Hematoma. Subacute subdural hematomas are also associated with contusions to underlying brain, the symptoms of which begin to appear between 2 days and 2 weeks after injury. Brain damage is usually less severe than with acute subdural hematoma, affording a better prognosis. Subacute subdural hematomas are often associated with intracerebral bleeding. These hematomas are commonly located over the hemispheric areas. They may cause progressive changes in the level of consciousness with irritability and confusion; ipsilateral pupillary changes may become evident along with ophthalmoplegia; and hemiparesis may occur along with Babinski's sign. Seizure activity may become evident.

The diagnosis of subacute subdural hematoma depends on the patient's initial signs and symptoms and findings on CT scan. Surgery may be deferred if no midline shift of cerebral structures is observed on CT scan, and if the patient remains neurologically stable. Recovery may be possible without surgical intervention.

Chronic Subdural Hematoma. Chronic subdural hematomas evolve very slowly over several weeks or months. By the time changes are observed in the patient's behavior, the initial injury may have been forgotten. This type of hematoma is especially prevalent in the elderly. The patient may be unable to remember the circumstances of the initial trauma, and the presence of vague symptoms (e.g., headache, lethargy, slowed mentation, mood or personality changes) may be attributed to the aging process, cerebral atrophy, or the misdiagnosis of Alzheimer's disease. Elderly patients who present to the emergency department with a Colles' (wrist) fracture should be assessed for possible head injury.

As the blood clot resolves, the consequent coagulum, or fluid formed, spreads diffusely over the brain within the subdural space, congeals, and becomes walled off. The resultant viscous, highly concentrated jellylike substance draws fluid from the surrounding tissue, and gradually the fluid mass expands. Symptoms induced by this expanding lesion include headache, which gets progressively worse; behavioral changes (e.g., giddiness, drowsiness, confusion, slow cerebration); pupillary changes; hemiparesis; and seizures. With progressive enlargement, the encapsulated mass may cause further bleeding by tearing surrounding tissue, membrane, or blood vessels.

Diagnosis of a chronic subdural hematoma is based on the patient's age and clinical history, and is confirmed by CT scan. Treatment involves surgical aspiration of the clot via burr holes or craniotomy. If symptomatology is minimal, surgery may be deferred and the clot is allowed to resolve over time.

Intracerebral Hematoma. *Intracerebral* hematoma (see Fig. 29–5) refers to bleeding into the brain parenchyma and is often associated with injury to small blood vessels in response to rotational or shearing forces. These hematomas may occur singularly or as multiple lesions. They are found most frequently in the frontal and temporal lobes and are frequently accompanied by serious contusions and laceration of brain tissue. Because intracerebral hematomas are not compartmentalized by the meninges as are epidural and subdural hematomas, they can cause more direct brain damage and be more difficult to evacuate surgically.

The clinical course of a serious intracerebral bleed is characterized by rapidly developing coma, a contralateral hemiplegia, and dilatation of the ipsilateral pupil. As intracranial pressure increases, evidence of developing supratentorial herniation becomes apparent, and the prognosis is very grave. CT scan and angiography studies may help to diagnose the condition, but surgical intervention has met with limited success. Mortality rates are high. (For additional information on hematomas, refer to Table 32–3.)

Secondary Head Injury

Secondary head injury occurs as a consequence of the primary injury when the body responds physiologically to the actual insult. Examples of secondary injury include cerebral edema, intracranial hypertension with a consequent reduction in cerebral perfusion pressure (CPP) and cerebral blood flow, cerebral ischemia, and cellular hypoxia. If unrelieved, the increasing ICP can precipitate brain herniation (see Fig. 29–4).

CLINICAL MANAGEMENT OF THE PATIENT WITH ACUTE HEAD INJURY

Clinical management of the patient with acute head injury involves a collaborative effort on the part of nurses, physicians, and other healthcare providers. The initial concern is with sustaining life and minimizing brain damage. An attempt is made to diagnose the type of underlying lesion (e.g., epidural versus subdural hematoma); to localize the level of brain function (e.g., hemispheric, diencephalic, midbrain, or lower brainstem; see Fig. 27–10); and to implement the appropriate course of treatment, medical and/or surgical intervention).

The major goal of management is to control and/or prevent further secondary injury, and in so doing, to optimize the patient's neurologic recovery. Therapeutic interventions are concerned with minimizing cerebral edema and reducing and/or maintaining ICP within the acceptable physiologic range.

Intracranial pressure monitoring (ICPM) is initiated and maintained to monitor the patient's status, to evaluate the patient's response to therapy, and to serve as a guideline for the patient's overall care. In the patient with actual or potential intracranial hypertension, treatment is directed toward *controlling* ICP, and maintaining it as close to baseline as possible. Ideally, ICP should be maintained at less than 10 mmHg; 15 mmHg is considered to be the upper limit of normal.

Ventilatory and circulatory support are initiated. Hyperventilation therapy is directed toward maintaining a $PaCO_2$ of 28 to 32 mmHg, and a PaO_2 of greater than 80 mmHg. Circulatory support is directed toward maintaining a mean systemic arterial blood pressure (MAP) of 80 to 100 mmHg, to ensure a CPP of at least 60 to 70 mmHg, and ideally 80 and 90 mmHg.

Selected pharmacologic therapy is also initiated. This includes the use of a variety of agents, including those designed to prevent and/or minimize cerebral edema, control ICP, minimize brain activity, relax muscles, prevent seizures, control body temperature, and prevent stress-related gastric ulcerations (see Table 30–1). For intracranial hypertension that does not respond to other therapeutic interventions, barbiturate coma therapy may be implemented.

Additional supportive therapies include measures to maintain normothermia and to facilitate drainage of blood and CSF from the cranial vault. These latter measures include maintenance of optimal patient positioning, and avoidance of Valsalva-type maneuvers. In addition, CSF drainage may be employed when indicated, to prevent and/or treat intracranial hypertension. (For a detailed discussion of these therapies see Chapters 29 and 30.)

Surgical intervention is employed in emergency situations to stop intracranial hemorrhage, evacuate clots, and prevent an increase in ICP that may precipitate brain herniation. Techniques include craniotomy, (i.e., surgical opening of the skull), craniectomy (i.e., surgical excision of part of skull), and cranioplasty (i.e., repair of defect in the skull).

Nursing Management

Implementation of nursing process in the care of the patient with acute head injury involves the following interventions:

1. Perform a thorough ongoing neurologic assessment comparing findings and trends with established baseline data.
2. Establish and/or maintain a patent airway.
3. Implement prescribed hyperventilation therapy, carefully monitoring the patient's clinical status and arterial blood gas values, so as to maintain $PaCO_2$ at 28 to 32 mmHg.
4. Provide hemodynamic support necessary to stabilize mean arterial pressure at a value sufficient to maintain a cerebral perfusion pressure greater than 60 mmHg.
5. Maintain fluid and electrolyte balance to sustain the patient in a slightly dehydrated state.
6. Minimize anxiety and discomfort, and promote rest and relaxation.
7. Provide nutritional support.
8. Maintain urinary and bowel elimination.
9. Prevent infection.
10. Prevent stress-related gastrointestinal complications.
11. Prevent complications associated with physical immobility.
12. Maintain skin integrity and musculoskeletal function.
13. Establish a working rapport with patient, family, and/or significant others.
14. Provide emotional and psychological support to patient, family, and/or significant others.

Nursing Diagnoses, Desired Patient Outcomes, and Nursing Interventions

Pertinent nursing diagnoses, desired patient outcomes, and nursing interventions in the care of the patient with acute head injury are presented in the care plan at the end of this chapter. Additional pertinent nursing diagnoses also include the following:

1. Alteration in cerebral perfusion pressure (CPP) related to increased ICP associated with intracranial and/or cerebral insult
2. Breathing Pattern, ineffective, related to brainstem compression associated with cerebral edema
3. Airway Clearance, ineffective, related to:
   a. Compromised cough
   b. Thick, tenacious secretions
4. Alteration in fluid and electrolyte balance, related to:
   a. Fluid volume excess associated with cerebral edema
   b. Fluid volume deficit associated with diuretic therapy and diabetes insipidus
   c. Altered electrolytes associated with diuretic and corticosteroid therapies, and acid-base imbalance
5. Injury, risk for seizures, related to:
   a. Cerebral hypoxia associated with increased ICP and reduced CPP
   b. Cerebral irritation associated with craniocerebral trauma, surgical manipulation of fragile brain tissue, cerebral edema, and infection (e.g., meningitis)
6. Infection, risk for meningitis related to:
   a. Craniocerebral trauma
   b. Surgical disruption of integrity of the meninges
   c. Invasive procedures
7. Body Temperature, altered, risk for, related to cerebral edema with altered hypothalamic function, and/or infection
8. Pain, acute, due to headache, related to:
   a. Meningeal irritation
   b. Surgical scalp incision and dressing
9. Skin Integrity, impaired, risk for, related to:
   a. Immobility associated with intracranial hypertension and altered state of consciousness
   b. Altered nutritional state

CASE STUDY WITH SAMPLE CARE PLAN: PATIENT WITH ACUTE HEAD INJURY

TN, a 19-year-old with no previous medical history, was accidentally struck in the head by a baseball bat during a softball game. He was unconscious momentarily (his friends said about 5 seconds), then awakened and was alert and responsive. T returned home complaining to his mother of a "splitting" headache and some nausea. An ice pack was applied to the injury site, and T fell asleep for the night.

When T awoke the next morning, the headache had increased in severity and T vomited several times. As the day wore on, T became increasingly drowsy and lethargic, and his mother had difficulty in waking him. His mother also noted that T seemed very confused. She immediately brought him to the local hospital emergency department.

Within the treatment area, T's condition was stable. A cervical spine film was taken to rule out cervical injury, and it was negative. On assessment, T was noted to have an altered state of consciousness; he was confused and became combative when aroused. T's respiratory pattern was eupneic, with occasional sighs and yawns. His pupils were 2 mm bilaterally and reacted sluggishly to light. Eye movements were slightly divergent; oculocephalic reflexes were intact. There appeared to be some weakness in T's left arm and leg; a Babinski's sign was noted bilaterally.

As T was prepared to have a CT scan of his head, his condition appeared to deteriorate. His verbal responses became inappropriate, spontaneous eye opening occurred only to speech or when prodded, and there was a gross withdrawal response of the right arm to a painful stimulus (pressure applied over a nailbed).

The results of the CT scan revealed a large subdural hematoma on the right side of the brain, with a shift of the falx cerebri and lateral ventricle to the left. Upon consultation with the neurosurgeon, the decision was made to evacuate the hematoma surgically, and T was prepared for surgery.

Initial Nursing Diagnoses

See sample care plan. Refer also to the care plans in Chapters 29 and 30.

SAMPLE CARE PLAN FOR THE PATIENT WITH ACUTE HEAD INJURY

Nursing Diagnoses

Nursing Diagnosis #1
Alteration in cerebral perfusion pressure, related to:
1. Large, right-sided acute subdural hematoma
2. Potential cerebral edema formation
(See also care plans in Chapters 30 and 31.)

Desired Patient Outcomes

Patient will:
1. Maintain:
   • Cerebral perfusion pressure > 60 mmHg
   • Intracranial pressure < 15 mmHg
   • Arterial blood pressure ~80 mmHg (mean)
2. Exhibit intact level of consciousness and mentation:
   • Oriented to person, place
   • Memory intact
3. Demonstrate intact sensorimotor function:
   • Distinguish pinprick from crude pressure
   • Purposeful motor response to painful stimulus

Nursing Interventions

• Assess: level of consciousness, mentation, respiratory rate and pattern, pupillary size and reactivity, sensorimotor function (muscle tone, deep tendon reflexes, posturing).

   ○ Assess vital signs: BP, pulse, body temperature.

• Maintain integrity of intracranial monitoring system: scrupulous hand-washing and aseptic technique; monitor system for leaks, avoid drainage of CSF.

• Obtain/record pressure readings using appropriate procedure/protocol:
   ○ Venting port of transducer at level of foramen of Monro.

   ○ Monitor waveform configuration/digital readouts.

• Implement measures to prevent and/or reduce ICP:
   ○ Maintain proper positioning; elevate head of bed; body in proper alignment.

   ○ Maintain controlled hyperventilation and oxygenation; prevent accumulation of tracheobronchial secretions; use meticulous suctioning technique.

Rationales

• Patient responses to increases in ICP can change rapidly from moment to moment; a sustained increase in ICP (>25–30 mmHg for greater than 15–20 minutes) can compromise cerebral perfusion pressure.
   ○ A rise in BP, widening pulse pressure, and slow bounding pulse are *late* occurring signs of increasing ICP.
• ICP monitoring is a highly invasive system with a high risk of infection.
   ○ Maintaining a closed system reduces risk of infection; ensures valid readings.

   ○ For every inch that the measurement is off, approximately 2 mmHg is added or subtracted from the digital readout.
   ○ Monitoring *trends* provides essential information regarding status of ICP and intracranial compliance.

   ○ Elevation of head facilitates drainage from cranium via gravity. Patients with sustained intracranial hypertension, in whom compensatory mechanisms are compromised, may experience a decrease in CPP and cerebral blood flow upon head elevation. In this circumstance, maintaining a flat, supine position may be indicated.
   ○ Hypercapnia causes cerebral vasodilation, increasing intracerebral blood flow, with potential risk of increasing ICP and decreasing CPP.
   ○ Proper suctioning technique reduces hypoxemia.

Nursing Interventions

• Monitor response to prescribed therapy to reduce cerebral edema:
   ○ Diuretic therapy/hyperosmolar therapy
   ○ Corticosteroid therapy
   ○ Strict control of intake and output
   ○ Laboratory data: BUN, creatinine, electrolytes, serum osmolality, urine specific gravity.

Rationales

• Fluid restriction coupled with pharmacologic therapy helps to reduce extracellular fluid volume; a mildly dehydrated state is maintained.

   ○ Craniocerebral insults frequently predispose to diabetes insipidus.
      □ Increased serum osmolality helps draw fluid from brain interstitium and reduce cerebral edema.

SAMPLE CARE PLAN FOR THE PATIENT WITH ACUTE HEAD INJURY (*Continued*)

Nursing Diagnoses

Nursing Diagnosis #2
Breathing Pattern, ineffective, related to expanding right-sided acute subdural hematoma with consequent brainstem compression

Desired Patient Outcomes

Patient will:
1. Demonstrate effective breathing pattern:
   - Respiratory rate <25 inspirations/min
   - Rhythm and depth eupneic
2. Maintain adequate pulmonary function:
   - Tidal volume > 7–10 mL/kg
   - Vital capacity >12–15 mL/kg

Nursing Interventions

- Assess respiratory functioning hourly:
  - Spontaneous breathing: rate/rhythm/depth.
  - Monitor arterial blood gases (serially).
- Implement measures to improve breathing pattern:
  - Maintain semi-Fowler's position.

  - Maintain nasogastric decompression.

  - Maintain mechanical ventilation and oxygenation: assess tidal volume and vital capacity at bedside.

Radionales

- Maintenance of adequate ventilation/oxygenation is imperative because hypercapnia and hypoxemia cause cerebral vasodilation.

  - Allows maximal chest excursion; facilitates drainage of blood and CSF from cranium.
  - Prevents abdominal distention, which can compromise diaphragmatic excursion.

Nursing Diagnoses

Nursing Diagnosis #3
Airway Clearance, ineffective, related to:
1. Compromised protective reflexes (e.g., gag, cough, epiglottal closure)
2. Altered state of consciousness

Desired Patient Outcomes

Patient will:
1. Maintain patent airway:
   - Normal breath sounds
   - Absence of adventitious breath sounds (e.g., crackles, wheezes)
2. Demonstrate secretion-clearing cough (unless contraindicated by intracranial hypertension)

Nursing Interventions

- Assess airway patency hourly:

  - Check status of protective reflexes (gag, cough).

  - Auscultate breath sounds.

  - Assess characteristics of sputum:
    - Color, tenaciousness, amount, odor.
  - Assess hydration status.
- Implement measures to maintain airway patency
  - Maintain hydration within prescribed limitations
    - Humidify oxygen administered.
  - Follow appropriate technique for tracheobronchial suctioning

Rationales

- Hypercapnia and hypoxemia increase cerebral blood flow.
  - Compromised protective reflexes place patient at risk of aspiration.
  - Presence of crackles, wheezes, and rhonchi suggests increased pulmonary secretions or inability to mobilize or clear secretions.

  - Dehydration causes tracheobronchial secretions to become thick, tenacious, and difficult to clear.

  - Reduces risk of hypercapnia and hypoxemia.
  - Reduces risk of infection.

SAMPLE CARE PLAN FOR THE PATIENT WITH ACUTE HEAD INJURY (*Continued*)

Nursing Diagnoses	**Desired Patient Outcomes**

Nursing Diagnosis #4
Gas Exchange, impaired, related to:
1. Widespread atelectasis
2. Potential neurogenic pulmonary edema

Patient will:
1. Be alert, oriented to person/place
2. Demonstrate appropriate behavior
3. Maintain optimal arterial blood gases:
   - $PaCO_2 \sim 30$ mmHg
   - $PaO_2 > 80$ mmHg
   - pH $\sim$ 7.35–7.45

Nursing Interventions	**Rationales**

- Assess cardiopulmonary function:
  - Heart rate, skin color
  - Hemodynamic parameters: systemic arterial BP, pulmonary capillary wedge pressure (PCWP), cardiac output
  - Presence of cardiac arrhythmias

- Hemodynamic parameters reflect tissue perfusion. Evidence of cyanosis is a late sign of altered perfusion usually occurring after >5 g hemoglobin become unsaturated.

  - Hypoxemia is associated with myocardial irritability.
    - Metabolic acidemia is associated with decreased tissue perfusion as the lack of oxygen predisposes to anaerobic metabolism with lactate production.
    - Metabolic acidemia may depress myocardial function predisposing to arrhythmias.

- Monitor laboratory data:
  - Arterial blood gases:
    - pH
    - PaO_2, $PaCO_2$
- Calculate PAO_2–PaO_2.

  - Most closely reflect effectiveness of gas exchange.

- Alveolar-arterial gradient <250 to 300 mmHg with a fraction of inspired oxygen (FIO_2) $\sim$ 60% in the presence of deteriorating pulmonary function is highly suggestive of adult respiratory distress syndrome (ARDS).

- Implement oxygen therapy as prescribed.
- Implement positive end-expiratory pressure (PEEP) therapy as prescribed. Monitor:
  - Arterial blood gases (ABGs), mixed venous oxygen tension ($P\bar{v}O_2$)

  - Lung compliance
  - Hemodynamic parameters (PCWP, pulmonary artery pressure, cardiac output)
- Monitor for complications of PEEP therapy:
  - Reduction in venous return to the heart and cardiac output; reduction in cerebral perfusion; barotrauma; increase in ICP

- O_2 concentration should maintain $PaO_2 > 80$ mmHg.
- PEEP therapy maintains airway opening pressure at end-expiration above the atmospheric pressure, thus increasing the functional residual capacity (FRC), preventing airway collapse, and enhancing gas exchange and oxygen transport.
  - Lung compliance is determined by dividing the peak inspiratory pressure (PIP) into the tidal volume.

  - The positive intrathoracic pressures generated reduce venous return via the great veins and can compromise outflow of blood and CSF from the cranial vault. For patients at risk of developing intracranial hypertension, close monitoring of ICP is imperative.
    - Overdistention and rupture of alveoli are major complications of PEEP therapy.

Nursing Diagnoses	**Desired Patient Outcomes**

Nursing Diagnosis #5
Injury, risks for seizures, related to:
1. Cerebral hypoxia associated with an increase in ICP with consequent decrease in CPP
2. Cerebral irritation associated with cerebral trauma with bleeding
3. Surgical manipulation of fragile brain tissue and meninges

Patient will:
1. Remain seizure-free
2. Maintain effective serum levels of phenytoin
   - Usual serum levels: $\sim$10–20 μg/mL

Nursing Interventions	**Rationales**

- Assess characteristics of seizure activity (Table 31–1):
  - Onset, influencing factors, duration
  - Type of movement: tonic-clonic

- Seizure activity can precipitate a significant increase in ICP; it increases cellular metabolism and the oxygen demand; it raises body temperature.

SAMPLE CARE PLAN FOR THE PATIENT WITH ACUTE HEAD INJURY (*Continued*)

Nursing Interventions	Rationales

Nursing Interventions

- ○ Associated changes in level of consciousness, respiratory status, pupillary size/reactivity
- ○ Vomiting, urinary/bowel incontinence
- • Implement measures to prevent seizure activity (Table 31–3):
  - ○ Avoid activities that cause a substantial sustained increase in ICP (>25–30 mmHg/15 to 20 min).
  - ○ Monitor for signs/symptoms of meningeal irritation: nuchal rigidity, photophobia, persistent headache, positive Kernig's and/or Brudzinski's signs.
- • Initiate and maintain seizure precautions:
  - ○ Oral airway; padded siderails and headboard, siderails in up position, bed in low position.
  - ○ Administer prescribed anticonvulsant therapy.
  - ○ Evaluate patient's response to anticonvulsant therapy (obtain serial blood levels of phenytoin).

Nursing Diagnoses

Nursing Diagnosis #6
Alteration in fluid and electrolyte balance (potential), related to:
1. Aggressive diuretic therapy and corticosteroid therapy
2. Diabetes insipidus

Desired Patient Outcomes

Patient will:
1. Maintain hemodynamic function:
   - • Mean systolic BP ~80 to 100 mmHg
   - • Heart rate at patient's baseline
   - • Regular rhythm without arrhythmias
2. Maintain balanced intake/output:
   - • Stable weight (unless contraindicated)
   - • Urine output: >30 mL, <200 mL/h
   - • Urine specific gravity: 1.010 to 1.025

Nursing Interventions

- • Assess hydration status:
  - ○ Daily weight if not contraindicated by the presence of a labile ICP
  - ○ Intake and output
  - ○ Status of skin/mucous membranes; edema
- • Implement fluid replacement regimen within limitations prescribed
- • Monitor for signs/symptoms of diabetes insipidus:
  - ○ Presence of polyuria, polydipsia
  - ○ Urine specific gravity ~ 1.005
  - ○ Presence of dehydration: poor skin turgor, sunken eyeballs
- • Monitor laboratory parameters: serum electrolytes, osmolality, BUN, creatinine, hematology profile.

Rationales

- • Patients at risk of developing cerebral edema, or an increase in ICP, are maintained in a slightly dehydrated state.

- • Diabetes insipidus may occur secondary to craniocerebral trauma, infection.

MENINGITIS

Meningitis is acute inflammation of the meningeal coverings of the brain and/or spinal cord and is usually due to infection by bacteria or viruses. Some infections may involve both the meninges and the brain parenchyma as well. Once having gained access to the subarachnoid space and the CSF contained therein, the infectious process can spread throughout the subarachnoid space to reach the ventricles of the brain. Meningitis is an extremely serious infection requiring prompt recognition and treatment if neurologic complications are to be prevented or minimized.

Pathogenesis

Bacteria implicated in the pathogenesis of meningitis include *Neisseria meningitidis* (one of the most contagious), *Staphylococcus aureus* (frequently after neurologic surgery), and *Streptococcus pneumoniae*. Meningitis associated with gram-negative bacilli (e.g., *Escherichia coli*, *Enterobacter*, *Serratia*, *Klebsiella*, *Proteus*, and *Pseudomonas*) is usually seen in patients who are immunosuppressed, including those with AIDS and advanced cancers. The most common viruses causing meningitis are the enteroviruses—coxsackievirus and echovirus; herpesviruses, particularly cytomegalovirus (also seen frequently in the immunosuppressed); mumps virus; and arbovirus.

Mechanisms of Pathogenesis

Meningitis may occur as a primary focal infection or as a secondary infection following hematogenous dissemination (e.g., systemic bacteremia). It may occur directly as a result of craniocerebral trauma when the dura has been disrupted, or secondary to infections involving other adjacent cranial structures, such as the ears (e.g., otitis media, mastoiditis), the orbits, or nasal sinuses (e.g., sinusitis). Meningitis caused by gram-negative bacteria (e.g., *Serratia, Pseudomonas, Klebsiella, Escherichia coli*, and *Proteus*) and viruses (e.g., cytomegalovirus) is usually seen only in immunosuppressed patients.

Pathophysiology

Clinically, meningitis is classified, largely on the basis of CSF examination, into two types: suppurative and nonsuppurative. In *suppurative* meningitis, the CSF is characteristically turbid (i.e., cloudy) in appearance; there is pronounced leukocytosis, with neutrophils as the predominant cell type; and there is an increased protein level with a low to normal glucose content. In *nonsuppurative* meningitis the CSF is clear; the leukocyte count is low with a predominance of lymphocytes; the protein is increased, but the glucose is within normal limits.

Suppurative meningitis is associated with infections of bacterial origin, and usually occurs subsequent to an upper respiratory infection. Nonsuppurative meningitis, or aseptic meningitis, is primarily viral in origin.

Clinical Presentation

Clinically, the early signs and symptoms of meningitis reflect meningeal irritation and may include severe headache, photophobia, nuchal rigidity, paresthesias, and the classic Kernig's and Brudzinski's signs (see Chapter 28). The patient may complain of general malaise and may appear to be lethargic, with a shortened attention span. In the presence of a bacteremia, signs and symptoms may include hyperpyrexia, shaking chills, hypotension, and tachypnea. Alterations in the level of consciousness and mentation are common. A rash (meningococcal meningitis) may also be observed.

Clinical Management of the Patient with Meningitis

Therapy ultimately depends upon identification of the causative organism. The mainstay of medical intervention is the administration of large doses of antibi-

otic therapy. Initial therapy involves administration of penicillins; penicillin G is the antibiotic of choice as it easily crosses the blood-brain barrier. Gram-negative organisms may require an aminoglycoside (e.g., gentamicin), or third-generation cephalosporins. Institution of other supportive therapeutic modalities depends on the severity of the patient's clinical status. Analgesics (usually non-narcotic) are prescribed for headache and pain relief; an antipyretic for control of fever.

Nursing Management

Meningitis is an infectious disease, and it is necessary to consult with the infectious disease officer/nurse to determine what precautions need to be instituted. Meningococcal meningitis *(Neisseria meningitidis)*, for example, requires fecal and oral precautions.

The patient's response to antibiotic therapy is monitored closely, and supportive care is instituted. Environmental stimuli are reduced, and the patient's bedside area is kept darkened and as quiet as possible. Patient care activities should be planned so that the patient has extended rest periods. Seizure precautions should be in effect (Table 31–3).

Any illness involving the nervous system can be especially distressing to patient and family. The presence of neurologic deficits can be frightening, since they raise the concern of permanent neurologic complications, and even death. It is important to keep both patient and family informed as to the patient's status and to give them the opportunity to ask questions, discuss their perceptions of the situation, and to vent fears, anger, and concerns.

Tentative Nursing Diagnoses: Basis for Managing the Patient with Meningitis. Specific nursing diagnoses in managing the patient with meningitis may include:
1. Alteration in comfort: Severe headache, photophobia, related to meningeal irritation
2. Anxiety, related to:
   a. Presence of neurologic deficits
   b. Fear of permanent neurologic sequelae, i.e., complications
   c. Fear of dying
3. Injury, risk for, associated with seizures, related to meningeal irritation
4. Thought Processes, alterated, related to:
   a. Altered level of consciousness and mentation
   b. Changes in tissue perfusion in the brain
5. Fluid and electrolyte balance, altered, related to:
   a. Nothing-by-mouth (NPO) status
   b. Hyperpyrexia
6. Knowledge deficit, related to meningitis and implications for recovery

SEIZURES

A seizure is a spontaneous paroxysmal episode of excessive and disorganized electrical activity, involving neurons within the brain; it interrupts the ongoing mental and behavioral activities of the individual. It is manifested clinically by transient alterations in the level of consciousness, impairment of mentation, and disturbances in sensorimotor function.

Pathophysiology

In a seizure, neurons begin to discharge rapid, repetitive electrical impulses without inhibition; simultaneously, they recruit other nearby neurons to form a focus of excessive electrical activity. This focus of increased electrical excitability can originate deep within the central core of the brain, or it may arise from focal areas and spread to other brain structures. Consciousness is disrupted when the excessive electrical activity involves the reticular activating system (see section on reticular formation in Chapter 27).

Seizures increase overall cerebral metabolism severalfold. In the scenario of repeated seizures (as in status epilepticus), increased oxygen and glucose consumption due to skeletal muscle contraction, coupled with periods of apnea, rapidly deplete oxygen and nutritive stores and lead to hypoxemia, hypercapnia, and hypoglycemia. The increase in cellular lactate associated with anaerobic metabolism further complicates the pathophysiologic state. In the critically ill brain-injured patient, the primary concern is that uncontrolled seizures can increase the risk for secondary brain injury.

Types of Seizures and Clinical Presentation

Seizures are classified as generalized or partial. Generalized seizures reflect involvement of the entire brain and are characterized at the onset by a sudden loss or lapse of consciousness. An *absence*, or *petit mal* seizure is a generalized seizure characterized by short lapses of consciousness lasting but a few seconds. There may be a vacant stare, a brief pause in conversation, or rapid eye blinking.

The *tonic-clonic*, or *grand mal* seizure is the classic epileptic seizure that begins with a sudden loss of consciousness, accompanied by generalized contraction of muscles throughout the body (tonic phase). This phase is followed by violent, rhythmic jerking movements, accompanied by strenuous and loud hyperventilatory, stertorous-type respirations (clonic phase). The face is contorted, the eyes roll back, and there is excessive salivation, with frothing from the mouth. Profuse sweating and tachycardia may be evident. The clonic jerking movements, the result of simultaneous contraction and relaxation of opposing muscle groups, eventually subside.

Partial seizures are usually unilateral, involving a localized or focal area of the brain. These seizures occur without loss of consciousness and involve one category of symptoms, sensory or motor. *Jacksonian* epilepsy is an example of a partial seizure. It is characterized by a focal onset, as, for example, a twitching of the fingers, and progressively increases in a stepwise fashion. The seizure is said to "march along" as the successive parts of the body become involved, and this activity is reflective of the spread of seizure activity within the brain.

Most seizures are idiopathic (i.e., of unknown cause). In the critical care setting, however, it is often possible to identify the underlying disorder that either directly, or indirectly, gives rise to the seizure. Precipitating and/or contributing factors include craniocerebral trauma, cerebrovascular disease; infections, particularly of the brain or its supportive structures (e.g., meningitis); cerebral tumors, metabolic derangements, arteriovenous malformations of the brain, or an abrupt withdrawal of anticonvulsant medication or chronically used sedatives.

Status Epilepticus

Status epilepticus is a state of recurrent, successive, and/or prolonged seizure activity or convulsions without intervening periods of physiologic recovery by the patient. The patient experiences successive tonic-clonic seizures, with each succeeding seizure occurring before the preceding seizure has ended. Because of the potential for developing anoxia, cardiac arrhythmias, and acidemia, the occurrence of status epilepticus is a life-threatening medical emergency.

Seizures: Assessment Considerations

In assessing the patient with seizures, an initial consideration is to determine whether the signs and symptoms are, in fact, seizures or a disorder that mimics seizures. Table 31–1 lists major factors to be considered when assessing seizure activity. A thorough history obtained from the patient, family, and/or significant others may help to characterize the seizure type, cause, duration, prior treatment, and current status.

As information regarding seizure activity is examined, it is important to appreciate that seizures are dynamic and changing. Information derived regarding one seizure episode may not apply to succeeding episodes. In the critical care setting, assessing for seizure activity is made more difficult because therapeutic measures instituted to manage neurologic complications may mask manifestations of seizures. For example, patients who are mechanically ventilated and are paralyzed with pancuronium, a skeletal muscle relaxant may exhibit only minor muscle twitching during a seizure episode. In these instances, seizure activity may be reflected by a marked increase in ICP.

Clinical Management of Seizures/Status Epilepticus

Controlling seizure activity requires that the underlying cause and precipitating factors be determined and that appropriate treatment be implemented. In

TABLE 31–1
Assessing Seizure Activity: Major Considerations

Major factors to be considered when assessing seizure activity include the following:
1. The time of day the seizure(s) occurred and the frequency of occurrence.
2. The activity the patient was involved in when the seizure occurred.
3. The precipitating event/other precipitating factors.
4. A description of any warning signs or aura experienced by the patient.
5. A detailed description of the onset of the seizure:
   a. Was there a shrill cry?
   b. Was there loss of consciousness? Did the patient fall?
   c. In what part of the body did seizure activity begin? How did it proceed?
   d. What type of movement occurred?
6. A description of the phases of the seizure and the progression from one phase to another.
7. Notation of any changes in the size and reactivity of the pupils; evidence of dysconjugate or deviant gaze.
8. Presence of urinary or bowel incontinence.
9. The duration of the apneic period if present; evidence of cyanosis of lips, mucous membranes, and nailbeds.
10. The duration of the entire seizure, as well as that of each specific phase.
11. Evidence of altered level of consciousness; or state of unconsciousness throughout the entire seizure.
12. Notation of patient's behavior after seizure:
    a. Alert, drowsy, confused?
    b. Evidence of weakness or paralysis—unilateral or bilateral?
    c. Fatigue, muscle aching?
    d. Length of sleep after seizure?

the critical care setting, this may mean the diagnosis and treatment of secondary metabolic disturbances associated with head trauma, intracranial surgery, drug overdose, or toxicity related to anticonvulsant therapy. In the brain-injured patient, seizures may be attributed to secondary brain injury (e.g., intracranial hypertension, cerebral edema, cerebral ischemia), which may be the *cause* or the *result* of seizure activity.

Pharmacologic Therapy

All types of seizure activity should be prevented and/or stopped *immediately*. Pharmacologic therapy includes the use of a short-acting benzodiazepine (e.g., diazepam) to halt seizure activity, followed by a loading dose and then maintenance doses of longer-acting anticonvulsants (e.g., phenytoin or phenobarbital). The drug of choice in the emergency treatment of status epilepticus is diazepam. Table 31–2 describes drugs used to treat status epilepticus, and includes dosage and administration, adverse reactions, and nursing implications.

It is important to note that respiratory depression is a major adverse reaction of these anticonvulsant drugs. Respiratory arrest and laryngospasm have been identified with diazepam and pentobarbital, respectively. Thus, patients treated with these drugs are usually intubated, and mechanical ventilation initiated. Cardiac arrhythmias have been associated with diazepam and phenytoin, so that use of these drugs requires continuous cardiac monitoring. If anticonvulsant therapy is unsuccessful in the treatment of status epilepticus, general anesthesia (usually induced with pentobarbital) may be necessary because the seizures *must be stopped if the patient is to survive*.

Nursing Management

Goals of nursing management in the care of the patient with seizures are focused on airway management, patient safety, and maintenance of cardiovascular, metabolic, and psychological and emotional integrity.

Airway Management. Maintenance of patent airway is of primary concern because *hypoxemia* predisposes to brain damage. During a seizure, support the head in a manner that allows secretions to drain out of the mouth rather than down into the pharynx. This reduces risk of aspiration. If possible, remove dentures, food, or other substances from the mouth and insert an oral airway. *Do not try to force* any objects into the patient's mouth during a seizure. *Do not try to pry* the mouth open when the teeth are clenched. *Do not insert* fingers into the patient's mouth.

Loosen any constricting clothing from the neck and chest to allow for respiratory excursion and observation. Assess breathing pattern, length of apneic period, cyanosis, labored breathing. If necessary, use suction to help maintain airway patency; ventilate and oxygenate with a hand resuscitator. Anticipate endotracheal intubation and initiation of mechanical ventilation. Appropriate equipment for these modalities should be available at the patient's bedside. Obtain a sample for arterial blood gas analysis.

Seizure Precautions: Patient Safety. There is always the potential for patient injury related to seizure activity. A major nursing responsibility is to protect the patient from possible injury. Factors concerned with seizure precautions and patient safety are listed in Table 31–3. Neurologic assessment and observation for seizure activity should be ongoing, and findings should be documented accordingly.

TABLE 31–2
Drugs Used to Treat Status Epilepticus*

Drug	Description	Dosage and Administration	Adverse Reactions	Nursing Implications
Diazepam (Valium)	Drug of choice in treatment of status epilepticus A short-acting anticonvulsant; seizures may recur within 30 min Frequently given in conjunction with phenytoin for treatment of status epilepticus	Intravenous administration *Dose Range:* 5–10 mg IV; may repeat every 10–15 min to total of 30 mg; may repeat regimen again in 2–4 h	Respiratory: Depression and possible respiratory arrest Cardiovascular: Hypotension, tachycardia Eyes: Blurred vision, diplopia, nystagmus Renal: Urinary retention CNS: Drowsiness, fatigue, headache, slurred speech	Do not mix or dilute with other drugs or solutions. Do not add to IV fluids. Have resuscitative equipment in readiness.
Phenytoin (Dilantin)	Formerly, diphenylhydantoin Often used in conjunction with phenobarbital	Initial dose: ~500 mg IV at 50 mg/min, slow intravenous infusion Maintenance dose: 3–7 mg/kg per day PO, IV, or IM in 1 to 3 individual doses Use of IV line containing normal saline (phenytoin precipitates in dextrose solutions)	Cardiovascular: Potential for arrhythmias— bradycardia, heart block, and ventricular fibrillation Respiratory depression CNS: Nystagmus, diplopia, drowsiness, lethargy Hypersensitivity: Pruritus, fever	For parenteral administration use only special diluent. Margin between therapeutic and toxic doses is very small. ECG continuous monitoring. Solubility of phenytoin is pH-dependent; avoid mixing with other drugs or solutions. Filter within IV line should be used.
Phenobarbital (Luminal) Phenobarbital sodium (Luminal sodium)	Used to control status epilepticus when diazepam and phenytoin have failed Most widely used anticonvulsant Often given in conjunction with phenytoin	Intravenous administration for management of acute seizures *Dose:* 200–600 mg IV push Rate for IV doses not to exceed 60 mg/min	Respiratory depression Decreased effects of other drugs, due to induction of hepatic microsomal activity by barbiturates Overdosage: Respiratory depression, pupillary constriction, oliguria, circulatory collapse, pulmonary edema Associated with IV use: Coughing, hiccoughing, laryngospasm Contraindications: Sensitivity to barbiturates, severe respiratory disease	Monitor respiratory rate and rhythm. Solutions for injections should not be used if a precipitate is present or if the solution is not clear. Constantly assess patient during IV use; have resuscitation equipment available. Increased secretions; patient may need suctioning.
Pentobarbital (Nembutal)	A rapidly acting barbiturate	Dose in treatment of seizures: 100–500 mg by slow IV push not to exceed 50 mg/min	Laryngospasm, respiratory depression, and hypotension precipitated by doses exceeding 50 mg/min Additive effects when given with other central nervous system depressants	Pentobarbital is highly alkaline; extravasation may cause local tissue injury. Prepare solutions for IV infusion in dextrose 5% in water. Patient must be mechanically ventilated.

*General anesthesia considered if anticonvulsant therapy is unsuccessful.

TABLE 31–3
Seizure Precautions: Patient Safety

Nursing care considerations concerned with seizure precautions and patient safety include:
1. Side rails padded and kept in up position.
2. Bed placed in low position.
3. Oral airway conspicuously placed at head of bed.
4. Laryngoscope and resuscitative equipment available nearby.
5. Suction equipment available and ready for use.
6. Drugs used for treatment of seizures immediately available.
7. Oxygen source available and ready for use.
8. Use of rectal rather than oral thermometer.
9. Removal of all potentially harmful objects and unnecessary furniture from bedside.

Maintenance of Cardiovascular Function. Continuous cardiac monitoring is essential because of possible cardiac arrhythmias associated with hypoxemia and administration of phenytoin. Phenytoin has a narrow therapeutic index, and elevated levels of the drug can predispose to serious cardiac arrhythmias. It is essential that serial levels of phenytoin be ascertained and monitored. Vital signs should also be monitored closely. Drugs used to treat seizures can have a hypotensive effect. Adequate hydration is essential. Urine output should be closely monitored to ensure adequate renal perfusion.

Maintenance of Metabolic Functions. Metabolic activity associated with seizures include acid-base and electrolyte disturbances. The sustained contractions of skeletal muscle and cessation of respirations associated with the tonic phase of grand mal seizures place the patient at risk of developing acidemia. Laboratory and clinical parameters reflective of the patient's acid-base and electrolyte status must be meticulously monitored. Intake and output should be closely monitored in conjunction with serum electrolyte levels.

Serial serum glucose levels also need to be monitored. Motor activity associated with seizure activity can be very energy-consuming. Hypoglycemia needs to be avoided because it can predispose to altered neurologic function and seizure activity.

Maintenance of Psychological and Emotional Integrity. The occurrence of seizures can be a frightening experience for patient and family. The nurse plays an especially important role in helping the patient and family to understand the underlying disease, its clinical course, and expectations for full recovery. Timely and appropriate explanations help to dispel fears and misconceptions, while reassuring patient and family that they are active participants in the healthcare process.

Tentative Nursing Diagnosis: Basis for Treating Patient with Status Epilepticus. Tentative nursing diagnoses that provide the basis for the nursing treatment of the patient with status epilepticus include:
1. Breathing pattern, ineffective, related to altered respiratory mechanics associated with tonic phase of grand mal seizure
2. Airway clearance, ineffective, related to inability to handle secretions during seizure
3. Injury, risk for related to:
   a. Seizure activity
   b. Aspiration
4. Knowledge deficit, related to:
   a. Understanding of seizure activity
   b. Medication regimen and follow-up care
5. Communication, impaired, related to seizure activity and altered state of consciousness
6. Coping, ineffective, individual and family, related to misconceptions regarding seizure disorder

SUGGESTED READINGS

Caine, RM: The cutting edge in neuroscience. Supplement to Critical Care Nurse, June 1993, p. 6.
Coburn, K: Traumatic brain injury: The silent epidemic. AACN Clinical Issues in Critical Care Nursing 3(1):9, 1992.
Guin, PR and Freudenberger, K: The elderly neuroscience patient: Implications for the critical care nurse. AACN Clinical Issues in Critical Care Nursing 3(1):98, 1992.

CARE PLAN FOR THE PATIENT WITH ACUTE HEAD INJURY

Nursing Diagnoses

Nursing Diagnosis #1
Gas Exchange, impaired, related to neurogenic pulmonary edema (i.e., ARDS of neurogenic origin):
1. Right to left shunting
2. Ventilation/perfusion mismatch
3. Diffusion defect
(See Chapter 25)

Desired Patient Outcomes

Patient will:
1. Be alert and oriented to person, place, time
2. Demonstrate appropriate behavior
3. Maintain effective cardiovascular hemodynamics:
   - Mean arterial blood pressure within ~10 mmHg of baseline
   - Cardiac output ~4–8 L/min
   - Hematocrit >30–35%
   - Hemoglobin > 10 g/100 mL
4. Maintain optimal arterial blood gases:
   - Pa_{CO_2} ~ 30 mmHg
   - Pa_{O_2} > 80 mmHg
   - pH 7.35–7.45

Nursing Interventions

- Implement positive end-expiratory pressure (PEEP) as prescribed, carefully monitoring effect on intracranial pressure.
  - Perform ongoing intracranial and arterial pressure monitoring.
  - Assess effectiveness of interaction of intracranial and hemodynamic phenomena in terms of maintaining adequate cerebral perfusion pressure (>60 mmHg; ideally 80–90 mmHg).

Rationales

- Consequent increase in intrathoracic pressure impedes venous outflow from the cranial vault via the venous sinuses, internal jugular veins, and superior vena cava; the resulting increase in intracranial volume may cause a precipitous rise in intracranial pressure in patients with unstable intracranial pressure dynamics and reduced brain compliance.

Nursing Diagnoses

Nursing Diagnosis #2
Oral Mucous Membranes, altered, related to:
1. Dehydration (diabetes insipidus)
2. Compromised nutritional intake

Desired Patient Outcomes

Patient will maintain oral mucous membranes that are intact, moist, and free of infection.

Nursing Interventions

- Assess for evidence of dehydration including the following parameters:
  - Vital signs; intake and output; skin turgor over forehead or sternum; presence of sunken eyeballs
  - Mouth and oropharynx for dryness, cracking, fissures, bleeding, or other lesions

- Provide supportive care:
  - Maintain hydration within prescribed limitations.

  - Provide oral hygiene at frequent intervals.

  - Apply Vaseline or swabs with glycerin.

Rationales

  - Dry, cracking, or fissured mucous membranes reflect dehydrated state. Ongoing assessment assists in determining changes in the mucosa and response to fluid therapy.

  - Ideally, the patient is maintained in a slightly dehydrated state to minimize risk of cerebral edema.
  - Provides comfort, is aesthetically appealing, reduces risk of oral infection in compromised patient (e.g., *Candida albicans*).
  - Prevents cracking and fissure formation.

Nursing Diagnoses

Nursing Diagnosis #3
Nutrition, altered, less than body requirements, related to:
1. Catabolic state
2. Compromised nutritional intake associated with:
   - Altered state of consciousness
   - Compromised protective reflexes (i.e., cough, gag, and epiglottal closure).
(See Chapter 9).

Desired Patient Outcomes

Patient will:
1. Maintain body weight within 5% of patient's baseline
2. Maintain total serum proteins: 6–8.4 g/100 mL
3. Maintain laboratory data within acceptable range: BUN, serum creatinine, electrolytes, fasting serum glucose, hematology profile, total protein (albumin)

CARE PLAN FOR THE PATIENT WITH ACUTE HEAD INJURY (*Continued*)

Nursing Interventions

- Arrange consultation with nutritionist and collaborate to perform nutrition assessment.
  - Assess specific parameters: general state of health; baseline body weight.
    - Physiologic factors: age, height, weight.
    - Caloric requirements of the critically ill patient
    - Laboratory data: fasting serum glucose; BUN, creatinine, serum electrolytes, total protein (serum albumin); hematology profile
- Maintain optimal nutrition with prescribed enteral and/or parenteral feedings.
  - Special considerations:
    - Methods of enteral and parenteral administration
    - Mechanical complications associated with enteral feeding tubes or with parenteral lines
- Place patient in optimal position for enteral feedings (semi-Fowler's position).
  - Assess status of protective reflexes.
  - Assess for bowel sounds.

  - Confirm placement of nasogastric tube in stomach before initiating enteral feedings.
- Provide frequent mouth care and other comfort measures.

- Assess bowel function: last bowel movement; presence, type, and location of bowel sounds; presence of abdominal distention; diarrhea.
- Implement prescribed bowel regimen.
  - Gastrointestinal decompression
  - Adequate fluid intake
  - Use of stool softeners
- Monitor daily weight (unless contraindicated because of intracranial hypertension) and fluid intake and output.

Rationales

- For details regarding the nutrition assessment, see Chapter 9.
- Adequate nutritional intake is essential to meet the metabolic needs of the catabolic state.

    - Nutritional deficiencies (especially in the elderly) are often associated with underlying chronic disease.

  - Patients receiving mechanical ventilation therapy are highly stressed and require additional nutritional supplements to meet hypermetabolic needs.

- Proper patient positioning and intact protective reflexes reduce risk of aspiration.

  - The presence of a paralytic ileus is a contraindication for enteral approach because of increased risk of aspiration; abdominal distention may compromise diaphragmatic excursion.
  - Proper placement of nasogastric tube helps prevent aspiration.
- May be aesthetically pleasing to patient and family; reduces risk of oral infection (e.g., *Candida albicans*) in the compromised patient; keeps mucous membranes moist and intact.
- Presence of a paralytic ileus may predispose to fecal impaction; measures need to be employed to minimize straining at stool because Valsalva's maneuver can increase intracranial pressure.

Nursing Diagnoses

Nursing Diagnosis #4
Physical Mobility, impaired, related to:
1. Altered state of consciousness
2. Restricted activity associated with intracranial hypertension
3. Sedation
4. Neuromuscular impairments (e.g., hemiparesis)
5. Pain

Desired Patient Outcomes

Patient will:
1. Maintain full range of motion
2. Remain without contractures
3. Verbalize and/or indicate comfort

Nursing Interventions

- Assess neuromuscular function.
  - Assess for limitations in range of motion, incoordination of movement, and presence of sensorimotor dysfunction.
  - Assess for the presence of pain, fear, and anxiety.

- Implement measures to improve mobility:

  - Include passive range-of-motion exercises in planning care.

Rationales

- It is important to determine how specific musculoskeletal activity affects intracranial pressure.

  - Fear of precipitating pain or causing injury can significantly compromise musculoskeletal function.
- In the patient at risk of developing an increase in ICP, all activities should be guided by ICP monitoring measurements.
  - Prevents pooling of blood in extremities.

CARE PLAN FOR THE PATIENT WITH ACUTE HEAD INJURY (*Continued*)

Nursing Interventions

○ Avoid cumulative effect of activities; too many activities within a short time span predispose to increases in ICP.
○ Provide rest periods between patient care activities.
○ Use hand/wrist splints as prescribed.
○ Maintain optimal positioning.

○ Avoid crossing one leg over the other; avoid pillows under knees.

Rationales

○ Exercise periods should be incorporated into daily care and planned around other patient care activities.

○ Positioning is important in patients with reduced brain compliance to allow free flow of blood and CSF from cranial vault.
○ Minimizes risk of thrombophlebitis or thromboembolic episodes.

Nursing Diagnoses

Nursing Diagnosis #5
Injury, risk for abrasions, to eyes, related to inability to close eyes, or keep eyes closed, associated with:
1. Altered state of consciousness
2. Neurologic deficit (cranial nerves)
3. Periorbital edema

Desired Patient Outcomes

Patients's eyes will remain intact without inadvertent abrasions.

Nursing Interventions

• Assess patient's ability to close eyelids and keep them closed.

○ Assess for corneal reflex.
• Implement measures to protect eyes.
○ Administer lubricants for the eyes (e.g., Tearisol).
○ Gently tape eyes in closed position if necessary.
○ Cleanse around eyelids to prevent crusting of secretions.

Rationales

• Disturbance in cranial nerve function can place eyeballs at risk of injury.
○ Cranial nerve III dysfunction causes ptosis of upper eyelid on ipsilateral side.
○ Cranial nerve VII dysfunction alters ability to close eyelid on ipsilateral side.
○ Cranial nerve V dysfunction impairs corneal reflex.
• Help to protect eyes and minimize risk of infection.

Nursing Diagnoses

Nursing Diagnosis #6
Thought Processes, altered, related to:
1. Cerebral ischemia and hypoxia
2. Sedation

Desired Patient Outcomes

Patient will demonstrate improvement in thought processes:
1. Oriented to person, place, time
2. Improved memory
3. Increased attentiveness
4. Improved ability to problem-solve and make decisions

Nursing Interventions

• Assess for alterations in mentation and thought processes.
○ Assess the following parameters:
□ State of awareness or cognition
□ Behavior: restlessness, irritability, reduced attentiveness
□ Impaired memory, confusion
□ Ability to problem-solve
• Confirm recent behavioral or personality changes with family members/significant others.
• Implement measures to assist patient in thought processes:

Rationales

• Disruption in thought processes suggests hemispheric lesion; alterations in arousal and cognition reflect disruption of reticular activating system.

• Helps to ascertain patient's baseline capabilities and to plan care.
• Thought processes are a component of an individual's overall mentation, which requires the integration of cognitive activities served by all parts of the brain. In addition to thinking, other components of mentation include memory, attention, language, feeling, and spatial perception, and problem solving.

CARE PLAN FOR THE PATIENT WITH ACUTE HEAD INJURY (*Continued*)

Nursing Interventions

- Reorient patient as follows:
  - Reorient to person, place, and time.
  - Call by name when talking with patient.
  - Orient to immediate environment, but minimize stimuli at any given moment.
- Repeat instructions and information, allowing adequate time for communication, explanations.
  - Encourage patient to ask questions; use clear simple sentences.
- Plan patient's activities and write out schedule for patient to refer to:
  - Involve patient in problem solving.
  - Monitor patient's readiness and ability to learn.
  - Ascertain patient's comprehension.
- Provide continuous encouragement and feedback, and praise positive gains made by patient.
- Involve family members and/or significant others in care plan.
- Offer reassurance regarding alterations in intellectual and emotional functions.
- Be realistic when offering explanations and providing information.

Rationales

- Implementing measures to assist the patient in thinking helps to stimulate the reticular activating system as well as other areas of the brain.

- Writing out instructions or schedules reinforces verbal communication.

- Assists in motivating patient.

- Depending on magnitude of insult and secondary injury, the patient may have memory loss and personality changes, which may persist for several months or longer.

Nursing Diagnoses

Nursing Diagnosis #7
Sensory/Perceptual alterations, related to:
1. Sensory deprivation:
   - Restricted environment
   - Altered communication capabilities
2. Sensory overload due to complexity of intensive care environment

Desired Patient Outcomes

Patient will:
1. Demonstrate appropriate interactions with people and environment using sensory perceptions
2. Verbalize restfulness and relaxed feeling

Nursing Interventions

- Assess patient's ability to interact with environment.

  - Identify specific sensory deficits:
    - Visual perception: need for glasses or contact lenses
    - Auditory perception: presence of language disorder (e.g., receptive dysphasia, expressive dysphasia), need for hearing aid
    - Tactile perception: hyperesthesia, hypoesthesia

  - Identify previous coping abilities and influence on behavior.
- Provide usual necessary aids (e.g., glasses, hearing aid).

- Arrange environment to compensate for deficits:
  - Reorient to environment as needed.
    - Keep articles and equipment in the same place.
    - Remove unnecessary materials from bedside.
    - Use safety measures to prevent accidents.
- Implement measures to reduce sensory deprivation:
  - Encourage communication by the patient as tolerated.
    - Allow visits by family members as tolerated.
  - Provide frequent, undisturbed rest periods.

  - Ask family members about the patient's preferences, likes and dislikes.
  - Provide occasional changes in routine and sensory stimuli.

Rationales

- Depending on the extent and location of insult, a disruption in sensation might be anticipated.
  - Major sensory capabilities include: visual, auditory, kinesthesia (spatial sense, perception of movement), tactile, gustatory, and olfactory.

    - *Hyperesthesia* is an overly acute sensitivity to touch, pain, temperature, or other stimuli.
    - *Hypoesthesia* is a diminished sensitivity to sensory stimuli.

- A patient's comprehensive clinical history helps to identify the patient's baseline capabilities and limitations.

  - Fatigue may compromise the patient's capabilities, leading to frustration, withdrawal, and depression.
  - Minimizes fatigue and conserves strength.
  - Familiar stimuli may motivate increased participation.

CARE PLAN FOR THE PATIENT WITH ACUTE HEAD INJURY (*Continued*)

Nursing Interventions	Rationales
□ Provide soothing music/other radio programs.	
□ Provide diversional activities depending on patient's status (e.g., reading, television).	
□ Encourage conversations with the client; update patient on what's happening, and other conversational topics of interest to the patient.	
• Implement measures to reduce sensory overload:	• Minimizing distractions enables the patient to concentrate on more pertinent stimuli. Ability to problem solve and tolerate frustration decreases as the number of stimuli impacting on the individual increase.
○ Set priorities in care.	
□ Arrange patient care activities to allow for undisturbed rest periods.	
□ Provide periods of uninterrupted sleep with lights off and minimal noise.	
□ Alter environmental activities (e.g., avoid constant use of radio or television).	
□ Encourage verbalization regarding concerns, annoyances.	
□ Allow patient to decide on care activities and environmental stimuli.	
□ Maintain continuity of care.	

Clinical Management of Patients with Potentially Life-Threatening Cerebrovascular Disease

Joan T. Dolan

CHAPTER OUTLINE

LEARNING OBJECTIVES

After completing this chapter, you should be able to:

1. Define cerebrovascular disease in terms of its mortality and morbidity.
2. Identify risk factors implicated in cerebrovascular disease.
3. Define cerebral artery syndrome, and list key clinical neurologic manifestations reflective of middle cerebral artery syndrome.
4. Identify cerebrovascular disorders most likely to disrupt consciousness and thus require critical care.
5. Contrast features of hypertensive cerebral hemorrhage and cerebral aneurysm with subarachnoid hemorrhage in terms of underlying pathology, clinical presentation, complications, recurrence, and clinical management.
6. Discuss vasospasm and rebleeding including patients at high risk, clinical manifestations, preventive measures, and treatment.
7. Implement the nursing process in the management of the patient with potentially life-threatening cerebrovascular disease: assessment, diagnosis, and planning of desired patient outcomes and nursing interventions.

CEREBROVASCULAR DISEASE

Cerebrovascular disease encompasses two clinical syndromes: *ischemic* cerebrovascular disease, and *hemorrhagic* cerebrovascular disease. Ischemic disease includes what is commonly referred to as a cerebrovascular accident (CVA), or stroke. The most common causes of stroke are cerebral thrombosis and cerebral embolism. Hemorrhagic disease encompasses hypertensive intracranial hemorrhage and ruptured cerebral aneurysm with subarachnoid hemorrhage.

Most ischemic cerebrovascular disorders (e.g., transient ischemic attacks (TIAs), stroke in evolution, completed stroke, and cerebral embolism) do not require critical care. Only when massive hemispheric or brainstem strokes disrupt consciousness and vital functions is an intensive care setting indicated. Hemorrhagic cerebrovascular disorders (e.g., hypertensive intracerebral hemorrhage, or ruptured cerebral aneurysm with subarachnoid hemorrhage), however, usually disrupt consciousness and thus warrant critical care.

Mortality and Morbidity

Stroke remains the third leading cause of death in the United States, second to heart disease and cancer. The morbidity of this syndrome is reflected by the impact that its consequent disabilities have on the lives of patients and their families. The effect on their personal (physical, psychological, emotional), social (including the healthcare system and the cost of healthcare), and economic (loss of earnings and opportunities for self-expression and creativity) well-being can be devastating.

Risk Factors

Certain risk factors predispose a person to stroke (Table 32–1). Hypertension, age, diabetes mellitus, and heart disease are major contributors to the pathogenesis of stroke. Associated with these risk factors is the process of *atherosclerosis*, a disease process involving blood vessels which causes them to lose their distensibility and become easily ruptured. Development of atherosclerosis in smaller cerebral blood vessels is particularly influenced by hypertension. All these factors are interrelated in the evolution of cardiovascular disease.

ISCHEMIC CEREBROVASCULAR DISEASE

Major Cerebral Artery Syndromes

Clinical Manifestations

Cerebrovascular accidents, or strokes, are characterized by the sudden onset of focal neurologic deficits that result from cerebral ischemia or infarction of brain tissue nourished by a particular cerebral artery and its branches. The specific neurologic deficits presented clinically reflect the dysfunction of the portion of the brain to which blood supplied by that particular arterial distribution has been disrupted.

Major clinical syndromes have been attributed to pathology of specific areas of the brain served by major cerebral arterial systems (Table 32–2). Knowledge of specific areas of brain functions and their respective blood supplies assist in assessing, monitoring, and predicting specific neurologic deficits and selected human responses. It is important to appreciate that a wide variety and complexity of neurologic dysfunction can occur, depending on the cause of the stroke, the vessel or vessels impaired, the extent of collateral circulation, and the area of the brain that is affected (i.e., the area of the brain supplied by a particular cerebral artery).

The major clinical syndromes are reflective of pathology involving the *anterior* and *posterior* cerebral circulations. Pathology of the anterior circulation (i.e., via the internal carotids) includes the internal carotid artery syndrome and the anterior and middle cerebral artery syndromes. Pathology of the posterior cerebral circulation (i.e., via the vertebral arteries) include vertebral and basilar artery syndromes and the posterior cerebral artery syndrome (Table 32–2). The circle of Willis connects the anterior and posterior cerebral circulations and contributes to collateral circulation (see Fig. 27–7).

Middle Cerebral Artery Syndrome Because the middle cerebral artery syndrome is the most common, it is useful to examine this particular clinical syndrome more closely.

The middle cerebral artery is the largest artery to arise from the internal carotid artery as it enters the base of the brain. It accounts for about 80% of the blood supply to the cerebral hemisphere. The distribution of the middle cerebral artery is predominantly over the *lateral* surface of the hemisphere including the somesthetic cortex (see Fig. 27–18). Thus,

TABLE 32–1
Cerebrovascular Accident (Stroke): Risk Factors

Hypertension	A major risk factor, which, together with atherosclerosis, is highly implicated in the pathophysiologic processes underlying vascular disease.
Age	Incidence of stroke and deaths attributed to stroke increase with age. Individuals over 65 years of age are at great risk.
Diabetes mellitus	Associated metabolic disorders may contribute to atherosclerosis. *Hypercholesterolemia* and *hyperlipidemia* have been found to exist concomitantly in stroke patients and are implicated in the atherogenic process.
Heart disease	A major contributor to cerebral infarction: • Rheumatic heart disease with valvular pathology, and subacute bacterial endocarditis are widely recognized as precursors to the development of cerebral embolism. • Cardiovascular disease and hypertension predispose to left ventricular failure.
Use of oral contraceptives	This has been implicated in the development of stroke. The risk involves an alteration in blood clotting related to estrogen. New oral contraceptive preparations contain reduced doses of estrogen and are considered to be safer.
Other risk factors	Other risk factors implicated in the pathogenesis of cerebrovascular disease and stroke include: Cigarette smoking Obesity Sedentary lifestyle Arteritis Polycythemia vera Congenital vessel anomalies Family history: genetic predisposition

TABLE 32–2
Major Cerebral Artery Syndromes: Location and Clinical Manifestations of Neurologic Deficits

Syndromes	Internal Carotid Artery	Anterior Cerebral Artery	Middle Cerebral Artery	Vertebral Artery, Basilar Artery	Posterior Cerebral and Thalamic Syndrome
Occurrence Origin Gives rise to	Common Common carotid Ophthalmic artery Anterior cerebral Middle cerebral	Least common Internal carotid Anterior communicating	Most common Internal carotid Superficial cortical and deeper penetrating arteries	Less common Subclavian artery Both vertebral arteries unite to form the basilar artery in the area of the pons	Less common Basilar artery Basilar artery
Distribution of blood supply	Optic nerve, retina	Medial surface of frontal and parietal lobes Internal capsule (major route connecting cerebral cortex with brainstem and spinal cord) Corpus callosum (connects hemispheres)	Provides 80% of blood supply to cerebral hemisphere, including lateral aspects of frontal, parietal, and temporal lobes	Medulla including the pyramid where decussation of nerves occurs Medial lemniscus and lateral medullary area Posterior, inferior portions of cerebellar hemisphere	Diencephaon (thalamus); midbrain, visual (occipital) cortex; choroid plexuses of lateral and third ventricles

Neurologic deficits (signs and symptoms)	• Mimics middle cerebral artery syndrome,
	• Contralateral hemiplegia
	• Dysphasia (aphasia)
	• Headache
	• Alteration in sensory function
	• Altered state of consciousness
	• Retinal insufficiency with monocular blindness (*amaurosis fugax*)
	• May mimic some signs of anterior cerebral artery dysfunction
	• Possible optic nerve dysfunction
		• Motor dysfunction with hemiplegia of contralateral leg with foot-drop; impaired gait
		• Paresis of contralateral proximal arm with damage of internal capsule
		• Sensory dysfunction with sensory deficit over lower leg and foot on contralateral side
		• Frontal lobe dysfunction: primitive reflexes on contralateral side (grasp and sucking reflexes)
		• Decreased cerebration
		• Dementia with flat affect, lack of spontaneity, confusion
		• Urinary incontinence
		• Abulia (inability to make decisions or to perform acts voluntarily)
			Classic picture of:
			• Contralateral hemiplegia involving face, arm, and leg
			• Hemianesthesia (loss of tactile sensibility)
			• Homonymous hemianopsia (loss of sight in corresponding lateral halves of both eyes)
			• Dysphasia (aphasia) with lesion of left cerebral hemisphere (Broca's speech center in left hemisphere)
			• Expressive and receptive aphasias
			• Apraxia (right hemisphere)
			• Unilateral spatial and visual neglect
			• Anosognosia
			• Disturbances in affect
			• Communication and language deficits
			• Altered state of consciousness, coma
			• Depending on extent and severity of cerebral infarction, alteration in neurologic function may
				Vertebral artery:
				• Clinical manifestations vary considerably from one individual to the next
				• Lateral medullary syndrome:
				  ○ Paresthesias with numbness, tingling, and burning sensations over face
				  ○ Ataxia
				  ○ Cranial nerve dysfunction: vertigo, nausea, vomiting (VIII)
				• Dysphagia, hoarseness, impaired gag reflex (IX, X)
				Basilar artery:
				• Supplies pons, cerebellum, and posterior cerebral area
				• Signs and symptoms: weakness of all extremities, paralysis with complete occlusion
				• Visual disturbances: diplopia, various degrees of alteration in conjugate gaze;
					Homonymous hemianopsia; visual field defects (the patient may be unaware of visual field defects and may be described as "bumping into objects")
					Thalamic syndrome:
					• Contralateral sensory diminution or loss
					• Alterations in proprioception (position sense) and tactile sensation

TABLE 32–2
Major Cerebral Artery Syndromes: Location and Clinical Manifestations of Neurologic Deficits (*Continued*)

Syndromes	Internal Carotid Artery	Anterior Cerebral Artery	Middle Cerebral Artery	Vertebral Artery, Basilar Artery	Posterior Cerebral and Thalamic Syndrome
			reflect changes in: ○ Respiratory rate and breathing pattern ○ Pupillary size and reactivity ○ Extraocular movements ○ Motor function with abnormal flexor or extensor responses	visual field defects; blindness • Vestibular and auditory disturbances (horizontal and/or vertical nystagmus, dizziness, tinnitus, and deafness) • Bilateral cerebellar ataxia; bilateral motor and sensory dysfunction	

hands, fingers, thumb, face, lips, and so forth, receive their blood supply through the middle cerebral artery.

Occlusion of the middle cerebral artery at its origin (the internal carotid artery) causes infarction of those areas of the brain concerned with motor and sensory function as represented by the somesthetic cortex. Clinically, the underlying pathology is reflected as the classic picture of contralateral hemiplegia (paralysis of one side of the body including face, arm, and leg opposite to that of the lesion), hemianesthesia (loss of tactile sensibility), and homonymous hemianopsia (loss of sight in corresponding halves of both eyes).

If the lesion occurs in the dominant hemisphere—commonly the left cerebral hemisphere—the patient may also experience aphasia (dysphasia), that is, difficulty in or impairment of the ability to communicate through speech, writing, or symbols. Patients with a nondominant hemispheric lesion—commonly the right cerebral hemisphere—may present clinically with apraxia rather than dysphasia. Apraxia refers to a disturbance in the execution of learned movements or the manipulation of objects in space. Other neurologic deficits associated with middle cerebral artery syndrome are listed in Table 32–2.

Patients with a middle cerebral artery syndrome, who experience *extensive* tissue injury and infarction, present clinically with corresponding physiologic changes, and the level of brain functioning is reflected by changes in the level of consciousness, alterations in breathing pattern, pupillary size and reactivity, extraocular movements, and the presence of abnormal flexor or extensor responses. These patients, as well as those with strokes from any cause, which disrupt consciousness and become life-threatening, require critical care. The discussion that follows focuses on the potentially life-threatening cerebrovascular disorders commonly seen in critical care.

HEMORRHAGIC CEREBROVASCULAR DISEASE

The onset of cerebral hemorrhage is sudden, explosive, and lacking of any prior signs of neurologic dysfunction. The patient quickly becomes critically ill. Based on underlying pathologic mechanisms, two types of cerebral hemorrhage have been identified: hypertensive cerebral hemorrhage and hemorrhage associated with a ruptured cerebral aneurysm (subarachnoid hemorrhage).

Hypertensive Intracerebral Hemorrhage

Longstanding hypertension predisposes to alterations in the cerebral vasculature, which are characterized as degenerative changes in the vessel wall. Such changes cause blood vessels to lose their distensibility, become easily ruptured, and bleed. Over time, cerebral autoregulation mechanisms may become impaired as well. Frank, symptom-producing cerebral hemorrhage usually involves smaller cerebral arteries that penetrate the brain parenchyma. Thus, a hypertensive cerebral hemorrhage is *intracerebral*, as opposed to hemorrhage associated with rupture of aneurysms, which usually causes a *subarachnoid* hemorrhage (see the following section). In addition to hypertension, additional factors associated with intracerebral hemorrhage are blood dyscrasias, bleeding associated with some brain tumors, and, less commonly, anticoagulant therapy.

Because intracerebral hemorrhage involves a high-pressure system, such bleeds rarely seal off spontaneously. Rather, extravasation of blood into the brain parenchyma creates a mass lesion, which compresses and displaces adjacent brain tissue and thus precipitates signs of neurologic dysfunction (see Fig. 29–5). A massive intracerebral bleed can cause extensive infarction with displacement of intracranial contents, resulting in coma, herniation, and death. If the bleed is large enough, blood will probably seep into the ventricular system. Blood in the cerebrospinal fluid may be detected on lumbar puncture.

Hypertensive intracerebral hemorrhage occurs abruptly without any warning and usually while the patient is active. A thorough patient history may reveal subtle clues as to the evolution of the hemorrhage. Initially, the patient may have complained of a severe headache associated with nausea and vomiting, followed at some point by focal neurologic deficits involving sensory and motor function. The earlier symptoms may reflect an increase in intracranial pressure (ICP), whereas later symptomatology reflects disruption of sensory and motor pathways within the involved cerebral hemisphere. Hemorrhage may also occur into subcortical areas, basal ganglia, or the brainstem, disrupting sensory and motor pathways there as well.

Specific neurologic signs and symptoms exhibited by the patient depend on the location and extent of bleeding. Cerebral lesions may reflect symptomatology discussed earlier with respect to the major cerebral artery syndromes (Table 32–2). The deterioration in neurologic function may be exceedingly rapid. See Table 32–3 for additional features of hypertensive intracerebral hemorrhage as well as those of other cerebrovascular disorders causing intracranial bleeding. (Note: Epidural and subdural hematomas are discussed in Chapter 31.)

Medical management of intracerebral hemorrhage requires a definitive diagnosis as to whether the underlying pathologic process is one of hemorrhage or infarction. Supportive therapy to prevent secondary brain injury is implemented. Depending on the location and extent of the bleeding, surgical evacuation may be indicated.

Ruptured Cerebral Aneurysm: Subarachnoid Hemorrhage

An aneurysm is a thin-walled outpouching or localized dilatation of a blood vessel. The most common type of aneurysm is described as saccular, or berry-shaped. These aneurysms usually occur at bifurcations of blood vessels; the circle of Willis is the most common site with blood extruded into the subarachnoid space (see Fig. 27–7). Cerebral hemorrhage related to a ruptured aneurysm generally occurs in persons between 30 and 65 years of age who may have more than one aneurysm. The occurrence of such aneurysms may reflect a developmental defect or weakness in the vessel wall. Saccular aneurysms range from the size of a pinhead up to 2 or 3 cm.

Usually there is no clinical evidence of an aneurysm until the initial rupture. Occasionally, recurrent unilateral migraine headache is mentioned as being a sign of aneurysm. Very large aneurysms may cause symptoms by compressing adjacent structures. Minor leakage of blood may precede actual rupture and may cause a warning headache.

Rupture of a saccular aneurysm occurs most often while the individual is engaged in vigorous activity. Hemorrhaging of blood under arterial pressure into the subarachnoid space may be accompanied by excruciating headache and may result in loss of consciousness. There may be sudden loss of consciousness without other signs or symptoms. When present, other signs and symptoms may include vomiting, dizziness, vertigo, and sweating and chills.

A grading system for quantifying neurologic deficits and risk for surgery in patients with subarachnoid bleeding includes the following:

Grade I	Asymptomatic or minimal headache, slight nuchal rigidity
Grade II	Moderate-to-severe headache, nuchal rigidity, minimal neurologic deficits
Grade III	Drowsiness, confusion, mild focal neurologic deficits
Grade IV	Stupor, moderate-to-severe hemiparesis, early decerebrate posturing
Grade V	Deep coma, decerebrate rigidity, disruption of vegetative functions

Blood is especially irritating to brain tissue and may contribute to vasospasm (see following text). The patient may also exhibit signs of meningeal irritation with photophobia, fever, nausea, and vomiting. Focal neurologic signs may be observed, including motor weakness, sensory deficits, visual disturbances (diplopia), and seizure activity. In addition, the presence of blood in the subarachnoid space intensely stimulates constriction of cerebral blood vessels (vasospasm).

Vasospasm. Cerebral vasospasm is seen in about 40% to 60% of patients diagnosed with aneurysmal rupture and subarachnoid hemorrhage.[1] It is the most serious complication of a subarachnoid hemorrhage and contributes significantly to the mortality and morbidity of affected patients. Patients presenting clinically with lower grades of risk, who survive the initial hemorrhage, are more likely to develop vasospasm. Patients with pooling of subarachnoid blood in the basal cisterns, as predicted on the basis of a computed tomography (CT) scan, also have an increased likelihood of developing vasospasm. The vasospasm reflects prolonged contraction of one or more blood vessels and most frequently occurs within 4 to 12 days after the initial hemorrhage. Vasospasm alters cerebral blood flow and contributes significantly to *delayed* cerebral ischemia.

Initially, there is focal vasoconstriction of cerebral blood vessels adjacent to the area of insult. Eventually, vasospasm may become widespread, resulting in ische-

TABLE 32–3
Intracranial Bleeding—Cerebrovascular Disorders

Characteristics	Epidural Hematoma	Subdural Hematoma	Cerebral Thrombosis	Cerebral Embolism	Subarachnoid Hemorrhage/ Aneurysm	Hypertensive Intracerebral Hemorrhage
Age	Any age	Any age	Most common CVA > 65 years	Any age, frequently young	30–65 years	40–60 years
Etiology	Trauma—blunt blow to squamous portion of temporal bone with fracture or closed head injury; laceration of middle meningeal artery	*Acute*—skull fracture; high-impact closed head trauma; contusions *Subacute/chronic*— seemingly mild head trauma; elderly; alcoholic; anticoagulation therapy	Inflammatory artery disease; atherosclerosis, prolonged vasospasm TIAs with gradual pathologic progression	Atherosclerosis; rheumatic heart disease; myocardial infarction Hypertensive heart disease; bacterial endocarditis	Trauma—rupture of an aneurysm	Fractured skull; penetrating skull injury; contrecoup injury; severe contusion and laceration of brain tissue
Location	Bleeding into potential space between periosteal dura and inner table of skull	Bleeding into space between dura and arachnoid, usually laceration of bridging veins	Occlusion of internal carotids, middle cerebral artery or its branches; basilar-vertebral system; anterior cerebral artery	Brain tissue nourished by branches of middle or anterior cerebral arteries	Bleeding into subarachnoid space between pia and arachnoid	May be widely dispersed; bleeding into brain parenchyma
Onset	Rapid—minutes to hours	*Subacute/chronic*— insidious	Minutes to hours, sometimes days	Sudden	Sudden and acute	Rapid, minutes to a few hours
Duration	Brief period of unconsciousness followed by lucid period; thereafter, rapid deterioration	*Acute*—hours *Subacute/ chronic*— months	Permanent with infarction; reversible with minimal damage and collateral circulation	May improve rapidly if collateral circulation is established	Variable; reversible neurologic deficits may improve with time	Large bleed = permanent damage; small bleed = reversible
Associated factors	Predisposition to trauma	Alcoholism Trauma	Atherosclerosis Hypertension Diabetes mellitus and other risk factors	Heart disease	Aneurysms, arteriovenous malformation, tumor, abscess, trauma	Hypertension Atherosclerosis
Pathology with loss of autoregulatory mechanisms	1. Usually arterial bleed = increase in cerebral blood volume = increase in ICP = cerebral ischemia = cerebral infarction and cerebral edema = further increase in ICP, and so on 2. Displacement of intracranial structures with compression and ischemia	Venous bleeding more common 1. Usually venous bleed = increase in cerebral blood volume = increase in ICP = cerebral ischemia = cerebral infarction and cerebral edema = further increase in ICP, and so on 2. Displacement of intracranial structures with compression and ischemia	Formation of atheromatous plaques with progressive vessel occlusion = cerebral ischemia with infarction	Sudden occurrence— collateral circulation may be minimal— increased tissue ischemia and infarction	Hemorrhage into subarachnoid space; Hydrocephalus	Hemorrhage into brain parenchyma; expanding mass causes compression of adjacent tissues with cerebral ischemia, edema, and infarction
Blood vessels involved	Middle meningeal artery	Bridging blood vessels in subdural space	Internal carotids; basilar-vertebral systems; anterior and middle cerebral	Middle cerebral artery	Circle of Willis	Middle cerebral artery

continued

TABLE 32–3
Intracranial Bleeding—Cerebrovascular Disorders (*Continued*)

Characteristics	Epidural Hematoma	Subdural Hematoma	Cerebral Thrombosis	Cerebral Embolism	Subarachnoid Hemorrhage/ Aneurysm	Hypertensive Intracerebral Hemorrhage
Relation to activity	Usually sudden with trauma	Depends on force of impact; may be acute	Frequently occurs at rest or sleep	Occurs at any time	May occur at any time	During activity
Clinical features:						
• Level of consciousness	After a lucid period, rapid deterioration to coma	*Acute*—rapid deterioration to coma *Subacute*—confusion, disorientation, progressive to coma *Chronic*—may resemble organic brain syndrome with impairment of consciousness, orientation, memory, intellect, judgment and insight; defects evolve over time (months)	Usually conscious, may be confused and disoriented TIAs	Depends on the extent of damage; usually conscious; coma rare	Explosive onset of headache; coma common	Rapidly developing coma
• Respiratory pattern	Cheyne-Stokes initially = central neurogenic hyperventilation	→ Same	Signs and symptoms depend on site and extent of infarction and collateral circulation; and the specific arterial system involved	→ Same	→ Same	→ Same
• Pupillary reaction	Ipsilateral pupil dilatation; sluggish to unreactive	Depends on location of lesion; may be pinpoint to moderately dilated, sluggishly reactive	Usually equal in size and reactive	Usually equal in size and reactive depending on location of lesion	Variable response depending on location of lesion	→ Same
• Eye movement	Varies—conjugate to dysconjugate; sluggish oculocephalic reflex	→ Same	Homonymous hemianopsia	→ Depends on site and extent of insult	Depends on site and extent of insult	→ Same
• Motor response	Contralateral hemiparesis or hemiplegia; posturing	→ Same	Contralateral hemiplegia	→ Depends on site and extent of insult	Contralateral hemiparesis and hemiplegia	Depends on site and extent of insult
• Nuchal rigidity	Possible but rare	Possible but rare	Absent	Absent	Usually present	Frequent
• CSF	Usually normal	Usually normal	Usually normal	Usually normal	Grossly bloody	Frequently bloody
• Convulsions	Frequent	Infrequent	Infrequent	Rare	Common	Common
• ICP	Increased—aggravated by hypercapnia and hypoxia	Probably increased	Not usually elevated	Not usually elevated	Frequently elevated	Frequently elevated
Complications:						
• Herniation	Uncal or lateral transtentorial	Uncal (lateral transtentorial) and/or central (transtentorial)	Uncommon	Uncommon	Common	Very common

TABLE 32–3
Intracranial Bleeding—Cerebrovascular Disorders (*Continued*)

Characteristics	Epidural Hematoma	Subdural Hematoma	Cerebral Thrombosis	Cerebral Embolism	Subarachnoid Hemorrhage/ Aneurysm	Hypertensive Intracerebral Hemorrhage
• Cerebral ischemia	Secondary change related to initial trauma	Occurs in response to compression from expanding mass with displacement of intracranial contents	Depends on area of brain affected and presence of collateral circulation	→ Same	Secondary to vasospasm as well as primary insult	Secondary to vasospasm and primary insult
• Cerebral infarction	Occurs secondary to progressive ischemia	→ Same	→ Same	→ Same	→ Same	→ Same
• Cerebral edema	Secondary to trauma, hypoxia; dysfunction of blood-brain barrier	→ Same	→ Same	→ Same	→ Common	→ Common
• Infection (cerebral)	Possible with extensive scalp injury and/or lacerated dura	Increased as dura is opened or invasive ICP monitoring	Uncommon	Uncommon	More frequent with invasive procedure	Same
• Vasospasm	Infrequent	Infrequent	Uncommon	Uncommon	Frequently present	Usually present
Recurrence	Uncommon with appropriate and timely therapy	Possible after surgery	Common	Common	Very common	Very common
Mortality	80%	*Acute*: high	If patient survives initial episode, there is gradual improvement	Increased mortality due to minimal collateral circulation		

CSF = cerebrospinal fluid; ICP = intracranial pressure.

mia, injury, and infarction of brain tissue. These alterations are manifested by the appearance of focal or diffuse neurologic deficits. Depending on the extent of the insult and the area of brain affected, these deficits may include an alteration in the level of consciousness, visual disturbances, hemiparesis, hemiplegia, and seizures.

A major consequence of vasospasm is the impairment or loss of cerebral autoregulation. The inability of the cerebral vasculature to regulate cerebral perfusion causes cerebral blood flow to fluctuate with mean systemic arterial blood pressure. Such fluctuations compromise cerebral blood flow and predispose to cerebral ischemia. The associated cerebral acidemia alters the integrity of the cerebral microcirculation, leading to vasogenic edema and an increase in ICP (see Chapter 29). Without intervention, the progressive increase in ICP leads eventually to cerebral infarction and death.

Current treatment of cerebral vasospasm involves hemodilutional hyperperfusion therapy, pharmacologic therapy, and cerebral angioplasty. *Hemodilutional hyperperfusion* is therapy designed to optimize cardiac output and blood pressure and, in so doing, to augment cerebral perfusion pressure and cerebral blood

flow during the vulnerable period in which vasospasm occurs. This therapy is achieved through the use of hypervolemia, supportive hypertension, and hemodilution. Hypervolemia, that is, intravascular volume expansion, is achieved through the use of fluid and volume expanders (e.g., crystalloids, plasma, hetastarch), administered in conjunction with hemodynamic monitoring (including monitoring of pulmonary artery and pulmonary capillary wedge pressures, cardiac output, and cardiac index). Systolic blood pressure is maintained between 150 and 160 mmHg to increase perfusion to vasospastic areas. Continuous serial assessments of neurologic function are essential to evaluate the response to therapy.

Hypervolemic hypertension therapy is used safely after surgical aneurysmal clipping, when the risk of hypertension-induced rebleeding has been reduced or eliminated. Close monitoring of hemodynamic parameters is essential to avoid the risk of pulmonary edema associated with the hypervolemic state.

Hemodilution is an essential adjunct to hypervolemic hypertensive therapy. This therapy reduces blood viscosity and facilitates cerebral perfusion. Without hemodilution, hypervolemic hypertension therapy has not been found to be effective in increasing cerebral blood flow to ischemic areas. Recommended target hematocrit levels range from 30% and 35%.

Pharmacologic therapy for the treatment of vasospasm includes the use of calcium channel blockers. Calcium channel blockers act on vascular smooth muscle, causing relaxation and thus vasodilation. The benefit of calcium channel blockers in the treatment of cerebral vasospasm may be to dilate cerebral blood vessels surrounding the areas of vasospasm, thereby increasing collateral circulation to ischemic tissues.[2]

Cerebral angioplasty is a new treatment option indicated for selected patients experiencing delayed cerebral ischemia unresponsive to hemodilutional hyperperfusion therapy or treatment with calcium channel blockers. This procedure involves isolating spastic cerebral arteries under angiography, followed by temporary balloon insertion to dilate affected vessels. Reperfusion has been found to be immediate.[3] Although this approach appears promising, complications can be catastrophic, such as cerebral infarction and vessel dissection or rupture. (For additional information on the treatment of vasospasm, refer to Suggested Readings at the end of this chapter.)

Rebleeding. All patients experiencing a ruptured cerebral aneurysm are at risk for rebleeding from the aneurysm site. Rebleeding may occur as early as 24 hours after hemorrhage; or it may occur within 7 days of the initial bleed in conjunction with the natural fibrinolytic process. While the clot, which formed initially to seal the rupture site, undergoes normal lysis or dissolution, the risk of bleeding increases. Hypertension, if present, may also play a role in clot dislodgement in the early course after the initial hemorrhage.

A deterioration in the patient's neurologic status may signal the occurrence of rebleeding. Profound changes in the level of consciousness, together with a sudden rise in blood pressure and ICP, may be observed. If alert prior to the rebleeding event, the patient may complain of a severe headache, which may be accompanied by nausea and vomiting.

The key to the clinical management of the patient at risk for rebleeding is surgical intervention, especially in patients presenting with grades I, II, or III subarachnoid bleeding. The timing of aneurysmal surgery is crucial. Surgery within the initial 48 to 72 hours of the initial bleed secures the aneurysm, thereby reducing the risk of rebleeding. In addition, early surgery enables aggressive hemodilutional hyperperfusion therapy to be implemented postoperatively to reduce the effects of vasospasm.

When treated medically to prevent rebleeding, pharmacologic therapy is a mainstay of therapy. Sedatives/analgesics are administered for patient comfort. Stool softeners are provided as part of a bowel regimen to prevent straining. Antihypertensives may be prescribed to control blood pressure. Such therapy requires diligent monitoring so that blood pressure is maintained at a level that is high enough for adequate cerebral perfusion and cerebral blood flow, but not high enough to cause rebleeding. The efficacy of antifibrinolytic agents, such as aminocaproic acid (Amicar), in reducing the risk of bleeding in the 2 weeks after the initial bleed has not yet been substantiated.

In addition to rebleeding, complications associated with subarachnoid hemorrhage include seizure activity, hypothalamic dysfunction, and hydrocephalus. Seizure activity may occur within the first 24 hours after the initial bleed. Anticonvulsant therapy may be initiated prophylactically.

Hypothalamic dysfunction is reflected by cardiac arrhythmias associated with enhanced sympathetic innervation, and by a salt-wasting hyponatremia. Continuous cardiac monitoring is indicated. Treatment of hyponatremia requires volume replacement usually with concentrated saline infusions.

Hydrocephalus refers to an increased accumulation of cerebrospinal fluid in the ventricles of the brain. It results from interference with normal circulation of cerebrospinal fluid caused by occlusion of the foramina of Magendie and Lushka or the arachnoid granulations (see Figs. 27–5 and 27–6), secondary to breakdown of blood products. Treatment of hydrocephalus may require temporary drainage of cerebrospinal fluid via a catheter placed in the lateral ventricle, or permanent drainage via a ventriculoperitoneal shunt.

MANAGEMENT OF THE PATIENT WITH A POTENTIALLY LIFE-THREATENING CEREBROVASCULAR DISEASE

Clinical management of the patient with an acute cerebrovascular insult sufficient to disrupt the level of consciousness is focused on the following therapeutic goals: (1) support of vital functions, (2) restoration and maintenance of adequate cerebral perfusion pressure and cerebral blood flow, (3) prevention of further neurologic damage, (4) maintenance of total body functioning, and (5) ongoing assessment to determine the impact of neurologic deficits, if present, on the patient's self-care capabilities and implications for rehabilitation. For a discussion of therapeutic modalities concerned with ventilatory and circulatory support, maintenance of intracranial pressure within the normal range, pharmacologic therapy, surgery, and other supportive measures, refer to Chapter 30.

Nursing Management

Rationales underlying nursing interventions in the care of the patient with a potentially life-threatening cerebrovascular event can be approached from the perspective of conserving or "keeping together" the patient's biologic, personal, and social integrity in the face of catastrophic illness.[4,5] Thus, interventions can be implemented to assist the individual or family in

(1) conserving energy to prevent further damage and promote recovery, (2) conserving the structural integrity of the individual by maintaining normal physiologic function and preventing and minimizing further disruption in neurologic and total body function, (3) conserving the personal integrity of the stroke patient who already may experience dysfunction in such areas as cognition, perception, feeling, sensation, and language, and (4) conserving social integrity of the individual so that, on admission, the rehabilitative process is initiated to assist the individual to return to family and community functioning at his or her utmost level or potential.

Implementation of nursing process in the care of the patient with a cerebrovascular insult involves the following interventions:

1. Establish patient's baseline neurologic function, including prior behavior and personality considerations, if possible.
2. Stabilize ventilatory function with prevention of hypercapnia, hypoxia, and aspiration of nasogastric secretions.
3. Stabilize cardiovascular dynamics: Maintain optimal blood pressure adequate to treat areas of vasospasm, but sufficiently low enough to prevent rebleeding; monitor for potential cardiac arrhythmias.
4. Stabilize cerebrovascular dynamics: Maintain adequate cerebral perfusion pressure and cerebral blood flow sufficient to prevent *delayed* cerebral ischemia; minimize bleeding, and prevent rebleeding and vasospasm.
5. Minimize pain: headaches, muscular aches, anxiety.
6. Monitor or prevent seizures.
7. Maintain urinary and bowel function.
8. Prevent physiologic injury associated with:
   a. Disruption of musculoskeletal and skin integrity
   b. Aspiration
   c. Ulcerogenic gastrointestinal bleeding
9. Maintain an anabolic nutritional state.
10. Initiate and establish a meaningful and trusting rapport with patient, family, and significant others; assist in identifying prior effective coping mechanisms.
11. Establish a system of communication in the intubated patient or the patient with dysphasia.

Nursing Diagnoses, Desired Patient Outcomes, and Nursing Interventions

Pertinent nursing diagnoses, desired patient outcomes, and nursing interventions in the care of the patient with a potentially life-threatening cerebrovascular insult are presented in the care plan at the end of this chapter. Refer also to the care plans in Chapters 29, 30, and 31 for additional nursing diagnoses. See also the following case study with sample care plan: patient with a carotid artery aneurysm and middle cerebral artery syndrome.

CASE STUDY WITH SAMPLE CARE PLAN: PATIENT WITH A CAROTID ARTERY ANEURYSM AND MIDDLE CEREBRAL ARTERY SYNDROME

Mrs. M, a 37-year-old mother of three children ages 5, 7, and 9, presented in the emergency room at University Hospital with a right hemiplegia and dysphasia. Although unable to speak, Mrs. M appeared to be aware of her surroundings. The patient's family stated that she was well and in good health until 2 weeks earlier, when she started to complain of headaches. The headaches persisted over the ensuing 2 weeks, and the family reported that Mrs. M had several episodes when she "seemed to lose her voice."

On physical examination, the patient was noted to open her eyes and interact with the examiner spontaneously. She was able to vocalize but could not verbalize. A right-sided hemiplegia was noted; a Babinski's sign was present on the right; a plantar reflex was intact on the left foot. Pupils were reactive, about 5 to 6 mm in size, with the right pupil slightly larger than the left. The right corner of the mouth drooped; no lid lag was noted. The patient had a weak gag reflex.

Examination of the skin and integument revealed good turgor, with no lesions or rashes. The chest was clear on auscultation. The heart rate was 72, rhythm regular sinus. Abdomen was soft and nontender; bowel sounds were present in all four quadrants.

Arteriogram revealed a left internal carotid aneurysm, with poor filling of the left middle cerebral artery and anterior communicating artery. The patient was admitted with a diagnosis of right hemiplegia secondary to cerebral infarction associated with carotid artery aneurysm and subarachnoid hemorrhage. Initial therapy included Decadron (dexamethasone), 4 mg every 6 hours; antihypertensives to maintain systolic BP less than 180 mmHg; hold the medication for BP less than 140 mmHg. Loading dose of Dilantin (phenytoin) was initiated.

A subsequent arteriogram performed 24 hours after admission revealed a large lobulated aneurysm of the left carotid (internal) artery. The treatment plan included a left pterional craniotomy with microsurgical dissection of basal cisterns.

Postoperatively, the treatment plan included hyperventilatory therapy via mechanical ventilation. The patient was pavulonized and sedated with morphine to keep stimuli to a minimum. Vital signs were monitored closely, with the systolic blood pressure allowed to find its own level within the range of 110 to 190 mmHg. The patient was monitored continuously for any increase in ICP. For ICP greater than 25 mmHg, mannitol was administered intravenously. Serum osmolality was closely monitored. A cooling blanket was prescribed to maintain the afebrile state.

The patient responded well to therapy. On the third postoperative day, the subarachnoid bolt was removed without difficulty, and the patient was weaned off the ventilator. On the fourth postoperative day, the patient was extubated successfully. Nutritional support was initiated. On overall assessment, the patient appeared to be regaining preoperative status. Through discussions with family members, the patient's usual behavior and personality were ascertained. They were pleased with the way Mrs. M "was coming around."

On physical examination, the eyes opened spontaneously; the patient was able to smile spontaneously with evident right facial palsy; the patient moved her left arm purposely, wiggled her fingers, and gripped the examiner's hand; movement of the left leg was also evident. A right hemiplegia with dysphasia persisted.

On the fourth postoperative day, the patient was alert and vocalizing and had regained preoperative level of motor and psychic activity; she was tolerating clear fluids. Hyperalimentation was continued. The dressing site over the left carotid artery was clean and dry with no exudate. Physical therapy program was initiated.

The patient was very concerned about her children. Her mother was caring for the family since the hospitalization. A social service consult was requested to evaluate the home situation and to plan for eventual placement of the patient in a rehabilitation center.

For initial nursing diagnoses, see sample care plan. Refer also to the care plans in Chapters 29, 30, and 31.

REFERENCES

1. MacDonald, E: Aneurysmal subarachnoid hemorrhage. J Neurosci Nurs 21:313, 1989.
2. Welty, TE and Horner, TG: Pathophysiology and treatment of subarachnoid hemorrhage. Clin Pharm 9:35, 1990.
3. Brothers, MF and Holgate, RC: Intracranial angioplasty for treatment after subarachnoid hemorrhage: Technique and modifications to improve branch access. AJNR 11:239, 1990.
4. Taylor, JW. Nursing management of stroke: Acute care—Part I. Cardiovasc Nurs 21(1): 1, 1985.
5. Taylor, JW. Nursing management of stroke. Acute care—Part II. Cardiovasc Nurs 21(2):7, 1985.

SUGGESTED READINGS

Biggs, J and Fleury, J. An exploration of perceived barriers to cardiovascular risk reduction. Cardiovasc Nurs 30(6):41–47, September/October 1994.
Cook, HA: Aneurysmal subarachnoid hemorrhage: Neurosurgical frontiers and nursing challenges. AACN Clinical Issues in Critical Care Nursing 2(4):665, November 1991.
Susi, EA and Walls, SK: Traumatic cerebral vasospasm and secondary head injury. Crit Care Nurs Clin North Am 2(1):15, March, 1990.
Wong, MC and Haley, EC. Calcium agonists: Stroke therapy coming of age. Current Concepts of Cerebrovascular Disease and Stroke 24(6):31–35, November–December 1989.

SAMPLE CARE PLAN FOR THE PATIENT WITH A CAROTID ARTERY ANEURYSM AND MIDDLE CEREBRAL ARTERY SYNDROME

Nursing Diagnoses

Nursing Diagnosis #1
Alteration in cerebral perfusion, related to:
1. Cerebral infarction with consequent cerebral edema
2. Vasospasm associated with subarachnoid bleeding

Desired Patient Outcomes

Patient will:
1. Maintain cerebral perfusion pressure >60 mmHg; ICP < 15 mmHg; mean arterial blood pressure ~80 mmHg
2. Remain without cardiac arrhythmias
3. Exhibit intact level of consciousness and mentation:
   • Oriented to person/place
   • Memory intact

Nursing Interventions
• Monitor for signs/symptoms of increasing ICP:

  ○ Establish baseline parameters for level of consciousness, mentation, respiratory rate and pattern, pupillary reactions, and sensorimotor function.
• Implement measures to prevent or reduce ICP:
  ○ Maintain proper positioning and body alignment; elevate head of bed; avoid head rotation or flexion on chest.
• Prevent increase in cerebral blood flow:
  ○ Initiate and maintain hyperventilation via mechanical ventilation to maintain $PaCO_2$ at 28–32 mmHg; PaO_2 > 80 mmHg.

Rationales
• Initial treatment is focused on stabilizing and supporting intracranial dynamics, and reducing or preventing rebleeding.
  ○ Baseline measurements are used to compare subsequent responses.

  ○ Correct positioning allows for optimal venous drainage from cranium via gravity. It prevents jugular vein compression or obstruction.
• Hypercapnia and hypoxemia predispose to cerebral vasodilation and increased cerebral blood flow.

SAMPLE CARE PLAN FOR THE PATIENT WITH A CAROTID ARTERY ANEURYSM AND MIDDLE CEREBRAL ARTERY SYNDROME (*Continued*)

Nursing Diagnoses

Nursing Diagnosis #2
Alteration in comfort: Headache, related to:
1. Meningeal irritation
2. Surgical incision

Nursing Interventions

- Assess for signs/symptoms of meningeal irritation:
  ○ Nuchal rigidity, photophobia, headache, positive Kernig's and Brudzinski's signs.
- Implement nursing measures to reduce headache and prevent bleeding:
  ○ Move patient carefully, minimizing head movement or sudden jarring of patient or bed; turn q2h

  ○ Dim the patient's bedside light, and maintain a quiet environment with minimal stimuli.
    □ Handle patient gently when providing care.
    □ Caution patient not to cough, sneeze, or strain.
- Administer analgesics as prescribed, and monitor effectiveness of medication in relieving pain and relaxing the patient.

Desired Patient Outcomes

Patient will:
1. Indicate (e.g., pointing finger) feeling relieved of pain
2. Demonstrate a relaxed demeanor

Rationales

- Intracranial bleeding is highly irritating to meningeal and brain tissues.

  ○ Turning helps to mobilize tracheobronchial secretions and redistribute pressure points to maximize circulation.
  ○ Dimming the lights helps reduce the discomfort of photophobia.

    □ These activities cause an increase in ICP.
- Headaches can be excruciating.

Nursing Diagnoses

Nursing Diagnosis #3
Potential for injury: Seizures, related to: Cranial cerebral insult (cerebral infarction and edema: intracranial bleeding)

Nursing Interventions

- Assess/monitor for seizure activity, documenting characteristics: onset, location, type of movement, associated changes in body function.
- Maintain seizure precautions as per protocol.
- Administer prescribed anticonvulsants.
  ○ Monitor serum levels of phenytoin (Dilantin) (serial)

Desired Patient Outcomes

Patient will:
1. Remain seizure-free
2. Maintain serum levels of phenytoin within the acceptable therapeutic range

Rationales

- Craniocerebral insults place the patient at risk of having seizures; anticonvulsant medications are usually prescribed prophylactically.

Nursing Diagnoses

Nursing Diagnosis #4
Nutrition, alteration in, less than body requirements, related to:
1. Altered state of consciousness
2. Compromised protective reflexes
3. Ineffective chewing or swallowing
4. Fatigue
5. Depression

Nursing Interventions

- Consult with nutritionist to determine caloric and nutritional needs.
- Initiate prescribed nutritional regimen:
  ○ Hyperalimentation; fluid restriction
- Monitor response to hyperalimination:
  ○ Intake and output
  ○ Laboratory parameters: BUN, creatinine, total protein, and albumin
  ○ Daily weight when patient's condition permits
- Maintain the integrity of the hyperalimentation system as per unit protocol.

Desired Patient Outcomes

Patient will:
1. Maintain an anabolic state:
   - Body weight within 5% of baseline
   - Total serum proteins within the acceptable range: albumin 3.5–5.0 g/100 mL
2. Exhibit having an appetite

Rationales

- Critical illness increases nutritional needs; these patients can rapidly experience a catabolic state when maintained on intravenous fluid replacement therapy. (One liter of dextrose and water contains 600 calories.)

SAMPLE CARE PLAN FOR THE PATIENT WITH A CAROTID ARTERY ANEURYSM AND MIDDLE CEREBRAL ARTERY SYNDROME (*Continued*)

Nursing Diagnoses

Nursing Diagnosis #5
Airway clearance, ineffective, related to:
1. Compromised cough
2. Need for minimizing activity of any kind during the acute phase
3. Limited mobility

Desired Patient Outcomes

Patient's airway will remain patent; breath sounds will be normal, without adventitious sounds (e.g., crackles, wheezes, rhonchi)

Nursing Interventions

- Assess breath sounds/adventitious sounds.
- Suction patient *only* when absolutely necessary, using meticulous technique.
  - Limit each pass to 15 sec or less.
  - Prevent accumulation of secretions.
- Maintain ventilation and oxygenation as prescribed.

Rationales

- Abnormal breath sounds or the presence of adventitious sounds suggests accumulation and pooling of secretions.
- Suctioning may increase ICP.
  - Pneumonia is a common complication and usually develops on the paralyzed side (in this case, the right upper and lower lobes). A decrease in thoracic excursion and altered pulmonary hemodynamics are contributory factors.

Nursing Diagnoses

Nursing Diagnosis #6
Communication impaired, related to: Dysphasia and dysarthria

Desired Patient Outcomes

Patient will:
1. Demonstrate use of alternative means of communication (e.g., nodding the head, pointing the finger, writing on a tablet, slate board)
2. Demonstrate ease and comfort when groping for words

Nursing Interventions

- Assess the patient's communication status:
  - Ask simple questions and determine patient's ability to answer.
  - Evaluate appropriateness of the answer, and the use of words, grammar, and syntax.
  - Evaluate the patient's understanding of the spoken word by asking the patient to follow simple instructions.
- Develop a system of communication that facilitates understanding, taking into consideration the patient's deficits.
- Encourage and reassure patient; anticipate needs; verbalize fears, frustrations for patient.
  - Convey acceptance of the patient's behavior.
- Approach to the patient:
  - Encourage verbalization.
  - Spend time with patient.
  - Assure patient that speech will improve over time and with rehabilitation.

Rationales

- Assessment identifies the skills that remain intact.
- Lesions of the left cerebral hemisphere frequently disturb Broca's area, resulting in an expressive aphasia.

- Loss of the ability to communicate can be devastating. A calm, reassuring approach and supportive manner are essential.

  - Feeling unhurried may be reassuring as the patient searches for words to express herself.

Nursing Diagnoses

Nursing Diagnosis #7
Anxiety, related to:
1. Fear of dying
2. Potential sequelae related to neurologic deficits

Desired Patient Outcomes

Patient will:
1. Write out needs and concerns on a slate board or tablet
2. Demonstrate relaxed demeanor and perform relaxation techniques as condition permits

Nursing Interventions

- Assess for signs/symptoms of anxiety:
  - Wide-eyed look, clenched fists, increased heart rate.
  - Identify cause, if possible, and treat.
- Initiate interventions to reduce anxiety: stay with patient to reassure; verbalize fears/frustrations the patient may be experiencing; indicate acceptance of the patient.

Rationales

- Severe anxiety can aggravate the patient's overall condition. Because Mrs. M is unable to communicate verbally, her anxiety level may be especially high.

CARE PLAN FOR THE PATIENT WITH A CEREBROVASCULAR ACCIDENT (STROKE)

Nursing Diagnoses

Nursing Diagnosis #1
Potential for injury: physiologic, related to: Diabetes insipidus associated with craniocerebral insult
• Hypothalamic/pituitary dysfunction

Desired Patient Outcomes

Patient will:
1. Maintain vital signs at baseline values
2. Maintain desired hydration status:
   • Urine output >30 mL and <200 mL/h
   • Urine specific gravity 1.010–1.025
3. Remain without clinical signs of dehydration
4. Maintain acceptable laboratory profile:
   • Serum electrolytes, BUN, creatinine
   • Serum osmolality, serum proteins
   • Hematology profile

Nursing Interventions

• Assess for signs and symptoms of diabetes insipidus.
   ○ Primary findings:
      □ Polyuria, polydipsia, dehydration, weight loss
      □ Urine specific gravity <1.010

   ○ Neurologic status: level of consciousness, mentation, cranial nerve and sensorimotor function and deep tendon reflexes
   ○ Hydration status: strict hourly fluid intake/output, body weight, urine specific gravity; signs/symptoms of fluid overload or dehydration; laboratory data: serum electrolytes, serum osmolality; hematology profile (i.e., hematocrit, hemoglobin)
   ○ Cardiopulmonary status: blood pressure, pulse, cardiac rate and rhythm
      □ Presence of adventitious sounds
      □ Ability to handle respiratory secretions; characteristics of sputum (e.g., thick tenacious)
• Identify patients at risk.

• Implement measures to maintain desired fluid status.

   ○ Administer prescribed medication regimen: vasopressin replacement therapy and corticosteroid therapy.
   ○ Administer prescribed fluid regimen.
• Monitor effectiveness of overall therapeutic regimen.

Rationales

• Diabetes insipidus is a common secondary complication of craniocerebral insult.
• Cerebral edema or intracranial hemorrhage may temporarily impair synthesis and release of antidiuretic hormone by the hypothalamus during the initial 48 h after insult.

   ○ Patient with diabetes insipidus can become dehydrated quickly.

• Clinical manifestations of diabetes insipidus after insult may be delayed because of limited endogenous stores of antidiuretic hormone.
• Patient is usually maintained in a slightly dehydrated state to minimize risk of cerebral edema and reduce blood pressure.
   ○ These drugs may be prescribed to heighten the efficacy of antidiuretic hormone.
   ○ Anti-inflammatory effect of corticosteroid therapy may help to minimize cerebral edema.

Nursing Diagnoses

Nursing Diagnosis #2
Impaired physical mobility, related to:
1. Comatose state
2. Restricted activity associated with risk of intracranial pressure or rebleeding
3. Hemostasis or dependent edema associated with immobility; neuromuscular impairment (e.g., hemiparesis)

Desired Patient Outcomes

Patient will:
1. Maintain full range of motion
2. Remain without contractures
3. Remain without incidence of thrombophlebitis

Nursing Interventions

• Consult with physician and physical therapist to assess neurologic and musculoskeletal status.

Rationales

• The risk of intracranial hypertension and rebleeding must guide the type and extent of an activity program. A major objective is to maintain optimal function as dictated by patient's overall condition.

CARE PLAN FOR THE PATIENT WITH A CEREBROVASCULAR ACCIDENT (STROKE)
(*Continued*)

Nursing Interventions	Rationales

• Plan and implement activity regimen:
  ○ Initiate schedule of range-of-motion exercises.
 	
  ○ Passive/active exercises should be performed as patient's condition warrants.
  ○ Allow rest periods before and after exercise routines.
  ○ Maintain optimal body alignment.
    □ Use hand/wrist splints as prescribed.
    □ Support affected extremities in functional position.
  ○ Use trochanter roll on outer aspects of thigh.
  ○ Initiate turning and positioning schedule.
    □ Encourage patient to deep breathe and cough (unless contraindicated).
	○ Exercise maintains muscle tone and prevents atrophy; stimulates circulation and prevents hemostasis.
	○ Immobility associated with hemiparesis predisposes to thrombophlebitis.
	○ Helps to conserve patient's energy.
	○ Proper alignment is essential to prevent development of contractures and dependent edema (sacral area, buttocks, extremities).
	○ This prevents external rotation.
	○ Turning, positioning, and deep breathing facilitate chest and lung expansion; mobilize oral and pulmonary secretions; prevent atelectasis.

Nursing Diagnoses	Desired Patient Outcomes

Nursing Diagnosis #3
Potential for physiologic injury: thrombophlebitis, related to: Hemostasis associated with immobility
	Patient will:
	1. Verbalize absence of calf tenderness
	2. Exhibit adequate peripheral circulation:
	  • Usual skin color; no cyanosis
	  • Extremities warm to touch
	  • Palpable pulses: pedal, popliteal, radial

Nursing Interventions	Rationales

• Assess for signs/symptoms of venous thrombosis.
  ○ Tenderness, pain, warmth, and peripheral pitting edema; Homan's sign, i.e., pain in calf upon passive dorsiflexion of toes and foot
  ○ Circumference of thighs and calves at designated points
 	
  ○ Skin color and temperature
    □ Observe extremities in both dependent and elevated positions.
 	
• Implement measures to minimize risk of thrombophlebitis/deep venous thrombosis.
  ○ Maintain desired hydration state.
 	
  ○ Apply antiembolic hose to both extremities; remove hose once per shift.
  ○ Assist patient to perform range-of-motion exercises as appropriate.
 	
  ○ Instruct responsive patient to avoid positions that compromise blood flow in the extremities (e.g., crossing of legs, prolonged sitting in one position, pillow under knees, or use of knee gatch).
	• Deep venous thrombosis (DVT) places patient at risk of pulmonary embolism.
	  ○ DVT is a characteristic manifestation of altered venous circulation.
	  ○ Evidence of DVT is best assessed and monitored by determining the circumference of calves and thighs at designated points (use tape measure) on a daily basis.
	  ○ With altered venous circulation, a bluish-red color of skin may be observed.
	  ○ Temperature of skin is assessed by touch; unusually warm temperature in the lowest extremities is commonly associated with venous thrombosis.
	
	  ○ While the patient with a cerebrovascular insult is usually maintained in a slightly dehydrated state, dehydration is to be avoided because it increases blood viscosity.
	
	  ○ Exercise enhances "skeletal-muscular" pump, which functions to prevent pooling of blood in lower extremities (venous stasis), and increases venous return to heart.
	  ○ Positions that compromise blood flow can cause circulatory stasis.

Nursing Diagnoses	Desired Patient Outcomes
Nursing Diagnosis #4 Communication impaired, related to: 1. Aphasia (dysphasia) 2. Dysarthria (i.e., disturbance in articulation) (left cerebral hemisphere involvement)	Patient will: • Use language to verbalize or communicate needs or answer questions

CARE PLAN FOR THE PATIENT WITH A CEREBROVASCULAR ACCIDENT (STROKE)
(*Continued*)

Nursing Interventions	Rationales

• Assess for difficulty in using language to verbalize needs and answer questions.
  ○ Consult with speech pathologist, if possible, to assess patient's clinical status and design a care plan.
• Implement measures that enhance communication:
  ○ Speak slowly, using simple sentences.
  ○ Repeat questions or directions.
  ○ Use supplemental gestures or pictures; blackboard or slate board.
  ○ Face the patient directly when speaking.
  ○ Avoid speaking too loudly.
  ○ Encourage patient to express his/her thoughts; avoid rushing the patient.
  ○ Minimize distractions.
  ○ Offer encouragement; praise the patient for his or her accomplishments.
• Anticipate patient's needs.
	• Primary speech center (Broca's) is predominantly in frontal lobe of left cerebral hemisphere. Cerebrovascular insult to this area can result in language deficits.
	
	• Directives here suggest some of the ways communication can be facilitated. In the clinical setting, ideally, speech therapy is conducted in collaboration with a speech pathologist so that specific communication problems can be addressed appropriately.
	
	  ○ A language problem doesn't mean that the patient can't hear.
	
	  ○ Assist the patient to concentrate on communicating.
	  ○ Assist the patient in gaining self-confidence.
	
	• May help to allay concerns regarding dependency on others.

Nursing Diagnoses	Desired Patient Outcomes
Nursing Diagnosis #5 Coping, alteration in: Patient and family, related to: 1. Situational crisis 2. Temporary family disorganization 3. Inability to problem-solve 4. Altered thought processes 5. Catastrophic illness with long-term effects	Patient/family will: 1. Identify useful coping mechanisms 2. Demonstrate ability to assess, problem-solve and make decisions 3. Express realistic expectations of each other

Nursing Interventions	Rationales

• Establish a rapport and trusting relationship with patient and family.
  ○ Observe family dynamics and interactions.
    □ Assess family relationships and communication pattern: usual coping mechanisms, usual decision-making process, especially during stressful or crisis situations.
    □ Assess response of patient/family to stressful situations: identify strengths/weaknesses.
• Implement measures to assist in coping:
  ○ Provide opportunity for patient and family members to express feelings and emotions:
    □ Encourage honest communication among family members.
  ○ Assist patient to prioritize daily activities.
  ○ Encourage patient/family to assist in decision-making process regarding care:
    □ Assist in identifying options and their consequences.
  ○ Advise patient/family regarding community resources.
	○ These observations may help to identify strengths and weaknesses and effective coping capabilities. Assisting patient/family to acknowledge their own strengths may help them cope more effectively.
	
	  ○ Recognizing feelings and emotions helps one to deal with them.
	
	  ○ Reduction in level of stress assists in coping.
	  ○ Assist patient/family to be responsible for self-care and level of health desired.
	
	  ○ Complications from cerebrovascular disease can be catastrophic; it is essential for the patient/family to identify family and community resources.

Nursing Diagnoses	Desired Patient Outcomes

Nursing Diagnosis #6
Unilateral neglect, related to:
1. Altered sensorimotor function associated with cerebrovascular accident
2. Alterations in thought processes: perceptual
	Patient will:
	1. Demonstrate awareness as to position or placement of all four extremities
	2. Demonstrate awareness of looking toward affected side in terms of:
	  • Self-care (personal hygiene, grooming, dressing)
	  • Safety measures
	  • Eating habits

CARE PLAN FOR THE PATIENT WITH A CEREBROVASCULAR ACCIDENT (STROKE)
(*Continued*)

Nursing Diagnoses

Nursing Diagnosis #7
Self-care deficits, related to:
1. Neuromuscular impairments (.e.g, paresis, apraxia, visual/sensory defects, anosognosia) (right cerebral hemisphere involvement)
2. Reduced attention span

Nursing Diagnosis #8
Potential for injury: Safety, related to:
1. Altered sensory/perceptual function
2. Altered musculoskeletal function

Nursing Interventions

- Assess sensorimotor function related to:
  - Special senses: visual field defects, dysphasia (aphasia)
  - General senses: pain and temperature, tactile sensations

- Implement measures to assist patient to learn what types of sensorimotor deficits exist and the extent of the deficits in terms of self-care.
  - Visual field deficits:
    - Teach patient to scan immediate environment and note the placement of objects and equipment.
    - Approach patient from intact side.
    - Position bed so that the intact side can fully visualize the doorway.
    - Keep bedside uncluttered.
  - Dysphasia:
    - Attempt to evaluate type of dysphasia. Enlist the assistance of speech pathologist, if available, to establish program for patient, family members, and healthcare professionals working with patient, designed to facilitate communication.
    - Speak slowly and face the patient.
    - Use short, simple sentences.
    - Repeat directions or explanations as necessary.
    - Use gestures to further clarify what is being said.
  - General sensorimotor functions: dressing and grooming:
    - Teach patient to care for affected side first when bathing or dressing and to undress the affected side last.
    - Use sensory stimuli to help patient become aware of affected part of body.
    - Use exercises that enable affected side to cross midline.
  - Reassure patient and family regarding progress:

    - Praise positive responses and activities.

Desired Patient Outcomes

Patient will:
1. Identify activities of daily living for which the patient requires some assistance
2. Verbalize feelings regarding dependency
3. Determine priorities
4. Plan activities of daily living, leaving ample time to accomplish tasks

Patient will remain free from falls or other injury.

Rationales

- It is essential to determine what deficits exist so that an appropriate approach to therapy can be individualized for the patient.
  - Often sensory deficits are permanent, necessitating that the patient learn what his or her deficits are, and how to accommodate actions and behaviors accordingly.
- It is important to involve patient and family members in patient care.

    - Prevents possible injury
  - Dysphasia (asphasia) is particularly associated with dominant cerebral hemisphere lesion (usually with the left hemisphere).

  - Apraxia, unilateral spatial and visual neglect, and anosognosia are neurologic deficits associated with nondominant cerebral hemisphere involvement (usually the right hemisphere involvement).

  - The patient's rehabilitation should begin during the acute phase; activities initiated during this period lay the foundation for patient/family participation in self-care.
    - Frequent praise encourages and motivates patient and family.

CHAPTER 33

Clinical Management of the Patient with a Spinal Cord Disorder

Joan T. Dolan

CHAPTER OUTLINE

LEARNING OBJECTIVES

After completing this chapter, you should be able to:

1. Define spinal cord injury and terminology used to indicate extent of injury and related sequelae (i.e., complications).
2. Differentiate mechanisms of vertebral and spinal cord injuries.
3. Differentiate incomplete spinal cord syndromes in terms of pathophysiology and clinical presentation.
4. Differentiate *primary* and *secondary* spinal cord injuries in terms of underlying pathophysiology, and implications for patient care.
5. Define neurogenic (spinal) shock and its clinical significance.
6. Discuss priorities of care in the early clinical management of the patient with spinal cord injury (cervical cord injury) for the following:
   a. Musculoskeletal integrity, including immobilization and stabilization
   b. Respiratory function, including initial airway assessment and management
   c. Cardiovascular function, including deep venous thrombosis and autonomic dysreflexia
   d. Body temperature instability
   e. Gastrointestinal function, including implications for bowel management
   f. Renal/urinary function, including implications for bladder management
   g. Nutritional status and implications for management
   h. Skin integrity and implications for management
   i. Physical, psychological, and social rehabilitation: Ultimate goal
7. Develop a plan of care reflective of nursing process for the clinical management of the patient with acute spinal cord injury during the acute phase.
8. Discuss Guillain-Barré syndrome, its etiology and pathophysiology.

9. Identify key clinical manifestations of Guillain-Barré syndrome, its clinical course, and potential life-threatening complications.
10. Develop a plan of care reflective of nursing process for the clinical management of the patient with Guillain-Barré syndrome during the acute phase.

SPINAL CORD INJURY

Spinal cord injury is a catastrophic event having far-reaching and devastating consequences for the victim, the family, the community, and today's society as a whole. More than 10,000 Americans sustain a traumatic spinal cord injury each year. Of this number approximately 80% are under the age of 40; the majority of these are between 15 and 25 years of age, and are predominantly male.

Motor vehicle accidents (MVAs) account for 50% of the total number of traumatic spinal cord injuries occurring each year, followed by falls (predominantly in the over-65 age group), sports accidents (i.e., contact sports and diving accidents), and violent trauma (e.g., use of guns). Strict enforcement of laws requiring use of seatbelts and use of car seats for young children has helped to reduce the risk and/or extent of injury sustained in a motor vehicle accident. Persons driving while impaired or intoxicated are one of the major contributing factors to the incidence of motor vehicle accidents and associated spinal cord injury.

Although the yearly incidence of spinal cord injury may be low, the cost of treating and maintaining the individual with spinal cord injury is phenomenal. Changes occur in virtually all body functions. The individual is subjected to a tremendous amount of stress—physically, emotionally, and psychologically—as he or she strives to survive the insult, eventually to adjust to and cope with a changed lifestyle, an altered body image and self-concept, and at times, a low self-esteem.

During the acute phase, the challenge to critical care nurses caring for patients with spinal cord injury is to sustain life, prevent further neurologic damage, and assist patients and their families to initiate the rehabilitative process. The goal of rehabilitation is to help these individuals to achieve their optimum level of functioning, within the limitations imposed by the injury. Care of patients with spinal cord injury requires a collaborative, interdisciplinary approach to provide effective, quality care and management from acute care through the ongoing rehabilitative process.

Spinal Cord Injury: Defined

Spinal cord injury refers to an acute pathologic insult to the spinal cord that interrupts sensory and motor communication within the central nervous system (CNS), and between the CNS and the peripheral nervous system (PNS). Depending on whether the lesion is complete or incomplete, the individual will experience a wide range of impairments to all body functions. Physiologically, all major organ systems are involved. Psychologically, complications emerge that are associated with lengthy and difficult adjustments and rehabilitation necessitated by physiologic dysfunction. The social, economic, and emotional ramifications of spinal cord injury are indeterminable.

Definition of Terms

Quadriplegia. Quadriplegia refers to paralysis involving all four extremities and the trunk. It results from injury to thoracic cord segment T-1 or above (see Fig. 27–15). Lesions at these levels impair autonomic nervous system function, especially that of the sympathetic system. Respiratory insufficiency is a significant concern (Table 33–1).

Complete Quadriplegia and Incomplete Quadriplegia. *Complete* quadriplegia describes loss of cord function above the C-6 cord segment. It leaves the individual with minimal or no potential for independence. An intact cord segment at C-6 is sometime referred to as the line of demarcation between complete dependence and the potential for independence. *Incomplete* quadriplegia describes loss of neurologic function below the C-6 spinal cord segment.

Respiratory Quadriplegia (Pentaplegia). Respiratory quadriplegia (pentaplegia) refers to lesions of the spinal cord involving the upper cervical cord segments C-1 through C-4 (see Fig. 27–15). The phrenic nerve which innervates the diaphragm has its origin in these cervical nerve roots. Consequently, individuals sustaining spinal cord injury at this level experience acute respiratory insufficiency characterized by possible lack of spontaneous respirations, reduced lung volumes and capacities, poor gas exchange, progressive decline in lung and thoracic compliance, and a loss of, or severely weakened cough, with inability to handle pulmonary secretions. Mechanical ventilatory support is required during the acute stage, and the patient remains ventilator-dependent with a permanent tracheostomy.

Paraplegia. Paraplegia refers to paralysis of the lower half of the body, which includes both lower extremities and may involve the trunk. Paraplegia occurs with injury to the 2nd thoracic cord segment (T-2) or below (see Fig. 27–15). Lesions at this level do not compromise upper body strength and full use of the upper extremities may be preserved. Functionally, the paraplegic individual has the potential of becoming independent in all aspects of daily living with wheelchair mobility (Table 33–2).

TABLE 33–1
Spinal Cord Injury—Functional Status of Quadriplegia

Level of Cord Injury		Motor Function	Sensory Function, Light/Deep Touch, Pain—Pinprick	Respiratory Function	Bladder and Bowel Function	Assessment—Movements Requested of Patient	Potential Outcomes
Vertebrae	Segment*						
C-1 to C-3	C-1 to C-3	• Partial function of accessory muscles of breathing; limited movement of head and neck • C-2 to C-7 innervate: sternocleidomastoid, scalenus muscles • Cranial nerve XI also innervates sternocleidomastoid muscles • Respiratory quadriplegia	• Full sensation to head and upper neck	• Respiratory quadriplegia • Lack of spontaneous respirations • Ventilator-dependent	• Loss of bowel and bladder control • Dependent on assistance • At risk for urinary tract infection	• C-2 to C-5 nerve roots form phrenic nerve, which innervates diaphragm. Loss of this innervation results in respiratory paralysis • Loss of intercostal muscle function • Tracheostomy • Mechanical ventilation • Maintain patent airway—removal of secretions	• Balance head, which assists in maintaining upright position in wheelchair; allows mouth stick activities • With development of accessory muscles, potential to remain off respirator for brief periods • Completely dependent for ADL • Reduced respiratory reserve; at risk for respiratory infection • Postural hypotension • At risk for autonomic dysreflexia
C-4	C-4	• Muscle function of head and neck as above • Some shoulder movement • Some diaphragm control	• As above • Shoulder tops (C-3 to C-4)	• As above • Compromised respiratory status	• As above	• As above • Shrug shoulders	• As above • Dependence for ADL and transfers
C-4 to C-5	C-5	• Complete control of head, neck, and shoulders • Elbow flexion • Trapezius muscle intact • Quadriplegia complete	• Full sensation to head, neck, and shoulder tops • Upper anterior chest and upper back • Lateral aspect of upper arms	• Phrenic nerve intact • No intercostal muscle function • Independent respiratory function but poor pulmonary capacity and reserve (tidal volume ~300 mL)	• Some independence with adaptive equipment and raised toilet seat	• As above • Request patient to take a deep breath; diaphragm should descend causing bulging of abdomen; upper chest does not move due to loss of innervation to intercostal muscles • Bend elbow	• As above • Independence with electric wheelchair and use of adaptive equipment to feed and groom self
C-5 to C-6	C-6	• Full elbow flexion • Some wrist extension • Possible incomplete quadriplegia	• As above • Thumb and index finger	• As above	• Independent with adaptive equipment	• Bend wrist up	• Independence in use of manual wheelchair • Independence in feeding and grooming using adaptive devices • Helps to dress self • Dependent for transfers

continued

TABLE 33–1
Spinal Cord Injury—Functional Status of Quadriplegia (*Continued*)

Level of Cord Injury		Motor Function	Sensory Function, Light/Deep Touch, Pain— Pinprick	Respiratory Function	Bladder and Bowel Function	Assessment— Movements Requested of Patient	Potential Outcomes
Vertebrae	Segment*						
C-6 to C-7	C-7	• As above, with elbow extension, some finger control • Quadriplegia incomplete	• As above • Middle finger • Part of ring finger	• As above	• As above	• Make a fist • Opposite thumb to each fingertip	• Independence in ADL • Use of wrist extensor splint to induce finger flexion • Some assistance in transfers • May be able to drive
C-7 to T-1	C-8 to T-1	• As above • Moderate to full control of arm, wrist, and fingers	• Full sensation to entire hand and medial aspects of upper and lower arm	• As above	• As above	• As above	• Independent in transfers with adaptive equipment • Can grasp and release hands voluntarily • Independent in ADL

*The cord segment level reflects the lowest cord level at which neurologic function is intact. Example: A C-5 quadriplegia means that the C-5 cord segment and roots are intact while C-6 is not.

Mechanisms of Spinal Injury

Mechanisms of Vertebral Injury

The vertebral column functions to support the skull and to provide protection for the spinal cord and spinal nerves (see Fig. 27–13). The relationship between the spinal cord and vertebral column is so intricate and unique that pathology to the vertebral column may have far-reaching implications with regard to spinal cord function and the functioning of the body as a whole.

Injury to the spinal cord occurs most frequently as a result of trauma to the vertebral column and/or ligaments. The irregular body structure and intervertebral articulations (see Fig. 27–13) are easily fractured and cause the vertebral column to be vulnerable to flexion, extension, and rotational forces. The degree, direction, and type of force applied to the vertebral column at the moment of impact determines the extent of injury.

Injury, when it does occur, most often involves those sections of the vertebral column that have the greatest mobility, namely, cervical lesions C-4 to C-7, and the thoracolumbar junction T-11, T-12, and L-1. The thoracic region is less vulnerable to injury as the articulating rib cage imparts a rigidity and stability to this area.

Major mechanisms of vertebral injuries include hyperextension, hyperflexion, vertical compression, and/or rotation of the vertebral column.

Hyperextension-Hyperflexion Injuries. Hyperextension-hyperflexion injuries result when strong forces impact the body causing the unsupported head, first to rapidly hyperextend, and then to hyperflex on the neck. The *acceleration* forces of a typical rear-end auto collision cause *hyperextension*-hyperflexion injuries.

Hyperextension injuries are seen in elderly persons who frequently have degenerative changes of the vertebral column and are prone to falls. Damage results if the force of the fall impacts the chin and snaps the head backward. In hyperextension-hyperflexion injuries, the greatest stress point is at vertebrae C-4 and C-5.

Hyperflexion-Hyperextension Injuries. The *deceleration* forces of a head-on auto collision result in *hyperflexion-hyperextension* injuries. On impact the head and body continue to move forward until they contact the dashboard or windshield. Forceful hyperflexion of the head on the neck occurs, followed by a forceful hyperextension as the head snaps backward. Diving accidents or blows impacting the back of the head frequently result in cervical injury due to hyperflexion. In *hyperflexion* injuries, the greatest stress points are cervical vertebral levels C-5 and C-6.

Hyperflexion injuries may also occur to the thoracolumbar junction (T-11, T-12, L-1). This region of the vertebral column has considerable mobility and, like the cervical area, is vulnerable to forces impacting this area. A classification of vertebral injuries is presented in Table 33–3.

TABLE 33–2
Spinal Cord Injury: Functional Status of Paraplegia

Level of Cord Injury		Motor Function	Sensory Function, Light/Deep Touch, Pain—Pinprick	Respiratory Function	Bladder and Bowel Function	Assessment—Movements Requested of Patient	Potential Outcomes
Vertebrae	Segment*						
T-2	T-3 to T-4 (nipple line)	• Full control of upper extremities • Some intercostal function	• Sensation intact to midchest including upper extremities (T-1 to T-2) and to nipple line (T-4)	• Some control of intercostal muscles • Pulmonary capacities within physiologic limits (tidal volume—500 to 700 mL)	• Independent with adaptive devices		• Completely independent in wheelchair and ADL • Potential for full-time employment • At risk for postural hypotension and autonomic dysreflexia
T-8 to T-9 T-11 to T-12 T-12 to L-1	T-10 (umbilicus) to T-12	• Full control of abdominal and trunk muscles • Hip rotation and some hip flexion (L-1 to L-3)	• Sensation intact below waist: T-10 supplies umbilicus, T-12 supplies groin area, L-1 pubis, L-2 hips. • Some sensation to anterior and medial thigh	• Full control of intercostals • No intereference with respiratory function	• As above	• Tighten abdomen • Flex hip	• As above with complete abdominal, back, and respiratory control • Participation in athletic activities
L-1	L-3 to S-1	• As above • Knee extension (L-3 to L-4) • Dorsiflexion of ankle (L-4, L-5, S-1) • Foot movement (L-4, L-5, S-1) • Knee flexion (L-4 to S-1) • Plantar flexion (S-1 to S-2)	• Sensation to upper legs (L-1 to L-3) • Anterior/posterior and lateral surfaces of lower leg and dorsum of foot (L-4 to L-5)	• As above	• Independent with or without adaptive devices	• Flex hip • Straighten (extend) leg • Bend and straighten toes	• As above • Optimal use of long leg braces • Note: Sympathetic innervaion largely intact
L-1 to L-2	S-2 to S-4	• As above; some foot control; reflex centers for bowel, bladder, and sexual function	• Note: *Lumbar* nerves innervate part of lower legs and feet • *Sacral* nerves innervate lower legs, feet, and perineum	• As above	• As above	• Tighten anal sphincter around examining finger • Sensorimotor assessment of perineal area is critical to determine extent of function	• Independent with or without short leg braces • Involvement of S-2 to S-4 can cause considerable disability related to bowel, bladder, and sexual dysfunction

*The cord segment level reflects the lowest cord level at which neurologic function is intact. Example: A T-12 paraplegia means that the T-12 cord segment and roots are intact while L-1 is not.

TABLE 33–3
Classification of Vertebral Injuries

Vertebral injuries may be classified as follows:
1. *Simple fracture*—involves spinous or transverse processes; vertebral body rarely affected; ligaments and spinal cord usually intact.
2. *Compression fracture (wedged fracture)*—involves compression of vertebral body anteriorly as occurs in hyperflexion injuries; intraspinous ligaments may be stretched but spinal cord usually remains intact.
3. *Comminuted fracture (burst fracture)*—involves an actual shattering of a vertebral body into many pieces; the spinal cord may sustain severe injury if bony fragments are driven into it.
4. *Dislocation*—disruption of vertebral alignment may result in injury to supporting ligaments. With impairment of ligaments the vertebral column becomes unstable, placing the cord at risk for injury. A partial dislocation is termed a *subluxation*.
5. *Sacral-coccygeal fractures*—these fractures are usually associated with falls onto the buttocks. Associated injury to the cord in this area is significant because the reflex centers for bowel, bladder, and sexual function occur in the spinal cord segments L-2 to S-5.

Mechanisms of Spinal Cord Injury

Mechanisms of spinal cord injuries include concussion, compression, contusion, laceration, partial section, or transection. As with injuries to the vertebral column, the extent and permanency of spinal cord dysfunction depend on the degree, direction, and type of injury. A classification of spinal cord injuries is presented in Table 33–4.

Spinal Cord Syndromes

Spinal cord syndromes are termed *incomplete* when there is partial preservation of neurologic function. The function preserved depends on the extent and severity of cord damage and includes varying degrees of motor, sensory, and autonomic function. The significance of incomplete cord syndromes is that there is the potential for recovery.

Incomplete spinal cord injuries having distinct patterns of neurologic dysfunction have been defined. It is unusual to see these syndromes in pure form, however; rather, there are characteristics of one or more forms in the patient with an incomplete lesion. Refer to Table 33–5 for details regarding specific spinal cord syndromes.

Spinal Cord Injury: Pathophysiology

Injuries to the spinal cord are often classified as primary and secondary. *Primary* neurologic injury is that sustained at the time of the initial trauma or mechanical insult. *Secondary* neurologic injury is that associated with an extension of the initial injury. Secondary injury occurs as a result of mechanical re-injury, altered hemodynamics, release of endogenous sub-

stances at the injury site, and localized cord edema, all of which predispose to tissue ischemia and necrosis.

Mechanical re-injury is that associated with inadequate or improper immobilization after spinal cord trauma. Altered hemodynamics are closely associated with spinal shock (see below). There is a decreased cardiac output associated with a reduction in venous return because of pooling of blood in the venous capacitant (i.e., distensible) vessels. Bradycardia is also present because of unopposed parasympathetic stimulation to the heart. Release of vasoactive substances (e.g., catecholamines, histamines, and endorphins) acts to further decrease blood flow to the injury site. The end result is a decreased blood supply to the spinal cord that contributes to tissue ischemia and necrosis. Proteolytic and lipolytic enzymes released at the site of injury disrupt blood supply by contributing to edema formation.

Most insults to the spinal cord predispose to edema formation. The localized inflammatory response to injury causes changes in the permeability of tissue cap-

TABLE 33–4
Classification of Spinal Cord Injuries

Spinal cord injuries may be classified as follows:
1. *Cord concussion*—defined as a momentary disturbance of cord function usually of a short duration without evidence of residual function loss.
2. *Compression*—associated with vertebral injury; may require surgery to relieve pressure on the cord; if relieved promptly before permanent cord damage is sustained, full function should be preserved. Underlying pathophysiology involves edema and/or direct pressure from malaligned or partially dislocated vertebrae; associated vascular injury can predispose to tissue ischemia/injury.
3. *Contusion*—associated with injury to vertebrae and/or disruption of ligaments resulting in an unstable vertebral column; major pathophysiologic concern is the possible impairment of collateral circulation predisposing to local cord ischemia.

   The blood supply to the vertebral column and spinal cord is not extensive; if the blood supply remains adequate, no major functional losses become apparent; poor collateral circulation may result in tissue injury and necrosis with permanent damage. The contused area reflects localized edema with microscopic hemorrhages and degenerative and demyelinated changes in spinal cord parenchymal tissue.
4. *Laceration (partial section)*, associated with fracture—dislocations of the vertebral column with severance or sectioning of spinal tracts resulting in a permanent loss of function since nerves within the CNS do not regenerate. Because the section of the cord is only partial, varying degrees of function are preserved.
5. *Transection*—involves severance of spinal cord with loss of neurologic function below the level of the lesion. (The cord segment identified reflects the lowest cord level at which neurologic function is intact. Thus, a C-5 quadriplegia means that the C-5 cord segment and roots are intact, while C-6 is not.)
   a. *Complete transection*—reflects a complete loss of neurologic function below the level of the lesion.
   b. *Incomplete transection*—reflects varying degrees of neurologic function or dysfunction below the level of the lesion depending on the severity of cord damage. (See laceration, above.)
6. *Hematomyela*—hemorrhage of blood into the spinal cord. Usually occurs as a post-traumatic lesion.

TABLE 33–5
Spinal Cord Syndromes

Syndrome	Mechanism of Vertebral Injury	Mechanism of Spinal Cord Injury	Motor/Sensory Pathways Disrupted	Clinical Manifestations
Anterior cord syndrome	• Flexion and dislocation injuries to cervical cord	• Direct injury; compression or vessel occlusion; infarction • Compromised anterior spinal artery	• Ventral and lateral corticospinal motor tracts • Ventral and lateral spinothalamic sensory tracts; spinal cerebellar tract • Pathways intact: dorsal columns	• Loss of all motor function below lesion; upper motor neuron disruption: positive bilateral Babinski's signs; spastic paralysis • Loss of pain and temperature sensation below lesion • Sensation intact: light touch, proprioception, vibration
Central cord syndrome	• Severe hyperextension injury to cervical cord • Spinal cord tumor	• Compression of cord between degenerated intervertebral disks • Centralized cord edema	• Centrally located nerve tracts, which innervate upper extremities, are disrupted	• Greater neurologic (motor/sensory) deficits in upper extremities than in legs • Varying degrees of bladder dysfunction • Occurs more often in elderly
Brown-Séquard syndrome (hemisection of spinal cord)	• Direct penetrating injury such as stab wound or gunshots	• Laceration and hemisection of spinal cord	• Lateral and ventral corticospinal tracts (ipsilateral side) • Ipsilateral dorsal columns	• Paresis or paralysis on ipsilateral side • Loss of tactile sensation, proprioception, and vibratory sense on ipsilateral side • Loss of pain and temperature on contralateral side
Conus medullaris–cauda equina injury	• Fracture dislocation	• Compression contusion, or laceration of conus and sacral spinal nerve roots	• Spinal nerve segments S-2 to S-4, which house the reflex centers for bowel, bladder, and sexual functions • Lower motor neuron disruption	• Neurologic deficits are variable • Nerve root injury commonly causes loss of both motor and sensory functions either unilaterally or bilaterally • Disruption of lower motor neuron causes loss of bowel, bladder, and sexual reflexes
Sacral sparing	• Direct trauma to major portion of cord • Spinal cord ischemia or infarction caused by disruption of spinal cord circulation • Radicular arteries remain intact	• Peripheral rim of cord tissue is preserved, including innervation to sacral area	• Sensation to sacral area is preserved in an otherwise completely paralyzed patient with loss of sensation below the level of the lesion	

illaries. This results in a disruption of osmotic gradients, thereby enabling fluid to move from the intravascular to the interstitial spaces. The resulting edema impairs circulation of blood to parenchymal tissues and may cause inhibition of spinal cord function.

The significance of edema formation involving the spinal cord becomes critical when the cervical region is affected. Edema may involve several cord segments above and below the level of the lesion. In the case of injury to cord segment C-5, for example, edema formation may advance to the C-3 to C-4 levels, where it may impair phrenic nerve function and precipitate respiratory insufficiency and/or arrest. Likewise, edema occurring at the C-1 to C-2 levels may progress upward to the medulla and impair other vital functions.

It is essential to establish *baseline* assessment data as to the *level of cord function* so that changes in function reflective of advancing edema formation can be readily identified and appropriate intervention can be initiated. Changes in breathing pattern, mental status, sensorimotor function, and reflex responses may provide clues to underlying pathophysiology and its progression. The nurse must be able to recognize changes indicative of deteriorating cord function. In the case of injury to cord segment C-5, for example, it may be important to intubate the patient prophylactically to ensure adequate respiratory function should further deterioration of spinal cord function occur.

Neurogenic Shock (Spinal Shock)

Neurogenic shock, or spinal shock, is a consequence of a sudden complete transection of the spinal cord at the level of T-4 to T-6, or above, causing immediate loss of all neurologic function below the level of the lesion, and an interruption of tonic impulses from the higher centers. There is complete cessation of motor, sensory, reflex, and autonomic function below the level of the lesion. Spinal shock may also occur in an incomplete transection of the cord, resulting in variable neurologic dysfunction. Spinal shock usually ensues within 30 to 60 minutes following cord injury.

Clinical Presentation

The syndrome of neurogenic shock, or spinal shock, presents clinically with motor, sensory, and autonomic dysfunction (Table 33–1) Motor dysfunction is characterized by flaccid, total paralysis of skeletal muscles below the level of injury and reflects interruption of descending pathways, including the upper and lower motor neurons of the corticospinal tracts (see Fig. 27–17). Loss of lower motor neuron (LMN) function is reflected by the absence of all skeletal muscle reflexes integrated within the cord (e.g., deep tendon reflexes).

Sensory dysfunction reflects interruption of ascending pathways (i.e., dorsal columns, spinothalamic tracts, etc.), which results in loss of all sensation below the injury. These include tactile sensation, vibratory sense, proprioception, pain, and temperature. There is an absence of somatic and visceral sensation below the level of the lesion.

Autonomic dysfunction is manifested by hypotension, bradycardia, warm dry skin, lowered body temperature, bowel and bladder dysfunction, and loss of sexual reflexes. Loss of sympathetic tone underlies the hypotension characteristic of neurogenic shock. Pooling of blood in the capacitant blood vessels of the lower extremities and splanchnic circulation decreases venous return to the heart. The result is a decreased cardiac output and arterial blood pressure. Venous blood pooling is particularly significant in that the patient becomes at increased risk of developing a deep venous thrombosis (see below). Vasodilation also accounts for the warm, dry skin and lowered body temperature, as body heat is lost via the dilated peripheral blood vessels. There is an inability to perspire below the level of cord injury.

Bradycardia occurs as a result of *unopposed* parasympathetic innervation to the heart via the vagus nerve. Heart rate in the patient with spinal cord injury may help to distinguish two types of shock sometimes encountered in cervical cord trauma, that is, *neurogenic* or spinal shock, and *hemorrhagic* or hypovolemic shock. The patient in neurogenic shock presents with hypotension and *bradycardia* because of loss of sympathetic tone below the level of the injury; the patient in hemorrhagic shock presents with hypotension and *tachycardia* because the body tries to compensate for the blood loss by increasing heart rate. Thus, in the patient with suspected spinal cord injury who is hypotensive and *tachycardic*, the patient should be examined carefully for signs of bleeding. Internal injuries may accompany spinal cord injuries, yet, because of loss of sensation below the level of cord injury, the patient may not experience the pain that might otherwise accompany a major internal hemorrhage.

The presence of a paralytic ileus largely reflects loss of parasympathetic tone. Bowel and bladder dysfunction and loss of sexual reflexes reflect the total loss of autonomic function.

The duration of neurogenic shock varies with each individual and may extend from days to weeks and even months. The average duration of spinal shock is 1 to 6 weeks. Recovery from shock may result in a state of hyperactivity. This is demonstrated by the *spastic* paralysis associated with loss of upper motor neuron (UMN) function. In the case of LMN function, reflexes remain hypoactive or absent with *flaccid* paralysis (Table 33–6).

TABLE 33–6
Clinical Manifestations of Upper and Lower Motor Neuron Dysfunction

	Upper Motor Neuron	Lower Motor Neuron
Muscle tone (Major effect)	Spasticity Spastic paralysis Contracture development	Flaccidity Flaccid paralysis
Reflexes	Hyperreflexia Babinski's sign	Hyporeflexia or areflexia No Babinski's sign
Fasciculations	Absent	Present
Muscle bulk	Slight atrophy (disuse) or no atrophy	Marked atrophy
Distribution of dysfunction	Decussation at medulla: Damage above— contralateral Damage below— ipsilateral	Specific muscles supplied by damaged nerve usually ipsilateral

PRIORITIES OF CARE IN THE EARLY CLINICAL MANAGEMENT OF THE PATIENT WITH SPINAL CORD INJURY (CERVICAL CORD INJURY)

Management of the patient who has sustained a spinal cord injury begins with stabilization of the patient at the scene of the accident. Goals of emergency care include prevention of death from asphyxia and/or mass hemorrhage, and prevention of further neurologic damage. Cardiopulmonary resuscitation (CPR), if necessary, is performed using the *jaw lift* as opposed to the *head tilt* (as per basic cardiac life support [BCLS] techniques).

Once airway, breathing, and circulation have been established, the major goal is immobilization and stabilization of the fracture and spinal cord to *minimize the extent of spinal cord injury* and consequent neurologic deficits. This is achieved by transporting the patient on a hard, flat surface with the head in a neutral position immobilized by a stiff cervical collar (preferably), with sandbags on either side, and/or by taping over the forehead to the transport board. Proper immobilization should prevent flexion, extension, and rotation of the cervical spine.

Any patient who has sustained a head injury must also be presumed to have a cervical spine injury until *definitively* ruled out by x-ray. Until this is accomplished, the head and neck must remain immobilized. Any inadvertent flexion, extension, or rotation of the cervical spine can result in secondary mechanical re-injury to the spinal cord.

The goal in the initial clinical management of the patient with spinal cord injury is to prevent irreversible neurologic deficits associated with secondary spinal cord injury. In addition, an effort is made to determine the level of cord functioning and to interpret how this functioning affects the other organ systems.

To prevent mechanical re-injury, the patient's head and neck remain immobilized while the status of the spinal cord injury is assessed more accurately. Transfer of the patient is avoided until the patient's condition is assessed and stabilized. If transfer or movement of the patient is necessary, a four-man lift technique should be used with one team member, skilled in such transfers, maintaining gentle, manual cervical traction, alignment, and immobilization.

A complete neurologic assessment is performed to establish a baseline as to the *level of cord function* so that any changes in the patient's neurologic function, whether an improvement or deterioration, can be readily identified and necessary therapy implemented. Special attention is given to an assessment of the four "p's"—paralysis, paresthesias, pain, and position. Assessment of motor function includes testing muscle strength using the 0 to 5 scale, where 0 indicates no evidence of muscle contraction, and 5 reflects full resistive strength (see Table 28–3) Testing of sensorimotor function can be guided by following the segmental dermatomal distribution of peripheral nerves (see Fig. 27–16). Baseline levels can be marked on the skin to aid in determining whether there are changes. X-rays, computed tomography (CT) scans, and magnetic resonance imaging (MRI) of the cervical spine, and other diagnostic studies are conducted at this time.

Initial medical management usually entails administration of high-dose methylprednisolone therapy. The effectiveness of steroid therapy is believed to be the result of stabilizing cell membranes and reducing edema formation. Naloxone, an endogenous opioid antagonist, has also been used after spinal cord trauma; however, significant neurologic improvement, both sensory and motor, has been primarily associated with trials involving high-dose prednisolone therapy.

Musculoskeletal Integrity

Surgical Stabilization

In the event of an unstable vertebral fracture, emergency surgery may be indicated to stabilize the spine and prevent mechanical re-injury. Surgical intervention is also indicated in unstable injuries of the cord (especially if cord transection is incomplete), in open injuries of the cord, and when there is evidence of progressive neurologic dysfunction. Surgical decompression and stabilization can be accomplished by a variety of surgical procedures. These include laminectomy with fusion, placement of rods (e.g., Harrington rod), and spinal fusion.

Nonsurgical Stabilization

Techniques of nonsurgical immobilization and stabilization are employed to: (1) prevent further neurologic damage and facilitate return of potential neurologic function, (2) maintain correct body alignment while ensuring necessary position changes to prevent skin breakdown, muscle fatigue, and contractures, (3) facilitate return of weakened musculature while promoting maximum function of unaffected muscles, and (4) minimize muscle spasms and promote patient comfort.

Cervical immobilization and stabilization may be achieved via the use of skeletal traction (e.g., Gardner-Wells tongs). Skeletal traction can achieve both reduction and immobilization of the fracture/dislocation.

Halo Immobilization Brace. An alternative method of achieving cervical immobilization, as well as traction, positioning, and alignment, is the application of the halo immobilization brace. It consists of a metal halo-ring attached to the skull via screws and to a metal frame of adjustable, interlocking metallic bars. These bars connect the ring to a rigid plastic vestlike jacket with a soft liner. It provides complete external immobilization for cervical instability, without flexion, extension, or rotational movements of the head.

The use of the halo brace has several advantages for the patient with spinal cord injury. These include (1) early application (can be placed on the patient in the emergency room if necessary) for prompt cervical reduction and alignment, (2) easy and safe patient transport, (3) timely institution of vigorous pulmonary toileting and physiotherapy, (4) pain reduction, (5) early mobilization and ambulation, reducing risk of such complications as pulmonary compromise (e.g., atelectasis, hypostatic pneumonia), impaired skin integrity, deep venous thrombosis, and sensory deprivation, among others, (6) ease of care and maintenance of the apparatus, and (7) decreased length of hospital stay and earlier, active participation of the patient in the rehabilitative process.

When caring for a patient with a halo immobilization brace, the nurse should be cognizant of ongoing nursing care management considerations including those listed in Table 33–7. Initially, the patient and family may be frightened because they may feel the halo brace is unsightly. The weight of the brace may make the patient feel "top-heavy" and awkward, and the patient may experience lightheadedness and nausea upon ambulating with the brace, commonly associated with postural hypotension. As the patient progresses from intensive to convalescent phase, a program of gradual ambulation can be implemented.

Respiratory Function

Initial Airway Assessment and Management

It is essential to maintain adequate tissue perfusion to protect the fragile, highly sensitive nerve tissue from ischemia, injury, and infarction. Airway obstruction is a frequent occurrence in cervical injury, particularly when head and facial trauma have also been sustained. Resuscitation efforts must avoid unnecessary manipulation of the fractured/dislocated neck to prevent mechanical re-injury.

To reestablish and maintain airway patency, the neck should be straightened without hyperextension (jaw-thrust maneuver) and an oral airway should be inserted. Ventilation via rebreather mask resuscitator should be initiated with oxygen concentrations of 8 to 12 L/min. To ensure effectiveness of the spontaneous ventilatory effort, arterial blood gases should be obtained while the patient is breathing *room air*. If the PaO_2 is less than 80 mmHg, the $PaCO_2$ is greater than 45 mmHg, and/or if the patient has a compromised ventilatory effort, intubation with mechanical ventilatory support may be indicated.

Intubation requires use of special techniques such as the jaw-thrust maneuver, to prevent hyperextension of the neck. Use of a nasotracheal tube may be preferred, or a tracheostomy may be performed. Early tracheostomy facilitates secretion clearance and is the primary choice when long-term use of an artificial airway is anticipated. Hyperventilation therapy is usually initiated to maintain $PaCO_2$ at 30 to 35 mmHg. By stimulating vasodilation, this therapy helps to maintain adequate blood supply to fragile nerve tissue.

Nasotracheal suctioning should be performed as necessary to maintain a patent airway. Management of pulmonary secretions is especially important if the patient has a weakened or absent cough reflex. Hypoxemia in the patient with spinal cord injury is most commonly caused by retained secretions. Humidified oxygen should be provided to keep secretions loose and to ensure adequate oxygenation.

The ability to cough requires the actions of intercostal and abdominal muscles, which build up pressure in the thorax and abdomen, so that air can be vigorously forced through the closed larynx. When the function of these muscles is lost, the patient is unable to cough up secretions and becomes susceptible to pulmonary complications. A moist-sounding but unproductive cough signals retention and pooling of pulmonary secretions.

Quad-assist coughing is a technique used to simulate the natural cough reflex. This method incorporates a Heimlich-type maneuver, wherein the nurse places a fist or the palm of the hand between the xiphoid process and umbilicus and vigorously applies a thrust during the coughing effort. This technique can be very

TABLE 33–7
Nursing Management Considerations for the Patient with a Halo Immobilization Brace

1. Avoid using the metal frame as a handle to turn, lift, or position the patient; avoid hitting the metal frame because bone conduction of the sound may be annoying to the patient.
2. Move the patient and halo immobilization brace as a unit to avoid undue stress on any one part.
3. Check pins and screws daily to ensure proper tightness.
4. Clean pin site areas twice daily with sterile normal saline and hydrogen peroxide followed by an application of povidone-iodine ointment.
5. Examine pin sites for any evidence of inflammation—pain, redness, swelling, drainage, increased body temperature, or headache, and report findings to patient's physician.
6. Examine skin under vest every 8 hours for pressure points and skin integrity. If possible, place patient in prone position to facilitate skin inspection and relieve pressure on scapulae and shoulders. Pressure points often occur over spinous processes T-1 to T-3. Be alert for unusual odors, which might indicate skin breakdown as, for example, the patient with diabetes mellitus or the severely debilitated patient. The paralyzed patient is unable to feel pain and requires diligent inspection and assessment after each position change.
7. Turn patient regularly to prevent skin breakdown and undue pressure on pin sites.
8. Maintain cleanliness with daily washing. Vest liners can be changed, and sheepskin padding can be applied to pressure areas.
9. All nurses caring for patient with a halo brace should know how to remove the anterior section of the brace in the event that cardiopulmonary resuscitation is needed. A wrench must be available at bedside to unlock the bolts that attach the anterior bars to the vest.
10. When the condition of the patient with a halo brace is stabilized, he/she may gradually be assisted into a sitting position, and eventually into a wheelchair. The transition to a sitting position is gradual to prevent postural hypotension.
11. When patient ambulates, caution patient to examine heights of doorways prior to entering them.

effective in raising pulmonary secretions when performed in conjunction with chest physiotherapy and nasotracheal suctioning.

Assessment and Promotion of Ventilatory Effort

The effectiveness of the patient's ventilatory effort needs to be carefully assessed and evaluated. Cervical cord transection at C-8 to T-1 and above, causes paralysis of intercostal and abdominal muscles and results in "paradoxical respiration." Clinically, the thoracic rib cage is observed to collapse passively on inspiration while the diaphragm descends and to expand on expiration as the diaphragm ascends. This is a reversal of normal ventilatory mechanics and reflects intercostal muscle paralysis. Paralysis of intercostal muscles (T-2 to L-1) prevents adequate expansion of the rib cage and decreases effective alveolar ventilation by as much as 60%.

Vital capacity is a useful measurement of the effectiveness of the patient's ventilatory effort. It is measured easily at the bedside using a spirometer. A lowered vital capacity (e.g., a trend leading to a vital capacity of <15 to 20 mL/kg), together with abnormal changes in the other assessment parameters, may signal the need for mechanical ventilatory support. Arterial blood gases (room air) also serve as a measurement of the effectiveness of the ventilatory effort.

The phrenic nerve, which innervates the diaphragm, arises from cord segments C-3 and C-4 (see Fig. 27–15). Injury to the cervical cord places the patient at risk of developing respiratory insufficiency or respiratory arrest; interruption of phrenic innervation causes paralysis of the diaphragm, and apnea results. Patients with cervical injuries (C-5 to C-6) frequently require mechanical ventilatory assistance until the edema resolves and the cord stabilizes. At this point, the patient can be weaned from the ventilator.

Prevention of Pulmonary Complications

Pulmonary complications are the major cause of death during the acute phase following spinal cord injury. Patient care is focused on maintaining a patent airway, preventing pooling of secretions, ensuring adequate chest expansion, and prevention or early recognition of major pulmonary complications. Such complications include atelectasis, hypostatic/aspiration pneumonia, pulmonary edema, and pulmonary embolism.

Preventive nursing measures include frequent turning and positioning, humidification, adequate hydration, pulmonary toileting and chest physiotherapy, application of antiembolic stockings, initiation of passive range-of-motion exercises, and patient teaching regarding breathing exercises when the patient's condition enables the patient to participate in these activities. The nurse and physical therapist need to work closely together to initiate a program designed to facilitate these measures, and to establish an exercise regimen to promote and maintain optimal cardiopulmonary function.

Cardiovascular Function

Alterations in the cardiovascular status of the patient with spinal cord injury are largely attributed, directly or indirectly, to autonomic dysfunction. Those examined here include neurogenic shock (see above), autonomic dysreflexia, and deep venous thrombosis.

Neurogenic, or spinal shock as discussed previously is characterized by loss of sympathetic vasomotor tone and vasomotor reflex activity below the level of the lesion. Consequent venous blood pooling and reduced venous return to the heart are treated by elevation of the lower extremities and application of antiembolic stockings. The patient is usually *not* hypovolemic and should not receive large amounts of fluid because this may aggravate edema formation at the site of injury. This type of shock may respond to vasopressor drug therapy, if the patient's clinical status necessitates this course of therapy to maintain adequate hemodynamics.

Autonomic Dysreflexia

Autonomic dysreflexia is defined as a clinical emergency characterized by an exaggerated sympathetic response occurring below the level of the spinal cord lesion and resulting in an uncontrolled paroxysmal hypertension (as high as 240 to 300 mmHg systolic and 150 mmHg diastolic). While it does not occur during the acute phase after cord injury, it is mentioned here because, when it does occur, its consequences can be life-threatening, leading to a fatal stroke, subarachnoid hemorrhage, and seizures.

Autonomic dysreflexia occurs in patients with spinal cord injury who have lesions at the T-4 to T-6 level or above. In patients with lesions at this level or lower, enough sympathetic innervation under the control of vasomotor centers in the brain is preserved to avoid this exaggerated abnormal response. Approximately 80% of individuals with spinal cord lesions above the T-4 to T-6 level experience autonomic dysreflexia within the first year after injury and after spinal shock has resolved. It may occur spontaneously several years after injury, even if the person has never experienced a prior episode.

Causes of autonomic dysreflexia are linked with nursing interventions and preventive aspects of daily care. They include a variety of abnormal stimuli arising from localized areas below the cord lesions, including the following:

Urinary
   Distended bladder due to urinary retention
   Kinking or plugging of catheter, if in place
   Genitourinary infection
   Calculus formation
   Pressure on genitals (testicles)
   Genitourinary procedures (e.g., cystoscopy)

Bowel
   Distended rectum
   Fecal impaction
   Digital examination
Skin
   Decubitus (pressure) ulcer
   Sharp object pressing into skin
   Drafts in room
Pain receptors
   Ingrown toenails
   Pressure on glans penis
   Inguinal rash
Abdominal problems
   Internal bleeding after instrumentation
Pregnancy
   Uterine contractions during labor

The clinical manifestations of autonomic dysreflexia can be explained as follows: Vasomotor tone to areas *above* the cord lesion can be enhanced by signals from higher brain centers. When blood pressure rises, the sympathetic tone is reflexly reduced and vasodilation occurs in vessels innervated by nerves above the cord lesion. This accounts for the profuse diaphoresis, headache, and flushing *above* the lesion. *Below* the lesion, an intense sympathetic response remains, since inhibition from higher brain centers is blocked. Blood vessels below the cord lesion, therefore, remain severely constricted, resulting in uncontrolled hypertension, and additional signs and symptoms, including pallor and coolness of the skin, pilomotor erection (i.e., goose bumps), and paralytic ileus.

Emergency Nursing Interventions. When an episode of autonomic dysreflexia is triggered, emergency treatment includes the following:
1. Place patient in an upright position to lower blood pressure.
2. Monitor blood pressure and heart rate.
3. Notify physician, if indicated (e.g., a severely elevated systolic blood pressure ≧240 mmHg and/or hypertension unresponsive to interventions).
4. Identify underlying cause and remove if possible.
5. Administer prescribed drug therapy (e.g., diazoxide, hydralazine) for persistent hypertension after removal of the triggering stimulus, or if the stimulus cannot be identified.
6. Stay with patient; provide reassurance, psychological and emotional support; recognize that anxiety and fright increase catecholamine secretion potentiating the mass sympathetic response.
7. Monitor patient's blood pressure every 4 hours for 24 hours after the crisis; should hypertension persist, an oral antihypertensive drug may be prescribed.

The best treatment of autonomic dysreflexia is *prevention*. The nurse plays a pivotal role in preventing the occurrence of this complication and in teaching patient and family about how to prevent it and what to do if it should occur. Specific nursing interventions are listed in Table 33–8.

TABLE 33–8
Autonomic Dysreflexia: Preventive Nursing Interventions

1. Identify patients at risk of developing autonomic dysreflexia, including patient with spinal cord lesions at T-4 to T-6 or above, and especially quadriplegics (C-6 to C-7 and above).
2. Avoid abnormal stimuli having the potential of triggering a mass sympathetic discharge.
   a. Avoid urinary retention and bladder distention.
      1) Monitor intake and output carefully.
      2) Avoid overhydration (increases risk of bladder distention/overdistention).
      3) Teach patient to avoid drinking a large amount of fluid at any one time.
      4) Maintain patency of indwelling catheter.
      5) Observe for bladder spasms.
   b. Avoid bowel retention or fecal impaction.
      1) Strict adherence to bowel regimen.
      2) Use dibucaine ointment (Nupercainal) for digital exam or removal of fecal impaction.
      3) Appropriate diet and fluid intake.
   c. Examine skin for pressure areas and imparied integrity.
      1) Special examination of sensitive perineal, perianal, and genital regions for pressure areas, excoriations, or rashes. Ascertain spontaneous body response to inadvertent sexual stimulation.
      2) Pressure areas of the skin require regular, consistent monitoring with appropriate position changes. Patients at risk of developing autonomic dysreflexia should not be placed in a flat, lying-down position because this might provide a triggering stimulus in the sensitive patient. Sitting positions lower blood pressure.
   d. Avoid drafts in rooms.
3. Recognize clinical manifestations.
   a. Specific signs and symptoms (*above* cord lesion)
      1) Sudden elevation in systolic blood pressure.
      2) Pounding headache, often associated with blurred vision.
      3) Profuse diaphoresis.
      4) Flushing above level of lesion.
      5) Nasal congesion.
      6) Nausea.
      7) Anxiety, fear.
      8) Bradycardia.
   b. Specific signs and symptoms (*below* cord lesion):
      1) Skin pallor, cold to touch.
      2) Chills, pilomotor erections (goose bumps).
      3) Intestinal relaxation (i.e., paralytic ileus).
4. Provide patient and family with education regarding autonomic dysreflexia: What it is, what triggers it, signs and symptoms, and treatment.
   a. Stress importance of reporting signs and symptoms.
   b. Assist patient/family to identify the triggering stimulus so that efforts can be made to avoid it.
   c. Recommend to patients prone to developing autonomic dysreflexia the importance of carrying identification cards that stipulate course of action for emergency care:
      1) Place in upright position.
      2) Monitor blood pressure, heart rate, pulse.
      3) Identify underlying cause and/or triggering stimulus.
      4) Remove triggering stimulus and/or correct underlying cause.
      5) Seek emergency medical assistance.
      6) Administer drug therapy for an episode of autonomic dysreflexia as prescribed.
      7) Stay with patient; offer reassurance; relieve anxiety.

Deep Venous Thrombosis— Pulmonary Embolism

The combination of vasomotor paralysis with pooling and stasis of blood, skeletal muscle paralysis, and immobilization, places the patient at risk of developing deep venous thrombosis and thromboembolic disease. Assessment and diagnosis of deep venous thrombosis in the patient with spinal cord injury are especially difficult because the patient is unaware of pain and tenderness, which might otherwise suggest the presence of deep venous thrombosis. Consequently, it is necessary to maintain a high degree of suspicion in this regard, and to regularly assess for signs of venous thrombosis. The skin color and temperature of lower extremities should be assessed. Bluish-red skin and an unusually warm temperature on palpation suggest a possible venous thrombosis. The circumference of thighs and calves should be measured at designated points daily, since a slowly increasing circumference suggests the possibility of underlying venous thrombosis.

The patient should be monitored for signs and symptoms of pulmonary embolism. The sudden onset of respiratory difficulties (e.g., tachypnea, dyspnea, cough with hemoptysis), alterations in cardiopulmonary function (e.g., tachycardia, hypotension, cyanosis), and neurologic findings (e.g., restlessness, lethargy, confusion), all suggest a pulmonary embolism.

Deep venous thrombosis prophylactic therapy includes measures to reduce the risk of venous stasis and to stimulate venous return to the heart. The risk of deep venous thrombosis is minimized by application of antiembolic stockings to lower extremities, passive range-of-motion exercises, including dorsiflexion of each foot, and maintenance of proper body alignment at all times. Other measures include avoiding situations and positions that compromise blood flow, such as placement of a pillow under the knees or use of a knee gatch, crossing of the legs, or prolonged sitting in one position. The patient who is breathing spontaneously should be encouraged to breathe deeply or to use the incentive spirometer hourly to expand the lungs and prevent atelectasis. Low-dose heparin may also be initiated prophylactically to prevent thromboembolic formation.

Body Temperature Instability

Disruption of sympathetic innervation following high cord injury also impairs regulation of body temperature. Vasodilation of peripheral blood vessels causes an increased heat loss. The disrupted homeothermia causes the patient's body temperature to fluctuate with that of room temperature.

Early management of the patient with spinal cord injury requires an ongoing assessment of the patient's temperature (every 2 to 4 hours), as well as that of the environment. Actions should be taken to minimize fluctuations of body and room temperature. Maintenance of a constant room temperature is probably the most effective way of controlling the patient's temperature, and drafts should be avoided. Use of extra blankets should be guided by the patient's temperature, and the use of excessive bedding should be avoided.

Gastrointestinal Function

The level of the spinal cord lesions largely determines the extent of gastrointestinal dysfunction. In cervical cord trauma, with the advent of neurogenic shock, the entire gastrointestinal tract becomes atonic, and paralytic ileus ensues. This usually occurs within the first 48 hours after trauma. There is loss of sensation, which complicates assessment of the patient. The patient does not experience pain, nor is there abdominal guarding in response to palpation, so that a tender area, if present, may go undetected. A high degree of suspicion is necessary to thoroughly assess the patient. Be especially alert for the presence of *referred* pain; auscultate the abdomen in all quadrants for bowel sounds; and initiate serial measurements of abdominal girth at the level of the umbilicus.

Associated with paralytic ileus is the danger of aspiration of vomitus due to acute gastric dilatation. Abdominal distention may limit diaphragmatic excursion and in this way predispose to respiratory complications (e.g., poor ventilatory effort with reduced vital capacity, and hypostatic pneumonia). Initial management involves insertion of a nasogastric tube to decompress the stomach and minimize abdominal distention. In a quadriplegia patient, unrecognized paralytic ileus coupled with a weak or ineffective coughing capability is the most common cause of sudden death within the first 48 hours after injury.

Stress-related gastric ulceration with the possibility for an acute gastrointestinal bleed, is always a potential complication for the patient with spinal cord injury, particularly during the first week after injury. Such pathology may be associated with endogenous release of corticosteroids and with an increased gastric secretion of hydrochloric acid resulting from unopposed vagal stimulation.

Serial assessments should be implemented for signs of gastrointestinal bleeding. Gastric contents should be tested for the presence of blood and to determine the pH; stools should be tested for occult blood with guaiac. Vital signs should be monitored for any drop in blood pressure or increase in heart rate. If indicated, daily hemoglobin and hematocrit levels should also be obtained. H_2 (histamine) antagonist therapy (e.g., ranitidine, nizatidine) is usually implemented prophylactically.

Bowel Management

Early management of bowel function is concerned with prevention of bowel distention and fecal impaction. The rectum should be checked daily for stool, which, if present, should be removed gently with a well-lubricated gloved finger. A lidocaine jelly should be used to minimize noxious stimuli. It is important to be alert for signs of constipation. Such signs may include a dull sound over the descending colon on percussion, and/or palpation of hard, rigid stool over different areas of bowel.

A major long-term goal of healthcare for the patient with spinal cord injury is to assist the patient to establish an effective bowel management program to ensure adequate elimination and maintain gastrointestinal function. During the acute phase of illness, bowel status is monitored and complications (e.g.,

constipation, diarrhea, intestinal obstruction) prevented. Information regarding the patient's pre-injury status is obtained, including diet tolerated, personal habits, and attitudes regarding bowel control. Such information can be helpful in establishing an effective bowel management program.

The level of spinal cord injury largely determines the extent of bowel control. Spinal injury above the conus medullaris (see Fig. 27–15), which contains the spinal defecation reflex center (S-2 to S-4) interrupts activity of the UMNs (Fig. 33–1). The result is loss of ability to voluntarily control the activity of the external anal sphincter. Ascending sensory information is also interrupted, resulting in the inability to feel fullness

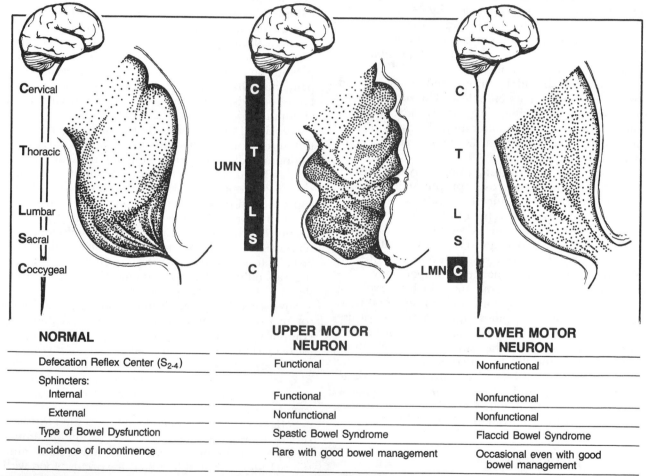

	NORMAL	UPPER MOTOR NEURON	LOWER MOTOR NEURON
Defecation Reflex Center (S₂-₄)		Functional	Nonfunctional
Sphincters: Internal		Functional	Nonfunctional
External		Nonfunctional	Nonfunctional
Type of Bowel Dysfunction		Spastic Bowel Syndrome	Flaccid Bowel Syndrome
Incidence of Incontinence		Rare with good bowel management	Occasional even with good bowel management

FIGURE 33–1. Innervation underlying bowel function and dysfunction, and potential for achievable bowel management. The level of spinal cord injury largely determines the extent of achievable bowel control. Interruption of UMN innervation results in the loss of voluntary control of the activity of the external anal spincter, which becomes completely dysfunctional, and an interruption of ascending sensory information resulting in the inability of the individual to feel fullness in the rectum or the urge to defecate. The spinal defecation reflex center (S-2 to S-4) remains functional and continues to exert a tone on the bowel and internal anal sphincter. This results in a *spastic* bowel syndrome, and bowel training is focused on using the intact defecation reflexes to evacuate the bowel on a regular basis (usually every other day). Prognosis for good bowel management with rare episodes of incontinence is excellent.

Interruption of LMN innervation to the bowel and internal anal sphincter results in an atonic, or *flaccid*, bowel syndrome. Prognosis for good bowel management in this instance is less favorable because in the presence of a nonfunctional spinal defecation relex center and internal anal sphincter, incontinence can occur at any time that a stool enters the rectum. Because innervation between the higher centers and external anal sphincter is also interrupted, the external anal sphincter is also nonfunctional. Even with good bowel management, incontinence can occur.

in the lower bowel and loss of the urge to defecate. In patients with spinal cord lesions above T-6, there is also an inability to contract abdominal muscles, a component of Valsalva's maneuver crucial to expelling stool. The significance of a UMN lesion is that the spinal defecation reflex center remains intact and continues to exert a tone on bowel and sphincters. The result is *spastic* bowel dysfunction. Bowel training in this instance is directed toward using the intact defecation reflexes to evacuate the bowel on a regular basis.

Injury to LMNs, whether directly to the defecation reflex center within the conus medullaris or to the sacral nerve roots in the cauda equina (see Table 33–5), results in *flaccid* bowel dysfunction (see Fig. 33–1). In this instance the reflex center and/or final nerve pathways are destroyed and no tonic activity exists. The presence of a flaccid sphincter means incontinence can occur at any time, without rectal or anal stimulation, provided stool is present in the rectum. In the case of a UMN lesion, defecation can be initiated at a convenient time so that bowel evacuation can be planned and incontinence prevented. Characteristics of these two neurogenic bowel dysfunction syndromes and implications for care are listed in Table 33–9.

TABLE 33–9
Neurogenic Bowel Dysfunction

	Spastic Bowel Dysfunction (Upper Motor Neuron; UMN)	Flaccid Bowel Dysfunction (Lower Motor Neuron; LMN)
Level of cord injury	Occurs above defecation reflex center (S-2 to S-4) located within the conus medullaris.	Involves defecation reflex center (S-2 to S-4) in the conus medullaris and/or sacral nerve roots in the equina.
Level of vertebral injury	Involves T-11 to T-12 vertebrae or above.	Involves T-12 vetebra or below.
Levels of innervation:		
1. Local	Intrinsic (myenteric plexus) intact; responsible for weak peristaltic activity, which is not of sufficient strength by itself to produce a large bowel movement.	Same as for UMN.
2. Spinal defecation reflex center S-2 to S-4	Defecation reflex intact; parasympathetic tone to descending and sigmoid colon, rectum, and internal anal sphincter intact.	Defecation reflex center in the conus medullaris and/or sacral nerve roots destroyed.
3. Brain/higher centers • Motor	• Nerve pathways between brain and spinal defecation reflex center (S-2 to S-4) interrupted: loss of inhibitory influences on spinal reflexes from higher centers.	• Loss of final common pathway for transmission of impulses between CNS and descending and sigmoid colon, rectum, and anal sphincters.
• Sensory	• Ascending sensory pathways interrupted: loss of sensation of fullness in bowel and urge to defecate.	• Same as for UMN.
Results of pathology	1. Loss of UMN innervation. 2. Intact spinal defecation reflexes. 3. Spastic bowel dysfunction with spastic contraction of bowel and anal sphincters.	1. Loss of LMN innervation. 2. Loss of spinal defecation reflexes. 3. Flaccid bowel dysfunction.
Prognosis for bowel control*	With intact defecation reflexes, bowel training is aimed at using these reflexes to evacuate the bowel. Bowel and anal sphincters respond to rectal/anal stimulation, enabling a planned bowel regimen, which empties the rectum and prevents incontinence. Prognosis is excellent for good bowel control.	With loss of spinal defecation reflex activity and LMN innervation, the bowel and anal sphincters are flaccid. They do not respond to planned rectal or anal stimulation. Arrival of feces in the rectum results in incontinence. Bowel training is deployed to evacuate stool from rectum. Presence of stool in rectum precipitates incontinence. Prognosis is favorable for bowel control providing a routine of regular bowel evacuation removes the stimulus for bowel emptying.
Bowel incontinence	Rarely occurs with good bowel management. Incontinence is due to spastic contraction. Diet is a significant factor in effective bowel management.	Occasionally occurs even with good bowel management, due to flaccid sphincters. As with spastic bowel dysfunction, diet is a significant factor in effective bowel management.
Bowel training program	Regularly scheduled evacuation, usually every other day.	Evacuation necessary on a daily basis to keep rectum clear of feces and prevent incontinence.
Use of medications including suppositories and laxatives	Responsive to a combination of laxatives (milk of magnesia), stool softener (dioctyl sodium sulfosuccinate [docusate, Colace]), and suppositories (Dulcolax).	Response to medications less effective than with spastic bowel dysfunction.
Digital stimulation	Used to initiate a planned reflex bowel evacuation.	Nonresponsive to digital stimulation; manual removal of stool from rectum may be required.

*Successful bowel training depends on many factors, such as level of injury, prior bowel habits, patient/family motivation, teamwork.

Renal/Urinary Function

Urinary Bladder Management

Micturition, or the act of emptying the bladder, becomes disrupted when injury to the spinal cord occurs. The significance of bladder emptying is reflected by the fact that renal dysfunction ranks high as a major cause of death in patients with spinal cord injuries. During the acute phase after spinal cord injury, the goals of care for the patient include maintaining adequate renal/urinary function; preventing complications of acute urinary retention that result in bladder overdistention and overflow incontinence; preventing infection due to stasis of urine, use of indwelling catheter, or urethral reflux of urine to upper urinary tracts and kidneys; and initiating assessment and data collection related to the patient's pre-injury status, for example, diet, personal habits, knowledge and attitude regarding urinary control, and prior coping capabilities.

The level of spinal cord injury largely determines the extent of urinary control. Spinal cord injury above the micturition reflex center (S-2 to S-4), located

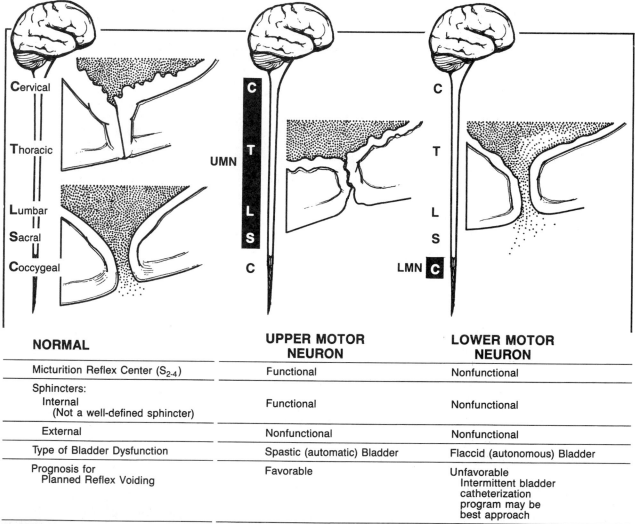

	NORMAL	UPPER MOTOR NEURON	LOWER MOTOR NEURON
Micturition Reflex Center (S$_{2-4}$)		Functional	Nonfunctional
Sphincters: Internal (Not a well-defined sphincter)		Functional	Nonfunctional
External		Nonfunctional	Nonfunctional
Type of Bladder Dysfunction		Spastic (automatic) Bladder	Flaccid (autonomous) Bladder
Prognosis for Planned Reflex Voiding		Favorable	Unfavorable Intermittent bladder catheterization program may be best approach

FIGURE 33–2. Innervation underlying bladder function and dysfunction, and potential for achievable bladder management. The level of spinal cord injury largely determines the extent of achievable urinary bladder control. Interruption of UMN innervation results in loss of voluntary, coordinated control of the external sphincter, which becomes completely nonfunctional, and an interruption of ascending sensory information resulting in the inability of the individual to feel bladder fullness or the urge to urinate. The micturition reflex center (S-2 to S-4) remains functional and continues to exert a tone on the bladder and internal sphincter, thereby resulting in a *spastic* bladder syndrome. In this instance, bladder training is focused on using the intact micturition reflexes to establish some regularity to bladder emptying, resulting in a favorable prognosis for planned reflex voiding.

Injury sustained to LMN innervation causes complete interruption of LMN innervation to the bladder and internal sphincter, resulting in an atonic or *flaccid* bladder. The bladder should be assessed on a regular basis to determine bladder overdistention. Prognosis for planned reflex voiding in this instance is unfavorable. Intermittent bladder catheterization may be the best approach.

TABLE 33–10
Neurogenic Urinary Dysfunction

	Spastic (Automatic) Urinary Dysfunction (Upper Motor Neuron; UMN)	Flaccid (Autonomous) Urinary Dysfunction (Lower Motor Neuron; LMN)
Level of cord injury	Occurs above micturition reflex center (S-2 to S-4) located within the conus medullaris.	Involves micturition reflex center (S-2 to S-4) in the conus medullaris and/or sacral nerve roots in the cauda equina.
Level of innervation: 1. Local	Stretch receptors in bladder wall and afferent neuron intact.	Same as for UMN.
2. Spinal micturition reflex (S-2 to S-4)	Micturition reflex intact. Parasympathetic innervation to detrusor muscle and bladder neck sphincter (internal) intact.	Micturition reflex center in conus medullaris and/or sacral nerve roots destroyed.
3. Sympathetic innervation cord segments T-11 to T-12	Reflexes may be intact depending on level of cord injury.	Same as for UMN.
4. Brain/higher centers • Motor	• Nerve pathways between brain and spinal micturition reflex center (S-2 to S-4) interrupted; loss of inhibiting influences on spinal reflexes from higher centers.	• Loss of final common pathway for transmission of impulses between CNS and detrusor muscle and bladder sphincters (internal and external).
• Sensory	• Ascending sensory pathways interrupted; loss of sensation of bladder distention and urge to urinate.	• Same as for UMN.
Results of pathology	1. Loss of UMN innervation. 2. Intact micturition reflexes. 3. Spastic bladder dysfunction.	1. Loss of LMN innervation. 2. Loss of micturition reflexes. 3. Flaccid bladder dysfunction.
Prognosis for bladder control*	Bladder training is aimed at using micturition reflexes and "trigger" stimulus to establish planned reflex voiding.	Unable to establish reflex voiding; intermittent bladder catheterization may be best method for bladder management.

*Bladder training depends on many factors, such as level of injury, prior bladder habits, patient/family motivation, and teamwork.

within the conus medullaris, interrupts ascending sensory pathways and UMNs (Fig. 33–2). Interruption of UMNs causes a loss of voluntary, coordinated control over the micturition reflex center in the cord. The reflex center itself remains intact so that a *spastic* automatic bladder results. This can be identified after spinal shock resolves. Patients with a spastic bladder are unable to sense bladder fullness or the urge to void due to interruption of ascending sensory pathways. As the bladder fills with urine, the micturition reflex is triggered, resulting in incontinence. The patient needs to be assessed frequently for bladder distention, which can occur if there is spasm of the bladder sphincter.

Injury to the LMNs (see Fig. 32–2), either directly to the micturition reflex center in the conus medullaris or to sacral nerve roots in the cauda equina, causes a *flaccid* autonomous bladder. In this instance, the reflex center and/or final pathways are destroyed and no tonic activity exists. As is the case with UMN paralysis, the patient is unaware of bladder distention and the need to void, due to interruption of ascending pathways. A primary concern is bladder overdistention. Characteristics of spastic urinary and flaccid urinary dysfunction are listed in Table 33–10.

Nutritional Status

Stress increases energy needs by as much as 50%. Glycogen stores within the body provide an immediate source of energy, but these stores are quickly used up (within 24 hours or less). Once carbohydrate stores are depleted, the body draws on its stores of fats and proteins to provide a source of energy. The catabolism of protein prevents its use for tissue building and repairs. There is an increased loss of nitrogen in the urine, and a negative nitrogen balance ensues. A nitrogen imbalance predisposes the patient with spinal cord injury to massive tissue wasting, severe weight loss, fluid and electrolyte imbalances, infections, and disruption of other body systems.

In the patient with spinal cord injury it is essential to maintain nutritional balance to promote wound healing and prevent complications. Early in the acute phase after spinal cord injury, the presence of paralytic ileus precludes oral nutrition. A nasogastric tube is usually placed for gastric decompression to reduce the risk of aspiration and to prevent gastric dilatation, which could compromise respiratory excursion. Intravenous fluid therapy alone is inadequate to meet the nutritional requirements of the patient with spinal cord injury and a state of malnutrition can develop within 3 to 5 days. Thus, total parenteral nutrition (TPN) has become an essential therapeutic modality in treating the patients with spinal cord injury.

TPN provides a source of essential amino acids, glucose, and additives, including electrolytes, vitamins, and minerals, and is administered via a central line. Administration of TPN requires careful, sophisticated patient care in initiating, maintaining, and monitoring the system. Prevention of sepsis requires very strict aseptic technique, and the patient must be evaluated daily to determine the response to therapy.

Skin Integrity

Loss of mobility and sensation, impaired circulation, and inadequate nutrition predispose patients with spinal cord injury to skin breakdown. The primary factor involved in the disruption of skin integrity is *pressure*. Continuous pressure occurs at specific sites when there is a lack of continuous movement and redistribution of body weight. It is most concentrated between bone and skin surfaces that support body weight. When unrelieved, pressure causes a "sustained ischemia," which disrupts cellular metabolism and leads to varying degrees of tissue injury and necrosis.

There is a definite relationship between the amount and duration of pressure and the development of a pressure ulcer. Weight-bearing bony prominences must be identified when the patient is placed in different positions. With each position change, the skin must be scrutinized carefully for any disruption of its integrity and for the presence of dependent edema, which contributes to the risk of skin breakdown. Reddened areas that do not blanch or fade within 20 to 30 minutes after a position change suggest that other positions need to be assumed, and the duration of time spent in a given position should be decreased. Pressure that is unrelieved at least every 2 hours places the patient at risk for pressure ulcer development. Use of specialty beds such as those providing kinetic therapy has significantly reduced the incidence of pressure ulcer development in patients with spinal cord injury.

Physical, Psychological, and Social Rehabilitation: Ultimate Goal

Rehabilitation is a dynamic process in which disabled persons are assisted in realizing their optimum physical, emotional, psychological, social, and vocational potential, so that they can maintain their dignity and achieve a sense of self-fulfillment. The ultimate goal of rehabilitation for individuals with spinal cord injury is to help them to achieve the highest level of personal independence possible within the restrictions and limitations imposed by their injuries. The concept of rehabilitation begins at the moment of injury, continues throughout the critical phase, and remains as a progressive ongoing, dynamic, and lifelong process for the individual.

In a collaborative effort with other members of the interdisciplinary health team, the nurse functions to prevent physical and psychological deterioration, to minimize suffering, and to engage the patient and family as integral, active participants of the health team. Such teamwork begins the moment the patient and family enter the healthcare system and enables all aspects of patient care to be approached collectively and simultaneously.

Rehabilitation must *not* be viewed as something that begins *after* the acute phase, but rather, the critical care nurse and colleagues in healthcare must learn to "think rehab" on initial patient contact and incorporate this concept into their daily practice.

NURSING MANAGEMENT: SUMMARY

Nursing care is crucial for the patient with spinal cord injury throughout the rehabilitative process. In assuming responsibility for the patient during the acute phase, nurses must be especially cognizant that events occurring early in the process of healthcare of the patient and family, be they physiologic, psychological, and/or sociological, may have considerable impact over the long term.

Therapeutic Goals

1. Stabilization of cardiopulmonary function
2. Prevention of further neurologic injury to the spinal cord
3. Determination of extent of neurologic injury
4. Establishment of baseline assessment data
5. Reduction in spinal cord edema
6. Maintenance of renal function and fluid/electrolyte balance
7. Prevention of complications related to gastrointestinal balance
8. Maintenance of anabolic nutritional state
9. Maintenance of intact skin integrity
10. Initiation and establishment of a meaningful and trusting rapport with patient and family or significant others
11. Initiation of rehabilitative process: physical, psychological, and social.

Nursing Diagnoses, Desired Patient Outcomes, and Nursing Interventions

For specific nursing diagnoses, desired patient outcomes, and nursing interventions related to the clinical management of the patient with spinal cord injury, refer to the care plan at the end of this chapter. Refer also to the following case study and sample care plan for the patient with acute spinal cord injury.

CASE STUDY WITH SAMPLE CARE PLAN: PATIENT WITH ACUTE SPINAL CORD INJURY

RT, a well-nourished, muscular, 21-year-old white man, sustained cervical spinal injury when thrown from his motorcycle, while on his way to morning classes at the university, at approximately 8:45 AM. He was admitted to the emergency room of University Hospital at 9:45 AM, where a diagnosis of transection of the spinal cord at cervical C-6 vertebral level was made. Following stabilization of his condition, Mr. T

RESEARCH APPLICATION: POWERLESSNESS IN CERVICAL SPINAL CORD INJURY PATIENTS
Mahon-Darby, J, Ketchik-Renshaw, B, Richmond, TS and Gates, EM. Dimensions of Critical Care Nursing 7(6), 346–355, 1988.

Purpose: Individuals suddenly overcome by acute spinal cord injury (SCI) are thrust into a state of unanticipated dependency and powerlessness. This paper identifies management goals in the critical care phase of injury and specifies nursing actions to assist in the reassumption of self-directed behavior and power.

Discussion: A case study of a patient with an acute SCI is presented. The authors relate five behavioral stages exhibited by individuals experiencing traumatic cervical SCI: numb, panic, egocentric, interactive, and directive. Nursing care initiatives are described as they relate to each of these five behavioral phases.

Stage 1. The "numb" stage is described as feeling powerless after the initial injury. "Numbness" is compounded by indirect communication between caregivers with the SCI victim. Nursing interventions during this stage should be directed toward building a rapport and trust with the patient. This includes demonstrated competency in care provision and an interest in the patient's individual reponse to the SCI.

Stage 2. The "panic" stage is described as a stage associated with overt fear and anxiety related to loss of sensory and motor function. During this stage, the patient needs to be aggressively assessed for pathophysiologic contributors such as shock or hypoxemia that may confound the clinical presentation. Stability in the patient's environment is essential; attempts to change care patterns (i.e., weaning from mechanical ventilation) should be avoided. The identification of specific triggers for the panic episode should be attempted. Methods for ensuring effective communication should be established.

Stage 3. The "egocentric" stage is associated with anger and depression related to the SCI. During this phase the patient may try to regain power through refusal to participate in activities. Caregivers should begin negotiation with the patient regarding care activities. Patients should be directed to enlarge their focus to include the outside world. This can be accomplished through involvement in family decision making and use of diversional activities such as television and radio.

Stage 4. In the "interactive" stage, the patient begins to pay attention to the way care is performed, questioning inconsistency in care and testing the environment. Consistency of assignment and fostering independent decision making is essential.

Stage 5. The "directive" stage is present when the patient exhibits social and verbal interaction with others, directing the manner in which care is provided. The patient becomes more knowledgeable about care needs and methods of care delivery. Successfully directing others without promoting anger is the hallmark of successful completion of this phase.

Practice Implications: Powerlessness is common in patients following acute cervical SCI. Recognition of the stages that commonly occur in this patient is essential to providing holistic care. Modifying the plan of care and communication style by team members plays an important role in facilitating successful completion of the five stages.

Reviewed by Anne W. Wojner, MSN, RN, CCRN.

---

was taken to the operating room for insertion of Crutchfield tongs.

7/16, 3:00 PM—Upon arrival in the intensive care unit, initial assessment reveals the patient on a Stryker frame with Crutchfield tongs maintained with 15 lb of cervical traction; the patient is aligned appropriately. Mr. T is lethargic, but arousable; oriented to person and place, but not time; pupils equal in size, round, and reactive to light and accommodation (PERRLA). The extremities are flaccid with no sensation or movement.

Vital signs on admission to the unit: blood pressure 90/60, heart rate 56, regular sinus rhythm, temperature 97.6°F (R). Skin pale, cool, and dry; patient complains of chilling. Intravenous fluid administration of 0.9% normal saline infusing at 100 mL/h. Respiration: patient on room air, breathing shallow at rate of 24/min. Arterial blood gases drawn: PaO_2 80 mmHg, $PaCO_2$ 44 mmHg, pH 7.35. Breath sounds diminished. Gastrointestinal: abdomen soft, nondistended, without bowel sounds. The patient is currently receiving nothing by mouth (NPO). Nasogastric tube to suction. Renal/urinary: straight catheterization in recovery room at 2:30 P.M. with 400 mL urine obtained. Urine specimen sent for culture/sensitivity. There is no evidence of bladder distention.

Mother at her son's bedside; Mr. T's surgeon spoke briefly with the patient and family, briefing them on the patient's current status and expectations.

Initial Nursing Diagnoses

See sample care plan. Refer also to the care plan at the end of this chapter.

SAMPLE CARE PLAN FOR THE PATIENT WITH ACUTE SPINAL CORD INJURY

Nursing Diagnoses

Nursing Diagnosis #1

Breathing Pattern, ineffective: alveolar hypoventilation, related to altered ventilatory mechanics: hypoventilation associated with paralysis of intercostal and abdominal muscles

Desired Patient Outcomes

Patient will:
1. Demonstrate effective minute ventilation with trend of improving:
   - Tidal volume >7–10 mL/kg
   - Respiratory rate <25/min
2. Achieve a vital capacity of >15–25 mL/kg
3. Verbalize ease of breathing

Nursing Interventions

- Perform a comprehensive respiratory assessment:
  ○ Airway patency; rate, rhythm, depth of breathing; chest and diaphragmatic excursion; use of accessory muscles; breath sounds and presence of adventitious sounds.
- Assess neurologic status: mental status, level of consciousness, status of protective reflexes (cough, gag, swallowing).
- Monitor serial pulmonary function tests: tidal volume, vital capacity.

Rationales

- Major goal of airway management is to establish/maintain adequate alveolar ventilation. Increased rapid, shallow respirations may signal deterioration of respiratory function.
- Hypoxia may be reflected by changes in mental status or behavior (restlessness, irritability).

- Serial monitoring enables trends to be identified in pulmonary function.

Nursing Diagnoses

Nursing Diagnosis #2

Airway clearance, ineffective, related to:
1. Ineffective cough associated with paralysis of intercostal and abdominal muscles
2. Immobility

Desired Patient Outcomes

Patient will:
1. Demonstrate a secretion-clearing cough
2. Maintain arterial blood gas values:
   - PaO_2 >80 mmHg
   - $PaCO_2$ ~ 35–45 mmHg
   - pH 7.35–7.45

Nursing Interventions

- Assess ability to cough and handle secretions.

- Monitor quality, quantity, color, and consistency of sputum; obtain specimen for culture/sensitivity.
- Implement measures to ensure adequate respiratory function:
  ○ Establish and maintain patent airway.
  ○ Monitor serial arterial blood gases; establish baseline function.
  ○ Initiate oxygen therapy to maintain arterial blood gases within acceptable range.
  ○

Rationales

- Loss of intercostal and abdominal muscles compromises the patient's ability to cough effectively.
  ○ Loss of protective reflexes places patient at increased risk of developing aspiration pneumonia.
- Airway obstruction frequently occurs with spinal cord injury or injuries involving head and neck.
  ○ Hypoxemia in the patient with spinal cord injury is most commonly associated with retained secretions.

Nursing Interventions

- ○ Initiate measures to handle secretions; provide humidified oxygen; maintain hydration; nasotracheal suctioning only when necessary.

  ○ Initiate chest physiotherapy when overall condition is stabilized: postural drainage; percussion and vibration; deep breathing and coughing exercises.
  ○ Instruct in use of incentive spirometry.

  ○ Use a calm, reassuring approach: anticipate needs, offer explanations, be accessible to patient/family.

Rationales

- ○ Suctioning increases risk of infection; suctioning-associated vagal stimulation may precipitate further bradycardia in the patient who may already suffer from bradycardia with spinal cord injury.
  ○ Loosens and dislodges secretions and enhances movement of secretions toward trachea, where they may be removed by coughing and/or suctioning.
  ○ Use of incentive spirometry encourages deep breathing, reducing risk of atelectasis.
  ○ Anxiety is a major problem in the patient with spinal cord injury.

Nursing Diagnoses

Nursing Diagnosis #3

Cardiac output, decreased, related to loss of systemic vasomotor tone (neurogenic shock)

Desired Patient Outcomes

Patient's vital signs will stabilize:
- BP >90 mmHg systolic (or within 10 mmHg of baseline)
- Heart rate ~60 beats per minute
- Body temperature 98.6°F

SAMPLE CARE PLAN FOR THE PATIENT WITH ACUTE SPINAL CORD INJURY (*Continued*)

Nursing Interventions

- Assess cardiovascular function and presence of neurogenic (spinal) shock:
  - Blood pressure, pulse, body temperature; skin temperature
  - Cardiac monitoring for arrhythmias
  - Hydration status

- Implement measures to stabilize cardiopulmonary function:
  - Initiate prescribed intravenous therapy ~75–100 mL/h
  - Monitor intake and output.
  - Initiate measures to minimize orthostatic hypotension: apply antiembolic stockings; abdominal binder.
  - Elevate lower extremities at regular intervals.

Rationales

- Spinal cord injury (T-4 to T-6 and above) precipitates spinal shock with loss of sympathetic autonomic reflexes: loss of sympathetic tone leads to hypotension; unopposed parasympathetic tone predisposes to bradycardia; interruption of sympathetic innervation underlies hypothermia with impaired temperature regulation.

  - Orthostatic hypotension results from venous stasis associated with impaired vasomotor tone and skeletal muscle paralysis.

Nursing Diagnoses

Nursing Diagnosis #4
Urinary elimination, altered, related to:
1. Loss of voluntary control of micturition
2. Compromised micturition reflex

Desired Patient Outcomes

Patient will maintain:
- Urine output >30 mL/h
- Weight within 5% of baseline
- Balanced intake and output
- Stable serum electrolytes, BUN, and creatinine
- Infection-free urinary tract

Nursing Interventions

- Monitor renal and hydration status:
  - Specific parameters to assess include body weight (daily), intake/output, serum electrolytes, BUN, and creatinine, hematology profile (Hct, Hb).

  - Implement straight catheterization protocol using aseptic technique and noting amount, color, clarity, and specific gravity of urine.
  - Assess for bladder distention at regular intervals and straight catheterize PRN.

Rationales

- Urinary retention predisposes to complications, such as urinary tract infection and autonomic dysreflexia (postacute phase).
- Accurate intake/output and daily weight assist in determining adequacy of renal/urinary function, and fluid balance.
- Adequate hydration functions to prevent urinary infection and urinary calculi.
  - Adequate renal perfusion maintains filtration and renal function; hemoconcentration may predispose to electrolyte imbalance; increased blood viscosity may cause thromboembolic complications.

Nursing Diagnoses

Nursing Diagnosis #5
Skin integrity, impaired, related to:
1. Immobility
2. Sensory loss

Desired Patient Outcomes

Patient will maintain:
- Intact skin with good turgor
- Body weight within 5% of baseline

Nursing Interventions

- Maintain skin integrity.
  - Assess skin carefully q2h for signs of compromised circulation especially at pressure points.

- Initiate therapeutic regimen:
  - Turn/position q2h; document rotation of positions.
  - Maintain proper body alignment.

  - Passive range-of-motion (ROM) exercises.

  - Monitor and evaluate response to therapy.
- Consult with nutritionist to initiate necessary nutritional regimen.

Rationales

- Pressure ulcer develops when there is lack of movement and distribution of weight; pressure is most concentrated between bone and skin surfaces that support body weight.
- Implementation of therapeutic regimen maximizes tissue perfusion, prevents venostasis and tissue ischemia.
  - Maintenance of proper body alignment prevents further neurologic damage.
  - Passive ROM exercises help to maintain muscle tone and to improve circulation.

- Breakdown of body proteins (gluconeogenesis) impairs tissue healing and places the patient at increased risk of pressure ulcer development and infection.

GUILLAIN-BARRÉ SYNDROME

Guillain-Barré syndrome (GBS) is a rapidly developing, progressive, and self-limiting condition distinguished by an inflammatory process involving the peripheral nervous system (PNS). It is characterized by demyelination and degeneration of the myelin sheath of peripheral nerves, including cranial and spinal nerves. The pathology of GBS is usually reversible, with good potential for complete recovery over a period of weeks to months in most cases. Mortality, when it does occur, is usually associated with respiratory complications, and it is for this reason, that patients with GBS require critical care.

Etiology

The underlying cause of GBS is thought to be an autoimmune process, wherein the body makes antibodies directed against the myelin sheaths of peripheral nerves. The illness is usually preceded by an infection (probably viral), usually of the upper respiratory tract and occurring 1 to 3 weeks prior to the onset of neurologic symptoms.

Pathophysiology

Many neurons throughout the nervous system have axons that are *myelinated*, that is, they have a lipid-protein substance, myelin, which is deposited along the axons to form a myelin sheath (see Fig. 27–1). The myelin sheath insulates peripheral nerves to facilitate rapid conduction of nerve impulses; it is interrupted at regular intervals called nodes of Ranvier.

In GBS, the autoimmune response directed against the myelin sheaths causes a segmental demyelination process that destroys the myelin and initiates an inflammatory response. This demyelination process affects both motor and sensory neurons, with sensory neurons affected to a lesser degree. Loss of myelin abolishes the *rapid* transmission of nerve impulses. This results in a slowing of conduction and/or conduction blockage, which underlies the muscle weakness and paralysis characteristic of GBS.

Demyelination classically begins in distal nerves and ascends in a symmetric manner, causing an ascending muscle weakness and/or paralysis and accompanying sensory deficits. The process may arrest at any point along the way or progress upward to involve the cranial nerves. Remyelination occurs gradually in a descending manner, with restoration of function to proximal areas first. Distal recovery follows.

Complete recovery occurs in the majority of cases. Residual neurologic deficits, if present, usually involve muscle weakness and/or an absence of tendon reflexes.

Clinical Presentation

The clinical presentation of Guillain-Barré syndrome is variable, with the extent of neurologic impairment depending on the intensity of the underlying pathophysiologic processes. Early on, the most prominent feature is muscle weakness occurring bilaterally, usually in the lower extremities. Walking becomes difficult. The weakness ascends to involve the trunk, upper extremities, and cranial nerve distribution. Muscle weakness may evolve into a full-blown flaccid paralysis within 48 to 72 hours, or it may develop more slowly over several days to weeks. Deep tendon reflexes may be diminished or absent.

Paresthesias may accompany the motor dysfunction. Sensory disturbances include numbness, tingling, prickling, or burning sensations, and occur over the extremities in a characteristic "glove and stocking" distribution. There may be complaints of headache, stiff neck, or photophobia. Pain is one of the most significant complaints made by the patient with GBS. It is usually described as a "deep aching and burning" muscle pain.

Potential life-threatening complications can occur when motor paralysis ascends to involve the muscles of respiration. The function of abdominal and intercostal muscles may become compromised with involvement of the thoracic nerve roots. The patient's respiratory effort may become impaired, and respiratory insufficiency may occur. As the paralysis ascends to include the cervical nerve roots and lower brainstem, all innervation to the diaphragm via the phrenic nerve ceases, and respiratory arrest ensues.

Despite the severity of the illness and the extent of paralysis, consciousness is preserved. Consequently, the patient experiences all the pain, fear, and physical devastation that is associated with this syndrome, yet may be able to communicate only by movement of the eyes.

Autonomic dysfunction may also become apparent. Disruption of cardiovascular function may be reflected by wide fluctuations in blood pressure and cardiac arrhythmias. The danger of asystole in some instances may require insertion of a temporary pacemaker. Other signs and symptoms include facial flushing, diaphoresis, and urinary retention. Complications may include hypostatic and/or aspiration pneumonia, paralytic ileus, thromboembolic disease, nosocomial infections, and impairment of skin integrity. Death can occur from respiratory or cardiac failure.

The clinical course of GBS is variable. Paralysis commonly peaks about 3 weeks after onset, followed by a short plateau period in which there is neither improvement nor deterioration in function. This is followed by the recovery phase, which may take months when nerve regeneration is required. There is no cure for this illness. It must simply run its course.

Clinical Management of the Patient with Guillain-Barré Syndrome

Major goals for treatment of the patient with GBS include supportive care and prevention of complications. During the critical phase, the major concern is maintenance of adequate respiratory function. If progressive respiratory failure becomes evident, early intubation and mechanical ventilation become necessary.

The use of corticosteroids to decrease the inflammatory process is controversial. Definitive evidence as to the efficacy of steroids in the treatment of GBS has not been demonstrated. If, however, the patient with GBS does not demonstrate significant improvement after an extended period of supportive care, use of steroids may be considered.

Plasmapheresis, or plasma exchange, has been instituted in certain instances, particularly in patients with extensive paralysis and respiratory dysfunction requiring long-term mechanical ventilation. The efficacy of this therapeutic modality in the treatment of GBS remains questionable.

Thromboembolic complications in the patient with GBS are a major concern, and use of prophylactic anticoagulation may be prescribed. Pain control may require the use of narcotics or other analgesics. Nutritional support is a major aspect of treatment in the patient who is immobilized. It is not unusual for the patient with GBS to lose upward of one half of total body weight during the course of prolonged paralysis. Supplemental feedings may be indicated to maintain sufficient caloric intake for energy, a positive nitrogen balance, and fluid and electrolyte balance. Nasogastric tube feedings may be instituted for the patient experiencing dysphagia. In the presence of paralytic ileus, TPN is the therapy of choice.

Nursing Management

During the acute phase of the illness, nursing care is directed toward maintaining life-support systems, preventing complications, providing comfort measures, and initiating a system of communication with patient and family, keeping them informed as to what they can expect over the course of the illness and assisting them to keep the goal of eventual recovery in proper perspective. The goals of nursing care are similar to those for the patient with a high cervical cord injury (see above). Major exceptions are the fact that the patient with GBS often retains sensory function and thus experiences all the discomforts of necessary life support systems and immobility. In addition, loss of motor function may make it impossible for the patient to communicate except by moving the eyes.

Implementation of nursing process in the clinical management of the patient with GBS involves the following nursing interventions:
1. Maintain adequate cardiopulmonary function.
2. Assess and monitor levels of neurologic function.
3. Establish an efficient means of communication.
4. Maintain fluid and electrolyte balance.
5. Maintain an anabolic nutritional state.
6. Maintain the integrity of the gastrointestinal system.

7. Prevent complications of immobility:
   a. Thromboembolic disorder
   b. Impairment of musculoskeletal function
   c. Impairment of skin integrity
8. Maintain the integrity of psychological and emotional processes:
   a. Establish a meaningful and trusting rapport with patient and family.
   b. Keep patient and family informed as to expectations and impact of clinical course of GBS.

Refer to the care plan presented at the end of the chapter for pertinent nursing diagnoses, desired patient outcomes, and nursing interventions in the care of the patient with GBS during the acute phase of the illness. Refer also to the following case study with sample care plan: patient with Guillain-Barré syndrome.

CASE STUDY WITH SAMPLE CARE PLAN: PATIENT WITH GUILLAIN-BARRÉ SYNDROME*

Mr. LL, a well-nourished, 21-year-old white man, arrived at the emergency room of University Hospital. His chief complaint was progressive weakness of all extremities (lower extremities weaker than upper) and difficulty speaking and swallowing. Further history revealed that the patient had had "the flu" approximately 4 weeks prior to this admission with symptoms of malaise, frontal headache, and a cough productive of greenish sputum. He visited his private physician 1 week ago, who treated him with amoxicillin without improvement. When he began to feel tingling in his fingers and toes, accompanied by progressive weakness, he decided to be examined in the hospital emergency room.

On physical examination, Mr. L was seen to be awake, alert, and oriented, with intact but depressed cranial nerve function. Motor strength in the lower extremity was rated 3/5; the upper extremity was rated 4/5. Sensation to light touch was intact. Deep tendon reflexes (DTR) were 1+ in lower extremities, 2+ in upper. Lumbar puncture revealed normal pressure, with a protein of 55 mg/100 mL (mildly elevated). While in the emergency room, the patient complained of becoming short of breath and was having difficulty speaking because of this. Mr. L was admitted to the medical ICU with a probable diagnosis of Guillain-Barré syndrome.

On the first day of admission Mr. L's condition deteriorated rapidly. He experienced increasing shortness of breath and fatigue. Arterial blood gases revealed a progressive hypercapnia and hypoxemia, and his vital capacity was 600 mL. The patient was intubated and mechanical ventilation initiated with an FIO_2 of 30%, on assist/control rate of 12/min, and a tidal volume

---

*This case study was prepared by Kathleen Daley White and Margaret Connelly.

of 700 mL. Motor strength in the lower extremities was 2/5; in the upper 3/5; there was increased numbness in the lower extremities to the waistline, and decreased sensation below T-12 level; deep tendon reflexes were absent in the lower extremities, and 1+ in the upper. A repeat lumber tap revealed a protein level of 152 mg/mL, and a cytomegalovirus titer of 1:64.

An examination of the cranial nerves on the second day after admission revealed cranial nerves III, IV, and VI grossly intact with the patient able to look up and down and to shut his eyes tightly (cranial nerve VII). He experienced decreased sensation over the maxillary and mandibular distribution of cranial nerve V, bilaterally; there was decreased facial tone symmetrically, and the patient was unable to show his teeth. Cranial nerve VIII was intact; IX and X were not examined (patient was intubated); motor function of muscles innervated by cranial nerve XI was 5/5; examination of XII revealed weakened motor activity of tongue. Nerve conduction studies done at this time revealed severe demyelinating neuropathy. A Keofeed tube was placed, and central feedings were started at this time.

On the third day of hospitalization, Mr. L was able to move his hands and arms slightly and to shrug his shoulders. There was slight movement of the toes; the legs were flaccid bilaterally. The patient was able to move his head from side to side. Mr. L was placed on a kinetic bed. He also complained of abdominal cramping, and his tube feedings were slowed.

On the 4th day of hospitalization, laboratory data revealed a serum albumin of 2.9, which was felt to be due to the interrupted Keofeed feedings because of abdominal cramping. ABGs were as follows: pH 7.39, $PaCO_2$ 42, PaO_2 64, and percent hemoglobin saturation 93%. An increase in the FIO_2 from 30% to 40% produced ABGs as follows: pH 7.41, $PaCO_2$ 42, PaO_2 106. The patient was incontinent of urine, and a Foley catheter was inserted. Physical therapy/occupational therapy program was initiated.

The patient's mother and father were with the patient almost 24 hours a day, and both the patient and family were becoming increasingly anxious and frightened. Referral was made to the psychiatric clinical nurse specialist, who became involved with the patient and family at this time.

The patient's motor function continued to deteriorate over the next several days. The vital capacity was 200 mL; the negative inspiratory force (NIF) generated was a −8. Enteral feedings were increased to 1800 calories/day, but remained far short of the 2900 calories/day required because of persistent abdominal cramping.

On the eighth hospital day the patient was found to have a vital capacity of 140 mL, and a tracheostomy was placed. Serum albumin stabilized at 3.7. The patient was very depressed, tearful, and constantly ringing the bell, afraid to be alone. An effort was made to expand the family support system by arranging for

visits by the hospital chaplain and volunteers; a schedule of visitors was set up to enable someone to be with the patient for the better part of the 24-hour day. A former patient with Guillain-Barré was invited to speak with the patient and family, an interaction that seemed to brighten and reassure both patient and family.

On the 10th day through the 18th day after admission, the patient experienced his most compromised level of function. His vital capacity was 60 mL; he was unable to close his eyes completely and developed diplopia. An eye patch was placed over one eye to decrease the diplopia during wakeful periods. Pupils were equal in size and reacted to light and accommodation (PERRLA); there was a reduced shoulder shrug, and motor function in all extremities was 0/5. Mr. L had some runs of supraventricular tachycardia (SVT), which was treated with verapamil 5 mg; blood pressure became labile with a scale of 120/80 to 210/90. Cytomegalovirus titer was 1:256, suggesting an acute CMV episode.

On the 20th hospital day there appeared to be some improvement in motor function; the patient was able to close his eyes completely; and motor function in the upper extremities ranged from 1 to 2+. Vital capacity improved to 100 mL and then to 270 mL; negatively generated inspiratory force increased to a −3 to −6 mmHg. The FIO_2 was decreased to 30% with ABGs: pH 7.4, $PaCO_2$ 42, and PaO_2 104 mmHg. The patient could move his right bicep and left little finger; there was increased facial and shoulder movement, and return of motor function continued to progress bilaterally.

Over the course of the next week the patient was able to wrinkle his forehead, squeeze his eyes shut, and smile. His dysphagia resolved, and he began to swallow clear fluids. He was now moving both hands and his right leg. Vital capacity improved to 350 mL, and the inspiratory force was measured at −8 mmHg.

By the 30th hospital day the vital capacity increased to 460 mL and the negative inspiratory force to −30 mmHg. A T piece was placed, and the FIO_2 was reduced to 21%. On the 34th day after admission, the vital capacity was 800 mL, inspiratory force was −30 mmHg. An active program of weaning continued until the tracheostomy could be plugged and the patient was able to mobilize and cough up pulmonary secretions.

The continued recovery of the patient enabled the tracheostomy to be removed, and he was transferred to a medical unit, awake, alert, and oriented, and worried about the possibility of a tracheostomy scar. Cranial nerves were intact; motor strength was 2/5 in lower extremities, 3/5 to 4/5 in the upper extremities; gross incoordination persisted, and the patient was unable to perform fine motor skills.

During the sixth week of hospitalization, the patient was able to move both lower extremities side to side horizontally and to wiggle his toes. He was still unable to move legs against gravity. Patient and family were both pleased and heartened by the patient's continued progress.

Mr. L was transferred to a progressive rehabilitation center during the seventh hospital week. After 4 months of intensive rehabilitation, the patient was able to function independently. He was discharged home with daily rehabilitation follow-up.

Initial Nursing Diagnoses

See the following sample care plan. Refer also to the care plan at the end of this chapter.

SUGGESTED READINGS

Coen, SD: Spinal cord injury: Preventing secondary injury. AACN Clinical Issues in Critical Care Nursing 3(1):44, 1992.

Hughes, MC: Critical care nursing for the patient with a spinal cord injury. Crit Care Nurs Clin North Am 2(1):33, 1990.

Mascarella, J and Hudson, D: Dysimmune neurologic disorders. AACN Clinical Issues in Critical Care Nursing 2(4):675, 1991.

Schlump-Urquhart, S. Families experiencing a traumatic accident: Implications and nursing management. AACN Clinical Issues in Critical Care Nursing 1(3):522–534, 1990.

Unkle, D, et al: Interpretation of the cervical spine x-ray: A simplified approach. Crit Care Nurse 10(8):48, 1990.

SAMPLE CARE PLAN FOR THE PATIENT WITH GUILLAIN-BARRÉ SYNDROME

Nursing Diagnoses

Nursing Diagnosis #1
Breathing Pattern, ineffective, related to:
1. Compromised function of respiratory musculature
2. Reduced diaphragmatic excursion
3. Anxiety

Desired Patient Outcomes

Patient will maintain adequate respiratory function:
- Respiratory rate ~14–18/min
- Respiratory rhythm eupneic
- Arterial blood gas values (room air):
  pH 7.35–7.45
  $PaCO_2$ ~35–45 mmHg
  PaO_2 >80 mmHg

Nursing Interventions
- Assess respiratory function hourly.
  - Specific parameters:
    - Rate, rhythm, depth, breath sounds, dyspnea; use of accessory muscles; status of pulmonary secretions; cough with sputum production.

  - Vital capacity and negative inspiratory force generated.

- Prepare patient/family for possibility of intubation and mechanical ventilation therapy.
  - Answer questions, take the time to explain what is happening.
  - Establish alternative means of communication: blinking eyes, wiggle of finger, use of slate board or picture cards.
- Implement kinetic (specialty bed) therapy.

- Maintain optimal body alignment:
  - Position patient so that chest is not restricted (e.g., if on his side, place arm slightly in front or back of patient).
  -

Rationales
- Progression of the underlying pathophysiologic process of Guillain-Barré syndrome is acutely reflected by increasing respiratory insufficiency.
  - Guillain-Barré syndrome is an ascending disease of motor function; it allows for the patient to be intubated prophylactically, rather than to have an emergency and potentially traumatic intubation.
  - Vital capacity and negative inspiratory force generated by the patient are especially crucial in identifying disease progression or improvement.
- Family and patient will accept initiation of mechanical ventilation therapy as part of the overall supportive therapy for patients with this syndrome.

- Use of kinetic therapy helps to prevent pooling of tracheobronchial secretions.

  - The weight of the patient's flaccid arms should be kept off his chest to allow for maximal chest wall excursion and lung expansion.

Nursing Interventions
- Notify physician of any changes in above assessment, and document trends.

Rationales
- By documenting data, trends can be followed and the stage of the disease progression can be pinpointed, facilitating good quality of care.

SAMPLE CARE PLAN FOR THE PATIENT WITH GUILLAIN-BARRÉ SYNDROME (*Continued*)

Nursing Diagnoses

Nursing Diagnosis #2
Airway Clearance, ineffective, related to:
1. Compromised protective reflexes
2. Weakness/paralysis of intercostal and abdominal muscles

Desired Patient Outcomes

Patient will:
1. Maintain patent airway:
   • Normal breath sounds
   • Absence of adventitious sounds (e.g., crackles, wheezes)
2. Demonstrate secretion-clearing cough.

Nursing Interventions

• Assess airway patency hourly:
  ○ Status of protective reflexes (cough, gag, epiglottal closure)
  ○ Ability to handle tracheobronchial secretions

• Maintain hydration state as prescribed. Humidify oxygen administered

Rationales

• Cranial nerve dysfunction is commonly involved in the pathophysiology underlying Guillain-Barré syndrome. Involvement of cranial nerves VII, IX, X, and XII predisposes to compromised chewing, swallowing, and speaking.
• Dehydration may cause tracheobronchial secretions to become inspissated.

Nursing Diagnoses

Nursing Diagnosis #3
Pain, related to sensorimotor dysfunction

Desired Patient Outcomes

Patient will be able to verbalize relief from pain, and demonstrate a relaxed demeanor.

Nursing Interventions

• Assess pain, including severity, location/radiation, and type or quality of pain.

• Provide comfort measures:
  ○ Assist patient into positions of comfort and correct body alignment.
  ○ Remain with patient to reassure.
  ○ Work with family members to help them understand what is happening and how they may best help their loved one.
  ○ Enlist hospital volunteers/chaplain or others to spend some time with the patient.
• Administer analgesics as prescribed; monitor effectiveness in relieving pain.

Rationales

• Pain is one of the most significant complaints made by patients with Guillain-Barré syndrome. It occurs in the most profoundly weakened muscles and is more intense at night.
• Maintaining body in appropriate alignment may help to ease some of the ache.

  ○ Families often feel helpless in this circumstance; allowing them to participate in the patient's care may be reassuring to both patient and family.

• Pain may become severe enough to require narcotics for relief.

Nursing Diagnoses

Nursing Diagnosis #4
Communication, impaired, verbal/nonverbal, related to:
1. Intubation
2. Weakened muscles of speech
3. Generalized muscle weakness/paralysis

Desired Patient Outcomes

Patient will:
1. Be able to demonstrate alternative means of communication
2. Verbalize feeling comfortable with alternative means of communication
3. Verbalize why alternative means of communication may be necessary

Nursing Interventions

• Assess for difficulty in speaking.

• Keep patient/family appraised of expectations.

• Constantly reassure patient that his needs will be met.
• Initiate alternative means of communication before dysfunction occurs.

Rationales

• Cranial nerve involvement may compromise muscles of speech; eventually, the patient may not even be able to blink his eyes; yet, throughout this ordeal, the patient remains conscious and aware.
• Keeping patient/family abreast of what is happening may help them to adjust to dysfunctional changes more easily.
• Mr. L's constant bell ringing reflected his frustration with his dependency and his fear of not having his needs met.

SAMPLE CARE PLAN FOR THE PATIENT WITH GUILLAIN-BARRÉ SYNDROME (*Continued*)

Nursing Diagnoses

Nursing Diagnosis #5
Self-Care deficit, related to:
dependent status necessitated by compromised
sensorimotor dysfunction

Desired Patient Outcomes

Patient will:
1. Be able to verbalize feelings about being dependent on others
2. Identify activities requiring assistance
3. Set priorities as to which dependent activities will be accomplished first

Nursing Interventions

- Identify with patient/family those activities over which the patient can have control (e.g., when to bathe, when to turn, when to have visitors).
- Work with family to assist the patient in some of his activities of daily living; assist the family to understand why they should respect the patient's need to maintain control of some of his care activities.
  - Encourage family members to verbalize thoughts and concerns.
- Allow patient to ventilate frustrations about dependency.

Rationales

- Allowing patient to make decisions over care will help the patient to maintain some control over his body.

- If the patient refuses to see family members or states he doesn't want them to do anything for him, the patient's family should be reassured that it's okay for the patient to do these things and they should not feel rejected.
  - The patient's illness places a tremendous strain on family relationships, interactions, and lifestyle.

CARE PLAN FOR THE INITIAL MANAGEMENT OF THE PATIENT WITH SPINAL CORD INJURY (CERVICAL CORD INJURY)

Nursing Diagnoses

Nursing Diagnosis #1
Breathing Pattern, ineffective, related to:
1. Altered ventilatory mechanics associated with paralysis of intercostal and abdominal muscles
2. Limited diaphragmatic excursion associated with paralytic ileus (abdominal distention)
3. Immobility

Desired Patient Outcomes

Patient will:
1. Demonstrate effective minute ventilation with trend of improving:
   - Tidal volume >7–10 mL/kg
   - Respiratory rate <25/min
2. Achieve a vital capacity >15–20 mL/kg
3. Verbalize ease of breathing

Nursing Diagnoses

Nursing Diagnosis #2
Airway Clearance, ineffective, related to:
1. Ineffective cough associated with paralysis of intercostal and abdominal muscles
2. Immobility

Desired Patient Outcomes

Patient will:
1. Demonstrate clear breath sounds on auscultation
2. Demonstrate a secretion-clearing cough
3. Maintain arterial blood gas values:
   - PaO_2 >80 mmHg
   - $PaCO_2$ 35–45 mmHg, if no head injury (<30 mmHg with injury)
   - pH 7.35–7.45

Nursing Interventions

- Perform a comprehensive respiratory assessment.
  - Airway patency
  - Rate, rhythm, depth of breathing

  - Chest and diaphragmatic excursion

Rationales

- Major goal of airway management is to establish and/or maintain adequate alveolar ventilation.
  - Increased rapid, shallow respirations may signal deterioration of respiratory function, as they contribute to alveolar hypoventilation.
  - C-3 to C-5 cervical cord injury may disrupt innervation of diaphragm; paralysis results in respiratory arrest.

CARE PLAN FOR THE INITIAL MANAGEMENT OF THE PATIENT WITH SPINAL CORD INJURY (CERVICAL CORD INJURY) (*Continued*)

Nursing Interventions	Rationales

Nursing Interventions

- ○ Use of accessory muscles
- ○ Auscultation of breath sounds

- ○ Monitoring of arterial blood gases (ABGs)

- Assess ability to cough and clear secretions.

- ○ Assess status of protective reflexes: cough, gag, and epiglottal closure.

- ○ Monitor quality, quantity, color, and consistency of sputum.

- ○ Assess secretions for state of hydration or need for mucolytic therapy.
- Monitor serial pulmonary function tests:
  - ○ Tidal volume
  - ○ Vital capacity
- Assess neurologic status:
  - ○ Level of consciousness; mentation
- Implement measures to ensure adequate respiratory function:
  - ○ Establish and maintain airway patency.
    - ▫ Provide endotracheal or tracheostomy care as per unit protocol.
  - ○ Maintain head and neck in straight alignment without hyperflexion or hyperextension.

  - ○ Implement intubation and mechanical ventilation as per unit protocol.

  - ○ Initiate oxygen therapy to maintain arterial blood gases within physiologically acceptable range (>80 mmHg).
  - ○ Initiate measures to clear secretions.
    - ▫ Provide humidified oxygen.
    - ▫ Maintain hydration.
  - ○ Implement nasotracheal suctioning as necessary to maintain airway patency.

  - ○ Initiate chest physiotherapy techniques as tolerated.
    - ▫ Postural drainage
    - ▫ Percussion and vibration
  - ○ Encourage deep breathing and coughing.

  - ○ Instruct patient in use of incentive spirometry.

  - ○ Ensure adequate hydration status.
  - ○ Monitor intake and output, daily weight.

Rationales

- ○ May detect evidence of secretion accumulation; airway obstruction.
- ○ Hypoxemia in the patient with spinal cord injury is most commonly caused by retained secretions.
- Loss of intercostal and abdominal muscles compromises the patient's ability to cough effectively.
  - ○ Loss of protective reflexes places patient at risk of developing aspiration pneumonia; a moist-sounding, unproductive cough signals retention and pooling of pulmonary secretions.
  - ○ Baseline data enable changes in sputum production and characteristics to be identified. Infection or other pulmonary insult may change quality and increase quantity of sputum; a pulmonary embolism may cause *hemoptysis.*
  - ○ Thinning of secretions facilitates mobilization and clearance of secretions.
- Serial monitoring enables trends to be identified; progressive decline in pulmonary function may signal need for elective intubation and mechanical ventilation.
- Hypoxia may be reflected by changes in patient's mental status or behavior (e.g., restlessness, irritability).

- ○ Airway obstruction frequently occurs with spinal cord injury or injuries involving head and neck.

- ○ Reduces risk of further neurologic damage; allows for unimpeded flow of blood and CSF from cranial vault; head injury often accompanies traumatic cord injuries.
- ○ Elective intubation and mechanical ventilation are often performed with cervical injury at C-4 to C-5, and above.

- ○ Note: vagal stimulation may cause severe bradycardia in the patient with spinal cord injury who already exhibits bradycardia.
- ○ Loosens and dislodges secretions and enhances movement toward trachea from where they can be removed by coughing and/or suctioning.
- ○ Quad-assist coughing method may be helpful in patients with weakened cough (see text for details).
- ○ Increase vital capacity; helps to more evenly match ventilation with perfusion.
- ○ Use of incentive spirometry encourages deep breathing, reducing risk of atelectasis.
- ○ Adequate hydration moistens, loosens, and liquefies secretions.

Nursing Diagnoses	Desired Patient Outcomes

Nursing Diagnoses

Nursing Diagnosis #3

Cardiac Output, decreased, related to:
1. Decreased venous return associated with spinal shock (pooling of blood in dilated vasculature)
2. Orthostatic hypotension
3. Bradycardia

Desired Patient Outcomes

Patient will maintain stable hemodynamics:
- Blood pressure within 10 mmHg of baseline
- Heart rate >60 < 100 bpm

CARE PLAN FOR THE INITIAL MANAGEMENT OF THE PATIENT WITH SPINAL CORD INJURY (CERVICAL CORD INJURY) (*Continued*)

Nursing Interventions	Rationales

• Assess for presence of neurogenic or spinal shock: blood pressure, pulse, body temperature, skin; orthostatic hypotension.	• Complete transection of spinal cord at T-4 to T-6 and above precipitates spinal shock with loss of sympathetic autonomic reflex activity.
	   ○ Hypotension occurs due to loss of sympathetic vasomotor tone with resultant vasodilation of systemic vasculature.
	   ○ Bradycardia occurs due to unopposed parasympathetic (vagal) tone to the heart.

• Rule out concomitant hemorrhagic, hypovolemic shock:
   ○ Neurogenic shock: hypotension, bradycardia, warm dry skin
   ○ Hemorrhagic shock: hypotension, tachycardia, thready pulse, cool clammy skin
      □ Assess for signs of bleeding in patient with spinal cord injury who exhibits tachycardia.
• Implement measures to stabilize cardiopulmonary function:
   ○ Initiate prescribed intravenous fluid therapy ~75–100 mL/h to maintain systolic blood pressure ~100 mmHg.
   ○ Monitor fluid intake and output.
   ○ Initiate activities to minimize orthostatic hypotension:
      □ Apply antiembolic stockings.
      □ Abdominal binder.
      □ Gradual increase to vertical position (sitting up at 90°) as tolerated.
	• Infrequently, spinal cord trauma may be accompanied by internal injuries with possible bleeding.
	
	   ○ Presence of internal bleeding may be difficult to detect in the insensate patient; a high degree of suspicion and meticulous assessment are essential.
	
	• Intact mental status, and acceptable urine outputs indicate adequate tissue perfusion.
	
	   ○ Orthostatic hypotension results from venous stasis associated with impaired vasomotor tone and skeletal muscle paralysis.
	   ○ Observe patient carefully when sitting up; syncopal episodes secondary to hypotension may occur.

Nursing Diagnoses	Desired Patient Outcomes
Nursing Diagnosis #4 Injury, potential for, related to: 1. Vertebral instability 2. Spinal cord edema 3. Stress	Patient will: 1. Maintain immobilization of head, neck, and back 2. Maintain and/or improve neurologic function

Nursing Interventions	Rationales

• Determine extent of injury and baseline assessment data.
• Patient history:
   ○ Obtain information regarding circumstances of injury/accident: Mechanism of injury? Neurologic status after injury?
      □ Did the patient lose consciousness? If so, for how long? Was there seizure activity? Was the patient incontinent—bowel? bladder?
      □ Type of treatment administered at scene of injury: Medications? Fluids?
      □ Mode of transporation to the hospital? How long a delay between occurrence of injury and admission to emergency department?
      □ Patient's status on arrival at the hospital?
• Physical examination:
   ○ Estimate extent of cord involvement. Level and areas of neurologic deficits can be delineated by checking sensation, muscular strength, and reflexes.
	○ Knowledge of mechanism/location of spinal cord injury assists in determining type and extent of spinal injury and the presence of other injuries.
	
	      □ Concomitant head injury is always a possibility especially with cervical cord injury.
	
	      □ Interview EMTs, and family member if present, about the circumstances of the injury.
	
	   ○ Knowledge regarding level of cord injury assists in determining level of function and in anticipating problems. *Example*: Impending danger of phrenic nerve dysfunction with cord injury at C-3 to C-5 or above.

CARE PLAN FOR THE INITIAL MANAGEMENT OF THE PATIENT WITH SPINAL CORD INJURY (CERVICAL CORD INJURY) (*Continued*)

Nursing Interventions	Rationales

○ Grade muscle strength with scale of 0–5:
  0 = no movement
  5 = movement against reflexes
	○ Organized approach ensures thorough testing of all major muscle groups.

○ Test for sensory function using touch and pinprick as stimuli.	○ To assist in demarcating areas of function from areas of altered sensation, progress from area of neurologic deficit to area where sensation is intact.
○ Assess patient's neurologic status every 1 to 2 h during initial 48–72 h after injury.	○ Neurologic deterioration with additional loss of function may be caused by spinal cord edema, hemorrhage, compromised blood supply, and tissue ischemia.
○ Examine patient thoroughly to determine if other injury has been sustained.	○ The neurologically compromised patient may not be able to tell you that other problems exist.
○ Look for signs of internal and/or external bleeding if tachycardia is present.	○ Traumatic spine injuries are frequently associated with internal abdominal complications caused by the violent force of such injuries.
• Obtain cervical spine x-rays.	• Patient should not be moved until cervical spine x-rays have been carefully evaluated and the patient's status has been determined. Cervical vertebrae: All seven must be definitively viewed.
• Implement measures to stabilize cervical spine. ○ Use principles underlying traction: □ Weights are never removed, but must be allowed to hang freely at all times.	• To prevent further neurologic damage.
○ When turning, positioning, or moving patient, obtain adequate assistance; patient should be lifted using a sheet.	○ Skeletal traction, if in use, must be in effect at all times.
○ Implement nursing measures in caring for the patient with a halo immobilization brace.	○ For details regarding the care of the patient with a halo brace see Table 33–7.
• Monitor for neurologic changes associated with spinal cord edema. ○ Assess respiratory function: rate, rhythm, depth, and pattern of breathing; arterial blood gas studies.	• In cervical spinal cord injury, ascending edema may compromise phrenic nerve innervation to diaphragm, precipitating respiratory arrest. It may be necessary to intubate the patient and initiate mechanical ventilation.
○ Monitor response of patient to corticosteroids.	○ Steroids have been found to be efficacious in incomplete cord transections. May reduce inflammation and edema.

Nursing Diagnoses	Desired Patient Outcomes
Nursing Diagnosis #5 Thermoregulation, ineffective, associated with autonomic dysfunction *Nursing Diagnosis #6* Body Temperature, altered, risk for	Patient will: 1. Maintain body temperature ~98.6°F (37.0°C) 2. Verbalize comfort and absence of chilling, or diaphoresis above level of lesion
Nursing Interventions	**Rationales**
• Monitor body temperature and complaints of chilliness or sweating. • Maintain a constant room temperature. ○ Use of extra blankets should be guided by patient's temperature. ○ Avoid drafts. □ Avoid use of excessive bedding.	• Impaired homeothermia causes the patient's body to assume environmental temperature. • This is the most effective way of controlling patient's temperature.

Nursing Diagnoses	Desired Patient Outcomes
Nursing Diagnosis #7 Urinary Retention, related to atonic bladder associated with spinal shock *Nursing Diagnosis #8* Urinary Elimination, altered, related to loss of voluntary control of external urethral spincter	Patient will: 1. Have a urine volume of <400–450 mL on intermittent catheterization program 2. Demonstrate absence of suprapubic distention 3. Balance intake with output

CARE PLAN FOR THE INITIAL MANAGEMENT OF THE PATIENT WITH SPINAL CORD INJURY (CERVICAL CORD INJURY) (*Continued*)

Nursing Interventions

- Monitor urinary function.

  ○ Assess for bladder distention

- Initiate intermittent catherization program as early as possible.
  ○ Establish necessary criteria: fluid intake <2000 mL/24 h; absence of urinary infection on culture and sensitivity.

  ○ Monitor fluid intake.
    □ Limit fluid intake after the evening meal.
    □ Avoid beverages that have a diuretic effect (e.g., caffeinated colas, tea, coffee).

Rationales

- Urinary retention predisposes to complications of infection.
  ○ During spinal shock, atonic bladder predisposes to urinary retention and urinary tract infection.
- Minimizes renal/urinary complications associated with infection.
  ○ Intermittent catheterization program should be initiated as early as possible, even during acute state if feasible. This simulates normal bladder filling and emptying and facilitates bladder training.
  ○ Efforts to establish effective urinary management require a collaborative approach involving patient, family and/or significant others, and healthcare providers.

Nursing Diagnoses

Nursing Diagnosis #9
Constipation, related to atonic bowel (paralytic ileus) associated with spinal shock.

Desires Patient Outcomes

Patient will:
1. Remain without constipation and fecal impaction
2. Establish regular bowel elimination management regimen

Nursing Interventions

- Prevent complications of gastrointestinal function.

  ○ Insert nasogastric tube to decompress gastrointestinal tract.
  ○ Assess patient with high degree of suspicion.
    □ Measure abdominal girth.
    □ Be alert for signs/complaints of "referred" pain.
    □ Auscultate in all quadrants.
  ○ Assess for signs of constipation: Dull sound over descending colon on percussion; palpation of hard, rigid stool over areas of bowel.
  ○ Be suspicious of diarrhea.
    □ Hematest gastric secretions, stool with guaiac.
- Initiate bowel continence program after spinal shock and resolution of paralytic ileus:
  ○ Establish regular routine: Dulcolax suppository inserted, digital examination.
    □ Same hour of day, usually after breakfast.
    □ Maintain appropriate diet.

Rationales

- Level of cord injury determines the extent of gastrointestinal and bowel dysfunction.
  ○ Entire gastrointestinal tract becomes atonic with onset of spinal shock 24 to 48 h after injury.
  ○ Prevents aspiration of gastric contents. Abdominal distention may limit diaphragmatic excursion.
  ○ With loss of sensation, patient may be unaware of signs of internal bleeding, ileus, impaction.

  ○ Diarrhea may signal presence of fecal impaction.

  ○ Critical care nurse can be instrumental in initiating and maintaining bowel and bladder program (see Fig. 33–1).

    □ Takes advantage of peristalsis initiated by eating.

Nursing Diagnoses

Nursing Diagnosis #10
Skin Integrity, impaired, risk for, related to:
1. Mechanical forces (pressure, friction, shear) associated with immobility
2. Urinary and bowel incontinence
3. Catabolic state

Desired Patient Outcomes

Patient's skin will remain intact.

Nursing Interventions

- Assess for alteration in skin integrity.

  ○ Identify areas at risk (weight-bearing bony prominences) depending on position assumed (i.e., supine, prone, and so forth).

Rationales

- Loss of mobility and sensation, impaired circulation, and inadequate nutrition predispose to skin breakdown.
  ○ Pressure develops when there is lack of continuous movement and distribution of weight.
  ○ Pressure most concentrated between bone and skin surfaces that support body weight.

CARE PLAN FOR THE INITIAL MANAGEMENT OF THE PATIENT WITH SPINAL CORD INJURY (CERVICAL CORD INJURY) (*Continued*)

Nursing Interventions	Rationales
○ Inspect skin after each position change.	○ Reddened areas should blanch within 20–30 min after a position change.
○ Inspect for open or ulcerated areas and localized edema (dependent edema).	○ Dependent edema is incriminated in the pathophysiology of skin breakdown; it interferes with cellular nutrition and increases susceptibility of tissues to the effects of pressure. Susceptibility increased during period of spinal shock.
• Implement measures to promote tissue perfusion.	• Meticulous systematic surveillance of all pressure points, from body position, bed, or traction equipment, is the key to maintaining intact skin integrity.
○ Turning and positioning at least every 2 h.	○ Prevents stasis and tissue ischemia.
□ Use kinetic therapy, if available.	
□ Use elbow and heel protectors.	
□ Use lift sheet.	□ Minimizes friction and shearing forces.
○ Maintain proper alignment.	○ Prevents further neurologic damage, contractures.
□ Passive ROM exercises with dorsiflexion of feet.	□ Minimizes risk of deep venous thrombosis.
○ Provide pressure relief device.	○ Helps to displace weight more evenly.

Nursing Diagnoses	Desired Patient Outcomes
Nursing Diagnosis #11	Patient will:
Injury, risk for deep venous thrombosis related to:	1. Exhibit adequate peripheral circulation:
1. Hemostasis associated with immobility	• Usual skin color; no cyanosis
2. Loss of skeletal muscle pump	• Extremities warm to touch
3. Pooling of blood in dilated capacitance vessels (e.g., absence of vasomotor tone during spinal shock)	2. Maintain consistent calf and thigh circumference measurements
	3. Maintain effective respiratory function
	4. Maintain stable vital signs

Nursing Interventions	Rationales
• Monitor for signs and symptoms of deep venous thrombosis.	• Venous stasis, skeletal muscle paralysis, and immobilization place patient at risk of developing deep venous thrombosis and pulmonary embolism.
○ Assess skin color and temperature.	○ Assessment for deep venous thrombosis is difficult because of sensorimotor deficits in patient with spinal cord injury.
○ Assess calf and thigh circumference.	○ A slowly increasing circumference suggests a possible underlying thrombosis.
• Monitor for signs and symptoms of pulmonary embolism.	
○ Assess sudden onset of respiratory difficulties (e.g., tachypnea, dyspnea, cough with hemoptysis); altered pulmonary function tests: tidal volume, vital capacity; neurologic findings; restlessness, lethargy.	
• Implement measures to minimize risk of deep venous thrombosis and pulmonary embolism.	
○ Maintain desired hydration.	○ Prevents increase in blood viscosity, which predisposes to a hypercoagulable state.
□ Monitor intake and output, daily weight.	
○ Apply antiembolic stocking to both lower extremities.	
○ Institute exercise program.	
□ Passive ROM exercises with dorsiflexion of feet.	
□ Maintenance of proper body alignment.	
–Use splints as directed.	
–Avoid crossing legs, using knee gatch, or pillow under knees.	
–Avoid prolonged sitting or lying in one position.	
○ Administer prophylactic heparin therapy as prescribed.	○ Prevents thromboembolic formation and aids clot dispersion.

CARE PLAN FOR THE INITIAL MANAGEMENT OF THE PATIENT WITH SPINAL CORD INJURY (CERVICAL CORD INJURY) (*Continued*)

Nursing Diagnoses

Nursing Diagnosis #12
Nutrition, altered, less than body requirements, related to:
1. Nothing-by-mouth (NPO) status during spinal shock associated with paralytic ileus
2. Weakened or absent protective reflexes (e.g., cough, gag, epiglottal closure)
3. Anorexia associated with depression, or inability to self-feed

Desired Patient Outcome

Patient will:
1. Maintain baseline body weight within 5% of baseline
2. Maintain triceps skinfold measurements within baseline range
3. Maintain laboratory parameters within acceptable physiologic range
4. Verbalize increase in appetite

Nursing Interventions

- Collaborate with dietician to obtain a complete nutritional assessment within 24–48 h of admission.
  - Baseline nutritional status
  - Nutritional requirements of the compromised state
  - Height and weight
  - Pre-injury nutritional status: dietary habits, likes, and dislikes
- Consult with nutritionist. Determine anthropometric data.
- Establish and maintain a balanced nutritional state—positive nitrogen balance.
  - Administer nutritional supplements: (as per unit protocol): parenteral nutrition (TPN and PPN) during period of spinal shock and paralytic ileus.
  - Initiate nasogastric tube feedings when paralytic ileus subsides but protective reflexes are still compromised.
    - Assess location/patency of nasogastric tube prior to each feeding.
  - Document daily caloric intake, fluid intake and output, daily weight.
  - Assess wound healing, skin integrity.
  - Assess patient's overall physical, mental, emotional state.

Rationales

- Baseline nutritional needs must be identified to ensure adequate nutritional intake; individualized care.

  - Stress increases energy needs by 50%.

  - Baseline data assist in planning a nutrition program specific to the needs and desires of patient.

- Balanced nutritional intake promotes wound healing and prevents complications.

    - To reduce risk of aspiration.

  - Depression can cause anorexia.

Nursing Diagnoses

Nursing Diagnosis #13
Sensory/Perceptual alteration: visual, tactile, related to:
1. Immobilization
2. Sensory deficits associated with disruption of ascending nerve pathways at level of cord lesion

Desired Patient Outcomes

Patient will:
1. Verbalize comfort in visualizing people and objects within immediate visual field
2. Verbalize areas where tactile sensation is perceived

Nursing Interventions

- Assess patient's view of immediate environment.
  - Consider type of spinal stabilization and use of specialized bed (e.g., Roto-Rest).
    - Skeletal traction
    - Halo immobilization brace
- Implement measures to make immediate environment accessible to patient's field of vision.
  - Arrange desired objects as patient requests.
  - Position mirrors to enhance patient's view.

  - Place self within patient's field of vision when speaking to patient. Direct others to do same.
- Assess patient's tactile and pain sensation.
  - Use touch and pinprick stimuli:
    - Test for sensory perception progressing from area of deficit to area of intact function.
    - Frequently touch patient in areas demarcated as having sensory perception intact.
    - Touch patient with different textured objects.

Rationales

- Viewing immediate environment from patient's perspective assists in arranging environment so desired materials are accessible to patient.

  - See Table 33–7.

  - Helps to provide increased visualization and stimulation.
  - Reduces sensory deprivation.

- Touching patient in areas of intact sensation helps to provide stimulation.

CARE PLAN FOR THE INITIAL MANAGEMENT OF THE PATIENT WITH SPINAL CORD INJURY (CERVICAL CORD INJURY) (*Continued*)

Nursing Interventions
- Implement measures to reduce sensory overload.
  - Set priorities in care.

  - Allow patient choices and options.
  - Encourage verbalization; carefully observe facial expression; provide a listening ear.

Rationales
- Minimizing distraction helps patient to concentrate on more pertinent stimuli, and on how best to perceive environment from a new vantage point.
  - Helps to give patient a feeling of some self-control.
  - What is not verbalized may be reflected in patient's facial expression.

Nursing Diagnoses

Nursing Diagnosis #14
Coping, alteration in: Patient and family, related to:
1. Situational crisis
2. Temporary family disorganization

Desired Patient Outcomes

Patient/family will:
1. Identify useful coping mechanisms
2. Demonstrate ability to assess, problem solve, and make decisions
3. Express realistic expectations of each other

Nursing Interventions
- Establish a rapport and trusting relationship with patient and family.
- Observe patient/family dynamics and interactions.

  - Assess family resources; usual coping mechanisms.

- Implement measures to assist in coping:
  - Provides opportunity for patient and family members to express feelings and emotions.
    - Encourage honest communication.
  - Provide emotional support and relieve anxieties by making appropriate explanations.
  - Keep patient and family informed:
    - Be honest and realistic.
    - Be accessible to patient/family.
    - Allow time for questions to be asked and feelings vented.
  - Increasingly include patient/family in decision-making process as they demonstrate a readiness to do so (e.g., the ability to verbalize and discuss feelings).

Rationales

- These observations may help to identify strengths, weaknesses, and effective coping capabilities.
  - Long-term rehabilitation places tremendous burden on family resources.

  - Recognizing feelings and emotions is the first step in dealing with them.

  - Support and reassurance assist patient/family to cope with catastrophic event.

  - Enables patient to feel useful, to have some control.
  - Promotes involvement in the rehabilitative process.

Nursing Diagnoses

Nursing Diagnosis #15
Social Isolation, related to:
1. Immobility
2. Prolonged hospitalization/rehabilitation
3. Depression

Desired Patient Outcomes

Patient will:
1. Demonstrate desire to interact and maintain relationships
2. Verbalize feelings of isolation
3. Participate in diversional activities

Nursing Interventions
- Assess patient's usual degree of social interaction.
- Assess for signs/symptoms suggesstive of social isolation.

- Encourage verbalization regarding patient's sense of isolation.
  - Assess patient's feelings about self: sense of being "out of control"; hopelessness.
- Develop a plan of action to decrease feelings of social isolation.

Rationales

- Specific signs/symptoms might include: Expression of loneliness or feelings of rejection: flat affect; depression; patient uncommunicative, withdrawn, preoccupied.
  - It is important to establish a therapeutic nurse–patient relationship, one in which the patient is able to comfortably air thoughts and concerns.

CARE PLAN FOR THE INITIAL MANAGEMENT OF THE PATIENT WITH SPINAL CORD INJURY (CERVICAL CORD INJURY) (*Continued*)

Nursing Interventions	Rationales
<ul><li>Provide effective alternative method of communication.</li><li>Encourage interactions with significant others.</li><li>Assist patient to set up visiting schedule with family/friends.</li><li>Encourage participation in diversional activities.</li><li>Initiate referral to appropriate resources (e.g., occupational, recreational therapist when feasible).</li></ul>	<ul><li>Helps to reassure patients that their needs are being met and that they have not been forgotten.</li><li>Knowing when to expect a visit or call can be reassuring.</li></ul>

UNIT FIVE

Renal/Urinary System

UNIT OUTLINE

CHAPTER 34

Anatomy and Physiology of the Renal/Urinary System

Jeanette G. Kernicki

CHAPTER OUTLINE

Role of Kidney in Removal of Waste
  Products, Toxins, and Excesses of
  Body Elements
Anatomic Structure of Kidney
  □ Gross Structure
  □ Microscopic Structure
Blood Supply to Kidney
Physiologic Property of Kidney
  □ Urine Production Processes

□ Homeostatic Mechanism for Fluid
  and Electrolyte Maintenance
Endocrine Influence on Kidney Function
Other Roles of Kidney
  □ Erythrocyte Production
  □ Vitamin D Activity Regulation
  □ Calcium-Phosphate Metabolism
References

LEARNING OBJECTIVES

After completing this chapter, you should be able to:

1. Identify the role of the kidney in removal of waste products, toxins, and fluid-
   particulate excesses.
2. Describe the gross structure of the kidney.
3. Describe the functional unit of the kidney.
4. Discuss the differences between the types of nephrons.
5. Identify the structures and processes of urine formation.
6. List the blood-supplying vessels to the kidney.
7. State the forces required for filtrate movement.
8. Discuss the influence of the endocrine system on renal function.
9. Describe the role of the kidney in erythrocyte production, vitamin D regulation,
   and calcium-phosphate metabolism.

ROLE OF KIDNEY IN REMOVAL OF WASTE PRODUCTS, TOXINS, AND EXCESSES OF BODY ELEMENTS

Metabolic waste products, toxins, drugs, and excesses of body elements must be removed from the human body, or disturbances in body homeostasis will occur. The major transport of metabolic wastes and excesses from the blood is accomplished through kidney function by the process of excretion and urine formation. Additionally, the kidneys play an important role in fluid volume control, electrolyte level maintenance, calcium-phosphate metabolism, acid-base balance, blood pressure regulation, erythrocyte production, and vitamin D activation.

Monitoring renal function is imperative for critically ill patients. Changes in body weight, blood chemistry,

and urine volume may herald clinical problems affecting the renal system. Medical and nursing interventions to minimize the consequences of dysfunction become more meaningful when the normal function of the kidney is understood. An extensive review of the renal system, however, is beyond the scope of this book, and the reader is advised to refer to a medical-surgical nursing text for an in-depth discussion of the system.

ANATOMIC STRUCTURE OF KIDNEY

Gross Structure

The paired, bean-shaped kidneys lie in the retroperitoneal space, slightly above the area of the umbi-

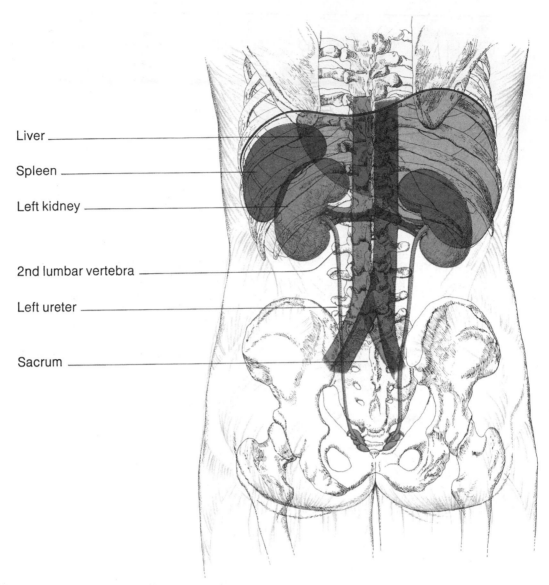

FIGURE 34–1. Location and size of the kidneys. Posterior view of the kidneys and related structures. The kidney is well protected by the overlying bone (ribs and vertebral column) and heavy posterior musculature. The right kidney is slightly lower than the left, because of the liver. The kidneys normally extend from the level of the T-11 or T-12 vertebra to that of the L-2 vertebra. Normal kidneys in a 70-kg man average 160 to 175 g in weight, and are approximately 10 to 12 cm long and 5 to 6 cm side. (From Wilson, RF: Critical Care Manual: Applied Physiology and Principles of Therapy, ed. 2, F.A. Davis, Philadelphia, 1992, p 568, with permission.)

licus, with the upper part of each kidney at about the level of the T-12 vertebra and the lower part at the L-2 vertebra (Fig. 34–1). The right kidney is lower than the left because the right lobe of the liver lies above it. A longitudinal section shows two areas in the kidney: the outer structure, the cortex, and the inner structure, the medulla (Fig. 34–2). In the medullary part of the kidney are from eight to eighteen pyramids, which project into a cup-shaped minor calyx. Several minor calyces open into the major calyces, in a funnel-shaped structure, the renal pelvis in the hilum of the kidney. Urine, which is formed and trans-

ported by way of the collecting ducts entering the medullary pyramid, exits the papillary pyramid, drains from the minor calyces to the major calyces, and flows into the renal pelvis, to the ureter and then the bladder.

Microscopic Structure

About one fourth of total cardiac output is delivered to the kidney by way of the renal artery and subsequent interlobar, arcuate, and interlobular arteries, which

Cortex

Renal pyramid

Minor calyx

Major calyx

Medulla

Renal pelvis

Ureter

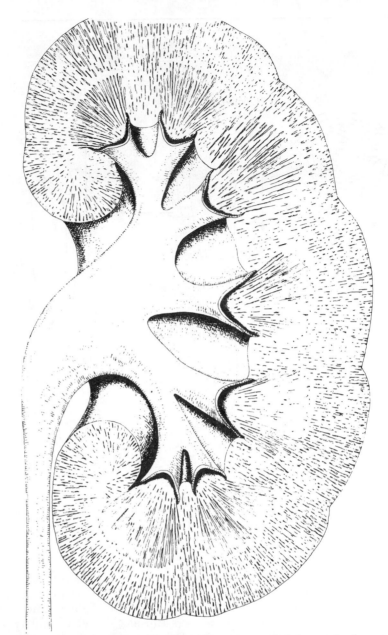

FIGURE 34–2. Sagittal section of the kidney. The cortex is located peripherally with portions called the renal columns running centrally between the medullary pyramids. The cortex is composed mainly of glomeruli and the convoluted portions of the proximal and distal tubules. The medulla contains the loops of Henle and collecting system portions of the nephron. The core of the kidney is occupied by the renal pelvis into which the collecting system empties. (From Wilson, RF: Critical Care Manual: Applied Physiology and Principles of Therapy, ed. 2, F.A. Davis, Philadelphia, 1992, p 569, with permission.)

give off the nutrient afferent arterioles terminating in the glomerulus. As a result, several processes are set in motion within the microscopic functional unit of the kidney, the nephron. Each kidney contains from 1 to 1.5 million nephrons, which are composed of a vascular and tubular system (Fig. 34–3). There are two types of nephrons: those in the innermost part of the cortex, the juxtamedullary nephrons, and those in the outer two thirds of the cortex, the cortical nephrons. Striations within the pyramidal structures are repre-

sentative of parallel, microscopic long nephron loops and blood vessels.[1]

BLOOD SUPPLY TO KIDNEY

About 90% of renal blood flow is directed to the renal cortex, and the remaining 10% to the medulla. The glomerular filtration rate is reduced when any marked reduction in renal blood flow occurs.[2]

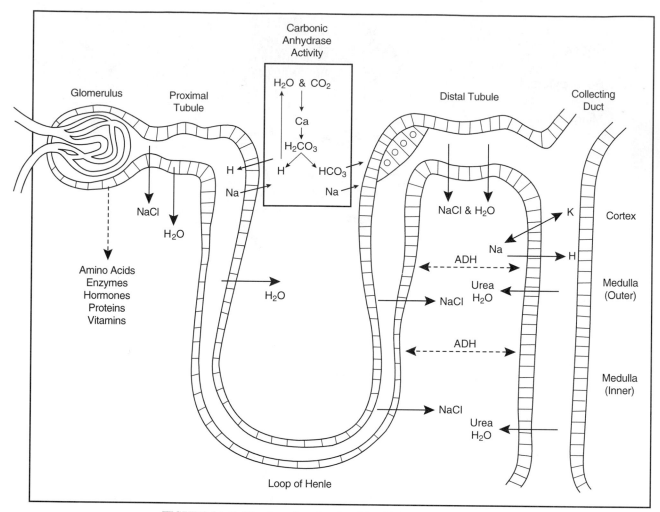

FIGURE 34–3. The functional unit of the kidney—the nephron.

A network of capillary branches of the afferent arteriole forms the glomerulus, which is invaginated in a funnel-like structure called Bowman's capsule. Extending from Bowman's capsule is the renal tubule, consisting of several segments: the proximal convoluted tubule, the loop of Henle, the distal convoluted tubule, and the collecting duct. The latter merges with larger tubules to form one tube entering the small calyces by way of the renal papilla.

PHYSIOLOGIC PROPERTY OF KIDNEY

Not all of the delivered cardiac output is excreted as urine. Important electrolytes and solutes (amino acids, enzymes, hormones, proteins, and vitamins), as well as volume, must be returned to the bloodstream if homeostasis is to be maintained. Leaving the glomeruli are the efferent arterioles, smaller in diameter than the afferent arterioles. The efferent arterioles are responsive to tubular changes associated with urine

flow and sodium content. In the outer cortex of the kidney, a network of capillaries, known as the peritubular capillary plexus, extends from the efferent arteriole and surrounds the tubular system. This arrangement differs somewhat in the juxtamedullary glomeruli. Straight vessels, vasa recta, follow the loops of Henle and return to the cortex, where they enter the venous system (Fig. 34–4). The vasa recta play an important role in urine concentration, eliminating more waste products and yet conserving body water, which is necessary when water intake is severely limited.[3]

Urine Production Processes

The maintenance of normal blood and body fluid composition is the primary function of the kidney. The kidney accomplishes this through the process of filtration through the glomerulus, reabsorption of water and essential substances by the tubular system, and secretion of hydrogen and ammonium ions from the blood into urine (Table 34–1). The glomerular filtrate is essentially an ultrafiltrate of plasma, and it enters the renal tubular system. It contains wastes, excess materials, and substances the body must conserve. The glomerular filtration rate averages about 120 mL/min. Filtration at the glomerulus delivers fluid to the proximal convoluted tubule, the loop of Henle, the distal convoluted tubule, and the collecting duct. About 65% of the filtered load can be reabsorbed in the proximal tubule, 25% in the loop of Henle, and 5% in the distal convoluted tubule. The composition of glomerular filtrate is modified either by reabsorption, which occurs in all parts of the nephron, or by secretion only by tubular cells, or by a combination of both. The greater the amount of sodium transported to the distal convoluted tubule, the greater the exchange for potassium (K^+) or hydrogen (H^+) ions. The extracellular fluid concentration of the ions influences the secretion of (K^+) or (H^+) ions.[4]

Homeostatic Mechanism for Fluid and Electrolyte Maintenance

Essential to the entire process of kidney function is the delivery of blood at an optimal mean arterial pressure (about 80 to 100 mmHg) to the small afferent arteriole (Fig. 34–4). The mean arterial pressure then drops within the glomerulus to about 45 to 55 mmHg. A further drop in mean pressure to about 10 to 15 mmHg is noted as blood flows from the glomerulus to the efferent arterial and subsequent peritubular capillary.[5] The efferent arteriole is narrower than the afferent arteriole. The difference in the caliber of the vessels serves as one of the sites of resistance that adjusts the pressure in the kidney.[6]

Filtration, a passive process, is essentially the same as the passage of fluid through the wall of body capillaries. The driving force of the blood (hydrostatic pressure) is opposed by the retaining force, the osmotic pressure of plasma proteins, and the pressure in Bowman's capsule (Table 34–2). Because the plasma proteins are in greater concentration, they do not filter through the pores of the glomerular capillary membrane, and therefore, they exert an osmotic pull or retaining force within the glomerular tuft. The osmotic back pressure normally amounts to about 25 mmHg. Also opposing the filtration of material through the glomerulus are the renal interstitial and the intratubular pressures.

ENDOCRINE INFLUENCE ON KIDNEY FUNCTION

Autoregulatory and hormonal properties of the kidney provide for pressure and volume adjustments. Hormone secretion by endocrine glands aids the kid-

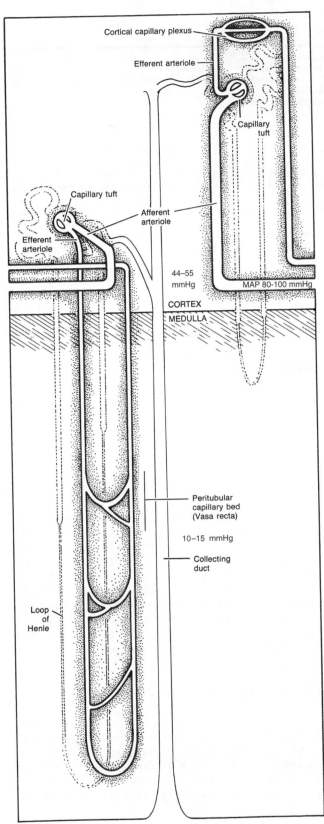

FIGURE 34–4. Vascular component of the nephron. Blood supply to the cortical and juxtamedullary nephrons is differentiated. In each case, afferent arterioles carry blood to the glomeruli, where they give rise to the capillary tuft; these capillaries converge to form the efferent arterioles, which carry blood away from the glomeruli. Each afferent arteriole, in turn, gives rise to a second bed of capillaries: the cortical capillary plexus and the vasa recta, or peritubular capillaries.

TABLE 34–1
Summary of the Processes Occurring in Urine Formation

Process	Where Occurring	Force Responsible	Result
Filtration	Renal corpuscle	Blood pressure, opposed by osmotic, interstitial, and intratubular pressures	Formation of fluid having no formed elements and low protein concentration
Tubular transport Reabsorption	Proximal tubule Distal tubule Loop of Henle	Active transport	Return to bloodstream of physiologically important solutes
Secretion	Proximal tubule Distal tubule	Active transport	Excretion of materials Acidification of urine
Acidification (acid and base regulation)	Distal tubule	Active transport and exchange of alkali for acid	Excretion of excess H^+ Conservation of base (sodium, Na^+, and bicarbonate, HCO_3^-)
Countercurrent multiplier and exchanger	Loop of Henle and vasa recta	Multiplier—active transport Exchanger—diffusion	Creates conditions for hypertonic urine formation
Antidiuretic hormone (ADH) mechanism	Collecting tubule and papillary ducts	Osmosis of water under permissive action of ADH	Formation of hypertonic urine

Source: From McClintic, J: Physiology of the Human Body, ed 3. John Wiley & Sons, New York, 1985, with permission.

TABLE 34–2
Forces of Fluid-Ion Transference

Glomerular Blood	Capsular Filtrate
Hydrostatic pressure = 55 mmHg	Hydrostatic pressure = 10 mmHg
Effective hydrostatic pressure = 45 mmHg →	
Osmotic pressure = 25 mmHg	Osmotic pressure = −0 to 1 mmHg
Effective osmotic pressure = 25 mmHg ←	
Net driving force = 20 mmHg →*	

*Filtered plasma crosses the membrane to Bowman's capsule.

ney in formation of urine and regulation of the composition of blood leaving the kidney. In the event of a decrease in cardiac output or pressure, or decrease in sodium delivery to the distal tubule, the enzyme renin is released from granules within the juxtaglomerular cells. The release of renin into the blood initates a series of reactions, one of which is the production of angiotensin II, an octapeptide that has a major effect upon blood pressure and electrolytes.[7] Renin acts upon a protein substrate (angiotensinogen) secreted by the liver to release the decapeptide angiotensin I. A converting enzyme released primarily from the lungs removes two amino acids from angiotensin I to produce angiotensin II, which has two effects: (1) raising blood pressure by increasing systemic resistance and (2) promoting sodium reabsorption from the tubules by stimulating the release of aldosterone from the cortex of the adrenal gland (Fig. 34–5).

OTHER ROLES OF KIDNEY

Although the kidney is an organ of excetion and urine production, regulation of fluid and electrolyte balance, and blood pressure control, it has several other functions.

Erythrocyte Production

The hormone renal erythropoietic factor is secreted by the kidneys when there is a decrease in oxygen delivery to the kidneys. Inadequate blood flow to the renal artery, as in hypotension and hypoxic and anemic states, serves as a stimulus for secretion of the hormone, which then enzymatically acts on a globulin secreted by the liver to form erythropoietin. The latter stimulates the bone marrow to increase erythrocyte production. It is not uncommon for patients with advanced renal disease to become anemic.[8]

Vitamin D Activity Regulation

The kidneys secrete and regulate the action of vitamin D. The activated form of vitamin D (1,25-dihydroxy vitamin D) stimulates absorption of calcium and phosphate by the intestine, promotes renal tubular reabsorption of calcium and phosphate, and enhances bone resorption. Vitamin D_3 is formed by irradiation of precursors in the skin.[9]

Calcium-Phosphate Metabolism

Prolonged hypocalcemia and hypophosphatemia decrease bone mineralization. The lack of calcium and phosphate triggers a series of events to correct the deficit. The kidney in the presence of parathormone, secreted by the parathyroid gland, converts vitamin D to its activated form (1,25-dihydroxyvitamin D_3 or dihydroxycholecalciferol) and allows for calcium to be absorbed from the gastrointestinal tract, thus restoring the plasma level of calcium.[10] (Please see Chapter 36 for further discussion of calcium and phosphate metabolism.)

REFERENCES

1. Farley, FH: Assessment of Urinary Function. In Phipps, W, Long, B, Woods, N, and Cassmeyer, V (eds): Medical-Surgical Nursing: Concepts and Clinical Practice, ed 4. Mosby Year Book, St Louis, 1991, pp 1385–1390.
2. Luckmann, J, and Sorensen, KC: Medical-Surgical Nursing. WB Saunders, Philadelphia, 1987, p 1149.
3. Hudak, CM, Gallo, BM, and Benz, JJ: Critical Care Nursing: A Holistic Approach. JB Lippincott, Philadelphia, 1990, p 339.
4. McClintic, JR: Physiology of the Human Body, ed 3. John Wiley & Sons, New York.
5. Wilson, RF: Critical Care Manual: Applied Physiology and Principles of Therapy, ed 2. FA Davis, Philadelphia, 1992, pp 577–578.
6. Krieger, JN, and Sherrard, DJ: Practical Fluids and Electrolytes. Appleton & Lange, Norwalk, Conn, 1991, pp 17–19.
7. Rose, BD: Clinical Physiology of Acid-Base and Electrolyte Disorders, ed 4. McGraw-Hill, New York, 1994, pp 27–28.
8. Guyton, AC: Textbook of Medical Physiology, ed 7. WB Saunders, Philadelphia, 1986, pp 946–948.
9. Anthony, CP, and Thibodeau, GA: Textbook of Anatomy and Physiology, ed 12. CV Mosby, St Louis, 1987.
10. Holloway, NM: Nursing the Critically Ill Adult, ed 4. Addison-Wesley, Redwood City, Calif, 1993, p 417.

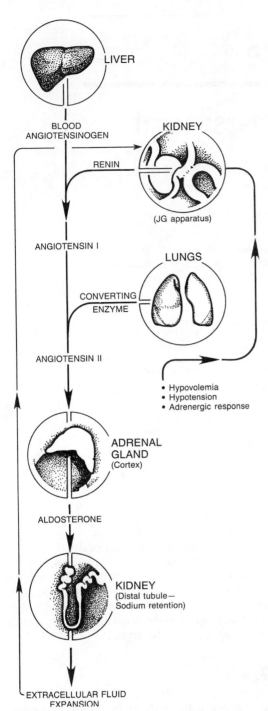

FIGURE 34–5. The renin-angiotensin-aldosterone system is depicted, including the roles played by the liver, kidneys, lungs, and adrenal glands, which culminate in the secretion of aldosterone.

CHAPTER 35

Renal/Urinary Assessment

Jeanette G. Kernicki

CHAPTER OUTLINE

Components of Assessment
□ Clinical History
□ Inspection
□ Auscultation

□ Additional Findings
Laboratory—Diagnostic Evaluation
References

LEARNING OBJECTIVES

After completing this chapter, you should be able to:
1. Identify the key components of the assessment process.
2. Discuss the rationale for use of a systematic format in renal/urinary assessment.
3. Explain the rationale for obtaining a clinical history.
4. Discuss the importance of assessing the skin, body weight, and hydration status.
5. Relate pitting edema to degree of severity.
6. Discuss the rationale for inspection of the urine sample.
7. State the importance of auscultation relative to blood pressure findings and characteristics of breath sounds in renal system dysfunction.

COMPONENTS OF ASSESSMENT

Observation of the patient for characteristic signs of renal impairment is a vital role of the critical care nurse. Monitoring the status of the renal system as an integral part of homeostasis and identifying clues to impending dysfunction is paramount in the care of any critically ill patient. The assessment of renal and urinary status incorporates history taking, inspection, and auscultation as modalities for baseline data collection.

Clinical History

Assessment of the patient is generally begun by obtaining the history of the present illness, associated medical problems, medications currently taken, and clinical findings. Obtaining a medical history of the client is an integral part of the assessment process. Baseline data include information about the onset of signs and symptoms associated with the present condition (frequency, urgency, incontinence, dysuria, hematuria, oliguria, polyuria, and flank tenderness), past medical problems, and familial tendency toward renal system dysfunction.[1]

A rapid and thorough assessment of the patient's chief complaint is possible through the use of the SLIDT mnemonic (Table 35–1).

Identifying clues that may pinpoint the nature of the problem is vital, particularly in clients who do not complain or from whom it is difficult to obtain information. Pain is not an uncommon complaint of individuals experiencing renal problems. The source of pain may be related to urinary obstruction, renal capsular swelling, or renal infarction.[2]

Inspection

Observation of the patient for potential or characteristic signs of renal impairment is vital in any clinical setting. Simply noticing the amount, color, and odor of urine and correlating the findings with laboratory data can be important in detecting signs of impending disasters such as congestive heart failure or frank renal failure. The patient's general appearance, skin texture, color, body weight fluctuation, and areas of edema may serve as clues to impending physiologic problems.[3]

The patient with chronic renal failure (CRF) is generally pale, has a yellow-gray cast or hue to the skin, and may complain of a dry and itchy skin. The paleness is related to deficiency of erythropoietin, whereas

TABLE 35–1
Assessment Tool: SLIDT*

S = Severity—How severe or intense is the symptom?
L = Location—Where is it located? Does it radiate to other parts of the body?
I = Influencing factors
  Precipitating—What causes or predisposes to the symptom?
  Ameliorating—What relieves symptoms?
  Aggravating—What makes it feel worse?
  Associated—What else happens at the same time (e.g., nausea, vomiting, blurred vision)? What is the setting in which it occurs (e.g., home, workplace, during exercise, or at rest)?
D = Duration—Timing of symptom in terms of events and patterns surrounding the patient. When does it occur? How long does it last? Does it come and go?
T = Type—The quality or characteristics of the symptom. What does it feel like (e.g., "throbbing," "constricting," "pounding like a sledgehammer," "knife-like")?

* This assessment tool can be applied to a variety of symptoms, including pain, bleeding, cough, and sputum production.

the yellow-gray cast or hue is thought to be due either to the deposition of a carotene-like substance within the skin or to a problem of the melanocyte-stimulating hormone.[4] Deficiency of erythropoietin or depression of the clotting mechanism activity may predispose the individual to easy bruising.

Clues indicative of the hydration status become important indices for assessing renal system function. The presence of engorged neck veins, particularly while the patient is in a semi-Fowler position, is highly suggestive of an expanded blood volume secondary to sodium retention or to the failure of the heart as a pump.[5] Weighing the patient at the same time of the day, with the same amount of clothing, can provide clues that body fluid retention is present, particularly when coupled with the existence of pitting edema. The latter may not be evident until a substantial body weight gain has occurred. Normally when the skin surface is indented by fingertip pressure, it will return to normal within 30 seconds. If it does not, pitting is present. The degree of pitting can be gauged by use of a number scale, with +1 indicating minimal pitting, and +4 maximal pitting. It is important both to assess the most dependent body parts for edema and to observe the patient for the presence of periorbital edema.[6]

Fluctuation in body weight over 1 or 2 days may indicate fluid gain or loss. A weight gain of 1 kg, or 2.2 pounds, suggests the accumulation of approximately 1 liter of body fluid.[7]

Essential to the inspection phase is the evaluation of urine for amount, color, and odor. The amount of urine voided by an adult within a 24-hour period may range from 750 mL to 1800 mL, depending upon intake and other circumstances. A copious amount of urine does not always imply good renal function. Polyuria is frequently a response to conditions such as diuretic therapy or an excessive amount and type of fluid intake. Coffee, tea, and alcohol tend to promote more diuresis than do other fluids.

The voiding of a large volume of urine can also be associated with disease states such as diabetes mellitus and diabetes insipidus. The urine specimen of an individual with diabetes mellitus will reveal an elevated specific gravity caused by the presence of glucose. However, an actual fluid volume deficit can also cause an elevated specific gravity. Urine osmolality is a better indicator of fluid imbalance since the osmolality is not influenced by the presence of glucose. A dilute urine can also be seen in the early stages of chronic renal failure, wherein there is loss of the concentrating ability of the kidney. A small output of urine may be related to a decrease in fluid intake, excessive loss of fluids through perspiration, vomiting, diarrhea, extensive body burns, and other pathologic or surgical conditions causing an abnormal seepage or drainage of body fluids.

The color of urine may vary from being straw-colored to dark amber. A by-product of hemoglobin destruction—urobilinogen—gives urine the amber color.[8] The color variations are related to freshness of urine, fluid and food intake, ingestion of medications, and other conditions. For example, smoky, dark appearance may be caused by blood in the urine, while purulent matter or pus may give the urine a cloudy appearance.

Freshly voided urine having a foul odor may be suggestive of infection within the urinary tract. Old urine has an ammonia smell, which is related to the breakdown of urea molecules. Additionally, ingestion of certain foods and medications can produce a foul-smelling urine. The characteristic fruity odor of an individual with diabetic mellitus is thought to be related to ketone spillage in the urine.[9] For additional characteristics of urine, see Table 35–2.

Auscultation

The art of listening for specific sounds within the heart and lung can provide information about volume overload or deficit in the extracellular fluid space. The presence of a third and fourth heart sound when accompanied by hypertension could suggest fluid overload. A rapid pulse rate associated with a low blood pressure reading may reflect a hypovolemic state. Additionally, a drop in blood pressure reading (20 mmHg), combined with a change in position from lying or sitting to standing, indicates an orthostatic change designated as orthostatic hypotension. One of the causes of orthostatic hypotension is fluid volume deficit. In the change of position from recumbent to sitting or standing, there may be an insufficient preload to fill the venous circuit.[10]

Volume overload can also be detected by auscultation of the lungs with the diaphragm of the stethoscope. Crackles (rales) and gurgles (rhonchi) are associated with many conditions; however, in patients with renal problems the presence of an adventitious sound generally indicates overloading of the circulatory sys-

TABLE 35–2

Urine Analysis: Constituents and Characteristics of Significance in Renal Function

Constituent Characteristics	Values/Volume/ Descriptions	Clinical Significance
Volume (per 24 h)	1200–1800 mL/day	
	Polyuria > 1800 mL/day	Excess fluid intake, osmotic diuresis, diuretic phase of acute renal failure (ARF), early chronic renal failure (CRF)
	Oliguria < 400 mL/day	Severe dehydration, ARF (e.g., acute glomerulonephritis)
	Anuria < 50 mL/day	Obstructive uropathy; oliguric ARF (rarely)
Gross characteristics:		
Color	Clear, amber	Reflects osmolality, degree of concentration; color changes—may be diet- or drug-related
Clarity	Clear	Cloudy urine may reflect infection; foamy, if albumin is present
Odor	Mildly fragrant or aromatic (fresh specimen)	Pungent on standing, in dehydration, drug-related, or urinary tract infection
pH	Range: 4.4–8.0	Usually slightly acidic from excretion of acid by-products of metabolism; decreased glomerular filtration reduces excretion of acid load
		Alkaline: urinary tract infection, diet-related, respiratory/ metabolic alkalemia, other
		Acidic: high-protein diet, pyrexia, respiratory/metabolic acidemia, other
Specific gravity*	Range: 1.005–1.035	Higher in dehydration or when the kidneys conserve water (concentrated urine)
		> 1.030: proteinuria, glycosuria, x-ray contrast media, severe dehydration
		Lower in fluid volume excess or when kidneys excrete water (dilute urine)
		< 1.010: diabetes insipidus, overhydration
		Fixed: in severe renal disease, urine specific gravity becomes fixed at ~ 1.010, the same as the glomerular filtrate prior to tubular activity
Osmolality	Range: 270–900 mOsm/kg; mean ~ 550 mOsm/kg	Depends on serum osmolality and overall hydration status
		Severe renal disease causes urine osmolality to be fixed, or the same as the glomerular filtrate prior to tubular activity
Urine chemistry:		
1. Electrolytes Sodium	Range: 43–217 mEq/L/24 h	Electrolytes in urine occur as a result of selective tubular reabsorption and secretion
Potassium	27–123 mEq/L/24 h	In renal failure, renal tubular regulation of electrolytes becomes compromised, altering electrolyte excretion
Chlorides	170–250 mEq/L/24 h	
Calcium	50–300 mg/24 h	Calcium excretion decreases because of reduced synthesis and secretion of activated vitamin D metabolite
Phosphorus	Varies with intake ~ 1g/ day	
Magnesium	< 150 mg/24 h	Analysis for electrolytes requires 24-h urine specimens
2. Glucose	Negative	Filtered glucose is normally totally reabsorbed in tubules
		Glucose appears in urine when renal threshold is exceeded
3. Acetone	Negative	Frequently seen in urine during starvation states and diabetic ketoacidosis (DKA)
		A false-positive result occurs in patients taking salicylates
4. Protein	Negative to trace, < 10 mg/100 mL	Protein molecules are usually too large to be filtered, all filtered protein is normally reabsorbed in tubules
		Heavy proteinuria is usually associated with altered glomerular function (e.g., glomerulonephritis) and/or renal tubule pathology
		A 24-h urine specimen is required
5. Creatinine	15–25 mg/kg/day	Concentration in urine decreases in renal disease
Microscopic elements:		
1. Red blood cells (RBC)	None to very minimal cell count	Hematuria indicates renal and/or urinary tract pathology (e.g., renal disease, tumor, ureteral calculi, infection, other)
2. White blood cells (WBC)	None to minimal cell count	Elevated WBC count suggests renal/urinary tract infection
3. Crystals: Urates (acidic urine)	Usually none	Seen in nephrolithiasis or following certain intoxications (e.g., oxalate calculi of ethylene glycol)
Phosphates (alkaline urine)		Composition of crystals may provide clue as to calculus formation

TABLE 35–2
Urine Analysis: Constituents and Characteristics of Significance in Renal Function (*Continued*)

Constituent Characteristics	Values/Volume/ Descriptions	Clinical Significance
4. Casts: Hyaline	Few (<5000)	Casts are precipitates of proteinaceous material formed in the tubules and collecting ducts by agglutination of protein, cells, or cellular debri, and flushed loose by flow of urine
RBC casts	None	Present in glomerular disease (e.g., glomerulonephritis)
WBC casts	Few	Reflect infection or inflammation (e.g., pyelonephritis)
5. Bacteria: Culture and sensitivity	> 100,000 organisms/mL	Indicates renal and/or urinary tract infection
Creatinine clearance	104–125 mL/min 150–180 L/day	This test is used to determine presence or progression of renal disease and to estimate percentage of functioning nephrons $$\text{Equation: } \frac{Ucr \times V}{Pcr} = Ccr$$ where: Ucr = amount of urinary creatinine excreted V = urine volume/min Pcr = plasma creatinine level Ccr = creatinine clearance

*Whitaker, AA: Acute renal dysfunction: Assessment of patients at risk. Focus Crit Care 12(3):12, 1985.

TABLE 35–3
Diagnostic Studies and Procedures for Evaluating Renal Dysfunction

Test/Study	Description	Clinical Significance and Nursing Implications
Radiography: KUB	Flat plate x-ray of kidneys, ureters, and bladder	Reveals kidney position, size, and structure; gross malformations, renal calculi No special preparation and follow-up care required
Excretory urography (intravenous pyelography) (IVP)	A series of radiographs taken following intravenous administration of contrast media, and before and after voiding	Allows visualization of renal parenchyma, major and minor calices, renal pelvis, ureters, bladder, and urethra Reveals altered renal anatomy, renal calculi, residual urine after voiding Procedure: 1. Rule out iodine sensitivity 2. Nothing by mouth (NPO) or clear liquids 12 h prior to test unless contraindicated 3. Evacuate bowel 4. Obtain informed consent 5. Following procedure, encourage fluids and monitor for dehydration and signs of delayed sensitivity to contrast media
Retrograde pyelography	Series of radiographs taken following injection of contrast media by cystoscope	Allows visualization of renal collecting system including calices, pelvis, and ureter May reveal obstruction to flow of urine in collecting system caused by calculi, neoplasms, blood clot, stricture, or adhesions Procedure: (see cystoscopy below) 1. Determine iodine sensitivity
Renal angiography	Series of radiographs taken after injection of contrast media into renal vasculature during phases of arterial, nephrographic, and venous filling Vascular access: Femoral artery most commonly used	Delineates renal vasculature and may reveal renal tumors, renal cysts, renal artery stenosis, aneurysm, or fistula; renal abscess; or trauma. Procedure: (see excretory uropathy above) Follow-up care: 1. Bed rest for several hours 2. Observe venipuncture site for evidence of bleeding (hematoma formation); puncturing of peripheral artery with consequent hematoma, embolism, and thrombosis are serious complications 3. Monitor peripheral pulses 4. Monitor for delayed reaction to contrast media
Intravenous digital subtraction angiogram (DSA)	Allows visualization of main renal arteries	Less invasive than renal arteriography, but false-negative rate is about 10%–12%
Voiding cystogram (cystourethrography)	Instillation of contrast media through a catheter introduced through the urethra and into the bladder; fluoroscopic films and overhead radiographs demonstrate bladder filling and emptying as patient voids	May reveal urinary tract abnormalities, such as ureteral stricture or stenosis; ureteral reflux; measures residual urine volume after voiding Procedure: 1. Rule out iodine sensitivity 2. Establish baseline vital parameters (e.g., blood pressure, heart rate, respiratory rate, temperature)

Continued

TABLE 35-3

Diagnostic Studies and Procedures for Evaluating Renal Dysfunction (*Continued*)

Test/Study	Description	Clinical Significance and Nursing Implications
Retrograde cystography	Radiographic examination following instillation of contrast media into bladder	Assists in diagnosing bladder rupture, presence of neurogenic bladder, residual urine volume, suspected vesicoureteral reflex, tumors, other Procedure: (see voiding cystogram above)
Retrograde urethrography		Provides information about status of urethra and visualization of membranes, bulbar, and penile portions in males
Cystoscopy	Passage of rigid flexible cystoscope into bladder and ureters under local or general anesthesia, and under strict aseptic techniques	Facilitates calculi removal Procedure: 1. NPO 2. Evacuate bowel 3. Obtain informed consent 4. Sedation as prescribed Follow-up care: 1. Encourage fluids 2. Monitor fluid intake and urine output 3. Monitor for urine retention, bleeding, infection
Renal computed tomography (CT) scan	A series of tomograms, or cross-sectional slices, translated by a computer and displayed on an oscilloscope screen Density of the image reflects the amount of radiation absorbed by renal tissue Renal CT scan may be performed after administration of contrast media, which accentuates the density of the renal parenchyma and assists in differentiating renal masses	Permits identification of masses and other lesions of different densities, as, for example, renal cysts, renal tumors, and other abnormalities (e.g., polycystic kidney disease, congenital anomalies, calculi, and other obstructions) Procedure: 1. Determine sensitivity to contrast media
Nuclear magnetic resonance (NMR)		Provides same information as CT scan but has the advantage of not using x-rays
Renal scan (radionuclide imaging)	Injection of nuclide followed by scintiphotography	Allows identification of structure of kidneys and can demonstrate lesions, intrarenal masses, and traumatic injury Dynamic scans assist in evaluating renal perfusion and can identify compromised circulation in patients with renovascular hypertension and abdominal aortic pathology Abnormalities of the collecting system (e.g., ureteral obstruction) can be detected Follow-up care: handle urine with gloves for 24 h after procedure; encourage fluid intake
Renal ultrasonography	High-frequency sound waves transmitted from a transducer through the kidneys and surrounding structures Resulting echoes amplified and converged into electrical impulses and displayed on an oscilloscope screen as anatomic images	Differentiates between solid and cystic structures and localized fluid collections Assists in visualizing renal anatomy, structure of perirenal tissues, location of urinary obstruction, abnormal accumulation of fluid; and in assessing and diagnosing complications after renal transplantation Noninvasive; no special preparation or aftercare is required
Renal biopsy	With visualization of kidney by fluoroscopy or ultrasound, an insertion of biopsy needle is performed percutaneously or by open incision	Highly invasive procedure Assists in diagnosis of renal disease that cannot be definitively determined by other methods Procedure: 1. NPO for 6–8 h prior to procedure 2. Maintain patent intravenous access 3. Obtain informed consent 4. Sedation as prescribed 5. Assess for hypertension, bleeding, or coagulation disorders Follow-up care: 1. Serial vital signs until stable 2. Monitor for complaints of pain and hematoma formation 3. Monitor hematocrit 4. Bed rest for 24 h 5. Encourage fluids; monitor hourly urine output; observe for hematuria 6. Chest x-ray as prescribed to rule out iatrogenic pneumothorax For open biopsy, follow unit postoperative protocols

tem. The patient may complain of shortness of breath with mild exercise or when in a recumbent position.

Shallow, gasping breaths associated with periods of apnea may reflect an acid-base problem.[11]

Additional Findings

Complaints of nausea, vomiting, inflammatory areas within the oral cavity (stomatitis), and anorexia are suggestive of the secondary involvement of the gastrointestinal system in patients with renal system dysfunction.

Hypertension may occur as a result of compensatory mechanisms initiated when blood volume is reduced to the renal artery. Occasionally, long-standing elevated blood pressures may be the cause of renal system problems.[12]

LABORATORY—DIAGNOSTIC EVALUATION

Many laboratory and diagnostic test procedures are available to confirm renal system dysfunction (Table 35–3). The critical care nurse's involvement in the diagnostic workup varies from collecting a urine specimen to preparing the patient for the diagnostic test to assisting with the procedural testing. Each laboratory or institution has a specific protocol to be followed prior to the diagnostic evaluation. Understanding the rationale for the specific test or procedure

enables the nurse to respond knowledgeably to questions the patient may have regarding the procedure, allaying some of the fears inherent with unfamiliar procedures.

REFERENCES

1. Metheny, NM: Fluid and Electrolyte Balance: Nursing Considerations, ed 2. JB Lippincott, Philadelphia, 1992, pp 253–254.
2. Becker, GJ, Whitworth, JA, and Kincaid-Smith, P: Clinical Nephrology in Medical Practice. Blackwell, Boston, 1992, p 94.
3. Roberts, S: Physiological Concepts and the Critically Ill Patient. Prentice-Hall, Englewood Cliffs, NJ, 1985, pp 359–360.
4. Becker, GJ, Whitworth, JA, and Kincaid-Smith, P: Clinical Nephrology in Medical Practice. Blackwell, Boston, 1992, p 144.
5. Hudak, CM, Gallo, BM, and Benz, JJ: Critical Care Nursing: A Holistic Approach. JB Lippincott, Philadelphia, 1990, p 408.
6. Lehman, MK, Soltis, B, and Cassemeyer, VL: Fluid and Electrolyte Imbalance. In Phipps, W, Long, B, Woods, N, and Cassmeyer, V (eds): Medical-Surgical Nursing: Concepts and Clinical Practice, ed 4. Mosby Year Book, St Louis, 1991, p 548.
7. Metheny, NM: Fluid and Electrolyte Balance: Nursing Considerations, ed 2. JB Lippincott, Philadelphia, 1992, p 41.
8. McClintic, JR: Physiology of the Human Body, ed 3. John Wiley & Sons, New York, 1985, p 492.
9. Corbett, JV: Laboratory Tests and Diagnostic Procedures with Nursing Diagnoses, ed 2. Appleton & Lange, Norwalk, CT, 1987, p 59.
10. Becker, GJ, Whitworth, JA, and Kincaid-Smith, P: Clinical Nephrology in Medical Practice. Blackwell, Boston, 1992, p 144.
11. Schrier, RW, and Gottschalk, CW: Diseases of the Kidney, ed 5. Little, Brown, Boston, 1993, p 1376.
12. May, RC, Stivelman, JC, and Maroni, BJ: Metabolic and Electrolyte Disturbance in Acute Renal Failure. In Lazarus, JM, and Brenner, BM (eds): Acute Renal Failure, ed 3. Churchill Livingstone, New York, 1993, p 107.

CHAPTER 36

Fluid and Electrolyte Physiology and Pathophysiology

Jeanette G. Kernicki

CHAPTER OUTLINE

Body Fluid Volume and Composition
Body Water Regulation
Fluid and Electrolyte Imbalances
  □ Aging and Fluid and Electrolyte
    Problems

□ Assessment of the Fluid State
□ Electrolytes
References

LEARNING OBJECTIVES

After completing this chapter, you should be able to:

1. Identify body fluid compartments.
2. Describe the composition and volume of the fluid compartments.
3. Explain the process of intercompartmental transference.
4. Discuss the concept of serum osmolality and be able to calculate it.
5. Understand tonicity of solutions.
6. Explain the role of electrolytes in maintaining homeostasis.
7. Identify the role and regulation of electrolytes.
8. Compare and contrast fluid and electrolyte imbalances.
9. Delineate the nursing interventions in patients with fluid volume and composition imbalances.

The prevention of fluid and electrolyte imbalance is frequently a part of the therapy in a hospitalized patient. The imbalance can be the primary reason for hospitalization and treatment, as may be seen in a severely dehydrated patient, secondary to vomiting, diarrhea, and/or restricted intake, or the imbalance can occur secondary to medical treatments, such as radiation therapy, or as a result of a disease process wherein there is a great loss of body fluids. Restoration of body fluids and electrolytes is essential to avert disturbance in body function. An understanding of the physiologic dynamics that maintain body fluid and electrolyte balance is an integral part of critical care nursing and helps one to understand the disruptive nature of pathologic processes.

BODY FLUID VOLUME AND COMPOSITION

Cells, as integral components of the human body, function best when the fluids and electrolytes within and around them remain relatively constant in volume and composition (homeostasis—intake must equal output). Body fluids consist of water and important dissolved substances—electrolytes and nonelectrolytes (dextrose, urea, and creatinine)—and are distributed among two main divisions, intracellular and extracellular, which are further divided into the intravascular and interstitial compartments. A minor subdivision of the extracellular fluid (ECF, transcellular fluid compartment) represents fluid found in the cerebrospinal, intraocular, pleural, peritoneal, and synovial fluid spaces.[1] The transcellular compartment can become a source of fluid retention, known as "third spacing." The fluid becomes trapped in the interstitial space and cannot be returned into the circulation. Conditions under which third spacing can occur are high capillary pressure (heart failure), low plasma proteins (liver disease, nephrosis, burns, malnutrition, and inflammation), blockage of the lymphatic system (lymph node blockage), and increase in capillary permeability (allergic reactions, burns, and shock).

TABLE 36–1
Distribution of Electrolytes Across the Capillary According to the Gibbs-Donnan Equilibrium

	Plasma mEq/L	Interstitial Fluid mEq/L
Diffusible		
cations	156	152
anions	140	144
Protein anions	16	8
Total	312	304

Source: From Wilson, RF: Critical Care Manual: Applied Physiology and Principles of Therapy, ed 2. FA Davis Company, Philadelphia, 1992, p 657, with permission.

In an average adult, 65% to 70% of body weight is water. The variability of volume is related to age and to the amount of body fat. With advancing age or obesity, total body water is reduced (a 40% to 60% reduction). Women have a greater amount of adipose tissue than men; therefore, the proportion of body water in the adult woman is lower. In an infant, the proportion of body weight represented by water averages about 70% to 83%. ECF provides a constant environment vital to cells and serves the function of transporting substances to and from cells. Intracellular fluid (ICF) facilitates chemical reactions necessary to maintain life.

The solute portion of body fluids consists of electrolytes, such as potassium, phosphate, sodium chloride, calcium, and sulfate, and of nonelectrolytes, such as creatinine, urea, and glucose. Body water serves as the solvent necessary to make up solutions of the solutes.

Electrolyte function is related to the physiologic processes of acid-base balance, water distribution, osmotic pressure, and neuromuscular irritability. Each fluid compartment varies in terms of volume and electrolyte composition. The major extracellular cation is sodium, and the anion, chloride. Calcium and bicarbonate are also a part of the extracellular compartment. Intracellular potassium is the major cation, and phosphate is the anion. Additionally, the intracellular compartment contains magnesium, protein, and a small amount of sodium, calcium, chloride, and bicarbonate. The major difference between the composition of interstitial and intravascular fluid is the presence of protein in plasma (Table 36–1). Mechanisms that maintain equilibrium of body fluids and electrolytes are regulatory processes (autoregulation of glomerular filtration rate, renin-angiotensin-aldosterone system), hormones (aldosterone, antidiuretic, atrial natriuretic), receptors (baro-, osmo-, volume), and the blood urea nitrogen (BUN) to creatinine ratio.

To maintain homeostasis, fluid movement between compartments is governed by the Gibbs-Donnan equilibrium and the Frank-Starling curve. Fluid moves freely between the compartments, generally from a less to a more concentrated area. It does so by the process of osmosis wherein molecules pass through vascular and cellular membranes permeable to small ions and molecules but impermeable to plasma proteins and large particles. The disparity between diffusible ions in the compartments accounts for the differences in osmotic pressure (Gibbs-Donnan forces). Thus the concentration of electrolytes and other osmotically active particles (fluid osmolarity) regulates the passage of fluid between body water compartments. When body fluids are in balance, blood serum has the same osmolarity as other body fluids—from 275 to 290 mOsm.

A serum osmolarity below 275 mOsm may suggest dilute intravascular fluid and fluid overload. A higher serum osmolarity would suggest hemoconcentration and dehydration. Plasma osmolarity can readily be estimated by using the values of the major osmoles—sodium, urea (BUN), and glucose—in the following equation:[2]

$$\text{Plasma osmolality} = 2 \times \text{plasma sodium} + \frac{\text{BUN}}{2.8} + \frac{\text{Glucose}}{18}$$

Thus, given the values Na 135 mEq/L, BUN 9 mg/dL, and glucose 100 mg/dL, plasma osmolality equals 278.8 mOsm/kg.

Discrepancies between body fluid gains and losses are responsible for clinical fluid imbalances. Normally the body gains water from fluids, solid food, oxidation of food, and body tissues, and loses water through the lungs, skin (insensible perspiration), urine, and feces (Table 36–2). The homeostatic property of the body maintains equilibrium between fluid loss and gain (Fig. 36–1). Excessive fluid losses can occur with fever, increased respiratory or metabolic rate, a hot and dry environment, diarrhea, fistulas, gastric suctioning, and ileostomies.

BODY WATER REGULATION

The volume and concentration of body water is maintained by thirst, neurohypophyseal, and renal mechanisms. The thirst mechanism within the anterior portion of the hypothalamus is stimulated by intracellular dehydration. In response to this state, an individual generally will ingest water to satiate thirst, experiencing temporary relief.

The posterior pituitary gland controls the release of the antidiuretic hormone (ADH) and is responsive to ECF, osmolality, and sodium concentration (Fig. 36–2).

TABLE 36–2
Fluid Gains and Losses

Fluid Gain Sources	Fluid Loss Sources
Water from fluids ingested	Water vapor loss (lungs, skin)
Water from solid food	Water loss through urine
Water from oxidation of food	Water loss through feces

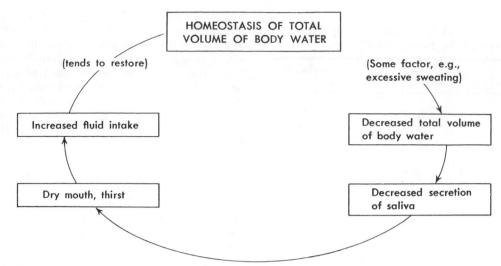

FIGURE 36–1. Homeostasis of the total volume of body water. A basic mechanism for adjusting intake to compensate for excess output of body fluid. (From Thibodeau, G and Patton, K: Anatomy and Physiology, ed 2. CV Mosby, Philadelphia, 1993, p 567, with permission.)

The control of ADH secretion is plasma osmolarity. When serum osmolality is increased, osmoreceptor cells in the hypothalamus are stimulated and transmit a message along the neurohypophyseal tracts, causing release of ADH from the posterior pituitary gland. Water reabsorption in the distal convoluted tubules and collecting ducts of the kidney nephron occurs in an attempt to restore body fluid volume (Fig. 36–3). Fluid volume is also restored by aldosterone, which is released by the adrenal glands and helps the kidneys conserve sodium. The aldosterone mechanism acts on the distal convoluted tubule of the nephron to

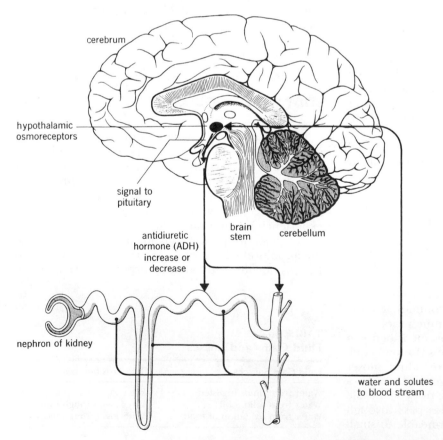

FIGURE 36–2. The antidiuretic hormone (ADH) mechanism for control of extracellular fluid volume and osmotic pressure. (From McClintic, J: Physiology of the Human Body, ed 3. John Wiley & Sons, New York, 1985, p 437, with permission.)

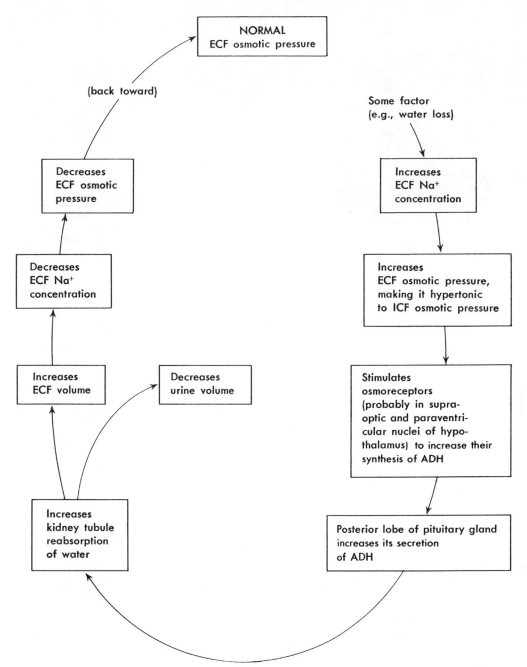

FIGURE 36–3. Antidiuretic hormone (ADH) mechanism for extracellular fluid (ECF) homeostasis. ADH mechanism helps homeostasis of ECF colloid osmotic pressure by regulating its volume and thereby its electrolyte concentration, that is, mainly ECF sodium concentration. (From Thibodeau, G and Patton, K: Anatomy and Physiology, ed 2. CV Mosby, Philadelphia, 1993, p 578, with permission.)

increase sodium reabsorption, which is accompanied by the simultaneous reabsorption of water (Fig. 36–4).

The resultant urine formed under these conditions is hypertonic. The hypertonicity of urine is the result of the countercurrent multiplier and exchange mechanism of the kidney nephron (see Chapter 34).

The atrial natriuretic peptide (ANP) also contributes to regulating body fluid volume. It increases the glomerular filtration rate and is thought to limit the reabsorption of sodium in the distal convoluted tubule

and collecting duct of the kidney.[3,4] An increase in ANP secretion responds to atrial stretch, secondary to volume and/or pressure.

FLUID AND ELECTROLYTE IMBALANCES

Assessing the hydration status of a high-acuity patient can be both challenging and rewarding to the critical care nurse. Direct and indirect measurements

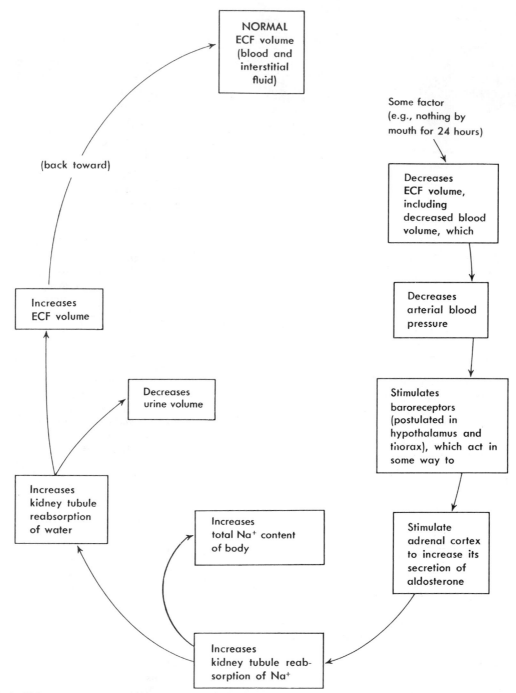

FIGURE 36–4. Aldosterone mechanism for extracellular fluid (ECF) homeostasis. The aldosterone mechanism tends to restore normal ECF volume when it decreases below normal levels. Excess aldosterone, however, leads to excess ECF volume (edema) and to an excess of the total sodium content of the body. (From Thibodeau, G and Patton, K: Anatomy and Physiology, ed 2. CV Mosby, Philadelphia, 1993, p 566, with permission.)

are generally made to detect imbalances from mild to severe. Although imbalances can occur in both the ICF and ECF fluid compartments, the focus of the following discussion is fluid volume imbalance of the extracellular body water compartment.

Actual ECF volume deficit (hypovolemia leading to

hypernatremia) occurs when an insufficient amount of water exists within the extracellular compartment and the compartment becomes contracted. Hypernatremia occurs when water loss exceeds sodium loss. Conditions that may predispose the patient to a contracted extracellular compartment are burns, gastro-

TABLE 36–3
Contrast: Extracellular and Intracellular Fluid Excess Disorders

	Extracellular Fluid Volume Excess	Intracellular Fluid Volume Excess
Definition	*Hypervolemia:* expanded ECF compartment, ECF volume excess	TBW excess; *hyponatremia*
Etiology	Cardiovascular dysfunction: congestive heart failure with pulmonary edema may result in reduced renal perfusion with decreased glomerular filtration and increased retention of fluid in intravascular space Too rapid administration of intravenous saline (overhydration) may precipitate congestive heart failure Renal dysfunction: primary renal disease; renal failure: reduced renal filtration, reabsorption, and secretion cause increasingly larger amounts of fluid to be held in circulation Serum protein depletion and hyponatremia cause ECF volume to become hypotonic to ICF; fluid shifts to intracellular compartment Cirrhosis with ascites and portal hypertension—alters renal blood flow; increased capillary fragility Endocrine dysfunction: hyperaldosteronism	Renal dysfunction: renal disease is major cause of ICF volume excess; renal parenchymal damage disrupts renal handling of water, resulting in fluid overload Syndrome of inappropriate secretion of antidiuretic hormone (SIADH) Excessive oral or intravenous intake
Clinical presentation	*Weight gain:* in excess of 5% of total body weight or >0.5 kg/day *Neurologic:* changes in mental status and level of consciousness; seizures, paralysis *Cardiovascular:* hypertension, tachycardia with bounding pulse initially, possibly progressing to bradycardia if treatment is delayed; neck vein distention; increased CVP and pulmonary pressures (associated with increased intravascular volume) *Edema:* reflects expansion of interstitial ECF volume; periorbital, presacral, extremities, *true pitting edema indicates ECF excess;* skin—taut and shiny *Respiratory:* shortness of breath, tachypnea, dyspnea, cough; rales, pulmonary edema *Renal:* urine output is disproportionately less than fluid intake	Classic manifestations of ICF volume excess reflect central nervous system dysfunction. Increase in intracranial pressure associated with swelling of brain cells accounts for the following symptomatolgy: *Neurologic:* changes in level of consciousness, mental status; headache; weakness, muscle cramps, muscle twitchings; seizure activity; nausea and vomiting frequently accompanying the headache
Laboratory data	No electrolyte parameter (by itself) is indicative of an extracellular fluid disorder; contributing data are reflective of hemodilution	• Serum sodium is an excellent indicator of ICF volume deficit: serum sodium level <130 mEq/L (hyponatremia) strongly suggests ICF volume excess
Serum:		
Hematocrit	Normal to low	• Normal
Hemoglobin	Normal to low	• Normal
Proteins	Normal to low	• Normal to low
Osmolality	~285–295 mOsm/kg	• <285 mOsm/kg
BUN	Normal to low	• Normal to low
Urine:		
Sodium	Reduced	• Reduced
Osmolality	<500 mOsm/kg	• <500 mOsm/kg
Specific gravity	<1.010	• <1.010
Treatment	1. Reduce fluid retention by salt and fluid restriction 2. Diuretics to increase fluid excretion: • Osmotic diuretics • Salt-poor albumin 3. Treat underlying cause	1. Reduce total body water by strict fluid restriction: • Initially fluid replacement is equal to urine output only • As symptoms abate and sodium returns to within normal limits, fluid replacement therapy is increased to include insensible losses in addition to urine output 2. Treatment underlying cause

Continuous assessment of patient's condition and response to therapy, and evaluation of laboratory data are essential to prevent fluid deficit and hypovolemic shock.

intestinal and insensible losses, excessive use of diuretics, diabetes insipidus, diabetic ketoacidosis, hyperglycemic hyperosmolar nonketotic coma, and third spacing. Defining characteristics will vary according to the severity of depletion.

Fluid volume excess (hypervolemia leading to hyponatremia) can occur in the presence of cardiac, renal, or hepatic disease; with the rapid administration of intravenous fluids in the elderly and infants; and with the administration of intravenous infusions of saline solutions. Overhydration, or fluid volume excess, is generally manifested by serial weight gain. A gain of 1 kg of body weight may indicate retention of approximately 1 liter of fluid.[5] Monitoring weight daily and being alert for acute weight gain in high-acuity patients is extremely important. Additionally, the presence of ECF volume excess could be manifested by distended neck veins; moist rales in lungs; a bounding, full pulse; urine output less than fluid intake; slow emptying of peripheral veins; peripheral edema, and central venous pressure > 11 cm of water.

Laboratory data associated with fluid volume excess are decreased BUN and hematocrit. The chest x-ray may reveal pulmonary congestion. See Table 36–3 for additional defining characteristics, laboratory data, and treatment of ECF excess.

Fluid deficits in the hospitalized patient can be corrected by intravenous fluid replacement. The elderly or very young patient, however, generally does not tolerate rapid infusion of intravenous fluids. The type and amount of fluid replacement is governed by the type of deficit and can be a crystalloid or colloidal solution. Crystalloids (having the potential for forming crystals), which include electrolyte solutions, behave much like ECF when infused into the bloodstream. The concentration of osmotically active particles influences the direction of flow across the capillary membrane. If a solution is isotonic (osmolarity is within the normal range for ECF), the solution will be distributed between the intravascular and interstitial space.[6] Conditions such as diarrhea and vomiting can deplete both the intravascular and interstitial volume; therefore, administration of an isotonic, crystalloid solution would replenish both of the fluid compartments. Isotonic fluid replacement solutions include lactated Ringer's, normal saline (0.9%), and dextrose (5%) in water, which, although it is considered to be isotonic while in the bottle, becomes hypotonic in the bloodstream as a result of cellular uptake of glucose.[7]

Fluid therapy with a hypotonic fluid solution (osmolarity less than serum osmolarity) would hydrate the interstitial space to a greater degree than the intravascular space. Solutions considered to be hypotonic in relation to body fluids include 0.45% saline, 0.33% saline, and 2.5% dextrose.

Hypertonic crystalloid solutions (osmolarity greater than serum osmolarity) are seldom used as a means of fluid replacement because of the inherent problems of rapidly expanding the intravascular compartment and depleting the intracellular compartment, causing

cellular dehydration.[8] Hypertonic saline (3% to 5%) has been used to decrease edema in patients with head trauma, sepsis, syndrome of inappropriate antidiuretic hormone (SIADH), and other conditions resulting in hyponatremia.

The infusion of colloids into the bloodstream (albumin, dextran, or hetastarch—Hespan) increases the intravascular colloid osmotic pressure, which tends to pull fluid from the interstitial to the intravascular fluid compartment by means of osmosis. The decision to use colloids for fluid resuscitation depends upon the integrity of the capillary endothelium. Once infused into the bloodstream, colloids remain there until they are metabolized by the liver and eventually excreted. However, if the capillary endothelium is compromised (as can occur in adult respiratory distress syndrome [ARDS], septic shock, and blunt trauma), the colloids can leak into the interstitial space and draw fluid into it from the intravascular to space.

Aging and Fluid and Electrolyte Problems

The elderly population is particularly prone to imbalances of fluids and electrolytes. The physiologic cause for impaired homeostatic mechanisms regulating fluid volume and composition is related primarily to changes within the renal system. In the elderly, there is

1. A decline in renal concentrating ability of the kidney
2. Alteration in sodium balance maintenance—sodium conservation capability declines
3. A diminution of thirst perception
4. An increase in ADH activity, causing a greater degree of water retention[34]

Assessment of the Fluid State

Measurements to identify composition or imbalance of body fluids may be direct (bedside evaluation) or indirect (laboratory tests). Knowing which patients require intake and output records, knowing which are more prone to develop imbalances, and being alert to clues of impending fluid-electrolyte imbalances are vital in assessing the hospitalized patient. An imbalance in fluid and electrolyte status may be the result of excessive losses secondary to the following:

1. Fever and an increase in respiratory rate—a patient with a temperature of 104°F and a respiratory rate of 30 to 40 respirations/minute can lose as much as 2500 mL of fluid over 24 hours.
2. Burns—a loss of fluids through the skin can amount to 1000 to 2000 mL/day.
3. Open wounds—a loss of water, sodium, calcium, and protein can occur.
4. Perspiration—with mild perspiration, a loss of 500 mL/day can occur, while with profuse perspiration, an individual can lose approximately

1000 mL of fluids per day, causing a deficit in water and sodium.

5. Activities and environment—fluid losses can occur with activities that increase the metabolic rate of the body and with a hot, dry environment.
6. Gastrointestinal losses—sodium, potassium, magnesium, and chlorides are lost to the body. Metabolic alkalosis may also occur.
7. Inadequate intake—in a conscious patient, the deficit may occur as a result of anorexia, apathy, lethargy, and difficulty in swallowing. Other patients cannot make their needs known, for example, feeble elderly and infants. In central nervous system disorders, the sense of thirst may be impaired.

Bedside Measurements

Observation of the patient for cues suggestive of fluid and electrolyte derangement is mandatory for critical care nursing. Baseline information can be obtained during the daily assessment and monitoring of patient responses to illess.

1. Body weight—a most sensitive measure. A gain or loss of 1 kg of body weight is comparable to a gain or loss of 1 liter of fluid. The use of the same scale at the same time of the day is essential to determine variability in body weight.
2. Intake and output records.
3. Stool—number and consistency.
4. Vital signs:
   a. Temperature—elevation in a dehydrated patient can reflect a decrease in total body weight (TBW).
   b. Pulse
      (1) *Increased* may indicate sodium excess or volume depletion (either isotonic or hypertonic loss).
      (2) *Bounding* may reflect volume excess.
      (3) *Easily obliterated* may suggest impending circulatory collapse.
   c. Respirations
      (1) Rapid and deep can indicate potential for fluid loss.
      (2) Shortness of breath can indicate fluid excess in absence of cardiopulmonary problems.

Laboratory Tests

The laboratory tests considered to be the most accurate means of assessing the patient's hydration status are serum osmolality, serum sodium, BUN, hematocrit, and urine osmolality (Table 36-4).

Patients who are at risk for a fluid volume deficit must be assessed frequently to prevent complications inherent with a deficit in body fluid volume. At the end of this chapter is a typical nursing care plan for the patient experiencing fluid volume deficit.

TABLE 36-4
Diagnostic Tests

Test and Reference Values[9,10]	Clinical Significance
Serum osmolality 275–295 mOsm/kg H$_2$O	Increases with fluid volume deficit or increase in solute load Decreases with fluid volume excess or decrease in solute load
Serum sodium 135–145 mEq/L	Increase > 145 mEq/L (hypernatremia) seen in dehydration, exchange transfusion with stored blood, impaired renal function, uncontrolled diabetes insipidus Decrease < 135 mEq/L (hyponatremia) seen in loss of sodium from vomiting, diarrhea, gastrointestinal drainage, profuse sweating, use of diuretics, diabetic acidosis, Addison's disease, renal disease
BUN Adult—8–25 mg/100 mL	Elevated with kidney disorders, renal perfusion deficit, dehydration, diet high in protein (tube feeding), gastrointestinal tract bleeding Low during pregnancy and in newborn
Hematocrit: Adult male—45%–52% Adult female—37%–48% Newborn—up to 60%	Increased with severe dehydration, polycythemia Decreased with overhydration; abnormal erythrocyte loss, destruction, and production; bone marrow suppression
Urine Osmolality 500–800 mOsm	Increased with kidneys conserving water, volume deficit, increased production of ADH Decreased with volume excess inappropriate secretion of ADH

An excess in body fluid volume is likewise dangerous in that it can increase the workload of the heart, specifically, an increase in preload. Some conditions are more prone to produce fluid retention, thus resulting in overload. Nursing care is directed toward the identification of priority nursing diagnoses and determining a plan of care to meet the needs of the patient. See the care plan for fluid volume excess at the end of this chapter.

Electrolytes

Electrolytes are substances that when immersed in water dissociate into negatively charged ions (anions) and positively charged ions (cations). They are expressed as milliequivalents per liter. Body fluids and electrolytes are interdependent. Electrolytes are found in all fluid compartments, body secretions, and wastes. Total cations always equal total anions. As diffusible substances, electrolytes readily cross semipermeable membranes of the fluid compartments. Fluid balance cannot be maintained without electrolyte balance.[11] Discussion of electrolytes in this section begins with those that are most commonly measured in the laboratory—sodium, potassium, chloride, and bicarbonate—and follows with those that are less commonly measured—calcium, phosphate, and magnesium.

Sodium

Reference values: Serum sodium 135 to 145 mEq/L

FUNCTIONS

1. Regulates the fluid volume of extracellular fluid compartments. Sodium does not easily cross the cell membrane.
2. Maintains plasma volume and regulates size of vascular compartment.
3. Aids in nerve impulse conduction.
4. Helps control muscle contractility, especially heart muscle.
5. Assists in maintenance of neuromuscular irritability.

Regulation. Because the kidneys can conserve sodium when necessary, serum sodium level is not entirely diet-dependent. A decrease in serum sodium concentration will prevent water retention by means of ADH inhibition. An increase in serum sodium concentration stimulates water retention (ADH release), thus diluting sodium.[12] Aldosterone is thought to have minimal influence upon serum sodium concentration because of the simultaneous water reabsorption effect of the hormone.[13]

Sodium imbalances may be referred to as hyposmolar and hyperosmolar imbalances, or as hyponatremia and hypernatremia[14] (Table 36–5). In hyponatremia, there is an actual sodium loss or fluid volume excess. Hypernatremia reflects either a sodium excess or body water loss. It is important to remember that natremias refer only to serum concentration levels and not to the amount of sodium in the body and that states of water deficit or excess, that is, dehydration and overhydration, frequently are associated with the conditions of sodium excess or deficit.

See the end of this chapter for a nursing care plan for patients with sodium imbalances.

Potassium

Reference values: Serum potassium 3.5 to 5.0 mEq/L

FUNCTIONS

1. Major cation within the cell, contributing to intracellular osmotic pressure.
2. Essential for neuromuscular transmission—by maintaining cellular transmembrane electrical balance, affects the resting membrane potential, especially in the conduction system of the heart.
3. Assists in maintaining acid-base balance.

4. Plays a role in cell metabolism, thereby regulating protein and glycogen synthesis.[15]

Regulation. Potassium has been depicted as being at times a villain and at other times lifesaving—a "Dr. Jekyll and Mr. Hyde" in relation to electrolyte composition of the body.[16] For a cardiac patient in particular, too high a plasma potassium concentration can cause bradycardia, heart block, or cardiac arrest, and too low a plasma potassium level can predispose the individual to an increased sensitivity to digitalis, resulting in digitalis intoxication or lethal dysrhythmias, such as ventricular tachycardia and ventricular fibrillation.[17]

The plasma potassium concentration serves as a guide to the needs of a patient. High serum potassium levels suggest potassium excess while low serum potassium levels reflect depletion. The average diet supplies 60 to 100 mEq of potassium, found in a variety of foods. Rich sources of potassium are found in concentrated meat broths, bananas, boiled meat, skim milk, orange juice, and tomato juice. The kidneys, however, are unable to conserve potassium, excreting 80% to 90% of body potassium. Therefore, daily replenishment is essential.[18]

Intracellular and extracellular potassium distribution is primarily influenced by the sodium-potassium-ATPase pump, aldosterone, catecholamines, plasma potassium levels, insulin, and exercise. Additionally, chronic conditions can also affect the ratio of intracellular and extracellular potassium. The sodium-potassium pump maintains the distribution of the two electrolytes across the cell membrane, keeping potassium within the cell and sodium outside. Because the pump requires metabolic energy for the movement of sodium out of the cell and potassium into the cell, an electrical gradient or electrical potential difference (resting membrane potential) is produced, giving cells the potential for action.[19,20]

The system is protected from an elevated level of potassium by aldosterone, which promotes greater renal excretion of potassium. The role of catecholamines is promoted by receptor type: α-receptors limit the entrance of potassium into the cells, and β-2 receptors promote the uptake of potassium by the cell. Thus patients who are on a β-blocker, such as propranolol, may have a higher plasma potassium level as a result of blocking the cellular uptake of potassium. However, the release of epinephrine during stressful states can lower plasma potassium concentration.[21] In addition, β-2 adrenergic activity serves as a stimulus for pancreatic secretion of insulin. Potassium is thought to be a cofactor with insulin in promoting cellular uptake of glucose.

The role of exercise in potassium regulation is thought to be related to the degree of exercising. The greater the degree of exercise, the higher the plasma concentration of potassium. Physical conditioning tends to attenuate the effects of the large amount of potassium released into the plasma.

Potassium Imbalance. Hypokalemia and hyperkalemia can occur as a result of many conditions. The clin-

TABLE 36–5
Contrast: Hypernatremia and Hyponatremia

	Hypernatremia	Hyponatremia
Definition	Serum sodium levels >148 mEq/L	Serum sodium levels <134 mEq/L
Pathophysiologic mechanisms*	Water loss in excess of sodium loss: dehydration (most common) may occur as a combined ECF and ICF volume deficit Sodium excess without proportional increase in water intake	Sodium loss (depletional): characterized by contraction of the ECF volume Water excess (dilutional, water intoxication): characterized by an ECF volume excess and an ICF volume excess

Etiology	Inadequate fluid intake—elderly or postoperative patient whose water intake is not perceived to be insufficient
	Water loss in excess of sodium: diabetes mellitus—water loss by high serum glucose osmotic diuresis
	Chronic renal failure—inability of kidneys to respond to volume contraction by reducing urine volume
	Diaphoresis—fluid lost in sweat is relatively hypotonic to serum
	Gastrointestinal losses—diarrhea
	Diabetes insipidus
	Sodium excess:
	• Salt craving—high sodium intake without water supplement
	  ○ Hyperaldosteronism
	  ○ Cushing's syndrome ⎱ Excessive sodium
	  ○ Excessive steroid ⎰ reabsorption in
	    administration excess of water
		Depletional (sodium deficit)
		• Diuretics
		• Salt-poor diet
		• Excessive gastrointestinal losses: Severe vomiting, nasogastric suctioning, diarrhea
		• Renal disease with impaired ability to conserve salt when necessary
		• Adrenal insufficiency with altered aldosterone secretion
		• Use of water only to replace sodium and water losses associated with sweating, blood loss, or by transudation of fluid into transcellular spaces (e.g., pleural or peritoneal cavities)
		Dilutional
		• Water excess commonly seen in cardiac failure, hepatic insufficiency, and nephrotic syndrome (inability to excrete free water)
		  ○ Excessive water ingestion or administration of hypotonic electrolyte-free intravenous solutions; excessive tap water enemas and gastric irrigations in which water is used rather than a saline solution
		  ○ Syndrome of inappropriate secretion of ADH

Clinical presentation	Specific symptomatology depends on underlying mechanism
	• Water loss in excess of sodium: A state of dehydration
	• Alterations in neurologic function associated with increased neuronal excitability from increased sodium concentrations: changes in mental status, restlessness, irritability, agitation, lethargy, confusion, coma, tremors, seizures
	• Sodium excess: sodium gain in excess of water (when both are increased) constitutes an extracellular fluid excess (refer to symptomatology of extracellular fluid excess presented in Table 36–3)
		Specific symptomatology depends on underlying mechanism
		• *Depletional* (sodium deficit)
		  ○ Contracted ECF volume with dehydration
		  ○ Altered cerebral function: mental status changes, headache, lethargy, confusion, seizures, coma
		  ○ Cardiovascular: hypotension, postural hypotension; reduced jugular venous pressure
		• *Dilutional* (water excess)
		  ○ Cardiac, hepatic, or renal disease (non-SIADH)
		  ○ Expansion of ECF and ICF volumes (refer to symptomatology of fluid excess presented in Table 36–3)
		  ○ Cardiovascular: no postural hypotension; possible increased jugular venous pressure
		  ○ SIADH: there is an increase in fluid volume but an absence of edema formation; there is no postural hypotension and jugular venous pressure is usually normal
		  ○ Neurologic/cerebral functions are altered by dilutional hyponatremia

Laboratory data	Hemoconcentration
	• Hematocrit: increased
	• Hemoglobin: increased
	• Serum osmolality >295 mOsm/kg
	• Serum sodium >148 mEq/L
	Urine
	• Urinary solution <20 mEq/L
	• Urine osmolality >500 mOsm/kg
	• Urine specific gravity >1.015
		• *Depletional vs. Dilutional*
		  ○ Serum sodium <134 mEq/L; serum sodium levels should be scrutinized carefully in determining type and severity of hyponatremia
		  ○ In depletional hyponatremia, serum sodium falls very slowly until the condition becomes severe; in dilutional states, the fall in serum sodium is more rapid
		  ○ Serum osmolality <285 mOsm/kg
		    Depletional—delayed fall
		    Dilutional—markedly reduced from onset
		  ○ Urine sodium
		    Depletional <20 mEq/L (excludes depletion from primary sodium loss)
		    Dilutional >30 mEq/L

Continued

TABLE 36–5
Contrast: Hypernatremia and Hyponatremia (*Continued*)

	Hypernatremia	Hyponatremia

		○ SIADH
		    Serum sodium <134 mEq/L
		    Serum osmolality <285 mOsm/kg
		    Urine sodium >20 mEq/L
		    Urine osmolality >500 mOsm/kg
		○ Note that urine sodium and urine osmolality are inappropriately high despite a reduced serum sodium and serum osmolality

Treatment	*Hypernatremia/dehydration* (water loss in excess of sodium loss) • Fluid replacement therapy usually with an isotonic or hypotonic intravenous solution. 5% dextrose solution is commonly given over first 48 h depending on severity of dehydration (cerebral edema may occur if hypernatremia is corrected too rapidly) • Electrolyte replacement therapy should begin as fluid loss is corrected *Sodium excess* • Sodium and fluid restriction • Administration of hypotonic intravenous fluids • Diuretics	• *Depletional* (sodium loss) ○ Fluid and sodium replacement therapy using intravenous normal saline (avoid undue haste to correct the abnormality) • *Dilutional* (water excess) (excluding SIADH) ○ Diuretics (furosemide) ○ Treat underlying cause: cardiac, hepatic, or renal disease ○ Spironolactone may be given to reverse secondary hyperaldosteronism • *Dilutional SIADH* Fluid restriction Diuretics (furosemide); demeclocycline to block action of ADH Urinary fluid losses replaced with normal saline

*Data from Metheny, N: Fluid and Electrolyte Balance: Nursing Considerations. JB Lippincott, Philadelphia, 1987, p 57, with permission.

ical picture as well as treatment varies. Potassium and calcium are two electrolytes that affect the function of the heart. Alterations in potassium or calcium balance are reflected electrocardiographically. Therefore, the critical care nurse who is well versed in the interpretation of the electrocardiogram may identify very early changes associated with potassium imbalances (Table 36–6).

Potassium Deficit (Hypokalemia). Hypokalemia generally occurs as a result of renal and gastrointestinal losses and use of loop diuretics. Patients receiving furosemide (Lasix) or other loop diuretics should be monitored carefully by the critical care nurse for potassium loss. The potassium level must be checked prior to administration of potassium-losing diuretics. Additionally, a fall in serum potassium level will occur in the presence of alkalosis because of plasma bicarbonate excess: in the presence of metabolic alkalosis, K^+ ions move into the cell and H^+ ions leave the cell.[22]

Hypokalemia potentiates the action of digitalis; therefore, the patient who has been on a maintenance dose of digitalis must be observed carefully for digitalis toxicity. This is particularly true of the patient who is likewise receiving a diuretic associated with potassium loss. Electrocardiographic changes associated with hypokalemia are flat or inverted T waves, prolongation of the PR interval, and widening of the QRS complex. Rhythms commonly seen in digitalis toxicity are ectopic beats and tachycardia.

Potassium Excess (Hyperkalemia). The most common cause of dangerously high levels of plasma potassium concentrations is renal failure accompanied by oliguria and metabolic acidosis. As the pH falls in acidosis, there is less intracellular exchange of potassium for H^+ ions; therefore, K^+ ions are predominant in plasma. Progressive electrocardiographic changes associated with hyperkalemia are tall, peaked, symmetric T waves; ST depression; PR interval prolongation; flattening to disappearance of the P wave; and widening and eventual merging of the QRS complex with the T wave (sine wave). Sinus bradycardia and heart block are commonly seen rhythms with hyperkalemia.

Nursing care of the patient with a potassium imbalance is both challenging and critical to the recovery of the patient. The nursing care is tailored to the needs of the individual, as presented in the care plan at the end of this chapter.

Chloride

Reference values: Serum chloride 100 to 106 mEq.

FUNCTIONS

1. Maintains the osmolarity of respiratory gases through the "chloride shift," which plays an important part in the buffering action when oxygen and carbon dioxide exchange in the red blood cells. When blood is oxygenated, chloride moves from the red blood cells to the plasma, and bicarbonate leaves the plasma. Changes in acid-base status secondary to altered bicarbonate are reflected by changes in chloride concentration.
2. Presence in parietal cells of stomach is essential for the secretion of gastric hydrochloric acid.
3. Plays an important role in body water balance.

TABLE 36–6
Contrast: Hyperkalemia and Hypokalemia

	Hyperkalemia	Hypokalemia
Definnition	Serum potassium levels >5.5 mEq/L	Serum potassium levels <3.5 mEq/L
Etiology	Acute renal failure, oliguric phase; chronic renal failure, later stage	Inadequate dietary intake: contributory
	Disruption of cellular integrity: crushing injury, trauma, burns	Gastrointestinal disorders: persistent vomiting contributes to hypokalemia by loss of potassium-containining secretions or marked urinary loss of potassium from metabolic alkalosis
	Potassium-sparing diuretics: spironolactone, triamterene	• Persistent diarrhea contributes to hypokalemia by direct loss of potassium or reduced gastrointestinal absorption of potassium caused by increased peristalsis
	Acidosis	Renal losses:
	Aldosterone deficiency (Addison's disease)	• Diuretics
	Overly aggressive potassium replacement therapy (iatrogenic)	• Hyperaldosteronism: hormonal imbalance causes reabsorption of sodium and enhanced secretion of potassium
	Factitious hyperkalemia: hemolysis of RBCs in blood sample; thrombocytosis; hemoconcentration; use of tight tourniquet when drawing blood	• Renal tubular disorder: tubular dysfunction causes loss of fluid and electrolytes
	Medications high in potassium (e.g., penicillin)	Resistance to ADH
		Drugs: gentamicin and carbenicillin cause increased urinary excretion of potassium
Clinical presentation	Signs and symptoms highly nonspecific	Signs and symptoms highly nonspecific
	Neuromuscular irritability; weakness; cramps, progressing to an ascending flaccid paralysis; paresthesias of face, tongue, extremities; symptoms of hyperkalemia often similar to those of hypokalemia	Reduction in overall muscle tone
		Skeletal muscles: fatigue, weakness, hyporeflexia, flaccid paralysis
	Gastrointestinal *Neurologic* } See hypokalemia *Respiratory*	*Gastrointestinal:* anorexia, nausea, vomiting, constipation, abdominal distention, paralytic ileus
	Cardiovascular: hypotension, dysrhythmias	*Neurologic:* apathy, depression, irritability, drowsiness, lethargy, paresthesias
	ECG changes: tented, symmetrical T waves (shortened repolarization); widened QRS, reduced R-wave amplitude, depressed ST segment; prolonged PR interval flattening to absent P waves	*Respiratory:* respiratory muscle weakness, compromised respiratory excursion, respiratory muscle paralysis, respiratory arrest with anoxia leading to cardiac arrest
	• Heart block	*Cardiovascular:* hypotension, dysrhythmias; digitalis toxicity—interplay between digoxin, diruetics, and hypokalemia, a potentially dangerous combination
	• Cardiac arrest	*ECG changes:* Peaked P wave, prolonged PR interval; flattened T wave; depressed ST segment, and elevated U wave (see Fig. 15–40)
		Evidence of digitalis toxicity: paroxysmal atrial tachycardia with Wenckebach (digitalis creates entrance block at AV node slowing ventricular response in atrial fibrillation); AV nodal block may result in junctional escape rhythms; exit block to His-Purkinje system; ventricular tachycardia
Treatment	Therapeutic goals: 1. Correct underlying cause 2. Avoid overly aggressive or too rapid correction of the potassium imbalance	
	Treatment will vary with the severity of the imbalance	Potassium replacement therapy dictated by severity of deficit and presence of dysrhythmias
	Serum K$^+$ level 5.5–6.5 mEq/L with adequate renal function: sodium polystyrene sulfonate (Kayexalate) 15–30 g orally or by enema, two to three times/ daily	Serum levels 2.5–3.5 mEq/L: oral potassium therapy; increased dietary potassium; oral potassium supplements. Relief of gastrointestinal disturbances (nausea/ vomiting) may be necessary
	Serum K$^+$ level >6.5 mEq/L and/or severely imparied renal function:	Serum levels <2.5 mEq/L coupled with cardiac dysrhythmias may require more aggressive potassium replacement therapy: intravenous KCl at concentrations not exceeding 40 mEq/L. If fluids need to be restricted: intravenous KCl 10–20 mEq via buretrol over 1 h, or as prescribed
	• Emergency measures: 10% calcium gluconate is usually administered with continuous cardiac monitoring	
	• 500 mL 10% glucose with 10 units regular insulin, IV over 30 min	
	• Sodium bicarbonate 2–3 amps, in 500 mL glucose, IV over 1–2 h or as prescribed	

Continued

TABLE 36–6
Contrast: Hyperkalemia and Hypokalemia (*Continued*)

	Hyperkalemia	Hypokalemia
	• Kayexalate (as above) • Diuretics (furosemide) • Hemodialysis, especially in cases of impaired renal function	Additional considerations: • Correct alkalosis and/or prevent its occurrence • Monitor serum potassium closely • Monitor renal function: urine output >30 mL/h • Monitor ECG continuously • Patients allowed NPO (e.g., after surgery) should receive minimal potassium maintenance dosage in intravenous fluids • A burning sensation at IV site may indicate that the KCl concentration is overly toxic and the rate should be slowed and/or the dosage decreased

Regulation. Chloride, the chief negative ion in the ECF, is found in a variety of foods. The intake of the anion occurs when sodium chloride is added to food. Chloride is reabsorbed with sodium throughout the nephron; however, the greatest reabsorption takes place in the proximal tubule. The kidneys excrete chloride and sodium and retain bicarbonate when body fluids are acidic.

Chloride Imbalances. An increase in serum chloride level is generally evaluated in relationship to an increase in sodium level or a decrease in bicarbonate. It is rarely the primary abnormality.[23] A loss of chlorides is usually associated with the loss of other electrolytes. See Table 36–7 for the identifying features of high and low serum chloride levels.

Serum Bicarbonate (HCO₃)

Reference values: Serum bicarbonate 24 to 28 mmol/L
Base excess + 2 to −2.

TABLE 36–7
Contrast: Hyperchloremia and Hypochloremia

	Hyperchloremia	Hypochloremia
Definition	Serum chloride level >106 mEq/L	Serum chloride level <96 mEq/L
Etiology	Metabolic acidemia associated with normal anion gap (hyperchloremic) • Gastrointestinal loss of HCO_3^-: diarrhea, small bowel, biliary, or pancreatic drainage/fistula; ureterosigmoidostomy • Renal loss of HCO_3^-: carbonic anhydrase inhibitors (acetazolamide); renal tubular acidosis Other	Metabolic alkalemia associated with: • Direct chloride ion loss (HCO_3^- is reabsorbed with chloride depletion) • Direct H^+ ion loss • Gastrointestinal: vomiting, gastric drainage, villous adenoma of colon Diuretic therapy: conditions that increase sodium loss with chloride following: • Osmotic diuresis • Excessive diaphoresis • Other
Clinical presentation	Symptomatology largely reflects that of metabolic acidemia *Neurologic:* drowsiness, lethargy, headache, weakness, tremors *Cardiovascular:* dysrhythmias *Respiratory:* tachypnea, dyspnea, Kussmaul's breathing with pH <7.20, hyperventilation	Symptomatology nonspecific; largely reflects that of metabolic alkalemia *Neuromuscular:* irritability, muscle cramps, weakness, hyperactive deep tendon reflexes, tetany-alkalemia decreases freely ionized serum calcium. *Cardiovascular:* dysrhythmias associated with hypokalemia *Respiratory:* depressed function
Treatment	Therapeutic goals: 1. Treat the underlying cause 2. Restore fluid and electrolyte balance Treat underlying cause of metabolic acidemia Emergency treatment: intravenous administration of bicarbonate to increase pH Intravenous fluid therapy with Ringer's lactate—liver converts lactate to bicarbonate, further increasing base and pH	Treat underlying cause of metabolic alkalemia Intravenous fluid replacement therapy with sodium chloride and potassium chloride

Serum bicarbonate levels are a part of blood gas analysis and electrolyte evaluation. The term "base excess" refers to the combination of bicarbonate and other base substances that have the ability to bind the excess H^+ ions within the blood.

An indirect measure of bicarbonate is reflected in the carbon dioxide (CO_2) combining power or CO_2 content.[24] CO_2 content (dissolved CO_2 gas) differs from partial pressure, P_{CO_2}, which is a measurement of arterial blood gases. The normal CO_2 content value of 25.2 mEq/L consists of an HCO_3 of 24 mEq/L and of CO_2 content of 1.2 mEq/L, which is equivalent to 40 mmHg P_{CO_2}, with a 3% conversion factor for changing millimeters of mercury to milliequivalents per liter. A P_{CO_2} of 40 mmHg equals 1.2 mEq/L CO_2 content. The ratio of bicarbonate to carbonic acid then would be 20:1. Therefore, if laboratory results do not contain the HCO_3 value, one can look at the CO_2 content value.

FUNCTIONS

1. The bicarbonate anion plays a major role as a buffer of blood, maintaining the pH from 7.35 to 7.45.
2. Metabolic acidosis and metabolic alkalosis are determined by the concentration of the bicarbonate ion.

Regulation. Bicarbonate supply is always present secondary to the production of carbon dioxide—the end product of metabolism. The concentration depends on kidney function in its regulation of available cations to combine with bicarbonate. The anion is filtered at the glomerulus and reabsorbed in the proximal and distal tubules, portions of the loop of Henle, and collecting ducts. See Chapter 23 for additional discussion of the bicarbonate ion.

Anion Gap

Occasionally in the laboratory results involving the electrolytes, there may be a disparity between the number of cations and anions, that is, more positive ions than negative ions. As mentioned previously, chemical neutrality is maintained when the total concentration of cations and anions is equivalent in milliequivalents per liter. The difference between the plasma concentrations of the major cation and the major measured anions is called the "anion gap."

Unmeasured anions such as plasma proteins, phosphates, sulfates, and organic acids may be involved in creating the gap.[25] Clinically the anion gap is helpful in complicated acid-base imbalances, such as acidosis, in terms of identifying the type of acidosis present.

The following formula is generally used to calculate the anion gap:

$$\text{Anion gap} = Na - (Cl + HCO_3)$$

Because of the low concentration and narrow range of fluctuation, potassium is frequently omitted from the calculation of the anion gap. The ionic composition of the major fluid compartments is such that overall body fluids are essentially electroneutral, that is, the number of cations matches the number of anions. See Chapter 35 for discussion of the anion gap in relation to acidosis.

Calcium

Reference values: Serum calcium 8.5 to 10.5 mg/dL or 4.3 to 5.3 mEq/L.

Versatility is the unique feature of the cation calcium.

FUNCTIONS

1. Serves as a framework for bones and teeth.
2. Essential for blood clotting.
3. Plays a major role in the transmission of nerve impulses.
4. Maintains neuromuscular irritability.
5. Exerts a sedative effect upon nervous system cells.
6. Regulates muscle contraction and relaxation, which is very important in myocardial cells.
7. Activates enzymes, which are essential for chemical reactions of the body.
8. Essential for secretion of many hormones.
9. Strengthens capillary membranes.

Regulation. Calcium is the most abundant cation within the body, found primarily within the structure of the bone (over 99%). Less than 1% of total body calcium is in the extracellular fluid compartment, where it exists in two forms: free, ionized calcium and bound calcium, which is bound to proteins, mainly albumin. In plasma, only one half of calcium exists as free ionized calcium (Table 36–8).

Calcium enters the body by way of the intestines. Dietary calcium requires vitamin D for absorption. Of the about 25 mmol ingested daily, only 25% are absorbed. The other source is the bone pool of calcium that can be used to keep serum calcium levels within normal range.[26]

Two hormones control serum calcium levels:
1. Calcitonin—a hormone secreted by the thyroid gland that prevents body calcium excess.
2. Parathormone (PTH)—a parathyroid gland secretion that functions to keep a sufficient level of calcium in the bloodstream. An increase in parathormone raises serum calcium levels while decreasing phosphate levels.[27]

See Table 36–9 for additional information about hormonal effects on calcium metabolism and Table 36–10 for information showing how calcium imbalances can occur as a result of many conditions.

Because calcium is a key participant in so many critical physiologic processes, any disturbance or alteration in calcium metabolism can cause profound, far-reaching, and even life-threatening effects on total body function. The occurrence of hypercalcemia or hypocalcemia is not uncommon in the critically ill patient, who often experiences multiorgan disease

TABLE 36–8
Regulation of Calcium Metabolism

Factors Affecting Parathyroid Hormone (PTH)	Factors Affecting Vitamin D Metabolites	Factors Affecting Calcitonin (CT)
Free, Ionized Serum Calcium Levels ↑ Serum calcium = ↓ PTH secretion ↓ Serum calcium = ↑ PTH secretion		↑ Serum calcium = ↑ CT release ↓ Serum calcium = ↓ CT release
Actions of ↑ PTH Enhances conversion of vitamin D to its highly active form (1,25-$(OH)_2D$) in the kidney PTH increases bone resorption PTH increases calcium reabsorption in distal tubules and collecting ducts within the kidneys	*Actions of Vitamin D* 1,25-$(OH)_2D$ greatly increases calcium absorption by intestinal mucosa Active metabolites inhibit release of PTH possibly by direct stimulation of calcium uptake by cells within the parathyroid glands. Sensory receptors within these glands interpret the increased calcium uptake as an increase in serum calcium levels even though actual serum levels of free, ionized calcium may not have changed	*Actions of Calcitonin* Calcitonin exerts an antagonistic effect on PTH Calcitonin decreases serum calcium by inhibiting calcium mobilization from bone
Permissive Effects PTH requires permissive effect of vitamin D to exert its effect on bone resorption and maintenance of serum calcium levels within physiologic range	PTH is required to convert vitamin D to its highly active metabolite, 1,25-$(OH)_2D$. This function requires unimpaired renal integrity PTH potentiates action of vitamin D metabolite on intestinal mucosa	
Serum Magnesium Levels Hypermagnesemia inhibits PTH release; alterations in serum magnesium may interfere with PTH secretion		Hypermagnesemia = ↑ CT release

Serum Phosphorus Levels
 	
↑ Serum phosphorus:
• Enhances PTH secretion
	↓ Serum phosphorus:
	   Enhances conversion of vitamin D in kidney
	   Increases absorption of calcium from gut
	   Net effect: increase in free, ionized serum calcium
	↑ Serum phosphorus:
	   Decreases conversion of vitamin D in kidney
	   Net effect: decrease in free, ionized serum calcium levels
		Calcitonin decreases phosphate levels by inhibiting bone remodeling and possibly by increasing urinary loss of phosphates

Other Factors Catecholamines } Cortisol } ↑ PTH secretion Arterial pH: • Influences free, ionized calcium	Serum levels of lesser vitamin D metabolites = decreased by barbiturates, phenytoin, chronic liver disease *Alkalemia* *Acidemia*	↑ Gastrin, pancreozymin hormonal secretions in gastrointestinal tract = ↑ CT release Calcium binding to protein increases Free, ionized calcium decreases Calcium binding to protein decreases Free, ionized calcium increases

Effect of Anabolic Hormones
• Growth hormone: indirect involvement in bone formation; influences liver to synthesize somatomedin whose action increases cartilage growth
• Thyroid hormones: exert an anabolic effect on bone formation
• Sex hormones:
   Estrogen }
   Testosterone } promote bone growth and development

Effect of Catabolic Hormones
• Glucocorticoids:
  1. Act to break down bone by removing bone matrix with secondary loss of hydroxyapatite
  2. Interfere with intestinal calcium absorption

TABLE 36–9
Hormonal Effects on Calcium Metabolism

	Parathyroid Hormone (PTH)	Vitamin D	Calcitonin (CT)
Primary function	Regulation/maintenance of free, ionized serum calcium concentration within physiologic range	Stimulation of intestinal calcium absorption	Reduction in free, ionized serum calcium concentration; a weak hypocalcemia agent
Prohormone (precursors)	Preproparathyroid and proparathyroid hormones	Vitamin D_2 (ergocalciferol)—dietary source, fortified milk; vitamin D_3 (cholecalciferol)—skin sterols	
Stimulus for hormone release	1. Decreased free, ionized serum calcium levels. 2. Increase in circulating catecholamines 3. Increase in circulating levels of cortisol 4. Elevated serum phosphate levels: hypophosphatemia induces increased renal synthesis of $1,25\text{-}(OH)_2D$,* which increases the intestinal absorption of phosphate as well as calcium	Decreased free, ionized serum calcium levels stimulate release of active metabolite	Large increases in free, ionized serum calcium levels stimulate calcitonin release
Inhibition	PTH inhibited by increased serum calcium and severely reduced serum magnesium		Decreases in free, ionized serum calcium levels inhibit calcitonin release
Metabolites		Highly active metabolite $1,25\text{-}(OH)_2D$ Lesser metabolites: $25\text{-}(OH)D$, $24,25\text{-}(OH)_2D$	
Actions Bone	1. Immediate effects: Stimulates osteoclastic activity in pre-existing bone cells to mobilize calcium and phosphates from exchangeable calcium pool Transiently depresses osteoblastic activity 2. Long-term effects: Stimulates proliferation of new osteoclastic resorption of bone matrix in addition to calcium and phosphate salts 3. Requires permissive influence of $1,25\text{-}(OH)_2D$ to effectively act on bone	Highly active metabolite of vitamin D $[1,25\text{-}(OH)_2D]$ may be required for mineralization of the organic matrix of bone; this form of vitamin D also helps to maintain stores of calcium in mitochondria of bone cells Lesser metabolites of vitamin D: $25\text{-}(OH)_2D$ and $24,25\text{-}(OH)_2D$ enhance synthesis of bone matrix and its mineralization, possibly to a greater extent than does $1,25\text{-}(OH)_2D$	Decreases activity of osteoclasts in bone resorption Decreases formation of osteoclasts Net effect on bone: Bone resorption Bone deposition by osteoblasts Hypermagnesemia = increase in release of calcitonin
Kidney	1. Immediate effect: Stimulates rapid loss of phosphate by a greatly diminished proximal tubular reabsorption of phosphate ions 2. Long-term effect: Stimulates increase of calcium reabsorption 3. Essential for conversion of vitamin D to its most potent metabolite, $1,25\text{-}(OH)_2D$ Increases urinary excretion of sodium, potassium, and bicarbonate Decreases urinary excretion of magnesium, hydrogen, and ammonium ions	Lesser metabolite $[25\text{-}(OH)D]$ stimulates renal tubular reabsorption of calcium and phosphate [possibly to a greater extent than does $1,25\text{-}(OH)_2D]$	Increases excretion of sodium, chloride, and calcium Increases phosphate excretion Inhibits renal conversion of vitamin D to its highly active metabolite, $1,25\text{-}(OH)_2D$

Continued

TABLE 36–9
Hormonal Effects on Calcium Metabolism (*Continued*)

	Parathyroid Hormone (PTH)	Vitamin D	Calcitonin (CT)
Intestines	Enhances both calcium and phosphate ion absorption from the intestines Potentiates action of vitamin D on intestinal calcium absorption Thus, indirectly increases calcium absorption by the intestines by increasing 1,25-(OH)₂D synthesis in the kidneys	Primary function of 1,25-(OH)₂D: potent stimulator of intestinal calcium-ion absorption	No definitive action on intestines. Increased levels of gastrointestinal hormones, gastrin, and pancreozymin, stimulate calcitonin release

*Vitamin D: 1,25-dihydroxycholecalciferol [1,25-(OH)$_2$D].

usually accompanied by a diminished nutritional state. The recognition and timely treatment of a calcium imbalance can be essential to patient survival. Yet, the early clues as to its presence may be so subtle as to go unnoticed to the unsuspecting healthcare provider. See the care plans for hypercalcemia and hypocalcemia at the end of this chapter.

Phosphorus/Phosphate

Phosphorus exists in the blood as phosphate.

Reference values:
Adult—2.5 to 4.5 mg/dL (1.7 to 2.3 mEq/L).
Child—4.5 to 5.5 mg/dL (2.3 to 2.6 mEq/L).

Phosphate is the only electrolyte that is markedly different in value for children and adults. The higher value in children may be partially explained by the increased amount of growth hormone available prior to puberty.[28] Phosphorus/phosphate is the major anion within the cell. It exists in the extracellular fluid in two major forms: monohydrogen phosphate (HPO_4) and dihydrogen phosphate (H_2PO_4).

The proportion of phosphate forms is determined by the pH of the extracellular fluid. At a pH level of 6.8, monohydrogen phosphate is in equilibrium with dihydrogen phosphate. However, at a pH level of 7.4, there is a greater proportion of monohydrogen phosphate than dihydrogen phosphate.[29]

FUNCTIONS

1. Safeguards the cells.
2. Gives rigidity to bone.
3. Essential to acid-base equilibrium of body fluids.
4. Plays a role in the metabolism of carbohydrates and fats.
5. In the compounds adenosine triphosphate (ATP) and adenosine diphosphate (ADP) takes part in many biochemical reactions to provide energy for cellular action.
6. Promotes nerve and muscle activity.

7. Primary role—releases oxygen from hemoglobin in the form of 2,3-diphosphoglycerate.[30]

Regulation. Phosphate is found in practically all foods. Vitamin D is required for phosphate absorption from the gastrointestinal tract. On a daily basis, 60% of phosphate is excreted through the urine and 40% through the feces. Factors affecting urinary output of phosphate are dietary intake, acid-base regulation, and endocrine influence. The electrolyte is controlled by the parathyroid hormone. Phosphate (HPO_4^{2-}) ions produce a buffering effect, primarily in the ICF compartment.

A reciprocal relationship exists between phosphate and calcium. When the level of phosphate increases, serum calcium levels decrease, and when phosphate decreases, calcium levels increase. The exception to this relationship is in the presence of neoplastic bone disease.[31]

Phosphate Imbalances. Hypophosphatemia and hyperphosphatemia are generally evaluated in relation to the calcium level.

Hypophosphatemia. Among the more common conditions that can cause hypophosphatemia are hyperparathyroidism, diuresis, malnutrition or malabsorption conditions, increased glucose metabolism, and excessive use of antacids.

Nursing measures in patients with hypophosphatemia include safety precautions since a low serum level of the electrolyte is associated with central nervous system disturbances, such as confusion and irritability. The potential for injury is ever-present. Additionally, observing the patient for signs of anorexia and complaints of pain in the muscles and bone is important.[32]

Hyperphosphatemia. The lack of parathyroid hormone decreases renal excretion of phosphates. Childhood diseases in which there is an increase in growth hormone can cause phosphate levels to increase. Vitamin D intoxication can also be a source of high levels of phosphate.

Nursing measures include the observation for signs and symptoms of tetany, which is associated with the presence of hypocalcemia, a consequence of a high

TABLE 36–10
Contrast: Hypercalcemia and Hypocalcemia

	Hypercalcemia	Hypocalcemia
Definition	Hypercalcemia is defined as an increase in total serum calcium above 10.5 mg/100 mL Symptomatic hypercalcemia may occur when total serum calcium levels exceed 11.0–12.0 mg/100 mL	Hypocalcemia is defined as a decrease in total serum calcium below 8.5 mg/100 mL Symptomatic hypocalcemia may occur when serum calcium levels drop below 7.0–7.5 mg/100 mL
Major concern	Progressive suppression of cardiac function by abnormally high levels of free, ionized serum calcium	Increased neuromuscular excitability is caused by increased neuronal membrane irritability Enhanced excitability of nerve fibers causes them to discharge spontaneously and rapidly, generating impulses that pass to neuromuscular junctions (skeletal muscle), where they elicit tetanic contractions
Pathophysiology	Underlying pathophysiologic basis may reflect: 1. Abnormal calcium input into the circulation 2. A decreased removal or output of calcium from the circulation Increased resorption of calcium from bone: 1. Hyperparathyroidism 2. Immobilization 3. Hyperthyroidism (Graves' disease) Abnormally large dietary intake of calcium and/or excessive intake of vitamin D Altered renal tubular reabsorption of calcium Hypercalcemia may also reflect an increase in free, ionized calcium; because approximately one half of total serum calcium is bound to serum proteins, factors affecting the amount of protein-bound calcium must be considered 1. Dehydration increases serum protein concentration, which may reflect an increase in total serum calcium without an increase in the free, ionized fraction 2. Acidemia decreases the amount of protein-bound calcium resulting in an increase in its free, ionized fraction	Underlying pathophysiologic basis may reflect: 1. Inadequate calcium input into circulation 2. Excessive losses of calcium Excessive losses of calcium: 1. Gastrointestinal disorders—diarrhea 2. Secondary to diuretics 3. Increased lipoprotein levels Inadequate intake: 1. Malabsorption syndromes—vitamin D deficiency
Etiology	Primary hyperparathyroidism associated with benign adenoma and resulting in increased tubular reabsorption of calcium Malignancy (metastatic carcinoma), which releases calcium into circulation Prolonged immobilization, resulting in increased resorption of calcium from bone, teeth Alkalemia increases calcium binding to protein, which decreases free, ionized serum levels; potent stimulus for PTH release, with resulting increase in serum calcium Excessive administration of vitamin D resulting in increased intestinal calcium absorption Hypophosphatemia Hyperthyroid crisis Long-standing thiazide diuretic therapy Renal tubular acidosis Use of sex hormonal therapy in the treatment of disseminated breast cancer is known to precipitate acute hypercalcemia Acidemia: aggressive correction of acidemia may reveal an underlying hypocalcemia	Most frequently encountered in patients following removal of, or damage to, parathyroid glands during neck surgery; hypoparathyroidism may occur within 2 days following surgery Malignancy: 1. Osteoblastic metastasis depletes calcium stores caused by abnormal bone formation 2. Thyroid carcinoma with abnormal secretion of calcitonin stimulates osteoblastic activity Alkalemia may independently increase neuronal excitability; patients with chronic hypocalcemia may develop tetany if they become alkalotic Akalosis from vomiting, alkali ingestion, or hyperventilation may precipitate asymptomatic hypocalcemia Chronic renal failure: 1. Hyperphosphatemia precipitates peripheral deposition of calcium phosphate salts in soft tissues 2. Vitamin D resistance caused by alterations in vitamin D—mediated intestinal calcium absorption 3. Vitamin D deficiency resulting from inadequate metabolism of vitamin D prohormones to active metabolites caused by chronic hepatic and renal failure

Continued

TABLE 36–10
Contrast: Hypercalcemia and Hypocalcemia (*Continued*)

	Hypercalcemia	Hypocalcemia
		Chronic malabsorption states associated with: Gastrectomy
		High-fat diet: fat impairs intestinal calcium absorption
		Small bowel disorders with inability to absorb dietary sources of vitamin D (prohormone)
		Hypomagnesemia: inhibits PTH secretion and use; hypomagnesemia must be corrected before normal serum calcium levels can be achieved
		Acute pancreatitis with precipitation of calcium in inflamed pancreas, and intra-abdominal lipids
		Idiopathic hypoparathyroidism
Diagnostic workup/history	*What is chief complaint?* *History of present illness?*	
	Onset / Course / Current status } General state of health? Easy fatigability: muscle weakness—proximal and lower extremity?	
	Neuromuscular: headache?	Neuromuscular: tingling or twitching around mouth? Extremities? Evidence of lowered sensory/motor excitability thresholds?
	Lethargy, drowsiness, paresthesias?	Cramping, stiffness, clumsiness?
	Emotional lability, apathy, depression, personality changes?	Seizure activity, convulsions?
	Visual disturbances or photophobia related to calcium deposits in the eye, conjunctivitis?	Evidence of autonomic ganglia hyperirritability: Alterations in gastrointestinal functions: nausea/vomiting, diarrhea, abdominal pain?
	Renal status: polyuria, kidney infections, renal calculi?	
	Abdominal status: anorexia, thirst, nausea, vomiting, epigastric distress, abdominal discomfort, constipation?	
	Past health history? Pertinent family history?	
	Previous illnesses, hospitalizations?	
	Endocrine illness, obesity?	
	Hyperthyroidism or hypothyroidism?	
	Bone disease?	
	Prolonged immobilization?	
	Tumor or malignancy?	
	Cataracts?	
	Mental retardation?	
	Previous neck surgery and/or irradiation?	
	Previous gastrointestinal surgery: gastrectomy, small bowel resection?	
	Recent malabsorption syndrome?	
	Nutritional derangements: high-fat or -protein diets?	
	Recent massive infection?	
	Renal disease?	
	Rickets?	
	Acute pancreatitis?	
	History of alcohol abuse?	
	Associated hypomagnesemia?	
	Recent massive blood transfusions?	
	Current medications?	
	Anticonvulsants? Antibiotics? Aminoglycosides?	
	Vitamin D supplements—excessive intake?	
	Corticosteroid therapy? Chronic thiazide diuretics?	
	Phosphate binders?	
	Phenobarbital? Heparin? Cimetidine?	
	Theophylline? Cytotoxic agents?	
	Functional health patterns? (See Appendix C.)	
Physical examination (also see section on clinical manifestations)	*Neuromuscular status:*	*Neuromuscular status:*
	Skeletal: pathologic fractures, extraosseous calcifications in soft tissues (hyperparathyroidism).	Mild hypocalcemia: muscle spasms, tremors.
	Ocular/visual status: metastatic calcifications with calcium deposition in cornea; band keratopathy.	Severe hypocalcemia: tetany, grand mal tonic/clonic seizures.
		Classic manifestations: tetany.
		Overt tetany may vary from muscle cramps, abdominal cramping, and pain, to

TABLE 36–10
Contrast: Hypercalcemia and Hypocalcemia (*Continued*)

	Hypercalcemia	Hypocalcemia
	Cardiovascular considerations: increased serum calcium levels can potentiate digoxin effect and predispose to dysrhythmias and/or cardiac arrest.	laryngospasms and bronchospasms, to grand mal tonic-clonic seizures. Latent tetany detected via: 1. Chvostek's sign: elicited by tapping cheek over facial nerve: observe for twitching of upper lip and facial muscles on the side stimulated. This sign is not specific for hypocalcemia. 2. Trousseau's sign: elicited by inflating blood pressure cuff to just above systolic pressure for 3 min. A positive response consists of paresthesias followed by tetany in the occluded extremity. *Pulmonary status:* compromised function related to bronchospasm and airway obstruction: Labored, shallow breathing; hypoventilation; adventitious breath sounds; wheezes; limited thoracic cage movement with involvement of muscles of respiration; use of accessory muscles. Neuromuscular irritability may precipitate laryngeal spasm with airway obstruction and respiratory arrest.
	Gastrointestinal status: vomiting; predisposition to peptic ulcer disease from increased gastric acid secretion in response to elevated calcium Smooth muscle hypotonicity with inadequate peristalsis, constipation, paralytic ileus, abdominal distention, and pain *Renal status:* renal calculi may occur with flank pain	*Gastrointestinal status:* Vomiting, paralytic ileus; abdominal pain and tenderness, distention.
Diagnostic studies: Serum studies	Serum calcium: 8.5–10.5 mg/100 mL (normal physiologic range) Serum calcium >10.5 mg/100 mL Symptomatic >11.0–12.0 mg/100 mL	Serum calcium <8.5 mg/100 mL Symptomatic <7.0–7.5 mg/100 mL
Rule-out studies	Specific laboratory tests: Creatinine, BUN = renal function Liver enzymes, total protein = liver function Alkaline phosphatase: evaluate liver and bone isoenzymes Amylase = pancreatic function Phosphorus: hyper- or hypophosphatemia Magnesium: hyper- or hypomagnesemia	Parathyroid hormome (PTH)—serum levels. This value will help to distinguish hypocalcemia caused by PTH deficiency from that caused by skeletal resistance
Urine test X-ray studies Rule-out studies	Sulkowitch's urine test for calcium Renal calculi Nephrocalcinosis (calcium deposition in the renal parenchyma)	Skeletal bone survey to rule out: Pseudofractures Pseudohypoparathyroidism Osteomalacia Osteoblastic lesions Cancer-induced hypocalcemia
ECG studies	Reveals shortened ST segment and QT interval Dysrhythmias	Reveals prolonged ST segment and QT interval; findings may reflect impaired myocardial contractility, predisposing to cardiac arrest Dysrhythmias
Clinical manifestations	Signs and symptoms of hypercalcemia or hypocalcemia depend on the rapidity of its development, and the extent and duration of the abnormality. Neurologic, cardiac, and renal function are those primarily affected	
Neurologic function	*Mental status:* lethargy, depression, emotional lability; poor recent memory; stupor, coma (severe) Personality changes depending on duration Headache, generalized muscle weakness; fatigue; neuromuscular weakness progressing to flaccidity	*Mental status:* Irritability, restlessness, limited attention span Acute hypocalcemia: Enhanced motor nerve excitability characterized by: muscle twitching; neuromuscular irritability; paresthesias; numbness and tingling of extremities, lips, and mouth; carpopedal

Continued

TABLE 36–10
Contrast: Hypercalcemia and Hypocalcemia (*Continued*)

	Hypercalcemia	Hypocalcemia
		spasm; stridor; seizures; and tetany; the occurrence of bronchospasm and laryngospasm may rapidly precipitate respiratory arrest Chronic hypocalcemia: predisposes to changes in integumentary system with pigmented dry, scaly skin; alopecia; and psychiatric complaints ranging from mild depression to clear-cut psychosis
Cardiovascular function	Increase in extracellular calcium levels predisposes to myocardial irritability, dysrhythmias with increased incidence of heart block, and cardiac arrest Increased peripheral vascular resistance; hypertension	Major concern: decrease in cardiac contractility predisposing to cardiac arrest
Renal function	Early clinical manifestations: 1. Diminished ability to concentrate urine because of a form of ADH resistance* that causes polydipsia, polyuria, and nocturia 2. With sustained hypercalcemia, glomerular filtration rate is diminished from hypovolemia and nephrocalcinosis (i.e., calcium deposits in renal parenchyma). There is the potential for nephrolithiasis from hypercalciuria Flank and thigh pain may be associated with the presence of calcium calculi in the urinary system	Hypocalcemia related to PTH resistance may predispose to pathophysiologic defects in the kidney; patients with PTH resistance are believed to have impaired formation of $1,25\text{-}(OH)_2D$
Skeletal function	Deep bone pain: pathologic fractures	Prolonged hypocalcemia predisposes to osteoporosis
Gastrointestinal function	Anorexia, weight loss, nausea Constipation due to decreased smooth muscle contractility of intestinal wall Activation of pancreatic enzymes or plugging of pancreatic ducts may predispose to acute pancreatitis	Diarrhea from smooth muscle irritability
Integument	Soft tissue calcification	
Eyes	Band keratopathy (i.e., linear deposits of calcium in the cornea)	
Treatment	Acute symptomatic hypercalcemia (>12.0 mg/100 mL) requires immediate therapy to prevent life-threatening ventricular dysrhythmias and altered neural excitability and transmission, leading to coma. A combination of approaches to therapy are used and include[†]: 1. Forced saline diuresis: urinary excretion of calcium is linked to that of sodium. Administration of normal saline and furosemide accelerates calcium excretion. Potassium and magnesium depletion may occur and require careful monitoring. Patients with diminished cardiac reserve require close monitoring for signs of congestive heart failure and pulmonary edema. A fluctuating fluid state may require hemodynamic pressure monitoring. 2. Mithramycin, a cytotoxic antibiotic, is a potent hypocalcemic agent especially indicated in the treatment of malignancy-related hypercalcemia. One dose is found to normalize the serum calcium of most patients within the first 48 h. Its calcium-lowering activity is variable, requiring close monitoring of serum calcium levels. Rarely is it associated with toxic effects	Acute symptomatic hypocalcemia (<7.0 mg/100 mL) of any cause must be treated aggressively with intravenous calcium because of the immediate danger of seizures, laryngospasm, tetany, and respiratory and cardiac arrests Dosage: urgent treatment includes: 1. 10–20 mL of 10% calcium gluconate intravenously, not to exceed 0.5 mL/min. 2. Subsequent calcium may need to be supplied by a slow intravenous infusion while the threat of tetany remains. 3. Oral calcium supplementation can commence as soon as necessary requirements can be tolerated. —Caution must be exercised in patients taking digitalis because calcium's inotropic effects can potentiate the action of digitalis and precipitate digitalis toxicity. Serum magnesium should be measured and monitored because hypomagnesemia inhibits both the release and action of PTH. Correction of hypomagnesemia can be made with magnesium sulfate, which has a rapid onset of action. The dose administered is magnesium sulfate 1–2 g

TABLE 36–10
Contrast: Hypercalcemia and Hypocalcemia (*Continued*)

Hypercalcemia	Hypocalcemia

such as renal/hepatic toxicity; and thrombocytopenia.
3. Glucocorticoids function to decrease intestinal calcium absorption and increase renal excretion. They are especially effective in the treatment of hypercalcemia associated with malignancies and sarcoidosis, the highest success rate being observed in patients with multiple myeloma, lymphosarcoma, and breast cancer. Glucocorticoid therapy is used in conjunction with other therapeutic modalities because its maximum hypocalcemic effect may not be realized for several days.
4. Calcitonin therapy is administered concomitantly with glucocorticoid therapy and acts to decrease calcium release from bone while increasing its renal excretion. Its effect is rapid and without significant adverse reactions.
5. Phosphate administration may be prescribed for the treatment of hypercalcemia associated with a low-to-normal serum phosphate.
  • Short-term glucocorticoid therapy and growth hormone administration increase renal reabsorption of phosphates.
  • Controversy exists over whether phosphate therapy is appropriate. Administration of phosphates will decrease serum calcium, but such therapy may cause extraosseus calcifications with deposition of calcium in soft tissues including kidney and lung.
6. Peritoneal dialysis and hemodialysis efficiently remove calcium and can be used in life-threatening situations.
7. Administer potassium and magnesium supplements to prevent depletion of these electrolytes.
	every 4–6 h intramuscularly, depending on the extent of hypomagnesemia and the clinical status of the patient.
	Long-term replacement therapy may include: oral calcium and vitamin D supplements as prescribed.

*Griffin, JE: Manual of Clinical Endocrinology and Metabolism. McGraw-Hill, New York, 1982, p 178.
†Metz, R and Larsen, E: Blue Book of Endocrinology. WB Saunders, Philadelphia, 1985, p 350.

serum level of phosphate. Urinary output should be monitored since a decrease in output can increase the serum phosphate level.

Magnesium

Reference values: Serum magnesium 1.7 to 2.3 mEq/L.

Magnesium is in an intracellular cation.

FUNCTIONS

1. Coenzyme in the metabolism of carbohydrate and protein.
2. Essential for the functional integrity of the neuromuscular system. Exerts a sedative effect on the nervous system.
3. Has been shown to slow the rate of atrial flutter, to abolish toxic rhythms produced by digoxin.[33]
4. Responsible for transport of sodium and potassium across cell membranes. A refractory hypokalemia may be related to hypomagnesemia.

Regulation. Thirty-five percent of the ion is bound to protein. There is a higher concentration of magnesium in the cerebrospinal fluid than that of serum. Magnesium is abundant in all foods. It is absorbed from the intestinal tract, and what is not absorbed is excreted primarily in the feces, with a small amount eliminated by the kidney. Renal reabsorption is regulated by the parathyroid hormone. See Table 36–11 for a comparison of hypomagnesemia and hypermagnesemia.

TABLE 36–11
Contrast: Hypermagnesemia and Hypomagnesemia

	Hypermagnesemia	Hypomagnesemia
Definition	Serum magnesium levels >2.5 mEq/L	Serum magnesium levels <1.5 mEq/L
Etiology	Renal failure, oliguric phase, resulting in decreased urinary excretion of magnesium Excessive use of magnesium-containing compounds: laxatives—milk of magnesia; antacids—Gelusil, magnesium oxide; Epsom salts Overdose of magnesium replacement therapy; excessive parenteral administration Hemoconcentration (dehydration)	Gastrointestinal losses: malabsorption syndrome: severe diarrhea, steatorrhea; long-term gastrointestinal suctioning; intestinal fistula; malnutrition; pancreatitis secondary to alcoholism Renal disorders: renal failure—diuretic phase; after administration of diuretics (e.g., furosemide) Hyperaldosteronism Hyperparathyroidism, thyrotoxicosis Toxemia of pregnancy Chronic alcoholism (increased urinary loss and probably decreased intake) After-drug use: aminoglycosides, cisplatin, digoxin, ethyl alcohol
Clinical presentation	Symptomatology reflects CNS depression with coma, lethargy, decreased respiratory rate, and bradycardia, which can progress to cardiac arrest There is depressed neuronal activity and transmission of neuromuscular impulses; muscle weakness and an ascending flaccid paralysis may occur Hypotension frequently occurs ECG changes similar to those occurring in hyperkalemia (e.g., peaked T wave) may become evident; prolonged PR and QRS duration	Symptomatology reflects increased neuromuscular excitation characterized by muscle weakness, tremors, muscle spasms Severe hypomagnesemia may present with generalized tetany, and seizures Other signs and symptoms may include: confusion, coma, dizziness, gastrointestinal symptoms, including anorexia and nausea ECG changes: flat or inverted T wave; possible ST-segment depression; prolonged QT interval
Treatment	Therapeutic goals: 1. Correct underlying disorder 2. Restore and maintain fluid and electrolyte balance 3. Identify high-risk patients In renal failure, dialysis may be indicated: hemodialysis or peritoneal dialysis Calcium gluconate may be administered to antagonize the effects of hypermagnesemia Observe for respiratory distress while efforts are made to reduce the magnesium levels Monitor continuous ECG and magnesium levels Magnesium toxicity can be treated with calcium gluconate, diuretics; tapering of magnesium-containing drugs; and by dialysis	Emergency treatment: • Magnesium sulfate 1–2 g 10–20% solution IV not to exceed 1.5 mL/min; kidney function should be assessed • Observe patient for signs of magnesium toxicity: flushing from peripheral vasodilation, hypotension, weakness, diminished to absent deep tendon reflexes, drowsiness, lethargy Maintenance magnesium dosage: 10 mEq/day Establish seizure precautions Note that hypomagnesemia will enhance digitalis effect predisposing to digitalis toxicity; monitor ECG

REFERENCES

1. Krieger, JN, and Sherrard, DJ: Practical Fluids and Electrolytes. Appleton & Lange, Norwalk, CT, 1991, pp 104–108.
2. Rose, BD: Clinical Physiology of Acid-Base and Electrolyte Disorders, ed 4. McGraw-Hill, New York, 1994, pp 639–644.
3. Vander, AJ: Renal Physiology, ed 3. McGraw-Hill, New York, 1991, p 127.
4. Rose, BD: Clinical Physiology of Acid-Base and Electrolyte Disorders, ed 4. McGraw-Hill, New York, 1994, pp 173–178.
5. Holloway, N: Nursing the Critically Ill Adult, ed 4. Addison-Wesley, Redwood City, CA, 1993, p 456.
6. Gasparis, L, Murray, E, and Ursomanno, P: I.V. solutions: Which one's right for your patient? Nursing '89, 19(4):62–64, April 1989.
7. Sommers, M: Rapid fluid resuscitation: How to correct dangerous deficits. Nursing '90 20(1):52–58, January 1990.
8. Mathewson, M: Intravenous therapy. Crit Care Nurse 9(2):23, February 1989.
9. Kee, JL: Laboratory and Diagnostic Tests with Nursing Implications, ed 2. Appleton & Lange, Norwalk, CT, 1987, pp 5–6.
10. Corbett, JV: Laboratory Tests and Diagnostic Procedures with Nursing Diagnoses, ed 2. Appleton & Lange, Norwalk, CT, 1987, pp 648–652.
11. Sprauve, D: Fluids, electrolytes, and acid-base balance. Nursing '90 20(3):103, March 1990.
12. Krieger, JN and Sherrard, DJ: Practical Fluids and Electrolytes. Appleton & Lange, Norwalk, CT, 1991, pp 103–105.
13. Guyton, AC: Textbook of Medical Physiology, ed 7. WB Saunders, Philadelphia, 1986, p 911.
14. Kee, JL: Laboratory and Diagnostic Tests with Nursing Implications, ed 2. Appleton & Lange, Norwalk, CT, 1987, p 300.
15. Rose, BD: Clinical Physiology of Acid-Base and Electrolyte Disorders, ed 4. McGraw-Hill, New York, 1994, pp 346–347.
16. Rice, V: The role of potassium in health and disease. Crit Care Nurse 2(4):54, May/June 1982.
17. Krieger, JN and Sherrard, DJ: Practical Fluids and Electrolytes. Appleton & Lange, Norwalk, CT, 1991, p 144.

18. Kee, JL: Laboratory and Diagnostic Tests with Nursing Implications, ed 2. Appleton & Lange, Norwalk, CT, 1987, p 262.
19. Phipps, WJ, Long, BC, Woods, NF, and Cassemeyer, VL: Medical-Surgical Nursing, ed 4. Mosby–Year Book, St Louis, 1991, p 1710.
20. Rose, BD: Clinical Physiology of Acid-Base and Electrolyte Disorders, ed 4. McGraw-Hill, New York, 1994, p 348.
21. Rose, BD: Clinical Physiology of Acid-Base and Electrolyte Disorders, ed 4. McGraw-Hill, New York, 1994, p 349.
22. Kokko, JP and Tannen, RL: Fluids and Electrolytes, ed 2. WB Saunders, Philadelphia, 1990, pp 22–23.
23. Corbett, JV: Laboratory Tests and Diagnostic Procedures with Nursing Diagnoses, ed 2. Appleton & Lange, Norwalk, CT, 1987, p 118.
24. Corbett, JV: Laboratory Tests and Diagnostic Procedures with Nursing Diagnoses, ed 2. Appleton & Lange, Norwalk, CT, 1987, p 120.
25. Krieger, JN and Sherrard, DJ: Practical Fluids and Electrolytes. Appleton & Lange, Norwalk, CT, 1991, pp 171–172.
26. Metheny, NM: Fluid and Electrolyte Balance: Nursing Considerations, ed 2. JB Lippincott, Philadelphia, 1992, p 96.
27. Kinsey, E and Smith, M: fluids and Electrolytes: A Conceptual Approach. Churchill Livingstone, New York, 1991, pp 130–133.
28. Corbett, JV: Laboratory Tests and Diagnostic Procedures with Nursing Diagnoses, ed 2. Appleton & Lange, Norwalk, CT, 1987, p 164.
29. Kinsey, E and Smith, M: Fluids and Electrolytes: A Conceptual Approach. Churchill Livingstone, New York, 1991, pp 134–35.
30. Seshardi, V and Meyer-Tettambel, O: Electrolyte and drug management in nutritional support. Crit Care Nurs Clin North Am 5(1):33, March 1993.
31. Kinsey, E and Smith, M: Fluids and Electrolytes: A Conceptual Approach. Churchill Livingstone, New York, 1991, pp 136–137.
32. Corbett, JV: Laboratory Tests and Diagnostic Procedures with Nursing Diagnoses, ed 2. Appleton & Lange, Norwalk, CT, 1987, p 165–166.
33. Kee, JL: Laboratory and Diagnostic Tests with Nursing Implications, ed 2. Appleton & Lange, Norwalk, CT, 1987, p 230.
34. Miller, M: Fluid and electrolyte balance in the elderly. Geriatrics 42(11):66, November 1987.

CARE PLAN FOR THE PATIENT WITH FLUID AND ELECTROLYTE IMBALANCE: FLUID VOLUME DEFICIT

Nursing Diagnoses

Nursing Diagnosis #1
Fluid volume deficit:
Actual, related to:
1. Extracellular dehydration (hypovolemia).
2. Intracellular dehydration (hypernatremia).

Desired Patient Outcomes

Patient's condition will stabilize:
1. Neurologic status: Oriented to person, place, date; deep tendon reflexes brisk.
2. Hemodynamic status will stabilize as follows:
   - Heart rate >60 but <100 beats/min.
   - Arterial BP within 10 mmHg of baseline.
   - CVP mean 0–8 mmHg.
   - PAP <25 mmHg (systolic).
   - PCWP mean 8–12 mmHg.
   - CO 4–8 L/min.
3. Body temperature ~98.6°F (37.0°C).
4. Body weight will stabilize within 5% of baseline.
5. Serum osmolality will stabilize at 275–295 mOsm/kg.
6. Serum sodium >1351 but <145 mEq/L.
7. Serum glucose, BUN, creatinine, hematocrit stabilized at optimum levels for patient.
8. Hourly urine output: >30 mL/h.

Nursing Interventions

- Assess impact of fluid volume deficit on body processes.

- Assess neurologic status.
  - Level of consciousness.
  - Behavioral changes: irritability, restlessness, listlessness, lethargy.
- Assess status of hemodynamic function.

  - Heart rate; peripheral pulses (quality—weak, thready).
  - Tachypnea, "air hunger."

Rationales

- Decreased intravascular volume triggers three compensatory mechanisms:
  - Renin-angiotensin-aldosterone system.
  - Thirst mechanism.
  - ADH secretion in response to serum hyperosmolality.
- Hyperosmolar state associated with severe dehydration usually reflects ICF deficit as well as contraction of the ECF volume; alterations in neurologic status primarily reflect *ICF* volume deficit (see below).
- Alterations in hemodynamic function primarily reflect *ECF* volume deficit.
  - Hypovolemia causes tachycardia (heart rate >100 bpm); the increase in heart rate is a compensatory mechanism to maintain cerebral and renal perfusion in the presence of a depleted intravascular blood volume.

CARE PLAN FOR THE PATIENT WITH FLUID AND ELECTROLYTE IMBALANCE: FLUID VOLUME DEFICIT (*Continued*)

Nursing Interventions

- ○ Postural (orthostatic) hypotension.

- ○ CVP reduced: <1 mmHg.

- ○ PCWP reduced: <4 mmHg.

- • Monitor body temperature: fever.

- • Assess renal function.

  - ○ BUN serum creatinine, serum osmolality, BUN-creatinine ratio.
  - ○ Urine output—decreased; specific gravity—increased (>1.030).
  - ○ Total fluid intake and output including urine output, insensible losses by lungs and skin, gastric suctioning, gastrointestinal losses by vomiting, diarrhea, wound drainage, iatrogenic losses (blood sampling).
  - ○ Assess gastrointestinal function: anorexia; nausea; vomiting; abdominal cramps and distention; diarrhea or constipation.
- • Assess body weight (daily).

- • Monitor laboratory values.

  - ○ Total serum protein.
  - ○ Hematocrit, hemoglobin, and serum electrolytes.
- • Monitor other parameters.

  - ○ Mucous membranes.
  - ○ Skin turgor over sternum and forehead; sunken eyeballs.
  - ○ Third spacing, fluid accumulation.

- • Collaborate with physician to correct underlying cause of fluid imbalance.
  - ○ Causes of ECF volume deficit:
- • Infection with hyperpyrexia and diaphoresis.
    - □ Renal: overly aggressive diuretic therapy.
    - □ Gastrointestinal dysfunction.
- • Third spacing fluid accumulation.
  - ○ Causes of ICF volume deficit:
    - □ Insufficient water intake (comatose patient; postoperative patient).
    - □ Excessive water loss (fever with profuse diaphoresis, gastroenteritis with diarrhea, diabetes mellitus, diabetic ketoacidosis, diabetes insipidus).
- • Implement fluid replacement regimen.
  - ○ ECF: saline deficit.

    - □ Implement prescribed treatment: saline fluid replacement orally or intravenously until oliguria is relieved, hemodynamic parameters stabilize, and neurologic status is intact.

Rationales

- ○ A drop in systolic blood pressure >10 mmHg from supine to upright position signals compromised hemodynamics.
- ○ Reduced CVP reflects decreased venous return to heart caused by hypovolemia.
- ○ PCWP reflects status of left ventricular function and ECF volume.
- • Profuse diaphoresis associated with fever aggravates underlying dehydrated state; dehydration decreases the amount of body water available for cooling, and, thus, body temperature rises.
- • Reduced renal perfusion associated with hypovolemia may compromise renal function; reduced glomerular filtration rate predisposes to oliguria.
  - ○ When BUN-creatinine ratio increases in favor of BUN (>10:1), conditions such as hypovolemia or reduced renal perfusion may be present.

- • Change in body weight is best indicator of fluid state; weight should be measured daily under the same conditions.
- • These values may be elevated in part from severe volume contraction with intravascular hemoconcentration.
  - ○ Hypoproteinemia may require replacement if protein loss is from the intravascular space; colloidal intravascular osmotic pressure is essential for maintaining intravascular volume.
  - ○ Dry mucous membranes reflect dehydrated state.
  - ○ Loss of interstitial (ECF) fluid reduces elasticity of skin. Fluid accumulation in third spaces is lost to body use; a tape measure can be used to determine expansion of body parts from progressive fluid accumulation as, for example, abdominal girth (ascites). Mark areas clearly, and measure at the same point using same tape measure.
- • Correction of the underlying cause contributing to the fluid loss is essential if hypovolemia is to be successfully treated and normovolemia restored.

  - ○ Results in excessive loss of Na, Cl, and H_2O.
  - ○ Gastrointestinal secretions contain large amount of Na, Cl, and H_2O.

  - ○ Unable to respond to thirst stimulus; NPO without adequate intravenous replacement.

- • Goal of fluid replacement therapy is to restore volume without rapid fluid shifts or alteration in electrolyte concentrations.
    - □ Rapid rehydration with isotonic saline is treatment of choice in fluid volume deficit caused by ECF imbalance.
    - □ Guideline: one half of estimated fluid deficit is replaced within first 12 h; remaining fluid deficit replaced over subsequent 24 h.

CARE PLAN FOR THE PATIENT WITH FLUID AND ELECTROLYTE IMBALANCE: FLUID VOLUME DEFICIT (*Continued*)

Nursing Interventions	Rationales
	□ Fluid volume and rate of administration will depend on severity of dehydration and effectiveness in relieving underlying cause. Isotonic saline (0.9N saline) or lactated Ringer's solution is usually prescribed.
□ Monitor rehydration closely: careful documentation of all fluid intake and losses; fluid losses include urinary output, gastric suctioning, insensible losses by lungs and skin, iatrogenic losses.	□ Overly aggressive fluid replacement therapy may precipitate fluid excess, with its attendant danger of congestive heart failure/pulmonary edema and cerebral edema.
□ Insert Foley catheter to monitor urine output closely.	□ Accurate assessment of urinary output is essential to assess renal function and to determine fluid and electrolyte therapy.
□ Monitor for signs of fluid excess: elevated hemodynamic parameter; neck vein distention in upright position (45 degrees); dependent or pitting edema.	□ Edema reflects an extracellular imbalance.
○ ICF deficit: water deficit (hypernatremia).	○ Loss of ICF (as opposed to ECF loss discussed above) causes a shrinkage in cell size from loss of water; shrinkage of brain cells in this manner underlies the symptomatology associated with ICF loss.
□ Assess neurologic function: weakness, restlessness, irritability; hyperpnea with danger of sudden respiratory arrest; tetany.	
□ Implement: water replacement orally or intravenously with 5% dextrose in water IV, and avoid further water loss: keep patient and environment cool; use of antipyretics may be indicated for fever.	□ Rapid rehydration with 5% dextrose in water is treatment of choice in fluid volume deficit caused by ICF imbalance.
□ Monitor serum sodium levels, serum proteins, urinary sodium, and urine specific gravity.	□ A sodium level >145 mEq/L indicates ICF deficit. Urinary sodium may be detectable in measurable amounts; urine specific gravity is elevated.

Nursing Diagnoses	Desired Patient Outcomes
Nursing Diagnosis #2 Oral mucous membranes, alteration in.	1. Mucous membranes will remain clean, moist, and without cracking or fissures.

Nursing Diagnoses	Desired Patient Outcomes
Nursing Diagnosis #3 Skin integrity, impairment: potential.	1. Skin warm and dry; turgor over forehead and sternum elastic.

Nursing Interventions	Rationales
• Implement supportive nursing care measures.	
○ Assist with oral hygiene.	
□ Maintain hydration as prescribed.	□ Keeps mucous membranes moist.
□ Assess mouth and pharynx for lesions, fissures, bleeding.	□ Assists in determining changes in the mucosa and the effectiveness of therapy.
□ Apply Vaseline or swabs with glycerin.	□ Prevents cracking and fissure formation.
□ Offer fluids as indicated/tolerated.	
○ Maintain skin integrity.	
□ Assess skin for edema, breakdown, dryness.	□ Daily inspection helps in recognizing potential problem area, enabling timely intervention to prevent complications.
	□ In illness, tissues are more easily impaired.
□ Provide comfort measures: massaging, turning, positioning, protecting bony prominences.	
○ Involve patient/family in daily care when appropriate.	○ Participation in self-care enables patient/family to assume responsibility for their health.
○ Prescribe appropriate level of activity:	○ Progressive increase in activity as tolerated promotes general well-being and reduces risk of complications associated with immobility (e.g., impairment of skin integrity and thromboembolic complications).
□ Bed rest while while orthostatic (postural) hypotension and heart rate changes are significant; progressive activity as tolerated.	

Arterial BP = systolic/diastolic; CO = cardiac output; CVP = central venous pressure; PAP = pulmonary artery pressure; PCWP = pulmonary capillary wedge pressure.

CARE PLAN FOR THE PATIENT WITH FLUID AND ELECTROLYTE IMBALANCE: FLUID VOLUME EXCESS

Nursing Interventions

Nursing Diagnosis #1
Fluid volume, alteration in: excess, related to:
1. Extracellular overhydration (hypervolemia) (circulatory overload).
2. Intracellular overhydration (hyponatremia).

Rationales

Patient's condition will stabilize:
1. Neurologic status:
   - Oriented to person, place, time; deep tendon reflexes brisk.
2. Hemodynamic status will stabilize as follows:
   - Heart rate >60 but <100 beats/min.
   - Arterial BP within 10 mmHg of baseline.
   - CVP $\overline{mean}$ 0–8 mmHg.
   - PAP <25 mmHg (systolic).
   - PCWP $\overline{mean}$ 8–12 mmHg.
   - CO 4–8 L/min.
3. Body temperature ~98.6°F (37°C).
4. Body weight will stabilize within 5% of baseline.
5. Serum osmolality will stabilize at ~285–295 mOsm/kg.
6. Serum sodium: >135 but <148 mEq/L.
7. Serum glucose, BUN and creatinine, hematocrit stabilized at optimum for patient.
8. Hourly urine output: >30 mL/h.
9. Respiratory status:
   - Lung fields resonant and without rales (crackles).

Nursing Interventions

- Assess impact of fluid volume excess on body processes.
  - Assess neurologic status: level of consciousness; mental status changes; confusion, lethargy; behavioral changes: irritability, restlessness, listlessness; headache; weakness, muscle twitchings, convulsions, coma.

  - Assess status of hemodynamic function: pitting or dependent edema reflects expansion of interstitial fluid volume; skin pale, moist, and cool to touch in edematous areas; heart rate: tachycardia; peripheral pulses; bounding quality; elevated systolic blood pressure.
    - CVP increases >6–8 mmHg.

    - PCWP increases >15 mmHg.
    - Neck vein distention in upright position (45 degrees).
    - Heart sounds: an S_3 and S_4 frequently occur in the setting of fluid overload with congestive heart failure.
  - Assess pulmonary function: tachypnea, dyspnea, increased respiratory rate, moist rales, productive cough.
  - Assess gastrointestinal function: anorexia, nausea, vomiting, constipation.
  - Assess renal function: oliguria, periorbital edema, BUN, serum creatinine, urine output, urine specific gravity.

  - Assess body weight (daily); weight gain >5% of baseline weight is significant.

  - Monitor laboratory data:
    - Serum sodium <135 mEq/L.
    - Serum proteins, albumin decreased.
    - Hematocrit: Low in ECF volume excess; normal in ICF volume excess.

Rationales

  - Hypo-osmolar state (excess of water or sodium depletion) usually reflects intracellular fluid volume excess, which is characterized by alterations in neurologic function.
  - An increase in intracranial pressure is related to swelling of brain cells from water excess.
  - Alterations in hemodynamic function primarily reflect ECF volume excess.
  - Elderly patients may develop dependent edema with relatively little fluid excess (e.g., mild congestive heart failure).

    - Increased CVP reflects the increased venous return caused by hypervolemia.
    - PCWP reflects left ventricular function and its effectiveness in handling increased fluid volume.

    - Congestive heart failure with pulmonary edema may be precipitated when the increased fluid volume is in excess of the amount of fluid the heart can effectively pump.

  - ECF volume excess is commonly associated with primary renal disease or with conditions that reduce renal perfusion (e.g., congestive heart failure, liver disease).
  - Body weight measurement is an excellent indicator of total body water. Rule: 1 kg (2.2 lb) equals 1 L fluid; weight should be measured daily under same conditions.

  - Reduced serum sodium is the best indicator of ICF volume excess.
  - Number and size of red blood cells remain unchanged in increased plasma volume.

CARE PLAN FOR THE PATIENT WITH FLUID AND ELECTROLYTE IMBALANCE:
FLUID VOLUME EXCESS (*Continued*)

Nursing Interventions	Rationales

• Collaborate with physician to correct underlying cause of the fluid imbalance.
   ○ Causes of ECF volume excess:
	○ Correction of underlying cause contributing to fluid gain is essential if the hypervolemia is to be successfully treated and normovolemia restored.
	   □ Decreased renal perfusion with decreased glomerular filtration rate predisposes to oliguria.

□ Cardiac insufficiency, congestive heart failure.
    □ Cirrhosis, hepatic insufficiency; hypoproteinemia; overly aggressive intravenous fluid therapy.
   ○ Causes of ICF volume excess:
    □ Parenchymal renal disease most common cause; iatrogenic (e.g., excessive administration of hypotonic fluid); syndrome of inappropriate antidiuretic hormone secretion.
	□ Diseased kidneys unable to excrete water load.

• Implement treatment for ECF volume excess.
   ○ Implement prescribed treatment of sodium (saline) and fluid restriction.
    □ Intravenous therapy is usually prescribed in amounts to cover sensible (urine) and insensible (skin and lungs) fluid losses only (initially).
    □ Hypertonic intravenous solutions may be used:
    –Osmotic diuretic agents include mannitol, 10% and 50% dextrose in water, and urea preparations.
	• Goal of therapy is to reduce fluid volume without rapid fluid shifts or alteration in electrolyte balance.
	   □ Goal of fluid restriction is the loss of about 0.5 kg of body weight per day.
	   □ Hypertonic solutions increase osmotic gradient favoring the movement of fluid from interstitial to intravascular space; excess fluid is excreted by the kidneys.

□ Oral fluid intake and/or intravenous therapy must be monitored very carefully to ensure an overall decrease in ECF volume.
 	
   ○ Implement prescribed diuretic therapy.
	□ Diligent monitoring of fluid intake and output must continue until the body has compensated for the fluid imbalance and body weight again approaches the ideal value for the patient.
	   ○ Diuretics are prescribed to increase excretion of extra fluid.

○ Monitor the following:
    □ Serum potassium; metabolic alkalosis.
 	
    □ Elevation of BUN; ECF volume depletion.
 	
    □ ECG.
	□ Most diuretics cause an increased excretion of potassium; a concomitant metabolic alkalosis can predispose to hypokalemia and hypochloremia.
	   □ Overly aggressive diuretic therapy may predispose to fluid volume deficit.
	   □ Changes in electrolyte concentrations can predispose to altered ECG.

• Implement major nursing interventions.
   ○ Measure and carefully document:
    □ Fluid intake: oral, intravenous; piggyback administration of medications; ice chips.
    □ Fluid output: urine, gastrointestinal losses by vomiting, gastric suctioning, diarrhea; wound or fistula drainage; insensible losses by skin and lungs; iatrogenic losses (blood sampling).
    □ Daily body weight.
   ○ Assess for signs of fluid overload.
    □ Neurologic: confusion.
    □ Cardiovascular: tachycardia, bounding pulse; elevated blood pressure and hemodynamic parameters; neck vein distention in upright position (45 degrees).
    □ Edema (pitting/dependent).
    □ Respiratory: Dyspnea, tachypnea; productive cough; rhonchi and rales.
 	
   ○ Assess for signs of fluid volume deficit associated with overzealous fluid restriction and diuretic therapy.
	○ Accurate intake and output is essential to determine fluid therapy and the effectiveness of therapy.
	   ○ Avoid overly rapid infusions of intravenous fluids.
	
	   □ Dependent edema may result in unobservable fluid retention (e.g., as much as 4–8 L of fluid can be retained in a supine position without detectable edema).
	   ○ See care plan for fluid volume deficit, nursing diagnosis #1.

CARE PLAN FOR THE PATIENT WITH FLUID AND ELECTROLYTE IMBALANCE: FLUID VOLUME EXCESS (*Continued*)

Nursing Interventions	Rationales
• Implement treatment regimen for ICF volume excess. 　○ Restrict water intake as prescribed: 　　□ Administration of oral and/or intravenous fluid therapy should be planned for each 12- to 24-h period. 　　□ Rate of administration of intravenous fluids should be carefully regulated to avoid too rapid or too slow administration. 　　□ Assess neurologic status frequently for changes in sensorium and level of consciousness. 　　□ Monitor serum sodium carefully. 　○ Implement nursing actions. 　　□ Offer explanations to patient and family regarding the significance of fluid restriction. 　　　–Fluid restrictions that may be as low as 500 mL/24 h require cooperation of patient and family. Constant reassurance is important; offer praise for each accomplishment. 　　□ Prescribe appropriate level of activity as tolerated by patient.	○ Initially, fluid replacement is restricted to the amount of urine output and insensible losses; as patient outcomes are achieved and fluid state approaches normalcy, adjustments can be made in fluid intake. □ Neurologic findings reflect ICF excess. □ A serum sodium <130 mEq/L is diagnostic of ICF volume excess. □ An understanding of the reasons for strict fluid restriction may assist patient and family to comply with treatment regimen. □ Progressive increase in activity as tolerated promotes general well-being and reduces risk of complications associated with fragile, edematous tissues, and immobility (e.g., impaired skin integrity).

Arterial BP = systolic/diastolic; CO = cardiac output; CVP = central venous pressure; PAP = pulmonary artery pressure; PCWP = pulmonary capillary wedge pressure.

CARE PLAN FOR THE PATIENT WITH A SODIUM IMBALANCE

Nursing Diagnoses

Nursing Diagnosis #1
Electrolyte imbalance, related to:
1. Hypernatremia.
2. Water deficit.
　(See care plan for fluid volume deficit, nursing diagnoses #1, #2, and #3.)

Desired Patient Outcomes

Patient's condition will stabilize:
1. Neurologic status: alert, oriented to person, place, date; absence of: headache, muscle cramps, convulsions, coma.
2. Hemodynamic status will stabilize as follows:
　• Heart rate >60 but <100 beats/min.
　• Arterial BP = within 10 mmHg of baseline.
　• CVP $\overline{\text{mean}}$ 0–8 mmHg.
　• PAP <25 mmHg (systolic).
　• PCWP $\overline{\text{mean}}$ 8–12 mmHg.
　• CO 4–8 L/min.
3. Body weight will stabilize within 5% of patient's baseline.
4. Serum studies will stabilize as follows:
　• Osmolality 275–290 mOsm/kg.
　• Sodium >135 to <148 mEq/L.
　• Potassium 3.5–5.5 mEq/L.
　• Chloride >100 to <106 mEq/L.
　• Proteins, glucose, BUN, creatinine, hematocrit, and osmolality will stabilize at optimum levels.
5. Urine studies:
　• Urine output >30 mL/h.
　• Specific gravity 1.010–1.025.
　• Sodium 50–130 mEq/L.
　• Osmolality 500–800 mOsm/kg.

CARE PLAN FOR THE PATIENT WITH A SODIUM IMBALANCE (*Continued*)

Nursing Interventions

- Assess impact of hypernatremia and hyperosmotic state on body processes. (See care plan for fluid volume deficit, nursing diagnosis #1.)

  - Assess neurologic status:
    - Level of consciousness, mental status.
    - Behavioral changes: irritability, restlessness, listlessness, lethargy.
    - Deep tendon reflex.
  - Assess hemodynamic function:
    - Heart rate increased.
      −Pulses, weak and thready.

    - Postural hypotension.

    - All hemodynamic parameters are reduced, including: CVP <1 mmHg; PCWP <4 mmHg.
  - Monitor body temperature.

  - Assess renal function:
    - Urine output: <400 mL/24 h suggests acute renal failure.
    - Urine specific gravity >1.030.
    - BUN, serum creatinine, and osmolality all elevated.
    - Total intake and output.
  - Assess gastrointestinal function:
    - Anorexia, nausea, vomiting, abdominal distention, diarrhea, constipation.
  - Assess body weight.

  - Monitor laboratory studies:
    - Serum sodium >145 mEq/L.
    - Serum protein.
    - Hematocrit/hemoglobin.

  - Monitor other parameters.
    - Mucous membranes.
    - Skin turgor.
    - Third spacing.
- Collaborate with physician to correct underlying cause of hypernatremia.
  - Fluid volume deficit.
  - Sodium excess.
  - Implement treatment program as prescribed:
    - Treatment of hypernatremia and dehydration (water loss) involves water replacement therapy:

      −Hypotonic or isotonic solutions are administered intravenously. 5% dextrose in water is frequently the solution prescribed.

      −Oral fluids are administered as tolerated using salt-free fluids.
    - Treatment of hypernatremia (sodium excess) involves salt restriction.
      −Hypotonic intravenous solutions and salt-free oral fluids are administered as described above.

Rationales

- Hyperosmolar state associated with severe dehydration reflects primarily an ICF volume deficit.
  - Hypernatremia is usually caused by a water deficiency rather than an actual increase in sodium concentration.
  - Alterations in neurologic function reflect an ICF volume deficit.

  - Hypovolemia causes tachycardia (heart rate ≥100/min), a compensatory measure to maintain cerebral and renal perfusion.
    - A drop in systolic BP >10 mmHg from supine to upright position signals compromised hemodynamics.
    - These parameters reflect diminished venous return to heart and left ventricular function.
  - Fever and associated diaphoresis contribute to the dehydrated state.
  - A reduction in renal perfusion and glomerular filtration rate predisposes to oliguria.

    - Hemoconcentration related to hypovolemic state.

  - Body weight most closely reflects fluid changes; weight should be measured daily under the same conditions.

    - Serum sodium most closely reflects ICF volume deficit.
    - Serum parameters may expect to be elevated from hemoconcentration associated with hypovolemic state.

  - See care plan for fluid volume deficit, nursing diagnosis #1.
  - Therapeutic approach depends on underlying pathophysiologic mechanisms (e.g., water loss in excess of sodium, or excess sodium intake without supplemental water intake).
    -Hypotonic or isotonic solutions serve to reverse hypertonicity of body fluids.
    - A hypotonic sodium solution is considered safer because it allows a gradual reduction in the serum sodium levels and reduces risk of cerebral edema.*
    - Avoid offering salty fluids, such as bouillon, tomato or V-8 juices, cocoa beverages, among others.

CARE PLAN FOR THE PATIENT WITH A SODIUM IMBALANCE (*Continued*)

Nursing Interventions	Rationales

• Nursing care considerations:
  ∘ Implement nursing treatments in caring for the patient with ICF volume deficit and sodium excess:
    ▫ Establish baseline data (e.g., vital signs, laboratory data).
	∘ Such data provide a framework for evaluating effectiveness of therapy.

▫ Document fluid intake and output from all sources: fluid intake including oral and intravenous fluids; intravenous piggyback medications; irrigation of gastric tube; saline used for endotracheal suctioning; humidified oxygen therapy; enemas.	∘ These measurements provide a basis for prescribing therapy.
▫ Fluid output including urine; gastrointestinal losses—vomiting, diarrhea, gastric suctioning; wound, fistula, or ostomy drainage; iatrogenic losses (blood sampling); insensible losses by lungs and skin; third spacing.	∘ A considerable amount of body fluid can be lost from iatrogenic causes, including blood samples for electrolyte assessment and arterial blood gases.
▫ Estimates of third spacing are critical; careful measurements of abdominal girth or diameter of thighs should be performed; appropriate markings and the use of the same tape measure contribute to consistency, accuracy, and usefulness of the data.	▫ Fluid accumulation in third spaces is unavailable for body use and thus contributes to fluid deficit.
∘ Assess weight daily.	∘ For accuracy, the same scale and conditions should be used with each measurement.
∘ Monitor serum sodium (>148 mEq/L indicates hypernatremia).	
∘ Monitor neurologic, cardiovascular, and respiratory parameters at regular intervals.	∘ Overly aggressive fluid replacement therapy can predispose to fluid overload. ∘ Cerebral edema, congestive heart failure, and pulmonary edema are associated with fluid overload.

▫ Patient, family interaction:
    ▫ Offer appropriate explanations regarding therapy and course of the illness.
    ▫ Elicit expectations of underlying illness and its impact on family lifestyle.
    ▫ Involve in decision-making process.
	∘ Insight and understanding breeds cooperation and compliance.

∘ Supportive care:
    ▫ Oral hygiene.
    ▫ Skin integrity.	

Nursing Diagnoses	Desired Patient Outcomes
Nursing Diagnosis #2 Electrolyte imbalance, related to 1. Hyponatremia. (Depletional hyponatremia = sodium deficit. Dilutional hyponatremia = water excess. [See care plan for fluid volume deficit, nursing diagnosis #1].)	Patient's condition will stabilize: 1. Neurologic status: alert, oriented to person, place, time; deep tendon reflexes brisk; seizure-free. 2. Hemodynamic status will stabilize within patient's baseline values. 3. Body weight will stabilize within 5% of patient's baseline. 4. Serum and urine parameters will stabilize at optimum levels for patient. (See nursing diagnosis #1, for specific hemodynamic and laboratory parameters.)

Nursing Interventions	Rationales
• Assess impact of hyponatremia on body processes:	• For assessment and management, see care plan for fluid volume deficit, nursing diagnosis #1 (depletional); and care plan for fluid volume excess, nursing diagnosis #1 (dilutional).
∘ Neurologic status.	∘ Altered fluid states associated with sodium imbalances predispose to neurologic dysfunction.
∘ Hemodynamic status.	∘ Major concern is to provide appropriate fluid therapy to maintain cerebral, renal, and peripheral perfusion without precipitating fluid volume overload.
▫ CVP, PCWP.	▫ Monitoring of these parameters guides fluid and electrolyte replacement therapy.

CARE PLAN FOR THE PATIENT WITH A SODIUM IMBALANCE (*Continued*)

Nursing Interventions	Rationales
○ Respiratory function: respiratory rate and pattern; evidence of adventitious breath sounds.	○ Continuous assessment of cardiopulmonary status helps to prevent complications (e.g., fluid overload with congestive heart failure and pulmonary edema).
○ Renal status. □ Urine output and specific gravity.	○ A reduction in renal perfusion and glomerular filtration rate (depletional) predisposes to oliguria and acute renal failure.
	□ Most closely reflects hydration status.

□ Body weight.
  □ Fluid accumulation in third spaces.
○ Monitor laboratory data:
  □ Serum sodium.	

	□ Serum sodium levels should be scrutinized carefully to determine type and severity of hyponatremia.
□ Serum osmolality. □ Urine sodium, osmolality.	□ Monitoring of laboratory data assists in evaluating response to fluid and electrolyte therapy.
• Collaborate with physician to correct underlying cause of hyponatremia. (See Table 36–5 for possible etiology.)	• Therapeutic approach depends on underlying pathophysiologic mechanism.
○ Implement treatment program as prescribed and monitor response to therapy.	
□ Treatment of *depletional* hyponatremia (sodium loss) involves fluid and sodium replacement therapy. Intravenous isotonic saline is commonly prescribed. An increase in dietary sodium may also be prescribed if tolerated.	□ See care plan for fluid volume deficit, nursing diagnosis #1. □ Intravenous normal saline replaces sodium as well as water. Avoid undue haste in correcting the abnormality to prevent fluid overload.
□ Treatment of *dilutional* hyponatremia (water excess) involves modalities to reduce water concentration, diuretic therapy (furosemide), treatment of underlying cause.	□ Dilutional hyponatremia has a higher incidence than the depletional form. □ See care plan for fluid volume excess, nursing diagnosis #1. □ Underlying cardiac, hepatic, or renal disease may require aggressive therapeutics.
• Nursing care implications: See nursing diagnosis #1, above): ○ Document and interpret baseline data: intake and output, daily weight.	○ Provide a basis on which to determine fluid therapy and to evaluate the effectiveness of therapy.
○ Implement measures to reduce water intake in treatment of dilutional hyponatremia: □ Avoid excessive water intake: tap water orally, or by enema; electrolyte-poor intravenous fluid; or irrigation of gastric tube with distilled water.	□ Excessive water intake by these routes will further complicate the fluid excess associated with dilutional hyponatremia or water intoxication state.
○ Monitor neurologic status closely: □ General cerebral function, mental status, level of consciousness, cranial nerve function, deep tendon reflexes, sensorimotor function.	○ Close monitoring of the neurologic status is essential to prevent complications associated with fluid dehydration/overhydration states, depending on whether the underlying cause is depletional or dilutional hyponatremia.

○ Monitor cardiovascular function:
  □ Hemodynamic parameters: CVP, PCWP.
  □ Heart rate and rhythm; presence of neck vein distention, quality of peripheral pulses (bounding, or weak and thready on palpation).
	○ Data provided by hemodynamic parameters and meticulous serial assessments assist in determining the status of venous return to the heart and left ventricular function.

○ Assess respiratory function: rate, rhythm, effort, presence of adventitious breath sounds.	○ In the setting of fluid overload, especially from chronic cardiac, hepatic, or renal disease, it is critical to perform ongoing assessment of neurologic and cardiopulmonary function to prevent and/or recognize signs of impending cardiac failure.
• Initiate efforts to obtain a comprehensive patient/family history including the functional health patterns.	• Family history may assist in assessing potential problems, including coping capabilities and stress tolerance.
○ How does patient/family perceive the impact of the illness on individual and family lifestyles? Coping capabilities? Stress tolerance? ○ Can the patient/family identify family support systems?	○ Fluid and electrolyte imbalances are often the result of serious underlying cardiac, hepatic, or renal disease requiring intensive care and follow-up. Knowing how to cope and how to assume responsibility for self-care may assist in minimizing impact of illness on individual and family lifestyles.

CARE PLAN FOR THE PATIENT WITH A SODIUM IMBALANCE (*Continued*)

Nursing Interventions

- Teach patient/family the importance of maintaining prescribed fluid intake restriction. Enlist their assistance in keeping a meticulous intake and output. Encourage to participate in decision-making regarding care.

Rationales

- In patients on strict fluid intake (e.g., 500 mL/24 h), it is essential to assist patient/family to adjust to this critical limitation. Decisions regarding when to drink may be left for the patient/family to decide. Such participation may ensure better compliance with the therapeutic regimen. (See Chapter 42.)

Arterial BP = systolic/diastolic; CO = cardiac output; CVP = central venous pressure; PAP = pulmonary artery pressure; PCWP = pulmonary capillary wedge pressure.

*Metheny, N: Fluid and Electrolyte Balance: Nursing Considerations. JB Lippincott, Philadelphia, 1987, p 57.

CARE PLAN FOR THE PATIENT WITH A POTASSIUM IMBALACE

Nursing Interventions

Nursing Diagnosis #1
Cardiac output, alteration in: decreased, related to dysrhythmias associated with *hyper*kalemia (>5.5 mEq/L).

Rationales

Patient's status will stabilize as follows:
1. Neuromuscular status: muscle strength intact; absence of muscle twitching or seizures; deep tendon reflexes brisk.
2. Cardiovascular status:
   - Heart rate >60 but <100 beats/min.
   - Arterial BP = within 10 mmHg of patient's baseline.
   - CVP = 0–8 mmHg.
   - PCWP = 8–12 mmHg.
   - CO = 4–8 L/min.
3. ECG: Regular sinus rhythm.
   - Rounded P wave.
   - PR interval 0.12–0.20 seconds.
   - QRS duration 0.06–0.12 seconds.
   - ST segment = isoelectric.
   - Rounded, asymmetrical T wave.
4. Serum potassium 3.5–5.0 mEq/L.
5. Arterial blood gases:
   - pH = 7.35–7.45.
   - P_{CO_2} = 35–45 mmHg.
   - HCO_3^- = 22–26 mEq/L.
6. Respiratory status: lung fields resonant; no rales (crackles).
7. Gastrointestinal function intact.
8. Renal function: urine output >30 mL/h.

Nursing Interventions

- Assess impact of hyperkalemia on physiologic processes:

  - Elicit comprehensive patient history:
    - Current cardiopulmonary status.
    - Past medical history: hypertension, coronary artery disease, angina, myocardial infarction, medications.
    - Family history: obesity, diabetes mellitus, hypertension, coronary artery disease, renal disease.
  - Assess neuromuscular status: evidence of twitching or seizure activity; muscle strength; deep tendon reflexes.

  - Assess cardiopulmonary dynamics:
    - Heart rate, peripheral pulses.
    - Arterial blood pressure.

Rationales

- Assists in differential diagnosis of underlying pathophysiology; altered cardiopulmonary dynamics may reflect a compensatory response to some other primary diagnosis.
  - May help to identify patient at risk of developing a potassium imbalance.

  - Potassium is intricately involved in establishing and maintaining cellular excitability; alterations in serum potassium are reflected by signs and symptoms of neuromuscular irritability.
  - Establishment of baseline data provides a basis for comparison and evaluation of effectiveness of therapy.

CARE PLAN FOR THE PATIENT WITH A POTASSIUM IMBALACE (*Continued*)

Nursing Interventions

- □ CVP.
- □ PCWP.

- □ Respiratory rate and pattern; breath sounds: adventitious (rales or crackles).
- □ Fluid volume intake-output.

- □ Neck vein distention (45 degrees).

- ○ Assess renal function.
  - □ Urine output per hour.
- ○ Assess gastrointestinal function: abdominal distention, paralytic ileus.
- ○ Evaluate arterial blood gases: pH, $Paco_2$, HCO_3^-.

- Collaborate with physician to correct underlying cause of hyperkalemia (see Table 36–6, Etiology).
  - –Metabolic acidosis.
  - ○ Implement treatment regimen (see Table 36–6, Treatment):
    - □ Emergency measures: serum potassium >6.5 mEq/L and/or severely impaired renal function:
      - –10% calcium gluconate, as prescribed, with continuous cardiac monitoring.

    - –500 mL 10% glucose (hypertonic) with 10 units regular insulin IV over 30 min.

    - –Sodium bicarbonate, 2–3 amps in 500 mL glucose IV, or as prescribed.

- ○ Additional therapy to correct hyperkalemia:
  - □ Sodium polystyrene sulfonate (Kayexalate) 15–30 g orally or by enema, 2–3 times daily.
- Nursing implications in hyperkalemia:
  - ○ Monitor cardiac function continuously.
    - □ Electrical activity (ECG) (see Table 36–6 for list of specific ECG changes associated with hyperkalemia).

    - □ Mechanical activity (cardiac contractility) as reflected by: arterial blood pressure, pulmonary pressures, cardiac output.
  - ○ Monitor arterial blood gases: pH, $Paco_2$, HCO_3^-, Pao_2, O_2 saturation of hemoglobin.

  - ○ Monitor serum electrolytes: notify physician of significant changes in serum electrolytes; serum potassium.
    - □ Decreased serum sodium.
  - ○ Monitor renal function:
    - □ Urine output >30 mL/h.
    - □ Accurate documentation of intake and output.
    - □ Daily weight.

Rationales

- □ Reflects volume of venous return.
- □ PCWP reflects the effectiveness of left ventricle in handling the volume of venous return to the heart; dysrhythmias associated with potassium imbalance decrease cardiac output.
- □ The occurrence of rales may reflect left heart failure.

- □ Fluid overload may cause cardiac failure in compromised heart.
- □ Neck vein distention reflects high central venous pressures associated with fluid overload and/or congestive heart failure.
- ○ Reduced renal perfusion related to decreased cardiac output may predispose to oligura and fluid overload.
- ○ Altered serum potassium disrupts smooth muscle excitability in gastrointestinal tract.
- ○ Metabolic acidosis drives H^+ ions into cells in exchange for K^+ ions; the result is hyperkalemia.
- Correction of the underlying cause is essential to establish potassium homeostasis.

- ○ Treatment will vary with the severity of electrolyte imbalance.

- □ Calcium is given to stimulate the heart; it should not be administered to patients taking digitalis preparations because the combined treatment may precipitate dysrhythmias.
- □ Potassium is driven into cells along with insulin-facilitated movement of glucose intracellularly (by K/Na pump).
- □ Bicarbonate therapy relieves acidemia, causing potassium to move into cells in exchange for H^+ ions; overall result is a decrease in serum potassium levels.

- □ Kayexalate functions as an exchange resin absorbing potassium in the gastrointestinal tract and eliminating it in the feces.

- □ K^+ is the primary intracellular ion; alterations in potassium concentration predispose to neuromuscular irritability and dysrhythmias.
- □ Electrical-mechanical asynchronization leads to reduced cardiac output, reduced arterial blood pressure, and reduced tissue perfusion.
- ○ Acidemia predisposes to hyperkalemia as H^+ ions move into cells in exchange for potassium.
- ○ O_2 administration may be indicated if $Paco_2$ >45 mmHg; an increase in CO_2 further contributes to acidemia.
- ○ It is important to follow trends in arterial blood gases and serum electrolytes to evaluate effectiveness of therapy.
  - □ May also contribute to hyperkalemia.
  - □ Potassium should not be administered in the presence of oliguria.
  - □ Fluid restriction may be necessary in presence of compromised cardiac function.

CARE PLAN FOR THE PATIENT WITH A POTASSIUM IMBALACE (*Continued*)

Nursing Interventions
- Auscultate lung fields.
  - Maximize ventilatory effort: semi-Fowler's position reduces pressure on diaphragm.
- Comfort measures: provide frequent rest periods; provide reassurance to patient and family; keep them informed.
- Monitor effectiveness of prescribed medications and potential drug interactions:
  - Diuretics (furosemide).

  - Digitalis preparation.

  - Morphine.

Rationales
- Presence of rales may suggest congestive heart failure.

  - Reduces intravascular volume and increases potassium excretion.
  - Stimulates contractility, slows heart rate, and increases cardiac output.
  - Alleviates anxiety, decreases venous return to the heart by decreasing peripheral vascular resistance.

Nursing Diagnoses

Nursing Diagnosis #2
Cardiac output, alteration in: decreased, related to dysrhythmias associated with *hypo*kalemia (<3.5 mEq/L).

Desired Patient Outcomes

Patient's condition will stabilize as follows:
1. Neurologic status: alert, oriented to person, place, date.
2. Neuromuscular status: muscle strength intact; deep tendon reflexes brisk.
3. Respiratory function: respiratory rate and pattern maintain arterial blood gases within acceptable physiologic limits:
   - pH 7.35–7.45.
   - $PaCO_2$ 35–45 mmHg
   - HCO_3^- 22–26 mEq/L.
   - PaO_2 >60 mmHg.
   - O_2 Sat >90%.
4. Cardiovascular function and ECG (see Patient Outcomes for Nursing Diagnosis #1).
5. Serum electrolytes maintained as follows:
   - Potassium 3.5–5.5 mEq/L.
   - Sodium 135–148 mEq/L.
   - Chloride 100–106 mEq/L.
   - Bicarbonate (as above).
6. Renal function: urine output >30 mL/h.
7. Gastrointestinal function intact.

Nursing Interventions
- Assess impact of hypokalemia on physiologic processes (see Nursing Interventions for Nursing Diagnosis #1, above). Additionally:
  - Evaluate arterial blood gases: pH, $PaCO_2$, HCO_3^-.

- Collaborate with physician to correct underlying cause of hypokalemia (see etiologies listed in Table 36–6).
  - Metabolic alkalemia.

  - Metabolic acidemia.

  - Implement treatment regimen (see Treatment in Table 36–6). Additionally:
    - Identify patient at risk.
    - Prevent conditions that may contribute to hypokalemia. For example, diuretic abuse (e.g., furosemide, thiazides).

Rationales

  - Metabolic alkalemia contributes to hypokalemia by driving potassium into cells in exchange for H^+ ions.
- Correction of the underlying cause is essential to establish potassium homeostasis.
  - Shift of potassium into cells in exchange for hydrogen may contribute to hypokalemia.
  - A normal serum potassium in the presence of an acidemia indicates a potassium deficit.
  - Treatment will vary with the severity of electrolyte imbalance.

    - Serum potassium should be closely monitored because these diuretics increase potassium excretion.

CARE PLAN FOR THE PATIENT WITH A POTASSIUM IMBALACE (*Continued*)

Nursing Interventions

- ▫ Minimal maintenance dose should be prescribed for patients with restricted oral intake of potassium:
  - –NPO preoperative; diagnostic studies.
  - –NPO postoperative.
  - –Nasogastric suctioning.
- ▫ Administer potassium replacement therapy as prescribed: 40 mEq/L KCl in 1000 mL of 5% dextrose in water.
  - ▫ A variety of potassium supplements are available for oral use.
- ▫ The occurrence of gastrointestinal symptomatology (nausea, vomiting, abdominal pain, distention, or bleeding) signals that oral potassium should be discontinued.

  - ▫ Potassium therapy should not begin until renal function has been evaluated.
  - ▫ Intravenous potassium administration requires continuous cardiac monitoring.

- • Other nursing considerations:
  - ○ Maintain accurate intake/output.
  - ○ Evaluate neuromuscular status hourly during acute phase of illness.
  - ○ Monitor cardiac status continuously (see Clinical Manifestations listed in Table 36–4 for specific ECG changes associated with hypokalemia).
  - ○ Monitor serum electrolytes and arterial blood gases:
    - ▫ Metabolic alkalemia, symptomatology: nausea, vomiting, diarrhea, shallow breathing.

  - ○ Anticipate potential cardiac dysrhythmias in patients receiving digitalis and diuretics.
    - ▫ Assess patient for digitalis toxicity; anorexia, nausea, vomiting, diarrhea; all types of dysrhythmias: paroxysmal atrial tachycardia, multifocal premature ventricular beats, atrioventricular conduction blocks, ventricular dysrhythmias.

Rationales

- ▫ Additional losses of potassium associated with tissue injury, vomiting, and diarrhea, for example, should be replaced.

- ▫ When potassium losses cannot be prevented, it is critical that they be replaced.

  - ▫ Oral potassium supplements must be administered cautiously as these preparations cause gastric irritation; oral preparations should be administered completely dissolved to prevent gastrointestinal irritation.
  - ▫ Serum potassium must be monitored closely to prevent hyperkalemia.
  - ▫ The kidneys are the major potassium-excreting organs.

- ○ Urine output should be maintained at >30 mL/h.

- ○ Alkalemia predisposes to hypokalemia as potassium moves into cells in exchange for H^+ ions.
  - ▫ Shallow breathing is a compensatory mechanism to increase CO_2 retention so as to help relieve alkalemic state.

- ○ Digoxin normally slows conduction through atrioventricular node (junction); potential digitalis toxicity results in heart blocks.

Arterial BP = systolic/diastolic; CO = cardiac output; CVP = central venous pressure; PAP = pulmonary artery pressure; PCWP = pulmonary capillary wedge pressure.

CARE PLAN FOR THE PATIENT WITH HYPERCALCEMIA

Nursing Diagnoses

Nursing Diagnosis #1

Electrolyte imbalance: hypercalcemia, related to:
1. Impaired renal function (renal tubular acidosis).
2. Alkalemia.
3. Prolonged immobilization.
4. Hypophosphatemia.
5. Hyperparathyroidism.
6. Others.

Desired Patient Outcomes

Patient's condition will stabilize as follows:
1. Neurologic status:
   - Alert, oriented to person, place, time.
   - Absence of fatigue, mood appropriate, memory intact.
   - Verbalizes comfort, without pain or headache.
2. Cardiovascular status:
   - Heart rate >60 but <100 beats/min.
   - Arterial BP within 10 mmHg of patient's baseline.
   - ECG: Regular sinus rhythm, ST segment isoelectric, QT interval within normal range.
3. Serum studies:
   - Calcium 8.5–10.5 mg/100 mL.
   - Phosphorus 3.0–4.5 mg/100 mL.
   - Sodium 135–148 mEq/L.
   - Potassium 3.5–5.5 mEq/L.
   - Magnesium 1.5–2.0 mEq/L.
   - Proteins (total) 6.0–8.4 g/100 mL.
4. Renal status: Urine output >30 mL/h (depends on status of renal function).
5. Serum studies:
   - BUN 8–25 mg/100 mL.
   - Creatinine 0.6–1.5 mg/100 mL.

Nursing Interventions

- Assess impact of hypercalcemia on physiologic processes.
  - Elicit pertinent aspects of patient/family history (see Table 36–8).

  - Perform physical examination.

    - Neurologic status: mental status, level of consciousness, alertness, orientation to person, place, time.
    - Lethargy, confusion, memory status; emotional lability; personality changes (as per family/significant others); headache, pain.
    - Cranial nerve function.
    - Neuromuscular function: extreme fatigue; decreased muscle strength; generalized muscle weakness; muscle hypotonicity, flaccidity; muscle twitchings, spasms; neuromuscular hypoactivity; diminished deep tendon reflexes; bone pain; flank pain.
    - Cardiovascular status: heart rate and rhythm; arterial blood pressure; pulmonary artery and capillary wedge pressures; cardiac output.

    - Assess for exaggerated, inotropic effect of increased serum calcium levels on cardiac contractility.
    - ECG.

    - Respiratory status.
      – Respiratory rate and rhythm.
    - Hydration status: evidence of congestive heart failure and pulmonary edema: tachypnea, dyspnea; adventitious breath sounds (crackles, rales, wheezes); cough, productive of frothy, pink-tinged sputum.

Rationales

- Personal characteristics and state of health play a crucial role in determining the ability of the patient/family to cope with the stress of hypercalcemia and its underlying cause.
  - Although many signs/symptoms may accompany hypercalcemia, they are usually nonspecific and difficult to recognize. The patient's assessment requires a high degree of suspicion and a meticulous examination of laboratory data.
  - Establish baseline data with which subsequent assessments can be compared.
    - Calcium is a key factor in cellular permeability, and in the transmission of electrical impulses.

    - Hypercalcemia causes depression and sluggishness of central and peripheral nervous systems; it alters neuromuscular responses.

    - Prolonged immobilization increases movement of calcium from bone into the bloodstream, contributing to hypercalcemic state.

    - Hypertension associated with high cardiac output and extremely enhanced cardiac contractility has been known to occur in the scenario of hypercalcemia.
    - The potent inotropic effect of elevated serum calcium predisposes to cardiac dysrhythmias, conduction delays, and cardiac arrest. There is an increased incidence of heart blocks in such clinical states.

      – Shortness of breath may reflect weakened state.
    - Fluid volume overload increases risk of congestive heart failure and pulmonary edema, especially in patients with prior limitations in cardiac reserve.

CARE PLAN FOR THE PATIENT WITH HYPERCALCEMIA (*Continued*)

Nursing Interventions

- ▫ Acid-base status—arterial blood gases: pH, $PaCO_2$, HCO_3^-.

- ○ Renal status and fluid and electrolyte status:

  - ▫ Determine fluid intake/output.
  - ▫ Determine body weight.
  - ▫ Assess hematocrit/hemoglobin.
  - ▫ Assess BUN and creatinine levels.
  - ▫ Establish baseline electrolyte levels:
    - –Calcium.
    - –Sodium.

    - –Phosphorus.
    - –Proteins (total and albumin).

- ○ Assess urine output for stones.

- • Collaborate with other healthcare providers to implement therapeutic regimen to restore serum calcium to within physiologic range.
  - ○ Initiate fluid and drug therapy to reduce serum calcium to appropriate physiologic range. (Refer to section on Treatment in Table 36–8 for specific therapies.)
  - ○ In addition:
    - ▫ Administer prostaglandin inhibitors, as prescribed.

- ○ Initiate efforts to determine and treat underlying cause of hypercalcemic state.
  - ▫ Treatment of underlying cause should be initiated once the acute phase is under control.
  - ▫ Precipitants of hypercalcemia, especially prolonged immobilization and volume depletion, should be diligently avoided.
- ○ Anticipate the occurrence of hypocalcemia with too rigorous antihypercalcemic therapy.
  - ▫ Be alert for signs of increased neuromuscular excitability: muscle twitchings and spasms; seizure activity; tetany.
- ○ Implement measures to restore and maintain fluid and electrolyte balance.
- ○ Establish and maintain hydrated state.

- ○ Administer normal saline infusion in conjunction with administration of furosemide (diuretic therapy).

- ○ Avoid use of thiazide diuretics.

- ○ Strain urine for stones.
- ○ Assess for signs/symptoms associated with passage of stones: severe, colicky flank pain; hematuria.
- ○ Consider acid-ash diet to keep urine acidic and avoid renal calculi formation.

Rationales

- ▫ Metabolic alkalemia increases binding of calcium to serum proteins; the net effect—hypocalcemia.
- ▫ Metabolic acidemia increases freely ionized serum calcium fraction.
- ○ Polydipsia and polyuria are frequently associated with an increased or forced calcium excretion.
- ○ Baseline data are essential to evaluate the patient's response to therapy.
  - ▫ Aggressive fluid therapy can predispose to fluid overload with congestive heart failure.

  - –Highly bound to serum proteins.
  - –Calcium excretion is largely dependent on concomitant excretion of sodium.
  - –Exhibits a reciprocal relationship with calcium.
  - –Approximately one half of serum calcium is freely ionized; the remainder is bound to proteins and organic molecules.
- ○ Renal calculi formation can be a major complication because of the increased excretion of high concentrations of calcium by the nephrons.

- ○ Goal of fluid and drug therapy is to attain an asymptomatic serum calcium level and to reverse process causing the hypercalcemia.

  - ▫ Prostaglandin inhibitors, as for example, indomethacin or aspirin, may lower serum calcium when hypercalcemia is associated with prostaglandin-producing tumors.

- ○ Wide fluctuations in serum calcium levels may occur and require very close monitoring.

- ○ Patient may be unable to conserve free water because of ADH resistance. Rehydration = dilutional effect on serum calcium.
- ○ Combination of normal saline and diuretic therapy increases glomerular filtration rate and renal excretion of calcium.
- ○ There is a concomitant decrease in urinary calcium excretion when thiazide diuretics are administered.
- ○ Elevated renal excretion of calcium predisposes to renal calculi formation.

CARE PLAN FOR THE PATIENT WITH HYPERCALCEMIA (*Continued*)

Nursing Interventions

○ Correlate serum electrolytes with clinical status.

 □ Carefully monitor serial serum calcium and phosphorus levels.

○ Carefully monitor total serum proteins to determine state of free, ionized serum calcium.
 □ ↑ In serum proteins = ↓ in free, ionized calcium.
 □ ↓ In serum proteins = ↑ in free, ionized calcium.
○ Carefully monitor serum potassium and magnesium.
 □ Replace urinary losses.

○ Monitor cardiovascular function.
 □ Cardiac rate and rhythm (continuously).
 □ Administer digitalis carefully in patients with hypercalcemia.
 □ Monitor arterial and pulmonary capillary pressures.

○ Implement peritoneal or hemodialysis in life-threatening situations.

Rationales

○ Following the trend of serum calcium levels assists in determining the effectiveness of therapeutic regimen.
 □ Close monitoring of serum calcium levels helps to anticipate and prevent hypocalcemia.
 □ A reciprocal relationship between these two ions usually exists. Hypophosphatemia frequently occurs in hypercalcemia.
 □ Approximately 45% to 50% of serum calcium is protein-bound.

 □ Depletion of serum potassium and magnesium levels frequently occurs, and their monitoring is mandatory to prevent alterations in cardiac function.
 □ Combination of hypercalcemia and hyperkalemia causes cardiac irritability.
 □ Ultimate goal of therapy is to establish an asymptomatic serum calcium level without alterations in neuromuscular or cardiac functions.

 □ Calcium will enhance digitalis effect and may precipitate digitalis toxicity.
 □ Assist in managing fluid status: fluid volume overload must be avoided because patients are at increased risk of congestive heart failure and pulmonary edema.
○ Either peritoneal or hemodialysis is capable of efficiently removing calcium from blood; the mode of dialysis depends on several considerations, as for example, the acuteness of the situation, age, and clinical status of patient.

Nursing Diagnoses

Nursing Diagnosis #2
Bowel elimination, alteration in: constipation, related to:
1. Smooth muscle hypotonicity with inadequate peristalsis, associated with hypercalcemia.

Nursing Diagnosis #3
Potential for injury: peptic ulcer disease, related to:
1. Increased gastric acid secretion, associated with elevated serum calcium levels.

Desired Patient Outcomes

Patient will establish and maintain effective bowel function:
1. Bowel pattern to return to patient's baseline.
 • Stool soft and formed.
 • Absence of constipation, abdominal distention, fecal impaction with diarrheal incontinence.
2. Bowel sounds appropriate and heard throughout all quadrants.
3. Absence of epigastric pain; relaxed facial expression and demeanor.
4. Stool/gastric secretions negative for occult blood.
5. Gastric pH >4.5.

Nursing Interventions

• Assess gastrointestinal function:
 ○ Ascertain bowel habits/pattern; establish pre-illness diet; presence of anorexia, nausea, vomiting; constipation, diarrhea.
 ○ Determine attitudes of patient/family regarding nutrition.
 ○ Perform abdominal examination: bowel sounds; evidence of tenderness or guarding; distention.
 ○ Determine hydration status.
 ○ Assess for potential complications.

Rationales

○ Hypercalcemia causes a decrease in smooth muscle contractility of the gastrointestinal tract; the bowel becomes hypoactive with reduced muscle tone.

CARE PLAN FOR THE PATIENT WITH HYPERCALCEMIA (*Continued*)

Nursing Interventions
- □ Peptic ulcer disease.
- □
- □ Acute pancreatitis.

- • Initiate comprehensive approach to reducing calcium absorption from the intestines.
  - ○ Diet (as per nutritionist).
    - □ Calcium restriction.
    - □ Fruit and fiber.
    - □ Avoid caffeine-containing foods/fluids.
  - ○ Medications (as prescribed).
    - □ Stool softeners.
    - □ Judicious use of laxatives.

    - □ Histamine antagonists (cimetidine, ranitidine).
    - □ Antacids
    - □ Administer phosphates to increase calcium excretion.
  - ○ Maximize exercise activity as tolerated.

Rationales
- □ Enhanced gastric secretions in the presence of hypercalcemia predispose to peptic ulcer disease.
- □ Associated with activation of pancreatic enzymes or plugging of pancreatic duct.

- □ Bulk stimulates peristalsis.
- □ Reduces hydrochloric acid secretion.

- □ Prevent constipation.
- □ Diarrhea must be avoided because of associated fluid and electrolyte imbalance.
- □ Presence of diarrhea may suggest fecal impaction in patients with constipation.
- □ Inhibit gastric secretions.
- □ Reduce gastric acidity.

- ○ Exercises (abdominal) assist to increase peristalsis and increase overall muscle tone.

Nursing Diagnoses

Nursing Diagnosis #4
Mobility, impaired physical.
Nursing Diagnosis #5
Activity intolerance, potential.

Desired Patient Outcomes

Patient will:
1. Achieve maximum mobility without discomfort, weakness, or fatigue.
2. Demonstrate maximum range of motion.

Nursing Interventions
- • Implement therapeutic regimen to restore/maintain mobility and activity tolerance.
  - ○ Maintain proper body alignment.

  - ○ Establish a progressive exercise program, as tolerated (per physical therapist).
    - □ Encourage range-of-motion exercises to all joints.
    - □ Initiate passive exercises when appropriate, and progress to active exercises.
    - □ Avoid rough handling; support joints to minimize pain and prevent trauma.
    - □ Avoid overfatigue; provide rest periods.

Rationales

- ○ Pathologic fractures are often associated with hypercalcemia and its underlying cause.
  - □ Exercise and mobilization reduce resorption of calcium from bone, maintain muscle strength, and prevent contractures and fractures.

- □ Providing a quiet, safe environment with frequent rest periods helps to conserve energy.

Nursing Diagnoses

Nursing Diagnosis #6
Skin integrity impaired, potential for, related to:
1. Immobilization.
2. Altered nutrition.

Desired Patient Outcomes

Patient will:
1. Maintain intact skin and mucous membranes.

Nursing Interventions
- • Maintain skin integrity.
  - ○ Turn and position every 2 h.
    - □ Lubricate skin.
    - □ Initiate pressure relief device (e.g., air mattress).
    - □ Assess nutritional status.
    - □ Assess pressure area at planned intervals to determine status.
    - □ Perform local site care as per unit protocol and/or physician's orders.

Rationales

- ○ Reddened areas that do not blanch within 20–30 min of position change dictate that the position be avoided or that the duration in that position be reduced.

CARE PLAN FOR THE PATIENT WITH HYPERCALCEMIA (*Continued*)

Nursing Diagnoses

Nursing Diagnosis #7
Potential for injury: Thrombophlebitis, related to:
1. Immobilization.

Desired Patient Outcomes

Patient will:
1. Remain without evidence of thrombophlebitis:
   • Increased calf/thigh circumference.
   • Pain upon dorsiflexion of foot.
   • Absence of redness or swelling of extremities.

Nursing Interventions

• Establish precautions related to thrombus formation and thrombophlebitis.
  ○ Apply antiembolic stockings.
  ○ Assess for redness, pain, and swelling of calves; measure circumference of extremity.
  ○ Perform range-of-motion exercises as above.

Rationales

• Immobility contributes to venous stasis and increases risk of thromboembolic disease.

  ○ Provides a measure to evaluate for presence of thrombophlebitis.

Nursing Diagnoses

Nursing Diagnosis #8
Knowledge deficit regarding follow-up/preventive care.

Desired Patient Outcomes

Patient will:
1. Verbalize knowledge of underlying disease process and therapy.
2. Verbalize understanding of therapeutic regimen:
   • Medications: indication, dosage, administration, schedule for taking, potential side effects.
   • Diet.
   • Exercise.

Nursing Interventions

• Assess patient/family knowledge regarding disease process and therapy.

  ○ Assess readiness to learn.

• Implement program to teach the following topics:
  ○ Pertinent anatomy and physiology of calcium metabolism.
  ○ Underlying pathophysiology.
  ○ Identification of precipitating stressors or other factors.
  ○ Recognition of signs and symptoms of the hypercalcemia state.
  ○ Appreciation of the importance of seeking timely assistance when the stressful event occurs, or with the first sign/symptom of hypercalcemia.
  ○ Understanding of medication regimen for disorders underlying the occurrence of hypercalcemia.
    □ Dosage and administration.
    □ Adverse side effects.
  ○ Understanding the importance of continuous healthcare follow-up.
  ○ Initiation of self-care, health-oriented practices to prevent recurring episodes.
  ○ Nutritional counseling.

Rationales

• Understanding of underlying disease processes assists the patient/family to cope with, and to adjust to, the limitations imposed by the disease.
  ○ Depending on the underlying causes, hypercalcemia may impact on all members of the family. Interested and supportive family members should be included in the educational process.

CARE PLAN FOR THE PATIENT WITH HYPOCALCEMIA

Nursing Diagnoses

Nursing Diagnosis #1
Electrolyte imbalance: hypocalcemia, related to:
1. Alkalemia associated with vomiting, alkali ingestion, or hyperventilation.
2. Chronic renal failure with hyperphosphatemia.
3. Vitamin D deficiency state.
4. Chronic malabsorption state.
5. Hypomagnesemia.
6. Acute pancreatitis.
7. Idiopathic hypoparathyroidism.

Desired Patient Outcomes

Patient's condition will stabilize as follows:
1. Neurologic status:
   • Alert, oriented to person, place, and time.
   • Absence of muscle spasms or cramping, tremors, seizure activity, or tetany.
2. Respiratory status:
   • Eupnea, unlabored respirations.
   • Full chest wall excursion.
   • Absence of adventitious breath sounds: rales, crackles, wheezes.
   • Absence of laryngospasm, airway obstruction (bronchospasm).
3. Cardiovascular status:
   • Heart rate >60 but <100 beats/min.
   • Arterial BP within 10 mmHg of patient's baseline.
   • ECG regular sinus rhythm:
     ST segment isoelectric.
     QT interval within normal range.
4. Renal status:
   • Urine output >30 mL/h (depends on status of renal function).
   • BUN 8–25 mg/100 mL.
   • Creatinine 0.6–1.5 mg/100 mL.
5. Serum studies:
   • Calcium 8.5–10.5 mg/100 mL.
   • Phosphorus 3.0–4.5 mg/100 mL.
   • Sodium 135–148 mEq/L.
   • Potassium 3.5–5.5 mEq/L.
   • Magnesium 1.5–2.0 mEq/L.
   • Proteins (total) 6.0–8.4 g/100 mL.

Nursing Interventions
• Assess impact of hypocalcemia on physiologic processes:
  ○ Elicit pertinent aspects of patient/family health history. (See section on Diagnostic Workup in Table 36–8.)

• Collaborate with other healthcare providers to implement therapeutic regimen to restore serum calcium to within physiologic range.
  ○ Administer calcium replacement therapy: 10–20 mL of 10% calcium gluconate, intravenously, not to exceed 1.5 mL/min. (See section on Treatment in Table 36–8.)

  ○ Use intracath for intravenous administration, and dilute method versus IV push.

  ○ Administer calcium slowly to patients receiving digitalis therapy.

Rationales

  ○ Personal characteristics and state of health play a crucial role in determining the ability of the patient/family to cope with the stress of hypocalcemia and its underlying cause.
  ○ Unlike *hyper*calcemia where the clinical presentation may be so nonspecific as to require laboratory confirmation, hypocalcemia is characterized by definitive diagnostic findings upon history and physical assessment.
  ○ Based on these assessment data, a decision must be made about whether the progress of the illness represents an immediate threat to life.
• Therapeutic goal is to raise serum calcium levels to >8.5 mg/100 mL. Reduced serum calcium levels precipitate neuromuscular irritability and seizure activity.
  ○ Goal of calcium replacement therapy is to attain an asymptomatic serum calcium level with absence of neuromuscular and cardiac alterations.
  ○ Calcium gluconate (or calcium chloride) preparation must be administered slowly to avoid high serum calcium concentrations and associated cardiac conduction delays.
  ○ Calcium preparations can cause vein irritation and inflammation; calcium chloride causes tissue necrosis and is associated with an increased incidence of thrombophlebitis.
  ○ In patients on digitalis therapy, a rapid infusion of calcium may potentiate digitalis effect and precipitate cardiac dysrhythmias and cardiac arrest.
  ○ Cardiac monitoring of rate and rhythm must be continuous.

CARE PLAN FOR THE PATIENT WITH HYPOCALCEMIA (*Continued*)

Nursing Interventions

- ○ Avoid simultaneous administration of calcium and sodium bicarbonate in the same line.
- ○ Avoid use of saline for infusions.
- ○ Monitor serum calcium, phosphorus, and total protein.

- ○ Monitor 24-h urine for calcium as total body calcium approaches an equilibrated physiologic state.
- ○ Administer vitamin D or its active metabolites:

  - □ Monitor for hypercalciuria.
  - □ Monitor serum calcium levels closely to prevent hypercalcemia.
- ○ Correct hypomagnesemia if present: magnesium sulfate 1–2 g every 4–6 h intramuscularly depending on state of hypomagnesemia.
- ○ Initiate efforts to determine and treat underlying cause of hypocalcemic state:

- Consider nursing implications related to the care of the patient with hypocalcemia.
  - ○ Identify patients at risk of developing seizures.
  - ○ Assess neurologic status: mental status and level of consciousness; status of cranial nerve function; presence of hyperreflexia.
  - ○ Presence of:
    - □ Chvostek's sign.

    - □ Trousseau's sign.

  - ○ Implement measures to minimize neurologic and neuromuscular stimulation:
    - □ Maintain cool, quiet environment; limit stressors; avoid drafts, bright lights, and sudden noise or movements.
  - ○ Institute seizure precautions:
    - □ Maintain at bedside: suction, oropharyngeal airway, oxygen source, and access.
    - □ Emergency drugs and equipment: anticonvulsants, diazepam.
    - □ Tracheostomy set, endotracheal airways.
    - □ Side rails padded and maintained in up position; bed in lowest position; call light accessible to patient.
  - ○ Monitor (record) seizure activity: Precipitating event? How initiated? Part of body involved? Unilateral or bilateral? Level of consciousness? Pupillary size and reactivity? Urinary/bowel incontinence?
  - ○ Protect patient from injury during seizure.
    - □ Turn on side if possible.

  - ○ Implement measures to maintain effective respiratory function.
    - □ Assess for and anticipate bronchospasm: Respiratory rate, rhythm; dyspnea, tachypnea; use of accessory muscles; auscultate all lung fields.
    - □ Assess effectiveness of cough and handling of secretions.
    - □ Monitor pulmonary function: tidal volume; vital capacity.

Rationales

- ○ Calcium will precipitate in an alkaline solution.

- ○ Saline increases calcium excretion by the kidneys.
- ○ Monitoring of serum values assists in evaluating effectiveness of therapeutic plan. (See fluid and electrolyte interventions, following).
- ○ It is important to monitor total body calcium to prevent the occurrence of a hypercalcemic state.
- ○ Vitamin D preparations increase intestinal calcium absorption.
  - □ Hypercalciuria and associated calculus formation may occur with doses of vitamin D sufficient to relieve tetany and normalize serum levels of calcium.
- ○ Magnesium deficit may inhibit PTH release and use.

- ○ Treatment of underlying cause should be initiated once the acute phase is under control.

- ○ Establish baseline data with which subsequent assessment can be compared.

  - □ Chvostek's sign is not specific for evaluating the effect of the hypocalcemic state on neuromuscular function because it is present in approximately 10% of normal individuals.
  - □ Trousseau's sign can be helpful in evaluating the patient's response to therapy.
- ○ Reduction in stimuli helps to prevent exacerbation of neuromuscular hyperexcitable and hyperirritable state; reduces risk of seizure activity and tetany.

- ○ Hypocalcemic state increases risk of laryngo-bronchospasm.

  - □ Reduces risk of aspiration of airway obstruction from tongue falling to back of throat.

- ○ The hypocalcemic state increases sensitivity and excitability of laryngeal and bronchial musculature, placing patient at risk of developing laryngo-bronchospasms.
- ○ Laryngeal stridor and wheezing reflect a compromised airway.

CARE PLAN FOR THE PATIENT WITH HYPOCALCEMIA (*Continued*)

Nursing Interventions

- Monitor for hyperventilation associated with stress.
  - Evaluate arterial blood gases and implement measures to correct:
    –Alkalemia (pH >7.45).

    –Acidemia (pH <7.35).

- Maintain effective cardiovascular function:
  - Assess the effect of heightened neuromuscular activity on cardiac function.
  - Monitor all vital signs: temperature, heart rate, blood pressure; hemodynamic parameters if indicated: pulmonary artery pressure (PAP), pulmonary capillary wedge pressure (PCWP), cardiac output.
  - Continuous cardiac monitoring of rate and rhythm.
- Implement measures to maintain fluid and electrolyte balance:
  - Correlate serum electrolytes with clinical status:
    –Follow serum calcium and phosphorus.

  - Monitor total serum protein.

  - Monitor serum magnesium levels.

  - Monitor serum potassium.

  - Assess for signs and symptoms of altered fluid state.
  - Monitor intake and output; daily weight; serum osmolality and urine specific gravity; serum electrolytes; hematocrit and hemoglobin.

Rationales

- Hyperventilation induces an alkalemia.

  –Alkalemia increases serum protein-binding of calcium, causing a further drop in free, ionized calcium levels, which may precipitate tetany.
  - Acidemia decreases serum protein-binding of calcium, causing an increase in levels of free, ionized calcium.
  - When correcting the acidemic state, monitor for signs of hypocalcemia, because as the pH rises toward alkalemia, more calcium becomes protein-bound, reducing levels of free, ionized calcium.

- Symptomatic hypocalcemia weakens myocardial contractility; impaired myocardial contractility can predispose to heart failure and cardiac arrest.

- Alterations in serum electrolytes can exacerbate neuromuscular irritability.
  - There is a natural reciprocal relationship between serum levels of calcium and phosphorus: when one is elevated, the other is usually low.
  - The presence of hypophosphatemia requires replacement therapy prior to administration of calcium.
  - Hypophosphatemia induces increased renal synthesis of 1,25-(OH)$_2$D, which increases intestinal absorption of both calcium and phosphate.
  - Hyperphosphatemia attributed to phosphate therapy or reduced renal excretion may be associated with hypocalcemia and deposition of calcium in bone and soft tissues.
  - Approximately 45%–50% of serum calcium is protein-bound.
  - Hypomagnesemia decreases PTH release and utilization, aggravating an already hypocalcemic state. (PTH functions to raise serum calcium levels.)
  - Hyperkalemia potentiates myocardial irritability in the presence of hypocalcemia.
  - If the tourniquet is left in place too long when obtaining blood specimens for serum calcium studies, the total calcium level may be falsely elevated by hemoconcentration.
  - Transfusions of citrated blood may predispose to hypocalcemia from chelation of circulating calcium.
  - Dehydration may accompany disturbances in gastrointestinal function (e.g., vomiting, diarrhea); hemoconcentration or hemodilution may predispose to an electrolyte imbalance.

CARE PLAN FOR THE PATIENT WITH HYPOCALCEMIA (*Continued*)

Nursing Diagnoses

Nursing Diagnosis #2
Injury, potential for: trauma, related to:
1. Seizure activity associated with hypocalcemia.

Desired Patient Outcomes

Patient will:
1. Remain seizure-free and injury-free.
2. Maintain serum calcium levels: 8.5–10.5 mg/100 mL.
3. Verbalize understanding of potential for seizure activity and necessary safety precautions.

Nursing Interventions

• Perform injury-potential assessment of patient's immediate environment.
• Minimize neurologic and neuromuscular stimulation.
• Institute seizure precautions.
• Instruct patient/family regarding potential for seizure activity and necessary precautions to be taken to prevent injury.

Rationales

• Environmental assessment helps to reduce risk of injury by removal of potentially hazardous objects.
• Refer to nursing interventions listed under nursing diagnosis #1.

Nursing Diagnoses

Nursing Diagnosis #3
Nutrition, alteration in: less than body requirements (calcium intake), related to:
1. Malabsorption syndrome (e.g., vitamin D deficiency).
2. Increased lipoprotein levels.
Nutrition, alteration in: less than body requirements (calcium loss), related to:
1. Gastrointestinal disorders: diarrhea.
2. Secondary to diuretics.

Desired Patient Outcomes

Patient will:
1. Maintain adequate nutritional status:
   • Body weight within 5% of baseline for patient.
   • Serum proteins within acceptable range.
   • Serum electrolytes within acceptable range.
   • Hematology profile stable.
2. Demonstrate increased strength and activity tolerance.
3. Remain without signs of infection.

Nursing Interventions

• Provide nutritional and supportive care:
  ○ Assess nutritional needs: dietary habits of patient/family; attitudes regarding nutrition.
  ○ Nutritional needs of hypocalcemic state: low-phosphorus and high-calcium diet.
  ○ Perform an abdominal assessment: presence of bowel signs; evidence of tenderness, abdominal distention.

• Collaborate with nutritionist to incorporate dietary instructions in overall patient/family education.
• Assist patient/family to coordinate medication around dietary intake.

• Establish a progressive exercise program tolerated by patient.
  ○ Begin with passive range-of-motion exercises with progression in activity as tolerated.

Rationales

  ○ Bowel hyperactivity associated with hypocalcemia may predispose to diarrhea; bowel hypoactivity is associated with hypercalcemic state.
• Oral calcium supplements should be taken to decrease gastrointestinal upsets; oral calcium supplements should not be taken with dairy products because the phosphorus content of these foods will decrease intestinal calcium absorption by causing calcium to precipitate in the intestinal tract and be excreted in the feces.
• Immobilization increases calcium resorption from bone.
  ○ Gentle handling and positioning reduce muscle spasms; reassuring and relaxing approach reduces unnecessary stimuli.

Nursing Diagnoses

Nursing Diagnosis #4
Coping, ineffective: individual.

Desired Patient Outcomes

Patient will:
1. Express willingness to participate in self-care activities.
2. Identify prior effective coping mechanisms (individual and/or familial).
3. Verbalize feelings of self-confidence.

CARE PLAN FOR THE PATIENT WITH HYPOCALCEMIA (*Continued*)

Nursing Interventions
- Assess psychological status of patient/family.
  - Identify prior coping mechanisms; familial and community resources.
- Implement measures to assist patient/family in coping.

  - Explain all ongoing procedures and reasons for care.

  - Encourage verbalization of fears, questions, concerns.

- Be accessible to patient/family.

Rationales

- Patient/family should be encouraged to participate in self-care.
  - Appropriate explanations may help to alleviate heightened anxiety.
  - The occurrence of tetany or seizures is a frightening experience for patient/family.

Nursing Diagnoses

Nursing Diagnosis #5
Knowledge deficit regarding follow-up/preventive care.

Desired Patient Outcomes

Patient/family will:
1. Verbalize knowledge of underlying disease process.
2. Verbalize understanding of therapeutic regimen:
   - Medications: indications, dosage, and administration, potential side effects.
   - Diet.
   - Exercise.

Nursing Interventions
- Provide patient/family education to assist in developing and implementing prophylactic healthcare practices.
  - Assess patient/family knowledge of the disease process and therapy.

  - Assess readiness to learn.

- Implement teaching program to include the following:
  - Pertinent anatomy and physiology of calcium metabolism.
  - Pertinent underlying pathophysiology.
  - Identification of precipitating stressors.
  - Recognition of signs/symptoms of hypocalcemic state (tetany).
  - Appreciation of the significance of seeking timely assistance when stressful event(s) occur, or with the first signs/symptoms of hypocalcemia.
  - Knowledge of medical regimen for the disorder underlying the hypocalcemia.
  - Knowledge of medication regimen: dosage and administration; adverse side effects.
  - Understanding importance of continuous healthcare follow-up.
  - Initiation of self-care, health-oriented practices to prevent reoccurring episodes.
  - Nutritional counseling.

Rationales

- Understanding of underlying disease processes assists the patient/family to cope with, and to adjust to, the limitations imposed by the disease.
- Hypocalcemia and its underlying course affect all members of the family; interested and supportive family members should be included in the educational process.

C H A P T E R   3 7

Nursing Management of the Patient with Acute Renal Failure

Jeanette G. Kernicki

CHAPTER OUTLINE

LEARNING OBJECTIVES

After completing this chapter, you should be able to:

1. Differentiate the primary basis for each of the forms of acute renal failure (ARF): prerenal, renal (parenchymal), and postrenal failure.
2. Relate concepts of renal physiology to volume disturbances and electrolyte and acid-base imbalances in the case of ARF.
3. Identify clues suggestive of ARF, based upon history and physical examination.
4. Differentiate prerenal and renal (parenchymal) failure on the basis of urinalysis and blood chemistry.
5. Discuss changes in urine output associated with each phase of ARF.
6. Describe the systemic consequences of ARF.
7. Identify priority goals for the patient experiencing ARF.

The renal system is instrumental in facilitating major body processes. The kidney plays a multifaceted role in maintaining acid-base balance, blood pressure regulation, calcium-phosphate metabolism, electrolyte level composition, erythrocyte production, transport of metabolic waste and excesses, and vitamin D activation. Thus, the internal environment for cellular activity is maintained and held constant by the role of the kidney.

Acute disruption of kidney function affects all body systems. Therefore being attentive to clues manifesting early derangements in kidney function and knowing what to do is particularly important in the care of the critically ill patient, whose body systems may have been compromised by disease or trauma. Early treat-

ment of ARF may prevent prolonged hospitalization and reduce the mortality risk. Knowing which patient is at risk for renal failure and the pathologic processes involved in preventing the kidney from performing its vital functions is an important aspect of critical care nursing.

TERMINOLOGY

For this chapter, only the more commonly used terms in relation to ARF will be defined.

1. Acute renal failure (ARF): the abrupt fall or cessation of urine volume and the retainment of metabolic waste products.[1]

2. Acute tubular necrosis (ATN): clinical syndrome of ARF secondary to ischemia or toxic injury to the renal tubules.[2]
3. Azotemia: an excess of metabolic waste products in the blood: urea, nitrogen, and creatinine.[3]
4. Oliguria: urine volume less than 400 mL per 24 hours for a nontrauma, nonsurgical adult male. The volume represents the average amount required generally to rid the body of metabolic wastes.[4]
5. Renal insufficiency: a compromised state of kidney function in the absence of clinical manifestations. Laboratory tests indicate deterioration of nephronic function.[5]

TYPES OF ACUTE RENAL FAILURE

Prerenal Failure

Prerenal failure occurs when there is a decrease in effective arterial blood volume perfusing the kidney. The result is a decrease in the glomerular filtration rate, thus compromising kidney function, as reflected by abnormal laboratory data but not by clinical manifestations.

CAUSES:

1. Volume depletion secondary to hemorrhage or fluid losses from skin, gastrointestinal tract, and diuretics.
2. Decreased cardiac output resulting from heart failure, pericardial tamponade, arrhythmias, or third space fluid sequestration.
3. Altered vascular resistance secondary to vasodilating drugs, calcium channel blockers, angiotensin-converting enzyme inhibitors, or sepsis. Failure to correct the problem can lead to renal (parenchymal) failure.

Renal Failure

Renal (parenchymal, or intrinsic) failure is a problem existing in the blood vessels, glomeruli, interstitium, or tubules. Renal function loss occurs secondary to structural damage within the kidney.

CAUSES:

1. Glomerulonephritis caused by an infection or an immunologic problem. The individual forms antibodies against circulating antigens or against renal tissue, resulting in the formation of antigen-antibody complexes that lodge within and damage the kidney.[6] Damage to the basement membrane allows red blood cells (RBCs) and protein to cross the more permeable membrane into the filtrate and to the urine.
2. Vascular lesions (atheromatous, inflammatory, and thromboembolic). Renal artery stenosis has been reported to be a common independent fea-

ture in patients with peripheral vascular disease. The prevalence tends to increase with the increasing severity of the peripheral vascular disease.[7]
3. Interstitial nephritis (infectious or allergic). An allergic reaction associated with the use of certain drugs. Carbamazepine, a drug mostly used in partial seizures with complex symptoms, has been reported to cause tubulointerstitial nephritis.[8]
4. ATN, the most common cause of ARF. The insult occurs most often in settings associated with renal perfusion compromise or nephrotoxin exposure. The former can be associated with a surgical procedure wherein hemodynamics may be altered, intraoperative fluid losses occur, and/or antidiuretic hormone (ADH) secretion is increased. Additionally, the general effects of an anesthetic may add insult to kidney function.

Nephrotoxicity associated with antibiotics, chemicals, and intravascular hemolysis is the second most common cause of ATN. Therefore, patients undergoing diagnostic testing in which contrast media is used or those on antibiotic therapy have the potential for ATN.[9]

Nephrotoxicity has been associated with ethylene glycol poisoning, the solvent commonly used in antifreeze solutions. It has been postulated that renal function is impaired as a result of calcium oxalate deposition and renal edema development, which compromises intrarenal blood flow.[10] ATN has likewise occurred in bone marrow transplant patients. Failure of kidney function occurs as a result of basement membrane inflammation and scarring associated with intrarenal ischemia or toxicity from drugs, free hemoglobin, or free myoglobin. Additionally, radiation-related intrarenal injury has been known to develop following toxic doses of radiation.[11]

Postrenal Failure

Postrenal failure is caused by conditions that obstruct urine flow. Although it occurs much less frequently than prerenal and renal failure, nonetheless when the patient has an unexplained drop in urine volume, recommendations are that, first, one seek out potential mechanical causes for the urine volume decline and, second, the functional causes of the problem. Failure to correct the blockage can result in renal system damage. Therefore, it is important to observe and report a diminished volume or absence of urine in the critically ill patient. Whether the patient becomes anuric as a result of the obstruction depends on the nature and location of the obstruction. With partial obstruction, the result may be a state of oliguria; whereas in the presence of complete obstruction, the individual may become anuric.

CAUSES:

1. Urinary calculi, collecting system clots, stricture, or hypertrophied prostate.
2. Mechanical obstruction by kinking of the indwelling cathether may also interrupt urine flow.

PHASES OF ACUTE RENAL FAILURE

Oliguric Phase

In the oliguric phase, the absence of urine may last for days or weeks. This phase is characterized by daily urine output of less than 400 mL, and it is generally caused by ischemia. An important nursing responsibility is to be aware of the onset of oliguria so that appropriate action may be taken immediately to prevent complications. The priority during the oliguric phase is effective treatment of the underlying condition.

Complications associated with the oliguric phase are overhydration accompanied by cardiac failure, pulmonary edema, acidosis, hyperkalemia, and uremic symptoms.[12]

ARF may occur in the absence of diminished output. About one fourth to one third of ARF patients may have the nonoliguric form typical of nephrotoxic acute tubular necrosi.[13]

Diuretic Phase

The oliguric phase generally merges into the diuretic phase, in which urine volume increases. The physiologic basis for the high volume of urine is the osmotic diuresis associated with high levels of retained urea and the inability of the kidneys to conserve sodium and water. This phase is not seen as frequently today as in the past because of the advent of early dialysis intervention.[14]

Complications secondary to diuresis are marked sodium wasting and pronounced electrolyte depletion.

Recovery Phase

During this phase the filtrating and concentrating properties of the kidney are gradually restored. There are some patients, however, in whom the glomerular filtration rate is permanently reduced.[15]

CLINICAL DATA

Laboratory Tests

The preliminary tests used to determine renal function are urinalysis, blood urea nitrogen (BUN), and serum creatinine.

Urinalysis is performed to check kidney and endocrine function. The following are generally measured during a urinalysis: color of urine, pH, specific gravity, glucose, protein, and the presence of blood cells.

Urinalysis and urine electrolytes are helpful in determining whether the cause of renal failure is prerenal or renal (parenchymal/intrinsic): urinalysis mirrors the structural integrity of kidney tubules and urine electrolytes, the functional integrity. Since the tubules are intact in prerenal failure, urinary sediment is normal; therefore, coarsely granular casts, white blood cells (WBCs), and RBCs are rarely found in the urine sample. In an attempt to correct a suspected volume deficit, the kidneys retain sodium and water; therefore, specific gravity and urine osmolality are high, and urine concentration is low. In renal failure, tubular function of the kidney is impaired; therefore, urine sodium values will be high, and specific gravity and urine osmolality values will be low.[16] Urinary sediment in renal failure will reveal the presence of coarse granular casts and numerous WBCs and RBCs.[17]

See Chapter 35 for nursing assessment of renal function and Table 35–2 for a more detailed description of urine analysis, its constituents, and its significant characteristics in renal function.

Blood Urea Nitrogen (BUN) measures the quantity of urea nitrogen found in the blood. Urea, a by-product of protein metabolism, is the most abundant solute in urine. The normal value for BUN in adults is 8 to 25 mg/100mL. A higher value may be seen with the aging process because of loss of the functional ability of the kidney to get rid of waste products. Kidney blood flow and changes in protein metabolism affect BUN levels. The BUN may be high in prerenal, renal, and postrenal failure. Hydrating the patient should return the BUN to normal in prerenal failure secondary to volume deficits. Failure to do so generally implies the presence of other causative factors. A low BUN may be associated with overhydration, severe liver damage, a diet low in protein, or drug influence.[18]

Creatinine (reference value of 0.6 to 1.2 mg/100 mL) is a by-product of creatine phosphate metabolism in skeletal muscle. The creatine phosphate serves as a storage depot for energy. Creatinine is released into plasma at a constant rate; therefore, it is a reliable indicator of kidney function.[19]

Comparing the constant rise of creatinine to the patient's normal level can give one information relative to the degree of nephron loss. A creatinine level twice the norm suggests a 50% nephron loss, and a level eight times the norm, a 75% loss of nephronic function.[20]

BUN levels are measured in conjunction with creatinine values. The normal BUN to creatinine ratio is 10:1. A rise in BUN without a concomitant rise in creatinine suggests either a volume depletion (from diuresis, vomiting, diarrhea, surgery, or burn), a perfusion deficit of the kidney (from cardiac insufficiency or sudden hypotension in a hypertensive patient), or an increase in protein metabolism (from excessive protein intake, starvation, infection/fever, or bleeding into the gut). A rise in both BUN and creatinine levels is highly suggestive of kidney disease.

Diagnostic Tests

A variety of confirmatory tests can be used to identify the source of renal dysfunction. Although an extensive discussion of these procedures is beyond the scope of this chapter, a brief statement of the purpose of the more commonly ordered tests follows.

Cystoscopy is used to visualize the bladder wall, to remove calculi from the bladder or urethra, to obtain a urine specimen directly from the kidney, to remove small lesions, or to obtain tissue for biopsy.

Intravenous pyelography (IVP), an injection of dye (a radio-opaque contrast medium) with a series of x-rays taken, is used to visualize the kidneys, kidney pelvis, ureters, and bladder to determine kidney dysfunction and to locate tumors and calculi.

The *kidney, ureter, bladder (KUB) x-ray* is used to identify the position, size, and shape of the kidneys, ureters, and/or bladder.

Renal angiography, an injection of contrast medium into the renal artery with rapid sequence x-ray filming, is used to detect renal vascular stenosis, nonfunctioning kidney, kidney masses, and obstructive uropathy.

In *renal ultrasound, or ultrasonography,* high-frequency sound waves are passed through a transducer to the kidneys and perirenal area. This test is used to detect masses and cysts, and is frequently performed to clarify findings from other tests.[21]

SYSTEMIC CONSEQUENCES OF ACUTE RENAL FAILURE

Electrolyte Imbalances

Hyperkalemia is the most critical electrolyte imbalance associated with ARF. Abnormalities in serum calcium and phosphorus may also occur. However, because of the short duration of ARF before treatment is initiated, the grave sequellae associated with calcium and phosphorus imbalances are not generally seen. The pathogenesis of hyperkalemia in the presence of ARF varies, but less efficient function of the kidney leads to less effective excretion of potassium. For the purposes of this chapter, only the more common causes contributing to hyperkalemia in the presence of acute renal failure are discussed.

The onset of acidosis and the increased catabolism related to impaired kidney function both contribute to a hyperkalemic state. The distribution of intracellular and extracellular potassium is influenced by changes in arterial pH. Cells are effective buffering systems that can either accept or donate hydrogen (H^+) ions. In metabolic acidosis (unrelated to lactic acidosis and ketoacidosis), H^+ ions move into the cell while potassium (K^+) ions move out, raising plasma potassium concentration. During alkalosis, the cation shifts are reversed.

An additional source of high concentrations of extracelluar potassium may be related to tissue breakdown, trauma, administration of cytotoxic drugs, and massive hemolysis, conditions frequently seen in critically ill patients.[22] Restrictive dietary intake (particularly glucose restriction) in critically ill patients may be another contributing factor leading to hyperkalemia. Normally, glucose is transported intracellularly with potassium in the presence of insulin. Unavailability of glucose because of restrictive intake hinders potassium from entering the cell, resulting in a high plasma potassium level in the extracellular fluid, that is, the plasma level. The diabetic patient particularly may be prone to hyperkalemia because of the inherent lack of insulin.

Some drugs can also contribute to hyperkalemia. β-adrenergic blockers interfere with the facilitation of potassium entry into cells. Therefore, the prescription of β-blockers for patients with ARF is generally avoided. In addition, ingestion of massive doses of digitalis has been implicated in hyperkalemic states. Digitalis inhibits the sodium-potassium-ATPase pump in the cell membrane; therefore, potassium cannot reenter the cell.[23]

Metabolic Acidosis

The metabolic processes of the body generally produce excess acid content. Normally, as acids are produced in the body, the bicarbonate-carbonic acid buffering system neutralizes the acids, which are then excreted by the kidneys. In ARF, the kidneys can no longer excrete H^+ ions or acids or reabsorb bicarbonate effectively. Central nervous system symptoms (shortened memory and attention span, drowsiness, confusion, and progression to stupor or coma) may occur if metabolic acidosis is continuous. Additionally, if the pH continues in the acidotic range, cardiovascular effects, such as a fall in cardiac output, drop in blood pressure, and/or a propensity for arrhythmias, can occur.[24]

Infection

Infection from staphylococcus and pseudomonas is a frequent cause of death in the patient with ARF. The debilitated state of the patients can predispose them to infection. Additionally, the patient has less resistance to infection because of a decrease in macrophage activity secondary to uremic toxins.[25]

Uremia

Uremia implies a decrease in the ability of the kidney to eliminate waste products of metabolism. Urea and nitrogenous waste product retention may lead to the clinical syndrome of uremia. Manifestations of the uremic state are as follows:

1. Neurological signs: confusion, convulsions, coma, and change in sensorium.
2. Gastrointestinal disturbances: anorexia, vomiting, bleeding secondary to uremic gastritis.
3. Infections.
4. Bruising and bleeding: result of blood coagulation factor dysfunction.
5. Anemia: secondary to a decrease in the erythropoietin factor, or erythrocyte destruction.[26]

Volume Overload

The inability of the kidney tubules to regulate sodium and water predisposes the individual to fluid overload. In addition, a compensatory response to ineffective glomerular filtration pressure during prerenal failure can promote volume excess by retaining sodium and water to fill what is perceived as a volume deficit. If volume overload is severe, the fluid overload can lead to edematous states manifested as peripheral, pulmonary, periorbital, or sacral edema, or to congestive heart failure. Hypertension, if present, is secondary to the hypervolemia.

GOALS OF ACUTE RENAL FAILURE MANAGEMENT

Medical Management

The medical management of the patient with ARF is dictated by the cause and phase of the failure of the kidney to perform its regulatory and excretory functions. During the oliguric phase, the aim of treatment is to control fluids, to prevent tissue catabolism, to enhance waste product excretion, and to regulate electrolyte composition. Therapy, therefore, may include dialysis, fluid and dietary restrictions (a low-potassium, low-protein, high-carbohydrate diet), high amino acid and glucose total parenteral nutrition preparations during dialysis, Kayexalate as an exchange resin for potassium excretion, sodium bicarbonate to raise pH, appropriate antibiotics, and minimal use of invasive lines and catheters. Therapy during the diuretic phase is directed toward regulation of electrolytes, maintenance of fluid volume, and dietary restrictions of protein until normalization of the BUN value occurs.

Nursing Management

Astute observation and monitoring are mandatory in the care of the patient with ARF. A plan of care is directed to remedy or offset complications inherent with the failure of the kidney to perform its function. See Chapter 35 for nursing assessment and the care plan for priority nursing diagnoses of a patient with ARF.

REFERENCES

1. Hagland, MR: The management of acute renal failure in the intensive therapy unit. Intensive Crit Care Nurs 9(4):237, December 1993.
2. Toto, KH: Acute renal failure: A question of location. Am J Nurs 2(11):47, November 1992.
3. Holloway, NM: Nursing the Critically Ill Patient, ed 4. Addison-Wesley, Menlo Park, Calif, 1993, p 424.
4. Wilson, RF: Critical Care Manual: Applied Physiology and Principles of Therapy, ed 2. FA Davis, Philadelphia, 1992, p 608.
5. Phipps, WJ, Long, BC, Woods, NF, and Cassemeyer, VL: Medical-Surgical Nursing, ed 4. Mosby–Year Book, St Louis, 1991, p 1461.
6. Roberts, SL: Physiological Concepts and the Critically Ill Patient. Prentice-Hall, Englewood Cliffs, NJ, 1985, pp 351–352.
7. Missouris, CG, Buckhenham, T, Cappucio, FP, and MacGregor, GA: Renal artery stenosis: A common and important problem in patients with peripheral vascular disease. Am J Med 96(1):10, January 1994.
8. Jubert P, Almiral, J, Casanovas, A, and Garcia, M: Carbamazepine-induced acute renal failure. Nephron 66(1):121, January 1994.
9. Solez, K and Racusen, L: Acute Renal Failure: Diagnosis, Treatment, and Prevention. Marcel Dekker, New York, 1993, p 481.
10. Hatchett, R: A severe and fatal case of ethylene glycol poisoning. Intensive Crit Care Nurs 9(3):183, September 1993.
11. King, CR, Hoffart, N, and Murray, ME: Acute renal failure in bone marrow transplantation. Oncol Nurs Forum 19(9):1327, September 1992.
12. Hudak, C, Gallo, B, and Benz, JJ: Critical Care Nursing: A Holistic Approach, ed 6. JB Lippincott, Philadelphia, 1994, p 582.
13. Toto, KH: Acute renal failure. Am J Nurs 92(11):52, November 1992.
14. Boulton-Jones, M: Acute and Chronic Renal Failure. MTP Press Limited, Lancaster, England, 1981, p 35.
15. Kee, JL: Laboratory and Diagnostic Tests with Nursing Implications, ed 2. Appleton & Lange, Norwalk, CT, 1987, p 84.
16. Ganong, WF: Review of Medical Physiology, ed 15. Appleton & Lange, Norwalk, CT, 1991, pp 276–277.
17. Stark, JL: BUN/creatinine: Your keys to kidney function. Nurs '80 10(5):36, May 1980.
18. Kee, JL: Laboratory and Diagnostic Tests with Nursing Implications, ed 2. Appleton & Lange, Norwalk, CT, 1987, pp 456–457.
19. Rose, BD: Clinical Physiology of Acid-Base and Electrolyte Disorders, ed 4. McGraw-Hill, New York, 1994, p 830–831.
20. Phipps, WJ, Long, BC, Woods, NF, and Cassemeyer, VL: Medical-Surgical Nursing, ed 4. Mosby–Year Book, St Louis, 1991, p 1462.
21. Toto, KH: Acute renal failure: a question of location. Am J Nurs 92(11):51, November 1992.
22. Roberts, SL: Physiological Concepts and the Critically Ill Patient. Prentice-Hall, Englewood Cliffs, NJ, 1985, p 356.
23. Rose, BD: Clinical Physiology of Acid-Base and Electrolyte Disorders, ed 4. McGraw-Hill, New York, 1994, p 831.
24. Phipps, WJ, Long, BC, Woods, NF, and Cassemeyer, VL: Medical/Surgical Nursing, ed 4. Mosby–Year Book, St Louis, 1991, p 1462.
25. Toto, KH: Acute renal failure: A question of location. Am J Nurs 92(11):52,
26. Roberts, SL: Physiological Concepts and the Critically Patient. Prentice-Hall, Englewood Cliffs, NJ, 1985, p 356.

CARE PLAN FOR THE PATIENT WITH ACUTE RENAL FAILURE

Nursing Diagnoses

Nursing Diagnosis #1
Fluid volume deficit: actual (extracellular dehydration, hypovolemia).
Fluid volume deficit: actual (intracellular dehydration, hypernatremia).

Nursing Diagnosis #2
Fluid volume, alteration in: excess (extracellular overhydration, hypervolemia, circulatory overload). Fluid volume, alteration in: excess (intracellular overhydration, hyponatremia).

Desired Patient Outcomes

(For patient outcomes, see care plan for fluid volume deficit, Chapter 36.)

(For patient outcomes, see care plan for fluid volume excess, Chapter 36.)

Nursing Interventions

* For pertinent information related to total body fluid and electrolyte status, see:
  Tables 36–2, 36–3, 36–4, 36–5, 36–8, and 36–9.

* For pertinent nursing interventions and their rationales in the care of the patient with fluid deficit or excess disorders, see care plan for fluid volume deficit and care plan for fluid volume excess.

Rationales

Nursing Diagnoses

Nursing Diagnosis #3
Electrolyte imbalance, related to:
1. Water deficit
2. Hypernatremia
Electrolyte imbalance, related to:
1. Water excess
2. Hyponatremia

Desired Patient Outcomes

(For patient outcomes, see care plan for potassium imbalance, Chapter 36.)

Nursing Interventions

* For pertinent nursing interventions and their rationales in the care of the patient with sodium imbalance, see care plan for sodium imbalance.

Rationales

Nursing Diagnoses

Nursing Diagnosis #4
Cardiac output, alteration in: decreased, related to:
1. Dysrhythmias associated with hyperkalemia (> 5.5 mEq/L).
2. Dysrhythmias associated with hypokalemia (< 3.5 mEq/L).

Desired Patient Outcomes

(For patient outcomes, see care plan for potassium imbalance, Chapter 36.)

Nursing Interventions

* For pertinent nursing interventions and their rationales in the care of the patient with potassium imbalance, see care plan for potassium imbalance.

Rationales

CARE PLAN FOR THE PATIENT WITH ACUTE RENAL FAILURE (*Continued*)

Nursing Diagnoses

Nursing Diagnosis #5

Acid-base balance, alteration in: metabolic acidemia (acidosis).

Desired Patient Outcomes

Patient's condition will stabilize as follows:
1. Arterial blood gases will normalize to baseline values:
   - pH > 7.35, < 7.45
   - $PaCO_2$ optimal level for patient (normal range 35–45 mmHg)
2. Anions will stabilize as follows:
   - Bicarbonate (HCO_3^-) 22–26 mEq/L
   - Chloride 100–106 mEq/L
   - Anion gap 12–15 mEq/L
3. Neurologic: alert, oriented to person, time, place; deep tendon reflexes—brisk
4. Serum potassium level: 3.5–5.5 mEq/L
5. Hemodynamic status will stabilize as follows:
   - Arterial BP within 10 mmHg of baseline
   - CVP = $\overline{mean}$ 0–8 mmHg
6. Ventilatory effort maintain blood gas values at optimal level for patient
   - Respiratory rate: 12–18/min
   - Tidal volume: > 5–7 mL/kg

Nursing Interventions

- Monitor neurological status: level of consciousness, mental status; cranial nerve function; deep tendon reflexes, seizure activity.

- Monitor arterial blood gases.

- Monitor serum potassium levels.

- Monitor respiratory rate and rhythm.

Rationales

- Alterations in neurologic function are commonly associated with severe metabolic acidosis and may include confusion, headache, seizures, coma, and other manifestations.
- Reflect effectiveness of ventilatory effort and gas exchange; blood gas levels and pH provide essential data for assessing acid-base and electrolyte balance.
- Severe metabolic acidemia can predispose to hyperkalemia as excess H^+ ions are moved into cells in exchange for K^+ ions, which enter intravascular space (circulation); hyperkalemia may predispose to cardiac dysrhythmias and cardiac arrest.
- Hyperventilation (Kussmaul's breathing): deep and rapid breathing—the body's compensatory response to severe acidemia (pH < 7.20).

- For pertinent information about acid-base abnormalities, including definition, pathophysiology, etiology, clinical presentation, treatment, and nursing diagnoses, see:
  Table 23–2. Respiratory Acid-Base Abnormalities
  Table 23–3. Metabolic Acid-Base Abnormalities

Nursing Diagnoses

Nursing Diagnosis #6
Nutrition, alteration in: less than body requirements.

Desired Patient Outcomes

Patient will:
1. Maintain body weight between 2–5% of patient's baseline.
2. Maintain serum albumin within physiologic range: 3.5–5.0 g/100 mL.
3. Tolerate oral feedings without nausea, vomiting, diarrhea, or stomatitis.

CARE PLAN FOR THE PATIENT WITH ACUTE RENAL FAILURE (*Continued*)

Nursing Interventions

- Collaborate with nutritionist to perform comprehensive nutritional assessment.

  - Weigh daily under same conditions.
  - Monitor intake and output.
    - Monitor electrolytes closely.

- Implement prescribed dietary regimen:
  - Caloric intake: 2000–3000 calories/24 h

  - Low protein intake: ~ 1 g/kg of body weight/24 h.
    - Protein sources high in essential amino acids.

  - Avoid foods high in potassium.
    - Offer oral high caloric supplements, vitamin and mineral supplements.
- Implement measures to enhance mealtimes:
  - Provide frequent oral care.

  - Limit fluids with meals; provide more frequent small feedings.
  - Encourage family to bring appropriate home-cooked foods; encourage visiting during mealtimes.
  - Encourage rest periods before and after meals.

Rationales

- Provides baseline for planning nutrition that will provide sufficient calories to prevent protein catabolism, and sufficient protein intake to meet body needs while avoiding excess production of urea nitrogen.
  - Body weight is best indicator of fluid gain or loss.
  - Diligent monitoring of fluid state is essential to prevent fluid excess during oliguric phase and fluid deficit during diuretic phase.

  - The number of calories depends on age, size, and level of activity.
  - Low protein intake helps to control azotemia associated with compromised renal excretion of nitrogenous waste. Goal of therapy: maintain body weight and prevent protein breakdown.
  - Acute renal failure and associated metabolic acidemia place the patient at risk of developing hyperkalemia.

  - Prevents stomatitis; decreases foul taste; improves appetite.
  - Smaller volume at mealtimes may facilitate gastric emptying and reduce gastrointestinal upsets.
  - Favorite foods may enhance appetite. Helps to provide a mealtime atmosphere conducive to good eating.
  - Avoids undue fatigue.

Nursing Diagnoses

Nursing Diagnosis #7
Knowledge deficit: dietary regimen in renal disease.

Desired Patient Outcomes

Patient will:
1. Verbalize knowledge of prescribed diet, specify dietary restrictions and their significance.

Nursing Interventions

- Initiate patient/family education regarding prescribed diet and meal preparation. Stress those foods permitted versus those foods restricted.
- Implement alternative approach to providing nutrition as dictated by patient's overall condition:
  - Nasogastric or enteral feedings
  - Total parenteral nutrition

Rationales

- Compliance with long-term dietary restriction requires that patient/family understand the relationship between renal disease, diet, and medication regimen.
- Ensures adequate intake of essential amino acids for maintaining and repairing body tissues; sufficient carbohydrate caloric source to reverse gluconeogenesis and catabolic state.

Nursing Diagnoses

Nursing Diagnosis #8
Infection, potential for: depressed immunologic system.

Desired Patient Outcomes

Patient's condition will stabilize as follows:
1. Nonfebrile.
2. WBC within physiologic range.
3. Patient will verbalize a general feeling of well-being.
4. Absence of infection.
   - Negative cultures
   - Absence of redness, swelling, pain

CARE PLAN FOR THE PATIENT WITH ACUTE RENAL FAILURE (*Continued*)

Nursing Interventions	Rationales
• Assess for signs of infection: ○ Vigilant assessment of all invasive lines and wound dressings is critical. ○ Observe for redness, pain, swelling at all invasive sites; dressing changes as per unit protocol. ○ Monitor body temperature, WBC; obtain cultures as indicated: sputum, blood, urine, wound. ○ Pulmonary function: encourage deep breathing and coughing. ○ Auscultate lungs for adventitious sounds of pulmonary congestion or increased secretions; encourage frequent position changes. ○ Urinary function: monitor use of Foley catheter; perform perineal care and cleansing around catheter as per unit protocol; maintain the integrity of the closed drainage system; examine urine for cloudiness or unusual odor.	• Uremic state depresses the body's immunologic defenses and increases patient's susceptibility to infection. ○ Infection is the most common cause of death in patients with ARF. ○ Patient care activities are directed toward prevention of accumulation of pulmonary secretions and atelectasis. ○ Assists in evaluating ventilatory effort; patients with ARF are at high risk of developing pneumonia. ○ Use of indwelling Foley catheters in patients with ARF is associated with a high incidence of urinary tract infection (nosocomial infections). If an indwelling catheter is necessary, its insertion and ongoing care require *strict* aseptic technique. ○ Indwelling catheter should be removed as soon as feasible as determined by the patient's overall condition.

Nursing Diagnoses	Desired Patient Outcomes
Nursing Diagnosis #9 Injury, potential for: uremia-induced gastrointestinal disorders.	Patient will: 1. Tolerate oral feedings. 2. Verbalize having an appetite. 3. Maintain usual bowel routine. 4. Exhibit nasogastric secretions and stool negative for occult blood.

Nursing Interventions	Rationales
• Monitor gastrointestinal function: assess abdomen for distention, tenderness; bowel sounds in all quadrants. ○ Monitor for nausea, vomiting, and diarrhea; test vomitus and nasogastric aspirate and stool for occult blood. ○ Monitor Hct and Hgb.	• Patients with ARF are susceptible to gastrointestinal upsets, resulting in part from the chemical irritation caused by bacteria that hydrolyze urea to ammonia in the gut. • Administration of antibiotics or other drugs alters the intestinal flora, placing the patient at increased risk of infection.

Nursing Diagnoses	Desired Patient Outcomes
Nursing Diagnosis #10 Skin integrity, impairment of: potential.	Patient will: 1. Maintain intact skin; no breaks, lesions, or infection. 2. Exhibit warm, dry skin, with good turgor and absence of interstitial edema. 3. Verbalize/demonstrate measures for optimal skin care.

Nursing Interventions	Rationales
• Maintain skin integrity. ○ Inspect skin on each shift, especially reddened areas over bony prominences where skin is thin. ○ Institute measures to prevent skin breakdown: frequent position changes, use of sheepskin or egg crate mattress (pressure relief device), frequent lubrication of skin, active/passive exercises as tolerated. ○ Teach patient/family the essentials of skin care.	• A comprehensive assessment of skin can assist in early detection of alterations in skin. ○ Deposition of phosphate crystals in the skin causes troublesome itching, which can lead to excoriation and infection. ○ Patient/family can be taught to rub a lanolin-base lotion on the skin to avoid scratching and to stimulate circulation.

CARE PLAN FOR THE PATIENT WITH ACUTE RENAL FAILURE (*Continued*)

Nursing Diagnoses

Nursing Diagnosis #11
Oral mucous membrane, alteration in.

Desired Patient Outcomes

Patient will:
1. Verbalize/demonstrate measures for optimal oral hygiene.

Nursing Interventions
- Maintain integrity of oral mucous membranes: provide oral hygiene, instruct patient/family on measures to enhance oral hygiene.

Rationales
- Changes in overall health status are often reflected in the status of the oral mucous membranes and the skin. Poor oral hygiene places the patient at risk of developing stomatitis; it decreases the patient's appetite and can seriously curtail oral intake.

Nursing Diagnoses

Nursing Diagnosis #12
Comfort, alteration in: pain (pericarditis).

Desired Patient Outcomes

Patient will:
1. Verbalize when in pain.
2. Identify appropriate pain relief measures.
3. Verbalize comfort.
4. Discuss origin of chest pain and significance in ARF.

Nursing Interventions
- Evaluate pain and stress tolerance.

  ○ Assess presence of chest pain: severity, location, duration, quality (type) of pain, influencing factors.

  ○ Assess presence of: fever, chills, pericardial friction rub, gallop rhythm.
  ○ Administer analgesic as prescribed, and evaluate its effectiveness in relieving pain.
  ○ Instruct patient to lean forward over a pillow or bedside table.
  ○ Perform comfort measures: repositioning, relaxation techniques.
  ○ Manipulate the environment and daily routines to provide rest periods.
- Identify patients at risk and predisposing factors: bacterial/viral infections associated with invasive lines, respiratory and gastrointestinal dysfunction, or wounds; poor dietary intake; depressed immunologic function.
  ○ Assess for cardiac failure and tamponade.

- Discuss underlying cause of pericarditis and its potential impact on patient/family lifestyle.

Rationales
- Pericarditis is frequently precipitated during the uremic state; fear of "heart attack" on the part of patient/family may complicate therapy and recovery.
  ○ Use SLIDT tool (Table 35–1).
  ○ Chest pain associated with pericarditis can be sudden onset, sharp and intermittent, located substernally with radiation to neck and back.
  ○ Diligent monitoring is essential because myocarditis and tamponade can lead to cardiac failure.

  ○ This positioning frequently relieves chest pain associated with pericarditis.
  ○ Comfort measures may decrease pain by promoting relaxation.

- Prevention and/or prophylaxis is the best treatment.

  ○ These complications must be anticipated and can create an acute emergency situation. The focus of diligent, ongoing assessment is to avoid these complications.
- An informed patient/family facilitates their participation in the care process.

Nursing Diagnoses

Nursing Diagnosis #13
Activity, alteration in: fatigue and anemia.

Desired Patient Outcomes

Patient will:
1. Verbalize decrease in fatigue.
2. Exhibit willingness to pace activities.
3. Maintain Hct and Hgb within realistic range based on renal function.

CARE PLAN FOR THE PATIENT WITH ACUTE RENAL FAILURE (*Continued*)

Nursing Interventions	**Rationales**
• Evaluate activity tolerance—impact of anemic state:	
○ Assess onset, time of day, and duration of fatigue, and clinical circumstances in which it occurs.	○ Fatigue is a major clinical manifestation attributed directly to the uremic state.
○ Monitor laboratory data to determine presence and extent of anemia: hematocrit and hemoglobin; complete blood count (CBC), platelet count; blood urea nitrogen (BUN), serum creatinine.	○ Anemia is often seen early in ARF and is associated with an inadequate synthesis of erythropoietin factor by the kidneys. Uremia may predispose to bleeding tendencies.
○ Assess skin for bruising or petechiae; nasogastric aspirate and stool for occult blood.	○ Diligent, ongoing assessment is essential to prevent anemia and/or a major bleeding disorder.
○ Minimize iatrogenic blood loss. Draw minimal blood samples for laboratory study; handle patient carefully to prevent bleeding; avoid hypodermic injections.	○ Efforts to minimize blood loss are essential in the presence of compromised hematologic function associated with uremia.
○ Use stool softeners to prevent constipation and hemorrhoidal bleeding; use soft small-lumen nasogastric tube to minimize gastric mucosa irritation; monitor vital signs and watch carefully for signs of anemia, hemorrhage, and occult bleeding from whatever source.	
○ Incorporate rest periods into daily routines. Assist patient/family to set priorities and to pace exercise and other activities alternating with timely rest periods.	○ Conservation of strength may improve endurance.

Nursing Diagnoses	**Desired Patient Outcomes**
Nursing Diagnosis #14	
Knowledge deficit, impact of renal disease on patient/family lifestyle when the course of ARF is extended over several weeks or months.	Patient and family will: 1. Verbalize understanding of ARF. 2. Verbalize willingness to make adjustments in lifestyle as necessitated by the course of the illness.

Nursing Interventions	**Rationales**
• Address knowledge deficit–health perceptions.	• ARF may require weeks to months for recuperation and often becomes chronic.
○ Assess patient/family baseline knowledge and readiness to learn.	○ An informed patient/family can participate in care and make adjustments in lifestyle as necessitated by the course of the renal disease.
○ Establish a rapport with patient and family.	○ An environment of mutual respect and trust can enhance the learning process.
○ Determine appropriate teaching strategies to facilitate learning:	○ Learning should occur at a rate that is meaningful and tolerable to patient and family.
□ Encourage open discussions regarding renal disease: etiology, clinical presentation, complications, treatment, and prognosis.	
□ Assist patient/family to relate dietary restrictions and exercise activities to status of renal disease.	
□ Encourage patient/family to verbalize concerns regarding renal disease and expectations of its outcome.	
○ Reinforce learning and provide feedback for patient/family progress and achievements.	○ Learning is an ongoing process; praise for one's accomplishments stimulates self-motivation, and assists in determining directions for further growth.

Nursing Diagnoses	**Desired Patient Outcomes**
Nursing Diagnosis #15	
Coping, ineffective individual/family: potential.	Patient will: 1. Verbalize feelings regarding renal disease. 2. Identify strengths and coping capabilities. 3. Make decisions regarding matters of importance to the patient/family. 4. Identify resources available in family and community.

CARE PLAN FOR THE PATIENT WITH ACUTE RENAL FAILURE (*Continued*)

Nursing Interventions	Rationales
• Evaluate coping capabilities: ○ Assess patient's ability to solve problems and set priorities.	○ Problem-solving capability enables patient to assume control and make decision regarding own actions and behaviors.
○ Establish a trusting and caring rapport: patient advocacy; accessibility to patient.	○ A definitive, dependable support system assists the patient to assume responsibility for the level of health desired.
○ Encourage verbalization of perceptions, concerns, and feelings.	○ Unexpressed and unresolved fears and concerns may compromise ability to cope effectively.
○ Assist patient to identify past coping capabilities. Emphasize strengths; offer praise for accomplishments; encourage development of new coping mechanisms.	○ Active participation in self-care assists the individual to gain a new sense of dignity and feelings of self-worth.
○ Assist to identify community resources and encourage patient to enlist assistance when necessary.	○ Additional resources may assist patient to gain increased awareness of self in the interaction among patient, family, and environment.

Arterial BP = systolic/diastolic; CVP = central venous pressure.

C H A P T E R   3 8

Nursing Management of the Patient with End-Stage Renal Disease

Christine M. Chmielewski,
Jo-Ann Murray-Schluckebier, and
Marcia Goldstein

CHAPTER OUTLINE

LEARNING OBJECTIVES

After completing this chapter, you should be able to:

1. Define *end-stage renal disease (ESRD)*.
2. Identify the etiologic and pathophysiologic mechanisms underlying ESRD.
3. Describe the stages of ESRD with respect to clinical presentation and treatment.
4. List the various body system manifestations associated with ESRD.
5. Review medications commonly used in the treatment of ESRD.
6. Describe the therapeutic interventions employed in the treatment of ESRD:
   a. Conservative management
   b. Dialytic therapy
7. Identify the types of renal transplants.
8. Specify the immunosuppressants used post-transplant.
9. Identify the pathophysiologic mechanisms of transplant rejection.
10. State the major complications of renal transplantation.
11. Describe the various types of dialysis access and the basic nursing care for each.
12. Use the nursing process to organize the care of the patient with ESRD.

One needs only to review the many functions performed by the kidneys in order to fully appreciate what happens to the patient in the course of ESRD. As the excretory, regulatory, and hormonal function of the kidneys are lost, the disease disrupts virtually every system of the body.

Decreased kidney function, appearance of uremic symptoms, and the loss of urinary output affect the renal patient physically, psychologically, and socially. These bodily changes cause the patient to experience symptoms such as nausea, weakness, fatigue, irritability, confusion, and erratic memory, among others. These symptoms, in turn, have a major impact on the patient's psychological and social states. Difficulties and disruption occur no matter what stage of renal failure the patient is in because all affect the activities of daily living. Chronic renal disease forces a certain amount of dependency on the patient. As a result, the patient may experience an altered self-image and self-worth.

Although uremic symptoms are alleviated with dialysis and transplantation, new problems occur as a result of these treatments. The renal patient, whether controlled by diet and medications or treated by maintenance dialysis, is not well, but rather is "suspended in a state of limbo between the world of the sick and the world of the well, belonging to neither yet a part of both."[1]

DEFINITIONS

ESRD is defined by Lancaster and Pierce as "irreversible kidney disease causing chronic abnormalities in the internal environment and necessitating treatment with dialysis or kidney transplantation for survival."[2] Without either of these interventions, the patient will die.

Azotemia refers to the accumulation and retention of nitrogenous waste products in the blood. *Uremia* refers to the complex multisystem alterations that occur when the level of kidney function can no longer support the internal milieu.

Progression of renal failure occurs at a variable rate, depending on such factors as etiology or additional insults to an already compromised renal status. Although the patient with type I diabetes mellitus may not show evidence of clinical symptoms of renal involvement for 10 years or longer,[3,4] the patient with rapidly progressive glomerulonephritis may follow a course of renal deterioration in weeks to months.[5]

CLASSIFICATION

The etiologic mechanisms underlying the development of ESRD are both numerous and varied. Yet despite this etiologic diversity, the eventual outcome is the same, though the course of the disease processes may vary.

There is no one accepted set of categories for the classification of ESRD; many exist. One such system groups the disease processes under the four major anatomic portions of the kidney: the glomeruli, tubular system, vascular system, and interstitium. Differential diagnosis is often made by biopsy to correlate the suspected underlying etiology with morphologic and hematologic changes. Another common approach is to classify etiology in the same manner as that used for acute renal failure, namely, prerenal (vascular), intrarenal (parenchymal), and postrenal (urologic) causes.

Descriptive categories that take into account the pathophysiologic basis for the particular disease entity include glomerular, infectious or interstitial, vascular, tubular, obstructive, collagen-related, metabolic, congenital, and nephrotoxic-induced diseases.[6,7] These categories are not meant to be exclusive but rather to serve as a guide for systematic arrangement of etiologies, as they do in this chapter.

Glomerular diseases account for nearly half of all cases of ESRD. Although the primary defect occurs in the glomeruli, the damage eventually spreads to include the other renal structures. Glomerular changes include cellular proliferation, leukocyte exudation, basement membrane thickening, and sclerosis or hyalinization.[8] These changes may be described further as focal (involving only some glomeruli), segmental (involving only certain regions of the glomeruli), or diffuse (involving either the entire glomerulus or all glomeruli).

Glomerular disease occurs most frequently as a result of *immunologic-mediated* processes. The presence of antigen—exogenous or endogenous—stimulates the production of antibody. The resultant effect is antigen-antibody complex deposition within the glomerulus. There are two separate mechanisms by which the immune-complex deposition takes place. First, the antigen-antibody complex circulates and becomes lodged within the glomerular capillary tuft. Second, as in the case of Goodpasture's syndrome, the antibody is directed against the glomerular basement membrane.

Glomerular damage allows passage of substances, such as red blood cells (RBCs) and plasma proteins, which normally cannot be filtered through the intact glomerular epithelium. Therefore, two of the major clinical manifestations of glomerular disease are *hematuria* and *proteinuria*. As proteinuria persists, hypoalbuminemia occurs. This, coupled with alterations in the sodium and water handling by the damaged kidneys, contributes to the edema seen in these patients. The renin-angiotensin-aldosterone system reacts to the physiologic cues it receives. Because the cues are released incorrectly by the damaged kidneys and because the feedback mechanisms are lost, hypertension occurs. As the number of functioning nephrons decreases, urine output falls, and the oliguria is accompanied by azotemia and uremic symptoms.

Interstitial diseases are characterized by changes that

occur primarily in the renal interstitium. Inflammation of the interstitium, often with accompanying cellular exudate, progresses on a course of renal tissue destruction. As fibrosis, hyalinization, and scarring occur, the tubular and vascular systems are affected. The most common interstitial disease category is pyelonephritis caused by the presence of long-standing, recurrent urinary tract infections. Other causes of interstitial disease are analgesic nephropathy, injury from irradiation, and certain metabolic and hereditary diseases.

The *vascular* diseases of the kidney involve changes in the renal vessels, primarily in the arteries and arterioles. Narrowing results from atherosclerotic plaque formation, hyaline deposits, endothelial inflammation with scarring, or fibrous tissue formation. Occlusion can occur from emboli, thrombus formation, or simply from the progression of the vessel narrowing to total occlusion.

The major site of renal injury can occur in the *tubular* system. Diseases that affect the proximal tubules primarily alter the reabsorptive capabilities of the kidneys, while defects in the distal tubules affect secretion and excretion. Urinary loss of electrolytes, retention of acids, and eventual inability to concentrate urine are just some of the results of tubular damage.

Obstructions found above the level of the bladder must be bilateral unless one kidney is already nonfunctional, congenitally absent, or surgically removed. Otherwise, the second kidney compensates for the loss in the contralateral organ.

Obstruction of urinary outflow predisposes the patient to infection and also causes dilation of the collecting system. Hydronephrosis creates a back pressure that is greater than glomerular filtration pressure. Consequently, filtration ceases. Increased and prolonged pressure further compresses kidney tissues, thereby decreasing renal blood flow. Ischemic changes occur, and a multifactorial basis for irreversible kidney damage ensues.

The collagen-related diseases are multisystem diseases. Systemic lupus erythematosus (SLE), polyarteritis nodosa, and systemic sclerosis affect not only the renal system but also the cardiovascular, respiratory, musculoskeletal, and neurologic systems. Renal damage occurs as the result of antigen-antibody complex deposition (as in SLE) and vascular changes such as inflammation, necrosis, and narrowing of the arteries.

Metabolic disorders affect the kidneys in a number of ways. Changes can occur in any or all of the renal structures. Diabetes mellitus causes structural change in the blood vessels and tubular system, while amyloidosis primarily affects the glomeruli by causing basement membrane thickening. The hallmark of *hyperoxaluria* is calcium deposition, not only in the renal tissue, but also in the blood vessels, myocardium, and other body tissues.

While some *congenital* disorders such as renal agenesis and renal aplasia are fatal, others may not cause renal dysfunction until later in life. The presence of structurally nonfunctional tissue decreases renal reserve, and altered renal status may eventually occur. Polycystic and medullary cystic diseases destroy renal tissue by displacement and compression. Infection of the fluid-filled cysts is common, and hematuria occurs secondary to the rupture of these cysts.

The toxins frequently encountered in *nephrotoxic-induced disorders* include heavy metals, chemicals, pesticides, and poisonous mushrooms. Chronic and prolonged use of phenacetin-containing analgesics is a recognized cause of renal damage. The hospitalized patient is also exposed to a number of potentially nephrotoxic agents. The most common agents are radiographic contrast media and the aminoglycosides. Renal damage caused by these agents include glomerular, vascular, tubular, and interstitial changes. Although these changes may be acute in nature and, therefore, theoretically reversible, there may also be residual renal impairment leading to eventual ESRD.

STAGES

Patients who present with renal dysfunction may do so in a number of ways. The patient may or may not feel ill and may be seen at any time during the course of renal disease. For instance, the patient with type I diabetes mellitus under close and continued medical supervision may be followed throughout the course of gradual but steady decline in renal function. Another patient may be seen with complaints of headache, fluid retention, shortness of breath, nausea, vomiting, and changes in mental status only to find that the patient's level of renal function is so compromised that the need for dialytic therapy is imminent. Still another patient, totally asymptomatic, may be found to have abnormal urine or serum results on a routine physical examination.

The clinical course of renal disease progresses through three stages: diminished renal reserve, renal insufficiency, and, finally, ESRD.

Diminished Renal Reserve

In diminished renal reserve, the glomerular filtration rate (GFR) is about 50% to 90% of normal. The nephrons hypertrophy, and homeostasis is maintained. The blood urea nitrogren (BUN) and serum creatinine levels are within normal limits, and usually the patient remains asymptomatic. A nephrotoxic dehydration or infection could cause an elevation in the BUN and serum creatinine, but removal of the offending agent allows laboratory values to return to baseline.

Renal Insufficiency

As the GFR drops to 20% to 50% of normal, renal insufficiency occurs. One half to three fourths of the nephrons have been destroyed. The patient may still remain relatively asymptomatic, but the BUN and serum creatinine are elevated. Changes in urine output occur. The kidneys can no longer concentrate the urine, and the patient experiences nocturia and polyuria. Urine osmolarity approaches that of the serum, and specific gravity remains fixed in the range of 1.008 to 1.012. Exposure to a stressful event at this stage of renal failure results in further elevation of blood values and appearance of related symptoms.

End-Stage Renal Disease

With a GFR 5% to 10% of normal, the kidneys lose their ability to regulate the internal environment. The BUN and serum creatinine continue to rise. The patient is symptomatic, the outcome of myriad alterations in the body systems. The patient is now in the final stage, that is, ESRD.

BODY SYSTEM MANIFESTATIONS

The body system alterations that occur with ESRD range from annoying to life-threatening, from easily controllable to persistently incapacitating. A brief overview of the changes the renal patient experiences is presented here. Of all of these changes, the effects of uremia on the cardiovascular and respiratory systems are, by far, the most serious encountered by the patient.

Cardiovascular

Hypertension is seen in most ESRD patients. The two major contributory factors are the retention of sodium and fluid and the inappropriate function of the renin-angiotensin-aldosterone system. Congestive heart failure is frequently seen in patients with fluid overload. Pericardial disease, ranging from pericarditis to tamponade, appears to result most frequently in highly uremic individuals.

Coronary artery disease is a condition found in many patients with renal disease. Hypertension, hyperlipidemia, atherosclerosis, and lack of physical activity contribute to the development of heart disease. Arrhythmias may occur from electrolyte imbalances, metabolic acidosis, volume overload, and dialysis-related problems. Angina may occur during hemodialysis treatments.

Arterial calcification, although rare, results from the calcium-phosphorus imbalance. As calcium and phosphorus bind and precipitate, they form deposits in the tissues. With adequate control of dietary intake of phosphorus and the prescribed use of phosphate binders, tissue calcification is prevented.

Respiratory

Pulmonary edema is an emergency that often requires hemodialysis for fast and effective fluid removal. Altered sodium and fluid handling by the body is the precipitating factor. Noncompliance with respect to fluid and salt restrictions may be the cause, although, in the hospital, intravenous therapy and fluid replacement in the face of oliguria may take the blame. Pleuritis is seen in the patient with a high BUN and serum creatinine level. If left untreated, it can progress to a pulmonary effusion. Depressed cough reflex, altered white blood cell (WBC) response, and sputum changes make the lungs more susceptible to infection. Calcifications in the lungs are a rare occurrence in the individual with adequate control of calcium-phosphorus metabolism.

Neurologic

The neurologic complications associated with ESRD are categorized into two types. The first is peripheral neuropathy, which, in most cases, affects the lower extremities. It tends to be bilateral and occurs as uremia worsens. The two most common neuropathies are the restless leg syndrome and the burning feet syndrome. Discomfort, burning, paresthesia, numbness, and a jumpy feeling in the legs are just some of the ways that patients describe these conditions. These conditions are worse at night and interfere with the patient's comfort and rest. Both syndromes tend to improve and eventually dissipate after dialysis is instituted.

Encephalopathy is the second category of neurologic alteration. One type of encephalopathy is seen in the patient whose uremia requires dialytic intervention. Changes in mental activity and personality occur. Irritability, insomnia, and headaches are frequent complaints. If left untreated, somnolence, seizures, coma, and eventual death would ensue. For the most part, these symptoms disappear when the person is adequately dialyzed.

The *dialysis disequilibrium syndrome* may be seen with the patient who is newly started on hemodialysis. As uremic toxins are removed from the bloodstream more rapidly than across the blood-brain barrier during the course of dialysis, fluid shifts occur. Fluid moves from the intravascular space into the cerebrospinal space where solute concentration is higher. The result of this fluid shift is cerebral edema. The patient may suffer from headaches, nausea, and vomiting. If not corrected, seizures and coma could result. Shorter dialysis time, less rapid solute removal, and use of mannitol have prevented this once common occurrence.

Another neurologic problem is a condition referred to as *dialysis dementia*. Seen in long-term hemodialysis patients, this condition appears to be due to aluminum toxicity. The sources of this aluminum are the water source used for the dialysis treatment and the aluminum hydroxide gels used as phosphate binders. Aluminum toxicity is treated with desferoxamine, which binds with the aluminum and allows for its removal during dialysis.[9]

Gastrointestinal

Gastrointestinal alterations occur anywhere within the alimentary tract. Changes in taste and smell contribute to an already decreased appetite caused by anorexia, nausea, and vomiting. Thirst may be ever present. *Uremic fetor* is the term used to describe the urinelike odor of the patient's breath. Irritation by uremic toxins causes oral, esophageal, gastric, and intestinal inflammation and ulcerations.

Hiccups may occur and are thought to be due to the uremia. Sometimes intractable, they contribute to discomfort and loss of rest. Sedatives and tranquilizers, although sometimes successful in stopping the hiccups, cause the patient to become somnolent. Hiccups usually disappear with the start of dialysis.

The most common gastrointestinal complaint is constipation. Decreased fluid intake, a change in eating habits forced by diet restrictions, phosphate binders, and less physical activity all contribute to the problem.

Because the renal patient has a propensity toward bleeding and because gastrointestinal irritation can add to further blood loss, it is important to check for the presence of occult blood in vomit or stool.

Hematologic

Hematologic abnormalities include anemia, bleeding tendencies, and altered WBC function. There are multiple mechanisms underlying the anemia associated with ESRD. As functional renal mass decreases with the progression of the disease, erythropoietin is affected and RBC production falls. Deficiencies in body iron stores and folic acid, likewise, contribute to inadequate RBC production. Survival of circulating RBCs is affected by the presence of uremic toxins. Blood loss occurs as the result of hemodialysis where some blood remains in the dialyzer, frequent and numerous blood samples, subclinical bleeding, and damage to the RBCs from the roller pump on the hemodialysis machine. Also, the lowered hematocrit, in part, may be a reflection of volume overload and, therefore, may be dilutional. Blood transfusions are not routinely given unless the patient is symptomatic, showing such symptoms as dyspnea, tachycardia, and fatigue.

The bleeding tendency in the renal patient is due to a qualitative rather than a quantitative platelet defect. The platelet count is normal, but the presence of uremia seems to interfere with the release of platelet factor III, an integral component of the clot-

ting sequence. As a result, bleeding time is elevated.

Although the WBCs appear to be normal in number and configuration, they have a slower response time. Renal patients are more prone to both bacterial and viral infections. The WBC count falls within minutes after hemodialysis is started, because there is a temporary migration of these cells to the lungs. Within a few hours, the count returns to its baseline. A complete blood count (CBC) drawn early in the dialysis run will provide spurious results.

Musculoskeletal

Muscle weakness may occur secondary to electrolyte imbalances, atrophy, and uremic toxins. Joint discomfort may result from calcification from calcium-phosphorus precipitation, gout, and bone changes. Altered calcium-phosphorus metabolism is at the root of the skeletal changes. A decrease in the functional renal tissue leads to an altered and ineffective synthesis of vitamin D. As a result, calcium cannot be absorbed as readily from the gastrointestinal tract. The serum calcium level falls, and this, in turn, triggers the secretion of parathyroid hormone (PTH). PTH causes bone resorption in order to elevate the low calcium levels.

PTH, in normal conditions, also causes the kidneys to excrete the extra phosphorus. In renal failure, this excretion cannot be accomplished. The constant effect of the low serum calcium on the parathyroid glands results in secondary hyperparathyroidism, which sometimes requires surgical intervention. If calcium continues to be extracted from the bones, renal osteodystrophy and osteoporosis occur. Bone pain, bone deformities, and pathologic fractures are all outcomes of bone resorption. Dietary phosphate restriction and phosphate binders instituted early in the course of renal failure help to stop this chain of events.

Integument

Although less serious than other body system changes, the alterations in the integumentary system, nevertheless, are cause for physical and psychological discomfort. The patient's skin, hair, and nails change in appearance. The skin takes on a tan to bronze color, the result of retained pigments in the body. Pallor from the anemia also contributes to the skin color change. The skin becomes dry and scaly as oil and sweat glands atrophy. Pruritus develops from the increased dryness and from the deposition of calcium-phosphorus crystals. Excoriation and infection may result from patients scratching their skin. Ecchymotic areas appear with the most minor of trauma because of the capillary fragility. The nails and hair become dry and brittle, the result of protein wasting. Hair may fall out and may even change color.

Acid-Base and Electrolyte

The acid-base disorders and electrolyte abnormalities seen in ESRD are metabolic acidosis, hyperkalemia, hypocalcemia, hyperphosphatemia, hypermagnesemia, and hyponatremia or hypernatremia. All are due to the inability of the diseased kidneys to excrete or reabsorb these substances.

Endocrine

Renal disease is responsible for a number of endocrine abnormalities, namely, thyroid dysfunction, pituitary-gonadal dysfunction, altered carbohydrate metabolism, and changes in lipid metabolism.

CONSERVATIVE THERAPY

Conservative management of ESRD involves diet therapy, fluid restriction, and medications. The goals of this management are threefold: to preserve renal function, to alleviate symptoms, and to prevent multisystem complications.

Diet Therapy

Diet therapy is used to control metabolic alterations and to replace lost nutrients. Special attention is given to protein intake, caloric requirements, fluid and electrolyte restrictions, and vitamin and mineral requirements.

As the GFR approaches 10 mL/min, protein intake and its subsequent breakdown play a major role in the accumulation of nitrogenous waste products (azotemia). At this point, a protein restriction, usually 0.5 to 1 g/kg of body weight per day, is instituted. This restriction keeps the BUN and other end-products of protein metabolism at a tolerable level and results in an overall improvement in the way the patient feels. However, an important consideration is that the patient's intake of protein, although restricted, must be adequate to prevent a negative nitrogen balance and, hence, muscle wasting. This is accomplished by the intake of high biologic value protein, which contains the essential amino acids. High biologic value foods include eggs, fish, meats and poultry, milk, and milk products.

Caloric intake should be in the range of 2000 to 3500 calories per day, depending on the patient's age, size, and level of activity. The goals are to maintain body weight and to prevent protein breakdown. Intake of carbohydrates and fats permits this protein-sparing effect. Control of sodium, potassium, and phosphorus intake is a necessary part of diet therapy. Sodium restriction is based on the overall evaluation of the patient's condition. As long as the kidneys are able to excrete sodium, problems are not encountered. How-

ever, certain renal conditions may cause the patient to lose excessive amounts of sodium in the urine. In these cases, hyponatremia can lead to dehydration, and sodium supplementation is a must. Later in the course of renal disease, however, sodium retention occurs, leading to fluid overload and its concomitant effects. Restriction at this time is imperative to prevent these complications, some of which are life-threatening.

Hyperkalemia tends to occur later in the course of renal disease, when the GFR falls below 10 mL/min. Dietary restriction poses a difficult problem because potassium is found in most foods. Even with adequate dietary control, other factors contribute to hyperkalemia and, therefore, must be carefully monitored. These include the use of salt substitutes (which contain potassium chloride), medications that contain potassium (such as potassium penicillin), metabolic acidosis, gastrointestinal bleeding and other sources of hemolysis, blood transfusions, and, finally, any catabolic state (such as trauma or infection).

Decreased renal function causes decreased excretion of phosphorus. The retention of phosphorus, coupled with the lack of vitamin D synthesis and consequent impairment of calcium absorption from the gastrointestinal tract, leads to the bone disease seen in ESRD. In an effort to halt these skeletal changes, therapy has a twofold approach: first, dietary restrictions of phosphorus and, second, the use of phosphate binders. Because some phosphorus will remain in the diet, these binders are taken after meals to prevent hyperphosphatemia.

Fluid Restriction

Fluid intake is restricted when the kidneys can no longer maintain the body's fluid balance. Allowances range from 1000 to 2000 mL/24 h. Those patients who maintain some urine output are permitted a more liberal intake and are less likely to suffer from overhydration. Thirst and habit make this restriction a difficult one for the patient to follow. It is important to keep this fact in mind, especially for the hospitalized patient whose meager oral fluid allowance is further decreased when intravenous therapy is instituted.

Medication Therapy

Medications commonly used in patients with ESRD may include any or all of the following: antihypertensives, diuretics, phosphate binders, stool softeners and laxatives, antiemetics, antipruritics, cardiotonics, antianemics, vitamins, calcium, iron, and cation exchange resins.

Both fluid overload and inappropriate renin secretion play a role in the development of the hypertension seen in ESRD. Blood pressure control can sometimes be difficult to attain, and it is not uncommon for the patient to be on more than one antihypertensive medication.

Diuretic therapy, often used in conjunction with antihypertensives, is used in the patient who maintains a urine output. Besides ridding the body of excess fluid, some of these drugs also enhance renal excretion of sodium and potassium. It must be kept in mind, however, that certain diuretics are potassium-sparing and, therefore, can lead to hyperkalemia.

Phosphate binders are used to prevent the bone disease of ESRD. Taken with meals, these medications bind with the dietary intake of phosphorus, thereby preventing an increase in serum phosphorus. The major side effect noted with phosphate binders is constipation.

Stool softeners and laxatives (usually bulk-forming) can be used, provided they do not contain magnesium or phosphorus.

To combat the nausea and vomiting, antiemetics can be prescribed. With the institution of dialysis, these symptoms usually subside.

Dry skin and abnormal calcium-phosphorus metab-

RESEARCH APPLICATION: RECOMBINANT ERYTHROPOIETIN ALFA (r-HuEPO) AS A TREATMENT FOR ANEMIA OF END-STAGE RENAL DISEASE

Erythropoietin is a glycoprotein hormone that stimulates bone marrow to produce RBCs. The hormone was first identified in the early 1900s, but it was not until the late 1950s that further studies showed that the kidney was the source of approximately 90% of erythropoietin, with the liver contributing the remaining 10%.

The significance of this hormone was realized when patients with chronic renal failure began receiving dialytic therapy. Those chronically ill patients were plagued with varying degrees of anemia, which contributed to their symptoms of a chronic illness.

Blood transfusions with their inherent risk of transmission of viral illnesses, such as hepatitis and human immunodeficiency virus (HIV), were often required. Patients awaiting transplantation often developed antibodies, which decreased their chances of getting a kidney transplant. Other patients developed iron overload, or hemochromatosis, from frequent transfusions.

In the 1980s, medical research progressed to the point where genetic technology made it possible to produce a molecule identical to the endogenous human erythropoietin hormone. During clinical trials in the 1980s, ESRD patients were given r-HuEPO either intravenously or subcutaneously, either two or three times weekly. The results were dramatic improvements in hemoglobin and hematocrit levels, to a low-normal range. With this decrease in anemia, patients reported decreases in angina and dyspnea and an increase in their well-being, less fatigue, better appetite, and overall increase in energy level. Objectively, there was a dramatic decrease in the use of blood products. There have also been studies documenting a decrease in hospitalization for angina and symptoms of severe anemia.

Since June 1989, r-HuEPO has been available commercially under the trade names Epogen (Amgen) or Procrit (Ortho Pharmaceuticals).

The available literature recommends a starting dosage of 50 to 100 U/kg, intravenously, three times per week, near the end of each dialysis session. When the patient's hematocrit reaches a target range of 30% to 33%, or rises more than 4% in any 2 weeks, it is recommended that the dose be reduced by 25 U/kg. Patients on peritoneal dialysis are given subcutaneous injections of EPO twice weekly. Dosages may be adjusted every 2 to 6 weeks, with either an increase or decrease of 25 U/kg to maintain hematocrit in the target range.

Prior to initiating EPO therapy, patients must have adequate iron stores, with a serum ferritin $\geq$ 100 mg/mL and a transferrin saturation of > 20%. To accomplish this, all patients must receive either oral iron supplements or intravenous iron. It is also important that the patient receive folic acid supplements and that serum folate level is checked. Serum aluminum levels should also be checked, and if elevated, the patient may have to be treated with a chelating agent, such as Desferal, prior to EPO therapy.

There are relatively few problems or complications with EPO therapy. However, patients with moderate to severe hypertension may need to change or increase doses of antihypertensive medicines.

There have also been reports of increased seizure activity in patients who are seizure-prone when their blood pressure and hematocrit increase. EPO is very rarely the cause of allergic reactions in patients with a hypersensitivity either to products derived from cells or to human albumin.

Currently, Medicare is paying approximately $11.00 per thousand units of EPO administered to patients with ESRD and receiving dialysis. This reimbursement only covers the cost until patients reach a target hematocrit of 30% to 33%.

Further studies are under way to determine whether some patients would do better if their hematocrits were in a normal range of about 42%.

olism contribute to pruritus. When meticulous skin care and control of serum phosphorus are ineffective, the use of antipruritics becomes necessary for patient comfort.

Cardiac medications are often found in the patient's drug regimen. Atherosclerosis, coronary artery disease, hypertension, cardiac hypertrophy, congestive heart failure, and angina pectoris are some of the cardiac-related conditions associated with ESRD. Because many of these conditions contribute significantly to renal patient mortality, it is the goal of drug therapy to prevent or treat cardiac disease.

Vitamin supplements consist of multivitamins, folic acid, and vitamin D. These fill the void left by inadequate intake secondary to dietary constraints. Once dialysis is employed, water-soluble vitamins are lost during treatment and must be replaced. An important point to remember is that serum phosphorus must be within normal limits before vitamin D is given. Otherwise, the increase in serum calcium will interact with an already elevated phosphorus, leading to potential tissue calcifications and worsening bone disease.

Oral calcium supplements are given when hypocalcemia occurs, when vitamin D has been ineffective used alone, and when serum phosphorus levels are normal. If vitamin D and calcium supplements are given concomitantly, careful monitoring of the serum calcium is necessary.

Iron supplements play a role in the correction of anemia, provided the anemia is related to depleted iron stores in the body. Usually administered in oral form, iron can be rendered inactive by phosphate binders and, therefore, should not be given at mealtime. Synthetic erythropoietin is currently used to stimulate RBC production.

Use of a cation exchange resin is most commonly seen as an emergency treatment for hyperkalemia. It works by releasing sodium (Na^+) ions in exchange for potassium (K^+) ions. The net result is a lowered serum potassium. The route of administration is by mouth or by retention enema. Because the site of action is in the large intestine, administration by enema achieves results in approximately 30 to 60 minutes, whereas the oral dose can take from 1 to 2 hours.

DIALYTIC THERAPIES

As renal failure progresses to end-stage and the GFR falls below 5 mL/min, the kidneys lose their compensatory capabilities. With the loss of the excretory and regulatory functions, the kidneys cannot rid the body of metabolic waste products, acids, electrolytes, or fluids. The uremia affects every system of the body and threatens the life of the patient. Conservative therapy is no longer an effective treatment option.

The patient has one of three choices to make: dialysis, transplantation, or no further treatment at all. Because refusal of or discontinuation of treatment can, in and of itself, be a lengthy topic of discussion, it will not be covered here.

There is no cure for ESRD. Although dialysis is able to sustain life, it falls short when compared to the work performed by the kidneys. While dialysis can remove some of the uremic toxins and maintain some semblance of fluid and electrolyte balance, it cannot replace the kidney's other important functions. The patient continues to follow diet and fluid restrictions, and medications continue to play a role in the control of the disease and its manifestations.

There are two basic types of dialytic therapy: hemodialysis and peritoneal dialysis. The principles of both are the same: each involves a blood compartment and a dialysate compartment separated by a semipermeable membrane. Movement of fluid and solutes across this membrane is governed by the processes of diffusion, filtration, and osmosis.

Hemodialysis

Although the technical aspects of hemodialysis require the mastery of certain knowledge and skills, the process of hemodialysis is not difficult to understand. The semipermeable membrane in this case is in the dialyzer (also known as the artificial kidney). A concentration gradient exists between the blood and dialysate compartments, and solute movement occurs in both directions. The electrolyte composition of the dialysate solution is similar to that of normal extracellular fluid. However, potassium, sodium, and calcium concentrations can vary to meet the needs of the patient.

Bicarbonate is commonly used to combat metabolic acidosis. Those substances, such as the metabolic waste products, that need to be removed from the patient are not found in the dialysate.

As the patient's blood is pumped through one compartment (hollow fibers or cellulose sheets, depending on the design of the dialyzer), the dialysate is pumped through the other compartment in a countercurrent direction. This flow pattern allows fresh dialysate to circulate continuously, thereby maintaining a constant concentration gradient between the two compartments.

Because blood has a tendency to clot in the extracorporeal circuit, an anticoagulant, most commonly heparin, is used. The goal of anticoagulation is to prevent clotting in the dialyzer and blood lines while, at the same time, preventing bleeding problems in the patient. Clotting times are performed throughout the dialysis procedure to monitor the anticoagulation effects. In some patients, most notably those with decreased hematocrits, thrombocytopenia, or prolonged partial thromboplastin time (PTT), it is possible to dialyze the patient without an anticoagulant.

The major function of the dialysis machine is to allow for both a safe and an effective treatment. Besides pumping the blood and delivering the proper concentration of dialysate solution and water, it monitors a variety of factors: blood and dialysate flow rates, the temperature and conductivity of the dialysate, and arterial and venous blood line pressures. It checks for the presence of blood in the spent dialysate (which signifies a rupture in the dialyzer) and, therefore, a source of blood loss. It also monitors the blood as it returns to the patient to be sure that there is no air in the line, a potentially fatal complication.

Auditory and visual alarms alert the dialysis nurse to the presence of a potentially harmful condition or to a change in one of the parameters on the machine. Conditions that are harmful to the patient, such as air in the blood or a change in the dialysate temperature, will automatically stop the machine and, subsequently, protect the patient.

Hemodialysis requires access to the patient's vascular system. This access may be external (shunt, subclavian catheter, femoral catheter) or internal (fistula, graft). Some, as is the case with the femoral catheter, are used only as a temporary access. The need for a special vascular access is dictated by the fact that blood flow rates up to 350 to 400 mL/min are required during dialysis.

The arteriovenous (AV) shunt was a major breakthrough that made chronic hemodialysis a possibility.[10] Its use today, however, is limited. Now rarely used, the shunt consists of two pieces of Silastic tubing, each connected to a sturdy Teflon tip. One tip is inserted surgically into an artery, the other into a vein. A special connector holds the Silastic tubing together so that the blood flows from the artery to the vein. Placement is usually in the wrist area of the nondominant arm, with ankle placement as a second choice. Complications include infection, clotting, skin erosion, dislodgement, and hemorrhage.

Subclavian catheters are seen more frequently in the patient with acute renal failure but are also used in the ESRD patient. Indications include temporary access for short-term dialysis before a scheduled living, related donor transplant or for use until a fistula matures. Also, if a problem with a fistula or graft occurs, the catheter may be used in the interim. A permanent, surgically placed subclavian dialysis catheter is available for use in the chronic hemodialysis patient. Complications seen with subclavian catheters are of two types: those secondary to insertion and those after the catheter has been in place. Those associated with the former include hemothorax, pneumothorax, laceration of the subclavian artery, and hematoma. The latter are clotting, emboli, subclavian vein thrombosis, and sepsis.

There are two kinds of femoral dialysis catheters. The Shaldon catheter is a single-lumen catheter that requires a second access (or a special device called a single-needle device) to avoid recirculation of the blood leading to inadequate dialysis. If two Shaldon catheters are used, they may be placed bilaterally or in the same femoral vein. The second type of femoral catheter has a double lumen so that blood can be taken from one port and returned through the other during dialysis without any mixing of dialyzed and nondialyzed blood. The complications seen with the femoral catheters include hematoma, retroperitoneal bleeding, and laceration of the femoral artery; infection; embolus; and femoral vein thrombosis.

With the advent of the AV fistula, another major step occurred in hemodialysis. Using the patient's own vessels, Cimino and Brescia were able to create the internal vascular access.[11] The anastomosis between the artery and vein directs arterial blood flow into the vein, resulting in venous distention. The creation of this high-flow vessel allows for direct and repeated venipunctures in the venous side of the access. The AV fistula is the most common vascular access route used. It has a lower incidence of complications (clotting and infection).

In some instances, it is not possible to create a fistula using the patient's own vessels. The vessels may be too small, injured, or rendered unusable by previous procedures. A graft is then used. Anastomosed between an artery and a vein, it serves as the conduit for blood flow and the site for needle placement during dialysis. As with the fistula, complications involve clotting and infection.

Two complications occur soon after surgical creation of the vascular access that require immediate attention and surgical intervention. The *steal syndrome*, which is responsible for ischemic changes in the extremity distal to the access, is caused by the shunting of blood through the access and away from the distal circulation. At first, subtle changes occur in the skin temperature and sensation. Later, pain, paresthesia, swelling, and absence of pulses ensue. If allowed to continue, gangrene and limb loss are the sequelae.

High-output cardiac failure also results from the large volume flow through the access. Increased venous return to the heart cannot be tolerated by some individuals and leads to pulmonary congestion and heart failure. Surgical intervention includes a procedure called banding, in which the lumen of the high-flow vessel is narrowed. If this intervention is ineffective in alleviating the problem, surgical ligation of the vessel is usually necessary.[12]

Peritoneal Dialysis

Peritoneal dialysis (PD), once the mainstay of acute renal failure therapy, has gained in popularity as a treatment modality for ESRD. There are several methods of peritoneal dialysis: continuous cyclic peritoneal dialysis and continuous ambulatory peritoneal dialysis.

Continuous cyclic peritoneal dialysis (CCPD) is automated. Treatments are usually performed at night for 8 to 10 hours. During the last exchange, the fluid is allowed to dwell in the peritoneal cavity, remaining there until the next night.

Continuous ambulatory peritoneal dialysis (CAPD) does not involve automated equipment. Three to five exchanges are performed manually every day. The last exchange is performed at bedtime, and the fluid is allowed to dwell overnight.

There are two pieces of equipment used with peritoneal dialysis patients that the nurse may encounter.

The first is the cycler. This automated machine is able to perform hourly (or longer) exchanges. By and large, it has replaced the old method of changing bags every 1 to 2 hours. Not only does it save time, but its major advantage is that fewer breaks occur in the system, thereby allowing fewer opportunities for contamination. Solution can be set up for up to 36 hours. The machine heats and delivers the solution; controls the inflow, dwell, and outflow cycles; and monitors the amount of fluid delivered and returned.

Because peritonitis is the major complication of CAPD (often from touch contamination), various methods have been designed to decrease the risk of contamination. One such device is the ultraviolet light. This small, easy-to-use piece of equipment uses light to sterilize both the catheter spike and the outlet port of the new bag. It must be used with each CAPD exchange.

The process of peritoneal dialysis involves both blood and dialysate compartments separated by a semipermeable membrane, in this case, the peritoneum. Dialysate is infused by way of a special catheter into the peritoneal cavity. To maintain a concentration gradient between the two compartments, exchanges are performed every 1 to 6 hours, depending on the mode of the treatment.

The effectiveness of peritoneal dialysis is influenced by a number of factors, some related to the dialysate and the others to the patient. Dialysate-related factors are the amount, concentration, and temperature of the fluid, the flow rate, and the volume of dialysate in the peritoneal cavity. The other factors are blood flow to the peritoneum and effective surface area of the peritoneal membrane. The last of these can be especially influenced by the presence of peritonitis.

Access to the peritoneal cavity is achieved by means of a catheter surgically implanted when the patient is in the operating room. This catheter serves as the conduit for the inflow and outflow of the dialysate. Although there are some differences in catheter design, usually involving the intraperitoneal section, each performs the same function. Care of the PD access, like the vascular access, must be meticulous. It is the patient's only means for treatment of ESRD.

Peritonitis is the most serious infectious complication associated with PD. The outcome of peritonitis ranges from quick resolution to less favorable outcomes, including the formation of an intraperitoneal abscess, the loss of effective membrane from scarring, the necessary removal of the catheter (usually because of unresolved peritonitis), and death of the patient. Cloudy effluent (from the presence of WBCs and fibrin) is the hallmark sign of peritonitis. Other signs and symptoms include abdominal pain, rebound tenderness, fever, and chills. A culture and Gram's stain of the effluent identify the causative organisms. Antibiotics are given intraperitoneally to combat infection, and heparin is added to the dialysate to prevent catheter blockage and adhesion formation. Two other infectious complications seen with PD are subcutaneous tunnel infection and exit site infection.

The dialysate is composed of a dextrose solution with added electrolytes and minerals. The dextrose concentration is available in three standard concentrations: 1.5%, 2.5%, and 4.25% solutions. Because the dialysate is hypertonic, it removes fluid by osmotic pull. As the fluid is removed by this force, it is accompanied by small molecules. This process is called solvent drag and, in addition to diffusion, plays a role in solute removal.

Because movement occurs between both compartments, substances can be added to the dialysate that the patient will absorb. Insulin, potassium, and antibiotics are just some of the common additives. Some diabetics can even be maintained solely on intraperitoneal insulin. However, because of the high glucose load and its subsequent absorption into the bloodstream, blood sugar control may sometimes be more difficult.

NURSING CARE OF THE PATIENT WITH END-STAGE RENAL DISEASE

For nursing diagnoses, desired patient outcomes, and nursing interventions in the care of the patient with ESRD, see the care plan at the end of this chapter.

RENAL TRANSPLANATION

Renal transplantation is an accepted and proven method of treatment for ESRD (see also Chapter 49). Several thousand transplants are performed annually in this country alone and are available at most major medical centers. Significant advances in the field of immunology have been made since the first transplants between identical twins in the 1950s. The ability to better control the immune response with potent specific immunosuppressants and refinements in both surgical techniques and organ preservation have established renal transplantation as a major medical intervention.

Data demonstrate dramatic improvements in both patient and kidney graft survival. The 1-year, living, related donor patient survival rate has increased from 84% in 1968 to 97% in the 1990s. During the same period, the 1-year survival rate for patients receiving cadaveric transplants went from 60% to 93%. The probability for 1-year graft survival for transplants from cadaveric donors is 79% now, as compared to 55% in 1968. Graft survival for living, related donor kidneys has remained over 90% throughout the years.[13]

Studies of ESRD patients following transplantation often reveal successful physical and occupational rehabilitation. Transplant patients reported a higher objective and subjective quality of life than did patients undergoing any form of dialysis.[14]

The benefits, however, should be weighed against the risks of major surgery and the need for long-term chemical immunosuppression. Further disadvantages of transplantation include the risk of potentially overwhelming fungal, bacterial, or viral infections; aseptic necrosis of the bone; and an increased incidence of malignancies, hypertension, and ulcer disease.[15]

Donor Evaluation

Donor kidneys for transplantation come from three sources. The first is a living, related donor, either sibling, parent, child, or more distant relative. Donors undergo a series of examinations and studies ensuring that two normal kidneys are present and that no underlying systemic disease or infection exists. It is important for the transplant team and family to openly discuss this donation. Although it has been shown that there is little risk to the donor aside from surgery itself, nothing should be undertaken that would adversely affect the potential donor's well-being.

The second donor source is a living person, nonrelated to the recipient, usually a spouse or close friend. Although not genetically related, the donor and recipient are considered emotionally related. If a living, related donor is unavailable and a cadaver kidney is difficult to obtain, a living, nonrelated donor who is properly motivated and medically stable may be considered.

The third and most common donor for kidney transplants is the cadaver donor. Patients who were previously in good health but have suffered brain death and are ventilator-dependent with intact circulation may be organ donors, with the following limitations:

1. *Age limitations:* persons between 0 and 75 years of age are suitable organ donors; however, older donors are sometimes accepted.
2. *Contraindications:*
   a. History of invasive cancer, with the exception of primary intracranial brain tumors.
   b. Presence of untreated systemic bacterial, viral, or fungal infections.
   c. Positive tests for HIV antibody, HBsAg.

Care of the donor in the intensive care unit focuses on the maintenance of cardiorespiratory and renal function. Adequate intravenous hydration prevents hypovolemia and should promote sufficient diuresis. The use of vasopressors is acceptable but should be weaned if vasoconstriction occurs with subsequent decreased renal perfusion. Laboratory studies are done routinely. Baseline serum creatinine levels are often helpful because serum creatinine elevations may result from trauma. The acceptance of brain death is extremely difficult, and supporting the patient's family at this time is an integral aspect of nursing care. Following donor nephrectomy, the kidneys are flushed and preserved in a cold electrolyte solution. Because graft survival has been related to cold ischemic time, most institutions prefer to transplant the organ within 48 hours of the donor surgery.[16] Efforts to promote increased awareness of the need for more organ donors should further expand organ availability.

Recipient Evaluation

The evaluation for renal transplantation is necessary to identify any potential problems resulting from preexisting conditions. The presence of malignancy or active infection is a contraindication to transplantation. Generally, the evaluation includes a review of all the body systems, with special attention to the cardiovascular system and with psychological and immunologic evaluations. Extensive information about transplantation, the need for long-term follow-up, and patient reliability are discussed in depth with the patient, family members, and the transplant team.

Upon successful completion of the evaluation, potential recipients are placed on a waiting list through the United Network for Organ Sharing (UNOS). This national computer registry allocates organs on a point system based on criteria such as the human leukocyte antigen (HLA) matching between donor and recipient, the preformed antibody levels of the recipient, and the length of time on the waiting list.

A potentially successful match is determined by blood group (ABO) compatibility and a negative T-cell crossmatch. The crossmatch is performed by mixing donor lymphocytes with serum from the recipient. If the recipient has preformed cytolytic antibodies to the donor, a positive crossmatch will ensue, and transplantation is contraindicated.

Transplant Immunology

The human immune system is responsible for recognizing and resisting foreign substances, such as bacteria, viruses, toxins, and cells unrelated to itself.[17]

The two types of acquired immunity are cellular immunity (T lymphocytes) and humoral immunity (B lymphocytes or antibodies). A cellular immune response involves the sensitization of the patient's T lymphocytes to the transplanted kidney tissue. These T cells proliferate and infiltrate the kidney, resulting in tissue damage, disruption of normal renal blood flow, and rejection.

Humoral, or B-cell, immunity involves antigen-antibody reactions. The presence of antigen or foreign tissue elicits the formation of specific antibodies, which function to attack the antigen. Antigen-antibody reactions are responsible for hyperacute and accelerated rejection as well as chronic rejection.

Medications that suppress the immune system are required for as long as the transplanted kidney functions. Immunosuppressants, however, interfere with the normal immune response and predispose the patient to infections, opportunistic pathogens, and possibly malignancies.

Transplant Rejection

Despite the use of immunosuppressive medications, allograft rejection remains one of the most plaguing problems for transplant recipients. Rejections can be categorized as follows:

Hyperacute rejection usually occurs within minutes to hours after the surgical anastomoses are completed. It results from the reaction of preformed cytotoxic antibodies in the recipient's body with the foreign antigen. Intrarenal vascular thrombosis results, and the kidney must be removed.[18]

Accelerated rejection occurs within the first week after transplant and also results from preformed antibodies. This form of rejection does not respond to immunosuppressive therapy, and the kidney is removed.

Acute rejection, a cell-mediated response, is the most common form of rejection and is often reversed with vigorous immunosuppression. The classic signs and symptoms of an acute rejection are as follows:

Elevated temperature
General malaise
Tenderness over graft
Elevated blood pressure
Decreased urine output
Rapid weight gain
Peripheral edema

Patients may have several, all, or even one of these symptoms. An elevation in the serum creatinine level is often the first indication of rejection. The majority of patients undergo at least one acute rejection episode, usually in the first 6 months. Differential diagnosis is facilitated by renal scans and ultrasounds, which demonstrate changes in kidney function and size. A transplant biopsy is helpful in distinguishing this cell-mediated process. Following treatment of the rejection, the patient continues on standard immunosuppression.

Chronic rejection, a humoral response, is characterized by a progressive deterioration of renal function, which may occur over a period of months to years. This form of rejection does not generally respond to treatment and is responsible for eventual failure of the graft. As renal function decreases, the patient may be placed on diet restrictions and medications to control the symptoms. When graft failure occurs, dialysis or retransplantation is necessary.

Immunosuppression

Successful renal transplantation depends on the ability to suppress the immune system judiciously.

Chemical immunosuppresion is achieved through various combinations of medications. The actions of each of these medications differ, and their simultaneous use yields a multifaceted attack on the reacting cells (Fig. 38–1).

Cyclosporine is a potent and specific immunosuppressant that prevents the replication of T lymphocytes by inhibiting the production of interleukin-2 (Fig. 38–1). The use of cyclosporine has significantly

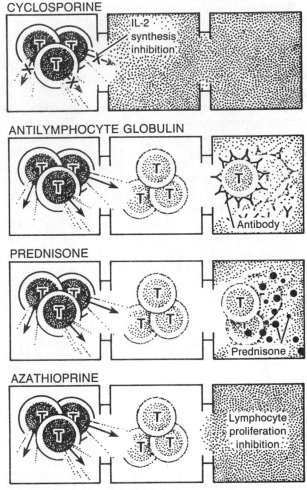

FIGURE 38–1. Pharmacologic immunosuppression in renal transplant therapy. Cyclosporines act on T lymphocytes, inhibiting the synthesis and secretion of interleukin-2 (indicated by X in top frame) that are essential for the proliferation of T lymphocytes. Hence, cyclosporine prevents lymphocytic replication. Antilymphocyte globulin (ALG) is an antiserum of lymphocytic antibodies (Y-shaped structures in frame 2) that is used to treat rejection by destroying circulating white blood cells. Prednisone (black dots in frame 3) acts nonspecifically as a lymphocytic agent, causing the destruction of circulating lymphocytes. Azathioprine interferes with cell synthesis, thereby inhibiting lymphocyte proliferation.

improved cadaver graft survival rates. Therapeutic blood level monitoring is necessary to ensure adequate immunosuppression to minimize toxicity and its side effects.

Antilymphocyte globulin (ALG) is an antiserum used to treat acute rejection by destroying the abundant circulating WBCs (Fig. 38–1). ALG may be used prophylactically after operation. Administration of ALG requires the use of a high-flow vessel. The nurse must monitor the patient for anaphylaxis, fever, chills, joint pain, or symptoms of infection. Symptomatic relief is achieved through administration of hydrocortisone, acetaminophen, and diphenhydramine prior to infusion of ALG.

Prednisone is a glucocorticoid whose anti-inflammatory action is cytolytic and whose immunologic action impairs the recognition and processing of foreign tissue by the immune system. Its lymphocytic action results in the destruction of circulating lymphocytes (Fig. 38–1). The nonspecific actions of this medication yield untoward systemic effects.

Azathioprine interferes with cell synthesis, thereby inhibiting proliferation of lymphocytes. However, its action is not specific and it also inhibits myelogenous cells, often resulting in bone marrow toxicity (Fig. 38–1).

Monoclonal antibody, an immunoglobulin, prevents antigen recognition by altering the T lymphocytes and yielding impaired function.

Administration of monoclonal antibody (OKT3) preparations requires special precautions. Upon receiving the initial dose, the patient may experience dyspnea, wheezing, tachycardia, fever, chills, possible anaphylaxis, and bronchospasm. Pulmonary complications have been avoided by ensuring that the patient's chest x-ray is negative for infiltrates and pulmonary congestion. Nursing care focuses on assessment for fluid volume overload prior to initiation of

therapy and diligent patient monitoring, and on symptomatic relief.[19]

Clinical Management

Preoperative Period

Preparation for transplantation includes assessment of the need for dialysis prior to surgery, initiation of immunosuppressants, and cleansing of the operative site. Patient teaching and support are vital now because events take place rapidly and may be overwhelming.

Intraoperative Period

The donor kidney is placed within the right or left iliac fossa. The donor renal vein is anastomosed to the external iliac vein. The donor renal artery is anastomosed to the hypogastric artery or to the iliac artery. The donor ureter is tunneled into the bladder by means of a ureteroneocystostomy. Once the vascular clamps are removed, the kidney should become pink

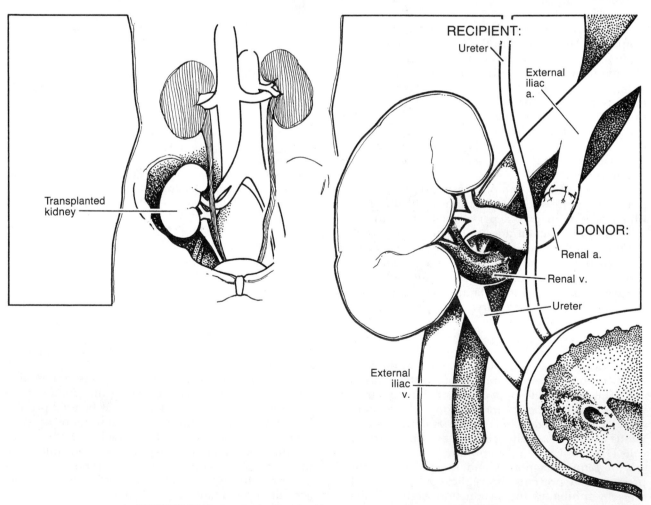

FIGURE 38–2. Surgical transplantation of donor kidney into recipient.

and firm, denoting adequate blood flow to the organ. It is important to avoid circulating volume deficit because hypovolemia interferes with renal function (Fig. 38–2).

Postoperative Period

In the immediate period following operation, the patient's vital signs and hemodynamic parameters are monitored frequently. Intake and output are measured hourly to assess the patient's fluid status, and laboratory specimens are used to evaluate the patient's electrolyte and acid-base status. Complications seen in this early postoperative period include fluid volume overload or deficit, metabolic acidosis, hyperkalemia, or hypokalemia.

Fluid replacement is determined both by the patient's hourly urine output and central venous pressure (CVP) readings. Excessive diuresis may sometimes occur, and with it hyponatremia and hypokalemia. This polyuria occurs secondary to diminished reabsorption in the proximal tubules. Intravenous fluids (usually a dextrose solution with 0.45% normal saline) may contain additives to combat metabolic acidosis and/or hypokalemia.

Hyperkalemia may occur as the result of tissue trauma intraoperatively, blood transfusions administered during the surgery, or nonfunction of the transplanted kidney. Because hyperkalemia is life-threatening, emergency measures are employed to bring the serum potassium near normal until either the transplanted kidney begins to function or the need for dialysis is ascertained. These emergency measures include the intravenous administration of glucose and regular insulin to facilitate the movement of the K^+ ions into the cells, and intravenous calcium chloride is given to protect the myocardium against the deleterious effects of the elevated serum potassium on the heart. Because these measures are temporary in nature (they do not lower the number of the K^+ ions but redistribute them), they are followed up with the administration of Kayexalate, which may be given either by mouth or by retention edema. This medication binds with the K^+ ions and, therefore, removes them from the body. Continued or recurrent hyperkalemia is an indication for dialysis.

The patient may be anuric or oliguric, the result of acute tubular necrosis (ATN) that develops from ischemic changes in the graft. ATN may never resolve or could last for as long as 6 weeks with reported full recovery of renal function.[20] The anuric patient must be supported with dialysis and monitored for infection because sometimes increased doses of immunosuppressive medication will be required. The patient must be given realistic encouragement. Fluid and dietary restrictions are usually required.

A sudden decrease in established urine flow indicates potential complications and mandates further assessment. The urinary catheter should be checked for patency and irrigated only under strict aseptic technique. Decreased urine flow could represent

hypovolemia, ureteral leaks, or an obstruction. A vascular thrombosis (e.g., renal artery thrombosis) may cause partial or complete infarction of the transplant. Observe for abdominal distention, tenderness, or leakage from the incision. Fluid challenges with diuretics and colloids may be given. Renal scans and ultrasounds usually assist in determining the source of the problem and establishing diagnosis.

An ongoing head-to-toe assessment is performed by the nurse. Because of the propensity for infectious complications (caused by the immunosuppressive medications), the patient requires diligent monitoring for the signs and symptoms of infection. Prevention of these infectious complications is of tantamount importance and should serve as the focal point in rendering bedside care. In all other respects, the renal transplant recipient is treated as all other patients after operation.

Nursing Responsibilities

Thorough assessment and monitoring of the transplant patient cannot be overemphasized. As long as a transplanted kidney is in place, these patients will require immunosuppressants. Immunosuppressed patients with compromised cell-mediated immunity are at increased risk for developing fulminant bacterial, viral, and fungal infections. Infections are treated with antibiotics and, if the infection is life-threatening, immunosuppression may be discontinued to save the patient.

Assessment of a renal transplant recipient for either infection or rejection includes physical examination and laboratory work, including cultures and radiographic results. Other parameters of kidney function include daily weight, intake and output, and vital signs.

An elevated temperature is rarely insignificant and may indicate infection or rejection. Fevers should be recorded, reported, and followed with bacterial, viral, and fungal cultures. Hepatitis profile is also to be considered. It is important to remember that large doses of steroids may mask an elevated temperature and a normal WBC response to an infectious process.

The surgical incision should be examined for swelling, erythema, or tenderness. Drainage should be cultured immediately, and an ultrasound should be obtained. Intravenous access areas should be inspected, cleansed daily, and changed frequently. Upon removal of the intravenous access in the presence of fever, the catheter tips should be inspected and sent for cultures. The mouth and mucous membranes are inspected often for herpetic lesions and monilial infections. Changes in mental status, headaches, or confusion could mean central nervous system involvement and necessitate a spinal tap for cultures of cerebrospinal fluid.

The urinary catheter predisposes the transplant recipient to urinary tract infections and should be removed as soon as possible. Symptoms of a urinary tract infection warrant immediate urine cultures. Patient education on recognition of the signs and symptoms of a urinary tract infection and the principles of good hygiene is vital.

Shortness of breath, tachypnea, cough, or sputum production may reveal a pulmonary infection and should be followed with sputum cultures and chest x-rays. Viral cultures should be sent, in addition to bacterial cultures.

Hypertension is a common problem for transplant recipients, and its causes are varied. It has been correlated with higher dosages of prednisone and cyclosporine. Intrinsic changes resulting from rejection episodes or recurrence of disease lead to a renal vasculitis and diminished renal blood flow. Subsequently, there appears to be a renin-angiotensin-aldosterone component to the hypertension.

The forms of transplant hypertension that respond to surgical intervention are renal artery stenosis (appearing in 5% to 10% of all transplant patients) and native kidney hypertension, which is induced by vasoconstrictive hormones secreted into the bloodstream. Finally, because many patients were maintained on dialysis prior to surgery, there is a higher incidence of atherosclerosis.[21]

Careful monitoring of the blood pressure is required, especially if antihypertensive medications are being adjusted. Patients are taught to check their blood pressure at home and to restrict their dietary intake of sodium.

Discharge Planning

There is a major need for education and emotional support in this particular patient population. These patients and their families must understand the full implications of a compromised immune response and the basic physiology of transplant rejection before they leave the hospital.

The nurse must serve as patient advocate and educator to ascertain that patients know how to administer their medications safely, care for themselves, and recognize potentially serious signs and symptoms, as well as understand the need for continuing medical supervision. Patients and their families will need assistance adjusting to new fears, concerns, and feelings of dependency. Increased activity and rehabilitation are encouraged.

The role of the transplant nurse is an ever-expanding one—one that changes and advances as rapidly as the progress made in the field of transplantation today.

REFERENCES

1. Landsmarr, MK: The patient with chronic renal failure: A marginal man. Ann Intern Med 82:268, 1975.
2. Lancaster, LE and Pierce, P: Total body manifestations of end-stage renal disease and related medical and nursing management. In Lancaster, LE (ed): The Patient with End Stage Renal Disease, ed 2. John Wiley & Sons, New York, 1984.
3. Knowles, HC: Magnitude of the renal failure problem in diabetic patients. Kidney Int 6:S2–S7, 1985.
4. D'Elia, JA, et al: Diabetic nephropathy. Compr Ther 5:47, 1979.
5. Leaf, A and Cotran, R: Renal Pathophysiology. Oxford University Press, New York, 1985, p 284.
6. Netter, F: Kidneys, Ureters and Urinary Bladder, Vol. 6. In The CIBA Collection of Medical Illustrations. CIBA Medical Education Division, West Caldwell, NJ, 1974, p 113.
7. Renal and Urologic Disorders. In Nurse's Clinical Library Series. Springhouse Corporation, Springhouse, PA, 1984, p 87.
8. Leaf, A and Cotran, R: Renal Pathophysiology. Oxford University Press, New York, 1985, pp 268–269.
9. Linamegl, E: Aluminum toxicity. NAPHT News, May 1985, p 2.
10. Quinton, W, Dillard, D, and Scribner, BH: Cannulation of blood vessels for prolonged hemodialysis. Trans Am Soc Art Int Organs 6:104, 1960.
11. Cimino, JE and Brescia, MJ: Simple venipuncture for hemodialysis. N Engl J Med 267:608, 1962.
12. Krupski, WC, et al: Access for dialysis. In Cogan, MG and Garovoy, MR (eds): Introduction to Dialysis. Churchill Livingstone, New York, 1985, p 66.
13. Report of the Task Force on Organ Transplantation: Organ Transplantation Issues and Recommendations. US Dept. of Health and Human Services, Washington, DC, 1993.
14. Evans, R, et al: The quality of life of patient with end-stage renal disease. N Engl J Med 312:557, 1985.
15. Parfrey, P, Hutchinson, T, and Lowry, R: Dialysis and transplantation: Complementary forms of treatment. In Garovoy, M and Guttman, R (eds): Renal Transplantation. Churchill Livingstone, New York, 1986.
16. Terasaki, P: Clinical Kidney Transplants 1993. The Regents of the University of California, Los Angeles, 1993.
17. Irwin, B: Renal transplantation: Advances in immunology. A nursing perspective. AANNT J 10(4):1, June 1983.
18. Simmons, RL, et al: Clinical transplantation. In Simmons, RL and Najarian, JS (eds): Transplantation. Lea & Febiger, Philadephia, 1972, p 474.
19. Trusler, LA: OKT-3: Nursing considerations for use in acute renal transplant rejection. ANNA J 17(4), 1990.
20. Simmons, RL, et al: Clinical transplantation. In Simmons, RL and Najarian (eds): Transplantation. Lea & Febiger, Philadelphia, 1972, p 474.
21. Curtis, JJ: Hypertension: A common problem for kidney transplant patients. Kidney 18(2):7, 1985.

SUGGESTED READINGS

Advances in the treatment of anemia of end-stage renal disease. 1990. Paper based on a pre-ANNA Symposium and selections from the American Nephrology Nurses' Association Annual Meeting, Dallas, TX. (Available from Adverceutics, Inc., 9035 Baltimore Street, Savage, MD 20763.)

Amgen, Inc: Introducing the first treatment to end transfusion dependency and transfusion risks. 1989.

Becker, BN and Koury, MJ: Resistance to erythropoietin in dialysis patients: Factors that decrease erythropoietin responsiveness. Dialysis & Transplantation 22(11): 686–689, 706–707, 1993.

Harris, JS and Delone, PA: Allocation of cadaver kidneys. ANNA J 19(1), 1992.

Lundin, AP: Recombinant erythropoietin and chronic renal failure. Hosp Prac 45–53, 1991.

Szromba, C (ed): Understanding and Managing Anemia in the Chronic Renal Failure Patient. May 1992. (Available from Ortho-Biotech.)

CARE PLAN FOR THE PATIENT WITH END-STAGE RENAL DISEASE

Nursing Diagnoses

Nursing Diagnosis #1
Acid-base balance, alteration in: metabolic acidosis

Desired Patient Outcomes

Patient outcomes: See care plan for acute renal failure in Chapter 37.

Nursing Interventions

For pertinent nursing interventions and rationales, see care plan for acute renal failure (Chapter 37), Nursing Diagnosis #5.

Rationales

Nursing Diagnoses

Nursing Diagnosis #2
Nutrition, alteration in: less than body requirements

Desired Patient Outcomes

See care plan for acute renal failure in Chapter 37.

Nursing Interventions

For pertinent nursing interventions and rationales, see care plan for acute renal failure (Chapter 37), Nursing Diagnosis #6.

Rationales

Nursing Diagnoses

Nursing Diagnosis #3
Knowledge deficit: dietary regimen in renal disease

Desired Patient Outcomes

See care plan for acute renal failure.

Nursing Interventions

For pertinent nursing interventions and rationales, see care plan for acute renal failure (Chapter 37), Nursing Diagnosis #7.

Rationales

Nursing Diagnoses

Nursing Diagnosis #4
Knowledge deficit: medications in renal disease

Desired Patient Outcomes

Patient will:
1. Correctly identify medications.
2. Verbalize understanding of the purpose and side effects.

Nursing Interventions

- Develop teaching plan:
  - Assess patient's level of understanding.

  - Assess patient's level of anxiety.
  - Assess patient's readiness to learn.

  - Implement schedule that allows for short, effective teaching sessions.

Rationales

- Appropriate vocabulary and teaching method are necessary for learning.
- Anxiety interferes with learning.
- Patient must be ready to learn before teaching can be started.
- Patient can become easily overwhelmed with information.

Nursing Diagnoses

Nursing Diagnosis #5
Infection, potential for: depressed immunologic system

Desired Patient Outcomes

See care plan for acute renal failure.

Nursing Interventions

For pertinent nursing interventions and rationales, see care plan for acute renal failure (Chapter 37), Nursing Diagnosis #8.

Rationales

Nursing Diagnoses

Nursing Diagnosis #6
Infection, potential for: dialysis access

Desired Patient Outcomes

See care plan for acute renal failure.
1. Access insertion site will remain free of signs of infection.
2. Patient on PD will remain free of peritonitis.

CARE PLAN FOR THE PATIENT WITH END-STAGE RENAL DISEASE (*Continued*)

Nursing Interventions	Rationales
• Shunt care:	
○ Change dressing as circumstances may require.	○ Dressing routinely done by dialysis nurse. Procedure for dressing must be followed.
○ Assess insertion sites for redness, swelling, exudate, or other signs of infection.	○ Infection at insertion site can erode skin and vessel.
○ Use sterile gloves when handling the shunt.	○ Infection is major complication of shunt.
○ Do not disconnect shunt (e.g., to draw blood samples).	○ Shunt should be used only for dialysis and then only by dialysis nurse.
○ Monitor patient's parameters: temperature, WBCs, routine culture results.	○ Note: WBC count falls within minutes after hemodialysis is started.
○ Obtain cultures as necessary.	
• For pertinent nursing interventions and rationales, see care plan for acute renal failure (Chapter 37), Nursing Diagnosis #8.	
• Subclavian catheter:	
○ Dressing should be sterile and occlusive. Change as circumstances may require if soiled or nonocclusive.	○ Infection is major complication and requires removal of catheter.
○ Assess catheter insertion site. Note whether sutures are intact.	○ Sutures prevent migration of catheter.
○ Do not reinsert catheter if it has partially slipped out.	○ Introduces contaminated catheter into vessel.
○ Do not use the access (for blood drawing, intravenous route).	○ Access is meant only for dialysis. Heparin is used to keep catheter patent. Catheter must be aspirated to remove heparin and also to reduce risk of embolism.
• Femoral catheter (see procedure for subclavian catheter, above).	
• PD catheter (acute or newly inserted).	
○ Change dressing every 24–48 hr. Dressing must be sterile and occlusive. Must cover catheter insertion site. (Acute catheter dressing must cover catheter tubing junction.)	○ Infection can occur at insertion site or at catheter junction.
○ Assess site for signs of infection.	○ Infection can lead to catheter removal.
○ Use sterile gloves and masks during dressing change, when performing bag changes, or whenever system is open.	○ Airborne contaminants can cause infection.
○ Use antibacterial soap to scrub hands before disconnecting anywhere in the system.	○ Decreases number of microorganisms.
○ Check for presence of catheter clamp. Close it whenever system will be disconnected.	○ Prevents direct route into peritoneum.

Nursing Diagnoses	Desired Patient Outcomes
Nursing Diagnosis #7 Injury, potential for: uremia-induced gastrointestinal disorders	See care plan for acute renal failure in Chapter 37.

Nursing Interventions	Rationales
For pertinent nursing interventions and rationales, see care plan for acute renal failure (Chapter 37), Nursing Diagnosis #9.	

Nursing Diagnoses	Desired Patient Outcomes
Nursing Diagnosis #8 Skin integrity impairment of: potential	See care plan for acute renal failure in Chapter 37.

Nursing Interventions	Rationales
For pertinent nursing interventions and rationales, see care plan for acute renal failure (Chapter 37), Nursing Diagnosis #10.	

Nursing Diagnoses	Desired Patient Outcomes
Nursing Diagnosis #9 Oral mucous membrane, alteration in	See care plan for acute renal failure in Chapter 37.

Nursing Interventions	Rationales
For pertinent nursing interventions and rationales, see care plan for acute renal failure (Chapter 37), Nursing Diagnosis #11.	

CARE PLAN FOR THE PATIENT WITH END-STAGE RENAL DISEASE (*Continued*)

Nursing Diagnoses	Desired Patient Outcomes
Nursing Diagnosis #10 Activity, alteration in: fatigue, anemia	See care plan for acute renal failure in Chapter 37.
Nursing Interventions	**Rationales**
For pertinent nursing interventions and rationales, see care plan for acute renal failure (Chapter 37), Nursing Diagnosis #13.	

Nursing Diagnoses	Desired Patient Outcomes
Nursing Diagnosis #11 Noncompliance, potential for: diet and fluid restrictions	Patient will: 1. Maintain weight within 3–5 lb of dry weight. 2. Be free of signs of volume overload. 3. Have laboratory values that reflect compliance with medical regimen.
Nursing Interventions	**Rationales**
• Evaluate patient's knowledge base to rule out knowledge deficit.	• Knowledge deficit is treated differently. (See care plan for acute renal failure (Chapter 37), Nursing Diagnosis #14.)
• Reinforce teaching of diet and fluid restrictions and medications.	• Increased understanding may lead to improved compliance.
• Allow patient to choose foods and fluids when necessary, and reinforce good choices	• This allows patient to feel more in control of situation.
• Assess patient to discover factors contributing to noncompliance.	• Anger, denial, frustration, and subconscious death wish are common factors underlying noncompliance and should be treated.

Nursing Diagnoses	Desired Patient Outcomes
Nursing Diagnosis #12 Bowel elimination, alteration in: constipation	Patient will have regular bowel pattern.
Nursing Interventions	**Rationales**
• Assess patient's usual pattern and use of aids. • Document bowel pattern.	• Gives baseline for comparison. • Prevents patient from developing impaction by monitoring bowel status.
• Consult with dietitian to evaluate allowable fiber and roughage in restricted renal diet. • Check stools for presence of blood.	• Gastrointestinal complications occur frequently in ESRD. Heme-positive stool may indicate subclinical to active gastrointestinal bleeding. Stools will be dark if patient is on iron therapy.

Nursing Diagnoses	Desired Patient Outcomes
Nursing Diagnosis #13 Pain: skeletal changes	Patient will maintain serum calcium and phosphorus within normal limits.
Nursing Interventions	**Rationales**
• Monitor lab values. • Review patient's dietary intake of phosphorus. Have dietary consult, if necessary. • Administer phosphate binders immediately after meals.	• Binders and food must be present in the stomach at the same time to be effective.

Nursing Diagnoses	Desired Patient Outcomes
Nursing Diagnosis #14 Coping, ineffective individual/family: potential	See care plan for acute renal failure in Chapter 37.
Nursing Interventions	**Rationales**
For pertinent nursing interventions and rationales, see care plan for acute renal failure (Chapter 37), Nursing Diagnosis #15.	

UNIT SIX

Endocrine System

UNIT OUTLINE

CHAPTER 39

General Features of the Endocrine System

Anecita P. Fadol

CHAPTER OUTLINE

Major Endocrine Glands
Hormones
  □ Classification of Hormones

Regulation of the Endocrine Function
References

LEARNING OBJECTIVES

After completing this chapter you should be able to:

1. Define endocrine gland, hormone, and target cell.
2. Discuss the regulation of the endocrine function.
3. List the major endocrine glands, specific hormones, and their sites of action.
4. Identify the medical condition resulting from the abnormal functioning of the specific endocrine gland.

The body functions are regulated by two major control systems: the nervous system and the endocrine system. The nervous system controls body functions by releasing neurotransmitters that act on neuron receptors, resulting in an immediate response. The endocrine system produces its effects through chemical substances known as hormones that are released in the blood when the endocrine organs are stimulated. The hormones reach their target organs through blood circulation. The endocrine system acts more slowly and has a more prolonged effect than the nervous system.

MAJOR ENDOCRINE GLANDS

The endocrine glands are ductless glands, or glands of internal secretion, synthesizing and secreting chemical substances (hormones) directly into the bloodstream, instead of into ducts.

Six structures in the body are definitely known to be endocrine glands: the pituitary, thyroid, parathyroid, and adrenal glands; the gonads (testes and ovaries); and the islets of Langerhans in the pancreas (Tables 39–1 and 39–2). However, several other structures produce hormones, including the kidneys, gastrointestinal tract, liver, thymus, and pineal gland (Table 39–3).

HORMONES

Hormones are chemical substances secreted by the endocrine glands. The word "hormone" is derived from the Greek meaning to "set in motion." Hormones set in motion the various processes that govern our lives, such as metabolism, maintenance of homeostasis, and physical and intellectual growth.

Classification of Hormones

Hormones may be classified according to chemical structure, the nature of hormonal effect, and mechanism of action.

Chemical Structure. Guyton[1] describes the three basic types of hormones according to their chemical composition:

1. Steroid hormones have a chemical structure similar to that of cholesterol and are secreted by the adrenal cortex, the ovaries, and the testes.
2. Tyrosine derivatives include the thyroid (thyroxine and tri-iodothyronine) and the two principal hormones of the adrenal medulla (epinephrine and norepinephrine).
3. Proteins or peptides encompass all other important endocrine hormones.

TABLE 39–1

Major Endocrine Glands, Hormones, Target Cells, Actions, and Gland Dysfunction

Endocrine Gland/Hormone	Target Cell/Organ	Action	ABNORMAL FUNCTIONING	
			Hypersecretion	Hyposecretion
Hypothalamus				
• Releasing hormones	Pituitary gland	Stimulates release of hormones from pituitary gland		
○ Growth hormone–releasing hormone (GHRH)	Anterior pituitary	Stimulates secretion of growth hormones	Child—giantism Adult—acromegaly	Child—dwarfism Adult—Panhypopituitarism
○ Thyrotropin-releasing hormone (TRH)	Anterior pituitary	Stimulates secretion of thyrotropin-stimulating hormone and prolactin	Grave's Disease (hyperthyroidism)	Myxedema (hypothyroidism)
○ Corticotropin-releasing hormone (CRH)	Anterior pituitary	Stimulates secretion of ACTH	Cushing's disease	Addison's disease
○ Gonadotropin-releasing hormone (GnRH)	Anterior pituitary	Stimulates secretion of LH and follicle stimulating hormone (FSH)	Sexual precocity	Hypogonadism Impotence in male Amenorrhea in female
○ Prolactin-releasing hormone (PRH)	Anterior pituitary	Stimulates secretion of prolactin		
• Inhibiting hormones		Inhibit release of hormones from pituitary gland		
○ Growth-inhibiting hormone (Somatostatin)	Anterior pituitary	Inhibits secretion of growth hormone and other hormones		
○ Prolactin-inhibiting hormone (PIH)	Anterior pituitary	Inhibits secretion of prolactin		
• Other hormones				
○ Oxytocin	Posterior pituitary	Stimulates milk production and uterine contraction		
○ Antidiuretic hormone (ADH)	Posterior pituitary	Water balance, excretion of water via the kidneys	Syndrome of inappropriate antidiuretic hormone (SIADH)	Diabetes insipidus
Pituitary (hypophysis)				
• Anterior (adenohypophysis)				
○ Adrenocorticotropic hormone (ACTH)	Adrenal cortex	Stimulates adrenal cortex	Cushing's disease	Addison's disease
○ Growth hormone (GH)	All body cells	Promotes general body growth	Child—giantism Adult—acromegaly	Child—dwarfism Adult—panhypopituitarism
○ Thyrotropin-stimulating hormone (TSH)	Thyroid	Controls thyroid gland hormones	Hyperthyroidism (Grave's disease)	Hypothyroidism (myxedema)
○ Gonadotropic hormones—luteinizing hormone (LH)	Gonads	Stimulates primary and secondary sex characteristics	Sexual precocity	Hypogonadism
○ Prolactin	Mammary glands	Breast development and lactation		
• Posterior (neurohypophysis)				
○ Oxytocin	Breasts and uterus	Stimulates milk ejection and uterine contraction		
	Kidney tubules, collecting ducts	Controls permeability to water		
○ ADH (vasopressin)	Arterial wall, smooth muscle	Vasoconstriction	SIADH	Diabetes insipidus
Thyroid				
○ Thyroxine (T$_4$)	All body cells		Hyperthyroidism	Child—cretinism Adult—hyperthyroidism
○ Triiodothyronine (T$_3$)	All body cells	Stimulates metabolism		
○ Calcitonin	Bone cells	Stimulates use of calcium and phosphorus		
Parathyroid Parathyroid hormone (Parathormone)	Bones Kidneys Gastrointestinal tract	Stimulates use of calcium and phosphorus	Hyperparathyroidism	Hypoparathyroidism (tetany)

TABLE 39–1
Major Endocrine Glands, Hormones, Target Cells, Actions, and Gland Dysfunction (*Continued*)

Endocrine Gland/Hormone	Target Cell/Organ	Action	ABNORMAL FUNCTIONING	
			Hypersecretion	Hyposecretion
Adrenal			Cushing's syndrome	Addison's disease
• Cortex				
○ Glucocorticoids (cortisol)	All body cells	Increase gluconeogenesis		
○ Mineralocorticoids (aldosterone)	Renal tubules	Retain sodium, excrete potassium		
○ Androgens	Facial and pectoral hair (vocal cords)	Stimulate secondary sex characteristics		
• Medulla				
○ Epinephrine	Heart muscle, smooth muscle, arterioles	Increases heart rate, muscle contraction, vasoconstriction, glycogenolysis	Pheochromocytoma	
○ Norepinephrine	Blood vessels	Vasoconstriction		
Pancreas				
○ Glucagon	Hepatic muscle tissue	Gluconeogenesis, glycogenolysis	Hypoglycemia	Diabetes mellitus
○ Insulin	Skeletal, muscle, cardiac cell	Promotes use of glucose, fat, and protein		
○ Somatostatin	Pancreatic A and B cells	Inhibits secretion of both insulin and glucagon		
Gonads				
• Ovaries (female)				
○ Estrogen	Accessory sex organs, breasts	Stimulates secondary sex characteristics		
○ Progesterone	Uterus	Prepares uterus for fertilized ovum		
• Testes (male)	Male organs, accessory sex organs	Primary and secondary sex characteristics		
○ Testosterone				

Nature of Hormonal Effect. The effects of hormones may be local or general. For example, prolactin, a local hormone, specifically affects the mammary glands, resulting in breast development and lactation. Epinephrine and norepinephrine, which are secreted by the adrenal medulla, are examples of general hormones. They are transported to the blood vessels of the circulatory system, resulting in a systemic response of vasoconstriction and elevation of blood pressure. General hormones are transported by the vascular system to a specific, predetermined site. The site of action for a hormone is known as a target cell.

Mechanism of Action. Hormones that are synthesized and secreted by the hypothalamus are classified

TABLE 39–2
Location of the Principal Endocrine Glands

Endocrine Gland	Location
Pituitary or hypophysis (master gland)	Lies in the sella turcica above the sphenoid at the base of the brain
Thyroid	Located at or below the cricoid cartilage in the neck, anterior to the trachea
Parathyroid	Four small glands imbedded in the thyroid gland
Adrenal	Two small glands lying in the retroperitoneal region, capping each kidney
Pancreas	Long, soft gland that lies retroperitoneally with the head of the gland in the duodenal cavity and the tail lying against the spleen
Gonads	
• Ovaries (female)	Two almond-shaped organs located on either side of the uterus
• Testes (male)	Two ovoid, glandular organs located in the scrotum

---

Releasing and Inhibiting Hormones of the Hypothalamus

Releasing Hormones:
Growth hormone–releasing hormone (GHRH)
Prolactin-releasing hormone (PRH)
Thyrotropin-releasing hormone (TRH)
Corticotropin-releasing hormone (CRH)
Gonadotropin-releasing hormone (GnRH)
Inhibiting Hormones:
Growth hormone–inhibiting hormone (somatostatin)
Prolactin-inhibiting hormone

TABLE 39–3
Other Structures: Their Hormones and Major Regulatory Functions

Gland	Hormone	Major Regulatory Functions
Kidneys	Renin (enzyme) angiotensin	Alderosterone secretion by adrenal cortex, blood pressure
	Erythropoietin	Erythrocyte production
	1,25-dihydroxycholecalciferol	Calcium balance, gastrointestinal absorption of calcium
Gastrointestinal tract	Gastrin	Gastrointestinal function: liver, pancreas, and gallbladder
	Secretin	
	Cholecystokinin	
	Gastric inhibitory peptide	
	Somatostatin	
Liver	Somatomedrin	Bone growth
Thymus	Thymic hormone (thymosin)	Lymphocyte development
Pineal	Melatonin	Circadian rhythms, sexual maturation

either as releasing or inhibiting hormones[2] (see box on page 743). These hormones control the secretion of the anterior pituitary hormones, resulting in either stimulation or inhibition of the secretion of the adenohypophyseal hormones.

REGULATION OF THE ENDOCRINE FUNCTION

The hypothalamus, which lies at the base of the brain and is connected to the pituitary gland by the pituitary stalk, plays a major role in regulating endocrine function. It initiates many endocrine responses as a result of stimuli that are received, processed, and communicated by the neurotransmitters within the central nervous system.

The endocrine system, like most control systems, is controlled by the negative feedback mechanism.[3] An increased concentration in the bloodstream of the secreted substance inhibits the stimulus to secrete, and a decreased concentration increases the stimulus to secrete. For example, in the parathyroid gland, the secretion of parathormone is dependent upon the plasma calcium level, which constitutes the feedback mechanism that either stimulates secretion of parathormone if the calcium level is low or inhibits secretion of parathormone if the serum calcium level is high. The principle of negative feedback in achieving regulatory control is similar for all the hormones, except the hormones of the adrenal medulla (epinephrine and norepinephrine), which are under the control of the autonomic nervous system.

Hormonal effects are highly specific. Although all organs are exposed to hormones, only certain organs respond to specific hormones, because appropriate hormones bind to the receptors and collect in specific target organs. The receptors are highly specific for certain molecular configurations, and only slight changes in structure of the hormone may reduce or prevent the hormonal effect by preventing interaction of the hormone with the receptor.

REFERENCES

1. Guyton, A: Textbook of Medical Physiology, ed 8. WB Saunders, Philadelphia, 1991.
2. Dolan, J: Critical Care Nursing: Clinical Management Through the Nursing Process. FA Davis, Philadelphia, 1991.
3. Goodman, M: Basic Medical Endocrinology, ed 2. Raven Press, New York, 1994.

CHAPTER 40

Assessment of Endocrine Function

Anecita P. Fadol

CHAPTER OUTLINE

Health History
Physical Assessment

Diagnostic Assessment
Suggested Readings

LEARNING OBJECTIVES

After completing this chapter, you should be able to:

1. Discuss the essential components of nursing assessment related to evaluating endocrine function.
2. Identify through physical assessment the clinical manifestations observed as they pertain to endocrine function.
3. Identify abnormal findings in common diagnostic tests performed to evaluate endocrine function.

Assessment of the endocrine system presents a challenge to the critical care nurse. The location of the majority of the endocrine glands makes it impossible for the clinician to adequately assess the condition of the glands using the assessment techniques of inspection, palpation, percussion, or auscultation. In addition, the hormones have diverse systemic effects. Both hypofunction and hyperfunction can result in dysfunction in a wide variety of organs and organ systems. Assessment, therefore, is based on the clinician's understanding of the metabolic actions of the hormones on the target cell or organ.

HEALTH HISTORY

A complete health history should be obtained to form a comprehensive database to establish a baseline for making a diagnosis. Although this history could be obtained from an interview with the patient, sometimes the patient in the critical care unit cannot provide an adequate history because of changes in the level of consciousness and urgent medical/nursing procedures that hinder the patient from answering questions. In such cases, sources other than the patient (family, friends, significant others, or previous medical records) should be used to provide this vital information. The medical history should include information about past history and pertinent family history, because many endocrine disorders have familial tendencies.

Interview questions should request information about the following:

1. Chief complaint
2. History of present problem
   a. Onset
   b. Duration
   c. Signs and symptoms
   d. Treatments
3. Other significant symptoms
   a. Changes in energy level or stamina
   b. Changes in personal appearance
      1) Size of head, hands, or feet
      2) Weight, skin, or hair
      3) Secondary sex characteristics
   c. Increased sympathetic nervous system activity
      1) Tachycardia
      2) Systolic hypertension with widened pulse pressure
   d. Change in mental abilities
      1) Memory loss
      2) Difficulty concentrating
   e. Change in sexual functioning

TABLE 40–1
Guideline for the Physical Assessment of Endocrine Function

Assessment Technique/Observation	Possible Endocrine Dysfunction
1. Inspection	
a. Head	
1) Abnormalities in facial structure, features, and expression	Hypothyroidism (myxedema)
• Prominent forehead and jaw	
• Round or puffy face	
• Dull or flat expression	
2) Exophthalmos (protruding eyeball, retracted upper lids)	Hyperthyroidism (Grave's disease)
3) Hirsutism	Cushing's syndrome
4) Fine, silky hair	Hyperthyroidism
b. Neck	
1) Enlarged thyroid gland	Hyperthyroidism
c. Trunk	
1) Truncal obesity, supraclavicular fat pads, buffalo hump	Adrenocortical excess
d. Change in secondary sexual characteristics	Adrenocortical excess
1) Change in size, symmetry, pigmentation, and presence of discharge in the breasts	
2) Presence of striae in breasts and abdomen	
3) Distribution and quantity of pubic hair	Hypogonadism
e. Skin abnormalities	
1) Bruising/petechiae	Adrenocortical hyperfunction
2) Increased pigmentation (fingers, joints, elbows, knees)	Primary hypofunction of adrenal glands
3) Vitiligo (decreased pigmentation on face, neck, and extremities)	Secondary hypofunction of adrenal glands
f. Nails	
1) Malformation and thickness or brittleness	Thyroid gland difficulties
2. Auscultation	
a. Baseline vital signs, cardiac rate, and rhythm	
1) Systolic hypertension with wide pulse pressure; tachycardia	Hyperthyroidism, pheochromocytoma
2) Bradycardia, weak arterial pulse, distant heart sounds	Hypothyroidism
3. Palpation	
a. Thyroid gland is routinely palpated for size, symmetry, and general shape (if enlarged)	Goiter, hyperthyroidism

4. Past or family history
  a. Abnormal progression in growth and development
  b. History of head injury or neurologic disorders
  c. Recent severe infection or surgical trauma
  d. Use of preparation or over-the-counter drugs
  e. Family history
    1) Obesity, hypertension
    2) Growth and development difficulties
    3) Diabetes
    4) Infertility
    5) Thyroid disorders
    6) Kidney problems

PHYSICAL ASSESSMENT

The condition of the endocrine glands cannot be assessed directly because of their location within the human body. Instead the metabolic effects of the hormones on the target cell or organ demonstrate the functional status of the involved endocrine gland. Therefore, when performing the physical assessment, take a systematic approach to avoid missing important data. Using a head-to-toe approach in physical assessment is often effective. However, it is important to note that many clinical findings can be associated with more than one endocrine disorder and that these findings may be related to another pathologic process. The guideline in Table 40–1 may be used in the physical assessment of endocrine function.

DIAGNOSTIC ASSESSMENT

Diagnosis of endocrine dysfunction is not solely based on information obtained from the medical history and physical examination. Laboratory tests are an

TABLE 40–2
Common Diagnostic Tests for Endocrine Function

Diagnostic Test	Normal Findings	Abnormal Findings
Radiographic Test		
1. Adrenal angiography (x-ray with contrast dye)	Normal adrenal artery vasculature	Pheochromocytomas Adrenal adenomas Adrenal carcinomas Bilateral adrenal hyperplasia
2. Sella turcica x-ray	No abnormalities	Pituitary tumors Destruction of the sella turcica
3. Thyroid scanning (nuclear scan)	Normal size, shape, position, and function of the thyroid gland No areas of decreased or increased uptake	Adenoma Toxic and nontoxic goiter Carcinoma Thyroiditis Grave's disease Hashimoto's disease
4. Thyroid ultrasound (thyroid echogram, thyroid sonogram)	Normal size, shape, and position of thyroid gland	Cysts Tumors Thyroid adenoma Thyroid carcinoma
Blood Test		
1. Adrenocorticotropic hormone (ACTH, corticotropin)	AM 15–100 pg/mL or 10–80 ng/L PM <50 pg/mL or <50 ng/L	**Increased Levels** • Addison's disease (primary adrenal insufficiency) • Cushing's disease (pituitary-dependent adrenal hyperplasia) • Stress • Adrenogenital syndrome **Decreased Levels** • Secondary adrenal insufficiency (pituitary insufficiency) • Cushing's syndrome • Hypopituitarism • Adrenal adenoma • Steroid administration
2. Antithyroglobulin antibody	Titer less than 1:100	**Increased Levels** • Hashimoto's thyroiditis • Pernicious anemia • Thyrotoxicosis • Systemic lupus erythematosus • Rheumatoid arthritis • Hypothyroidism • Myxedema
3. Blood glucose [blood sugar, fasting blood sugar (FBS)]	70–105 mg/dL (increase in normal range after age 50)	**Increased Levels (Hyperglycemia)** • Diabetes mellitus • Hyperparathyroidism • Acute stress response • Cushing's disease • Pheochromocytoma **Decreased Levels (Hypoglycemia)** • Insulinoma • Hypothyroidism • Addison's disease • Extensive liver disease
4. Calcium	Total: 9.0–10.5 mg/dL Ionized: 4.5–5.6 mg/dL	**Increased Levels (Hypercalcemia)** • Hyperparathyroidism • Metastatic tumor to the bone • Sarcoidosis • Addison's disease • Acromegaly **Decreased Levels (Hypocalcemia)** • Hypoparathyroidism • Renal failure • Rickets • Osteomalacia • Hypophosphatemia secondary to renal failure • Vitamin D deficiency • Pancreatitis

Continued

TABLE 40–2
Common Diagnostic Tests for Endocrine Function (*Continued*)

Diagnostic Test	Normal Findings	Abnormal Findings
5. Blood cortisol (hydrocortisone, serum cortisol)	8:00 AM: 6–28 μg/dL 4:00 PM: 2–12 μg/dL	*Increased Levels* • Cushing's syndrome • Adrenal adenoma • Ectopic ACTH-producing tumors • Hyperthyroidism • Obesity • Stress *Decreased Levels* • Addison's disease • Hypopituitarism • Hypothyroidism • Liver disease
6. Blood osmolality (serum osmolality)	285–295 mOsm/kg H_2O	*Increased Levels* • Hypernatremia • Dehydration • Hyperglycemia • Hyperosmolar nonketotic hyperglycemia • Diabetes insipidus • Ketosis *Decreased Levels* • Hyponatremia • Overhydration • Syndrome of inappropriate ADH secretion (SIADH)
7. Parathyroid hormone (PTH, parathormone)	<2000 pg/mL	*Increased Levels* • Hyperparathyroidism • Hypocalcemia • Chronic renal failure • Malabsorption syndrome • Rickets *Decreased Levels* • Hypoparathyroidism • Hypercalcemia • Vitamin D intoxication • Grave's disease • Hypomagnesemia
8. Phosphorus (P; phosphate, PO_4)	3.0–4.5 mg/dL	*Increased Levels (Hyperphosphatemia)* • Hypoparathyroidism • Renal failure • Hypocalcemia • Liver disease *Decreased Levels (Hyphosphatemia)* • Hyperparathyroidism • Hypercalcemia • Chronic alcoholism • Vitamin D deficiency • Hyperinsulinism
9. Thyroid-stimulating hormone (TSH, thyrotropin)	2–10 μU/mL	*Increased Levels* • Primary hypothyroidism • Thyroiditis • Congenital cretinism *Decreased Levels* • Secondary hypothyroidism • Hyperthyroidism • Pituitary hypofunction
10. Thyroxine index, free (FTI, FT_4 index)	0.8–2.4 ng/dL	*Increased Levels* • Hyperthyroidism *Decreased Levels* • Hypothyroidism

TABLE 40–2
Common Diagnostic Tests for Endocrine Function (*Continued*)

Diagnostic Test	Normal Findings	Abnormal Findings
Urine Test 1. Catecholamines and vanillylmandelic acid (VMA)	Catecholamines Epinephrine: 0.5–20 μg/24 h Norepinephrine: 15–80 μg/24 h Dopamine: 65–400 μg/24 h VMA: 2–7 mg/24 h	*Increased Levels* • Pheochromocytomas • Neuroblastomas • Ganglioneuromas • Severe stress • Strenuous exercise
2. Urine cortisol	10–100 μg/24 h	*Increased Levels* • Cushing's syndrome • Stress • Pregnancy *Decreased Levels* • Addison's disease • Hypopituitarism
3. Urine glucose	Random specimen: negative 24-h specimen: <0.5 g/day	*Increased Levels* • Diabetes mellitus • Cushing's syndrome • Infection • Drug therapy • Pregnancy
4. Urine ketones (urine acetone)	Negative	*Increased Levels* • Uncontrolled diabetes mellitus • Starvation • Excessive aspirin ingestion • Anorexia • High-protein diets • Dehydration
5. Urine calcium	Vary with diet Normal diet: 100–300 mg/day	*Increased Levels (Hypercalciuria)* • Primary hyperparathyroidism • Cushing's syndrome • Renal tubular acidosis • Vitamin D intoxication *Decreased Levels (Hypocalciuria)* • Hypoparathyroidism • Vitamin D deficiency • Malabsorption disorders

essential part of the diagnostic workup for the client with suspected endocrine dysfunction (Table 40–2).

SUGGESTED READINGS

Bates, BA: A Guide to Physical Examination and History Taking, ed 6. JB Lippincott, Philadelphia, 1995.

Hurwitz, L and Porth, C: Alterations in endocrine control of growth and metabolism. In Porth, CM (ed): Pathophysiology: Concepts of Altered Health States. JP Lippincott, New York, 1994.

Pagana, K and Pagana, T: Mosby's Diagnostic and Laboratory Test Reference, ed 2. Mosby Year Book, St. Louis, 1995.

CHAPTER 41

Nursing Management of the Patient with Endocrine Pancreas Dysfunction: Diabetic Ketoacidosis; Hyperglycemic, Hyperosmolar, Nonketotic Coma; and Hypoglycemia

Joan T. Dolan

CHAPTER OUTLINE

LEARNING OBJECTIVES

After completing this chapter, you should be able to:

1. Describe the endocrine pancreas and its structure and function.
2. Define the metabolic states: absorptive and postabsorptive.
3. Describe the regulation and control of body metabolism and energy use.
4. List the major functions of insulin on specific metabolic processes.
5. Describe the regulation of insulin secretion.
6. List the major functions of glucagon on specific metabolic processes.
7. Describe the regulation of glucagon secretion.
8. Define diabetic ketoacidosis (DKA), and examine its precipitating factors, pathogenesis, signs and symptoms, initial laboratory values, and management.
9. Define hyperglycemic, hyperosmolar, nonketotic coma (HHNK), and examine its precipitating factors, pathogenesis, signs and symptoms, initial laboratory values, and management.
10. Define hypoglycemia, and examine its precipitating factors, pathophysiology, signs and symptoms, initial laboratory values, and management.
11. Delineate nursing process in the clinical management of patients with complications of endocrine pancreas dysfunction:
    a. Assessment
    b. Nursing diagnosis
    c. Planning: desired patient outcomes and nursing interventions

Metabolism reflects the ability of the body to capture and store the energy derived from foods and to make that energy available as needed for physiologic activities. Efficient management of energy resources within the body requires a precise control and integration of metabolic processes. The endocrine pancreas, through its release of the hormones insulin and glucagon, plays a major role in regulating metabolic processes and using energy.

ENDOCRINE PANCREAS: STRUCTURE AND FUNCTION

The endocrine pancreas makes up about 2% of the total mass of the pancreas. It is composed of small clusters of endocrine cells called the *islets of Langerhans*. These cells are responsible for releasing somatostatin, synthesizing the hormones insulin and glucagon, and secreting them directly into the circulating blood.

The islets of Langerhans contain distinct cell types. The alpha cells are the source of glucagon; the beta cells, which are the most numerous, are the source of insulin; and the delta cells are the source of somatostatin. While insulin and glucagon play significant roles in the regulation of carbohydrate, protein, and fat metabolism, the precise physiologic role of somatostatin is less well defined. It is known, however, to inhibit secretion of insulin and glucagon from the beta and alpha cells, respectively.

The islets of Langerhans are innervated by the sympathetic branch of the autonomic nervous system. Sympathetic innervation, together with circulating epinephrine from the adrenal medulla, stimulates glucagon secretion by alpha cells, while inhibiting the secretion of insulin by the beta cells. These systems, together with insulin, glucagon, and somatostatin, play a significant role in the regulation of body metabolism and energy use.

METABOLIC STATES: ABSORPTIVE AND POSTABSORPTIVE STATES

Overall body metabolism encompasses two functional states: the *absorptive* and *postabsorptive*. The absorptive, or eating, state reflects the digestive period, during which nutrients are ingested, digested, and absorbed from the gastrointestinal tract into the blood. Glucose is the major energy provider during this period, with only a very small fraction of ingested amino acids and fats used for this purpose. Most amino acids and fats, as well as carbohydrates not used for energy, are converted to fat and stored in adipose tissue for use as the energy source during the postabsorptive state.

The postabsorptive, or fasting, state reflects the nondigestive period occurring between meals, during which the gastrointestinal tract is empty and energy must be supplied by the oxidation of fat stored in adipose tissue. In contrast to the absorptive state, use of carbohydrates for this purpose is greatly reduced.

The shift from glucose use to fat use that takes place during the transition from the absorptive to postabsorptive state is essential to spare glucose stores and preserve blood glucose concentrations to meet the nearly exclusive continuous energy needs of neural, retinal, and germinal tissues, and of red blood cells. While other tissues of the body will readily use fat as their energy source during the postabsorptive state, glucose remains the major energy source for these tissues.

REGULATION AND CONTROL OF BODY METABOLISM AND ENERGY USE

The overall status of energy stores in the body at any given moment is largely controlled by the actions of the pancreatic hormones, insulin and glucagon, and is reflected by the ratio of insulin to glucagon. Normally, the insulin/glucagon (I/G) ratio is 2.3/1. As an anabolic hormone, insulin increases storage of glucose, amino acids, and fatty acids as glycogen, body proteins, and triglycerides, respectively. Glucagon, a catabolic hormone, breaks down these stores and mobilizes energy to fuel vital physiologic activities.

In the normal healthy individual maintaining a balanced diet, the I/G ratio is indicative of a net storage tendency and positive nitrogen balance that favors to a greater extent the anabolic effects of insulin. Elevation of the I/G ratio reflects an anabolic state with weight gain. Secretion of insulin is enhanced by the overfed state. A reduction in the I/G ratio reflects a catabolic state with weight loss. Secretion of glucagon is enhanced by fasting, or the underfed, state.

Other hormones in the body also influence metabolism. Thyroid hormones control the metabolic rates of anabolism and catabolism, and the transformation of energy into its various forms for cellular use. Glucocorticoids (e.g., cortisol) regulate intermediary metabolism and maintain blood glucose levels at concentrations necessary to meet metabolic needs. Growth hormone exerts a hyperglycemic effect, increasing serum glucose levels.

Other factors influencing metabolism include epinephrine, secreted by the adrenal medulla, and sympathetic innervation to the pancreas, liver, and adipose tissue. The sympathetic influence inhibits insulin secretion during periods of exercise and stress.

It is important to note that the glucagon, cortisol, growth, and epinephrine hormones are referred to as "counter-regulatory" hormones because they antagonize or counter the anabolic actions of insulin.

Insulin: Major Functions

Insulin acts to facilitate glucose uptake by most cells of the body. Notable exceptions include neural, retinal, and germinal tissues, pancreatic beta islet cells,

TABLE 41–1
Distinguishing Features and Functions of Insulin and Glucagon

	Insulin	Glucagon
Origin of hormones: synthesis/ secretion	Beta cells within the islets of Langerhans (pancreas)	Alpha cells within the islets of Langerhans (pancreas)
Overall effect on target tissues	Anabolic hormone functions to decrease serum glucose and fatty acid concentrations	Catabolic hormone functions to increase serum glucose and fatty acid concentrations
	Net increase in glycogen, body protein, and triglyceride stores	Net decrease in glycogen, body protein, and triglyceride stores
	Promotes absorptive state	Promotes postabsorptive state
Major stimulus for hormone release	Elevated serum glucose concentrations, as occurs during eating or absorptive state	Reduced serum glucose concentrations as occurs in fasting or postabsorptive state
	Elevated serum amino acids levels	Ingestion of amino acids: arginine, alanine
		Hormones: pancreozymin, epinephrine
Major inhibition of hormone release	Fasting or postabsorptive state; hypoglycemia	Eating or absorptive state; hyperglycemia and increased free fatty acid levels
Autonomic nervous system: Parasympathetic	Stimulates insulin secretion during eating or absorptive state	
Sympathetic	Inhibits insulin secretion	Stimulates glucagon secretion into bloodstream
Hormonal influence: Epinephrine (adrenal medulla)	Inhibits insulin secretion during exercise or stress	Stimulates glucagon secretion during exercise, stress, or postabsorptive state by its hyperglycemic effects: Increased glycogenolysis in liver Increased gluconeogenesis in liver Increased lipolysis in adipose tissue Enhanced use of fatty acids for energy by most cells
Cortisol (adrenal cortex)	Exerts a hyperglycemic effect via increased gluconeogenesis in liver; insulin antagonist	
Thyroid and growth hormones	Insulin acts in a synergistic capacity with these hormones to increase uptake of amino acids to promote growth	
Gastrointestinal hormones: Gastrin Cholecystokinin Gastric inhibitory peptide	Increased secretion of these hormones in response to eating and absorptive state stimulates insulin secretion	Gastrointestinal factors whose release is triggered by protein ingestion increase glucagon secretion
Target cells	Most cells, but primarily liver, muscle, and adipose tissue; major exceptions include neural tissue, retina, germinal tissue and red blood cells.	Target cells include liver and adipose tissue
Metabolism	Insulin is rapidly (within minutes) removed from blood and degraded by the liver	Glucagon is metabolized primarily by the liver
Serum glucose levels	Normal fasting: 70–110 mg/100 mL Hyperglycemia: >110 mg/100 mL Hypoglycemia: 40–70 mg/100 mL	
Renal threshold for glucose	Normal threshold: ~160–180 mg/100 mL Serum glucose: >180 mg/100 mL results in glycosuria	

and red blood cells. In addition to glucose uptake, insulin increases the active transport of amino acids into cells and enhances the uptake of glucose by adipose tissue.

Through its effects on enzymatic activities, insulin stimulates glycogen synthesis (glycogenesis) in the liver and skeletal muscle while inhibiting glycogen breakdown (glycogenolysis). Similarly, insulin acts to enhance body stores of fat in the form of triglycerides (lipogenesis) while inhibiting breakdown of fat stores (lipolysis). Insulin also inhibits enzymes that break down body protein and fat for conversion to glucose (gluconeogenesis). Unlike glucose (glycogen) and fatty acids (triglycerides), there is no storage form of protein. In the presence of insulin, excess protein is converted to triglycerides, the storage form of fat. Thus, during the absorptive state when insulin is the predominant hormone and glucose is used as the major source of energy, a net synthesis of glycogen, body proteins, and triglycerides ensues (Table 41–1).

Insulin has little to no direct effect on uptake and use of glucose by brain tissue. Brain cells are permeable to glucose without any mediation by insulin; they rely primarily on the concentration of glucose in the blood. Therefore, a certain minimal serum glucose level must be maintained at all times.

Regulation of Insulin Secretion

Regulation of insulin secretion occurs primarily by a simple negative feedback mechanism exerted by the serum glucose concentration on the pancreatic beta islet cells. Changes in serum glucose levels are sensed very quickly as entry into the beta cells is unaffected by insulin. When the serum glucose concentration is low, so is insulin secretion. When blood glucose levels increase, insulin secretion by the beta cells also increases. Insulin reduces serum glucose levels by stimulating rapid entry of glucose into cells and decreasing the glucose output by the liver. The consequent reduction in blood glucose levels removes the stimulus that initiated the increase in insulin secretion. The physiologic effects of insulin and the regulation of its secretion are so finely and precisely tuned that the serum glucose concentration is normally maintained within very narrow limits: 70 to 110 mg/100 mL (fasting).

An elevation in serum levels of certain amino acids also increases insulin secretion. Insulin promotes membrane transport of amino acids and increases protein synthesis. In this way, insulin acts as a protein sparer, preventing amino acids from being used as an energy source. Hormones (e.g., gastric inhibitory peptides) secreted by the intestinal mucosa in the presence of ingested glucose or amino acids account in part for the enhanced insulin secretion that is produced in response to oral ingestion, as opposed to intravenous infusion, of these nutrients. Other factors influencing insulin secretion include the activity of thyroid and growth hormones and the counter-regulatory hormones mentioned previously (glucagon, cortisol, and epinephrine).

Glucagon: Major Functions

The major effects of glucagon on body metabolism are antagonistic to those of insulin. Glucagon's overall effect is to increase serum glucose and fatty acid concentrations, and in this regard, it is a critically important hormone secreted during the postabsorptive, or fasting, state.

Most of the glucagon is secreted by the pancreatic alpha islet cells, although it is also released by intestinal mucosal cells. As a catabolic hormone, glucagon exerts its hyperglycemic effect by two mechanisms: it increases serum glucose levels by breaking down liver glycogen (glycogenolysis), and it largely stimulates

glucose synthesis in the liver from noncarbohydrate sources (gluconeogenesis). Glucagon also stimulates breakdown of triglyceride stores in adipose tissue (lipolysis), releasing glycerol (substrate for gluconeogenesis) and fatty acids, which are the major energy sources during the postabsorptive state (Table 41–1).

Regulation of Glucagon Secretion

The major stimulus for glucagon secretion is a decreasing serum glucose concentration. This decrease induces an increase in glucagon secretion from the pancreatic alpha islet cells, which by its catabolic effects on glycogen and triglycerides, serves to restore serum glucose levels, thereby removing the stimulus that initiated the glucagon secretion. However, unlike glucose entry into beta cells, which is not affected by insulin, alpha cells are unable to respond to elevated serum glucose levels unless insulin first facilitates glucose uptake by alpha cells. Thus, the presence of *both* insulin and glucagon is necessary to produce a negative feedback action on further glucagon secretion by alpha cells.

Glucagon secretion, like that of insulin, is also strongly stimulated by an increase in serum amino acid concentration. In this instance, glucagon secretion is necessary to maintain adequate serum glucose concentrations so that the amino acids will be used specifically for protein synthesis and not for energy (by gluconeogenesis). In this way, glucagon facilitates the protein-sparing and storage effects of insulin alluded to earlier.

DIABETES MELLITUS

Diabetes mellitus is a chronic disorder characterized by inappropriate hyperglycemia that is caused by a relative to absolute insulin deficiency or by a resistance to the actions of insulin in peripheral tissues. It commonly involves abnormalities in carbohydrate, protein, and fat metabolism. It is not a single disorder but is generally recognized to encompass a group of genetically and clinically heterogeneous disorders that have in common *glucose intolerance*. Individuals with diabetes have a marked propensity to develop microvascular, macrovascular, and neuropathic disorders, and it is widely assumed that chronic hyperglycemia is a major contributory factor.

Based on a 1990 survey,[1] the American Diabetes Association estimated that 13 million people had diabetes in the United States, including 6.5 million diagnosed cases, and about 6.5 million undiagnosed cases. Of those diagnosed, about 5% were type I insulin-dependent, and 90% were type II non–insulin-dependent. The remaining 5% included those with gestational diabetes, or diabetes secondary to pancreatic disease, hormonal disturbances, drug therapy, or genetic defects.

Clinical Subclasses of Diabetes Mellitus

In 1979 the National Diabetes Data Group established subclasses of diabetes, which have been endorsed by the American Diabetes Association. The two dominant forms of diabetes mellitus are type I, insulin-dependent diabetes mellitus (IDDM), and type II, non–insulin-dependent diabetes mellitus (NIDDM), described as follows:

Type I: insulin-dependent diabetes mellitus (previously juvenile diabetes, juvenile-onset diabetes, ketosis-prone diabetes):

Distinguishing characteristics: Relative to absolute deficiency of insulin; those with IDDM may be of any age but usually young (<30 years) and thin; abrupt onset of signs and symptoms, usually requires endogenous insulin upon diagnosis; prone to ketosis; dependent on insulin therapy to prevent ketoacidosis and to sustain life; without timely intervention, will result in DKA, coma, and death; probable underlying autoimmune response involving destruction of beta islet cells of pancreas, beta islet-cell antibodies often demonstrated; autoimmune process is believed to be triggered by exposure to the rubella or mumps viruses, or to the coxsackievirus.

Type II: non–insulin-dependent diabetes mellitus (previously adult-onset diabetes, maturity-onset diabetes, ketosis-resistant diabetes):

Distinguishing characteristics: Variable amounts of endogenous insulin available, and therefore, not prone to ketoacidosis except during periods of stress; onset is insidious; may be diagnosed at any age but usually after age 40; most are obese; not dependent on insulin therapy for survival, but may require it for adequate control of hyperglycemia; family history usually significant with strong genetic propensity; may involve impaired beta cell function and insulin secretion, decrease in tissue sensitivity to insulin, and/or a peripheral insulin resistance; hyperinsulinemia (elevated serum insulin levels) often demonstrated.

Pathophysiology of Diabetes Mellitus

The common denominator for all types of diabetes is *glucose intolerance* caused by a relative or an absolute lack of insulin. Without insulin, or in the presence of peripheral insulin resistance, glucose cannot be taken up by most cells of the body despite the presence of increasing levels of blood glucose. Consequently, glucose cannot be used as a source of energy, or as a substrate for glycogen synthesis.

In an attempt to meet energy needs, counter-regulatory hormones (glucagon, epinephrine, cortisol, and growth hormone) are reflexly secreted. Through hormone-stimulated processes of glycogenolysis and gluconeogenesis, the hyperglycemia is further aggravated and cellular energy needs persist. A shift from

glucose use to fat use becomes necessary. Glucagon stimulates increased lipolysis in adipose tissue releasing glycerol, a substrate used for gluconeogenesis, and fatty acids used as the energy substrate by most cells.

In addition, hepatic ketogenic pathways are activated wherein fatty acids are oxidized to form *ketone bodies*. These include β-hydroxybutyric acid, acetoacetic acid, and acetone. In the presence of insulin, ketone bodies circulating in the blood provide an important energy source for the body's peripheral tissues during the fasting state. When a deficiency or lack of insulin exists, as it does in diabetes, peripheral metabolism of ketones is impaired, and these organic acids accumulate in unusually large quantities in blood and body fluids, a condition called *ketosis*.

This impaired ketone metabolism associated with an insulin deficiency and coupled with the continued release of ketone bodies by the liver exhausts the compensatory capabilities of body buffers, and a severe metabolic acidosis evolves. If untreated, it can lead to coma and death. These events underlie the pathogenesis of DKA (see the following discussion).

ACUTE COMPLICATIONS OF DIABETES MELLITUS

Acute complications of diabetes are all life-threatening emergencies and include the following: diabetic ketoacidosis (DKA); hyperglycemic, hyperosmolar, nonketotic syndrome (HHNK); and hypoglycemia (hypoglycemic shock).

DKA is a complication resulting from uncontrolled IDDM or type I diabetes; or, rarely, from decompensated NIDDM or type II diabetes. HHNK is a syndrome more commonly found in elderly patients with mild or previously undiagnosed NIDDM. It often occurs in elderly patients who are taking oral hypoglycemic agents or who are inadequately monitored. It is often precipitated by illness or other stresses.

Hypoglycemia, or hypoglycemic shock, is the most commonly encountered acute complication of treatment of insulin-dependent patients with diabetes. It occasionally occurs as a complication of treatment with oral hypoglycemic agents, but the risk of severe hypoglycemia is greatly increased in patients with IDDM or type I diabetes, using intensive regimens designed to achieve consistently near-normal blood glucose levels.[2]

Diabetic Ketoacidosis

DKA is an acute metabolic disorder involving alterations in carbohydrate, protein, and fat metabolism, in which the underlying pathophysiologic processes are attributed to an absolute or relative lack of insulin. It most commonly occurs in patients with uncontrolled IDDM, or type I diabetes (Table 41–2).

Precipitating Factors. Precipitating factors of DKA vary from individual to individual and may include the

TABLE 41–2
Contrast: Diabetic Ketoacidosis (DKA) and Hyperglycemic, Hyperosmolar, Nonketotic Coma (HHNK)

	Diabetic Ketoacidosis	Hyperglycemic, Hyperosmolar, Nonketotic Coma
Definition	DKA is an acute metabolic disorder in which the major underlying hormonal abnormality is an absolute or relative insulin deficiency. DKA is a syndrome associated with severe, uncontrolled diabetes and characterized by hyperglycemia, ketonemia, fluid and electrolyte imbalance, and a negative nitrogen balance.	HHNK is a syndrome associated with a relative insulin deficit and characterized by marked hyperglycemia and minimal to absent ketonemia. The patient has sufficient insulin to prevent fatty acid breakdown but inadequate amounts for carbohydrate metabolism. Thus, this syndrome is characterized by severe hyperglycemia and hyperosmolality without significant ketoacidosis.
Clinical Setting/Epidemiology	Occurs most frequently in patients with type I IDDM	Occurs most frequently in patients with type II NIDDM
Age	Young population	Middle-aged or elderly
Onset	Sudden or gradual	Gradual, several days to weeks
Previous history of diabetes	85%	60%
Drug history	Usually take insulin	Use of oral hypoglycemics; insulin usually not necessary
Frequency of occurrence	DKA six times more common than HHNK	
Precipitating illness	Usually a factor	Usually a factor
Mortality	15% annually; more commonly in women and nonwhites; directly linked to degree of metabolic derangement	40% to 50% annually

Precipitating Factors	DKA occurs most commonly:
	1. In initial presentation of a previously undiagnosed patient with diabetes mellitus.
	2. In the type I IDDM patient who:
	  a. Omits an insulin dose or decreases the dose.
	  b. Has uncontrolled diabetes with inadequate insulin coverage.
	  c. Experiences a severe stress without appropriate adjustment in insulin coverage:
	    (1) Infection: respiratory, urinary tract
	    (2) Gastrointestinal illness with nausea/vomiting and diarrhea
	    (3) Trauma, surgery, pregnancy
		Precipitating causes of HHNK:
		• Acute illness: infection (e.g., pneumonia, sepsis, gastroenteritis), pancreatitis, cerebrovascular insult
		• Chronic illness: renal disease, compromised cardiovascular function
		• Drugs: thiazide, furosemide, Dilantin (phenytoin), propranolol, steroids (cortisol), diazoxide
		• Procedures:
		  ○ Peritoneal dialysis with hypertonic glucose solution
		  ○ Hemodialysis
		  ○ Total parenteral nutrition
		  ○ Intravenous glucose in patient with severe burns
		  ○ General anesthesia
		  ○ Hypothermia
		• Associated endocrinopathies:
		  ○ Cushing's syndrome
		  ○ Thyrotoxicosis

Laboratory Data		
Serum tests: Glucose (range)	300–800 mg/100 mL	600–1200 mg/100 mL
Electrolytes: Potassium	Early hypokalemia to normokalemia not uncommon; later, hyperkalemia; total body deficit always present	Usually normal to slightly elevated initially; then hypokalemia with total body deficit
Sodium	Initial hypernatremia, but more commonly hyponatremia as sodium is lost in the osmotic diuresis	May be elevated, normal or low initially; then total body sodium deficit
Mild	>135 mEq/L	Similar to values for DKA
Moderate	~130 mEq/L	
Severe	<130 mEq/L	
BUN	Elevated with severe dehydration	Often markedly elevated: >80 mg/100 mL BUN/creatinine ratio >1:10
Osmolality	<330 mOsm/kg	>330 mOsm/kg; mean ~400 mOsm/kg
Arterial blood gases	pH <7.20; mean 7.07; HCO_3^- <10 mEq/L; markedly lowered in severe DKA	pH >7.20; mean 7.25; HCO_3^- >10 mEq/L; normal to moderately lowered
Urine studies	Glycosuria	Glycosuria
Ketonuria	Acetone elevated	Acetone normal
Proteinuria	Trace	Trace
Specific gravity	Elevated >1.025	Elevated >1.025
Cultures	As indicated (throat, sputum, blood, urine, stool, invasive sites)	Similar to DKA
Differential Diagnosis	In the presence of altered level of consciousness or coma, consideration must be given to other etiologies including: hypoglycemia, cerebrovascular accident, drug intoxication, uremia, hepatic coma, hypertensive encephalopathy, head trauma, other central nervous system lesions, sepsis, severe lactic acidosis. If patient has abdominal pain, an acute, or surgical, abdomen must be ruled out; respiratory or urinary infection may also need to be ruled out. The presence of hyperpyrexia or hypopyrexia is variable and cannot be relied on exclusively as to the presence or absence of infection.	

following: an absolute insulin deficiency that exists when no insulin is available, as in the newly diagnosed patient with IDDM; inadequate insulin dosing when insulin therapy is deliberately or unintentionally omitted by the patient with established IDDM; or when the patient experiences severe stress without appropriate adjustments in insulin coverage. Major stressors include acute illness (e.g., infection, gastrointestinal upsets, myocardial infarction, cerebrovascular accident, and endocrine disorders), trauma, surgery, emotional stress, or pregnancy.

Other precipitating factors may be related to drug therapy, including the use of diuretics (e.g., thiazides and furosemide), antihypertensives, steroids, adrenergic agonists (e.g., epinephrine, isoproterenol), β-adrenergic blockers (e.g., propranolol), psychotropic agents (e.g., tricyclic antidepressants, haloperidol, lithium, and phenothiazines), and anticonvulsants (e.g., phenytoin). Total parenteral nutrition has also been cited as a precipitating factor for DKA.

Pathogenesis of DKA. The pathogenesis of DKA is largely attributed to insulin lack, and to an alteration in the balance between anabolic and catabolic hormonal influences. Although small amounts of insulin may be available, the presence of large amounts of the counter-regulatory hormones (glucagon, epinephrine, cortisol, and growth hormone) render the insulin less effective. Some of the hallmarks of DKA and their mechanisms of action follow.

Hyperglycemia:
- Following a meal, insulin deficiency impairs glucose uptake in the peripheral tissues (mainly muscle) and liver, causing hyperglycemia.
- Secretion of counter-regulatory hormones (glucagon, cortisol, and epinephrine) increases hepatic glucose production through enhanced glycogenolysis and gluconeogenesis, also contributing to hyperglycemia.

Glycosuria:
- The glucose load presented by hyperglycemia exceeds the renal threshold, resulting in osmotic diuresis, which causes hypotonic fluid losses with dehydration and electrolyte depletion.

Ketonuria:
- Excretion of ketone bodies contributes further to fluid loss and electrolyte depletion. (Cations must be eliminated along with the anionic ketone bodies to maintain electrical neutrality.)

Uncontrolled lipolysis:
- Excessive free fatty acid mobilization and release from triglyceride stores in peripheral adipose tissue occurs in the presence of counter-regulatory hormones. Increased amounts of glycerol, an important gluconeogenic substrate, are also made available as a result of uncontrolled lipolysis.

Ketogenesis:
- Increased availability of free fatty acids, in conjunction with suppression of fatty acid synthesis associated with insulin lack, leads to enhanced production of ketone bodies (β-hydroxybutyric acid and acetoacetic acid) in the liver. Insulin deficiency enhances certain critical hepatic enzymes that convert free fatty acids into ketone bodies.

Ketonemia (metabolic ketoacidosis):
- Because of insulin lack, peripheral tissues are unable to use excess ketones, leading to an accumulation of these organic acids in the blood with a consequent acidosis.

Negative nitrogen protein balance:
- Insulin deficiency impairs protein synthesis because amino acids are used as a gluconeogenic substrates rather than as building blocks for body tissue. This accounts for the loss of lean body mass seen in patients with uncontrolled diabetes.

Signs and Symptoms of DKA

DKA can be classified as mild, moderate, or severe, based on the clinical presentation (Table 41–3). Early on in the course of DKA, symptoms may mimic other diseases or illnesses. Nonspecific symptoms may include anorexia, weakness, fatigue, headache, malaise, somnolence, and lethargy. Early manifestations of hyperglycemia include complaints of polydipsia, polyuria, blurred vision, and polyphagia if insulin deficiency is prolonged (days to weeks).

The onset of gastrointestinal symptoms—nausea, vomiting, diarrhea, epigastric discomfort, and abdominal pain or cramping—may signal the onset of ketosis and/or acidosis. Abdominal pain may be so severe as to mimic that of a "surgical abdomen," requiring meticulous assessment and differential diagnosis.

Respiratory symptoms may include complaints of shortness of breath or inability to "catch one's breath." Later in the course, the patient may become aware of a very deep, and sometimes rapid breathing unrelated to exertion. This type of hyperventilatory breathing, termed "Kussmaul's breathing," demonstrates the body's attempt to correct the underlying metabolic acidemia.

Signs of DKA are nonspecific. The overall clinical presentation, however, should alert the clinician to the possibility of DKA. The patient's neurologic status may reflect a change in mental status, or an altered level of consciousness. The patient may be alert,

TABLE 41–3
Diabetic Ketoacidosis: Clinical Classifications

	Mild	Moderate	Severe
History	Increasing polyuria with excessive thirst Weakness, fatigue, lassitude Weight loss (recent)	"Can't catch breath," air hunger with marked hyperventilatory effort Marked weakness, unable to cope with physical exertion Excessive thirst, marked polyuria Nausea, vomiting, epigastric discomfort Somnolence, lethargy	Marked drowsiness and lethargy progressing to coma Deep and rapid Kussmaul's breathing through an open mouth

Physical examination	Skin flushed
	Tachycardia
	Hyperventilation: increased rate and depth of respirations
	Possible slight odor of acetone (fruity smell) to breath
		Drowsy, weak
		Respirations more vigorous, use of accessory muscles
		Signs of dehydration: dry mucous membranes, poor skin turgor (forehead or sternum), soft eyeballs, dry mouth (mouth breathing)
		Hypovolemia: narrowed pulse pressure
		Noticeable acetone breath
			Severe dehydration with hypovolemic shock: hypotension, tachycardia, reduced cardiac output
			Air hunger
			Lethargy
			Coma
			Temperature:
			  Subnormal—sepsis?
			  Vasomotor collapse?
			  Elevated—infection?

obtunded, stuporous, or semicomatose. Deep tendon reflexes may be diminished; Babinski's reflex may be present. Hyporeflexia, or diminished reflexes, if not present initially, may occur during treatment as the potassium level falls. Frank coma, flaccidity, uncoordinated extraocular movements, and fixed, dilated pupils are late signs that suggest a poor prognosis.

Signs of dehydration reflective of intracellular and extracellular fluid volume deficit are common. Dehydration can be assessed by the presence of dry, crusty lips and mucous membranes; poor skin turgor (over forehead or sternum); soft or sunken eyeballs; flattened neck veins with the patient lying in a supine position; and weak, thready pulses. Orthostatic hypotension (i.e., a fall in systolic blood pressure of >10 to 20 mmHg within 1 minute of a change in position, e.g., from lying to standing position) reflects a significantly reduced intravascular blood volume associated with total body dehydration.

Kussmaul's breathing, as mentioned previously, may be noted. A fruity odor to the patient's breath may be detected. This reflects the presence of acetoacetate, one of the ketone bodies, which is converted to acetone. Acetone is excreted by the lungs, and its presence is noted by the fruity odor. The clinical presentation of an acute abdomen is common. Diminished bowel sounds, tenderness on abdominal palpation, and muscle guarding are also common findings. Occasionally, a patient may come to the clinic with more severe signs such as absent bowel sounds, boardlike abdomen, or rebound tenderness, that might suggest a surgical emergency. However, these signs can usually be attributed to a profound DKA.

Assessment of cardiovascular function may reveal hypovolemic shock with hypotension, tachycardia, decreased cardiac output, decreased central venous and pulmonary artery pressures, and cardiac arrhyth-

mias. Reduced peripheral perfusion may be reflected by cyanotic, mottled-appearing, cold, clammy skin. Occasionally, a patient may have flushed skin, which may reflect vasodilation of the peripheral vasculature caused by elevated ketone levels. Hypothermia may be present, and if so, sepsis must be ruled out. The presence of hyperthermia suggests an underlying systemic infection.

The patient may have oliguria (i.e., <30 mL/h) in the presence of intravascular fluid volume deficit. The presence of glycosuria and ketonuria underlies the osmotic diuresis, accounting for the fluid volume deficit. In addition, oliguria may reflect reduced renal perfusion, also secondary to the profound total body dehydration with intravascular fluid volume deficit.

Initial Laboratory Values in DKA[3]

Once a diagnosis of DKA is made by clinical impression, initial laboratory studies should be performed to confirm the diagnosis before therapy is initiated.

The following are common findings in patients with DKA.

1. Serum studies
   a. Glucose concentrations: usually >300 mg/dL, with a range from 300 to 800 mg/dL. This value is not a good index of the severity of DKA. Lower levels are not uncommon especially in patients with severe vomiting.
   b. Ketone bodies: strong (in undiluted plasma). This test is only useful in determining the initial diagnosis of DKA because it only detects acetoacetate and not β-hydroxybutyrate.
   c. Electrolytes.
      1) Potassium: because of acidosis and ketonemia, the patient usually presents with hyperkalemia, but total body deficit is

always present. Potassium concentrations depend on the balance between what is lost in the urine and other factors that raise the potassium level, such as lack of insulin, which allows potassium to remain in the circulation; the metabolic acidemia; which causes potassium to move out of cells in exchange for hydrogen ions; or prerenal azotemia, associated with intravascular fluid volume deficit.

2) Sodium: low, normal, or high levels, but total body deficit usually develops as a result of the osmotic diuresis. Sodium levels at any given time will reflect the relative amounts of water and sodium lost and replaced. If water deficit is greater than that of sodium, sodium levels will be high; if the sodium deficit is greater than that of water, the sodium level will be low; if the deficits are approximately equal, the sodium level will be normal.

3) Phosphate and magnesium: usually elevated initially, but may decrease markedly after therapy is begun.

4) Calcium: usually within normal range, but with drop in phosphate level, hypercalcemia may occur.

d. BUN and creatinine: usually mildly increased prior to therapy because of total body dehydration and prerenal azotemia. With therapy, these values should return to normal.

e. Osmolality: significantly elevated prior to therapy (>330 mOsm/kg). (Normal serum osmolality is 275 to 295 mOsm/kg.)

f. Albumin and total proteins: may be mildly elevated initially because of dehydration and intravascular fluid volume deficit.

g. Liver enzymes: often mildly increased, eventually return to normal (over days to weeks).

h. Hemoglobin and hematocrit: may be mildly elevated initially because of dehydration and intravascular fluid volume deficit.

i. White blood cells (WBCs): may be elevated, occasionally very high. An increase may not indicate an infection because DKA often causes rise in count; however, the presence of $>10\%$ bands (immature WBCs), suggests severe underlying infection.

j. Arterial blood gases:
   1) pH <7.20 (mean 7.07) reflects metabolic acidemia.
   2) HCO_3^- <10 mEq/L reflects metabolic acidemia.
   3) $Paco_2$ <20 to 35 mmHg reflects ventilatory compensatory response to metabolic acidemia.

2. Urine studies
   a. Glycosuria.
   b. Ketonuria.
   c. Proteinuria.

d. Specific gravity >1.025 reflects osmotic diuresis.

3. Cultures: as indicated (throat, sputum, blood, urine, stool, and wound).

4. ECG (12-lead): ST-segment and T-wave abnormalities, cardiac arrhythmias especially with alterations in potassium levels. T-wave changes aid in determining the potassium status on admission, which allows for earlier treatment decisions about replacement therapy. Hyperkalemia causes bradycardia, peaked T waves, disappearance of P waves, widened QRS measurements, and if markedly elevated, idioventricular rhythm and asystole. Hypokalemia causes prolonged PR interval and QT interval, low or flattened T waves, and rhythm disturbances, including premature atrial and ventricular contractions and ventricular tachycardia.

Management of the Patient with DKA

In the acute setting, overall treatment is focused on the following goals:

1. Restore fluid and electrolyte balance.
2. Provide adequate insulin to restore and maintain normal glucose and to correct the underlying metabolic acidemia.
3. Diagnose and treat underlying cause.
4. Maintain function of related systems and prevent complications.
5. Assess patient/family knowledge of IDDM and its management. Initiate appropriate patient education about diabetes self-care and follow-up.

All patients with moderate to severe DKA who cannot retain oral fluids or who have an altered mental status or level of consciousness require immediate emergency treatment. Initial treatment of DKA is directed at correcting any life-threatening abnormalities and stabilizing the patient. Adequate ventilation should be established as necessary. Hypovolemic shock should be corrected with vigorous fluid resuscitation. Plasma expanders may be necessary for hypotension unresponsive to fluid therapy. Patients who are comatose should have nasogastric drainage to prevent aspiration. Ongoing treatment is based on fluid and electrolyte replacement and administration of insulin.

Fluid and Electrolyte Therapy. Fluid and electrolyte replacement therapy is based on specific needs. Replacement requirements, maintenance needs, and ongoing losses need to be taken into consideration. Fluid volume deficits in DKA can be estimated as follows:

Mild	1 to 2 liters
Moderate	3 to 4 liters
Severe	5 to 8 liters

Initial fluid replacement depends on the degree of dehydration and the patient's cardiovascular status. One to two liters of half-normal (0.45%) or normal (0.9%) saline is administered over the first 1 to 2 hours, and then the patient is reassessed. Frequently, it is necessary to administer 500 to 1000 mL of intravenous (IV) saline over each subsequent hour until hypotension is corrected and urine output is stable at 1 to 2 mL/min. When blood pressure is stabilized, 0.45% saline can be substituted for normal saline (0.9%).

When serum glucose levels are reduced to approximately 250 mg/dL, IV fluids should be switched to a dextrose solution, usually dextrose 5%/0.45% saline. The hyperglycemia can be corrected more quickly than the underlying acidemia. Therefore, serum glucose levels must be maintained along with adequate insulin, to prevent any further ketosis and to allow the underlying acidemia to resolve.

Treatment of metabolic acidemia with sodium bicarbonate ($NaHCO_3$) is controversial, even for pH values of 7.0 or less. One concern is the effect on serum potassium levels, which will drop much more quickly and require very close monitoring. The status of the patient's cardiac function is also a major concern when administration of $NaHCO_3$ in this scenario is contemplated.

Potassium replacement therapy is guided by ECG changes in addition to initial and serial serum potassium studies. If hypokalemia is present, potassium should be administered immediately. Because of the total potassium depletion associated with DKA, all patients with adequate urine output eventually require potassium replacement therapy. Depending on the potassium level, potassium is replaced at concentrations of 20 to 40 mEq/L, usually in the form of potassium chloride (KCl).

With rehydration, potassium levels must be monitored closely because a rapid decline in these levels can occur. This decline is attributed in part to the dilutional effect of an expanding intravascular fluid volume and to an increased renal excretion resulting from improved renal perfusion. Additionally, insulin therapy will cause an increased movement of potassium into cells, along with glucose, further reducing the serum potassium concentration.

Clinical signs of hypokalemia include the following: skeletal muscle weakness or cramping, diminished-to-absent deep tendon reflexes, lethargy, anorexia, nausea and vomiting, abdominal pain, paralytic ileus (with absence of bowel sounds), changes in breathing pattern (shallow, gasping respirations), cardiac arrhythmias, and coma.

Insulin Therapy. All insulin therapy regimens must be individualized for each patient with DKA. Regular (crystalline) insulin is used because it affords relatively quick adjustments in serum glucose levels. The usual approach is to administer an IV *low-dose* infusion of regular insulin through a piggyback system into an existing IV line. To ensure that the correct dosage of insulin is administered, preflush all IV tubing with at least 50 mL of the infusion to allow insulin to bind to the plastic prior to initiating the infusion.

Low-dose IV insulin therapy is the method of choice because the risks of hypoglycemia and hypokalemia are reduced, and because changes in the levels of glucose and potassium are more predictable. IV insulin therapy is usually initiated at a dose of 0.1 U/kg per hour, and the dose is titrated so that serum glucose levels drop at a rate of approximately 75 to 100 mg/dL per hour.

Blood glucose levels are monitored at the patient's bedside after the first hour, and every 1 to 2 hours thereafter. If the glucose level has not dropped by 10% over 2 hours, and the patient is being adequately hydrated, the insulin infusion rate may be doubled.

Diagnose and Treat Underlying Cause. A diligent and careful search may be necessary to identify the underlying cause of the DKA. Thorough patient/family assessment, including health history and physical examination, is crucial to the diagnostic process. The patient should be carefully assessed for the presence of intercurrent illness, including upper respiratory infection, pneumonia, bronchitis, urinary tract infection, or other illness that may not readily be apparent. Cultures of specimens of blood, urine, stool, throat, sputum, wounds, and drainage should be obtained prior to initiating any antibiotic therapy.

Prevent Complications. Mortality for patients with DKA is linked directly to the age of the patient and to the degree of metabolic derangement. Most deaths occur in older patients primarily because of medical complications other than DKA. Mortality rates are significantly greater in women and in the nonwhite population.

In addition, complications of treatment can occur, including hypoglycemia, aspiration pneumonia, infection, fluid overload, congestive heart failure with pulmonary edema, acute renal failure, and cerebral edema, among others (although cerebral edema, which occurs rarely, is seen to occur more often in children with IDDM). Death may also be attributed to the unsuccessful diagnosis and/or treatment of the precipiating cause.

Prevention of DKA. The best therapy for DKA is its prevention. For the newly diagnosed patient, the focus must be to educate the patient and/or family regarding their responsibility in diabetes self-care management and follow-up. The patient's knowledge and use of sick-day management skills must be evaluated following any episode of DKA. An evaluation of patient/family stress management skills is essential. Many individuals with diabetes fail to recognize the impact that stress (emotional, physical, psychological, social, and economic) plays on the effective management of their diabetes. A multidisciplinary healthcare team approach is critical, especially in caring for patients with recurrent episodes of DKA.

Nursing Management

Therapeutic Goals. The nursing process for the care of the patient with DKA focuses on the following therapeutic goals:

1. Identify the patient at risk of developing DKA.

2. Establish a thorough and comprehensive database, including clinical history, physical examination, and initial laboratory values.
3. Collaborate with other healthcare providers to assist in diagnosing the precipitating cause of DKA.
4. Implement measures to restore and maintain fluid and electrolyte balance.
5. Implement prescribed insulin therapy regimen to restore and maintain euglycemia and to correct the metabolic acidemia.
6. Provide supportive care to reduce the risk of complications (e.g., hypoglycemia, infection, aspiration pneumonia, fluid overload, and congestive heart failure with pulmonary edema).
7. Maintain the integrity of neurologic and psychological processes.
8. Collaborate with multidisciplinary healthcare providers to assist patient/family in the following:
   a. Stress management and coping skills
   b. Diabetes self-care management skills and follow-up care

Nursing Diagnoses, Desired Patient Outcomes, and Nursing Interventions. Pertinent nursing diagnoses, desired patient outcomes, and nursing interventions for DKA are presented in the care plan at the end of this chapter.

Hyperglycemic, Hyperosmolar, Nonketotic Syndrome (HHNK)

Hyperglycemic, hyperosmolar, nonketotic syndrome (HHNK) is associated with a *relative* insulin deficit that occurs most commonly in elderly patients with mild or previously undiagnosed NIDDM. In this way, HHNK differs from DKA, which occurs *only* in patients with IDDM. (See Table 41–2.) Clinically, HHNK is indicated by severe hyperglycemia, *absence* of ketosis, profound dehydration, and neurologic manifestations. Elderly patients on oral hypoglycemic therapy, who may be inadequately monitored, or who are often unable to communicate their fluid needs, are especially at high risk to develop HHNK.

The mortality rate for HHNK is 40% to 50% greater than that for DKA because these patients are older and frequently have other significant medical problems that either precipitate or are precipitated by HHNK. In addition, sometimes the diagnosis of HHNK is overlooked, thereby delaying diagnosis and treatment.

Precipitating Factors

The major precipitating factor is usually a stressful event. Identified stressors include infection (e.g., pneumonia, sepsis, and gastroenteritis); acute illness (e.g., gastrointestinal hemorrhage, pancreatitis, and cerebrovascular insults); surgery; or procedures such as hypertonic feedings (e.g., total parenteral nutrition and enteral feedings), hemodialysis, and peritoneal dialysis.

Conditions that precipitate massive fluid losses have also been implicated in HHNK. Osmotic diuresis secondary to hyperglycemia, administration of hypertonic feedings without sufficient free water, severe burns, intractable diarrhea, and the indiscriminate or poorly supervised use of certain diuretics (e.g., thiazides and furosemide) have been identified.

It is important to elicit a thorough drug history because other drugs, in addition to diuretics, have been implicated as causative factors in HHNK. Such drugs include oral hypoglycemic agents (mentioned previously), phenytoin (Dilantin), steroids, propranolol and some antihypertensives (e.g., diazoxide and Hygroton), and over-the-counter drugs.

Pathogenesis of HHNK

The hallmarks of HHNK include a severe hyperglycemia with marked hyperosmolality, profound volume depletion with total body dehydration, and consequent neurologic alterations. Significantly, there is an *absence* of ketosis. Unlike in DKA, the insulin deficiency in HHNK is not nearly as profound. The patient has sufficient insulin to *prevent* significant lipolysis and ketogenesis, but inadequate amounts for carbohydrate metabolism.

The absence of ketoacidosis is especially significant because it lessens the gastrointestinal symptoms experienced by these patients, who may not feel sick enough to seek medical assistance before a profound volume depletion ensues. Because of the longer clinical course, which may span several weeks, the hyperglycemia is more severe, the hyperosmolality more marked, and the total body fluid deficit more profound. Contraction of the intravascular fluid volume reduces renal perfusion, which in turn, allows glucose concentrations to increase further, while also causing a significant rise in the BUN levels. Serum osmolality values exceed 330 mOsm/kg (normal range of 275 to 295 mOsm/kg).

Normally, the body responds to a rising serum osmolality by triggering the thirst mechanism. However, in the elderly, this mechanism may be impaired, or the patient may be unable to respond. Often, the elderly live alone with impaired mobility, which does not allow them access to fluid sources. Or they may already be experiencing an altered sensorium, preventing them from meeting their fluid needs. Even in nursing home or otherwise hospitalized patients, fluid intake may be inadequate. The consequent total body fluid volume deficit involving intracellular and extracellular fluid compartments is what ultimately underlies the neurologic alterations experienced by patients with HHNK.

Signs and Symptoms of HHNK

Specific signs and symptoms of HHNK are similar to those of DKA, with several important exceptions. In the absence of ketosis, gastrointestinal symptoms are less severe. Respirations are usually not of Kussmaul's pattern seen in DKA, and the breath lacks the characteristic acetone or fruity odor.

Because of the longer clinical course, fluid volume deficits are more pronounced in HHNK. Thus, changes in mental status and an altered sensorium are more common. Lethargy and drowsiness are often identified, and the patient may also exhibit focal neurologic signs, such as transient hemiparesis, aphasia, and seizures. Often, the clinical picture mimics that of a stroke. In addition, hypovolemia, attributed to severe fluid and electrolyte losses, accounts for the extreme hypotension, tachycardia, and oliguria, often evident.

Initial Laboratory Values in HHNK

Initial laboratory studies in HHNK differ from those seen in DKA in several notable respects (refer to earlier section on initial laboratory values in DKA.)

1. Serum studies
   a. Serum glucose levels: usually more significantly elevated to >600 mg/dL, with range from 600 to 1200 mg/dL.
   b. Ketone bodies: absent to minimal.
   c. BUN: markedly elevated, usually in excess of 60 to 80 mg/100 mL (normal range of 10 to 20 mg/100 mL).
   d. Serum osmolality: markedly elevated to >330 mOsm/kg; may approach 400 mOsm/kg.
   e. Arterial blood gases
      (1) pH 7.20 (mean 7.25)
      (2) HCO_3^- normal to moderately lowered
      (3) $PaCO_2$ usually normal unless underlying pulmonary disease is present
2. Urine studies
   a. Glycosuria: markedly elevated.
   b. Ketonuria: absent, or only slightly elevated.
3. Cultures: as indicated (blood, urine, throat, sputum, stool, and wound/drainage); may help to determine the precipitating cause of HHNK.

Management of the Patient with HHNK

The general principles for the management of the patient with HHNK are similar to those for DKA (refer to earlier section on management of the patient with DKA):

1. Restore fluid and electrolyte balance.
2. Provide adequate insulin to normalize and maintain serum glucose levels.
3. Diagnose and treat underlying cause.
4. Maintain function of related systems and prevent complications.
5. Assess patient/family knowledge of NIDDM and its management. Initiate appropriate patient education about diabetes management and follow-up care.

The initial treatment of the patient with HHNK is similar to that discussed for the patient with DKA. Interventions are focused on correcting life-threatening abnormalities and stabilizing the patient. Subsequent treatment is directed at correcting the total body fluid volume deficit and interrupting the metabolic imbalance associated with the marked hyperglycemia.

Fluid and Electrolyte Therapy. Fluid and electrolyte replacement is individualized for each patient. In the elderly, who are at greater risk of compromised cardiovascular function, fluid replacement should be *gradual*, with close monitoring of the patient's hemodynamic parameters (i.e., central venous and pulmonary artery pressures and cardiac output). Patients with a previous history of cardiac disease are at especially high risk of developing congestive heart failure from fluid overload.

Initial fluid volume deficit can be as high as 15% of total body water, or as much as 6 to 10 liters. Fluid replacement in HHNK usually follows that discussed for DKA. Initially, 1 to 2 liters of normal saline (0.9%) is administered over the first 1 to 2 hours. Half-normal saline (0.45%) may be substituted for normal saline as the hemodynamic status stabilizes. Necessary potassium, phosphate, and other electrolytes are added as indicated. Large amounts of potassium are usually necessary because of a total body depletion, thereby requiring ongoing ECG monitoring. All vital parameters are closely monitored to evaluate the response to therapy and to prevent fluid overload.

Insulin Therapy. In general, insulin therapy in HHNK follows the same treatment guidelines as in DKA. However, because ketosis is usually not a major factor in HHNK, insulin therapy can be decreased and even discontinued when glucose levels reach acceptable levels. Subsequently, for patients with HHNK, continued insulin may not be required. This is in contrast to DKA, where virtually all patients require ongoing insulin therapy.

Diagnose and Treat Underlying Cause. Diagnosis of the underlying cause of the HHNK should be aggressively pursued. Thorough patient assessment, including comprehensive clinical history and physical examination, is of paramount importance. High-risk patients need to be identified.

Prevent Complications. Patients who develop HHNK are usually over 60. Often they have other medical problems. Consequently, these patients are at even greater risk of developing complications of treatment. Hypoglycemia, aspiration or hypostatic pneumonia, congestive heart failure, acute renal failure, deep venous thrombosis, and pressure ulcers are frequent occurrences in these patients. Meticulous monitoring of all body organ system functions and a high level of suspicion are critical to a positive outcome for these patients.

Prevention of HHNK. As is the case with DKA, the best therapy for HHNK is its prevention. Individuals at high risk of developing HHNK must be identified. These include patients with diagnosed NIDDM and individuals with a family history of diabetes and obesity. Patients with NIDDM who are taking oral hypoglycemic agents must be especially closely monitored, particularly if they live alone.

The adequacy of fluid intake for patients in nursing home facilities and acute care hospitals must also be closely monitored. Even in these settings, adequate hydration of elderly, debilitated patients may not be maintained. Subtle changes in mental status, listlessness, and lethargy may be the initial signs of a fluid volume deficit and/or electrolyte imbalance, and are not necessarily attributable to old age.

Those with NIDDM and significant family history should be assessed regarding their knowledge and management skills in diabetes self-care. Guidelines regarding self-management of diabetes, especially during intercurrent illness, should be provided.

Nursing Management

Therapeutic Goals. Implementation of the nursing process in the care of the patient with HHNK is focused on all of the therapeutic goals discussed previously for the patient with DKA (refer to the section on nursing management in the discussion of DKA).

Nursing Diagnoses, Desired Patient Outcomes, and Nursing Interventions. Pertinent nursing diagnoses, desired patient outcomes, and nursing interventions for the patient with HHNK include those discussed for the patient with DKA (see the care plan at the end of this chapter).

Hypoglycemia

Hypoglycemia (hypoglycemic coma, formerly, insulin shock) is the most commonly encountered acute complication of IDDM, but it can also occur in patients with NIDDM who are treated with oral hypoglycemic agents. Specifically, hypoglycemia is a symptom complex initiated by an alteration in glucose metabolism wherein serum glucose concentrations decline to levels insufficient to meet the metabolic demands of the nervous system. The diagnosis of hypoglycemia usually requires an abnormally depressed serum glucose level (usually below 50 to 55 mg/100 mL) and a distinct clinical presentation.

Clinically, hypoglycemia in persons with diabetes can usually be defined as occurring at three levels: mild, moderate, and severe. *Mild* hypoglycemia is usually associated with symptoms that are primarily *adrenergic* in origin (e.g., shakiness, nervousness, hunger, tachycardia, and palpitations); *moderate* hypoglycemia reflects symptoms associated with *neuroglycopenia* (e.g., inability to concentrate, confusion, irrational behavior, and slurred speech). In both mild and moderate hypoglycemia, the patient is able to recognize the need for, and to seek, food and/or assistance. In *severe* hypoglycemia, patients have neuroglycopenia that is so profound (e.g., altered level of consciousness, coma, and seizures) that the intervention of another person is required. As a result of a lack of recognition, confusion, or inability to eat or drink, these patients are unable to treat themselves.

Precipitating Factors

Hypoglycemia can be caused by a number of precipitating factors. The most common cause is *too much* diabetes medication. Inadvertent or deliberate, errors in dosing are a frequent cause of hypoglycemia. Whether an insulin excess or too much oral hypoglycemic therapy, hypoglycemia will occur unless there is an increased carbohydrate intake or unless the body is able to compensate by increasing serum glucose levels through the actions of the normal glucose counterregulatory hormones (primarily, glucagon and epinephrine).

Hypoglycemia occurs as a result of a mismatch in timing and amount of insulin in the circulation, food consumption, and physical activity. Changes in timing or schedule of insulin administration or meals, or inadvertent reversal of short- and intermediate-acting insulin can precipitate hypoglycemia. Delayed or skipped meals and the intake of meals low in carbohydrate content can predispose to hypoglycemia. Delayed gastric emptying or impaired carbohydrate absorption because of gastrointestinal neuropathy can be less obvious precipitating factors.

Strenuous exercise is commonly associated with hypoglycemia in IDDM. In the individual without diabetes, the normal compensatory response to exercise involves a *decrease* in serum insulin levels and a concomitant *increase* in the serum levels of counterregulatory hormones. Through consequent hepatic glycogenolysis, gluconeogenesis, and lipolysis processes, an increase in serum glucose levels occurs sufficient to match glucose use.

In the patient with IDDM, whose insulin source is *exogenous* in origin (i.e., from outside the body), the normal compensatory decrease in insulin during exercise does not occur. In fact, serum insulin levels may actually increase because of mobilization from subcutaneous depots. A high serum insulin level during exercise enhances glucose uptake and use in exercising muscles, and inhibits hepatic glucose output. The end results are a drop in serum glucose levels and hypoglycemia.

Additionally, late-onset hypoglycemia after exercise is a concern, particularly in patients with IDDM. It is usually associated with moderate to intense exercise for periods greater than 30 to 60 minutes. An increase in insulin sensitivity, ongoing glucose use, and exhaustion of glycogen stores are thought to underlie this type of hypoglycemia.

Other precipitating factors of hypoglycemia include drugs. Some β-blockers (e.g., propranolol) induce hypoglycemia by inhibiting glycogenolysis. These drugs may also mask adrenergic manifestations associated with hypoglycemia. Heavy alcohol consumption superimposed on an inadequate dietary intake may precipitate hypoglycemia. Ethanol decreases hepatic glucose output by directly blocking several steps in hepatic gluconeogenesis. Other drugs identified as precipitating factors of hypoglycemia include acetylsalicylic acid (aspirin), disopyramide (Norpace), haloperidol, phenylbutazone, and Coumadin.

Patients with chronic renal disease who also have IDDM may develop hypoglycemia associated with impaired inactivation of insulin by the kidneys. An excessive increase in endogenous insulin secretion associated with islet cell tumors (insulinomas) may precipitate hypoglycemia by inhibiting hepatic glucose production. Primary liver disease (e.g., hepatitis, cirrhosis, and cancer) may alter the ability of the liver to store and release glucose and in this way contribute to hypoglycemia.

Pathophysiology of Hypoglycemia

Hypoglycemia occurs when serum glucose levels are inadequate to meet tissue glucose demands. In particular, the metabolic demands of the nervous system are especially sensitive to reduced serum glucose levels because glucose is its major energy source. The brain uses glucose as its *primary* fuel, rarely using other energy substrates (such as fatty acids and ketones). Consequently, the processes involved in lowering serum glucose levels (insulin release) and those involved in raising glucose levels (release of counter-regulatory hormones) are carefully modulated.

Acute insulin-induced hypoglycemia triggers release of glucose counter-regulatory hormones, primarily glucagon and epinephrine, thereby increasing serum glucose to levels that match glucose use. In this way, recovery from insulin-induced hypoglycemia is achieved. An increase in glucagon secretion in response to insulin-induced hypoglycemia is frequently impaired in the early course of IDDM, starting within the first few years. An alpha islet cell dysfunction, it results in a failure of glucagon to be released in response to hypoglycemia, despite a normal or even exaggerated glucagon response to stress and other stimuli.

In patients with impaired glucagon secretion, epinephrine assumes the primary role in raising serum glucose levels. Epinephrine facilitates recovery from insulin-induced hypoglycemia by increasing hepatic glucose production; it also inhibits the release and action of insulin, thereby reducing glucose use. However, some patients with IDDM develop a diminished or absent release of epinephrine in response to hypoglycemia, a deficiency sometimes identified in patients with autonomic (sympathetic) neuropathy, or hypoglycemia unawareness (see following discussion). When it does occur, epinephrine deficiency usually occurs later in the course of diabetes than does glucagon deficiency.

In patients with a marked deficiency of *both* glucagon and epinephrine secretion in response to insulin-induced hypoglycemia, a condition referred to as *defective glucose counter-regulation*, there is a markedly increased risk for recurrent, severe hypoglycemia.[4]

Nocturnal Hypoglycemia. In patients who are insulin-dependent, over one half of all episodes of severe hypoglycemia occur during the night. Nocturnal hypoglycemia can occur for several reasons. First, patients, when asleep, may not be awakened by the warning signs of hypoglycemia; second, an underlying impaired response of glucose counter-regulatory hormones to insulin-induced hypoglycemia may be present; third, insulin requirements to maintain normal serum glucose levels are lower in the predawn hours (midnight to 3:00 AM); and lastly, intermediate-acting insulin, given before dinner, often produces a relative rise in insulin levels during the predawn period.

Somogyi Phenomenon. The *Somogyi* phenomenon is defined as a morning rebound hyperglycemia following an episode of nocturnal hypoglycemia associated with too much insulin. It is treated by reducing the dose of insulin.

Dawn Phenomenon. The Somogyi effect is sometimes confused with another form of morning hyperglycemia termed the "dawn" phenomenon, which is an abrupt increase in early morning (4:00 AM to 8:00 AM) serum glucose levels (fasting hyperglycemia) without antecedent nocturnal hypoglycemia. The causative mechanism has not been positively identified, but current data suggest a primary determinant involves the early dawn release of counter-regulatory hormones, growth hormone, and cortisol.[5] The dawn phenomenon affects the majority of individuals with IDDM. It peaks during adolescence and in young adulthood.

Hypoglycemia Unawareness. Hypoglycemia unawareness is a syndrome wherein patients with diabetes do not recognize signs of hypoglycemia and, therefore, do not initiate treatment. The underlying cause is thought to involve a blunted epinephrine response to hypoglycemia. As a result, these individuals tend to lack, or are unable to recognize, the adrenergic symptoms of hypoglycemia, and they may develop neuroglycopenic symptoms (see the following) and severe hypoglycemia without prior warning.

Signs and Symptoms of Hypoglycemia

Signs and symptoms of hypoglycemia comprise two major categories: (1) adrenergic symptoms reflective of autonomic nervous system stimulation, and (2) symptoms related to an inadequate glucose supply to neural tissues, referred to as neuroglycopenia. The *adrenergic* signs and symptoms are associated with a rising epinephrine level. These include shakiness, nervousness, irritability, tremulousness, hunger, tachycardia/palpitations, circumoral numbness, paresthesias, general weakness, dilated pupils, and pallor.

Although it is commonly observed, profuse diaphoresis that occurs during a hypoglycemic episode is attributed to *cholinergic* stimulation and not to the actions of epinephrine. Thus, the presence of diaphoresis is not necessarily indicative of sufficient epinephrine secretion to recover from the hypoglycemia. In fact, profuse sweating can be seen in some patients with hypoglycemia even in the absence of increased epinephrine levels.

Signs and symptoms of *neuroglycopenia* are those associated with the lack of adequate glucose supply to the brain. This may be observed when the decline in serum glucose levels is slower, more severe, and more prolonged, or when the epinephrine response to hypoglycemia is impaired. Signs and symptoms include headache, restlessness, inability to concentrate, slurred speech, visual disturbances, confusion, inappropriate behavior, seizures, severe lethargy, and coma. Neuroglycopenia almost always becomes recognizable in patients when serum glucose levels drop below 45 to 50 mg/dL. Occasionally, it may be observed at glucose levels only as low as 60 mg/dL.

Neuroglycopenia is not always preceded by adrenergic or cholinergic manifestations. Some patients may not experience adrenergic activity that would otherwise prompt treatment, but rather progress to frank neuroglycopenia. Others develop neuroglycopenia initially, followed by adrenergic and cholinergic responses.

Initial Laboratory Values in Hypoglycemia

The severity of hypoglycemia as reflected clinically is poorly correlated with laboratory values. Blood glucose levels that trigger symptoms and the severity of these symptoms are dependent on a variety of modifiable factors that may differ from one patient to the next, and from one episode to the next, within the same individual. For example, some patients may remain alert with few symptoms at a serum glucose level of 50 mg/dL, while others may become comatose at this same glucose level. Furthermore, an individual may tolerate a serum glucose level of 50 mg/dL on one occasion, but become significantly incapacitated at this same level on a different occasion. Thus, the precise serum glucose level at which patients develop symptomatic hypoglycemia is difficult to define. In general, however, symptoms do not occur until serum glucose levels become less than 50 to 60 mg/dL.

Management of the Patient with Hypoglycemia

The goals of management of hypoglycemia are the following:
1. To restore serum glucose to normal levels
2. To determine the underlying cause
3. To prevent recurrence of hypoglycemic episodes

Treatment is individualized for each patient and depends on the type of diabetes and its treatment and on the severity of associated symptoms. Immediate treatment of hypoglycemia is essential regardless of the severity.

Glucose Therapy. In both mild and moderate hypoglycemic episodes where the patient remains conscious, the best treatment is the immediate ingestion of a rapidly absorbed glucose source. For mild hypoglycemia, 10 to 15 grams of carbohydrate is recommended (e.g., 4 to 6 ounces of fruit juice or regular soda (not diet), five Lifesavers candies, or a cup of milk) followed by a resumption of usual activity.

Recovery from moderate hypoglycemia may require 15 to 30 grams of carbohydrates. To prevent recurrence, patients are advised to eat longer-lasting carbohydrate sources (e.g., milk and bread) or their planned meal or snack. Following treatment, the patient may need to wait for 15 minutes or more before resuming prior activity. In some cases, the neuroglycopenic symptoms may last for an hour or longer, even after serum glucose levels rise above 100 mg/dL.

Severe hypoglycemia usually impairs consciousness or the ability to swallow. These patients require emergent treatment with glucagon or intravenous glucose. In the home setting, severe hypoglycemia is best treated with glucagon 1.0 mg by intramuscular injection, if available. Administration of glucagon involves the same technique as that of insulin administration. Upon recovery (usually 10 to 15 minutes), the patient is then advised to seek medical assistance.

In the acute care setting, severe hypoglycemia is treated most rapidly by administering an ampule of 50% glucose by intravenous push. A continuous infusion of 50% glucose is then administered until consciousness returns or the serum glucose level rises to more than 200 mg/dL. Clinical improvement should occur within 1 to 5 minutes of intravenous glucose administration. However, if the hypoglycemia was prolonged or extremely severe, complete recovery of mental functions could take several hours.

Determine Underlying Cause. It is essential to work with the patient, family, and other healthcare providers to determine the cause of repeated hypoglycemic episodes. A thorough patient assessment, including in particular a close examination of diabetes self-care management skills, is necessary if the underlying causative factor is to be determined and recurrence prevented.

Prevention of Hypoglycemia. The key to preventing hypoglycemic episodes is educating the patient/family about the signs, symptoms, causes, and treatment of hypoglycemia. Knowedge base and management skills in diabetes self-care need to be re-evaluated because problems predisposing to hypoglycemia can involve any number of areas of diabetes care. Diet, including timing of meals and snacks in conjunction with diabetes medication, and adequacy of food intake are especially important. Over 50% of patients with diabetes fail to follow their prescribed diets.

Errors in taking diabetes medication, whether inadvertent or deliberate, are a frequent cause of hypoglycemia. Excessive dosing, reversal of morning or evening doses of short- and intermediate-acting insulins, or attempting to maintain too tight glucose control using intensive regimens can all precipitate hypoglycemia. More rapid absorption of insulin, as for example from an exercising limb, or unpredictable absorption from hypertrophied injection sites are also contributing factors of which the patient with diabetes needs to be aware.

Patients must also understand that unplanned exercise or prolonged duration or increased intensity of exercise without additional adjustments in diabetes medication and food intake can precipitate hypoglycemia. Patients should be taught to monitor blood glucose levels before, during, and after periods of vigorous exercise.

All patients with diabetes should be taught to recognize signs and symptoms that *they*, themselves, develop when glucose levels are low. Patients should be instructed to test their blood glucose levels when experiencing symptoms associated with hypoglycemia to verify blood glucose levels. To maintain hypoglycemia awareness, patients should also know that their symptoms of hypoglycemia may change over time, requiring recognition of even the most subtle signs of hypoglycemia. Patients should also be aware of steps to take to prevent nocturnal hypoglycemia.

All patients with diabetes, whether IDDM or NIDDM, should know that self-monitoring of blood glucose (SMBG) is the key to good diabetes control without the occurrence of hypoglycemic episodes.

Nursing Management

Therapeutic Goals. The nursing process for the care of the patient with hypoglycemia focuses on the following therapeutic goals:

1. Recognize that hypoglycemia is a potential complication in all patients with IDDM *and* NIDDM.
2. Assess thoroughly the patient's knowledge of diabetes and diabetes self-care management skills.
3. Collaborate with other healthcare providers to assist in diagnosing the precipitating cause of diabetes, especially when episodes of hypoglycemia recur frequently (e.g., on a daily basis).
4. Implement prescribed/indicated glucose therapy to restore serum glucose levels to normal.
5. Provide supportive care for the patient experiencing severe neuroglycopenia (e.g., seizures and coma), until consciousness returns and the patient's condition is stabilized.
6. Collaborate with multidisciplinary healthcare providers to assist in patient/family education about their diabetes self-care practices.

Nursing Diagnoses, Desired Patient Outcomes, and Nursing Interventions. Pertinent nursing diagnoses, desired patient outcomes, and nursing interventions for hypoglycemia are presented in the care plan at the end of this chapter.

CASE STUDY: PATIENT WITH DIABETIC KETOACIDOSIS

S.B., a 55-year-old white woman, was brought into the emergency room barely arousable. Her family reported that she had become ill 2 days ago with nausea and vomiting and complaints of abdominal cramping. The patient had long-term NIDDM, but had been dependent on insulin for the past 2 years. She was taking isophane insulin suspension, 30 U subcutaneously in the morning and 15 U in the evening.

Her family reported that her husband had had a sudden heart attack and passed away 5 weeks ago. They also stated that in the past S.B. had always been diligent about caring for her diabetes. She tested her blood sugar daily, was careful about her diet, and enjoyed jogging several times a week. However, since her husband's death, she seemed to become lax in all phases of her diabetes care and was experiencing a deep depression for which she refused any help.

On initial examination, the patient was difficult to arouse, but responded appropriately to pain. Her vital signs included a blood pressure of 80/50 mmHg; she was in a sinus tachycardia at a rate of 120 beats/min, and her respirations were deep and labored. Body temperature was recorded as 98.6°F. Mucous membranes were dry; skin turgor poor; and a fruity odor was detected on the breath. Examination of the abdomen revealed marked distention with hypoactive bowel sounds. There was no organomegaly. Deep tendon reflexes were hyperactive bilaterally in both lower extremities. The remaining physical examination was unremarkable.

Blood chemistry studies revealed a blood sugar level of 468 mg/dL, a BUN of 37 mg/dL, creatinine of 1.8 mg/dL, sodium of 130 mEq/dL, potassium of 3.4 mEq/dL, and bicarbonate of 6 mEq/dL. Serum osmolarity was 310 mOsm/dL, and the plasma was positive for ketones. Arterial blood gas determinations on room air revealed the following: PaO_2 of 90 mmHg, $PaCO_2$ of 24 mmHg, and a pH of 7.20. Urinalysis indicated glucose (4+) and ketones (3+). Complete blood count was found to be within acceptable range. Chest x-ray findings were unremarkable. An electrocardiogram displayed sinus tachycardia with occasional multifocal premature ventricular contractions (PVCs).

In the emergency room, 2 liters of IV saline (0.9%) was infused within the initial 2 hours. The patient was then given 8 U of regular insulin as an IV bolus, and an insulin drip of 1.0 U/kg per hour was started. A urinary catheter was inserted, and urine output averaged 60 mL/h. Plasma glucose levels were checked hourly, and serum electrolytes, arterial pH, and ketones were monitored at 2- to 4-hour intervals.

About 2 hours after arrival in the emergency department, the patient became arousable. Blood glucose levels had dropped to 364 mg/dL. Serum potassium was 2.8, and bicarbonate increased to 10 mEq/dL. The patient's blood pressure was 90/60, and the patient remained in a sinus tachycardia at a rate of 120 beats/min, with occasional multifocal PVCs. Aggressive hydration with potassium replacement was continued, and the patient was transferred to the intensive care unit.

With continued hydration and potassium replacement, the patient's blood pressure rose to 110/60, with a heart rate of 110 beats/min, and her cardiac rhythm remained sinus with only infrequent unifocal PVCs. Blood glucose levels dropped to 240 mg/dL over the ensuing 2 hours, and serum electrolytes began to normalize as follows: sodium of 138 mEq/

dL, potassium of 3.6 mEq/dL, and bicarbonate of 12 mEq/dL. At this time, an IV solution of dextrose 5%/0.45% saline with 30 mEq/dL of potassium was initiated at a rate of 200 mL/h. The insulin drip was reduced to 0.5 U/kg per hour, and the patient was given 10 U of regular insulin subcutaneously.

Approximately 8 hours after admission, the patient was awake, alert, and able to tolerate clear fluids. Her blood sugar level was 190 mg/dL; sodium, 135 mEq/dL; potassium, 4.1 mEq/dL; and bicarbonate, 20 mEq/dL. The patient was given her usual evening dose of 15 U of isophane insulin suspension, and the insulin infusion was discontinued. The patient tolerated an evening meal, but she appeared listless and withdrawn.

TENTATIVE NURSING DIAGNOSES

1. Fluid volume deficit related to osmotic diuresis caused by extreme glycosuria associated with hyperglycemic state.
2. Electrolyte imbalance related to the following:
   a. Osmotic diuresis caused by extreme glycosuria
   b. Acidemia and ketonemia
3. Alteration in acid-base balance related to the following:
   a. Ketoacidosis associated with insulin insufficiency
   b. Enhanced glycolysis
   c. Lactic acidemia associated with compromised tissue perfusion and tissue hypoxia
4. Potential for physiologic injury, hypoglycemia, related to the following:
   a. Stressful event
   b. Noncompliance with therapeutic regimen
5. Ineffective individual coping related to stress associated with husband's recent death.

REFERENCES

1. Lipsett, LF and Geiss, L: Statistics: Prevalence, Incidence, Risk Factors, and Complications of Diabetes (memorandum). American Diabetes Association Bulletin, April 9, 1993.
2. Cryer, PE: Iatrogenic hypoglycemia as a cause of hypoglycemia-associated autonomic failure in IDDM. Diabetes 41:255–260, 1992.
3. Peragallo-Dittko, V: A Core Curriculum for Diabetes Education, ed 2. American Association of Diabetes Educators and the AADE Education and Research Foundation, Chicago, 1993.
4. Haire-Joshu, D: Management of Diabetes Mellitus: Perspectives of Care Across the Life Span. Mosby–Year Book. St Louis, 1992, p 267.
5. Haire-Joshu, D: Management of Diabetes Mellitus: Perspectives of Care Across the Life Span. Mosby–Year Book, St Louis, 1992, p 272.

CARE PLAN FOR THE PATIENT WITH DIABETIC KETOACIDOSIS

Nursing Diagnoses

Nursing Diagnosis #1
Fluid volume deficit: actual (total body dehydration), related to:
1. Osmotic diuresis caused by extreme glycosuria associated with hyperglycemic state
2. Ketosis and ketonemia associated with enhanced lipolysis caused by insulin insufficiency

Nursing Diagnosis #2
Electrolyte imbalance, related to:
1. Profound osmotic diuresis caused by extreme glycosuria
2. Acidemia and ketonemia associated with enhanced lipolysis, and lactic acidosis associated with tissue hypoxia
3. Profound dehydration and hypovolemia
4. Nasogastric suctioning
5. Profuse diaphoresis

Desired Patient Outcomes

Patient will maintain stable:
1. Neurologic status:
   - Alert, oriented to person, place, date
   - Appropriate behavior
   - Usual personality (per family)
   - Sensorimotor function intact
   - Deep tendon reflexes brisk
2. Hemodynamic status:
   - BP within 10 mmHg of baseline
   - Heart rate >60, <100 beats/min
   - Cardiac rhythm: regular sinus
   Hemodynamic parameters:
   - CVP mean 0–8 mmHg
   - PCWP mean 8–12 mmHg
   - Cardiac output: 4–8 L/min
3. Renal status:
   - Body weight within 5% of baseline
   - Urine output >30 mL/h
4. Laboratory status:
   Serum:
   - Osmolality: 285–295 mOsm/kg
   - Sodium: 135–148 mEq/L
   - Potassium: 3.5–5.5 mEq/L
   - Glucose: 70–110 mg/100 mL
   Urine:
   - Specific gravity: 1.010–1.025
   - Negative for glucose and acetone

CARE PLAN FOR THE PATIENT WITH DIABETIC KETOACIDOSIS (*Continued*)

Nursing Interventions	Rationales
• Assess impact of osmotic diuresis on total body fluid and electrolyte status.	• Extreme glycosuria related to hyperglycemic state precipitates profound fluid loss via a glucose osmotic diuresis.

○ Assess neurologic status:
  □ Mental status, level of consciousness.
  □ Behavior and personality.
  □ Sensorimotor function.
  □ Deep tendon reflexes.
	○ Severe hyperosmolality related to hyperglycemia can predispose to alterations in neurologic function.

○ Assess fluid status:
  □ Body weight, vital signs.
  □ Intake and output.
  □ Skin turgor, signs of dehydration: dry, parched skin and mucous membranes; sunken eyeballs.
  □ Gastrointestinal fluid losses, nasogastric suctioning, diarrhea.
  □ Insensible fluid losses through lungs and skin
  □ Fever, excessive diaphoresis.
	○ Hypovolemic state is reflected by altered hemodynamics with decreased arterial and venous blood pressures; pulse may be rapid and thready; potential risk of hypovolemic shock must be anticipated and carefully assessed.

○ Laboratory tests: serum osmolality, electrolytes, serum glucose
  □ BUN and creatinine.
  □ Total protein (blood).
  □ Urine specific gravity.
	□ Excessive ventilatory effort of Kussmaul's breathing can lead to considerable fluid loss.
	○ Laboratory values may appear elevated because of hemoconcentration (i.e., severe volume contraction related to total body dehydration).
	○ Decreased renal perfusion diminishes the glomerular filtration rate, predisposing to oliguria and placing the severely dehydrated patient at risk of developing acute renal failure.

□ Urine glucose and acetone.
○ Assess sources of electrolyte loss:
  □ Profound osmotic diuresis with sodium loss.
  □ Losses of sodium and chloride occur with vomiting and nasogastric suctioning.
	○ Loss of sodium contributes to hyperkalemia because there is a decrease in potassium secretion in the distal renal tubules in the absence of sodium reabsorption.
	○ In the presence of acidemia, there is a shift of K^+ ions from the intracellular to extracellular space in exchange for H^+ ions, contributing significantly to hyperkalemia.
	○ It is estimated that for every 0.1 decrease in pH, the serum potassium concentration increases by 0.6 mEq/L.
	○ Serum electrolytes must be evaluated in terms of total body water status because such values, if assessed separately, may not reflect the true electrolyte status.

• Implement prescribed fluid replacement regimen:	• Rapid rehydration with isotonic saline (0.9 N saline) is the treatment of choice; overly aggressive use of hypotonic saline (0.45 N saline) may produce a precipitous fall in extracellular fluid osmolality, generating rapid intracellular fluid shifts and cerebral edema.
○ Administer aggressive fluid therapy.	○ Because patients with DKA manifest varying degrees of fluid and electrolyte imbalance, fluid and electrolyte replacement therapy must be individualized and guided by continuous monitoring and assessment.
○ Monitor for signs/symptoms of fluid excess: cardiac rate and rhythm; hemodynamic parameters—CVP, PCWP, CO. □ Physical signs: extra heart sounds (gallop rhythm), full bounding pulse, neck vein distention at 45 degrees (upright position), dependent edema.	○ Rapid fluid replacement necessitates close monitoring of vital signs and hemodynamic function to avert overhydration with its attendant danger of congestive heart failure and pulmonary edema. Patients with compromised cardiac and/or renal function are especially at high risk.
○ Closely monitor for hypoglycemia, hypokalemia, and cerebral edema. □ Serial serum glucose studies. ○ Insert Foley catheter during the acute phase to more closely monitor urine output.	○ When serum glucose levels approach 250 mg/100 mL, dextrose 5% in 0.45 N saline is substituted for normal saline to avoid precipitating a hypoglycemic reaction. ○ Accurate assessment of urinary output is essential to assess renal function and to determine fluid and electrolyte therapy.

CARE PLAN FOR THE PATIENT WITH DIABETIC KETOACIDOSIS *(Continued)*

Nursing Interventions

- Restore and maintain electrolyte balance.
  - Implement electrolyte replacement therapy.

    - Administer prescribed saline therapy.
    - Assess for signs and symptoms of *hyper*kalemia.
      - Monitor ECG for peaked T-wave and ST-segment changes; bradycardia, idioventricular rhythm, and cardiac arrest (particularly if serum potassium levels exceed 6.5 mg/dL)
      - Monitor serum electrolytes and pH.
    - Assess for signs and symptoms of *hypo*kalemia.
      - Monitor ECG for inverted or flattened T wave; appearance of U wave; prolonged PR interval and QT interval; and rhythm disturbances, including premature atrial and ventricular contractions and ventricular tachycardia.
      - Monitor serum electrolytes and pH.

    - Administer potassium replacement therapy as prescribed.
  - Continuous monitoring of ECG and serial serum potassium levels is critical.

- Implement prescribed insulin replacement therapy.

  - Low-dose regular insulin regimens are usually prescribed.

Rationales

  - Precise documentation of fluid intake and output is necessary to determine fluid replacement therapy and the patient's response to such therapy.
- Serum sodium and potassium concentrations are variable, but total body concentrations are severely depleted.
  - Provides necessary sodium and water replacement.
    - Hyperkalemia is associated with profound osmotic diuresis with hemoconcentration; shifting of K^+ ions from intracellular to extracellular space because of ketoacidemia; and retention of K^+ ions in intravascular compartment in the absence of insulin.

    - Hypokalemia becomes manifest within 2–4 h of initiation of insulin, fluid, and electrolyte replacement therapies. Physiology underlying the total body potassium deficit: dilutional factor with rehydration; reduction in ketoacidemia related to insulin therapy—shift from fatty acid to glucose metabolism; movement of K^+ ions into cells with glucose in the presence of insulin; increase in renal perfusion with consequent fluid and electrolyte loss.
    - Goal is to restore and maintain normal extracellular potassium concentrations during the acute period.
  - Close monitoring of serum potassium and ECG changes is essential because alterations in serum potassium can precipitate serious/lethal arrhythmias.
- Goal is to ensure a sustained, progressive reduction in serum glucose levels.
  - Insulin therapy requires that serum glucose be monitored at frequent intervals. In DKA, prolonged insulin therapy is required after serum glucose levels reach 250 mg/100 mL, because correction of ketoacidemia takes longer to resolve.

Nursing Diagnoses

Nursing Diagnosis #3

Acid-base balance, alteration in, related to:
1. Ketoacidosis associated with insulin insufficiency
2. Enhanced lipolysis
3. Lactic acidemia associated with reduced tissue perfusion and tissue hypoxia

Desired Patient Outcomes

1. Patient's arterial blood gases will normalize as follows:
   - pH: 7.35–7.45
   - $Paco_2$: 35–45 mmHg, or optimal for patient
2. Anions will stabilize as follows:
   - HCO_3^-: 22–26 mEq/L
   - Chloride: 100–106 mEq/L
   - Anion gap: <12–15 mEq/L

Nursing Interventions

- Implement measures to restore and maintain acid-base balance.
  - Monitor acid-base balance:
    - Serial arterial blood gases.
    - Serial electrolytes.
    - Calculation of anion gap: the major two anions are chloride (Cl^-) and bicarbonate (HCO_3^-). They account for all but 10–15 mmol/L of the total anion charge in the body. To calculate:
      Anion gap = $Na^+ - (Cl^- + HCO_3^-)$
  - Normal anion gap: <15 mmol/L.
  - Monitor ketoacidotic state:
    - Presence of prominent gastrointestinal symptomatology: epigastric distress, nausea, vomiting, abdominal pain, distention, ileus.
    - Heavy, labored breathing (Kussmaul's).
    - Flushed skin; fruity odor to breath.

Rationales

- Ketoacidemia is a major distinctive finding in DKA with marked depression of the arterial pH (<7.20) largely from ketosis.
  - Serum and urine are highly positive for acetoacetic acid, β-hydroxybutyric acid, and acetone. *Note:* Ketostix test for acetoacetic acid and acetone does *not* test for β-hydroxybutyric acid. Thus, in the patient with predominantly elevated levels of this latter ketone, a severe ketoacidemia may exist without a positive serum acetone.
  - An anion gap greater than 15 mmol/L indicates existence of another anion. In DKA, the source of these additional anions are the ketones, acetoacetic and β-hydroxybutyric acids, and acetone.

CARE PLAN FOR THE PATIENT WITH DIABETIC KETOACIDOSIS (*Continued*)

Nursing Interventions

- If pH is <7.0, bicarbonate therapy may be prescribed. Approach to therapy:
  - Administer 1 ampule of sodium bicarbonate (44.6 mEq/L) at a time; follow blood study results carefully. When pH is >7.0, discontinue bicarbonate therapy.

Rationales

- If bicarbonate therapy is initiated (for pH <7), caution must be taken to avoid too rapid restoration of pH; this may predispose to alterations in cerebral functions from paradoxical cerebrospinal fluid acidosis. *Remember:* Carbon dioxide penetrates the blood-brain barrier much more easily than the ion HCO_3^- does.

Nursing Diagnoses

Nursing Diagnosis #4

Breathing pattern, ineffective: hyperventilation (Kussmaul's breathing), related to:
1. Severe ketonemia and acidemia associated with excessive lipolysis in the absence of insulin (pH <7.20)
2. Tissue hypoxia associated with impaired perfusion.

Desired Patient Outcomes

Patient will:
1. Maintain ventilatory effort as follows:
   - <25–30 breaths/min
   - Tidal volume (TV): >5–7 mL/kg
   - Vital capacity (VC): >15 mL/kg
2. Demonstrate eupnea, without use of accessory muscles of breathing.
3. Avoid fatigue with reduced work of breathing.

The patient's parameters will stabilize as follows:
1. Arterial blood gases:
   - pH >7.35
   - PaO_2 >80 mmHg
   - $PaCO_2$ return to baseline (normally 35–45 mmHg)

Hemoglobin oxygen saturation: >95%
2. Neurologic status: oriented to person, place, date; protective reflexes (cough, swallowing) intact.
3. Skin and mucous membranes—no cyanosis.

Nursing Interventions

- Establish baseline assessment database:
  - Assess pertinent parameters of respiratory function:

    - Respiratory rate, rhythm and pattern of breathing.

    - Hyperventilation (Kussmaul's).
    - Tachypnea, dyspnea.

  - Use of accessory muscles of respiration.
  - Pleuritic pain.
  - Pulmonary function parameters:
    - Tidal volume.
    - Vital capacity.
  - Auscultation of breath sounds.

  - Arterial blood gases: trends.

  - Cyanosis of lips, mucous membranes, and nail beds.

  - Acetone odor to breath.
  - Neurologic status.

- Provide supportive therapy.
  - Administer humidified oxygen.

  - Assist patient to assume a position that facilitates breathing.

Rationales

- Goal of therapy is to maintain effective respiratory function as guided by arterial blood gas, tidal volume, vital capacity, and neurologic function.
  - Ineffective breathing pattern often associated with muscle weakness caused by hypokalemia; patient is at great risk of developing respiratory arrest.
  - Kussmaul's breathing associated with severe ketoacidemia; it is a compensatory response of the body to blow off excess CO_2 and thereby increase arterial pH.
  - Use of accessory muscles may cause undue fatigue.
  - Severely dehydrated state may predispose to pleuritic friction rub.

  - Adventitious sounds (rales, rhonchi, wheezes) may signal pulmonary congestion progressing to pulmonary edema; secretions.
  - A rising $PaCO_2$ suggests decreasing ventilatory capability. A PaO_2 <60 mmHg predisposes to tissue hypoxia.
  - Cyanosis reflects decreased tissue oxygenation related to altered ventilation.
  - Reflects ketogenesis.
  - Ongoing neurologic assessment is essential to detect alterations in cerebral function from paradoxic CSF acidosis.

  - May assist in relieving tissue hypoxia; prevents thick tenacious secretions of dehydrated state.
  - Efforts must be directed toward assisting patient to conserve strength.
  - Insertion of nasogastric tube may be necessary to prevent gastric dilation, which limits diaphragmatic excursion and increases the risk of aspiration, with consequent aspiration pneumonia.

CARE PLAN FOR THE PATIENT WITH DIABETIC KETOACIDOSIS (*Continued*)

Nursing Interventions

- ○ Encourage deep breathing.

- ○ Initiate ventilatory assistance if indicated (respiratory arrest).

Rationales

- ○ Deep breathing minimizes atelectasis.
- ○ Position changes minimize pooling of secretions.
- ○ Ventilatory support may be needed in presence of altered state of consciousness, ineffective breathing pattern, inability to handle secretions.

Nursing Diagnoses

Nursing Diagnosis #5
Self-concept, disturbance in: body image, self-esteem, related to chronic illness

Desired Patient Outcomes

Patient will feel comfortable talking about what diabetes means and how it will affect lifestyle and optimal level of health desired.

Nursing Interventions

- Encourage verbalization of fears and concerns.
- Explain all ongoing procedures.

- Involve patient/family in decision-making process.
  - ○ Support patient/family efforts in coping.
  - ○ Remain accessible to patient and family.
  - ○ Provide emotional support to patient and family.

Rationales

- It may help to identify problems or areas of concern.
- Appropriate explanations may help to alleviate heightened anxiety.
- Management of diabetes, a chronic disease syndrome, requires self-care health practices by patient and family; their active involvement is essential if they are to evolve a meaningful life within the constraints of the disease.

Nursing Diagnoses

Nursing Diagnosis #6
Nutrition, alteration in: less than body requirements, related to:
1. Catabolic state
2. Insulin lack

Desired Patient Outcomes

Patient's condition will stabilize as follows:
1. Body weight will stabilize within appropriate range.
2. Positive nitrogen balance will be maintained.
3. Combination of insulin, diet, and exercise therapies will maintain serum glucose levels within optimal range.
4. Abdominal discomfort will be minimized; gastric aspiration will be averted.

Nursing Diagnoses

Nursing Diagnosis #7
Knowledge deficit: diabetes self-care

Desired Patient Outcomes

Patient and family will:
1. Discuss underlying principles of diabetic diet therapy.
2. Specify dietary restrictions and their significance.
3. Relate how diet therapy coincides with insulin and exercise regimens.
4. Demonstrate proficiency in performing and interpreting tests for serum glucose.
5. Identify action to be taken in the event of gastrointestinal disorder or significant stressor.
6. Verbalize concerns about the disease syndrome and overall antidiabetes therapy regimen.

Nursing Diagnoses

Nursing Diagnosis #8
Injury, physiologic, potential for: hypoglycemia, related to:
1. Ineffective dietary/insulin regimen
2. Noncompliance with therapeutic regimen
3. Stressful event
(See care plan for hypoglycemia on pp. 772–774.)

Desired Patient Outcomes

1. Patient will maintain optimal serum glucose levels:
   - Fasting serum glucose: 70–110 mg/100 mL
   - 1–2 h postprandial: <160–180 mg/100 mL
2. Patient will be able to verbalize signs and symptoms of hypoglycemic and hyperglycemic states.

Nursing Interventions

- Assess nutritional status: nutritional history and physical examination.
  - ○ Perform an abdominal assessment:
  - ○ Subjective: anorexia, nausea, vomiting, epigastric discomfort, abdominal pain
  - ○ Objective: tender, distended abdomen, absence of bowel sounds, paralytic ileus; limitation of diaphragmatic excursion
- Monitor serum glucose, ketones, electrolyte levels, and arterial blood gases.
- Monitor intake, output; daily weight.

Rationales

- ○ Alterations in serum potassium and severe acidemia predispose to impaired gastric motility and abdominal discomforts and symptomatology.

- With initiation of insulin therapy, metabolism shifts from fatty acids to glucose with a resultant drop in serum glucose and ketones.

CARE PLAN FOR THE PATIENT WITH DIABETIC KETOACIDOSIS (*Continued*)

Nursing Interventions

- Initiate insulin drip and monitor response to therapy.
- Consult with nutritionist, physician, patient, and family to determine specific nutritional needs.

- Initiate teaching program regarding dietary therapy for the diabetic patient.
  - Involve patient/family in diet planning and decision-making.
    - Provide booklets and pamphlets to reinforce teaching.
    - Stress importance of regularity of diet and exercise; rest, sleep, and relaxation.
    - Encourage verbalization of feelings regarding impact of diabetes on family lifestyle and the integrity of each individual.
  - Teach the importance of, and how to document, significant data, including
    - Insulin dosage, time
    - Site of injection
    - Serum glucose: self-monitoring of blood glucose (SMBG)
    - Urinary acetone
    - Diet
    - Exercise
    - Stressors
  - Teach acute complications of diabetes (hyperglycemia, diabetes ketoacidosis, hypoglycemia)
    - Precipitating factors
    - Signs and symptoms
    - Actions to take to prevent
    - Actions to take to treat

Rationales

- Overall goals of nutritional therapy:
1. Meet the basic nutritional requirements.
2. Attain and/or maintain ideal body weight.
3. Prevent complications (e.g., hypoglycemia).
  - Therapeutic antidiabetes treatment regimen requires that diet therapy coincide with insulin and exercise regimen.

  - Self-care is an absolute requirement for successful management of diabetes. Participation in decision-making and planning increases motivation and compliance.

  - Data assist in evaluating response to therapy so that appropriate adjustments can be made as necessary.

Arterial BP = systolic/diastolic; CVP = central venous pressure; PCWP = pulmonary capillary wedge pressure; CO = cardiac output.

CARE PLAN FOR THE PATIENT WITH HYPOGLYCEMIA (HYPOGLYCEMIC SHOCK, FORMERLY INSULIN SHOCK)

Nursing Diagnoses

Nursing Diagnosis #1

Cerebral function, alteration in, related to hypoglycemia

Desired Patient Outcomes

Patient's condition will stabilize:
1. Neurologic status:
   - Mental status: oriented to person, place, date.
   - Level of consciousness: arousal and awareness intact.
   - Cranial nerve function intact.
   - Cerebellar function intact.
   - Sensorimotor function intact.
   - Deep tendon reflexes brisk.
2. Vital signs:
   - Arterial BP within 10 mmHg of patient's baseline.
   - Heart rate: >60, <100 beats/min.
   - Cardiac rhythm: regular sinus.
   - Respirations: <25–30 breaths/min.
   - Breathing pattern: eupnea.
3. Serum glucose: Stable at 70–110 mg/100 mL.

Nursing Interventions

- Implement patient care to stabilize glucose metabolism.
  - Establish baseline neurologic function: neuroglycopenia.
    - Mental status: changes in level of consciousness, disorientation, confusion; headache, lightheadedness, visual disturbances, irritability, lethargy; inappropriate behavior, convulsions, paralysis, coma
    - Cranial nerve function
    - Cerebellar function
    - Sensory/motor function: paresthesias, hemiparesis, paralysis, seizures, convulsions
    - Deep tendon reflexes
  - Establish baseline adrenergic function: vital signs—BP, heart rate, pulses, respiration, temperature.

  - Administer 50 mL of 50% dextrose in water intravenously as prescribed.
    - If venous access not available, administer glucagon 1 mg intramuscularly.
    - Infusion of 10% dextrose should be initiated to maintain serum glucose levels from 100–200 mg/100 mL, and until the patient can safely ingest oral intake.
  - Monitor all vital signs and ECG throughout acute phase.
  - Carefully monitor serum glucose levels.

Rationales

- Primary energy substrate for the brain is glucose. Serum glucose levels <55 mg/100 mL can produce alterations in cerebral functions; appropriate and timely treatment is necessary to avert permanent neurologic damage.

  - Appropriate cranial nerve and cerebellar functions reflect an intact brainstem.

- Adrenergic stimulation is a compensatory reaction by the body in response to hypoglycemia; it is largely responsible for symptomatology that occurs early in the course of hypoglycemia.
- Draw blood sample prior to administration of glucose for retrospective diagnosis.
- A rapid and dramatic response (1–5 min) should be expected upon glucose administration; if coma persists in spite of therapy, suspect cerebral edema.
- Establish that protective reflexes—gag, swallowing, cough—are intact before offering food/drink for oral consumption, to prevent aspiration.
- Assists in evaluating response to therapy.

Nursing Diagnoses

Nursing Diagnosis #2

Injury, potential for: seizures, related to altered neuronal cellular metabolism associated with hypoglycemia.

Nursing Interventions

- Implement measures to protect patient from potential injury associated with seizure activity and neuroglycopenia.
  - Identify patient at risk of developing seizures.

Desired Patient Outcomes

Patient will remain seizure-free and without injury.

Rationales

- Precautions can be taken to avert seizure activity and to protect the patient from injury.

CARE PLAN FOR THE PATIENT WITH HYPOGLYCEMIA (HYPOGLYCEMIC SHOCK, FORMERLY INSULIN SHOCK) (*Continued*)

Nursing Interventions	Rationales
○ Assess for seizure activity: 　□ Patient's activity at time of seizure 　□ Precipitating event 　□ Description of onset and progression 　□ Note any changes in pupil size and reactivity; urinary or bowel incontinence 　□ Duration of apneic periods if generalized seizure 　□ Duration of seizure activity 　□ Patient's behavior after seizure ○ Institute seizure precautions: 　□ Side rails padded and kept in up position 　□ Bed placed in low position if possible 　□ Oral airway at bedside 　□ Suction equipment available for emergency care 　□ Available oxygen source 　□ Removal of potentially harmful objects from bedside	○ An alteration in the level of consciousness may occur from a variety of circumstances. Careful assessment and description of seizure activity may be helpful in diagnosing and treating the underlying problem.

Nursing Diagnoses	Desired Patient Outcomes
Nursing Diagnosis #3 Knowledge deficit regarding underlying disease and overall therapeutic regimen: nutritional/insulin or hypoglycemic therapy/exercise *Nursing Diagnosis #4* Health maintenance, alteration in	Patient will be able to: 1. Relate hypoglycemia with level of health desired. 2. Specify major underlying principles regarding therapeutic regimen: diet, insulin or oral hypoglycemics, and exercise. 3. Explain why it is necessary to carry a rapid-acting sugar source and usefulness of wearing a Medic-Alert tag. 4. State the early signs and symptoms of hypoglycemia and actions to be taken. 5. Demonstrate self-care activities: monitoring blood/urine; self-medication.

Nursing Interventions	Rationales
• Determine the presence of knowledge deficit regarding overall treatment regimen and diet in particular. • Initiate teaching program about diet therapy with emphasis on self-care. 　○ Patient/family should become familiar with signs of hypoglycemia and institute treatment immediately on their appearance. • Assess patient/family knowledge regarding disease syndrome and its essential long-term therapy. 　○ Assess readiness to learn. • Implement teaching program on self-care healthcare practices.	 • Knowledge of overall therapeutic regimen will facilitate self-care and health management; complications will be minimized. 　○ Patient should verbalize the need to carry a rapid-acting sugar source on his or her person at all times; a Medic-Alert bracelet or wallet card is important to have at all times. • Understanding of underlying disease processes assists patient and family to cope with, and to adjust to, the limitations imposed by the illness.

Nursing Diagnoses	Desired Patient Outcomes
Nursing Diagnosis #5 Noncompliance: denial.	Patient will be able to: 1. Admit he/she has diabetes mellitus or a hypoglycemic disorder. 2. Ask pertinent questions regarding care. 3. Actively plan necessary changes in lifestyle to include self-care of underlying illness. 4. Verbalize need for continued and regular follow-up care. 5. Report on available resources within the family and community setting.

CARE PLAN FOR THE PATIENT WITH HYPOGLYCEMIA (HYPOGLYCEMIC SHOCK, FORMERLY INSULIN SHOCK) (*Continued*)

Nursing Interventions

- Assess patient's attitude regarding chronic illness.
- Allow patient and family to verbalize fears and concerns about underlying disease.

- Encourage patient to make decisions regarding care.
  - Have patient/family explain the significance of continued follow-up care.

Rationales

- Fostering a positive attitude helps to ensure compliance.
- Verbalization assists in identifying misconceptions and unwarranted fears; patient and family attitudes regarding the health state desired can be ascertained.
- When patient feels in control, he/she may readily assume responsibility for self-care.

U N I T   S E V E N

Gastrointestinal System

C H A P T E R   4 2

Anatomy and Physiology of the Gastrointestinal System

Linda Cole

CHAPTER OUTLINE

Gastrointestinal Tract: Basic
  Considerations
- Microstructure of the
  Gastrointestinal Tract
- Gastrointestinal Functions
- Circulatory and Lymphatic
  Distribution of Digestive
  Organs
- Control of Gastrointestinal
  Functions

Functional Anatomy of the Upper
  Gastrointestinal Tract
- Structural Components and Their
  Functions
Functional Anatomy of the Lower
  Gastrointestinal Tract
- Structural Components and Their
  Functions
Accessory Organs of Digestion
- Liver
- Pancreas
References

LEARNING OBJECTIVES

After completing this chapter, you should be able to:

1. Describe the structure of the gastrointestinal tract.
2. Identify the mechanisms underlying gastrointestinal motility and its functional
   significance.
3. Describe the mechanisms underlying digestion, absorption, and assimilation of
   digested foodstuffs.
4. Define the neural and hormonal control and regulation of gastrointestinal
   functions.
5. Describe the functional anatomy of the upper and lower gastrointestinal tract.
6. Differentiate digestive and absorptive pathways for the major nutrients.
7. Describe the structure of the liver and exocrine pancreas.
8. List the major functions of the liver and exocrine pancreas.

The major processes by which the gastrointestinal system functions to prepare nutrients for use by cells include digestion and absorption. Digestion is the preparation of ingested foods for use by the body and involves a number of physiologic activities, including chewing (mastication), swallowing (deglutition), gastrointestinal mobility, and secretion of various enzymes and hormones. Absorption involves the actual movement of digestive nutrients, vitamins, and minerals from the gastrointestinal tract into the bloodstream. The blood then transports these substances throughout the body, making them available to the cells for their metabolic activities.

GASTROINTESTINAL TRACT: BASIC CONSIDERATIONS

The gastrointestinal tract consists of a tube that extends from the mouth to the anus and includes the oropharynx, esophagus, stomach, and small and large intestines (Fig. 42–1). Each part of this tube is adapted for specific functions. In the mouth, chewing effectively breaks up large food particles and mixes these chewed particles with salivary secretions. The esophagus acts as a conduit of food from the oral cavity to the stomach; the stomach and colon act as storage chambers for food and end-products of digestion,

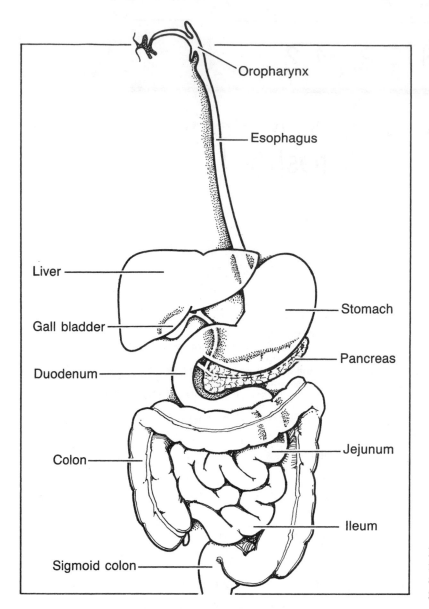

Oropharynx

Esophagus

Liver

Stomach

Gall bladder

Pancreas

Duodenum

Jejunum

Colon

Ileum

Sigmoid colon

FIGURE 42–1. The digestive system, including the gastrointestinal tract and accessory organs, pancreas, liver, and gallbladder.

respectively. The stomach and the entire small intestine are involved in the actual processes of digestion and absorption. The colon also functions in a limited but highly significant absorptive capacity.

The salivary glands, pancreas, liver, and gallbladder are accessory organs of the gastrointestinal system. They empty their secretions directly into the gastrointestinal tract at specific points.

Microstructure of the Gastrointestinal Tract

The overall microstructure of the gastrointestinal tract consists of four distinct layers of tissues. Proceeding from the lumen outward, they include the mucosa, submucosa, muscularis externa (circular and longitudinal smooth muscle layers), and the serosa. Structural modifications of these layers occur in different parts

of the gastrointestinal tract, depending on the underlying function (e.g., transfer, digestion, absorption, or storage).

Mucosa

The mucosa consists of the innermost lining of the epithelial cells and a mucosal layer (lamina propria) containing loose connective tissue and a fine network of elastic fibers for distensibility and structural support. Blood vessels contained within the lamina propria nourish the epithelial layer and serve as channels for water-soluble substances absorbed by the epithelial cells.

Submucosa

The submucosa consists of areolar connective tissue, elastic fibers, blood vessels that receive absorbed nutrients from the intestinal tract, and a network of nerve fibers called Meissner's plexus.

Muscularis Externa

The muscularis externa consists of circular and longitudinal smooth muscle layers. These layers occur throughout the gastrointestinal tract and facilitate gastrointestinal motility, which is a critical element of the digestive process. The stomach muscularis externa comprises three muscle layers, an outer longitudinal layer, a middle circular layer, and an inner oblique layer, making it differ from that found elsewhere in the gastrointestinal tract. This unique muscular arrangement facilitates the mixing, churning functions of the stomach, where semisolid food from the oral cavity is reduced to a fluid mass.

Serosa

The serosa is the outermost surface of the gastrointestinal tract. Its function is to anchor the gastrointestinal tract to surrounding tissues/organs by loose connective tissue.

Gastrointestinal Functions

Motility

Optimal digestion, absorption, and distribution of nutrients by the gastrointestinal tract require coordinated motor activity that facilitates an orderly intraluminal propulsion of ingested food at a rate that ensures maximal mixing of food with digestive secretions. Striated muscle is found within the pharynx, the upper one third of the esophagus, the upper esophageal sphincter, and the anal sphincter, giving voluntary control over these areas. The remainder of the gastrointestinal tract is composed of smooth muscle layers, which provide the basis for well-coordinated gastrointestinal motility.

Characteristically, the smooth muscle is arranged in two layers: an inner, thick circular layer and a thinner, outer longitudinal layer. Fundamental to smooth muscle cells is the presence of gap junctions, or nexi, between these cells to provide a low-resistance pathway for the movement of ions, thus assisting conduction of electrical impulses from cell to cell. These nexi are particularly seen in circular smooth muscle cells. The electrical and contractile properties of gastrointestinal smooth muscle yield three motility patterns: rhythmic segmentation, peristalsis, and tonic contractions.[1]

Rhythmic Segmentation. Rhythmic segmentation is attributed largely to the activity of the circular muscle layer. Distention of the intestinal wall caused by the food within it causes localized contractions to occur at intervals along the gastrointestinal tract, lasting for several seconds. As these contractions wane, similar rings of contractions appear in the previously inactive intervening segments. Occurring at a rate of 7 to 12 times per minute, these actions promote the progressive mixing of solid and semisolid food particles with digestive secretions.

Peristalsis. Peristalsis consists of waves of circular smooth muscle contractions responsible for the bulk of forward movement on gastrointestinal contents within the tract. Peristaltic waves also function to spread out the semifluid mass of partly digested food along the intestinal tract to increase the surface area of the gut to which it is exposed. This activity may also help to avoid areas of unusual hypertonicity and hypotonicity that might result in unexpected fluid shifts.

Tonic Contractions. Tonic contractions of sphincters alternating with their intermittent relaxation serve to regulate movement of intraluminal contents. The term "sphincter" is applied to specialized areas of muscle occurring at strategic points along the gastrointestinal tract. With the exception of the upper esophageal and external anal sphincters, which are voluntary muscle tissue, all other sphincters consist of smooth muscle fibers. These sphincters function to regulate movement of digestive contents between adjacent gastrointestinal sections.

Digestive and Absorptive Processes

Intestinal digestion and absorption are the physiologic processes by which essential foods, water, vitamins, minerals, and other substances are taken into the body and made available to cells for their metabolic activities.

An integral part of cellular metabolism is the biosynthesis of large molecules from more simple molecules, such as proteins from amino acids or polysaccharides from simple sugars, glucose, and fructose. Such metabolic activities require energy in the form of adenosine triphosphate (ATP), in addition to the basic building blocks.

Digestion is the process by which ingested foods are broken down into compounds small enough for absorption. Absorption involves the transfer of the end-products of digestion from the intestinal lumen into the blood and lymph circulation for uptake and use by the cells.

Digestion. The chemical basis of the digestive process is hydrolysis, which simply means the addition of a molecule of water to the substance undergoing digestion. The three major foodstuffs—carbohydrates, fats, and proteins—are derived from combinations of their building blocks (namely monosaccharides, fatty acids and glycerol, and amino acids, respectively) by the process of water removal known as condensation. Thus two monosaccharides, such as glucose and fructose, will combine to form the disaccharide, sucrose.

It follows, therefore, that if water is removed to produce these large molecules, then all that is necessary to break them down into simpler forms is the addition of water. As Guyton suggests, the chemistry of digestion is simple because in every case the same basic process of hydrolysis is involved.[2] The only difference involves the specificity of enzymes essential to the digestion of each food type.

Absorption. Once food is broken down by the various digestive enzymes, the end-products must be transported from the intestinal lumen into the blood and eventually metabolized by the cells. The route of absorption is determined by the characteristics of the substances, including molecular size, charge, and if present, the relative aqueous and lipid solubilities.

Mechanisms of Absorption. The basic processes involved in the absorption of nutrients from the gastrointestinal tract are diffusion and active transport. Diffusion is the passive process of movement of molecules through a membrane. Two subprocesses of diffusion are simple diffusion and facilitated diffusion.

Simple Diffusion. Simple diffusion involves the movement of molecules or ions through a membrane either directly through the lipid bilayer and/or by way of protein channels within the membrane. The rate of simple diffusion depends on molecular size, net charge on the molecule, concentration gradient across the membrane, lipid solubility, the total cross-sectional surface area for diffusion to occur, and the diffusion distance. Water molecules, for example, diffuse easily into membranes through the lipid bilayer and the protein channels, because of their small size. In contrast, hydrogen (H^+) ions and electrolytes, which, though very small in size, are repulsed by the charged ion's interaction with the positive and negative charges within the membrane. Consequently, transport of these ions occurs predominantly through protein channels.

Facilitated Diffusion. Facilitated diffusion, also referred to as carrier-mediated diffusion, requires a specific carrier protein to assist movement of the molecule across the membrane. Larger water-soluble molecules, for example, are unable to cross the membrane by simple diffusion and are obliged to use an alternative pathway involving carrier proteins within the membrane. These carriers facilitate the diffusion of these substances through the lipid portion of the membrane in which they would otherwise be insoluble.

As with simple diffusion, facilitated diffusion of molecules occurs in accordance with their concentration gradients. These processes differ in that facilitated diffusion depends on a fixed number of carrier sites, thus limiting the rate of diffusion. Once these sites become fully occupied with specific molecules, further diffusion is limited.

Active Transport. No substances can diffuse passively against either a concentration gradient or an electrical gradient. To move molecules through these gradients, energy is required. This process is termed active transport. Active transport differs from diffusion in that it can move substances against an electrochemical gradient with the expenditure of energy. Sodium and potassium movement across the cell membrane is an example of a primary active transport process in which the energy that fuels the process is derived from ATP.

Intestinal Absorption of Water. Water absorption from the gastrointestinal tract deserves special mention because up to 10 liters of water daily are normally transported from the gastrointestinal tract into the blood. Much of this water is absorbed in conjunction with osmotic pressure gradients created by electrolyte secretion, for example, the active transport of sodium.

Circulatory and Lymphatic Distribution of Digestive Organs

Perfusion of digestive organs plays an important role in that the processes of digestion and absorption involve the transport of large volumes of solute and fluids between the gastrointestinal tract and the blood. Three major arteries perfuse the digestive organs—the celiac, superior mesenteric, and inferior mesenteric arteries. The venous drainage from these organs empties directly into the portal vein that perfuses the liver.

Key features of the microcirculation of the digestive organs, which facilitate movement of large amounts of fluid, nutrients, and electrolytes between the blood and mucosal epithelial cells, include (1) the extensive surface area available for absorption and secretion, (2) the presence of fenestrated-type capillaries (i.e., characterized by having a large pore area for exchange of water and solutes), and (3) an increased permeability to smaller-sized molecules, while remaining relatively impermeable to macromolecules.

About 1 to 2 liters of lymph entering the thoracic duct every 24 hours are derived from the gastrointestinal tract. Lymph is the major pathway for fat transport into the systemic circulation.

Control of Gastrointestinal Functions

Innervation

The gastrointestinal tract is extensively innervated by the sympathetic and parasympathetic divisions of the autonomic nervous system (extrinsic innervation) and by a network of ganglia and nerve fibers located within the walls (intrinsic innervation). Additionally, motor fibers from the voluntary division of the peripheral nervous system control the skeletal muscles of the oropharynx; of the upper one third of the esophagus, including the upper esophageal sphincter; and of the external anal sphincter. This accounts for the voluntary control of such activities as chewing, initiation of swallowing, and defecation.

Gastrointestinal Hormones

Scattered throughout the gastrointestinal mucosa are cells that synthesize and secrete hormones. These hormones regulate important physiologic functions of the gastrointestinal tract. Cholecystokinin (CCK), for example, is synthesized and secreted from mucosal cells in the small intestine in response to ingestion of dietary fat. CCK reaches the gallbladder by way of the blood and stimulates it to contract and empty its bile contents into the duodenum. The presence of bile within the gut facilitates fat digestion.

Other major gastrointestinal hormones include gastrin, which is structurally similar to CCK but exerts its major influence on parietal cells of the stomach, and secretin, which stimulates pancreatic bicarbonate secretion. It is now recognized that the principal physiologic stimuli for release of gastrointestinal hormones are the carbohydrates, fats, and proteins in the gastrointestinal tract. As food is digested, blood levels fluctuate in accordance with the needs.

FUNCTIONAL ANATOMY OF THE UPPER GASTROINTESTINAL TRACT

Structural Components and Their Functions

Oral Cavity

Initiation of the digestive process begins with the oral ingestion of food. The activities of the cheeks, gums, teeth, palate, and tongue are coordinated primarily to prepare food for swallowing and transport to the stomach by the esophagus. The tongue, by virtue of its ability to change shape rapidly and extensively, plays a key role in various digestive activities.

Salivary Glands

The salivary glands include the parotid, sublingual, and submandibular glands and numerous small buccal glands widely scattered throughout the submucosal lining of the oral cavity. The salivary secretions produced and secreted by these glands are important to hygiene, comfort, and normal digestion. Mucin, secreted largely by the sublingual and submandibular glands, reduces frictional interaction between ingested food and the oral and esophageal mucosa and assist in chewing and swallowing. The enzyme ptyalin, secreted largely by the parotid gland, initiates carbohydrate digestion by converting much of the starch digested to the disaccharide form.

Saliva has the highest potassium level of any digestive juice. Clinically, it may be necessary to provide supplemental potassium therapy to patients with draining neck or facial fistulas who may be unable to eat.

The salivary glands are innervated by the autonomic nervous system. Parasympathetic stimulation promotes a copious secretion of watery saliva; sympathetic innervation causes a decreased secretion of a thick saliva. Atropine, an anticholinergic agent, reduces salivation greatly.

Pharynx

The pharynx consists of three sections—the oropharynx, nasopharynx, and laryngeal pharynx—all of which participate in swallowing.

Esophagus

Motility. The primary function of the esophagus is to transfer ingested solids and liquids from the pharynx to the stomach. Each end of the esophagus is guarded by sphincters. The cricopharyngeal muscle forms the upper esophageal sphincter and consists of skeletal striated muscle fibers. Its contraction relaxes the esophageal opening, allowing the bolus to enter the esophagus, while its relaxation facilitates peristaltic movement. Peristalsis is largely regulated by impulses from the vagus nerve.

The lower esophageal sphincter, while not anatomically distinct, nevertheless functions to prevent reflux of gastric contents into the esophagus. The normally alkaline environment within the esophagus is unable to tolerate highly acidic gastric secretions.

Secretions. The esophagus does not have any digestive or absorptive functions. Glands within the lamina propria and the submucosa secrete mucus, which serves to lubricate the food bolus as it passes into the stomach.

Stomach

The stomach is an expanded portion of the gastrointestinal tract that functions to store food and to process it in a preliminary manner to assist its transfer into the duodenum. The stomach initiates some definitive digestive processes that alter the foodstuffs chemically in preparation for further digestion and absorption in the small intestine. Although the absorptive function of the stomach is limited, some water and lipid-soluble substances are absorbed at this level of the gastrointestinal tract. The major role of the stomach is to regulate the rate at which the chyme is delivered to the duodenum.

The anatomic divisions of the stomach include the fundus, cardia, corpus (body), and the pylorus area. The pylorus area may be further divided into the pyloric antrum and pyloric canal (Fig. 42–2). The innermost surface throughout the entire stomach is formed into longitudinal folds, or rugae. These function to increase surface area for digestion and absorption, to enhance expansion/distention, and to provide friction to the movement of food, assisting the mechanical activities of food breakdown in the stomach.

The stomach is guarded at its two ends by sphincters: the lower esophageal sphincter at the upper end and the pyloric sphincter at the lower (Fig. 42–2). These two sphincters function to prevent retrograde reflux of digestive contents into the esophagus and stomach, respectively.

Gastric Motility. Gastric motility facilitates the mechanical functions of the stomach. These include

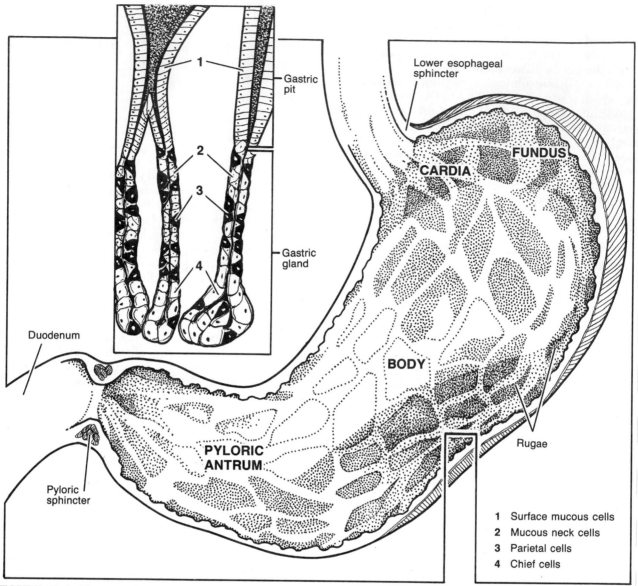

FIGURE 42–2. Macroscopic and microscopic anatomy of stomach. Grossly depicted are the major areas of the stomach, including the fundus, cardia, body, and pylorus; rugae occur throughout the inner lining of the stomach; the entrance to and exit from the stomach are guarded by the lower esophageal and pyloric sphincters, respectively. Microscopically, the gastric gland is depicted, and the major cell types included therein are identified.

the expansion and distention of the stomach to accommodate large volumes of ingested foods, the contraction of the gastric musculature to break down foodstuffs and mix them with gastric juices that initiate the digestive process, and the organized propulsion of the partially digested gastric contents into the duodenum. The upper part of the stomach temporarily stores the ingested semisolid food mass for a time following meals, while in the more distal areas of the stomach, the semisolid mass is reduced mechanically and chemically into chyme, which is the soft fluid consistency necessary for transport into the duodenum.

The unique motility characteristics of the stomach are a result of the arrangement of its three muscle layers in the muscularis externa: the outer longitudi-

nal, middle externa, and inner oblique layers. The circular layer is the most prominent and strongest of the three layers. It is found throughout the wall of the stomach and is intimately involved in forming the muscular ring that makes up the pyloric sphincter.

Regulation of Gastric Motility. Regulation of gastric motility involves neural and hormonal influences, including intrinsic signals from the stomach and the duodenum. These factors ensure that foodstuffs have been properly processed for delivery to the duodenum and that chyme is propelled into the duodenum only when it can be accommodated by it. Otherwise, gastric emptying is prohibited.

Hormonal Influences. The hormone gastrin, secreted by G cells in the antrum, influences gastric motility in several ways. Gastrin promotes a receptive relaxation of the stomach, which assists movement of ingested food into the stomach. It strongly influences gastric emptying by causing increased antral motility while relaxing the pylorus. Gastrin also prevents reflux of gastric contents into the esophagus during peak gastric mixing.

Duodenal influences on gastric motility are concerned primarily with duodenal distention and the physical and chemical consistency of the chyme itself. Feedback signals from a distended duodenum depress gastric emptying and ensure that chyme enters the duodenum at a rate that can be processed by the small intestine.

Chyme that is too acidic, is hyperosmolar, or has a high fat content upon entering the duodenum will initiate the enterogastric reflex, which inhibits both gastric acid secretion and gastric emptying. The enterogastric reflex in response to hypertonic fluids is especially important to prevent rapid flow of such fluids through the intestinal tract, thus preventing fluid and electrolyte imbalances.

Hormonal inhibition of gastric emptying includes the effect of CCK, which is released from the mucosa in the jejunum in response to fatty substances entering the duodenum. This hormone blocks the effect of gastrin. Secretin, secreted by cells in the duodenum in response to the presence of acidic chyme, also has a slowing effect on gastric motility.

Gastric Secretion. The epithelium of the gastric mucosa is concerned chiefly with the secretory and digestive processes of the stomach, and its distinctive structure is correlated with these functions. The mucosal surface is lined with mucus-secreting, simple columnar epithelium, occurring within numerous involutions and convolutions known as gastric pits. The gastric pits function to increase surface areas and give rise to the gastric glands that house the various secretory cells of the stomach.

Distinct Cell Types. Histologically, each major anatomic region of the stomach contains distinctive cell types that elaborate the gastric secretions. In the cardia, mucous neck cells secrete mucus, which serves to further moisten the foodstuffs entering the stomach and to protect the gastric mucosa from the highly acidic pH (pH 1 to 3). The pyloric antral region contains cells similar in both structure and function to the

mucous neck cells. In addition, the antrum contains numerous endocrine cells, the G cells, which secrete the hormone gastrin.

Two cell types characteristically found in the body of the stomach are parietal and chief cells. The parietal cells occur in the midportion of the gastric glands and secrete hydrochloric acid and intrinsic factor. Intrinsic factor is thought to combine with vitamin B_{12}, assisting its absorption in the ileum. A lack of intrinsic factor results in pernicious anemia, a condition that may occur after gastrectomy or in atrophic gastritis unless parenteral vitamin B_{12} supplement is provided.

Chief cells occur in the lower third of the gastric glands and secrete pepsinogen, the precursor to the enzyme pepsin. Pepsinogen is converted to the active enzyme pepsin, which is necessary for initiating protein digestion, in the presence of hydrochloric acid. When gastric contents are transported into the duodenum, pepsin activity ceases as the acidity of gastric contents is neutralized by alkaline pancreatic and duodenal secretions.

Control Mechanisms. Regulation of the digestive events in the stomach involves both nervous and hormonal mediation and can be subdivided into the cephalic, gastric, and intestinal phases. The cephalic phase, which is largely neurogenic, includes the secretory responses to sensory stimuli at the level of the cerebral cortex and/or appetite center. Sympathetic innervation of the stomach provides the mechanism whereby psychologic and emotional factors influence gastric secretions.

The gastric phase is so named because stimuli occur in the stomach itself and are of two types: mechanical and chemical. Distention, caused by the entrance of the food bolus into the stomach, provides the most significant mechanical stimulus. Chemical stimuli include the contents of ingested foods, alcohol ingestion, or the presence of an alkaline pH.

Both mechanical and chemical stimuli evoke gastric secretion by contact with pyloric antral cells, resulting in the secretion of gastrin. Although some vagal stimulation occurs, the gastric phase is considered primarily hormonal in nature because gastrin release is the primary stimulus for gastric secretion. Table 42–1 summarizes the major actions of gastrin in promoting digestion.

TABLE 42–1
Gastrin: Summary of Hormonal Actions

Stomach	Duodenum	Pancreas	Liver
↑ HCl secretion	↑ Intestinal motility	↑ Bicarbonate secretion	↑ Hepatic bile flow
↑ Pepsinogen/pepsin	↑ Bicarbonate secretion (Brunner's glands)	↑ Pancreatic enzyme secretion	
↑ "Receptive relaxation"			
↑ Lower esophageal tone	↓ Secretin secretion	↑ Insulin secretion	
↑ Pylorus sphincter tone	↓ CCK secretion		
↑ Gastric motility			
↑ Intrinsic factor secretion			

The intestinal phase of gastric secretion regulation is mainly inhibitory. This hormonal response causes a reduction in gastric secretion as chyme enters the duodenum.

Neural mediation does occur by the myenteric plexus and autonomic nerve fibers in response to distention of the small intestine. Stretch or increased tension in the intestinal wall initiates the enterogastric reflex, which inhibits gastric secretion and gastric emptying.

FUNCTIONAL ANATOMY OF THE LOWER GASTROINTESTINAL TRACT

Structural Components and Their Functions

Small Intestine

The bulk of digestion and absorption of essentially all major foodstuffs takes place in the small intestine. Its major divisions, based on structural and functional differences, include the duodenum, the jejunum, and the ileum. The pyloric sphincter separates the stomach from the duodenum. It allows entry of chyme into the duodenum and prevents retrograde reflux of duodenal contents into the stomach. The ileocecal valve occurs at the junction of the ileum with the cecum and allows exit of digested foodstuffs into the colon, while preventing reflux of colonic contents back into the small intestine.

The free surfaces of organs in the abdominal cavity are covered by peritoneum (lesser and greater omentum), which protects the abdominal contents and provides support for abdominal viscera. The mesentery is a fold of peritoneum that functions to suspend and support the small intestine and provides a rich blood and lymphatic supply to the jejunum and ileum. The manner in which it suspends the intestine allows for considerable motility of the bowel, which accentuates mixing actions and peristalsis.

Intestinal Motility. Intestinal motility of the small intestine is essential to the digestive and absorptive processes. Not only is it necessary for chyme to be moved through the gastrointestinal tract, but it must be thoroughly mixed so that all portions of it may be exposed to digestive enzymes and absorptive surfaces. Mixing and propulsive contractions characterize motility of the small intestine.

Characteristically, intestinal peristalsis is increased after a meal. This increase in intestinal activity is mediated by the gastroenteric reflex in response to gastric distention. Peristaltic waves within the ileum intensify, and this, accompanied by relaxation of the ileocecal valve, enables chyme to be emptied into the colon.

Control of Intestinal Motility. Control of intestinal motility involves a combination of neural and hormonal factors. Intrinsic innervation occurs throughout the intestinal tract so that activity in the upper gastrointestinal tract can affect that in the more distal areas. Parasympathetic (extrinsic) innervation increases muscle tone and stimulates intestinal motility; muscle tone decreases with sympathetic innervation to the point of blocking chyme movement through the gastrointestinal tract with a strong sympathetic effect.

Hormonal Influence. Gastrin, secreted by G cells in the stomach antrum, stimulates intestinal motility and promotes digestion. CCK, secreted in response to fat in the duodenum by jejunal endocrine cells, inhibits gastric motility. In addition, CCK stimulates contraction of gallbladder smooth muscle. Fat digestion and absorption are facilitated by CCK through limitation of gastric emptying and, thus, the volume of chyme in the small intestine, and through enhancement of bile secretion. The hormone secretin exerts a mild inhibitory effect on motility throughout most of the gastrointestinal tract.

Secretion. Digestive and absorptive functions of the intestinal tract are related to its unique structure. The duodenum is a critical segment because it is anatomically situated to receive the connecting ducts of the liver, gallbladder, and pancreas (Fig. 42–3). Endocrine cells within the duodenum and jejunum secrete hormones that aid digestion and absorption. The

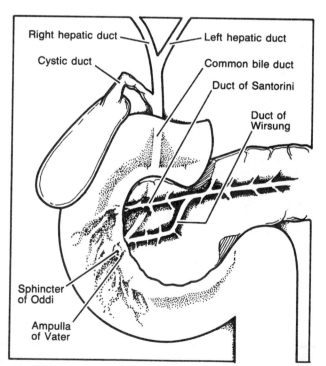

FIGURE 42–3. Depiction of structural relationships of biliary system, pancreas, and duodenum. The right and left hepatic ducts join to form the common bile duct, which eventually drains bile into the intestinal lumen (duodenum). Bile not used for digestion drains by way of the cystic duct into the gallbladder, where it is stored. Pancreatic secretions drain by way of the ducts of Wirsung and Santonni into the duodenum. The sphincter of Oddi guards the opening of the common bile duct as it enters the intestinal lumen.

ileum has enhanced absorptive capacities, including the absorption of nutrients, bile salts, and vitamin B_{12}.

Microstructure. The mucosal layer composing the luminal surface of the small intestine is structured to provide a large surface area for digestive and absorptive activities. It consists of three anatomic modifications called the plicae circulares: fingerlike projections called villi, depressions called crypts, and microvilli. The plicae circulares are permanent structures involving both the mucosal and submucosal layers and are found predominantly in the distal duodenum and proximal jejunum.

The intestinal villi are minute, fingerlike projections of mucosa covering the entire surface of the mucosa. The villus is considered to be the main structural and functional unit of the small intestine. There may be as many as 25 million villi throughout the small intestine, most numerous in the duodenum and proximal jejunum. In addition to the villous surface projections, the mucosal surface area is further increased by introverted layers of mucosa that form the crypts. The microvilli are projections of the luminal surface of absorptive cells. The combination of villi, crypts, and microvilli enhances total intestinal surface area by as much as 600-fold.

Digestion-Absorption. Upon arrival in the duodenum, chyme is mixed with a combination of intestinal secretions, including a viscous mucus, alkaline secretions, digestive enzymes, and bile.

Carbohydrate. Carbohydrate digestion is completed within the duodenum and jejunum by the pancreatic enzyme, amylase. The alkaline intestinal environment is conducive to amylase activity. As chyme enters the duodenum, secretin is secreted by endocrine cells, which then enhances pancreatic secretion of digestive juices with a high bicarbonate content. This hormone also stimulates Brunner's glands in the duodenum to secrete another bicarbonate-rich fluid.

The neutralization of acidic chyme protects the duodenal mucosa from the digestive action of the gastric juices and provides an appropriate pH for the pancreatic enzymes, which function best in an alkaline environment. This protective mechanism afforded by secretin is considered to be essential in preventing duodenal ulcers.

Final hydrolysis for carbohydrates takes place within the brush border of the enterocytes, which contain lactase, sucrase, and maltase. The action of these enzymes splits the appropriate disaccharide sugars into their monosaccharides. It is in their monosaccharide form that carbohydrates are absorbed into the blood. Once within the blood, these end-products of carbohydrate digestion are carried to the liver by the portal venous system.

Protein. Protein digestion is initiated in the stomach. Pepsin, secreted as pepsinogen by the chief cells within the gastric mucosa, is involved in the hydrolysis of protein. The activity of pepsin is optimal at a pH of 1 to 3. Its activity ceases when the stomach contents reach the alkalinity of the duodenum.

CCK stimulates pancreatic secretion of proteolytic enzyme precursors into the small intestine, where they are activated by enzymes located within the microvilli. The end-products of protein metabolism include free amino acids, dipeptides, and tripeptides. Absorption of peptides may constitute the predominant mechanism for intestinal assimilation of dietary protein.

Fat. Fat digestion and absorption occur in the small intestine and differ from that of carbohydrate and proteins by virtue of the size and lipid solubility of fat molecules. Triglycerides, cholesterol esters, phospholipids, and the lipid-soluble vitamins A, D, E, and K are the primary forms of dietary fat.

Hydrolysis of fats requires an initial process of emulsification. Emulsification assists fat digestion by increasing the total surface area available for the action of the pancreatic enzymes, which act only on the surface of the minute fat droplet. The presence of fat in the duodenum triggers secretion of CCK, which stimulates pancreatic secretion of lipase and other essential fat-digesting enzymes.

Absorption of the end-products of fat metabolism requires the solubilization or dissolution of these products in the aqueous phase of the intestinal contents. This is achieved by molecule aggregation in the presence of bile salts. Bile salts contain both hydrophilic (attracted to water) and lipophilic (attracted to lipids) properties. They promote molecule aggregation by positioning the lipid molecules so that their lipophilic portion faces the interior of the resultant aggregation, while the hydrophilic portion faces the aqueous phase of the intestinal contents within which it dissolves.

At the intestinal surface of the absorptive cells, fatty acids and monoglycerides leave the environment and diffuse passively across the plasma membrane into the cell. The bile salts remain within the intestine and continue to participate in the solubilization of fat. Eventually, the bile salts pass to the distal ileum, where up to 95% are absorbed.

Although some short-chain fatty acids are absorbed directly into the blood, the bulk of fatty acids and monoglycerides are resynthesized into triglycerides within the absorptive cell and packaged into complexes called chylomicrons. This new complex is thrust from the absorptive cell and passes into the intestinal villus. The chylomicrons ultimately gain access into the circulatory blood by way of the thoracic duct, which empties into the subclavian vein.

The absorptive cell also forms small lipoproteins called very low-density proteins (VLDL), which contain more cholesterol and protein than do the chylomicrons. The processes of VLDL synthesis and release are similar to those of the chylomicrons. The very low-density lipoproteins may be a major route of transport of dietary cholesterol into the blood.

Vitamins. Absorption of vitamins can be considered on the basis of their solubility properties. The fat-soluble vitamins are assimilated in much the same way as are fats. They are incorporated into the chylomicrons for transport into the villi, eventually reaching the systemic circulation. Any disorder causing a malabsorption of fat will likewise alter absorption of fat-soluble vitamins.

Absorption of water-soluble vitamins is less well defined but largely occurs within the duodenum and jejunum. Absorption of vitamin B_{12} occurs largely in the distal ileum and requires intrinsic factor secreted by the gastric parietal cells.

Water and Electrolyte Absorption. As much as 10 liters of fluid enters the gastrointestinal tract daily, with reabsorption of all but 200 to 300 mL, which is excreted in the feces. Movement of water through the intestinal mucosa occurs by passive diffusion that follows osmotic or hydrostatic pressure gradients. If the chyme is hypertonic, transport of water occurs from the blood into the intestinal tract; if the chyme is hypotonic, movement of the water occurs in the opposite direction. An osmotic equilibrium is established within the proximal intestine, and the chyme remains isosmotic with the blood during its transit through the gastrointestinal tract.

Factors that contribute to the driving force for water absorption include the permeability of intestinal mucosal cells to the movement of water and the osmotic gradients associated with active transport of electrolytes and solutes. Because water diffuses rapidly in both directions across the intestinal wall in response to changes in osmotic pressure gradients, the gastrointestinal tract has a tremendous capacity to move large volumes of water into and out of the intestine. This capacity can affect other organ systems. For example, movement of fluid out of the blood and into the intestinal tract in response to a hypertonic load may compromise cardiovascular dynamics by significantly reducing blood volume. Hypotension may rapidly occur. Alterations in electrolyte transport occur in the presence of intestinal obstruction. The resulting disruption in osmotic pressure gradients may predispose to retention and pooling of fluid in the gut, causing marked distention of the intestinal wall, which results in disruption of blood flow and then ischemia of visceral organs.[3]

Electrolytes and Trace Metals. Absorption of electrolytes and trace metals occurs by passive diffusion and active transport mechanisms. Active transport of an electrolyte creates an electrochemical gradient, which aids the passive diffusion of another electrolyte. Active transport of sodium, for example, facilitates chloride absorption by simple, passive diffusion. Other mechanisms may be involved. The active and selective absorption of calcium requires the presence of vitamin D and the influence of parathyroid hormone. In general, the amount of absorption of any one electrolyte or trace metal is related ultimately to the body's needs. Table 42–2 lists the absorption sites of the nutrients.

Control Mechanisms. Regulation of intestinal digestive secretions follows a similar pattern to that described for gastric secretion. The cephalic phase of intestinal digestion is mediated largely by neuronal pathways. Responses to sensory stimuli are generated within the cerebral cortical and subcortical levels and carried by the vagus nerve directly to stimulate the

TABLE 42–2
Gastrointestinal Absorption Sites of Major Nutrients

Duodenum-Jejunum	Ileum	Colon
Water	Water	Water
Electrolytes:		
Sodium, potassium	Chloride	Potassium
Chloride,		
bicarbonate		
Calcium (requires	Bile salts (95%	
vitamin D)	reabsorbed)	
Folic acid	Vitamin B_{12} (requires	
Water-soluble vitamins:	intrinsic factor)	
Thiamine, niacin,		
ascorbic acid		
Fat-soluble vitamins:		
(A, D, E, K)		
Simple sugars:		
Glucose, fructose		
Galactose		
Amino acids, small		
peptides		
Triglycerides, fatty		
acids		

pancreas to secrete digestive juices. Much overlap exists between gastric and intestinal phases, but the predominant control is hormonal, as reflected by the actions of gastrin, secretin, and cholecystokinin.

Large Intestine–Colon

The divisions of the colon include the cecum, ascending colon, hepatic flexure, transverse colon, splenic flexure, descending colon, sigmoid, rectum, and anus. The ileocecal valve separates the ileum of the small intestine from the proximal colon (Fig. 42–4). Internal and external anal sphincters guard the distal end of the colon and play an important role in defecation.

The most important function of the colon is water and electrolyte absorption. Of the ½ to 1 liter of water received daily, the colon absorbs 80% to 90%. This is a significant factor in reducing intestinal contents from a semifluid to a semisolid mass. If the amount of fluid within the colon exceeds its absorptive capacity of 2 liters or if inflammation and infection exist, diarrhea may develop, with an ensuing loss of both water and electrolytes. Because water and electrolyte losses can be significant, a predisposition to dehydration, electrolyte imbalances, and acid-base disturbances exists.

Intestinal Motility. As with the more proximal gastrointestinal tract, large intestine motility is characterized by mixing and propulsive movements. Mixing movements are very similar to the segmentation movements that occur in the small intestine. Combined contractions of longitudinal smooth muscle strips and the circular muscle layer cause different portions of the colon to bulge outward into sacs or segments, called haustrations. Such movements have a kneading and churning effect on the intestinal contents, which serves to mix fully and mold the stool as it travels anal-

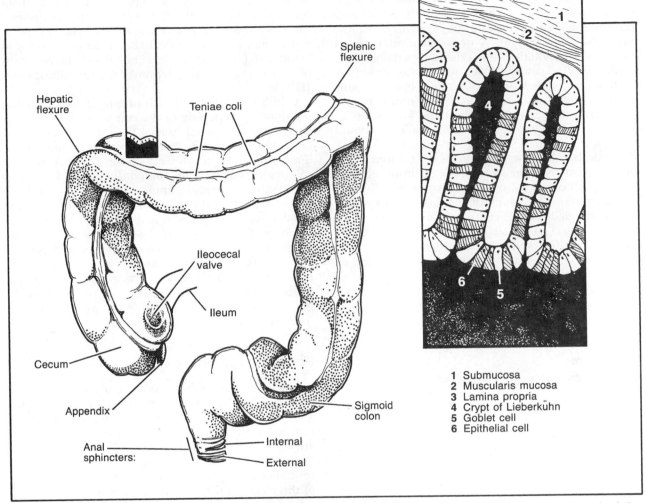

FIGURE 42–4. Macroscopic and microscopic anatomy of the large intestine. Its major divisions are depicted on the left, as are the ileocecal valve and anal sphincters. Microscopic structures are depicted on the right, including the crypts of Lieberkühn and specific cells contained therein. In contrast to the small intestine, the predominant cells lining the colon are goblet cells, which secrete mucus. The epithelial cells are fewer in number, and they contain no enzymes.

ward. The uncoordinated manner in which these movements occur in various parts of the colon serves to slow down intestinal movements, providing more time for absorption to occur.

Peristaltic waves of the type seen in the small intestine probably occur rarely in the large intestine. Most of the propulsive force is generated by the haustrations, which have some net forward movement. The movement is very slow, taking as much as 10 to 12 hours for the chyme arriving at the ileocecal valve to move into the transverse colon.

Propulsion of chyme over the distal half of the colon occurs by mass movement. These strong peristaltic movements may occur only a few times each day, most often during the hour after eating. They can move the colonic contents en masse over long distances. When feces are forced into the rectum from their storage depot in the sigmoid colon, the urge for defecation is experienced.

Secretions. Secretions of the large intestine are scant, with no digestive function. The epithelial cells lining the crypts are fewer in number than in the small intestine and contain no enzymes. The predominant cells lining the colon are goblet cells that secrete mucus. In the large intestine, mucus has several functions. It acts as a lubricant and protects the intestinal mucosa from injury or excoriation as the forming stool moves toward the rectum. It provides a viscous medium that helps to hold fecal matter together in a semisolid mass. In combination with a rich bicarbonate supply, mucus protects the mucosal wall from any acids that may be formed from bacterial activity within the feces. In the presence of inflammation, secretion of mucus may be increased greatly, causing a loss of protein in the stool.

The large intestine contains a flourishing bacterial flora, which makes a distinct contribution to body physiology. Vitamin K, essential for blood coagulation, is synthesized by bacteria within the intestinal flora. Any alteration in or destruction of the intestinal bacterial flora may cause a vitamin K deficiency. While a small amount of vitamin K does occur in ingested foods, it is not enough to meet the body's daily needs.

Malabsorption disorders can also lead to vitamin K deficiency, and deficiency of other fat-soluble vitamins as well. Folic acid and some of the B vitamins are also derived from bacterial metabolism and are subject to deficiency states when there is an alteration in bowel function.

Colonic bacteria are involved in continuous petrification activity that serves to break down undigested and/or unabsorbed substances. This process of petrification accounts for much of the gas present within the gut on a daily basis. Production of ammonia from the petrifiation of blood in the gut is a significant consideration in cirrhosis of the liver.

Other functions of the colon include excretion of heavy metals such as silver, zinc, and mercury and of unabsorbed substances like calcium and phosphate. The sigmoid portion of the colon acts as a storage chamber for feces until such time as defecation occurs.

ACCESSORY ORGANS OF DIGESTION

Liver

The liver, the largest gland in the body, is involved intricately in numerous and complex biochemical functions essential in maintaining the life processes of the body in an equilibrated state.

The functional unit of the liver is the liver lobule. Classically, the liver lobule is described as roughly hexagonal in shape and composed of rows or plates of hepatic cells called hepatocytes. These hepatocytes are arranged radially around the central vein, which drains the lobule with the blood, emptying into the hepatic veins and, thence, into the vena cava. The hepatocytes make up 70% to 80% of the total mass of the liver. The hepatocyte is the only cell in the liver responsible for many of the metabolic processes, both anabolic and catabolic, essential for life. Its close anatomic approximation to both biliary and sinusoidal vascular systems enables the hepatocyte to carry out many of its sophisticated metabolic functions. Major functions of the hepatocyte include carbohydrate, protein, fat, and drug metabolism; detoxification of endogenous and exogenous substances; hormonal metabolism; vitamin and mineral use and storage; storage of iron, copper, and calcium; bile synthesis; bilirubin metabolism; synthesis of coagulation factors; and blood filtration and storage.

Hepatic Biliary System

The bile duct drains bile produced by the hepatocytes. Bile flows through a system of tiny bile capillaries between the plates of the hepatocytes, moving from the central areas of the liver lobule to the periphery. All bile eventually empties into the main hepatic duct, which merges with the cystic bile duct from the gallbladder to form the common bile duct. The common bile duct enters the duodenum at the ampulla of Vater (Fig. 42–3).

Oddi's sphincter, a sheath of muscle fibers, guards the duodenal opening of the common bile duct as it enters the intestinal tract. The sphincter relaxes largely in response to the presence of chyme in the duodenum and to the effects of CCK. A relaxed sphincter, coupled with the contractions of the gallbladder, which is also stimulated by CCK, enables the appropriate amount of bile to be emptied into the duodenum, where it is available for the digestion of fat. When the sphincter is closed, bile is directed into the gallbladder, where it is concentrated and stored.

Bile salts aid digestion and absorption of fats by their role in emulsification and aggregation formation processes. Without the presence of bile salts in the gastrointestinal tract, up to 40% to 50% of the ingested fat would be lost in the stool.

Blood and Lymphatic Circulation

The liver enjoys a dual blood supply, accounting for up to 25% of the cardiac output each minute. Of this amount, approximately 1 liter is supplied by the portal vein while the remainder is supplied by the hepatic artery.

An important feature of the portal system is the low resistance to hepatic blood flow. Hydrostatic pressure of the blood in the portal system as it enters the liver is about 9 mmHg, while the pressure within the hepatic vein leaving the liver is about zero.

The portal vein, formed by the union of the splenic and superior mesenteric veins, carries nutrient-rich venous blood from the capillaries of the gastrointestinal tract into the liver. The uniqueness of the portal system is that the portal vein is interposed between two capillary beds: the gastrointestinal tract and the liver lobules.

Bilirubin Metabolism

In addition to secretory functions, the hepatocytes are also involved in the excretion of substances formed elsewhere in the body. One of the more important of these is bilirubin, a major metabolic end-product of the degradation of hemoglobin. As aging red blood cells are sequestered within cells of the reticuloendothelial system, hemoglobin is catabolized, with the heme portion converted first to biliverdin and subsequently to unconjugated bilirubin. In this reaction, the iron is liberated and enters the circulation by transferrin, a carrier molecule. It may be used in the production of new red blood cells or stored in a variety of tissues until needed.

Unconjugated bilirubin circulates in the blood

tightly bound to albumin. The concentration of conjugated bilirubin occurring in the blood is reflected by the indirect serum bilirubin level. Excessive hemolysis of red blood cells is often associated with elevated indirect serum bilirubin levels.

Eventually, unconjugated bilirubin is transported to the liver, where it is metabolized in a series of reactions to its conjugated form. The significance of the conjugation reactions is that the previously water-insoluble, unconjugated bilirubin is rendered water-soluble and capable of being excreted by the liver into the bile. Once delivered to the small intestine in the bile, bilirubin conjugates are acted on by the normal bacterial flora to form urobilinogen.

Urobilinogen is highly soluble, and some of it is reabsorbed into the bloodstream, where it is subsequently excreted in the urine as urobilin. A small amount of conjugated bilirubin does remain in the blood, and this is reflected by the direct serum bilirubin levels. The remaining urobilinogen found in the intestine is oxidized to stercobilin and excreted in the feces. Urobilin and stercobilin give the urine and stool their characteristic colors. Elevated direct serum bilirubin levels reflect either parenchymal liver disease or biliary obstruction.

Hyperbilirubinemia and Jaundice States

Jaundice refers to the yellowish tint or staining of the skin, sclerae, deeper tissues, and body secretions. It is usually due to the presence of large quantities of bilirubin in the extracellular fluid. The normal serum bilirubin concentration, including direct and indirect forms, averages 0.5 mg/100 mL. Jaundice may begin to appear at serum bilirubin levels greater than 1.5 to 2.0 mg/100 mL.

Four pathophysiologic mechanisms may lead to hyperbilirubinemia and jaundice. They include bilirubin overproduction, decreased uptake by hepatic cells, impairment of hepatic conjugation reactions, and decreased excretion of bilirubin into bile. The resulting disease states include hemolytic jaundice, hepatocellular jaundice, and obstructive or cholestatic jaundice.

Pancreas

Next to the liver, the pancreas is considered to be the largest gland connected with the gastrointestinal tract. It is located in the retroperitoneal space deep within the epigastrium at the level of the first and second lumbar vertebrae. The pancreas has no defined external capsule as does the liver; therefore, infections and other pancreatic disorders may not be well contained. Disease of surrounding tissue may directly involve the pancreas, causing inadvertent release of digestive enzymes into adjacent tissue, with consequent abscess formation.

Microstructure

Endocrine. The pancreas functions as both an endocrine and exocrine gland, with these functions carried out by different groups of cells. The endocrine pancreas consists of isolated clumps of cells called the islets of Langerhans, which are scattered throughout the organ. Functionally, these islet cells are unrelated to the exocrine pancreas; rather, as true endocrine glands, they secrete the hormones insulin and glucagon directly into the bloodstream. These hormones, which are essential for metabolism of fats, proteins, and carbohydrates, are discussed in detail in Chapter 41.

Exocrine. The exocrine pancreas consists of groups or clusters of cells called acini, which are responsible for the production of pancreatic digestive juices. Small ducts from these acini empty their contents directly into the main pancreatic duct, which extends throughout the length of the pancreas. Within the ampulla of Vater, it joins the common bile duct before entering the duodenum (see Fig. 42–3). The exocrine pancreatic glands produce approximately 1200 to 1500 mL of digestive juices each day.

Secretion

Pancreatic digestive juices contain enzymes for digesting carbohydrates, proteins, and fats. Trypsin is a pivotal enzyme because once it is activated it becomes responsible for activating other enzymes. The pancreas also contains specific enzymes for metabolism of nucleic acids.

Most proteolytic enzymes synthesized within the pancreatic acinar cells are secreted by the acini in an inactive form. They become activated only after they reach the alkaline environment of the duodenum. Perhaps this is nature's way of protecting the pancreas from self-digestion.

Two other important components of pancreatic juice are bicarbonate and water. This highly alkaline juice serves to neutralize the acidic chyme emptied into the duodenum from the stomach and thus protects the sensitive mucosal cells of the small intestine from the digestive action of gastric juice. Secretion of bicarbonate ions is essential to provide an appropriate alkaline pH for the catalytic activity of pancreatic enzymes.

Regulation of Pancreatic Secretion. Regulation of pancreatic secretion involves both neuronal and hormonal mechanisms. During the cephalic and gastric phases of stomach digestion, the pancreas receives parasympathetic stimulation by the vagus nerve to increase enzyme secretion. There is little concomitant secretion of water and electrolytes to facilitate movement of enzymes through the pancreatic ductal system. Therefore, pancreatic enzymes are stored in the acini during these phases of digestion.

After chyme enters the duodenum during the intestinal phase, pancreatic secretion becomes copious, mainly in response to hormonal innvervation by secretin and CCK. Secretion of secretin by intestinal mucosal cells in response to the presence of chyme in the duodenum triggers massive secretions of bicarbonate by the pancreas to neutralize the acidic chyme. Secretin also stimulates Brunner's glands within the duodenum to secrete a bicarbonate-rich fluid, thus further neutralizing the acidity.

CCK directly stimulates the pancreas to secrete digestive enzymes. This hormone also stimulates the musculature of the gallbladder to contract, propelling bile into the duodenum for the digestion of fats.

Gastrin also stimulates pancreatic secretion, but its effect is quantitatively less important than that of CCK.

REFERENCES

1. Granger, DN, Barrowman, J, and Kvietys, P: Clinical Gastrointestinal Physiology. WB Saunders, Philadelphia, 1985, p 17.
2. Guyton, AC: Textbook of Medical Physiology, ed 8. WB Saunders, Philadelphia, 1991, p 726.
3. Bryant, G: When the bowel is blocked. RN, 52(1), 58–67, 1992.

CHAPTER 43

Gastrointestinal Assessment

Linda Cole

CHAPTER OUTLINE

LEARNING OBJECTIVES

After completing this chapter, you should be able to:

1. Identify essential aspects of the clinical history as they pertain to gastrointestinal function and dysfunction.
2. List the cardinal symptoms of gastrointestinal dysfunction.
3. Elicit assessment data based on knowledge of functional health patterns.
4. Describe the four abdominal quadrants and the anatomic relationships of organs within each quadrant.
5. List the four techniques used in the physical examination of the abdomen in the order in which they are performed.
6. Define essential information to be obtained on inspection of the mouth and pharynx, neck, and abdomen.
7. Describe the techniques of auscultation of the abdomen and expected findings.
8. State the significance of percussion in determining size and location of abdominal organs, distribution of air in the gastrointestinal tract, and presence of solid or fluid-filled masses and ascites.
9. Describe key aspects of the palpatory examination of the gastrointestinal system.
10. Outline key diagnostic tests and studies for gastrointestinal disorders.
11. Identify key nursing considerations in the diagnostic workup for gastrointestinal disorders.

The critical care nurse assesses the patient with altered gastrointestinal function by collecting data from history-taking and astute observation, physical assessment, laboratory tests, and pertinent diagnostic studies. The assessment and diagnosis of gastrointestinal disorders can be perplexing and formidable tasks. It may be difficult to differentiate systemic manifestations of underlying gastrointestinal disease from systemic disease involving other organ systems that is complicated by gastrointestinal dysfunction. Such cardinal gastrointestinal signs and symptoms as anorexia, nausea, vomiting, diarrhea, or abdominal pain may be indicative of a number of markedly different etiologies (e.g., severe metabolic derangement, fluid and electrolyte imbalance, renal disease, cancer, and adverse drug reactions).

Often, what may appear to be an innocuous gastrointestinal symptom (e.g., heartburn or indigestion) may, in fact, signal the occurrence of a serious underlying pathology in another organ system (e.g., myocardial infarction). It is important to determine whether assessment data are related to the established diagnosis or reflect a change in the patient's condition. Establishing baseline assessment data is invaluable in differential diagnosis. It is essential to always consider the patient as a whole and to evaluate clinical manifestations and responses in terms of total body function.

CLINICAL HISTORY

In initiating the patient's gastrointestinal assessment, it is essential to consider the patient's immediate status and whether the patient is experiencing distress. The extent and comprehensiveness of the initial history and examination should be modified accordingly.

Components of the Clinical History

Chief Complaint

In eliciting the patient's history, it is necessary to establish the chief compliant (i.e., the single, most important reason the patient has sought health care at this time). The critical care nurse should ask about the duration of the complaint and what interventions have been tried and their success. Obtaining as much information as possible about the presenting symptoms will permit comprehensive medical and nursing care.

History of Present Illness

The history of the present illness serves to elaborate the details surrounding the chief complaint and should include its *onset*, the *course since onset*, and the *current status*. Use of the SLIDT tool (see Table 35–1) assists in eliciting specific information about the nature of the gastrointestinal complaint, which may otherwise seem vague. It is important to determine the *S*everity of the symptom; its *L*ocation (radiation); the *I*nfluencing factors, which include the precipitating event, factors that aggravate the complaint, and associated factors and events, including the setting within which it occurs; the *D*uration of the complaint and its timing in terms of events or patterns surrounding the patient; and the *T*ype or quality of the complaint, or its descriptive characteristics (e.g., bright red hematemesis).

Cardinal Symptoms of Gastrointestinal Dysfunction. The cardinal symptoms of gastrointestinal dysfunction include anorexia, nausea, vomiting, dysphagia, diarrhea, constipation, and abdominal and referred pain.

Anorexia. Anorexia is a nonspecific symptom associated with many acute and chronic illnesses. It is defined as an aversion to eating despite an existing hunger (i.e., craving for food). It is significant clinically in that it predisposes to malnutrition. Regulation of food intake occurs primarily within the hypothalamus and involves the interaction of the neural networks within the feeding (hunger) center and the satiety center. ("Satiety" is defined as the lack of desire to eat that occurs after food is ingested.)

Factors that stimulate the feeding center (increase the appetite) include hypoglycemia and the hormone insulin; factors that stimulate the satiety center (decrease the appetite) include hyperglycemia, gastric distention, and the hormone cholecystokinin. Emotional factors also affect appetite and eating patterns, probably by neuronal connections between the cerebral cortex, subcortical areas, and the hypothalamus.

Nausea. Nausea is the conscious awareness of the need to vomit. It occurs largely as a premonition of vomiting and is associated with distention and/or irritation of the gastrointestinal tract, motion sickness (brainstem neuronal activity), and/or altered autonomic system activity. It is usually accompanied by hypersalivation and a reduction in gastric tone with a concomitant increase in intestinal muscle tone. Diaphoresis, skin pallor, and hypotension may also occur.

Vomiting. Vomiting is the forceful expulsion of gastric and duodenal contents. Strong contractions of abdominal muscles increase intra-abdominal pressure, forcing the diaphragm and cardia portion of the stomach up into the thorax, which increases intrathoracic pressure. When intrathoracic pressure overcomes the resistance of the upper esophageal sphincter, gastrointestinal contents are expelled. Vomiting is thought to be controlled by a vomiting, or emetic, center within the brainstem (medulla), which is closely approximated, both anatomically and functionally, to respiratory and vasomotor medullary centers. The major stimulus for vomiting is gastric and duodenal overdistention and/or excessive irritation.

Clinically, major sequelae of severe vomiting include dehydration and malnutrition associated with reduced fluid and food intake, metabolic alkalemia and hypokalemia associated with loss of gastric secretions, and an increased risk of aspiration in patients who have compromised protective reflexes (e.g., gag and swallowing reflexes).

Documentation of the vomiting episode should include precipitating or associated factors, whether it was projectile, and the amount and characteristics of the vomitus (e.g., bright red blood, coffee-grounds, bilious, or feculent).

Dysphagia. Dysphagia is difficulty in swallowing. In assessing this symptom, it is important to appreciate that its clinical presentation will vary according to the anatomic location of the difficulty. Disturbances at the level of the oropharynx may result in nasal regurgitation, choking, aspiration, and the inability to move the bolus into the esophagus. Disruptions at the level of the esophagus may involve ineffective, diminished, or absent peristalsis, preventing movement of the bolus through the esophagus. The patient may complain of retrosternal fullness on swallowing. Dysfunction of the lower esophageal sphincter (achalasia) may disrupt esophageal motility, prevent movement of the bolus into the stomach, and result in the accumulation of food within the esophagus.

It is important to pinpoint where the discomfort occurs during swallowing and whether it occurs with liquids, solid foods, or both. The swallowing center in the medulla coordinates the highly complex and intricate nature of the events involved in swallowing. Most muscles involved in swallowing are innervated by the vagus nerve. Dysphagia is often a consequence of neurologic or neuromuscular disease.

Diarrhea. Diarrhea refers to an increase in frequency and fluidity of the stool. The stool should be assessed for the presence of abnormal constituents, such as blood (inflammation), mucus (irritable colon), or greasy, bulky, or foul-smelling stools (fat malabsorption). Influencing factors, such as pattern of bowel movements (e.g., constipation alternating with diarrhea); ingestion of foods that seem to precipitate the diarrhea; and associated symptoms, including abdominal cramping, pain, weakness, diaphoresis, and vomiting, should all be evaluated.

The significance of diarrhea is the impact it can have on fluid and electrolyte balance. Of the nearly 10 liters of fluid that enter the gastrointestinal tract daily, 2 to 3 liters come from exogenous sources (ingested foods and fluids), and the remainder, from endogenous sources (salivary, gastric, pancreatic, biliary, and intestinal secretions). All but a few hundred milliliters of this amount is reabsorbed. Active absorption of electrolytes (especially sodium) plays a significant role in establishing electrochemical, osmotic, and hydrostatic gradients, thus facilitating absorption of nutrients, vitamins, minerals, and water.

Any abnormal increase in gastrointestinal secretions and/or alteration in the absorptive efficiency of the gastrointestinal tract can predispose to diarrhea. *Secretory* diarrhea is characterized by a net loss of sodium and bicarbonate ions, and the 24-hour stool volume may exceed 1 liter. *Osmotic* diarrhea occurs when the absorptive capabilities of the gastrointestinal tract are exceeded. It is characterized primarily by potassium and water depletion. The 24-hour stool volume is usually less than 1 liter. Frequently, a combination of both types of diarrhea occurs. Hypermotility and excessive peristalsis throughout the gastrointestinal tract are often implicated as underlying causes.

Constipation. Constipation refers to a decrease in the usual frequency of bowel evacuation. It may imply excessive straining during a bowel movement and is usually characterized by a small volume of stone-hard stools. It is important to determine the patient's bowel routine before illness and how it may have changed. The acuity or chronicity of the constipation should be established. Chronic constipation is associated with a low-residue diet. It is a frequent occurrence in patients with a longstanding pattern of voluntary inhibition of the defecation reflex.

Documentation should include the size, volume, character, and frequency of bowel movements; the presence or absence of flatulence; the presence of associated symptoms such as abdominal cramps or pain and abdominal distention; and whether there has been any recent change in the patient's lifestyle.

Abdominal and Referred Pain. Pain is a factor in the clinical presentation of a variety of disorders. A thorough, comprehensive history is often helpful in differential diagnosis. Use of the SLIDT tool (see Table 35–1) is especially helpful when assessing pain.

Referred Pain. Referred pain is pain in a part of the body that is distant to the tissues in which the pain originates. Commonly, such pain is initiated in a visceral organ and referred to an area of the body surface. Branches of visceral pain fibers synapse in the spinal cord, with afferent neurons transmitting pain impulses from the skin surface along dermatomic distribution. The resulting pain sensation may be perceived as originating in the skin rather than in a viscus. Referred pain may be the only symptom of underlying visceral pathophysiology. It is usually described as sharp and is well localized.

Visceral Pain. Visceral pain originates in abdominal or thoracic viscera. It differs from body surface pain in that it is poorly localized. It is frequently described as a dull, gnawing, or cramping sensation. Widespread stimulation of visceral pain nerve endings, as occurs with ischemia, stretching, or overdistention of the gut, or with smooth muscle spasm of a hollow vicus (e.g., intestines, gallbladder, bile ducts, or ureter), can precipitate severe pain. Injury caused by chemical stimuli (e.g., leakage of proteolytic enzymes into surrounding tissues, as occurs in acute pancreatitis or perforated peptic ulcer) can cause extremely severe abdominal pain. Cramping pain may assume a rhythmic pattern, waxing and waning in severity in conjunction with relaxation.

Parietal Pain. Parietal pain is associated with inflammation of underlying viscera with extension to parietal membranes lining body cavities (e.g., pleura, pericardium, and peritoneum). These linings and adjacent tissues are richly endowed with pain nerve endings, which, when irritated, can cause very sharp pain (e.g., pleuritis and peritonitis).

Functional Health Patterns

Assessment of the patient's functional health patterns (see Appendix C) is essential to elicit information of significance to nursing diagnosis and treatment, including patient/family education and discharge planning.

Nutritional and Metabolic. The nutritional and metabolic assessment may reveal changes in the patient's general state of health. It involves asking questions such as the following:

- Has there been a weight gain or loss? How much, over how long a period of time?
- Is there loss of stamina? Does the patient tire easily?
- Is there an increased susceptibility to infection? Is wound healing sluggish?
- Has the patient experienced any intolerance to foods? Are there complaints of heartburn, indigestion, or belching associated with eating? An intolerance to foods high in fat content, for example, may suggest a gallbladder problem.
- Is there evidence of the pain-food-relief pattern commonly associated with peptic ulcer disease?
- Does the patient take antacid medications? Why, how much, how frequently, for how long? Are the symptoms relieved?

The nutritional assessment should help to determine patient/family attitudes regarding diet and eating and how they view themselves in terms of nutrition and weight. Questions such as the following can guide the assessment:

- What is a typical daily diet?
- Who prepares the food?
- Do socioeconomic constraints affect daily food intake?
- Are there emotional or psychological considerations that may affect the patient's nutritional status (e.g., depression)?

Elimination Pattern. Assessment of the patient's bowel function, diet, and bowel habits is essential. Such information may provide the initial, often subtle clues to the presence of underlying gastrointestinal pathophysiology. Important questions to be asked include the following:

- Have there been recent changes in the patient's bowel elimination pattern?
- Is excessive straining required to move the bowels?
- Are the bowel movements painful?
- Are there changes in the frequency and consistency of bowel movement—diarrhea? constipation?
- What is the appearance of the stool—bloody (hematochezia), tarry, fatty (steatorrhea), mucoid, clay-colored, foul-smelling?
- Is there use of enemas, laxatives, other medications? What medications—over-the-counter or prescribed? Reason for taking medications?
- Does the patient have hemorrhoids? For how long?

Assessment of urine elimination should include frequency, amount, and color. A dark or orange urine suggests hyperbilirubinemia.

Health Perceptions and Health Management. It is important to determine what the patient's overall status has been and whether there have been any significant changes in health or lifestyle. Patient/family attitudes about health and the optimal level of health desired can be helpful in planning care. The patient's use of medications—prescriptions and over-the-counter—should be ascertained. Data about use of such drugs as aspirin, steroids, and anticoagulants are critical in the patient who has gastrointestinal bleeding. Use of antibiotics can alter the intestinal bacterial flora, disrupting bowel motility and digestive and absorptive functions of the gastrointestinal tract. Alcohol or other drug use and abuse may provide a clue to underlying hepatic insufficiency.

Past Medical History

Ascertain if the patient has had any previous gastrointestinal surgery—dental surgery, cholecystectomy, gastric or intestinal resection, appendectomy, hemorrhoidectomy, other? Have there been previous hospitalizations—why, when? Is there a past history of any of the following: peptic ulcer disease (gastric, duodenal, or stress), gastrointestinal hemorrhage, hepatic disease (cirrhosis, hepatitis, blood transfusions, or jaundice), abdominal trauma, pancreatitis, renal disease (renal colic or lithiasis—calculi formation), or diabetes mellitus?[1]

Family History

It is important to determine if a predisposition exists for any disease that may be transmitted genetically or along ethnic lines. Examples of such diseases include peptic ulcer disease, ulcerative colitis, regional enteritis (Crohn's disease), diverticulitis, gastric or colonic cancer, pernicious anemia, malabsorption syndromes, lactose intolerance, and alcoholism.

PHYSICAL EXAMINATION

Components of the Physical Examination

Components of the physical examination of the gastrointestinal assessment include an examination of the mouth and pharynx, the neck, and abdomen.

Examination of the Mouth and Pharynx

Techniques used to examine the mouth and pharynx include inspection and palpation. The face, lips,

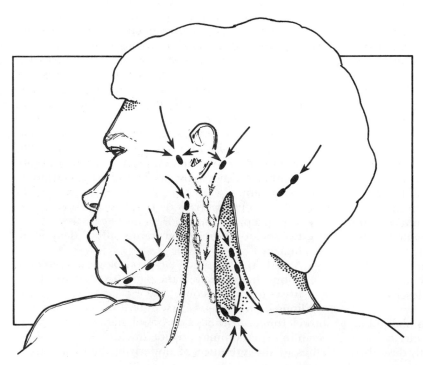

FIGURE 43–1. Lymph nodes of the head and neck. Arrows indicate regions drained by the lymph nodes.

and jaw are inspected for signs of swelling or asymmetry. While the patient opens and closes his or her mouth, the temporomandibular joint is examined for tenderness, crepitus, and limitation of movement.

The lips are inspected for any abnormal color, dryness, cracking, lumps, ulceration, or other lesions. Using a rubber glove, the nurse should inspect the inner lip, buccal membranes, and gums for color, pigmentation, inflammation (swelling and/or tenderness), excessive salivation, white patches, plaques, and ulceration. These tissues are palpated for lumps or nodules. Gums should also be examined for evidence of hypertrophy or retraction. Teeth are observed for malocclusion, dental caries, and general state of repair.

The tongue is inspected for color, moisture, unusual smoothness, abnormal movement, deviation, or paralysis (12th cranial nerve, hypoglossus). Grasping the tongue with a gauze pad enables inspection and palpation of the superior and lateral surfaces of the tongue for ulcerations or other lesions, lumps, or nodules. The floor of the mouth is inspected by asking the patient to touch the roof of the mouth with the tongue.

The pharynx can be examined by holding the tongue down with a tongue depressor and tilting the head backwards. When the patient is asked to say "ah," the uvula and soft palate should rise and remain in the midline (9th cranial nerve, or glossopharyngeus; 10th cranial nerve, or vagus). The anterior and posterior sections of the pharynx are examined for color, symmetry, inflammation, plaques, exudation, petechiae, and ulceration. Mouth odors, if unusual, should be described (e.g., sweet or fruity smell).

Examination of the Neck

Examination of the neck is performed under good lighting using inspection and palpation. The neck is inspected for symmetry, swelling, masses, and scars. Lymph nodes are systematically examined, noting size, shape, mobility, consistency, and tenderness. It is important to appreciate the regions drained by the lymph nodes (Fig. 43–1). The trachea should be inspected for any deviation from its midline position. The thyroid gland is palpated by an anterior or posterior approach, noting its size, shape, symmetry, tenderness, and the presence of any lumps or nodules.

The carotid arteries and jugular veins may be examined. The presence of jugular venous distention should be assessed with the patient in a sitting position. Auscultation may detect a thyroid or carotid bruit, or a jugular venous hum (see Chapter 13).

Examination of the Abdomen

Abdominal Quadrants. For descriptive purposes, the abdomen is usually divided into four quadrants by imaginary lines that cross at the umbilicus (Fig. 43–2).

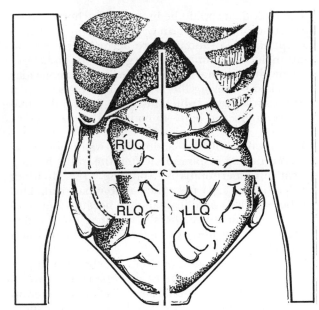

FIGURE 43–2. Abdominal quadrants: RUQ = right upper quadrant; RLQ = right lower quadrant; LUQ = left upper quadrant; LLQ = left lower quadrant.

It is important to visualize underlying organs and their structural relationships in each quadrant.

Techniques of Examination. The techniques of examination are inspection, auscultation, percussion, and palpation, *in that order.* A systematic approach ensures thoroughness. The examination should be conducted with the examiner at the patient's bedside.

To facilitate the examination, make appropriate explanations regarding the examination and help the patient relax. The patient should not have a full bladder. The supine position with a pillow under the head and knees and the arms placed at the patient's side enhances relaxation of abdominal musculature. The patient should be appropriately draped to ensure privacy, with full exposure of the abdomen. Good lighting is essential.

It is important to ask the patient to point to areas of pain or tenderness; these areas should be examined last. Throughout the abdominal examination, it is important to watch the patient's face and expression for clues to the presence of any discomfort.

Inspection. When inspecting the abdomen for pulsations or peristaltic movements, it is important to bend down so that the abdominal surface can be viewed at eye level. The nurse should visualize the underlying organs. The position of the umbilicus should be noted, and the contour of the abdomen should be observed. Normally, the abdomen should be flat; there should be no bulging of the flanks. The skin is inspected for scars, texture, color, wounds, masses, or lesions. Bluish discolorations, bruises, or petechiae should be viewed with suspicion.

Spider angiomas (i.e., small red blood vessels radiating from a central point) suggest liver disease. Veins are normally not visible or prominent. When veins are prominent, the direction of blood flow should be noted. Normally, blood flows away from the umbilicus.

The abdomen should be inspected for hernias (i.e., a protrusion of tissue or an organ through an abnormal opening). Locations where hernias are prone to occur include the umbilicus, surgical scars, and above or below the inguinal ligament. Small protrusions may be checked by having the patient strain or perform a Valsalva's maneuver, which increases intra-abdominal pressure. Palpation helps to confirm the presence of a hernia.

The motion of the abdominal wall should be observed during respiration. Often the initial finding indicative of peritonitis is "splinting" (i.e., holding the diaphragm still) to reduce abdominal pain. This may be especially significant in men because they tend to be "abdominal breathers" (i.e., they use the diaphragm to a greater extent than do women, when breathing).

Portions of the abdominal wall may be seen to pulsate at the same rate as the heart, usually reflective of pulsations of the abdominal aorta. This phenomenon is especially true of patients with thin-walled, flat abdomens. Occasionally, an abdomen distended by fluid (ascites) may also reflect pulsations. Peristalsis is not normally visible.

Auscultation. In the examination of the abdomen, auscultation precedes percussion and palpation techniques to minimize any alteration in the frequency of bowel sounds.[2] The sounds produced by the peristaltic movements of the intestine are normally of medium pitch, and best heard with the diaphragm of the stethoscope pressed lightly against the abdomen. The nurse should listen for bowel sounds in all four quadrants, noting their frequency and characteristics. The mixing and moving forward of liquid and air in the intestines produce brief bursts of gurgling, bubbling sounds, occurring at a frequency from 5 to 30 times/min. These sounds should be audible in all four quadrants. Occasionally, very active bowel sounds, or *borborygmi* (i.e., loud, prolonged gurgles of hyperperistalsis—"growling stomach"), may be heard.

Bowel sounds may be described as hypoactive or hyperactive. In the presence of a paralytic ileus, the frequency of bowel sounds may only be one per minute or less. This rate reflects abnormally slow bowel activity and is described as *hypo*active.

With increased bowel activity, as occurs in bouts of gastroenteritis, diarrhea, or partial intestinal obstruction, bowel sounds may be heard occurring every 2 to 3 seconds. These sounds are described as *hyper*active. In the case of obstruction, the character of bowel sounds also changes in that they become more high pitched than normal, taking on a tinkling quality.

It is important to listen for bruits in all four quadrants and over the midline in the epigastrium. A bruit in this area most often arises from lesions of the abdominal aorta, celiac artery, or the renal arteries. If a bruit is detected, the area should be palpated very gently so as not to injure atherosclerotic vessels. Occasionally, a cardiac murmur may be transmitted along the aorta. In this instance, it may be difficult to differentiate the murmur from the abdominal bruit.

A venous hum is a continuous sound that, when heard, may reflect an increase in collateral circulation from the portal system to the systemic venous system.

Percussion. Percussion is a useful technique for determining the size and location of organs, detecting air in the stomach and bowel, and identifying solid or fluid-filled masses, or ascites. The presence of a large amount of air (swallowed) in the stomach and intestines produces a hollow percussion note called tympany; dullness is the percussion note elicited over solid or fluid-filled masses, or ascitic fluid. Tympany usually predominates. Each of the abdominal quadrants should be percussed to ensure that tympany is present to a greater or lesser degree throughout the abdomen. If fluid has collected in the abdomen, there will be increased dullness to percussion in the flanks and shifting dullness. Dullness elicited over the suprapubic area suggests a distended bladder.

Percussion of Abdominal Organs: Liver, Spleen, and Stomach. In most adults, the liver is completely tucked up under the thoracic cage, with its superior surface under the dome of the right diaphragm and its inferior border at or above the right costal margin. The lower liver edge may normally be found to be several centimeters below the costal margin (see Fig. 43–2).

To estimate its size, the liver is percussed at the midclavicular line (MCL). The lower border of liver dullness is determined by starting at a level below the umbilicus in an area of tympany and lightly percussing upward toward the liver. The transition from a note of tympany to one of dullness marks the lower border of the liver. To determine the upper border of the liver at the MCL, lightly percuss downward from an area of lung resonance toward liver dullness. The transition from a note of resonance to dullness marks the upper border of the liver. Between its upper and lower borders at the MCL, the liver measures about 6 to 12 cm. If the liver appears enlarged, it may be necessary to outline the boundaries of liver dullness using the midsternal and right anterior axillary lines.

The presence of a right pleural effusion or consolidated lung adjacent to the liver may falsely increase the estimated size of the liver; gas in the overlying colon may produce a note of tympany in the right upper quadrant (RUQ) and may falsely decrease the estimated size of the liver.

Percussion over the left upper quadrant (LUQ) is usually performed to rule out enlargement of the spleen. The small area of splenic dullness near the left tenth rib posterior to the midaxillary line is often obscured by gastric or colonic air. A full stomach or feces-filled colon may exaggerate the area of splenic dullness.

Any increase in the size of the gastric air bubble (i.e., an increased area of tympany in the LUQ) accompanied by upper abdominal distention suggests gastric dilation.

Palpation. When eliciting the patient's clinical history, it is important to have the patient identify any area of pain. These areas are left for last in palpation to avoid producing spasm and rigidity of the abdominal wall, which would interfere with the abdominal assessment. It is important to observe the patient's expression throughout the examination.

Light Palpation. Light palpation assists in identifying muscle resistance, detecting areas of tenderness, and locating superficial organs and masses. It is performed by pressing the abdominal wall with the pads of the fingers, lightly, but firmly enough to indent the wall. No attempt should be made to press deeply. All areas of the abdomen should be palpated, comparing the resistance on one side to that on the other. Areas of tenderness should be palpated last and as gently as possible to avoid muscle guarding. If resistance is detected, determine whether it is voluntary or involuntary. An effort should be made to help the patient relax. The abdominal rectus muscle should be checked for relaxation, which occurs with expiration. If the abdominal wall remains rigid in spite of these maneuvers, it is probably involuntary. Involuntary spasm of the abdominal musculature indicates peritonitis.

Deep Palpation. Deep palpation helps delineate abdominal organs and masses and identify areas of deep pain or tenderness. The palmar surfaces of the fingers are used to explore all four quadrants. It is essential for the patient to be relaxed. Appropriate explanations regarding the examination should be made. The patient should know that deep palpation may cause some discomfort. Deep abdominal breathing may help the patient relax.

All areas of the abdomen should be examined thoroughly and systematically. If any masses are identified, it is important to note the location, size, shape, consistency, tenderness, pulsations, and mobility. If tenderness is detected, the abdomen should be checked for rebound tenderness. *Rebound tenderness* is elicited by firmly and slowly pressing into the abdominal wall, then quickly letting go. If pain is elicited during the quick release, rebound tenderness is present, indicating peritoneal inflammation.

Bimanual palpation (using two hands) can be used for deep palpation, particularly when there is obesity or muscle resistance. One hand is placed on top of the other. Pressure is applied with the outer hand, while the nurse concentrates on what the fingers of the inner hand are feeling.

Several approaches can be used in palpating the liver, spleen, kidneys, and abdominal aorta. The reader is referred to an appropriate text for a detailed discussion of the techniques. Normally, the spleen is not palpable unless it is three times its normal size. The kidneys are usually not palpable except in children or very thin adults. A blunt blow to the *costovertebral angle* is performed to elicit tenderness caused by inflammation of the kidney.

Summary of the Abdominal Assessment. To assess the abdomen thoroughly, the nurse must do the following:
1. Have a solid understanding of underlying anatomy and physiology.
2. Elicit a thorough clinical history.
3. Appreciate structural relationships of abdominal organs and their location in each quadrant.
4. Be skilled in the techniques of inspection, auscultation, percussion, and palpation.
5. Document the findings accurately and precisely.

Examination of the Rectum

The rectal examination is an essential component of the assessment of the gastrointestinal system in the adult. Omitting this part of the examination increases the risk of missing an asymptomatic carcinoma. The anus is inspected for inflammation, excoriation, hemorrhoids, fissures, and lesions. With a well-lubricated glove, the nurse should palpate the rectum for tenderness, nodules, masses, and fecal impaction. Appropriate explanations are made to the patient prior to the examination. The examination should be conducted with gentleness and a calm demeanor.

DIAGNOSTIC STUDIES

In patients with gastrointestinal disorders, the diagnosis can be elusive. Many types of studies may be employed to determine the underlying cause. These studies may include laboratory tests, radiologic studies, cytologic studies, and endoscopy procedures. In many instances, it is the nurse's responsibility to prepare patients for specific diagnostic studies. Appropriate explanations need to be made, dietary restrictions may be necessary, and bowel preparation and evacuation may be indicated. Tests may need to be scheduled so they do not conflict with one another and, thus, invalidate results.

Laboratory Tests

Blood and urine tests can be of considerable diagnostic value, especially in the presence of liver and pancreatic dysfunction, biliary disorders, and intestinal malabsorption. Serum enzyme studies assist in differential diagnosis. Each organ of the body contains its own characteristic enzymes, which function to catalyze numerous metabolic activities. In the presence of tissue injury or necrosis, these enzymes are released from the damaged tissues into the blood. Their concentrations in the blood provide inferential or confirmatory evidence of the underlying disease process.

The ability to differentiate *isoenzymes* (i.e., enzymes occurring in more than one organ and having a similar function but uniquely different structural and physical characteristics) further assists in the differential diagnosis. A list of these and other specific laboratory tests for gastrointestinal disorders is presented in Table 43–1.

Diagnostic Studies and Procedures

Other helpful diagnostic studies frequently used in gastrointestinal liver, biliary, and pancreatic disorders are listed in Table 43–2. Results of all of these diag-

TABLE 43–1
Laboratory Tests for Gastrointestinal Dysfunction

Test	Purpose	Clinical Significance
Liver Function Tests		
Biliary System		
Serum bilirubin	Measures the liver's ability to conjugate and excrete bilirubin, a product of hemoglobin degradation within the reticuloendothelial system	Hyperbilirubinemia is associated with hepatocellular disease; hemolytic jaundice, hepatic jaundice, and obstructive jaundice.
• Total	Normal level: 1.0 mg/100 mL	
○ Direct	Normal level: 0.4 mg/100 mL; reflects level of conjugated bilirubin in the blood	Increased in obstructive disease of the biliary system.
○ Indirect	Normal level: total minus direct bilirubin; measures concentration of unconjugated bilirubin in the blood	Increased in hemolytic disorders (increased erythrocyte destruction). Increased in hepatocellular disease.
Serum alkaline phosphatase	Normal levels: vary depending upon laboratory and procedure used	Increased in cholestasis (i.e., an arrest in bile flow); biliary obstruction; liver metastasis; viral, drug-induced, or chronic hepatitis.
	Enzyme most often measured to indicate bile duct obstruction	Increased in bone disease.
	Measures enzyme activity in bone and intestine, and in liver and biliary systems	Results must be evaluated in terms of complete clinical picture.
	Overall clinical picture usually sufficient for discriminative evidence of underlying pathology; can partition this enzyme into its isoenzymes if more definitive data are required for diagnosis	
Serum cholesterol	Normal levels: 120–220 mg/100 mL: measures liver metabolism and synthesis of this bile acid precursor	Increased with cholestasis resulting from biliary disease, bile duct obstruction, hepatitis, lipid disorder, and pancreatitis.
	Basic constituent of structural elements (e.g., plasma membrane) and hormones and other metabolites	Decreased levels may occur with hepatocellular damage, cirrhosis.
Urine bilirubin	Measures conjugated (water-soluble) form of bilirubin	Increased with liver disease and/or biliary obstruction; increased when levels of conjugated bilirubin are increased.
Urine bilinogen	Reflects patency of biliary ducts and the hepatocellular capacity to process and excrete bilirubin	Characteristically increased in hemolytic disorders and states of large hemoglobin turnover; increased in hepatocellular disease; absent in complete obstructive biliary disease.
Fecal urobilinogen	Reflects patency of biliary ducts, quantity of bilirubin processed.	Increased levels with hemolysis; or with soft-tissue bleeding requiring resorption and degradation of hemoglobin.
Hepatocellular Function: Serum Enzyme Studies		
Amino transferases	Stored in the liver and released when liver cells are damaged	The two enzymes SGOT and SGPT are most often associated with hepatocellular damage.
Serum glutamic oxaloacetic transaminase (SGOT)	Normal levels: 10–40 U/mL Also called aspartate aminotransferase (AST)	SGOT levels serve as an indication of the extent and severity of tissue damage. They need to be evaluated in terms of the complete clinical picture because this enzyme is also released from heart, kidneys, lungs, pancreas, and skeletal muscle.
Serum glutamic pyruvic transaminase (SGPT)	Normal levels: 6.0–36.0 U/mL Also called alanine aminotransferase (ALT)	SGPT is more specifically associated with the liver than is SGOT. It occurs in high concentrations in the liver; lesser concentrations occur in kidney, heart, and skeletal muscle. Increased SGOT and SGPT occurs in biliary obstruction, cirrhosis, acute or drug-induced hepatitis, liver metastasis, and pancreatitis.
Gamma glutamyl transpeptidase (GGT)	Active in amino acid transport Reflects enzyme activity in liver, biliary tract, epithelium, pancreas, and kidney tubules	Increased in acute liver disease, particularly that associated with chronic alcohol abuse; obstructive biliary disease; liver metastasis; acute pancreatitis. This test requires 24-hour alcohol abstention.
Lactic dehydrogenase (LDH)	Normal levels and distribution of isoenzymes: • LDH$_1$—heart, brain, RBC 18%–33% • LDH$_2$—heart, brain, RBC 28%–40% • LDH$_3$—lung, spleen, pancreas, thyroid, adrenals, kidneys, RBC 16%–30% • LDH$_4$—liver, skeletal muscle, brain, kidneys 6%–16%	This enzyme is found in nearly all cells with especially high concentration in liver, heart, brain, kidney, blood, and skeletal muscle. Isoenzymes provide more specific information about the source of LDH.

TABLE 43–1
Laboratory Tests for Gastrointestinal Dysfunction (*Continued*)

Test	Purpose	Clinical Significance
	• LDH$_5$—liver, skeletal muscle, kidneys 2%–13% Total LDH: 60 to 120 U/mL	
Hepatocellular Function: Protein Metabolism		
Serum total protein	Normal level: 6.0–8.4 gm/100 mL; reflects a quantitative measure of albumin and globulins in the blood	Longstanding hepatocellular dysfunction decreases levels of circulating serum proteins.
Albumin	Normal level: 3.5–5.0 g/100 mL; reflects capacity to synthesize protein	Hypoalbuminemia is associated with gradual progressive diseases, including cirrhosis, tumors; malnutrition; protein-wasting renal or gastrointestinal diseases; severe catabolic states such as burns; and acute and chronic infections. Hyperalbuminemia is associated with dehydration (prolonged vomiting or diarrhea) with hemoconcentration.
Globulins	Include alpha, beta, and gamma fractions; beta fraction also includes lipoproteins	Serum globulins frequently rise above normal values in chronic liver disease. Beta globulin fraction is elevated in viral hepatitis, biliary cirrhosis, and extrahepatic biliary tract obstruction.
Serum ammonia	Normal levels: 80–110 μg/100 mL Measures ability of liver to detoxify ammonia, an end-product of protein metabolism Normally metabolized to urea by hepatic cells; urea is then eliminated by kidneys	Increased in hepatic necrosis; hepatic failure accompanied by portal hypertension with its frequently occurring sequelae of esophageal varices and upper gastrointestinal bleeding, and hepatic encephalopathy; and cirrhosis.
Serum urea		Serum urea levels are reduced in severe liver disease. Impaired sodium and water metabolism, characteristics of hepatocellular and circulatory disorders of the liver, produce dilutional changes reflected by reduced serum urea levels. Severe liver disease reduces the capacity of the liver to degrade proteins, further reducing serum urea levels. Degradation of protein by intestinal bacteria generates ammonia, which readily enters the portal circulation to be normally converted to urea. In liver failure and/or portal hypertension, portal blood is diverted to collateral vessels, causing systemic ammonia levels to rise and urea levels to fall.* Elevated ammonia levels predispose patient to hepatic encephalopathy.
Prothrombin time	Normal values: <2-sec deviation from control; measures clotting time to determine activity of prothrombin and fibrinogen	Normal liver synthesizes clotting factors II (prothrombin), VII, IX, and X in the presence of adequate vitamin K (fat-soluble vitamin). Synthesis of these four factors declines with hepatocellular dysfunction or inadequate supply of vitamin K. Vitamin K is produced by the intestinal bacterial flora. It requires bile salts for absorption from the gut. Bile duct obstruction preventing bile salts from entering the duodenum may indirectly cause a reduction in vitamin K absorption. Prothrombin time is increased with vitamin K deficiency; a value >2½ times normal very likely reflects abnormal bleeding.
Other Liver Function Tests		
Serum alpha-fetoprotein (AFP)	Normal levels in nonpregnant patients: <30 ng/mL The major serum protein in early fetal life, with synthesis of large quantities through the 32nd week of gestation; thereafter synthesis declines, reaching its lowest concentrations during the first year of life	Synthesis of AFP is repressed in normal, resting hepatocytes after the first year of life, but may resume in rapidly multiplying and proliferating hepatocytes. Hepatocellular carcinoma may cause the AFP level to rise a thousand-fold or more. Lesser elevations (~500 ng/mL) may occur in active cirrhosis or in viral or toxic hepatitis. Demonstration of elevated levels of AFP may assist in the differential diagnosis of hepatomegaly, hepatocellular dysfunction, and the jaundice state.

Continued

TABLE 43–1
Laboratory Tests for Gastrointestinal Dysfunction (*Continued*)

Test	Purpose	Clinical Significance
Serum hepatitis B surface antigen	Used to screen for latent or active hepatitis B virus Normal results: negative	Highly sensitive for hepatitis B antigen (HBsAg); widely available and permits specific diagnosis of hepatitis B in mild, subclinical, or persistent cases.
Pancreatic Function Tests		
Serum amylase	Normal levels: 4–25 U/mL Measurement of pancreatic enzyme active in the digestion of starch; splits starch into smaller carbohydrate units Amylase activity in many cells, but pathologic elevations of serum amylase levels nearly always involve the pancreas; significant concentrations of amylase also in salivary gland secretions	Increased levels occur in acute pancreatitis and common bile duct obstruction. Elevations in serum amylase levels may be attributed to disruption of pancreatic secretory cells and to the absorption of extracellular enzyme from intestinal contents and ascites fluid through dilated permeable peritoneal lymphatic capillaries. Morphine and cholinergic drugs may alter serum amylase levels.
Serum lipase	Normal levels: 2 U/mL or less Measurement of pancreatic enzyme active in digestion of fats	Significant elevations occur with acute pancreatitis; carcinoma of the pancreas may produce a sustained moderate elevation. Levels may also be increased in pancreatic duct obstruction, biliary duct obstruction, and intestinal obstruction. Morphine and cholinergic drugs may alter serum lipase levels.
Secretin test	Measurement of pancreatic secretion	
Miscellaneous Tests for Gastrointestinal Disorders		
Serum glucose	Normal level: (fasting) 70–110 mg/100 mL Hyperglycemia: • Mild—120–150 mg/100 mL • Moderate—200–500 mg/100 mL • Marked: >500 mg/100 mL • Hypoglycemia: <70 mg/100 mL	Hyperglycemia reflects reduced insulin secretion by islet cells of pancreas, or a crude indication of the liver's capacity to store glycogen and mobilize glucose. Hypoglycemia may reflect excessive secretion of insulin, or it may occur in response to stress in which inadequate sugar is being consumed in proportion to the amount being metabolized. Other causes of hypoglycemia include extensive liver disease, insulin overdose, malnutrition.
Oral glucose tolerance test	Reflects metabolic response to glucose load Normal serum glucose: • 160–180 mg/100 mL in 30–60 min • Return to fasting levels within 2–3 h Normal urine glucose: negative	This test is affected by many physiologic variables with many different diagnostic interpretations.
Galactose	Reflects ability of liver to convert galactose to glycogen Normal result: negative	Absence of tolerance occurs with extrahepatic biliary obstruction or obstructive jaundice.
D-xylose test	Evaluates intestinal absorption of xylose, a pentose sugar normally passed through liver and excreted intact	Reduced levels occur in cirrhosis, regional ileitis, sprue, diverticula.
Schilling test	Helps to establish if vitamin B_{12} absorption is defective, or if intrinsic factor necessary for vitamin B_{12} absorption is deficient	Decreased absorption may occur in pernicious anemia (lack of intrinsic factor), pancreatic insufficiency, intestinal disorder.
Fecal Analysis		
Occult blood		Positive tests occur in upper gastrointestinal bleeding; gastritis, gastric carcinoma; bleeding varices; peptic ulcer disease; lower gastrointestinal causes: diverticulitis, colitis, carcinoma of colon.
Fat (lipids)	Stool analysis to quantitate fat excretion—test requires a known dietary intake and timed stool collection	Lipase deficiency, commonly associated with pancreatic disease, increases the proportion of neutral fat in stool. Steatorrhea can occur in liver and biliary tract disease, but jaundice and abnormal blood chemistries occur before steatorrhea becomes a significant diagnostic problem.

*Cohn, HO: Complications of portal hypertension. Current Hepatology 1:119–180, 1980.

TABLE 43–2
Diagnostic Studies and Procedures for Gastrointestinal Dysfunction

Test	Description	Clinical Significance/Nursing Implications
Radiography Abdominal series	A three-way view of abdomen: flat plate, erect position, decubitus position.	Useful in differentiating free air in the abdomen from that related to perforated bowel; can detect presence of bowel obstruction and ascites.
Contrast Radiography Oral cholecystography	A study of the gallbladder to detect gallstones, tumors, or inflammatory disease. A radiopaque dye is ingested, absorbed by the small intestine, removed from blood by the liver, excreted into the bile, and stored in the gallbladder.	This test should be performed prior to barium swallow; since contrast dye contains iodine, tests such as iodine uptake should be done prior to this study. • Whenever an iodine-based contrast medium is used, it is important to establish if the patient is allergic to iodine. • This test permits visualization of gallbladder and biliary system (extrahepatic); it reflects the capacity of the liver to conjugate and excrete the dye (intrahepatic). • Inability to visualize gallbladder suggests biliary duct obstruction, or an inability of the gallbladder to concentrate the dye.
Barium enema	Permits visualization of lower intestinal tract, including ileocecal junction, colon, and rectum.	This test should be performed prior to barium swallow because the slow passage of barium through the gastrointestinal tract may alter the findings. Preparation requires use of laxative and enemas; and appropriate explanation so that patient can cooperate in retaining the barium enema during the procedure. After the procedure, enemas may be required to prevent constipation associated with barium. • This study is of diagnostic value in structural changes of large intestine—diverticula, polyps, colorectal cancer—and in inflammatory disorders of the colon (ulcerative colitis).
Barium swallow (upper gastrointestinal series)	The patient swallows a thick barium sulfate mixture, and cineradiography and fluoroscopy are used to record esophageal and gastric action.	This test allows visualization of the upper gastrointestinal tract as the patient swallows • It is of diagnostic value in detecting esophageal irregularities such as polyps, tumors, diverticula and hiatal hernia; gastric pathology, including tumors; and intestinal abnormalities, such as altered motility, obstruction, masses, polyps, and diverticula.
Intravenous cholangiography	Allows direct visualization of cystic, hepatic, and common bile ducts.	This procedure can be performed before, during, and after surgery. The tests may be performed in patients unable to tolerate oral intake.
Percutaneous transhepatic cholangiography	This procedure is performed in the presence of mechanical obstruction of the biliary system causing bile ducts to be dilated. A long needle is used to inject dye directly into a dilated bile duct under fluoroscopy.	This study is used to assess biliary duct obstruction; it helps to differentiate extrahepatic from intrahepatic obstructive jaundice. • Hemorrhage and leakage of bile are potential complications requiring monitoring for 24 hours after procedure.
Angiography studies	Radiographic contrast study of the vascular system. A catheter is placed in either the superior or inferior mesenteric arteries, and dye is injected.	These studies are used to locate sites of gastrointestinal and mesenteric bleeding; they are especially helpful in defining aneurysms of the aorta. Areas of ischemia may also be determined.

Continued

TABLE 43–2
Diagnostic Studies and Procedures for Gastrointestinal Dysfunction (*Continued*)

Test	Description	Clinical Significance/Nursing Implications
Ultrasonography (Echography)	This is a noninvasive procedure wherein high-frequency sound waves are emitted from a transducer and spread throughout underlying tissues. Depending upon the density of the tissues, these sound waves bounce back (echo) and are converted by a receiver into a dot pattern. The dots reflect the location of an echo in the body.	This procedure helps to differentiate between obstructive and nonobstructive jaundice. It assists in the diagnosis of cholelithiasis and cholecystitis. • Ultrasonography of the liver can detect hematomas and metastasis. Pancreatic ultrasonography is helpful in detecting pancreatitis, pancreatic carcinoma, pseudocysts. • Ultrasonography can be used in conjunction with liver-spleen scanning to pick up "cold spots" (i.e., areas that do not pick up the radionuclide, e.g., tumors or abscesses).
Nuclear Imaging Liver/spleen scanning	An injection of a radionuclide is given to the patient, who is then positioned under a scanner that records the distribution of radioactivity in the liver and spleen.	Nuclear imaging is an efficient way to diagnose hepatocellular disease, liver metastasis, hepatomegaly, splenomegaly, and abdominal hematoma after trauma. • Local bleeding sites can also be detected using this technique.
Computed tomography (CT scan)	A computer-assisted cross-sectional x-ray that can be used with or without a contrast medium.	CT scan can detect biliary, liver, and pancreatic disorders. This study is helpful in differentiating between obstructive and nonobstructive jaundice; it can identify tumors, cysts, hematomas, and abscesses. Barium studies, when ordered, should be performed 4 days before or after CT scan.
Endoscopy Esophagogastroduodenoscopy	Procedure involves the passing of a fiberoptic endoscope through the patient's mouth, esophagus, stomach, and into the duodenum. Endoscopy enables taking photographs, obtaining biopsies and cytologic specimens, and removing polyps.	Enables visualization of luminal lining of upper gastrointestinal tract. The procedure can detect areas of inflammation, ulcerations, varices, hiatal hernia, mucosal lesions, and carcinoma. It helps to differentiate between gastric and duodenal ulcers, and between benign and malignant ulcers in conjunction with a barium swallow.
Endoscopic retrograde cholangiopancreatography (ERCP)	This procedure involves the passing of a catheter with the aid of a fiberscope into the common bile duct and pancreatic duct so that a contrast dye can be introduced and x-rays taken.	ERCP enables radiologic visualization of common bile and pancreatic ducts. The patient should be observed for possible complications after the procedure, including pancreatitis or cholangitis. This procedure is not without risks.
Colonscopy	This procedure involves insertion of a flexible fiberscope.	This procedure allows for direct visualization of the bowel; biopsy of lesions and/or excision of polyps can be performed.
Proctosigmoidoscopy	This procedure permits direct visualization of distal sigmoid colon, rectum, and anal canal.	This procedure is useful in detecting hemorrhoids, polyps, fissures, fistulas, and inflammatory, infectious, and ulcerative bowel disease.
Paracentesis (Peritoneal Tap with Lavage)		This procedure is useful to determine intra-abdominal hemorrhaging after trauma; to detect presence of pancreatitis by measurement of amylase and lipase levels in the peritoneal fluid aspirated; and to determine the presence of tumors through cytologic studies.

nostic tests, studies, and procedures must be evaluated in terms of the overall clinical presentation.

Nursing Considerations

A major nursing responsibility is to assist in preparing the patient for the diagnostic workup. Many of these tests are time-consuming, expensive, and not without risks and complications. Often, a series of tests is ordered, and these must be performed in a specific sequence to prevent one test from altering the results of another.

An understanding of the purpose of these tests and the actual procedures involved assists the nurse in better preparing the patient. Preparation begins with an assessment of the patient to determine if there are any contraindications to performing a test (e.g., an allergy to iodine in patients scheduled for tests requiring the use of a contrast medium). Many tests require dietary restriction, bowel preparations, and the administra-

tion of appropriate medications. All diagnostic procedures require that the patient have an adequate explanation of what to expect. The patient, then, will probably be more cooperative so that necessary procedures can be carried out.

Upon completion of the diagnostic workup, the nurse assists the patient and family in understanding results and their implications in terms of treatment, prognosis, and recovery. The nurse helps to reinforce and to clarify explanations made to the patient and family by the physician. The nurse supports the patient and family in the decision-making process regarding the ultimate level of health desired.

REFERENCES

1. Steel, RJC, Chung, SCS, and Leung, JWC: Practical Management of Acute GI Bleeding. Butterworth-Heinemann, Oxford, 1993, pp 8–9.
2. Jarvis, C: Pocket Companion for Physical Examination and Health Assessment. WB Saunders, Philadelphia, 1993, pp 138–139.

CHAPTER 44

Nursing Management of the Patient with Acute Upper Gastrointestinal Bleeding

Linda Cole

CHAPTER OUTLINE

Acute Upper Gastrointestinal Tract
  Bleeding
  □ Etiology and Pathophysiology
  □ Clinical Presentation
  □ Diagnosis
  □ Treatment and Management
Nursing Care of the Patient with Acute

Upper Gastrointestinal Tract Bleeding
and Hypovolemic Shock
  □ Therapeutic Goals
  □ Nursing Diagnoses, Desired Patient
    Outcomes, and Nursing
    Interventions
References

LEARNING OBJECTIVES

After completing this chapter, you should be able to:

1. Differentiate peptic ulcer disease, erosive bleeding, and esophageal/gastric
   varices in terms of etiology and pathophysiology.
2. Define classes of blood loss and consequent clinical manifestation based on the
   percentage of total blood volume lost.
3. Describe the essential aspects of the diagnostic evaluation of acute upper
   gastrointestinal (GI) hemorrhage.
4. Identify goals of emergency treatment and overall management of acute upper
   GI bleeding.
5. Describe implications for nursing care based on the nursing process:
   a. Assessment
   b. Specific nursing diagnoses
   c. Planning:
        Desired patient outcomes
        Nursing interventions and rationales.

ACUTE UPPER GASTROINTESTINAL TRACT BLEEDING

Acute upper gastrointestinal (GI) tract bleeding may be the primary reason for admission of a patient into the intensive care setting. Frequently, it occurs as a complication of a critical illness involving another organ system. Common causes of the majority of cases of upper GI bleeding include peptic ulcer disease, erosive gastritis, and variceal bleeding associated with portal hypertension.

Etiology and Pathophysiology

Peptic Ulcer Disease

Two major factors need to be considered in the pathophysiology of peptic ulcer disease. First, all areas of the GI tract exposed to gastric juice (acid pepsin) are well supplied with mucous glands. In the duodenum, added protection against the acidity of gastric juice is afforded by the alkalinity of small intestinal and pancreatic secretions. Second, the GI tract is

RESEARCH APPLICATION: RISK FACTORS FOR GASTROINTESTINAL BLEEDING IN CRITICALLY ILL PATIENTS

Cook, DJ, Fuller, HD, Guyatt, GH, Marshall, JC, Leasa, D, Hall, R, Winton, TL, Rutledge, F, Todd, T, Roy, P, Lacroix, J, Griffith, L, and Willan, A. N Engl J Med 330, 377–381, 1994.

Purpose: Stress ulceration resulting in GI bleeding is a significant complication in critically ill patients. This study was conducted to determine the incidence of clinically important GI bleeding in a group of critically ill patients. The study also identified risk factors for patients who developed clinically important GI bleeding.

Method: The study was a prospective multicenter cohort study in which potential risk factors for stress ulceration in critically ill patients were evaluated. The incidence of clinically important GI bleeding was obtained. Clinically important GI bleeding was defined as overt bleeding associated with hemodynamic compromise or blood transfusion.

Results: Clinically important bleeding occurred in 33 of 2252 patients enrolled in the study. Two independent risk factors for GI bleeding were noted: respiratory failure requiring mechanical ventilation for >48 hours (odds ratio 15.6, $P < .001$) and coagulopathy (odds ratio 4.3, $P < .001$). Mortality for the patients with clinically important bleeding was 48.5%, compared to 9.1% for all other patients.

Practice Implications: This study provides the critical care nurse with identifiable risk factors for patients who may develop stress ulceration to the point of clinically important GI bleeding. Close monitoring and assessment are needed in this high-risk group for the development of stress ulceration GI bleeding. The critical care nurse should seek medical intervention for prophylaxis against stress ulcers in this high-risk group and be prepared to intervene if GI bleeding develops.

endowed with a rich, submucosal blood supply with major arteries or branches so situated anatomically that they can be easily eroded in the presence of underlying pathology.

Disruption of the delicate balance between acidic gastric juices and the defensive mucosal barrier may result in duodenal and gastric ulceration, or peptic ulcer disease. Erosion of the peptic ulceration into a major artery or its branches is probably the most common cause of massive upper GI tract bleeding. Predominantly, the majority of these ulcers are situated in the proximal duodenum in an area called the duo-denal bulb. The proximity of the gastroduodenal and pancreaticoduodenal arteries in this area frequently results in bleeding if the ulcer erodes through the posterior wall. When a patient with a prior history of peptic ulcer has acute upper GI bleeding, the ulcer is the most probable site of bleeding.

Breakdown of the gastroduodenal mucosal barrier may be caused by a variety of factors, including stress (physiologic stress of trauma, burns, extensive surgery, or sepsis, or psychological stress),[1] ischemia, excess secretion of gastric acid, reflux of bile acids, drugs (aspirin, alcohol, caffeine, nicotine, corticosteroids, nonsteroidal anti-inflammatory drugs, phenylbutazone, and indomethacin), and helicobacter pylori infection. A back diffusion, or reflux, of hydrochloric acid (HCl) through the impaired mucosal barrier destroys mucosal cells and liberates histamine. Histamine stimulates further acid secretion and causes vasodilation of underlying blood vessels. The mucosa becomes edematous, and there is leakage of interstitial fluid into the lumen of the GI tract. Eventually, blood vessels (arterioles) are ruptured and bleeding occurs.

Erosive Gastritis

Erosive gastritis usually involves a combination of an increase in acid pepsin secretion coupled with another factor, such as drug ingestion or stress. Recent heavy alcohol consumption or a history of ingestion of salicylates, corticosteroids, indomethacin, and phenylbutazone has a direct effect on increasing acid secretions. Ingestion of such drugs may also alter the structural integrity of the mucosal layer. Trauma, burns, sepsis, and hypovolemic shock are examples of stressful situations that can predispose to GI bleeding. The consequent bleeding probably reflects ischemic cellular injury and disruption of the defensive mucosal barrier, which prevents neutralization of hydrochloric acid.

Variceal Bleeding Associated with Portal Hypertension

Esophageal variceal bleeding may result from dilation of lower esophageal venous plexi in the scenario of portal hypertension, whether associated with cirrhosis or portal venous thrombosis in the absence of cirrhosis. Variceal bleeding may also occur as a result of forceful vomiting, particularly on a full stomach, and as a result of an excess of alcohol in the system. Forceful vomiting under these circumstances can cause a traumatic tear of the lower esophageal mucosa into the submucosal layer, rupturing blood vessels in the process.

Commonly, variceal bleeding occurs in conjunction with alcoholic cirrhosis and, to a lesser extent, postnecrotic cirrhosis. Obstruction at the liver interface causes an increase in portal blood pressure, which opens up existing collateral channels. Included among these are the lower esophageal venous plexi, which soon dilate and become thin-walled veins easily eroded by reflux of the acidic gastric juices.

Bleeding from esophageal varices tends to be abrupt and frequently massive. Minor bleeding may occur for days prior to the acute episode.

Clinical Presentation

The clinical presentation of acute upper GI bleeding depends in large measure on the amount and acuity of the blood loss and the character of blood loss (i.e., whether it presents as bright red blood or coffee-ground material in vomitus [hematemesis], as bloody stool [hematochezia], or as tarry stools [melena]). Table 44–1 classifies blood loss according to the approximate amount of blood lost and the consequent clinical manifestations.

Diagnosis

In the diagnosis of acute upper GI bleeding, it is necessary to establish the site of the GI bleeding. This site will largely determine the type and sequence of various diagnostic procedures and the management of care. If blood loss has been extensive (>1200 mL), it may be necessary to stabilize the patient's cardiopulmonary function before initiating diagnostic steps. The orderly sequence of history-taking, diagnostic evaluation, and treatment frequently is adjusted to meet the emergent demands. A meticulous clinical history and physical examination, in conjunction with radiologic and endoscopic investigations, may be necessary to determine the underlying cause of the gastrointestinal bleeding.

Complete assessment of the patient's clinical status is necessary because of a variety of systemic diseases that may be associated with bleeding (e.g., aortic aneurysm, gastric carcinoma, mesenteric venous thrombosis, arterial embolic occlusion, blood dyscrasias such as leukemia, thrombocytopenic disorders, or a bleeding diathesis such as disseminated intravascular coagulation). If the patient has known heart, liver, renal, or other serious diseases, such information may be valuable in guiding medical and, if necessary, surgical decisions during the management of GI bleeding.

Clinical History

A history of known peptic ulcer or the existence of a *pain-food-relief* pattern suggests the possiblity of erosive bleeding. Epigastric pain is a cardinal symptom of peptic ulcer disease, and its assessment may be of assistance in differential diagnosis. The patient with a *duodenal* ulcer experiences epigastric pain about 2 hours after a meal and in the middle of the night. These episodes of pain are characteristically relieved by food and/or antacids, and the pain-food-relief pattern of peptic ulcer disease is established.

In the presence of a *gastric* ulcer, the patient may describe the onset of gnawing epigastric pain ½ to 1 hour after meals. Pain may or may not occur in the middle of the night, and often the pattern of *food-pain* is present, rather than pain-food-relief. Gastric cancer is often characterized by the onset of epigastric fullness or distress shortly after a meal.

A history of cirrhosis, hepatitis, jaundice, or chronic alcoholism suggests possible bleeding esophageal varices, and confirmatory signs of portal hypertension must be sought during the physical examination. Erosive gastritis is suggested by a history of recent con-

TABLE 44–1

Assessment of the Extent of Blood Loss and Clinical Manifestations

Blood Loss Classification	Approximate Amount of Blood Loss*	Percent (%) of Total Blood Volume Lost	Clinical Manifestations
Class I	500–750 mL	10–15	None
Class II	700–1200 mL	15–25	1. Anxiety, tachycardia, tachypnea 2. Orthostatic hypotension 3. Urine output normal
Class III	1200–1500 mL	25–35	1. Anxiety, tachycardia, tachypnea 2. Restlessness, agitation 3. Systolic blood pressure 90–100 mmHg in recumbent position (orthostatic hypotension) 4. Reduced urine output
Class IV	1500–2000 mL	35–50	1. Anxiety, tachycardia, tachypnea 2. Systolic blood pressure ~60 mmHg 3. Reduced tissue perfusion: • Cerebral—confusion, restlessness • Renal—oliguria (<30 mL/h) • Skin—diaphoresis, cool, clammy, pallor 4. Hypovolemic, hemorrhagic shock state

*All blood loss estimates are acute losses in 60–70 Kg individual.

Source: Kelton, JG: Management of the bleeding patient. In Sibbald, WJ (ed): Synopsis of Critical Care, ed 3. Williams & Wilkins, Baltimore, 1988, p 245.

sumption of large quantities of alcohol or drugs, such as aspirin, nonsteroidal anti-inflammatory drugs, and steroids.

Additional clinical history that may be of assistance includes information about the following: recent medication history, including the use of antacids and/or laxatives, in addition to those drugs previously mentioned; dietary habits, including complaints of anorexia, food intolerance, indigestion, dysphagia, belching, nausea, and vomiting; occurrence of changes in bowel habits, including the character of stools, flatulence, diarrhea, and constipation; significant weight change; and the presence of a precipitating cause related to stress.

While a thorough clinical history should be obtained if possible, it is important to be cognizant of the fact that this information may be misleading in determining the bleeding site. For example, nearly two thirds of patients with known esophageal varices who have acute upper GI bleeding will have another lesion in the upper GI tract.

Physical Examination

The findings on physical examination may reflect the acuity of blood loss. If bleeding is gradual, the patient may show weakness, fatigue, pallor, and a slightly increased heart rate. Changes in blood pressure and heart rate occur in response to acute blood loss. As intravascular volume is reduced, there is a decrease in venous return with a consequent decrease in cardiac output and systemic blood pressure. As a rule, if, when the patient sits up from a supine position, the heart rate increases more than 20 beats/min and the systolic blood pressure falls more than 20 mmHg, then it is likely that the blood loss has exceeded 1 liter. If bleeding is severe, signs of hypovolemic shock may quickly ensue, characterized by extreme apprehension; pallor; cold, clammy skin; rapid, thready pulse; rapid, shallow respirations; hypotension (systolic ~60 mmHg); and reduced urine output (~30 mL/h).

Abdominal rigidity and rebound tenderness suggest perforation, especially when preceded by an episode of markedly exacerbated abdominal pain, followed by sudden but temporary relief. The complete physical examination includes a rectal examination. Aside from information that can be obtained about the anus, perianal area, and possible rectal masses—polyps and nodules—the character of the stool can be confirmed.

Laboratory Tests

Laboratory investigation (see Tables 43–1 and 43–2) should include a determination of the hematocrit, hemoglobin, white blood cell count with differential, platelet count, prothrombin time, and coagulation studies. Establishing baseline parameters assists in monitoring the evolving clinical course of the GI bleeding. However, some patients bleed so rapidly that there is insufficient time for the blood volume to equilibrate, and the hematocrit and hemoglobin may be normal or only slightly reduced. In patients with acute bleeding, changes in vital signs coupled with direct evidence of profuse bleeding are better indicators than the hematocrit and hemoglobin for replacement of blood and electrolyte solutions because significant changes will not be seen for 4 to 6 hours.[2]

Extensive transfusion will dilute platelets and clotting factors, particularly factors V and VII. This condition can be treated by infusion of fresh-frozen plasma and platelets, as necessary.

Monitoring of the blood urea nitrogen (BUN) level may assist in evaluating upper GI bleeding. Because blood in the upper GI tract may be digested and absorbed, an elevated BUN level in a patient who has recently had a normal BUN level, or in whom the creatinine level is normal, may provide supportive evidence of GI bleeding. Increases in both BUN and serum creatinine levels may reflect impaired adrenal perfusion associated with the hypovolemia of acute blood loss.

Nasogastric Tube Insertion

The simple maneuver of nasogastric tube insertion can quickly confirm the presence of blood in the stomach. The presence of bright red blood confirms ongoing hemorrhage, while the presence of dark and clotted blood (coffee-grounds) is more indicative of an earlier hemorrhage that may have ceased. Once inserted, the nasogastric tube allows for continuous monitoring of the bleeding. It is also used to remove blood clots and to decompress the stomach. An empty stomach will allow the walls to collapse and may contribute to hemostasis.

Endoscopy

Endoscopy is the primary diagnostic step in the investigation of upper GI bleeding. It enables direct evaluation of the esophagus, stomach, and duodenum. It is especially helpful in diagnosing erosive gastritis, which is a superficial lesion not evident in radiology studies.

Radiology Studies

If the cause of upper GI bleeding is not determined endoscopically, a nuclear medicine examination known as a technetium Tc99m red blood cells (RBC) scan may be employed. The patient is injected with a radioactive isotope, and scans are performed at 1-, 4-, and 24-hour intervals. The tagged RBC scan is able to reveal bleeding rates as low as 0.1 mL/min.

If bleeding persists and endoscopic and nuclear medicine studies are inconclusive, emergency selective angiography may demonstrate the site of active bleeding. In addition, in the case of suspected esophageal varices, it may demonstrate the presence of varices as well as portal hypertension.

Treatment and Management

Overall goals in the treatment and management of the patient with acute upper GI bleeding involve the treatment of hypovolemia and hemorrhagic shock, assessment of the severity of blood loss, diagnosis and control of the source of bleeding, and planning for definitive treatment of the underlying disease.

Initial Management

The initial management in any patient with GI bleeding must be *hemodynamic stabilization* by replacement of blood, fluid, and electrolyte losses. Initial measures require establishing at least one, and if bleeding is profuse, multiple, large-bore intravenous access lines. Blood samples for appropriate laboratory studies and type and crossmatching are drawn at this time. Normal saline or Ringer's lactate solution is infused rapidly in volumes sufficient to maintain blood pressure and correct tachycardia, until blood for transfusion is available. Albumin or plasma may also be used. With ongoing and/or massive hemorrhage, stabilization requires use of whole blood or packed cells.

A nasogastric tube is placed to permit aspiration whenever upper GI tract bleeding is suspected or when the exact location of the bleeding cannot be determined. A nasogastric tube also allows monitoring of the amount of blood loss and gastric lavage in preparation for upper endoscopy.[3]

Patients with acute GI bleeding must be monitored continuously until bleeding has ceased or a decision has been made to intervene surgically. Frequently, a pulmonary artery catheter (Swan-Ganz) is inserted to evaluate closely the effects of fluid replacement.

Because gastric acidity plays a pathogenic role in most causes of upper GI bleeding, an approach to treatment is either to neutralize acid with antacids and/or to inhibit acid secretion with histamine$_2$ antagonists, which act to reduce the direct harmful effects of acid and pepsin on the bleeding lesion. They also create an environment in which platelets are more likely to aggregate, thus promoting clotting.[4]

The most efficacious approach to therapy is a combination of *antacid* and *histamine$_2$ antagonists*. The most common histamine$_2$ antagonists are ranitidine, nizatidine, and cimetidine. These may be given orally, intravenously (except nizatidine) on an intermittent or continuous basis, or mixed with hyperalimentation. A sample regimen might include 300 mg cimetidine every 6 hours (q6h), administered by continuous infusion with 600 mg in 1000 mL 5% dextrose in water (D$_5$W).[5]

Antacids, in amounts of 60 to 90 mL, can be administered every 2 hours (q2h), leaving the nasogastric tube clamped for 30 minutes. Monitoring the pH of the nasogastric aspirate prior to the next dose of antacid or histamine$_2$ antagonist therapy helps to evaluate the effectiveness of therapy. Diarrhea, hypermagnesemia, hypernatremia, and metabolic alkalosis are common side effects of antacid use.[6] Antacids low in sodium and not magnesium-based are preferred.

Though gastric alkalinization has proven to be an effective method in prevention and treatment of gastrointestinal bleeding, recent controversy has arisen related to this practice. The acid environment of the stomach provides a natural barrier to prevent bacterial colonization. When the pH is raised above 5, bacterial counts increase significantly. Translocation of gastrointestinal bacteria can occur via nasogastric tube or aspiration of gastric contents, leading to colonization in the respiratory tract and subsequent nosocomial pneumonias.[6] Although the gastrointestinal bleeding patient may be at risk for nosocomial pneumonia, that risk alone should not be the deciding factor for drug selection and treatment.

If *helicobacter pylori* is involved, combination therapy is required. Bismuth subsalicylate (two tablets with meals and bedtime) is given in conjunction with tetracycline (500 mg four times a day [qid]) or amoxicillin (500 mg qid) and with metronidazole (250 mg three times a day [tid]) or clarithromycin (500 mg tid) for at least 2 weeks.[7]

Definitive Treatment of Underlying Disease

Peptic Ulcer Disease and Erosive Gastritis. The majority of patients with peptic ulcer disease and erosive gastritis can usually be controlled with conservative antacid and histamine$_2$ therapy and require no other treatment than prevention of their recurrence. In patients who have a history of previous GI bleeding or whose conditions fail to respond to conservative medical treatment, other modes of therapy may be considered, including the following:[5]

Peptic Ulcer Disease
- Arterial embolization
- Freezing of the gastric mucosa
- Laser surgery
- Intragastric, intra-arterial, or intraperitoneal vasoconstrictors
- Surgical procedures such as vagotomy, pyloroplasty, and gastrectomy

Erosive Gastritis
- Angiography and vasopressin administration
- Total gastrectomy—because erosion is seldom limited to a particular region within the stomach, partial surgical resection even with vagotomy may not be effective

Esophageal Variceal Bleeding. Treatment of bleeding esophageal varices secondary to alcohol cirrhosis remains controversial. Current available therapies are less than ideal, primarily because of the underlying alcoholic cirrhosis. Mortality remains about 50%.

Special Therapeutic Considerations[8]

Esophageal Tamponade. Active bleeding should be controlled, if possible, by compression of gastroesophageal varices using balloon tamponade. The *Sengstaken-Blakemore* tube is the prototype of several tubes (including the triple-lumen Linton tube and the quadruple-lumen Minnesota esophagogastric tamponade tube) capable of applying direct pressure to the bleeding area, and thereby controlling the bleeding. It is a triple-lumen tube, wherein one lumen is made of a relatively large-bore gastric tube used to evacuate the stomach, and the second and third lumens lead to the gastric (distal) and esophageal (proximal) balloons, respectively (Fig. 44–1).

The gastric or distal balloon is round and should be situated in the stomach; the esophageal or proximal balloon is sausage-shaped and should lie in the esophagus. The gastric balloon is inflated with 100 to 150 mL of air, and traction is applied to pull it back into the gastroesophageal junction. The esophageal balloon is then inflated to 25 to 40 mm Hg pressure to tamponade the bleeding vessel. Tamponade should be maintained for 48 hours. See Table 44–2 for nursing considerations related to Sengstaken-Blakemore tubes.

Selective Angiography with Continuous Vasopressin (Pitressin) Infusion. When balloon tamponade fails to control bleeding, selective angiography of the left gastric and superior mesenteric arteries can be performed with initiation of a continuous arterial infusion of vasopressin, 0.2 to 0.4 U/min (in D_5W). An infusion pump is used, and vasopressin therapy is continued for 2 to 3 days, with slow decreases in rate over this time.

Nursing care requires extreme precautions to prevent dislodging of the arterial catheter, because arterial bleeding can occur. The leg used for the arterial line insertion should be kept straight and loosely restrained, if necessary. This leg should be assessed hourly for changes in pulse, temperature, and mottling. These signs suggest compromised perfusion to the extremity. The cutdown site should be examined for infection, clot, or hematoma formation, and possible infiltration. If infiltration occurs, immediate removal of the line is necessary to prevent tissue sloughing.

Ongoing monitoring of systemic blood pressure is necessary to recognize trends indicative of hypertension. Vasopressin is a potent vasopressor. In addition, it increases water reabsorption in the distal kidney tubules, contributing to an increase in intravascular volume, which, in turn, also contributes to an increase in blood pressure. Continuous cardiac monitoring is required to detect the development of arrhythmias and myocardial ischemic changes.

Sclerotherapy. In patients with uncontrollable bleeding who are poor surgical risks, sclerotherapy may be indicated. Sclerosing solutions may be administered directly to the bleeding site by catheters passed into the portal circulation, or such solutions may be applied by endoscopy. Sclerosing solutions function to create variceal thrombosis and, in this way, curtail bleeding.

Oral Propranolol Therapy. Propranolol has been found to lower portal venous hypertension and may be efficacious in the treatment of cirrhosis complicated by recurrent esophageal and gastric variceal bleeding.

Interventions for Bleeding Varices. The most common surgical interventions performed for the treatment of bleeding varices include portocaval or splenorenal shunts. The treatment goal is to decompress the portal venous system by shunting blood into nearby, low-pressure venous channels. In general, such surgical procedures have not been found to prolong life. Major complications of surgery include bleeding, shunt thrombosis, hepatic encephalopathy, ascites, and edema of lower extremities.

Interventional Radiography. The transjugular intrahepatic portosystemic shunt (TIPS) has proven to be a valid alternative to standard medical and surgical therapies. Patients with variceal bleeding caused by portal hypertension that has failed treatment with sclerotherapy and/or surgery are primary candidates for this procedure. Using fluoroscopy, a needle is directed from the hepatic vein to a branch of the portal vein along an intrahepatic tract. After dilation of the intrahepatic tract, stainless-steel stents are inserted

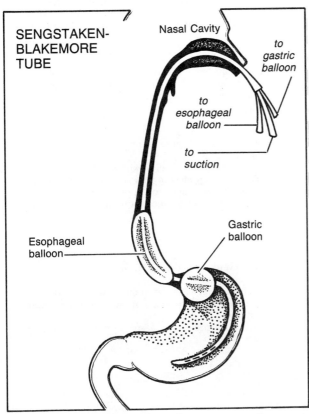

SENGSTAKEN-
BLAKEMORE
TUBE

Nasal Cavity

to
gastric
balloon

to
esophageal
balloon

to
suction

Esophageal
balloon

Gastric
balloon

FIGURE 44–1. Sengstaken-Blakemore tube used for esophagogastric tamponade.

TABLE 44–2
Sengstaken-Blakemore Tube: Nursing Care Considerations

Purpose
The Sengstaken-Blakemore tube is used for the emergency control of hemorrhage from esophageal and gastric varices. This tube affords the application of direct pressure to these bleeding blood vessels, thereby compressing them and controlling bleeding.

Description
The Sengstaken-Blakemore tube consists of a triple-lumen, double-balloon catheter. One lumen is used for gastric decompression, another for inflation of the gastric balloon, and the third for inflation of the esophageal balloon (see Fig. 44–1).

Nursing Actions	Rationales
1. Patient preparation. 　a. Appropriate explanations to patient and family.	Knowing what to expect may help patient to relax and cooperate.
b. Sedate before insertion 　　1) Morphine. 　　2) Diazepam.	Administration of sedatives must be done cautiously in patients with hepatic failure because such drugs can precipitate coma in these patients.
c. Position patient in left lateral and/or semi-Fowler's position.	Facilitates passage of gastric balloon into stomach. Semi-Fowler's position facilitates breathing and prevents aspiration.
d. Physician may attempt gastric lavage prior to insertion.	Minimizes risks of aspiration of stomach contents.
2. Equipment preparation. 　a. Inflate both balloons and hold under water to assess for air leaks.	Ensures proper function upon insertion.
b. Lubricate entire tube, including balloons, thoroughly with a water-soluble lubricant.	Reduces trauma to mucous membranes.
c. Have suction readily available.	Patient may vomit during insertion and aspiration is a danger.
Insertion and Tube Placement 1. Upon insertion, inflate gastric balloon with 50 mL air and clamp.	Prevents air leak.
2. Withdraw tube until gastric balloon sits snugly against cardia of stomach (see Fig. 42–2).	
3. Verify tube placement: 　a. Aspirate gastric contents. 　b. Auscultate over stomach while injecting air. 　c. Obtain abdominal x-ray to confirm position of gastric balloon	Verification of placement of gastric balloon is important to avoid inadvertent inflation of gastric balloon in the esophagus. This could precipitate respiratory distress, cardiac arrhythmias, tissue necrosis, and perforation.
4. Inflate gastric balloon with 100–150 mL air when tube placement is verified.	
5. Apply gentle traction by taping catheter to a piece of sponge rubber as it emerges from the nostril, or place football helmet on patient and tape tube to face guard.	Prevents movement of tube with peristalsis; maintains continuous pressure to varices. Use of sponge helps to minimize pressure on nostrils caused by traction.
6. Inflate esophageal balloon if bleeding persists. 　a. Maintain pressure of 25–40 mmHg with the use of a sphygmomanometer.	
b. Maintain pressure for up to 48 h.	Longer use could cause esophageal tissue injury, necrosis, and perforation.
c. Suction oropharynx and esophagus frequently: 　　1) Assist patient to suction her or his own secretions if the patient is alert and cooperative.	Patient is unable to swallow with esophageal tube inflated. Physician may elect to pass an accessory nasogastric tube into esophagus and apply continuous low suction to prevent fluid accumulation with its increased risk of aspiration.
Maintenance and Ongoing Care 1. Irrigate gastric tube as frequently as prescribed (q 30–60 min). 　a. Perform initial irrigation (with iced saline or water) until returns are clear.	This prevents clotted blood from plugging up gastric lumen.
b. Connect gastric lumen to continuous intermittent suction and monitor returns.	With initial evacuation of stomach, subsequent assessments can be made of the effectiveness of the tamponade.
c. Observe for persistent bleeding.	This may suggest erosive gastritis or bleeding peptic ulcer.
2. Maintain tamponade for prescribed time. 　a. Monitor vital signs frequently. 　b. Assess neurologic status: 　　1) Lethargy, drowsiness, confusion, unconsciousness. 　c. Assess for chest pain, back pain, respiratory distress. 　d. Record intake and output. 　e. Monitor serial electrolyte, BUN, hematocrit, hemoglobin, clotting factors. 　f. Monitor balloon pressure hourly.	

TABLE 44–2
Sengstaken-Blakemore Tube: Nursing Care Considerations (*Continued*)

g. Double clamp balloon parts.	This prevents air leaks and prevents gastric balloon from riding up into esophagus as air leaks out.
h. Keep scissors at bedside at all times.	Airway obstruction and esophageal perforation are major complications. Rupture of gastric balloon will cause entire tube to move up in the esophagus, with the danger of airway obstruction.
1) In a true emergency, e.g., airway obstruction, cut through the entire tube with scissors and remove it.	
2) Notify physician immediately.	Sudden upper abdominal and/or back pains and altered hemodynamics or shock suggest esophageal perforation.
i. Deflate/inflate esophageal balloon as prescribed.	
3. Provide comfort measures:	
a. Frequent and conscientious oral hygiene.	Prevents mucous membrane encrustation, dryness, and cracking; mouth breathing often becomes necessary because of large-bore nasal tube.
b. Examine nostrils frequently and keep cleansed and lubricated.	
c. Maintain on complete bed rest, avoiding any exertion, e.g., coughing or straining.	These activities increase intra-abdominal pressure and may predispose to further bleeding.
d. Maintain in semi-Fowler's position.	
e. Stay with patient because this may be a frightening experience.	
1) Provide reassurance.	
4. Continuous monitoring for the following complications:	
a. Aspiration of oral secretions or refluxed blood.	
b. Airway obstruction.	
c. Esophageal rupture.	
d. Cardiac arrhythmias from distended esophagus.	
5. Deflate balloons for a period of ~12 h prior to removal.	
a. Monitor for signs of rebleeding.	Evidence of any rebleeding can be assessed.

to maintain tract patency. A portosystemic shunt is created within the liver.[9]

NURSING CARE OF THE PATIENT WITH ACUTE UPPER GASTROINTESTINAL TRACT BLEEDING AND HYPOVOLEMIC SHOCK

Whether the underlying cause is a primary disease of the GI system or occurs as a complication of a critical illness involving another organ system, the critical care nurse plays a crucial role in the assessment, diagnosis, and management of the patient with acute upper GI tract bleeding complicated by hypovolemic shock.

The immediate goals are to treat the shock and control the bleeding. Hemodynamic function can be stabilized and maintained through timely and aggressive fluid and blood replacement therapy. It is essential to reestablish adequate circulatory fluid volume so that tissue perfusion can be maintained and the oxygen delivered to the tissues is sufficient to meet the metabolic demands of the cells. (See Chapter 21 for an in-depth discussion of shock.)

Monitoring of a patient with, or at risk of developing, acute upper GI bleeding should be ongoing and continuous. It is necessary to establish a baseline of assessment data so that the patient's responses to therapy can be assessed and the effectiveness of such therapy in meeting patient outcomes can be evaluated. Clinical findings are not considered separately, but rather, they are examined in terms of the patient's entire clinical status. Furthermore, it is the *trend* or series of responses rather than any single, isolated response that is of clinical significance.

Nurses caring for the patient must be alert for any changes in the patient's condition, however subtle they may be. It is important to appreciate the distinct classes or degrees of blood loss and the associated clinical manifestations (see Table 44–1). In the patient at risk, complaints of weakness, fatigue, apprehension, and shortness of breath, coupled with tachycardia and orthostatic hypotension, take on added clinical significance in terms of possible underlying GI bleeding. The extent of blood loss can sometimes be estimated based on the a patient's overall clinical presentation.

In patients receiving massive blood transfusions, the nurse has the added responsiblity of preventing complications associated with such therapy. An appreciation of the pathophysiology underlying blood incompatibility and transfusion reactions, dilutional coagulopathies, citrate toxicity with hypocalcemia and acidemia, hyperkalemia, and hypothermia is necessary for the prevention and/or early detection and treatment of such complications, should they occur.

For the patient with frank upper GI tract bleeding and his or her family, fear and apprehension are appropriate responses. The sight of blood can be upsetting regardless of how massive or minuscule the quantity. The critical care nurse provides a calming and stabilizing effect by encouraging the patient and family to ask questions and verbalize their fears, by offering appropriate explanations and reassurance, by being accessible to them, and by displaying a competent, efficient demeanor in providing overall patient care. The critical care nurse establishes a working rapport and trusting relationship with the patient and family, which assists them in coping with the immediate crisis situation and lays the foundation for assisting the patient and family to work through their problems, examine their lifestyles, and meaningfully consider the level of health desired.

Therapeutic Goals

Implementation of the nursing process in the care of the patient with acute upper GI tract hemorrhage and hypovolemic, hemorrhagic shock revolves around the following therapeutic goals:

1. Reestablish/maintain hemodynamic stability by restoring circulating blood volume, increasing cardiac output, and improving tissue perfusion.
2. Maintain a patent airway.
3. Prevent tissue hypoxia by providing oxygen therapy to maximize oxygen-carrying capacity of the blood and oxygen delivery to the tissues.
4. Establish a thorough, comprehensive assessment database, including clinical history and physical examination.
5. Maintain fluid and electrolyte balance.
6. Reduce anxiety and apprehension.
7. Maintain therapeutic milieu with optimum rest, comfort, and relaxation to minimize bleeding or rebleeding.
8. Provide nutritional support to maintain ideal body weight.
9. Prevent and/or monitor for complications of shock, including adult respiratory distress syndrome (ARDS), acute renal failure, and disseminated intravascular coagulation (DIC).
10. Prevent infection.
11. Provide emotional and psychological support to patient and family.
12. Initiate patient/family health education about the underlying disease process, the impact on performance of activities of daily living and overall lifestyle, and the decision-making process regarding the optimum level of health desired.

Nursing Diagnoses, Desired Patient Outcomes, and Nursing Interventions

Pertinent nursing diagnoses, desired patient outcomes, nursing interventions, and their rationales are presented in the care plan that follows. See Chapter 21 for an in-depth discussion of shock.

REFERENCES

1. Prevost, SS, and Oberle, A: Stress ulceration in the critically ill patient. Crit Care Nurs Clin North Am 8(1):163–169, 1993.
2. Wardell, TL: Assessing and managing a gastric ulcer. Nursing '91 21(3):34–42, 1991.
3. Cohen, LB, and Lewis, BS: Acute gastrointestinal bleeding. In Sachar, DB, Waye, JD, and Lewis, BS (eds): Gastroenterology for the House Officer. Williams & Wilkins, Baltimore, 1989, p 27.
4. Eastwood, GL: Core Textbook of Gastroenterology. JB Lippincott, Philadelphia, 1994, p 91.
5. Cohen, LB, and Lewis, BS: Acute gastrointestinal bleeding. In Sachar, DB, Waye, JD, and Lewis, BS (eds): Gastroenterology for the House Officer. Williams & Wilkins, Baltimore, 1989, p 35.
6. Prevost, SS, and Oberle, A: Stress ulceration in the critically ill patient. Crit Care Nurs Clin North Am 8(1):163–169, 1993.
7. McGuffey, E: H. pylori and ulcers. Am Pharm 34(7):21, 1994.
8. Steele, RJC, Chung, SCS, and Leung, JWC: Practical Management of Acute Gastrointestinal Bleeding. Butterworth-Heinemann, Oxford, 1993, pp 44–56.
9. Adams, L, and Saulen, M: A new alternative for variceal bleeder. Am J Crit Care 2(3): pp 196–201, 1993.

CARE PLAN FOR THE PATIENT WITH ACUTE UPPER GASTROINTESTINAL BLEEDING AND HYPOVOLEMIC SHOCK

Nursing Diagnoses

Nursing Diagnosis #1
Fluid volume deficit, actual, related to:
1. Acute blood loss—hematemesis, hematochezia
2. Gastric drainage (continuous)

Desired Patient Outcomes

Patient will:
1. Maintain an effective circulating blood volume and stable hemodynamic functions:
   - Heart rate (resting) <100 beats/min.
   - Central venous pressure 0–8 mmHg.
   - Pulmonary artery pressure <25 mmHg.
   - Pulmonary capillary wedge pressure 8–12 mmHg.
   - Cardiac output ~5 L/min.
   - Systemic arterial blood pressure within 10 mmHg of baseline, without orthostatic hypotension.
2. Remain alert, and oriented to person, place, time; without weakness and dizziness.
3. Maintain urine output >30 mL/h.
4. Remain without signs of rebleeding:
   - No hematemesis, hematochezia.
   - Gastric aspirate, blood-free.
5. Maintain body weight within 5% of baseline.

CARE PLAN FOR THE PATIENT WITH ACUTE UPPER GASTROINTESTINAL BLEEDING AND HYPOVOLEMIC SHOCK (*Continued*)

Nursing Diagnoses

Desired Patient Outcomes

6. Balance intake with output.
7. Exhibit good skin turgor, moist mucous membranes, minimal thirst.
8. Maintain laboratory parameters within acceptable physiologic range:
   - Hematocrit 37%–52%.
   - Hemoglobin 12–18 g/100 mL.
   - RBC and white blood cell (WBC) counts.
   - BUN, electrolytes, calcium.

Nursing Interventions

- Assess for signs and symptoms of hypovolemic shock:
  - Observe for signs of acute or subacute bleeding: hematemesis, hematochezia, melena, abdominal distention, epigastric pain.

  - Assess cardiovascular function:
    - Hypotension (orthostatic).

    - Resting pulse >100 beats/min. Characteristics— faint, rapid, thready.

    - Skin color—pallor, cyanosis; skin temperature; delayed capillary refill time (>3 sec).
    - Signs of dehydration—poor skin turgor, weakness, fatigue.
    - Cardiac monitoring: rate and rhythm.
- Assess renal function:
  - Urine output >30 mL/h.

- Establish baseline abdominal assessment data:
  - Presence or absence of bowel sounds (timing and characteristics).
  - Pain and tenderness (location, radiation, quality, severity, duration). (See Table 13–1.)

  - Hepatomegaly, ascites, spider nevi, splenomegaly.
  - Abdominal mass or bruit.
- Insert at least one or more (if bleeding is massive) large-gauge angiocatheters for rapid administration of blood and blood products, volume expanders, and fluids (Ringer's lactate and normal saline).
  - Obtain blood samples for baseline laboratory data.

- Monitor hematocrit, hemoglobin; RBC, WBC counts; electrolytes, serum calcium; blood glucose levels.

Rationales

- A baseline assessment is necessary to establish the stage of shock—initial compensatory, progressive, or final, and emergent measures indicated; it serves as a measure of the patient's response to therapy. (See Chapter 21 for a discussion of hypovolemic shock, including the stages of shock.)

  - A drop in blood pressure of 10–15 mmHg from supine to sitting position suggests blood loss of ~1 liter.
  - Blood loss and enhanced peripheral vasoconstriction underlie diminished to absent pulses, coolness of the extremities, and pallor of conjunctiva, mucous membranes, and nailbeds.

  - Skin turgor is best assessed over forehead or sternum.
  - Reflect effect of blood loss on cardiac function.
- Reduced circulating blood volume and hypotensive state compromise renal perfusion. The consequent reduction in glomerular filtration underlies the reduced urine output associated with hypovolemic shock.

  - Abdominal pain with muscle guarding and rebound tenderness is highly suggestive of peptic ulcer perforation, especially if preceded by an episode of severe abdominal pain, followed by sudden but temporary relief, in patients at risk.
  - Suggestive of cirrhosis with portal hypertension.
  - Questionable abdominal aneurysm.
- A single peripheral intravenous catheter may not be sufficient to provide adequate blood replacement in a profusely bleeding patient.
  - A central venous line or pulmonary artery catheter is needed to closely monitor the patient's response to volume replacement.
- In patients bleeding profusely, there may be insufficient time for the blood volume to equilibrate. Thus, hematocrit and hemoglobin may not be reliable indicators of the patient's status. In such patients, changes in blood pressure and pulse are better indicators for replacement of blood and blood products.
  - Rapid fluid shifts during GI bleeding, and subsequent infusion of blood, blood products, and other fluids, require frequent assessment of serum electrolytes— sodium, potassium, chloride, bicarbonate, and serum calcium. The serum calcium level may become depressed after several units of anticoagulate (citrate)-containing blood have been administered.

CARE PLAN FOR THE PATIENT WITH ACUTE UPPER GASTROINTESTINAL BLEEDING AND HYPOVOLEMIC SHOCK (*Continued*)

Nursing Interventions	Rationales
○ Monitor BUN and creatinine levels.	○ Metabolism of blood by intestinal bacterial, coupled with compromised liver perfusion, causes the BUN level to rise. □ A rising BUN in the presence of a normal creatinine is highly indicative of a massive upper GI bleed.
○ Obtain blood samples for type and crossmatch.	○ Even in acute emergencies, there is usually sufficient time to type and crossmatch blood for infusion properly. This reduces the incidence of blood incompatibility and transfusion reactions.
○ Monitor prothrombin time, clotting factors, fibrin degradation products.	○ Patients receiving massive fluid and blood replacement therapy are at risk of developing a dilutional coagulopathy; patients with profuse bleeding are at high risk of developing consumptive coagulopathies (e.g., DIC).
• Initiate aggressive infusion of electrolytes and volume expanders until blood is ready for administration.	
• Insert nasogastric tube.	• To decompress the stomach and assist (in conjunction with endoscopy) in determining site, amount, and rate of bleeding; to test gastric aspirate for blood and pH; and to administer antacids, iced saline lavage (as prescribed).
• Check for tube placement.	• Inadvertent placement of the nasogastric tube into the respiratory passage is always a potential complication of this procedure.
○ Auscultate over the gastric area while injecting 50 mL air into the nasogastric tube.	○ A rush of air should be heard if the tube is properly placed.
• Assess gastric aspirate. ○ Presence of fresh blood or a large amount of old blood (coffee-ground material) are indications for gastric lavage.	• Removal of as much clot and intragastric material as possible is important; it assists in evaluating continuous bleeding; an empty stomach will allow the walls to collapse and may contribute to hemostasis.
• Implement gastric lavage as prescribed.	• Irrigation with iced saline causes vasoconstriction of bleeding vessels; the efficacy of this treatment has yet to be substantiated.
○ Maintain patency of tube by irrigation and repositioning if necessary.	○ Use of saline for lavage minimizes sodium depletion through gastric mucosa.
• Maintain the patient on nothing by mouth protocol (NPO), and implement continuous gastric suction, as prescribed. ○ Monitor amount and characteristics of gastric drainage.	• Continuous gastric suctioning enables close monitoring of bleeding; it minimizes the amount of blood passing into the intestine, where the action of the intestinal bacteria metabolizes blood to ammonia.
• Maintain a strict intake and output. ○ Include amount of fluid lavaged and that removed by gastric suction. ○ Document amount and characteristics of any emesis.	
• Provide comfort measures: ○ Provide quiet, calm environment with frequent rest periods; minimize stimuli.	○ To promote physical and mental rest; stimulation may provoke vomiting, bleeding.
○ Provide mouth care with oral suctioning as necessary.	○ Aspiration is a potential complication.
○ Secure tube to patient's gown with adequate slack.	○ This prevents tugging on tube when patient moves, which can injure nose.
○ Lubricate nares; assess nares for pressure areas caused by nasogastric tube.	
○ Monitor body temperature. □ Provide extra blankets if appropriate.	○ Continuous iced saline lavage can lower body temperature.

CARE PLAN FOR THE PATIENT WITH ACUTE UPPER GASTROINTESTINAL BLEEDING AND HYPOVOLEMIC SHOCK (*Continued*)

Nursing Interventions	Rationales
• Transfuse blood and blood products as prescribed. 　○ Consider unit procedure and protocols for: 　　▫ Administering blood therapy. 　　▫ Monitoring patient's response to blood therapy. 　　▫ Recognizing early signs of adverse effects and transfusion reactions. 　　▫ Procedure to follow in the event of transfusion reaction.	
• Insert Foley catheter to measure hourly urine output.	• Hourly urine outputs assist in monitoring renal perfusion and function.
• Assist with insertion of hemodynamic pressure monitoring lines.	• Insertion of systemic arterial and pulmonary artery flotation (Swan-Ganz) catheters is needed in the setting of massive upper GI hemorrhage and massive blood and fluid replacement therapy. 　○ PCWP is a useful parameter for monitoring for fluid overload, a potential complication of massive, aggressive fluid replacement therapy.
○ Monitor hemodynamics: arterial, and pulmonary artery pressures—central venous pressure and pulmonary capillary wedge pressures (PCWP); and cardiac output. 　○ Monitor hydration status during fluid replacement therapy. 　○ Assess respiratory function: respiratory rate and rhythm; presence of adventitious sounds. 　○ Assess signs/symptoms of fluid overload. (See Chapter 36.) 　○ Monitor daily weight.	○ The detection of rales in previously clear lungs suggests possible overhydration. • Should be maintained within 5% of baseline.
• Assist with insertion of Sengstaken-Blakemore tube in setting of persistent variceal bleeding.	• See Table 44–2 for nursing care considerations for patients with a Sengstaken-Blakemore tube.

Nursing Diagnoses	Desired Patient Outcomes
Nursing Diagnosis #2 Gas exchange impaired: ventilation/perfusion imbalance, related to reduced circulating volume and compromised hemodynamics	Patient will: 1. Be alert and oriented to person, place, time. 2. Exhibit appropriate behavior. 3. Maintain effective cardiovascular function: 　• Blood pressure within 10 mmHg of baseline. 　• Cardiac output: ~5 L/min. 4. Maintain arterial blood gas parameters within acceptable physiologic range: 　• pH 7.35–7.45 　• Pa_{O_2} >60 mmHg 　• Pa_{CO_2} 35–45 mmHg 5. Maintain hematologic values within acceptable range. 　• Hematocrit 37%–52%. 　• Hemoglobin 12–18 g/100 mL. 　• RBC count.

Nursing Interventions	Rationales
• Perform neurologic assessment. 　○ Mental status; orientation to person, place, time; level of consciousness; appropriateness of responses/behavior.	• Hypoxemia coupled with hypovolemic shock can predispose to cerebral tissue hypoxia.
• Monitor cardiovascular function: 　○ Cardiac arrhythmias. 　○ Tachycardia; rapid, thready peripheral pulses.	○ Hypoxemia is commonly associated with myocardial irritability. 　○ Commonly associated with blood loss, and consequent reduced circulating blood volume and peripheral vasoconstriction.

CARE PLAN FOR THE PATIENT WITH ACUTE UPPER GASTROINTESTINAL BLEEDING AND HYPOVOLEMIC SHOCK (*Continued*)

Nursing Interventions
- ○ Cyanosis.

- • Monitor respiratory function:
  - ○ Respiratory rate and pattern, breath sounds: normal and adventitious breath sounds.
  - ○ Arterial blood gases: pH, PaO_2, $PaCO_2$; alveolar-arterial gradient ($AaDO_2$).
  - ○ Monitor hematologic profile: hematocrit, hemoglobin, RBC count.

- • Administer prescribed humidified oxygen therapy.
  - ○ Monitor arterial blood gas and hematologic parameter as indicated.
  - ○ Provide frequent rest periods.
  - ○ Evaluate effectiveness of oxygen therapy; assess neurologic function and vital signs.

Rationales
- ○ Late sign reflecting desaturation of at least 5 g/100 mL of hemoglobin; commonly associated with ventilation/perfusion mismatch and right-to-left shunting.

- ○ Presence of rales (crackles) may be indicative of fluid overload.
- ○ Most closely reflect effectiveness of gas exchange.

- ○ Reflects hemoglobin oxygen-carrying capacity within blood; reduced hemoglobin levels can compromise oxygen delivery to tissues.
- • Tissue hypoxia is a common consequence of hypovolemic shock from depleted blood volume and reduced number of RBCs.
- ○ To reduce oxygen demand by tissues.

Nursing Diagnoses

Nursing Diagnosis #3
Anxiety, related to:
1. Acute upper GI bleeding
2. Abdominal pain
3. Transfusion therapy
4. Intensive care setting

Desired Patient Outcomes

Patient will:
1. Verbalize feeling less anxious.
2. Demonstrate relaxed demeanor.
3. Perform relaxation techniques with assistance.
4. Verbalize familiarity with intensive care unit (ICU) routines and protocols.

Nursing Interventions

For specific nursing interventions and their rationales, see the care plan for pulmonary embolism, in Chapter 26, nursing diagnosis #4, Anxiety.

Rationales

Nursing Diagnoses

Nursing Diagnosis #4
Epigastric pain, related to:
1. Enhanced gastric acidity
2. Reflex muscle spasm

Desired Patient Outcomes

Patient will:
1. Verbalize pain relief.
2. Exhibit relaxed demeanor:
   • Relaxed facial expression and body posture.
Gastric aspirate: pH >4.5

Nursing Inteventions
- • Assess complaints of pain, including severity, location/radiation, influencing factors (e.g., what precipitates, aggravates, or ameliorates the pain? what signs and symptoms are associated with the pain?)
- • Assess for nonverbal clues to the presence of pain (e.g., restlessness, irritability, agitation, diaphoresis, tense facial features, and rapid, shallow breathing).
- • Implement measures to reduce pain:
  - ○ Administer the following medications as prescribed:
    - □ Antacids.
  - ○ Histamine₂ antagonists—cimetidine (Tagamet) or ranitidine (Zantac).

  - ○ Analgesics.
    - □ Encouarge patient to request medication when pain is first perceived, rather than waiting until it becomes severe.
    - □ Evaluate the effectiveness of medication in relieving patient's pain.

Rationales
- • Use of the SLIDT tool (see Table 35–1) assists in eliciting specific information about the nature of the complaints.

- □ Antacids neutralize gastric acidity.
- ○ Inhibit gastric acid secretion. The combination of antacids and histamine antagonist therapy is more efficacious than either therapy alone in reducing the harmful effects of acid and pepsin on the bleeding lesion.

CARE PLAN FOR THE PATIENT WITH ACUTE UPPER GASTROINTESTINAL BLEEDING AND HYPOVOLEMIC SHOCK (*Continued*)

Nursing Interventions
- ○ Mild sedation.

- • Determine how patient usually copes with pain or stress:
  - ○ Pain tolerance.
  - ○ Willingness to discuss pain, or stoically "keeping it in."
  - ○ Willingness to use medication for pain.
  - ○ Behavior used to reduce level of stress.

Rationales
- ○ It is absolutely essential to assist the patient to rest and relax, mentally and physically, to reduce danger of continued bleeding or rebleeding.
- • Details elicited at this time regarding patient/family attitudes about pain and stress may help lay the foundation for patient/family education.

Nursing Diagnoses

Nursing Diagnosis #5
Nutrition, alteration in: less than body requirements, related to maintenance on NPO with continuous gastric suctioning
(See Chapter 9, Nutritional Support of the Critically Ill Patient.)

Desired Patient Outcomes

Patient will maintain:
1. Body weight within 5% of baseline.
2. Total serum proteins 6.0–8.4 g/100 mL.
3. Laboratory data within acceptable physiologic range:
   - • BUN, serum creatinine.
   - • Electrolytes, serum calcium.
   - • Blood glucose levels.
   - • Serum albumin 4.5–5.5 g/100 mL.
   - • Hematology profile.
4. Triceps skinfold measurement within normal range.

Nursing Interventions
- • Consult with nutritionist in assessing overall nutritional status; and signs and symptoms of malnutrition.
  - ○ Major considerations: general state of health— weakness; body weight; physiologic factors—age, height, triceps skinfold; mid-upper arm circumference; food intolerance; allergies.
  - ○ Laboratory data: BUN, serum creatinine; fasting blood glucose; serum electrolytes, total protein (serum albumin); cholesterol; transfusion levels, hematology profile.
- • Maintain adequate nutrition with prescribed enteral and/or parenteral nutrition.

  - ○ Order prescribed feeding from pharmacy.

  - ○ Assist with placement of TPN central intravenous catheter.
    - □ Explain purpose of parenteral therapy.
    - □ Explain procedure for insertion:
    - –Use of Trendelenburg position and Valsalva maneuver.
    - □ Apply dressing.
  - ○ Prepare patient for chest x-ray.

  - ○ Assess patient for signs and symptoms of respiratory distress: dyspnea, decreased breath sounds, chest pain, hematoma formation.
  - ○ Initiate prescribed parenteral feedings.
    - □ Begin infusion at slow rate (60–80 mL/h); increase infusion by 25 mL/day.
    - □ Use flow control device or pump to administer feeding.
    - □ Weigh patient daily; record intake and output.
    - □ Monitor serum glucose; monitor for signs of hyperglycemia (polyuria, glycosuria, elevated serum glucose).

Rationales
- • Catabolic state associated with critical illness rapidly depletes body stores of nutrients.

- • The purpose of total parenteral nutrition (TPN) is to provide sufficient nutrients intravenously, to achieve anabolism, and to promote weight gain.
  - ○ Solution should be prepared in pharmacy under a laminar air-flow unit to minimize danger of contamination.

  - –Helps to avoid air embolism upon insertion.

  - ○ To confirm correct placement of catheter and rule out potential pneumothorax.
  - ○ Pneumothorax, hemothorax, air embolism, and sepsis are major complications.

    - □ Allows for physiologic adjustments in pancreatic insulin secretion; helps to avoid glucose intolerance.
    - □ This helps to prevevent fluid or glucose overload.

CARE PLAN FOR THE PATIENT WITH ACUTE UPPER GASTROINTESTINAL BLEEDING AND HYPOVOLEMIC SHOCK (*Continued*)

Nursing Interventions	Rationales
□ Wean from TPN therapy slowly.	□ This avoids danger of hypoglycemic reaction as pancreatic secretion of insulin is allowed to decline accordingly.

• Ongoing monitoring/maintenance:
  ○ Maintain catheter asepsis. Monitor body temperature at regular intervals and report any temperature elevation to physician. Follow unit protocol in obtaining specimens for culture and sensitivity.
  ○ Never use TPN catheter for anything other than parenteral feedings.
  ○ Provide catheter site care as per unit protocol.
	○ Consistent monitoring is necessary because there is no single febrile pattern associated with TPN sepsis. Temperature elevation may be low grade, constant, intermittent, or characterized by daily spiking.
	○ If catheter is used as a central access line in an emergency, it should not be reused for TPN.
	○ Cleaning catheter site minimizes potential complications of sepsis or mechanical disruption of catheter placement; it helps to preserve skin integrity at insertion site.

Nursing Diagnoses	Desired Patient Outcomes
Nursing Diagnosis #6 Sleep pattern disturbance, related to: 1. Frequent interruption for assessment and treatments 2. Intensive care environment and protocols 3. Psychological stress	Patient will: 1. Verbalize underlying concerns regarding inability to sleep. 2. Verbalize familiarity with ICU protocols and environmental stimuli. 3. Assist in planning for undisturbed rest periods within the constraints of ongoing monitoring and essential patient care. 4. Report a sense of well-being and restfulness.

Nursing Interventions	Rationales

• Assess sleep pattern and difficulty sleeping:
  ○ Encourage patient to verbalize concerns regarding sleeplessness.
  ○ Monitor the amount of time the patient is sleeping or napping.
    □ Identify times and circumstances during which sleep seems most restful.
    □ Identify factors particularly disturbing to the patient.
    □ Observe for signs and symptoms of fatigue, restlessness, apprehension.
• Administer prescribed medications for pain and sedation.
  ○ Monitor effectiveness of medications in relieving pain and relaxing the patient.
• Provide comfort measures:
  ○ Include personal hygiene, back massage, position changes.
  ○ Minimize room noise; dim the lighting during rest period (if possible); maintain comfortable room temperature.
• Assist patient to establish a pattern conducive to sleep.
  ○ Explain ICU protocols and procedures.
  ○ Encourage patient to verbalize feelings; provide an attentive, listening ear.
  ○ Stay with patient at times that are especially stressful.
  ○ Provide reassurance.
  ○ Allow patient to make some decisions regarding his or her care (e.g., when to rest, when to have visitors).
	• To minimize bleeding and prevent rebleeding, it is essential to provide a clinical milieu that is as calm and quiet as possible and is conducive to patient rest and relaxation.
	
	• Pain and anxiety undermine efforts to rest and relax.
	
	• Comfort measures aid muscle relaxation.
	
	○ Understanding what to expect and what is expected of the patient may help to relieve concerns and apprehension.
	○ Demonstration of caring, concern, and acceptance may be reassuring to patient.
	○ Enables patient to assume responsibility for some aspects of overall care.

CARE PLAN FOR THE PATIENT WITH ACUTE UPPER GASTROINTESTINAL BLEEDING AND HYPOVOLEMIC SHOCK (*Continued*)

Nursing Diagnoses

Nursing Diagnosis #7
Fear, related to possibility of bleeding to death

Desired Patient Outcomes

Patient will:
1. Verbalize fear of dying.
2. Verbalize knowledge of clinical status and proposed course of therapy.
3. Demonstrate behaviors indicative of lessened fear (e.g., relaxed facies and posture).

Nursing Interventions

- Assess degree of fear and patient's perceptions of the possibility of dying.
  - Encourage patient/family to discuss their perceptions and feelings regarding the patient's health status and to share subjective experiences.
  - Observe nonverbal and verbal responses.
  - Assess for accompanying changes in patient's physiologic status.
    - Vital signs.
  - Assess for accompanying changes in patient's psychological status.
    - Evidence of denial, anger, depression.

- Assist patient/family to deal with fear:
  - Stay with patient/family.
  - Allow time for and encourage expression of feelings and concerns.
  - Assist patient/family to identify feelings.
  - Clarify questions or misconceptions about illness or treatment.
- Assist patient/family to learn from this experience and to problem-solve:
  - Identify strengths of family members, individually and collectively.
  - Acknowledge usefulness of fear, denial, anger in coping.
  - Promote honest and open communication between family members.
  - Involve patient/family in problem-solving and decision-making.
- Referral to psychiatric liaison nurse and/or social worker as indicated and/or requested by patient and/or family.

Rationales

- An episode of massive upper GI bleeding can be perceived by patient/family as an imminent threat that the patient is going to bleed to death.

  - Recognize that sympathetic response to fear may actually aggravate bleeding and needs to be minimized.

    - These responses may assist patient/family to cope at least temporarily until patient/family have learned ways to reduce the threat.

- Recognizes that fear can be a motivating factor for learning only if the arousal of fear is accompanied by steps/actions to reduce the threat.

  - Assists patient/family in coping; this may help to increase self-confidence in their own capabilities.
- Patient/family may feel reassured that other resources are available to lend assistance and support.

Nursing Management of the Patient with Hepatic Failure

Marina Hamilton

CHAPTER OUTLINE

LEARNING OBJECTIVES

After completing this chapter, you should be able to:

1. Identify types and common causes of hepatic failure.
2. List the clinical manifestations of hepatic failure.
3. State the major complications of hepatic failure.
4. Define hepatic encephalopathy and the stages of its clinical course.
5. Identify treatment priorities in the management of hepatic failure.
6. Describe the nursing process in the care of the patient with hepatic failure, including the following:
   a. Assessment
   b. Nursing diagnoses
   c. Planning: Desired patient outcomes
          Nursing interventions and rationales.

TYPES OF HEPATIC FAILURE

Patients with liver disease are admitted to the intensive care setting with complications from either fulminant hepatic failure, associated with an acute onset of symptoms, or chronic hepatic failure caused by cirrhosis, with complications from a gradual and progressive degeneration of the liver.

Fulminant Hepatic Failure

Fulminant hepatic failure involves a rapid, progressive deterioration and degeneration of liver parenchyma, frequently with massive hepatocellular necrosis, resulting in severe hepatic dysfunction. Fulminant hepatic failure is typically viral in its etiology, primarily from hepatitis B, but there are numerous other possible causes (see box on p. 821).

Chronic Hepatic Failure

Chronic hepatic failure, or cirrhosis, is characterized by a gradual, insidious, and progressive degeneration of the liver parenchyma, with diffuse hepatocellular necrosis, widespread hepatic fibrosis, and nodular regeneration. Several clinically distinct forms of cirrhosis have been identified.

Laënnec's Cirrhosis. Laënnec's cirrhosis is the most commonly occurring chronic liver disease, and it is most closely associated with chronic alcohol abuse. The direct toxic effect of alcohol on hepatocytes, coupled with malnutrition, predisposes to fatty infiltration of the hepatic parenchyma.

CAUSES OF FULMINANT HEPATIC FAILURE

Viral:
Hepatitis B
Hepatitis C
Chemical:
Acetaminophen
Salicylates
Phenylbutazone
Halothane
Tetracycline
Sulfonamides
Isoniazid
Rifampin
Phenytoin
Ethanol
Carbon tetrachloride
Metabolic:
Malnutrition
Fatty liver of pregnancy
Reye's syndrome
Ischemic:
Hepatic necrosis

TABLE 45–1
Clinical Manifestations of Hepatic Failure

Body System	Clinical Manifestations
Neurologic	Hepatic encephalopathy
	Asterixis
	Sensory disturbances
Metabolic	Altered carbohydrate, fat, and protein metabolism
Endocrine	Increased estrogens ♂—testicular atrophy and gynecomastia
	Increased testosterone ♀—amenorrhea or menstrual irregularity
	Increased aldosterone
Fluid and electrolyte	Hyperaldosteronism
	↓ K
	↑ Na
	↑ H_2O
	Ascites
	Anasarca
Hematologic	Anemia
	Impaired coagulation
	↓ platelets
	↓ clotting factors
	Disseminated intravascular coagulation
	Hemorrhage
	Leukopenia
Gastrointestinal	Portal hypertension
	Abdominal pain
	Clay-colored stools
	Diarrhea
	Esophageal varices
	Fetor hepaticus
	GI bleeding
	Varices
	Nausea and vomiting
	Splenomegaly
Cardiovascular	Hypovolemia
	Cardiac arrhythmias
	Ascites
	Portal hypertension
Pulmonary	Limited expansion
	Dyspnea
	Hypoxemia
Renal	Hepatorenal syndrome
Dermatologic	Edema
	Pectoral and axillary alopecia
	Palmar erythema
	Jaundice
	Spider angiomas
	Moon faces
	Pruritis
	Caput medusae
	Striae

Postnecrotic Cirrhosis. Postnecrotic cirrhosis is characterized by a significant loss of hepatic cells, collapse of the framework of the liver parenchyma, and the presence of large, irregular nodules of regenerating and degenerating hepatic tissue. About 25% of patients with postnecrotic cirrhosis have a history of acute viral hepatitis. Intoxication with industrial chemicals, drugs, and poisons, and certain infections have been implicated in the etiology of this form of cirrhosis. Postnecrotic cirrhosis has been associated with primary hepatic neoplasm formation (hepatoma).

Biliary Cirrhosis. Biliary cirrhosis may develop secondary to decreased bile flow and cholestasis, as occurs in intrahepatic and/or extrahepatic biliary obstruction. Stasis of bile within the liver parenchyma and its accumulation result in destruction of hepatic cells.

Cardiac Cirrhosis. Cardiac cirrhosis is relatively rare and associated with severe right-sided congestive heart failure. Severe venous congestion predisposes to ischemia and anoxia, with consequent cellular injury and necrosis. Persistence of this process leads to generalized fibrosis.

CLINICAL MANIFESTATIONS AND MANAGEMENT OF HEPATIC FAILURE

The clinical manifestations seen in hepatic failure are diverse (Table 45–1). Understanding the various functions of the liver assists in anticipating and identifying the impending dysfunctions specifically related to the liver as well as those affecting other organ systems.

Neurologic

Hepatic encephalopathy is an alteration in mentation, consciousness, and motor function caused by liver disease. Table 45–2 outlines the four stages of hepatic encephalopathy, although clinical presenta-

TABLE 45–2
Stages of Hepatic Encephalopathy

Stage	Mental State	Neuromuscular State
I	Mild confusion, euphoria, depression, decreased attention, slowness of mentation, slurred speech	Mild incoordination, impaired handwriting
II	Drowsiness, inappropriate behavior, intermittent disorientation	Asterixis, ataxia, dysarthria
III	Sleeps most of the time but rousable, incoherent speech, marked confusion	Hyperreflexia, muscle rigidity
IV	Coma that is responsive to painful stimuli (IVA) or unresponsive to painful stimuli (IVB)	Decerebrate posturing, abnormal oculovestibular response

tion may vary from patient to patient. The hepatic encephalopathy seen in fulminant liver failure is similar to that seen in chronic liver failure, but there are some differences (Table 45–3). Asterixis (flapping tremor of the hand) and sensory disturbances, such as paresthesias or hallucinations, may be present. As a result of the altered level of consciousness, it is important that neurologic assessments be performed with attention to the patient's ability to maintain his or her airway open.

Pathophysiology of Hepatic Encephalopathy in Cirrhosis

The precipitating factors of hepatic encephalopathy are as follows:
- GI bleeding
- Systemic infections
- Drugs
- Dietary protein load
- Alkalosis
- Diarrhea or dehydration
- Constipation
- Azotemia

Altered ammonia metabolism is most closely identified with this type of hepatic encephalopathy. The majority of serum ammonia originates in the gastrointestinal (GI) tract, where it results from the metabolism of ingested proteins, breakdown of blood, or

degradation of urea secreted into the colon. The ammonia is usually detoxified in the liver by the synthesis of urea. When the liver is bypassed, as it is in portal-systemic shunting, the major site of ammonia detoxification is eliminated, and ammonia accumulates in the blood. The ammonia traverses the blood-brain barrier, where it has neurotoxic effects.

Management of Hepatic Encephalopathy

Lactulose. Lactulose is a synthetic disaccharide that is not absorbed but is metabolized by intestinal bacteria. It reduces the pH of the intestinal milieu and facilitates the conversion of ammonia (NH_3) to ammonium (NH_4^+). The NH_4^+ is trapped within the bowel and eliminated during catharsis. Lactulose speeds bowel evacuation; it also stimulates intestinal bacteria to take up ammonia and incorporate it into bacterial protein synthesis. The desired effect is to cause two to three bowel movements per day. Lactulose can be administered either orally, through a nasogastric tube, or in the rectum. Lactulose is a synthetic disaccharide and may cause increased glucose levels. Therefore, glucose levels should be monitored, and patients should be assessed for signs of hyperglycemia. In addition, lactulose should be used with caution in patients with diabetes mellitus.

Antibiotic Therapy. Antibiotics reduce the intestinal bacterial flora, thereby reducing the number available to convert urea and amino acids into ammonia and other toxic metabolites. Neomycin is the most commonly used antibiotic, and its nephrotoxic effects must be considered prior to its administration.

Protein Intake. Protein intake should be restricted or eliminated because dietary protein may be the source of various harmful substances, including ammonia, mercaptans, and amino acids. A reduction in protein intake (0.5 g/kg per day) diminishes a source of hepatotoxins.

Metabolic

Carbohydrate Metabolism

The pathology occurring in the liver may result in the liver's inability to store glycogen and to perform gluconeogenesis. This inability can result in hypoglycemia.

TABLE 45–3
Hepatic Encephalopathy in Fulminant and Chronic Hepatic Failure

Type	Onset of Symptoms	Pathophysiology	Additional
Fulminant	Within 8 weeks of the onset of liver-related symptoms	Increased levels of inhibitory neurotransmitter	Cerebral edema and ↑ intracranial pressure
Chronic	>8 weeks after the onset of liver-related symptoms	Portal systemic shunting, resulting in altered ammonia metabolism	Cerebral edema and ↑ intracranial pressure absent

Fat Metabolism

The liver is responsible for the synthesis of lipoproteins, cholesterol, and phospholipids. It also breaks down fat into glycerol and fatty acids and eventually acetyl coenzyme A. Abnormal lipid metabolism reduces the availability of triglycerides for energy and lipoproteins for transport. Abnormalities in cholesterol synthesis cause disruption of bile salt synthesis. Bile salts are required for the absorption of fats and fat-soluble vitamins (A, D, E, and K) from the GI tract.

Protein Metabolism

The liver synthesizes serum proteins, deaminates amino acids, and converts ammonia to urea. In liver failure, serum proteins such as albumin, alpha and beta globulins, and fibrinogen are not produced in sufficient quantities. Albumin is therefore not able to maintain serum colloid osmotic pressure. The alpha and beta globulins are not available to transport other proteins and act as cellular enzymes. Fibrinogen (factor I) is not accessible for the coagulation process. The deamination of amino acids results in their availability as an energy source. Since this function is altered during liver failure, energy cannot be obtained from this source. As previously discussed in relation to hepatic encephalopathy, the conversion of ammonia to urea normally occurs in the liver. An abnormally functioning liver cannot perform this process, causing exceptional levels of ammonia.

Management

Glucose Monitoring. The patient should be assessed for signs of hypoglycemia, and glucose levels should be monitored.

Glucose Administration. Glucose may be administered as a bolus ($D_{50}W$), as continuous infusion with 10% glucose, or as parenteral nutrition.

Albumin Administration. Albumin is administered intravenously to aid in maintaining serum colloid oncotic pressure.

Endocrine

The liver is responsible for the inactivation of estrogen, testosterone, aldosterone, and cortisol. Elevated testosterone levels are the culprit of amenorrhea, or menstrual irregularity, in women, whereas elevated estrogen levels are responsible for testicular atrophy and gynecomastia in men and for pectoral and axillary alopecia and palmar erythema in both sexes. Surpluses of cortisol precipitate moon faces, weight gain, and striae.

Fluid and Electrolyte

Hyperaldosteronism predisposes the patient to fluid and electrolyte imbalances by stimulating sodium reabsorption while secreting potassium and hydrogen ions. This action explains the hypokalemic, metabolic alkalemia associated with hepatic failure. The enhanced sodium reabsorption results in water reabsorption.

Generalized edema (anasarca) and ascites (accumulation of fluid in the peritoneal cavity) occur as a result of decreased serum colloid osmotic pressure. This third spacing is further influenced by the presence of hyperaldosteronism and portal hypertension. Intravascular fluid volume can also be depleted by hematologic abnormalities coupled with portal hypertension and varices, causing a GI hemorrhage (Fig. 45–1).

Management

Abdominal Paracentesis. Abdominal paracentesis involves the removal of fluid from the peritoneum for diagnostic purposes or decompression to relieve dyspnea. It is important that the urinary bladder is emptied prior to the procedure to avoid puncturing the bladder during the procedure. The usual position for the patient is supine with the head of the bed elevated 45 to 90 degrees.

Restriction of Sodium and Fluids. Restriction of sodium and fluids may be used to limit ascites. Sodium and fluid intake is restricted to between 500 to 2000 mg per day and 500 to 1500 mL, respectively, based on the severity of the ascites.

Diuretics. Diuretics are administered to decrease edema. They should be administered cautiously, and it is essential that serum potassium levels be monitored. Prior to the administration of diuretics, albumin is often administered to promote the shifting of fluids from the interstitial spaces to the intravascular space. Furosemide is next administered after about 1 hour to cause diuresis of the fluid now within the intravascular space. Spironolactone is a popular choice for long-term diuretic therapy, because it is potassium sparing and inhibits aldosterone.

Colloid and Crystalloid Administration. The administration colloids, such as albumin and blood products (packed cells, stored plasma, and fresh-frozen plasma), or crystalloids, such as hespan or hetastarch, act to correct the serum colloid oncotic pressure and aid in shifting fluid from the interstitial spaces into the intravascular compartment.

Hematologic

The patient with hepatic failure is predisposed to bleeding for several reasons. Fibrinogen is not produced in sufficient quantities since protein metabolism is affected. Vitamin K is decreased as a result of decreased bile salts production, and therefore, the clotting factors dependent on vitamin K (factors II, VII, IX, and X) are reduced. Splenomegaly is often present in this patient population as a result of the

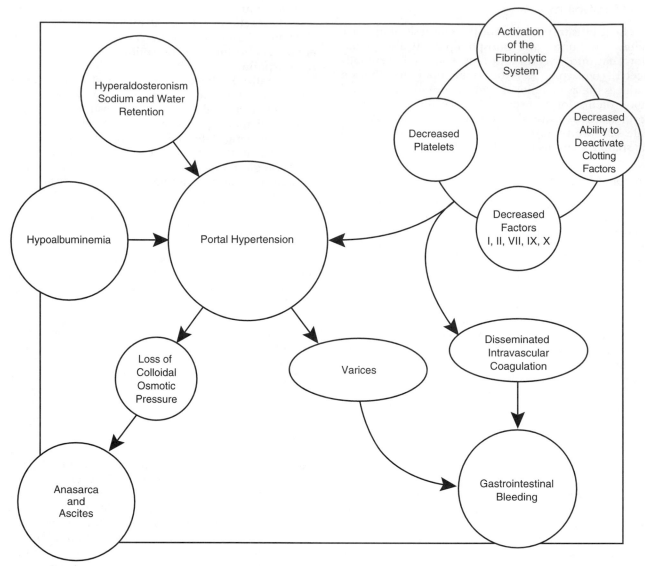

FIGURE 45–1. Intravascular fluid deficit.

portal hypertension and resulting distention of the splenic vein. The enlarged spleen removes platelets and white blood cells from the circulating blood volume, resulting in thrombocytopenia and leukopenia, respectively. Clotting factors, once activated, are typically inactivated by the liver. This function is not effective, precipitating the development of microthrombi and further consumption of platelets. The presence of microthrombi activates the fibrinolytic system and produces fibrin split products, which act as anticoagulants. These elements all play a role in the development of the disseminated intravascular coagulation that is often seen in patients with hepatic failure.

These patients are further predisposed to bleeding as a result of elevated pressures in the portal vein (portal hypertension). Venous blood from the stomach, spleen, intestines, pancreas, and mesentery ordinarily drains into the portal vein and passes through the liver. These organs are unable to adequately drain, resulting in elevated pressures and development of varices. Varices in the esophagus and lower GI tract are the culprits of GI bleeding.

Management

Administration of Blood Components. In the presence of active bleeding, packed red blood cells are administered to treat a low hemoglobin and hematocrit. Fresh-frozen plasma provides blood clotting factors, and platelet administration corrects thrombocytopenia.

Gastric Lavage. Gastric lavage involves the instillation and removal of normal saline through a nasogastric tube to control bleeding by inducing vasoconstriction of gastric vessels. This process removes toxins, blood clots, and old blood from the stomach.

Balloon Tamponade Therapy

Sengstaken-Blakemore Tube. The Sengstaken-Blakemore tube is a triple-lumen red rubber catheter inserted through the nose or the mouth (Fig. 45–2). The three lumens provide a port for gastric aspiration, inflation of a gastric balloon, and inflation of an esophageal balloon. The inflation of these balloons places direct pressure, or balloon tamponade, on bleeding esophageal or gastric varices. It is most important to closely monitor the patient's airway. Deflation or rupture of the gastric balloon will allow the tube to migrate upward, and the esophageal balloon may cause airway obstruction. Nursing considerations are as follows:

- Discuss elective intubation of the patient with the physician before insertion.
- Obtain a chest x-ray to verify placement.
- Maintain esophageal balloon pressure from 20 to 40 mm Hg. Excessive pressures can lead to esophageal necrosis.
- Inflate the gastric balloon with 250 to 300 mL air.
- Keep scissors at the bedside to allow immediate deflation of balloons by cutting the lumens. Upward migration of the esophageal balloon or rupture of the gastric balloon may result in airway occlusion.
- Deflate the esophageal balloon for 12 to 24 hours preceding tube removal. If there is no recurrence of bleeding, the gastric balloon is deflated and the tube is removed.

Minnesota Tube. The Minnesota tube is a quadruple-lumen tube providing ports for gastric and esophageal aspiration and inflation of gastric and esophageal balloons (Fig. 45–3).

Sclerotherapy. Sclerotherapy is performed as an endoscopic procedure. Sclerosing agents are injected into varices to thrombose and obliterate them, thus decreasing the frequency and severity of bleeding. Epinephrine injections may be used to cause vasoconstriction of bleeding varices. The potential complications of this therapy are as follows:

Mild retrosternal pain
Transient dysphagia
Esophageal perforation
Esophageal ulceration
Esophageal stricture
Aspiration pneumonia or pleural effusion

Vasopressin. Vasopressin is a posterior pituitary antidiuretic hormone. It may be administered through a central line or preferably into a local site, such as the superior mesenteric artery. Vasopressin acts as a potent vasoconstrictor and is a synthetic source of factor VIII. Its vasoconstrictive properties affect the splanchnic vessels, and it reduces blood flow and pressure in the portal vein. It also decreases coronary blood flow and increases blood pressure and, therefore, may be administered concurrently with nitroglycerin. However, vasopressin therapy does have side effects (see box on page 826).

Transjugular Intrahepatic Portosystemic Shunt (TIPS).[1] TIPS is typically performed under fluoroscopy as a radiologic procedure. A puncture needle is advanced in a catheter through the jugular vein and inferior vena cava into a hepatic vein. Then an intrahepatic branch of the portal vein is punctured, and an expandable stent of metallic mesh is implanted to establish a shunt between the portal vein and hepatic vein, thus reducing portal hypertension (Fig. 45–4).

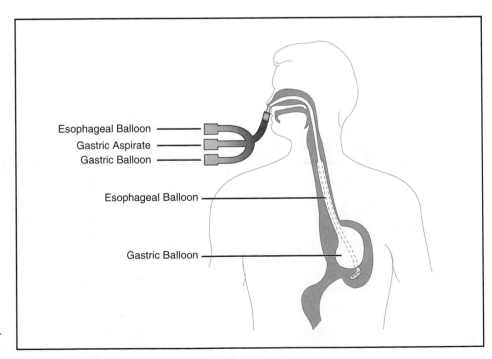

Esophageal Balloon
Gastric Aspirate
Gastric Balloon

Esophageal Balloon

Gastric Balloon

FIGURE 45–2. Sengstaken-Blakemore tube.

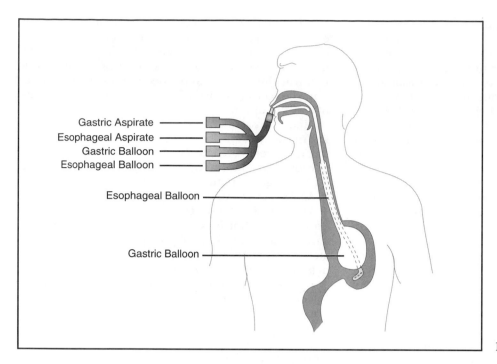

FIGURE 45–3. Minnesota tube.

Gastrointestinal

Anorexia, diarrhea, nausea, and vomiting are all early signs of hepatic failure. Complaints of dyspepsia, bloatedness, and gas pain are associated with impaired fat ingestion and absorption. Fetor hepaticus is a musty, sweetish breath odor that is thought to occur as a result of the liver's inability to metabolize methionine, an essential amino acid. Clay-colored stools occur because of obstructive jaundice.

Management

In treating symptoms, medications such as promethazine hydrochloride (Phenergan), prochlorperazine (Compazine), acetaminophen, and salicylates should be avoided, because these are hepatotoxic drugs.

SIDE EFFECTS OF VASOPRESSIN THERAPY

Cardiovascular:
Hypertension
Angina
Myocardial infarction
Peripheral cyanosis
Bradycardia
Gastrointestinal and Genitourinary:
Abdominal cramping
Nausea
Diarrhea
Decreased urinary output

Cardiovascular

Portal hypertension, ascites, bleeding, and overzealous diuresis can alter circulating fluid volume, resulting in hypotension. Sinus tachycardia may ensue in an effort to maintain an adequate cardiac output. Electrolyte disturbances, such as hypokalemia, may stimulate ventricular arrhythmias, such as premature ventricular contractions.

Management

Fluid Administration. Use of colloids, such as albumin, packed red blood cells, or plasma, or of crystalloids, such as hespan or hetastarch, assists in correcting colloidal osmotic pressures.

Potassium Administration. Potassium may be administered orally, nasogastrically, or intravenously to correct ventricular arrhythmias.

Hemodynamic Monitoring. Preload indicators may be evaluated through the use of central venous catheters. A desirable central venous pressure (CVP) is 2 to 6 mmHg. If a pulmonary artery catheter is used, the desired pulmonary artery wedge pressure (PAWP) is 6 to 12 mmHg with a cardiac index (CI) of greater than or equal to 2.5 L/min.

Pulmonary

Pronounced ascites can limit the patient's ability for respiratory expansion, resulting in dyspnea and hypoxemia.

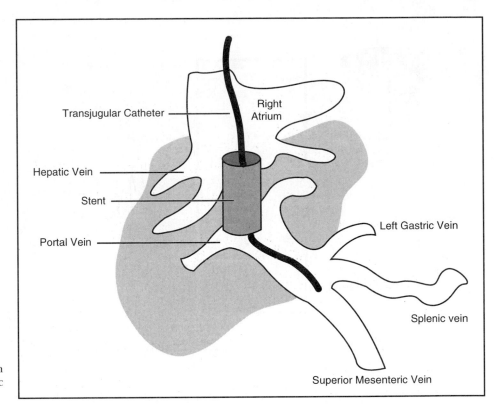

FIGURE 45–4. Implantation of a transjugular intrahepatic portosystemic shunt.

Management

Paracentesis. Paracentesis removes the fluid from the peritoneal cavity and relieves the pressure on the diaphragm and abdominal organs, resulting in easier breathing.

Position: Elevate the head of the bed 45 to 90 degrees to aid breathing.

Oxygen Therapy. Oxygen may be administered to the patient through nasal cannula or face mask to treat hypoxemia.

Intubation and Mechanical Ventilation. Intubation may be initiated for patients who are unable to maintain an airway because of severe hepatic encephalopathy or intense hypoxemia. It can also be used to protect the airway during balloon tamponade therapy.

Renal

Hepatorenal syndrome is renal failure without obvious cause in the presence of liver disease. It is believed to result from a decrease in plasma volume. The portal hypertension, ascites, and hypoalbuminemia may add to the diminished perfusion, with resulting acute tubular necrosis.

Management

Maintain Intravascular Volume. Crystalloids or colloids are used to maintain adequate intravascular volumes and prevent vasoconstriction of renal vessels. Adequate volume replacement is confirmed with a urinary output of greater than or equal to 30 mL/h, a CVP of 2 to 6 mmHg, a heart rate from 60 to 100 beats/min, and a blood pressure in normal limits for the patient.

Dermatologic

In the patient with hepatic failure, several dermatologic signs may be present. Jaundice occurs when bilirubin is deposited in the skin, mucous membranes, and sclera. Spider angiomas are vascular lesions that appear as central red bodies with radiating branches or legs and are associated with estrogen imbalances. Caput medusae are dilated abdominal veins radiating from the umbilicus in the presence of portal hypertension.

TREATMENT FOR HEPATIC FAILURE

Liver transplantation has been the primary option available for patients with hepatic failure. However, the future holds another option. An extracorporeal liver assist device (ELAD)[2] has been developed and is being implemented in patients. The device is a hollow fiber cartridge containing liver cells. The cells perform normal liver functions such as ureogenesis and gluconeogenesis, and they secrete clotting factors and

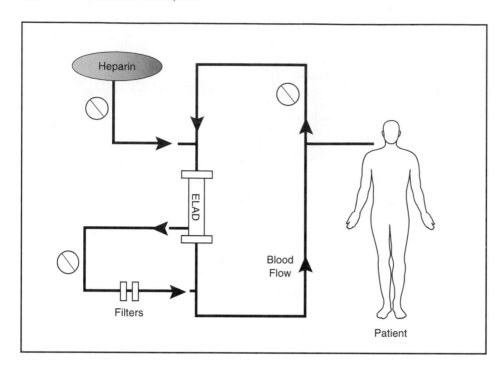

FIGURE 45–5. Extracorporeal liver assist device (ELAD) vascular access and blood flow.

other liver-specific proteins. The patient is vascularly accessed, and blood flows through the cartridge using a modified hemodialysis approach (Fig. 45–5).

NURSING CARE OF THE PATIENT WITH HEPATIC FAILURE

Nursing care of the patient with hepatic failure is especially challenging because the liver is involved in so many life-sustaining processes. Hepatic dysfunction affects every organ system in the body. Therefore, critical care nurses must have a keen understanding of basic physiologic and psychological processes and of the pathophysiologic responses underlying liver disease. Knowing what to expect in hepatic dysfunction helps the nurse to assess the patient thoroughly, to

identify actual and/or potential alterations in body processes, and to plan and implement timely and appropriate interventions.

Priority Nursing Diagnoses

Priority nursing diagnoses, desired patient outcomes, and nursing interventions and rationales are presented in the care plan at the end of this chapter.

REFERENCES

1. Rossle, M, et al: Transjugular intrahepatic portosystemic stent-shunt procedure for variceal bleeding. N Engl J Med 330:165, 1994.
2. Sussman, N, et al: Extracorporeal liver support. J Clin Gastroenterol 18:320, 1994.

CARE PLAN FOR THE PATIENT WITH HEPATIC FAILURE AND HEPATIC ENCEPHALOPATHY

Nursing Diagnoses

Nursing Diagnosis #1
Fluid volume deficit (intravascular, actual), related to:
1. Ascites and anasarca (third spacing)
   - Hypoalbuminemia
   - Portal hypertension
   - Hyperaldosteronism (secondary)
2. Bleeding.
   - Bleeding varices
   - Coagulopathy
(For fluid volume deficit related to hypovolemic, hemorrhagic shock, see care plan at the end of Chapter 44, nursing diagnosis #1.)

Desired Patient Outcomes

Patient will:
1. Maintain stable hemodynamics:
   - Heart rate (resting) 60–100 beats/min.
   - CVP 2–6 mmHg.
   - PCWP 6–12 mmHg.
   - CI >2.5 L/min.
   - Systemic arterial blood pressure within 10 mmHg of baseline.
2. Maintain baseline mental and neurologic status; deep tendon reflexes brisk.
3. Achieve resolution of ascites and anasarca.
   - Body weight within 5% of baseline.
   - Abdominal girth at baseline measurement.
   - Functioning peritoneovenous shunt (if inserted).
4. Balance intake and output.
5. Maintain urine output >30 mL/h.
6. Maintain laboratory parameters as follows:
   - Serum osmolality 285–295 mOsm/Kg.
   - Serum sodium >135 and <148 mEq/L.
   - Serum albumin 3.5–5.5 g/100 mL.
   - Hematocrit 37%–52%.
   - Hemoglobin 12–18 g/100 mL.
   - Platelet count >150,000 mm^3.

Nursing Interventions

- Assess for signs and symptoms of hypovolemia:
  - Assess cardiovascular function:
    - Heart rate (resting).

    - Hypotension (orthostatic).

    - Skin color—pallor, mottled appearance; cyanosis; cool to touch; peripheral edema (anasarca).

    - Assess for ascites—abdominal assessment:
      - Inspect for bulging of flanks or a protruding, misplaced umbilicus; skin tautness; new striae.
      - Percuss for shifting dullness.
      - Palpate for fluid wave.

    - Measure abdominal girth daily using markings indicated on abdomen.

    - Determine body weight.

    - Assess serum albumin levels.

Rationales

- Establish baseline assessment data with which to evaluate the patient's response to therapy.
  - An increase in heart rate reflects a compensatory response to maintain cardiac output.
  - A decrease in blood pressure of >10–15 mmHg from a supine to sitting position reflects a reduced circulatory (intravascular) volume.
  - Compensatory peripheral vasoconstriction shunts blood from skin and nonvital organs to the heart and brain.
  - Ascites results from a combination of low intravascular colloidal osmotic pressure (hypoalbuminemia), portal hypertension, and secondary retention of sodium and water.
    - When forces favoring movement of fluid from the intravascular space into the interstitium (portal hypertension) exceed forces favoring movement of fluid in the opposite direction (e.g., decreased intravascular colloidal osmotic pressure), fluid accumulates. When the capacity of the lymphatic system to return fluid to the circulating blood is exceeded, ascites results. Of central importance to the formation of ascites is renal sodium and water retention.
  - Measurement of abdominal girth assists in evaluating the status of the ascites. Markings made on the abdomen help to assure that repeated measurements are made at the same circumference; measure with patient in same position. Clinical findings of ascites are usually demonstrable after >1500 mL of ascites fluid has accumulated.
  - Daily measurement of body weight most closely reflects total body fluid volume.
  - Serum albumin is largely responsible for maintaining serum colloidal osmotic pressure.

CARE PLAN FOR THE PATIENT WITH HEPATIC FAILURE AND HEPATIC ENCEPHALOPATHY (*Continued*)

Nursing Interventions	Rationales
□ Cardiac monitoring.	□ Cardiac arrhythmias may occur in respone to ischemia or electrolyte imbalance.
□ Hemodynamic pressure monitoring parameters: CVP; pulmonary artery pressure; PCWP; CI; arterial pressure monitoring.	□ Monitoring of these parameters is indicated in the setting of hypovolemic shock, hemodynamic instability, and during massive fluid, albumin, and blood replacement, to monitor patient's response to therapy and prevent fluid overload.
○ Assess neurologic function: mental status, orientation; thought processes; motor responses.	○ Assists in assessing for encephalopathy or hypoxemia.
○ Assess renal function: intake and output; hourly urine output; monitor creatinine and BUN.	○ Hypovolemia can cause a decrease in renal perfusion; patients with hepatic failure are at risk of developing hepatorenal failure. Renal function is best monitored by serum creatinine; BUN may be altered by GI bleeding and impaired liver function.
○ Assess for signs and symptoms of electrolyte imbalance: hypokalemia—general malaise, fatigue, anorexia, nausea, vomiting, diarrhea; abdominal cramps; muscle weakness; hyporeflexia; cardiac arrhythmias.	○ Excessive sodium reabsorption and retention associated with increased aldosterone secretion and diuretic therapy can predispose to hypokalemia and metabolic alkalemia.
• Implement prescribed measures to reestablish normovolemia:	• Therapeutic goal is to gradually mobilize fluid back into the intravascular compartment and prevent further third spacing.
○ Maintain fluid restriction (~500–1500 mL/day).	○ To decrease ascites and generalized edema.
○ Maintain sodium restriction (500–2000 mg/day).	○ To reduce fluid retention as ascites and anasarca and to enhance mobilization of excessive fluids from the tissues.
□ Avoid use of saline for intravenous therapy, gastric lavage, or other irrigation.	
○ Administer diuretic therapy with necessary potassium replacement therapy.	○ Controlled diuresis decreases water load, with consequent reduction in ascites and edema; it minimizes the risk of renal failure.
□ Furosemide, thiazide diuretics.	□ Require monitoring of serum potassium with concomitant potassium replacement therapy.
□ Spironolactone therapy.	□ A potassium-sparing diuretic, it inhibits the action of aldosterone on the distal tubular cells, thereby increasing excretion of sodium, chloride, and water, while retaining potassium.
○ Administer inotropic agents and vasopressors (e.g., low-dose dopamine).	○ To increase cardiac output and maintain effective renal perfusion.
○ Administer protein supplementation.	○ To restore intravascular colloidal osmotic pressure to within acceptable physiologic range, and to enhance movement of ascitic and edema fluid into the intravascular space, promoting diuresis.
○ Administer salt-poor albumin intravenously.	○ Replaces albumin levels, restores intravascular volume, and maintains renal perfusion. Monitor for fluid overload.
• Assist with abdominal paracentesis:	• In patients with severe ascites, paracentesis may be necessary to relieve dyspnea and compromised respiratory excursion and/or urinary frequency.
○ Have patient urinate before procedure.	○ Reduces risk of nicking bladder with needle.
○ Provide necessary explanations.	○ May help patient to relax.
○ Position appropriately and as comfortably as possible.	
○ Remove fluid slowly.	○ Sufficient quantity of fluid is removed to decrease intra-abdominal pressure; altered hemodynamics, including hypotension and shock, can be precipitated by the removal of too large a volume of fluid.
○ Monitor vital signs before, during, and after paracentesis.	○ Assists in assessing possible intra-abdominal bleeding.
○ Measure abdominal girth before and after paracentesis, and daily thereafter.	○ Assists in assessing for further fluid accumulation.
□ Assess insertion site; monitor for complications of hypotension, bleeding, protein depletion, and infection.	

CARE PLAN FOR THE PATIENT WITH HEPATIC FAILURE AND HEPATIC ENCEPHALOPATHY (*Continued*)

Nursing Interventions

- Implement ongoing monitoring:

  ○ Cardiovascular status:
    □ Monitor heart rate, pulses, blood pressures, hemodynamic parameters.
  ○ Respiratory status:
    □ Monitor respiratory rate and pattern; respiratory excursion, breath sounds (normal and adventitious).

    □ Monitor arterial blood gases.

  ○ Renal status: assess urine output (hourly); BUN, creatinine.
  ○ Assess fluid and electrolyte status: accurate intake and output; daily weight; daily measurement of abdominal girth.
  ○ Serum studies: electrolytes; protein (albumin/globulin ratio); osmolality, glucose.
  ○ Urine studies: electrolytes, specific gravity.
- Assist in preparation of patient for:
  ○ Sclerotherapy
  ○ Sengstaken-Blakemore tube
  ○ TIPS procedure

Rationales

- Assists in evaluating the patient's response to therapy; reduces risk of complications.
  ○ Patients with cirrhosis, ascites, and bleeding potential are at high risk of complications.

  ○ Respiratory embarrassment caused by ascites can lead to pulmonary complications; e.g., compromised alveolar ventilation with CO_2 retention (CO_2 narcosis may complicate the clinical representation of hepatic encephalopathy); and pneumonia.
  ○ Assists in evaluating effectiveness of ventilation; and acid-base balance.

  ○ Assists in evaluating the patient's response to therapy.

Nursing Diagnoses

Nursing Diagnosis #2
Breathing pattern, ineffective, related to:
1. Ascites (abdominal distention)
2. Weakened, debilitated state
3. Hepatic encephalopathy

Desired Patient Outcome

Patient will:
1. Maintain baseline mental status.
2. Maintain effective respiratory function:
   - Respiratory rate <25–30/min.
   - Tidal volume (V_T) >5–7 mL/Kg.
   - Vital capacity (V_C) >12–15 mL/Kg.

Nursing Interventions

- Assess respiratory function: Assess specific parameters—rate, pattern, depth of breathing; symmetry of chest wall and diaphragmatic excursion.

  ○ Assess use of accessory muscles; breath sounds, evidence of adventitious sounds (rales, wheezes); dyspnea, tachypnea, orthopnea.
  ○ Assess effectiveness of cough; sputum production.

  ○ Assess pulmonary volume/capacity: tidal volume (V_T); vital capacity (V_C).
  ○ Monitor arterial blood gases: PaO_2, $PaCO_2$ pH
- Assess tissue perfusion and oxygenation.
  ○ Assess cerebral function: mental status—restlessness, apprehension, confusion; drowsiness.
  ○ Assess cardiovascular function: evidence of cyanosis—lips, mucous membranes, nail beds; vital signs—heart rate, blood pressure, peripheral pulses, cardiac arrhythmias.
  ○ Assess fluid status: intake and output; body weight.
  ○ Laboratory data: hematocrit, hemoglobin, serum electrolytes; BUN; serum osmolality.
- Assist patient to semi-Fowler's position.

Rationales

- Ascites causes pressure on diaphragm, limiting respiratory excursion and contributing to decreased alveolar ventilation and to atelectasis. The end result is hypoxemia.
  ○ Weakened, debilitated status may compromise patient's respiratory effort, reducing alveolar ventilation and predisposing to hypoxemia.
  ○ Accumulation of fluids and secretions reduces ventilation and predisposes to infection.

  ○ Reflect effectiveness of ventilation and gas exchange.
- These signs and symptoms may be reflective of hypoxemia and tissue hypoxia.

- This position allows for maximal respiratory excursion and lung expansion. Adequate lung expansion facilitates more even distribution of ventilation; it enhances ventilation/perfusion matching.

CVP = central venous pressure; PCWP = pulmonary capillary wedge pressure; CI = cardiac index.

CHAPTER 46

Nursing Management of the Patient with Acute Pancreatitis

Vivian Nowazek

CHAPTER OUTLINE

Acute Pancreatitis: Definition and
   Classification
Etiology and Pathogenesis
□ Pathophysiology
□ Clinical Presentation and Physical
   Findings
□ Diagnosis

□ Complications
□ Prognosis
□ Treatment
□ Nursing Care of the Patient with
   Acute Pancreatitis
References
Suggested Readings

LEARNING OBJECTIVES

After completing this chapter, you should be able to:

1. Define acute pancreatitis and its classifications.
2. Describe the etiology and pathogenesis of acute pancreatitis.
3. Examine the underlying pathophysiology associated with acute pancreatitis.
4. Describe the clinical presentation of acute pancreatitis based on underlying pathophysiologic processes.
5. Specify the essential components of the assessment of the patient/family health status.
6. List the potential complications of acute pancreatitis and the implications for nursing care.
7. Define the goals of treatment and the treatment priorities.
8. Describe the nursing process in the care of the patient with acute pancreatitis, including:
   a. Assessment
   b. Nursing diagnosis
   c. Planning: Desired patient outcomes
                   Nursing interventions and rationales.

ACUTE PANCREATITIS: DEFINITION AND CLASSIFICATION

Acute pancreatitis is an acute inflammatory process involving autodigestion of the pancreas by its own enzymes. The severity of acute pancreatitis varies, with classification occurring along a continuum, from mild to severe (Table 46–1). The reason for variation in severity is unknown.

ETIOLOGY AND PATHOGENESIS

The exact cause of acute pancreatitis remains unknown, but a number of factors and disease states

have been linked to its development (see box on page 833). The most common etiologic factors are biliary tract disease, with gallstones involving the common bile duct and the ampulla of Vater (see Fig. 42–3); chronic alcoholism (considered to be the most common cause of chronic pancreatitis); and idiopathic acute pancreatitis. Acute pancreatitis associated with cholelithiasis is more common among middle-agd females and the elderly, while acute pancreatitis associated with alcoholism is more common in men in their 40s.[1]

Normally, four barriers protect the pancreas from autodigestion: (1) the activation of proteolytic enzymes only after secretion into the intestines, (2) the secretion of pancreatic trypsin inhibitor, (3) an

TABLE 46–1
The 1992 Atlanta Classification System of Acute Pancreatitis (AP)

	Mild Acute Pancreatitis	Severe Acute Pancreatitis
Old terms	Edematous pancreatitis Interstitial pancreatitis	Hemorrhagic pancreatitis Necrotizing pancreatitis
Definition	Minimal organ dysfunction	Organ failure, pseudocyst, abscess, necrosis
Incidence of cases	About 75%	About 25%
Clinical signs/symptoms	Hypotension that responds to fluid resuscitation Suspect complications if no resolution in 48–72 h	Abdominal findings of increased tenderness, rebound or distention, hypoactive or absent bowel sounds
	Upper abdominal pain Vomiting	Presence of epigastric mass Rarely: flank or periumbilical ecchymosis
	Fever, tachycardia, leukocytosis Elevated pancreatic enzymes	≥3 Ranson criteria ≥8 APACHE-II criteria
		Organ Failure • Shock (systolic blood pressure <90 mmHg) • Pulmonary insufficiency (PAo_2 ≤60 mmHg) • Renal failure (creatinine >2 mg% after rehydration) • Gastrointestinal bleeding (>500 mL/24 h)
		Systemic Complications • Disseminated intravascular coagulation (platelets ≤100,000 mm^3) • Fibrinogen <100 mg/dL • Fibrin split products >80 μg/mL
		Severe Metabolic Disturbances • Calcium ≤7.5 mg/dL
		Local Complications • Acute fluid collections • Pseudocyst • Abscess • Necrosis
Pathology	Interstitial edema Microscopic areas of parenchymal necrosis Possible parapancreatic fat necrosis	Pancreatic necrosis

ETIOLOGIES OF ACUTE PANCREATITIS IN UNITED STATES

>80% of Cases:
Biliary tract stone disease
Chronic ethanol abuse
Idiopathic
10% of Cases:
Idiopathic
<10% of Cases, Other:
Pancreatic trauma
Pancreatic tumors
Infections
Pancreatotoxic drugs
Hyperlipoproteinemia
Postoperative state
Hyperparathyroidism
Hypercalcemia
Endoscopic cannulation of pancreatic duct

intraductal pressure gradient between the pancreatic and common bile duct, and (4) the sphincter of Oddi. Although the mechanism by which the etiologic factors bypass the protective barriers and initiate acute pancreatitis is uncertain, several theories have been proposed (Table 46–2). Current theories attribute acute pancreatitis to direct toxic effects on the acinar or ductal cells by proteolytic enzymes and ischemic damage secondary to changes in the microcirculation of the pancreatic gland.

Pathophysiology

Regardless of the etiology of acute pancreatitis, pancreatic enzymes are activated prematurely, causing digestion of pancreatic tissue. Trypsinogen is converted to trypsin, which activates phospholipase A, elastase, the kallikrein-kallidin-bradykinin system, and the renin-angiotensin system. Trypsin and chymotrypsin break down parenchymal tissue protein, causing edema and hemorrhage. Phospholipase A converts lecithin to lysolecithin, which digests the phospholipid constituents of the acinar cell membranes, producing

TABLE 46–2
Theories of Acute Pancreatitis (AP)

Theory	Process	Reason Negated
Common biliopancreatic channel	Bile refluxes into pancreatic duct, triggering AP.	• Normally, pancreatic secretory pressure exceeds biliary secretory pressure; therefore, stone creating common channel would favor reflux of pancreatic juice into biliary system rather than bile into pancreatic ductal system. • Many patients have too short a common channel, so an obstructing stone would not cause reflux. • Bile perfused through ductal system under physiologic pressure does not precipitate AP.
Duodenal reflux	Duodenal juice containing pancreatic digestive enzymes refluxes through incompetent sphincter of Oddi into pancreatic ductal system, triggering AP.	Division of sphincter of Oddi during sphincterotomy to create incompetent sphincter does not lead to AP.
Pancreatic ductal obstruction	Continued bile secretion into obstructed ductal system results in pancreatic ductal hypertension, triggering AP.	Bile reflux into pancreatic ductal system is not required for development of AP.
Toxic effect theory	Pancreatic enzymes and alcohol have toxic effect on acinar or ductal cells.	Current theory
Ischemic theory	AP is caused by changes in microcirculation of pancreatic gland.	Current theory

edema, fat necrosis, and coagulation. Microembolic and consumptive coagulopathy is thought to lead to the development of disseminated intravascular coagulation (DIC). Lipase triggers fat necrosis of the pancreatic and surrounding tissues by converting neutral fats into free fatty acids. The consequent liberation of large amounts of fatty acids is thought to predispose to hypocalcemia because calcium is taken up by these fatty acids in the form of calcium salts. Elastase digests collagen and the elastic fibers in blood vessel walls, leading to hemorrhage, ischemia, and necrosis.

Activation of the kallikrein-kallidin-bradykinin system (a system of serum proteins that amplifies the humoral immunologic response) predisposes capillary walls to edema, vasodilation with increased capillary permeability, infiltration of inflammatory cells, and pain. This inflammatory process results in devitalization of pancreatic parenchyma and loss of serum albumin in the exudates. The resulting hypoalbuminemia causes massive fluid shifts from the intravascular space into the interstitium (pancreatic ascites). As much as 5 to 6 liters of fluid can sequester in the interstitial spaces during the early phase of acute pancreatitis. If left untreated, the resulting hypovolemia, hypotension, and depressed cardiac function can lead to hypovolemic shock and death.

Complement factors activate polymorphonuclear leukocytes, which cause increased stickiness and formation of intravascular microaggregates. When lodged in the pulmonary microvasculature, microaggregates may release oxygen-free radicals, leukotrienes, prostaglandins, and lysosomal enzymes. More polymorphonuclear leukocytes are thought to be recruited to the site, causing further capillary membrane damage and increased vascular permeability.

Activation of the renin-angiotensin system causes the development of renal complications. Impaired renal function is also associated with hypoperfusion and microthrombi from the hypercoagulable state.

Autodigestion of the parenchymal tissue is a destructive cycle. As the enzymes digest the tissue, the acinar cells are damaged, leading to the release of more enzymes for activation, causing more tissue destruction. When proteolytic enzymes digest their way through the surface of the pancreas, pancreatic juice seeps into the peritoneal cavity, causing a chemical peritonitis. Zones of fat necrosis and calcium deposition may develop throughout the omenta, and possibly the mesentery. Large acute fluid collections, an acute pseudocyst, pancreatic abscess, or pancreatic necrosis (Table 46–3) may develop.

Clinical Presentation and Physical Findings

Clinical manifestations of acute pancreatitis depend on the extent of inflammation and destruction of pancreatic tissue (Table 46–4). Severe, persistent upper abdominal pain is the clinical hallmark of acute pancreatitis, occurring in about 95% of patients.[2] This pain is usually the reason patients seek medical attention. It is usually described as severe, relentless, knife-like, twisting, and deep in the midepigastric or periumbilical region, which may radiate around either costal margin, to the spine, flank, or left shoulder. The degree of pain correlates strongly with the extent of pancreatic involvement.[3] The pain becomes overwhelming as autodigestion generates inflammation and necrosis. To reduce the intensity of the pain, the

TABLE 46–3
Local Symptoms of Acute Pancreatitis (AP)

Local Symptom	Definition	% of AP Cases	Onset
Acute fluid collection (AFC)	Fluid collection in or near pancreas; lacks wall of granulation or fibrous tissue	40%–50%	Early in course of AP; about 50% regress spontaneously for unknown reason; common in severe AP
Acute pseudocyst	Collection of usually sterile pancreatic enzymes enclosed by well-defined, nonepithelialized wall	10%–15%	4 weeks or more after onset of AP
Pancreatic abscess	A circumscribed intra-abdominal collection of pus usually close to pancreas, with little or no pancreatic necrosis	1%–2%	4 weeks or more after onset of severe AP
Pancreatic necrosis	Diffuse or focal area(s) of nonviable, devitalized pancreatic parenchyma and parapancreatic fat necrosis: 1. Sterile pancreatic necrosis (lacks pancreatic enzymes and bacteria) 2. Infected pancreatic necrosis	About 20%	Early in course of AP
Phlegmon	Term no longer in use		
Infected pseudocyst	Term no longer in use		

TABLE 46–4
Clinical Manifestations of Acute Pancreatitis (AP)

System	Symptom	Cause(s)
Neurologic	Pain	Peritoneal chemical burn from pancreatic enzymes and kinin peptides, pancreatic edema and distension, biliary tree obstruction, duodenal obstruction, pancreatic acute fluid collection, pancreatic acute pseudocyst, pancreatic abscess, pancreatic necrosis
	Fever >102°F	Cholangitis, cholecystitis, peritonitis, intra-abdominal abscess
	Restlessness, agitation, confusion	Decreased cerebral perfusion secondary to hypoperfusion
	Toxic psychosis	Lipolytic demyelination of central nervous system
	Muscle tremors/weakness, lethargy, hyporeflexia	Hypocalcemia, hypomagnesemia
	Pancreatic retinopathy	Complement-induced embolization of leukocyte aggregates
Cardiovascular	Hypotension	Vasodilation, fluid sequestration, hemorrhage
	Anemia	Bleeding from wall of pseudocyst, effect of myocardial depressant factor, disseminated intravascular coagulation
Respiratory	Tachypnea	Anxiety, pain, hypermetabolic state
	Pleural effusion(s)	Pancreatic exudate crossing diaphragm and entering pleural cavity through lymphatic channels
	Pulmonary embolus	Complement-induced embolization of leukocyte aggregates
Gastrointestinal	Diminished/absent bowel sounds	Slowed peristalsis secondary to fluid sequestration in bowel
	Jaundice	Biliary tree obstruction
	Nausea/vomiting	Obstruction of pylorus or duodenum
	Dysphagia	High retrogastric obstruction
	Portal hypertension	Splenic vein obstruction
	Gray, greasy, foul-smelling stool	85%–90% loss of pancreatic ability to secrete digestive enzymes
	Hematemesis/melena	Gastritis, gastric, or esophageal varices
	Gray-blue flank/periumbilical area, marbled abdomen (Grey Turner's/Cullen's sign)	Pancreatic hemorrhage
Genitourinary	Oliguria	Hypoperfusion of kidneys and microemboli from hypercoagulable state
	Icteric, frothy urine	Biliuremia
Musculoskeletal	Tender subcutaneous nodules on buttocks, thighs, upper arms, thorax, pretibial, malleolar areas	Subcutaneous and periarticular fat necrosis

patient usually sits up in a flexed fetal position, because a supine position tends to exacerbate the pain.

Protracted vomiting is frequently present and is worsened by food or drink. Vomiting does not usually relieve the pain or nausea. On physical examination, abdominal tenderness, guarding, distention, and tympany are present. Peritoneal signs, such as abdominal rigidity, ascites, and rebound tenderness, may also be present. Hypoactive or absent bowel sounds are common. Steatorrhea may be present.

Fever, usually less than 102°F, is a common symptom. The presence of an elevated temperature greater than 102°F may indicate infectious complications. Infectious complications account for more than 80% of all deaths from acute pancreatitis.[3]

Hypovolemic shock may manifest as hypotension, tachycardia, respiratory alkalosis, cold mottled skin, restlessness, weakness, diaphoresis, and oliguria. The oliguria is usually associated with acute tubular necrosis. Hypovolemic shock occurs in 30% to 40% of patients with acute pancreatitis and is the leading cause of death in the first few days after the onset of symptoms.[1] The mortality rate approximates 80% if acute renal failure develops.[1]

Jaundice and mild elevation of liver enzymes, especially alkaline phosphatase, are usually transient, resolving within 1 week. Peritoneal ascites and/or palpable abdominal masses are associated with severe pancreatic disease and with the development of pancreatic and parapancreatic fat or hemorrhagic necrosis, pancreatic pseudocyst, or abscess.

Hemorrhage within and around the pancreas manifests as gray-blue discoloration of the flank (Grey Turner's sign) or around the umbilical region (Cullen's sign). These signs usually appear 1 to 2 weeks after the onset of hemorrhage. Pancreatic hemorrhage is associated with a high mortality.

Respiratory complications include elevation of the diaphragm, pleural effusion (usually left pleural effusion), atelectasis, alveolar collapse, hypoxemia, and carbon dioxide retention. A correlation has been documented between levels of phospholipase A_2 and the severity of respiratory failure.[4] Almost two thirds of patients with acute pancreatitis exhibit respiratory insufficiency within the first 48 hours, as evidenced by arterial hypoxemia with no clinical or radiographic abnormalities. The remaining one third exhibit clinical and radiographic abnormalities and require assisted ventilation. A 75% mortality rate has been associated with the need for mechanical ventilation.[5] Twenty percent of patients with acute pancreatitis will develop acute respiratory distress syndrome (ARDS) with ventilation/perfusion mismatching and inadequate oxygenation of the blood.[4]

Diagnosis

Clinical History

Functional Health Patterns. Assessment of the patient with possible acute pancreatitis requires a careful history. It is important to elicit information regarding the following functional health patterns.

Health Perception–Health Management. Establish overall health status and recent changes in the patient's health or lifestyle. Has there been a recent illness, significant weight change, anorexia, nausea, vomiting, or abdominal distention? Has there been recent abdominal surgery or endoscopic examination of the common bile duct? Has the patient sustained recent abdominal trauma? Has there been a recent infection? Is there a history of biliary tract disease, pancreatitis, hepatitis, peptic ulcer disease, hepatic or pancreatic cancer, hyperlipidemia, endocrine disorders, or a hereditary predisposition to any disease?

It is important to elicit a thorough history regarding patient/family use and/or abuse of alcohol and drugs. Medications such as oral contraceptives, corticosteroids, thiazide diuretics, antihypertensives, and opiates may precipitate pancreatitis. Data obtained should reflect the amount, type, and duration of alcohol or drug consumption. Patient/family attitudes about the use/abuse of alcohol and drugs and their significance in the patient/family lifestyle should be ascertained.

Coping–Stress Intolerance. Has there been any recent emotional upheaval or stress? It is important to identify how the patient and family cope with stress. What resources are available to assist them in handling stress?

Cognitive-Perceptual. The patient's perception of pain should be assessed. The location, radiation, and duration of the pain, its severity and quality, need to be established. How does the patient describe the pain? Is the pain accompanied by nausea and vomiting? Does vomiting relieve the pain? What position does the patient assume in an attempt to reduce the pain? What is the patient's response to analgesic therapy?

Nutritional-Metabolic. Is there a history of anorexia, weight gain or loss, or the inability to tolerate dietary intake? Is the abdominal pain aggravated by thoughts of food or by attempts to ingest food or drink? Is there a history of hyperlipidemia or fat intolerance?

Elimination. Has the patient recently experienced changes in bowel habits? Is constipation a problem? Is there steatorrhea? Are there complaints of abdominal bloating?

Laboratory Tests

Presently, there is no specific, single, accurate diagnostic laboratory test for acute pancreatitis. Serum amylase and lipase are the two most commonly performed tests that assist in the differential diagnosis of acute pancreatitis. A *serum amylase* level (>200 Somogyi U/100 mL), although a sensitive indicator of pancreatic cellular damage, may only be elevated early in acute pancreatitis (the first 24 to 72 hours) and can be elevated in a number of other conditions, such as perforated duodenal ulcer, acute cholecystitis, small bowel obstruction, or kidney stones. However, these conditions usually declare themselves rather quickly,

PROGNOSTIC LABORATORY TESTS FOR ACUTE PANCREATITIS

Tests No Longer Used:
Isoamylase
Macroamylase
Urinary amylase
Amylase/creatinine clearance ratio
Controversial Tests (Limited Clinical Validation):
Methemalbumin
Fibrinogen
α_2-Macroglobulin
α_1-Antiprotease
C-reactive protein (CRP)
Interleukin-6 (IL-6)
Granulocytic elastase (GE)
Tests Requiring Clinical Validation:
Carboxylic ester hydrolase (CEH)
Trypsinogen activation peptides (TAP)
Immunoreactive trypsin (IRT)
Elastase I
Macroglobulin
Ribonuclease
Complements 3 and 4
Phospholipase A_2

TABLE 46–5
Diagnostic Radiology Tests

Test	Purpose
Abdominal computed tomography (CT) scan with vascular enhancement	For direct visualization of pancreas and surrounding structures; to follow extent of pancreatic necrosis
CT-guided/ultrasound-guided aspiration	Fluid aspiration of pancreatic fluid collections and pseudocysts for gram stain and culture
Abdominal ultrasound	To rule out gallstones; to determine common duct size and contents; to detect/localize superficial fluid collection
Endoscopic retrograde cholangiopancreatography (ERCP)	For direct visualization of pancreatic ductal system
Chest x-rays	To diagnose basal atelectasis, pleural effusions, mediastinal abscess, elevated diaphragm, consolidation, infiltrates, acute respiratory distress syndrome
Abdominal x-rays	To diagnose paralytic ileus (gas-filled loops); and to free air from bowel perforation

ruling them out as the diagnosis. A *serum lipase* level is elevated within the first 24 to 48 hours of the disease and remains elevated for up to 5 to 7 days. A lipase concentration of greater than 5 URL (upper reference limit) is associated with acute pancreatitis. Other laboratory tests have either been found to be poor discriminators, to be too complicated or expensive to perform, or to need more study (see box above).

Nonspecific laboratory findings may include leukocytosis, elevated bilirubin, alkaline phosphatase, and serum triglyceride levels, decreased total serum protein and albumin levels, hypocalcemia, hypomagnesemia, and hyperglycemia. Hypocalcemia, hypomagnesemia, hypokalemia, and hyperglycemia usually occur in more severe cases of acute pancreatitis. Hypocalcemia occurs in 30% to 60% of patients with acute pancreatitis. Marked fat necrosis results in the release of free fatty acids. These fatty acids bind with calcium to form calcium soaps. Serum calcium levels are usually maximally depressed during the first 3 days after onset of pancreatitis.[4] A serum calcium level below 7.5 mg/dL reflects extensive disease and indicates an extremely poor prognosis.[3] Hyperglycemia (blood glucose >200 mg/dL) is another poor prognostic sign of acute pancreatitis.[4] Transient hyperglycemia may be seen in 50% of cases of acute pancreatitis, glycosuria in 30% of cases, and permanent diabetes in 2% to 10% percent of cases.[4]

Radiologic Studies

Several radiologic studies are used in diagnosing and stratifying the severity of acute pancreatitis (Table 46–5). Abdominal CT with contrast is the present gold standard used for diagnosing acute pancreatitis and classifying pancreatic necrosis.

Complications

Potential complications of acute pancreatitis are numerous and may be difficult to distinguish from clinical manifestations of the disease. The most serious complications include the development of hypovolemic shock, ARDS, acute renal failure, disseminated intravascular coagulation, malnutrition, and local symptoms (see Table 46–3). Complications occurring in the first 48 to 72 hours are a result of cardiovascular, pulmonary, and renal compromise. Later complications are usually the result of inflammation, infection, and necrosis in or immediately around the pancreas. The presence of necrosis, with or without fluid, is a grave prognostic sign.[6] In recent years, infection of devitalized pancreatic and parapancreatic tissue has become the leading cause of death and morbidity.[6] The two major groups of infective complications arising in the abdomen are pancreatic abscess and infected necrosis.

Prognosis

Early identification of life-threatening complications allows for appropriate monitoring and implementation of therapeutic interventions. Early prognostic signs associated with an increased risk of death or major complications were described by Ranson (Table 46–6).[7] If patients have three or more Ranson

TABLE 46–6
Prognostic Factors in Acute Pancreatitis

Time Frame	Factor	Value
On admission:	Age	>55 years
	Blood glucose	>200 mg/100 mL
	White blood cell count	>16,000 mm³
	Serum lactate dehydrogenase	>350 µg/mL
	Serum glutamic-oxaloacetic transaminase	>250 µg/mL
Within 48 hours of admission:	Hematocrit	>10% decrease
	BUN	>5 mg/100 mL increase
	Serum calcium	<8 mg/100 mL
	PaO₂	<60 mmHg
	Base deficit	>4 mEq/L
	Estimated fluid sequestration	>6000 mL
Classification of acuity of pancreatitis based on the number of prognostic factors present:		
	Mild pancreatitis	<3 factors
	Severe pancreatitis	≥3 factors

Source: Ranson, JH, Ritkin, KM, and Turner, JW: Prognostic signs and nonoperative peritoneal lavage in acute pancreatitis. Surg Gynecol Obstet 143:212, 1976.

TABLE 46–7
Treatment of Severe Acute Pancreatitis

Therapy	Description
Stabilization Therapies	
Fluid resuscitation	Crystalloids, colloids (albumin), blood
Electrolyte replacement	Potassium, calcium, magnesium
Respiratory support	Assisted mechanical ventilation with positive end-expiratory pressure (PEEP) with the earliest indication of respiratory distress
Supportive Therapies	
Pain management	Meperidine (Demerol)—analgesic of choice to prevent spasm of sphincter of Oddi and false elevation of amylase level
Measures to decrease pancreatic secretion	Bedrest; pancreatic rest (nothing by mouth; nasogastric tube with low continuous suction if paralytic ileus present)
Cardiovascular support	Inotropic support using intravenous dopamine drip
Nutritional support	Total parenteral nutrition (TPN); intrajejunal enteral feedings when bowel sounds present
Treatment of pancreatic infection	Use of quinolone antibiotics
Surgical Therapies	
Biliary procedures	Cholecystectomy, choledochojejunostomy, pancreaticojejunostomy (Roux-en-Y)
Pancreatic resection, drainage, debridement	For infected pancreatic necrosis only

---

DISCREDITED TREATMENTS FOR SEVERE ACUTE PANCREATITIS

Suppression of Pancreatic Secretion:
Anticholinergics
Calcitonin
Glucagon
Somatostatin
H₂ blockers
Inhibition of Pancreatic Enzymes:
Aprotinin
Gabexelate
Mesilate
5-Fluorouracil
Phospholipase A inhibitors
Antitoxic and Anti-Inflammatory Measures:
Prostaglandin inhibitors
Free radical scavengers
Reticuloendothelial system stimulators
Fresh-frozen plasma
Fibronectin
Steroids
Peritoneal Lavage
Total Pancreatectomy
Triple Tube Intubation (gastrostomy drainage of stomach, cholecystostomy drainage of biliary tree, jejunostomy feeding tube)

---

risk factors, they are at high risk of having a long, complicated, often fatal course. Because the method is too complex for routine clinical use, other means of predicting severity in acute pancreatitis are used, including APACHE-II (Acute Physiology and Chronic Health Enquiry) score, peritoneal lavage, and CT contrast imaging.

Treatment

There is presently no specific, clinically substantiated, efficacious treatment for acute pancreatitis. The current approach to medical management and nursing intervention focuses on hemodynamic stabilization, pancreatic rest, pain relief, oxygenation, and prevention and/or treatment of complications. Mild acute pancreatitis usually resolves within a few days of onset without any systemic complications after aggressive fluid resuscitation, elimination of oral intake, oxygen supplementation, and pain management.

Treatment of severe acute pancreatitis includes stabilization therapies, supportive therapies, treatment of systemic complications, and surgical therapies (Table 46–7). A number of initially promising treatments for severe acute pancreatitis have been discredited through clinical testing (see box above).

The definitive treatment for severe acute pancreatitis awaits the development of clinically validated drugs and therapies.

Nursing Care of the Patient with Acute Pancreatitis

Therapeutic Goals

Nursing management and care of the patient with acute pancreatitis focuses on attaining/maintaining optimal body functioning and on preventing complications. Because the clinical presentation of acute pancreatitis does not necessarily correlate with disease severity and/or outcome, care of the patient with acute pancreatitis requires continuous use of acute assessment and critical thinking skills.

Implementation of the nursing process in the care of the patient with acute pancreatitis centers around the following therapeutic goals:

1. Establish a thorough, comprehensive assessment database, including:
   a. Clinical history.
   b. Physical examination.
   c. Laboratory/radiologic data.
2. Promote/maintain fluid, electrolyte, and acid-base balance.
3. Alleviate/control pain.
4. Promote/maintain optimal oxygenation.
5. Promote/maintain optimal alveolar ventilation and tissue perfusion.
6. Implement measures to minimize pancreatic secretory activity.
7. Implement nutritional therapy to prevent malnutrition.
8. Prevent complications, including:
   a. Cardiovascular: shock, hemorrhage, cardiac arrhythmia, DIC.
   b. Pulmonary: atelectasis, hypoxia, pleural effusions, ARDS.
   c. Renal: acute renal failure.
   d. Metabolic: acid-base disturbance, hyper- or hypoglycemia, hypocalcemia, hypomagnesemia.
   e. Infection.

9. Provide emotional support to patient/family.
10. Assist patient/family with stress management.

Nursing Diagnoses, Desired Patient Outcomes, and Nursing Interventions and Rationales

Pertinent nursing diagnoses, desired patient outcomes, and nursing interventions and rationales are presented in the care plan at the end of the chapter.

REFERENCES

1. Brodrick, RL: Preventing complications in acute pancreatitis. DCCN 10(5):262, 1991.
2. Krumberger, JM: Acute pancreatitis. Crit Care Nurs Clin North Am 5(1):185, 1993.
3. Smith, A: When the pancreas self destructs. Am J Nurs 91(9):38, 1991.
4. Pitchumoni, C, Agarwal, N, and Jain, N: Systemic complications of acute pancreatitis. Am J Gastroenterol 83:597, 1988.
5. Smith, S and Wills Butler, R: Acute pancreatitis (a peer-reviewed article for self-study from the publisher of Critical Care Nurse). Aliso Viejo, CA: American Association of Critical-Care Nurses, 1993.
6. Bradley, EL (ed): Acute Pancreatitis: Diagnosis and Therapy. Raven Press, New York, 1994, 16, 170.
7. Ranson, JH, Ritkin, KM, and Turner, JW: Prognostic signs and nonoperative peritoneal lavage in acute pancreatitis. Surg Gynecol Obstet 143:212, 1976.

SUGGESTED READINGS

Bradley, EL: A clinically based classification system for acute pancreatitis. Arch Surg 128:586, 1993.
Clavien, P, Burgan, S, and Moossa, A: Serum enzymes and other laboratory tests in acute pancreatitis. Br J Surg 76:1234, 1989.
Noone, J: Acute pancreatitis: An Orem approach to nursing assessment and care. Crit Care Nurs 15(4):27–35, 1995.
Singh, M and Simsek, H: Ethanol and the pancreas. Gastroenterol 98:1051, 1990.
Steer, ML: Classification and pathogenesis of pancreatitis. Surg Clin North Am 69:467, 1989.
Thompson, C: Managing acute pancreatitis. RN 55(2):52, March 1992.

CARE PLAN FOR THE PATIENT WITH SEVERE ACUTE PANCREATITIS

Nursing Diagnoses

Nursing Diagnosis #1
Tissue perfusion, alteration in, related to fluid volume deficit/hypovolemia
1. Third spacing (pancreatic ascites)
2. Vasodilation
3. Dehydration
4. Hemorrhage

Desired Patient Outcomes

Patient will:
1. Maintain stable hemodynamics:
   - BP within 10 mmHg of baseline, or SBP >90 mmHg
   - HR <100, >60 beats/min.
   - CVP 0–8 mmHg.
   - PCWP 8–12 mmHg.
   - CO ~5 L/min.
   - Skin warm with usual color.
2. Demonstrate alert mental status, appropriate behavior and neurologic function:
   - Oriented to person, place, time.
   - Cranial nerves intact.
   - Deep tendon reflexes brisk.

CARE PLAN FOR THE PATIENT WITH SEVERE ACUTE PANCREATITIS (*Continued*)

Nursing Diagnoses

Desired Patient Outcomes
3. Maintain renal function:
   - Urine output >30 mL/h, or 0.5 mL/kg/min.
   - Balanced intake and output.
   - BUN, serum creatinine in acceptable physiologic range.

Nursing Interventions
- Perform ongoing cardiovascular assessment:

  ○ Continuous cardiac monitoring.
    □ Establish baseline rate, rhythm, ectopy.
  ○ Continuous hemodynamic pressure monitoring:
    □ Establish baseline values: CVP, PCWP, mixed venous saturation, oxygen saturation

  ○ Assess peripheral pulses: rate, rhythm, quality.
  ○ Assess skin temperature, moisture, color, turgor,

- Assess ongoing neurologic function: mental status, level of consciousness, appropriate behavior, cranial nerves, deep tendon reflexes.

- Monitor renal function: hourly intake and output.

  ○ Daily weight.

Rationales
- Establishing baseline data assists in evaluating patient status and subsequent responses to therapy.
  ○ Cardiac tissue hypoxia may predispose to arrhythmias.

  ○ Continuous hemodynamic monitoring provides an indication of the patient's intravascular volume status, which is a major factor in tissue perfusion.
  ○ Offers significant data about cardiopulmonary status; affords *trending*, that is, frequent serial measurements; trending more accurately reflects changes occurring in patient's condition and the patient's response to therapeutic measures.
  ○ Presence of cool, moist skin with pallor or cyanosis reflects compensatory peripheral vasoconstriction response to permit blood to be shunted to vital organs.
- Compromised hemodynamics (hypotension) and hypoxemia predispose to cerebral hypoxia, reflected by alterations in cerebral function, level of consciousness, responsiveness of cranial nerves, and deep tendon reflexes.
- Close monitoring of intake/output provides for early recognition of intravascular fluid volume deficits.
- Reduction in urine output suggests decreased renal perfusion commonly associated with hypovolemic shock. Acute renal failure is a major complication of acute pancreatitis.
  ○ Most closely reflects fluid balance.

Nursing Diagnoses
Nursing Diagnosis #2
Fluid volume deficit (intravascular), actual, related to:
1. Dehydration
   a. NPO
   b. Nasogastric suctioning
   c. Vomiting
2. Third spacing (pancreatic ascites)
   a. Hypoalbuminemia
3. Hemorrhage
   (See also Chapter 44 care plan, Nursing Diagnosis #1, and Chapter 45 care plan, Nursing Diagnosis #1.)

Desired Patient Outcomes

Patient will:
1. Achieve hemodynamic stability (BP, HR, CVP, PCWP, CO, urine output, as per Nursing Diagnosis #1.)
2. Achieve resolution of edema/ascites:
   - Body weight within 5% of baseline.
   - Abdominal girth at baseline measurements.

Nursing Diagnoses
Nursing Diagnosis #3
Electrolyte balance, alteration in, related to:
1. Diuretic therapy
2. Acid-base imbalance

Desired Patient Outcomes

Patient will:
1. Restore/maintain laboratory parameters in acceptable physiologic range:
   - Serum osmolality 285–295 mOsm/Kg.
   - Serum sodium >135 <148 mEq/L.
   - Serum potassium 3.5–5.5 mEq/L.
   - Serum albumin 3.5–5.5 g/100 mL.
   - Hematocrit 37%–52%.
   - Hemoglobin 12–18 g/100 mL.
   - CBC.
   - Urine electrolytes and specific gravity.
2. Demonstrate absence of signs and symptoms of electrolyte imbalance.

CARE PLAN FOR THE PATIENT WITH SEVERE ACUTE PANCREATITIS (*Continued*)

Nursing Interventions	Rationales
• Administer colloids/crystalloids as ordered to replace/ maintain intravascular volume.	• The inflammatory process of acute pancreatitis causes devitalization of the pancreatic parenchyma with loss of serum albumin in the exudate, which causes massive fluid shifts from the intravascular space to the interstitium (pancreatic ascites). Aggressive fluid replacement prevents hypovolemia, hypotension, depressed cardiac function, hypovolemic shock, and death.
• Perform frequent gastrointestinal assessment:	• Frequent gastrointestinal monitoring tracks clinical manifestations of acute pancreatitis. The extent of pancreatic involvement has been correlated to the severity of pain and other organ system involvement.
○ Abdominal assessment: abdomen—soft, rigid; rebound tenderness; presence of Cullen's or Grey Turner's signs; abdominal girth; guarding; presence of bowel sounds; palpable masses.	○ Compensatory vasoconstriction of splanchnic circulation (sympathetic response) may result in decreased peristalsis and ischemia of the gastric and intestinal mucosa.
○ Nausea/vomiting/constipation, hematemesis, melena.	□ *Cullen's* sign: Bluish umbilicus or faintly blue discoloration of skin associated with hemoperitoneum from any cause.
	□ *Grey Turner's* sign: Ecchymoses on abdomen and flanks possibly associated with infiltration of extraperitoneal tissues with blood.
• Monitor for signs of hypovolemia: hypotension, tachycardia, decreased CVP, PAP; decreased urine output, increased specific gravity; signs of dehydration—elevated body temperature, poor skin turgor, sunken eyeballs, and dry mucous membranes.	
• Assess for signs and symptoms of electrolyte imbalance:	• Acute pancreatitis usually predisposes to electrolyte imbalance. Nasogatric suctioning, vomiting, diarrhea, and extravasation of fluid account for much of the loss of sodium, potassium, and chloride.
○ Hypokalemia—cardiac arrhythmias; hypotension; weakness; fatigue; nausea, vomiting; lethargy, muscle weakness; paresthesias, hyporeflexia.	○ It is important to establish baseline blood chemistry values so that replacement therapy may be guided by serial studies, which should include total protein and serum osmolality, in addition to electrolytes.
○ Hyponatremia—nausea, vomiting, headache, lethargy, confusion, seizures, coma.	
○ Hypocalcemia—tremors, paresthesias, tetany, laryngospasm, convulsions, positive Chvostek's and Trousseau's signs.	
○ Hypochloremia: alkalemia.	
○ Monitor serial electrolyte levels.	
• Implement prescribed measures to reestablish and maintain normovolemia and electrolyte balance.	
○ Administer blood products and intravenous fluids.	○ To reverse hypovolemia/hypotension. Reestablishing intravascular volume improves circulation, tissue perfusion, and oxygenation. Replace fluid losses associated with NPO, vomiting, nasogastric suctioning, and third spacing.
	□ Irritating and inflammatory effects of acute pancreatitis on the pancreatic parenchyma and surrounding tissues cause extravasation of fluids, electrolytes, and protein into the interstitium and peritoneal cavity (third spacing).
○ Replace serum albumin.	○ Loss of plasma proteins from the intravascular space disrupts colloidal oncotic pressure, predisposing to even greater fluid loss with interstitial edema and ascites.
○ Monitor for signs of circulatory overload: generalized (dependent) edema, weight gain, increased blood pressure, bounding pulses; signs of pulmonary congestion—dyspnea, crackles (rales), elevation of CVP and PAP.	○ Fluid overload is a complication of aggressive fluid volume replacement.

CARE PLAN FOR THE PATIENT WITH SEVERE ACUTE PANCREATITIS (*Continued*)

Nursing Interventions	Rationales
○ Monitor for signs of hypovolemia: hypotension, tachycardia, decreased CVP and PAP, decreased urine output, increase in urine specific gravity; signs of dehydration—elevated body temperature, poor skin turgor, sunken eyeballs, and dryness of mucous membranes.	○ Hypovolemia may result after institution of diuretic therapy.
○ Administer prescribed inotropic and vasopressor therapy. □ Dopamine hydrochloride.	○ Increases cardiac output by increasing preload (venous return) and cardiac contractility; enhances tissue perfusion.
○ Replace serum electrolytes: □ Sodium. –Hyponatremia/hypernatremia: monitor hydration status, monitor serum/urine sodium levels.	□ Hyponatremia is a frequent occurrence in acute pancreatitis. –A decrease in total body sodium predisposes to hypovolemia. –Intravenous replacement of sodium needs to be carefully monitored to prevent sodium excess (hypernatremia) with consequent fluid overload.
□ Potassium. –Hypokalemia/hyperkalemia: monitor ECG for arrhythmias; monitor arterial blood gases (acid-base status); monitor serum potassium levels.	□ Potassium (K^+), an intracellular ion, is closely associated with acid-base balance: –Acidemia—hydrogen (H^+) ions are driven into cells in exchange for K^+; this increases serum potassium levels. –Alkalemia—H^+ ions move out of cells in exchange for K^+; this decreases serum potassium levels. –This reciprocal relationship between K^+ and H^+ ions also occurs in the distal tubules, necessitating that kidney function be closely monitored.
□ Calcium. –Hypocalcemia: Monitor serum total and ionized calcium levels, albumin, and total protein levels.	□ Deposition of calcium into areas of fatty necrosis occurs frequently in acute pancreatitis and requires close monitoring of serum calcium levels. Calcium replacement therapy requires careful administration to prevent complications: –Patent intravenous line needs to be maintained because tissue sloughing and necrosis can occur with extravasation of calcium preparations. –Need to monitor albumin level and ionized calcium level for accurate calcium level.
□ Magnesium. –Hypomagnesemia: Monitor serum magnesium levels.	□ May result from vomiting, nasogastric suction, and inadequate nutritional support. –Can cause hypokalemia and hypocalcemia.
○ Monitor ECG for arrhythmias.	○ Potentiation of digitalis effect by calcium can occur in patients receiving digitalis; this can predispose to digitalis toxicity. Continuous ECG monitoring is essential.
○ Monitor total serum protein and serum albumin levels.	○ Calcium is highly bound to serum proteins; alkalemia increases percent calcium bound to protein, thus reducing fraction of ionized calcium.
○ Chloride. □ Hypochloremia: monitor acid-base status; monitor serum chloride.	○ Chloride is necessary for gastric production of HCl; it plays a major role in acid-base balance. ○ Hypochloremia is associated with vomiting and nasogastric suctioning; it predisposes to metabolic alkalosis.

Nursing Diagnoses	Desired Patient Outcomes
Nursing Diagnosis #4 Breathing pattern, ineffective, related to: 1. Hypoventilation associated with severe abdominal pain 2. Atelectasis 3. Pleural effusion 4. Elevated left diaphragm	Patient will: 1. Demonstrate effective minute ventilation: • Tidal volume (V_T) >5–7 mL/Kg. • Respiratory rate <25–30 per min. >12/min. 2. Achieve vital capacity (V_C) >12–15 mL/Kg.

CARE PLAN FOR THE PATIENT WITH SEVERE ACUTE PANCREATITIS (*Continued*)

Nursing Diagnoses

Nursing Diagnosis #5
Airway clearance, ineffective, related to:
1. Cough suppression and failure to deep breathe because of severe abdominal pain
2. Immobility

Desired Patient Outcomes

1. Verbalize ease of breathing.
2. Demonstrate deep-breathing techniques and effective secretion-clearing cough.
3. Maintain arterial blood gases in acceptable physiologic range:
   - PaO_2 >60 mmHg, <100 mmHg.
   - $PaCO_2$ 35–45 mmHg.
   - pH >7.35 <7.45.
   - Base excess +2/−2.
4. Maintain appropriate responses on respiratory examination:
   - Tactile fremitus present on palpation.
   - Resonance throughout lung fields on percussion.
   - Vesicular breath sounds throughout peripheral lung fields on auscultation.
5. Demonstrate an absence of atelectasis, pleural effusion, and elevated left diaphragm on chest x-ray.

Nursing Interventions

- Monitor respiratory function frequently:
  - Rate, rhythm, depth, and pattern of breathing.
  - Symmetry of chest wall and diaphragmatic excursion.
  - Use of accessory muscles.
  - Auscultation of breath sounds.
  - Pulmonary lung volumes: total minute ventilation; V_T, respiratory rate; vital capacity.
  - Assess quantity, quality, color, odor, and consistency of sputum.
  - Assess arterial blood gases.
  - Chest x-rays: atelectasis, interstitial edema.
- Implement measures to improve respiratory function:
  - Administer prescribed medication for abdominal pain and monitor response.

    - Meperidine is drug of choice.

  - Perform measures to reduce anxiety:
    - Encourage verbalization of fears and concerns.
    - Provide a caring touch and listening ear.
    - Provide explanations and feedback about care and health status.
    - Identify patient/family coping strengths and resources.
  - Perform measures to facilitate chest wall expansion and diaphragmatic excursion:
    - Minimize abdominal distention associated with gastrointestinal gas and fluid accumulation.
    - Maintain proper placement and patency of nasogastric tube.
    - Encourage position changes every 1–2 h.
    - Maintain patient in semi- to high-Fowler's position unless contraindicated.

Rationales

- Frequent monitoring of respiratory status is imperative since almost two thirds of patients with acute pancreatitis exhibit respiratory insufficiency (arterial hypoxemia) in the first 48 hours.

  - Abdominal pain causes splinting and hypoventilation; hypoventilation predisposes to hypercapnia and atelectasis; atelectasis predisposes to ventilation/perfusion inequality.
    - Abdominal pain predisposes to cough suppression and immobility; pooling of secretions predisposes to pneumonia.
  - Relief of pain prevents splinting and hypoventilation by encouraging patient to breathe more deeply and to cough more vigorously.
    - Meperidine causes less spasm of sphincter of Oddi than does morphine.
  - A reduction in the level of anxiety or stress may help to reduce the level of pain and facilitate breathing.

  - Help to improve ventilation and oxygenation and to prevent atelectasis and pooling of secretions.

    - Nasogastric suction helps to reduce gastric distention.
    - Patient is inclined to assume a position of greatest pain relief and to remain in that position. Coughing, deep breathing, and position changes may best be performed following administration of analgesics.

CARE PLAN FOR THE PATIENT WITH SEVERE ACUTE PANCREATITIS (*Continued*)

Nursing Interventions	Rationales
□ Encourage patient to expel flatus whenever the urge arises.	□ Deep breathing and position changes may stimulate peristalsis and flatulence.
○ Monitor for signs and symptoms of pleural effusion: shortness of breath, pleuritic pain, splinting to reduce chest excursion, dullness on percussion, and diminished to absent breath sounds over the affected area on auscultation.	
○ Perform measures to minimize pancreatic secretory activity.	○ The pancreas is stimulated by gastric juice in the duodenum; a patent nasogastric tube with suction reduces delivery of HCl to duodenum.
○ Prepare patient and assist with thoracentesis (see Table 26–3).	○ Decompression of pleural effusion facilitates greater lung expansion.
○ Monitor coagulation studies	○ Complement-induced pulmonary emboli may be cause of ventilation/perfusion problems.
○ Prepare patient and assist with paracentesis.	○ Decompression of peritoneal fluid increases diaphragmatic excursion.
○ Implement prescribed respiratory support therapy: □ Oxygen therapy. □ Intermittent positive pressure breathing (IPPB). □ Chest physiotherapy.	○ Arterial hypoxemia is a major cause of respiratory insufficiency in acute pancreatitis.

Nursing Diagnoses	Desired Patient Outcomes
Nursing Diagnosis #6 Acute pain	Patient will: 1. Verbalize relief of pain. 2. Exhibit relaxed demeanor: • Relaxed facial expression and body posturing. • Ease of breathing. 3. Identify effective pain relief and coping mechanisms.

Nursing Interventions	Rationales
Refer to Chapter 10 for specific nursing interventions. The following interventions should be considered for the patient with acute pancreatitis:	
• Implement measures to reduce pancreatic stimulation.	• Stimulation of inflamed pancreatic acinar cells aggravates pain. ○ Pain and anxiety increase pancreatic secretory activity via enhanced parasympathetic stimulation.
○ Maintain status NPO.	○ It is necessary to minimize gastric secretions as they stimulate secretion of the hormones secretin and cholecystokinin, which stimulate pancreatic secretion.
○ Maintain patency of nasogastric tube with continuous nasogastric suction. □ Confirm tube placement every 2 hours.	○ Nasogastric suction also relieves nausea, vomiting, and intestinal distention.
○ Administer prescribed analgesic: □ Meperidine is usual analgesic of choice. Evaluate the effectiveness of the prescribed analgesic.	□ Morphine is avoided because it causes a greater degree of spasm of sphincter of Oddi than does meperidine.
○ Provide frequent comfort measures: □ Mouth care; position changes; time periods of quiet and sleep; spending more time with patient. –Provide a listening ear.	
○ Involve patient/family in quiet recreational activities.	○ This may help to distract the patient from thoughts of food and to avoid parasympathetic stimulation associated with the cephalic phase of digestive activity.
○ Minimize visitors.	○ Increased activity may aggravate pain.
○ Instruct family members and friends not to take food into the patient's room.	○ Sight of food can stimulate pancreatic secretory activity (cephalic phase of digestion).

CARE PLAN FOR THE PATIENT WITH SEVERE ACUTE PANCREATITIS (*Continued*)

Nursing Diagnoses

Nursing Diagnosis #7
Nutrition, alteration in, less than body requirements
(malnutrition), related to:
1. Nausea and vomiting
2. NPO status
3. Malabsorption (altered fat metabolism)
4. Altered carbohydrate and protein metabolism
   a. Hypoglycemia
   b. Hypoalbuminemia

Desired Patient Outcomes

Patient will:
1. Maintain body weight within 5% of baseline.
2. Maintain serum albumin in physiologic range:
   • 3.5–5.0 g/100 mL.
3. Maintain serum total protein in physiologic range:
   • 6–8.4 g/100 mL.
4. Maintain intact skin and mucous membranes.
5. Verbalize feeling of increased strength.
6. Maintain triceps skinfold in acceptable range.
7. Maintain laboratory parameters in acceptable range:
   • Hematology profile.
   • Cholesterol.
   • BUN, creatinine.

Nursing Interventions

Refer to Chapter 9 for details related to treatment and prevention of malnutrition.

Rationales

Nursing Diagnoses

Nursing Diagnosis #8
Infection, high risk for, related to:
1. Malnutrition
2. Invasive procedures/lines
3. Peritonitis associated with autodigestion of adjacent
   tissues by pancreatic juices

Desired Patient Outcomes

Patient will:
1. Maintain body temperature in acceptable physiologic
   range, ~98.6°F.
2. Maintain white blood count: ~5000–10,000/mm³.
3. Remain free of signs and symptoms of peritonitis.
4. Remain free of signs and symptoms of systemic
   infection.

Nursing Interventions

• Monitor for signs and symptoms of:
  ○ Respiratory tract infection: fever (spiking), dyspnea,
    tachypnea, pulmonary dullness, bronchial breath
    sounds, presence of crackles and rhonci, purulent
    sputum, chest x-ray indicating pulmonary
    consolidation
  ○ Intravascular catheter-related infection: swelling, pain,
    tenderness, warmth, and erythema at insertion site, or
    over an indurated vessel; elevated temperature

  ○ Urinary tract infection: urgency, frequency, dysuria,
    fever, chills, sweats.

  ○ Peritonitis: abdominal pain, rebound tenderness,
    abdominal muscle rigidity, nausea, vomiting, fever,
    chills, decreased or absent bowel sounds, decreased
    urinary output, hypotension, tachycardia, tachypnea

• Monitor for temperature > 102°F and WBC < 5,000 or
  > 10,000/mm³

Rationales

  ○ Ineffective breathing patterns related to
    hypoventilation, atelectasis, pleural effusion, elevated
    diaphram, cough suppression, and immobility
    predispose the patient to lung consolidation and
    pneumonia.
  ○ Intravascular catheters are inserted for fluid volume
    resuscitation/maintenance, hemodynamic monitoring,
    and parenteral nutrition.
  ○ Infection rate markedly increases 48 to 72 hours after
    intravascular catheter insertion.
  ○ Bacteremias are most commonly associated with
    hemodynamic pressure monitoring.
  ○ Phlebitis is highly implicated in intravascular infections
    and bacteremia.
  ○ Urinary catheters are frequently used to monitor
    hourly urine outputs.
  ○ The length of time a urinary catheter remains in the
    bladder is directly related to the incidence of urinary
    tract infection.
  ○ Acute pancreatitis involves autodigestion of pancreatic
    tissue and seepage of pancreatic juice into the
    peritoneal cavity.
  ○ Large acute fluid collections, an acute pseudocyst,
    pancreatic abscess, or pancreatic necrosis may develop.
  ○ Clinical signs and symptoms depend on the extent of
    inflammation and pancreatic tissue destruction.
• A fever >102°F may indicate infectious complications.
• A WBC <5,000 or >10,000/mm³ may indicate an
  infectious process.
• Infectious complications account for >80% of all acute
  pancreatic deaths.

CARE PLAN FOR THE PATIENT WITH SEVERE ACUTE PANCREATITIS (*Continued*)

Nursing Interventions
- Administer prescribed antibiotics in timely manner.
- Implement universal precautions and category-specific isolation precautions as necessary.

Rationales
- Maintains serum antibiotic levels.
- Controls the spread of nosocomial infections.

Nursing Diagnoses

Nursing Diagnosis #9
Knowledge deficit regarding:
1. Convalescence and follow-up care
2. Impact on lifestyle
   - Alcoholism
   - Stress

Desired Patient Outcomes

Patient will:
1. Verbalize importance of strict adherence to prescribed dietary regimen:
   - Total abstinence from alcohol
   - High carbohydrate and protein diet, low fat intake.
2. Verbalize alternatives in pain relief:
   - Medication therapy.
   - Relaxation exercises.
3. Identify effective coping mechanisms in stress management.

Nursing Interventions
- Establish a trusting rapport with patient and family members.

   ○ Verbalize fears and concerns for patient and family.

- Assess patient/family baseline knowledge and readiness to learn.
   ○ Encourage patient/family to assist in identifying needs and learning objectives.
- Assist patient/family in problem-solving techniques.
   ○ Help to identify family strengths and weaknesses.

- Determine appropriate teaching strategies to facilitate learning:
   ○ Encourage open discussions regarding illness and impact on family lifestyle.
      □ Consider role of alcohol in lifestyle, if appropriate.
- Initiate health teaching concerned with the following:
   ○ Diet management: emphasize importance of strict adherence to prescribed diet and abstinence from alcohol and high fat intake.
      □ Consider who in the family is responsible for meal preparation.
   ○ Pain management: advise patient as to alternatives in pain relief: medication therapy, surgery, relaxation exercises, recreational therapy.
      □ Support patient/family in their decision.
      □ Include the following teaching for prescribed medications: purpose, action(s), dosage, frequency, route of administration, and drug interactions.
   ○ Management of stress: assist patient/family to: identify sources of stress, identify effective and ineffective coping mechanisms; assist patient/family to identify and communicate their feelings to each other.

Rationales
- An environment of mutual respect and trust can enhance the learning process. Often a long convalescence follows recovery from acute pancreatitis. Discharge planning should begin as early as possible.
   ○ While the patient may be too ill initially to participate in learning, involvement of family members in the patient's overall care may affect the progress made by patient and family members alike toward the level of health and well-being desired.
- An informed patient/family can participate in care and make necessary adjustments in lifestyle.

   ○ Assisting patient/family to cope increases self-confidence in their own capabilities.
- Learning should occur at a rate that is meaningful to participants.

      □ It is essential for the family member who cooks to appreciate the patient's diet and its preparation.
   ○ Effective pain management promotes active patient involvement in care.

   ○ Effective stress management may be helpful in reducing pain.

CARE PLAN FOR THE PATIENT WITH SEVERE ACUTE PANCREATITIS (*Continued*)

Nursing Interventions
- Initiate referrals to appropriate resources:
  - Dietician.
  - Social worker.
  - Psychiatric liaison nurse.
  - Other.

Rationales
- Successful recovery of all family members from the stress of acute illness and continued health maintenance requires timely and ongoing support.

*BP = blood pressure; SBP = systolic blood pressure; HR = heart rate; CVP = central venous pressure; PCWP = pulmonary capillary wedge pressure; CO = cardiac output; BUN = blood urea nitrogen; CBC = complete blood count; PAP = pulmonary artery pressure; NPO = nothing by mouth; ECG = electrocardiogram.

UNIT EIGHT

Immune System

UNIT OUTLINE

C H A P T E R   4 7

Functions and Responses of the Immune System

Kristin Kane Ownby and Diane Ragsdale

CHAPTER OUTLINE

Anatomy
Classification of the Immune System
□ Nonspecific/Innate Immunity

□ Specific Immunity
Immunologic Disorders
Suggested Readings

LEARNING OBJECTIVES

After completing this chapter, you should be able to:

1. Describe the overall organization of the immune system, including the cellular and humoral components.
2. Describe the major functions of the immune system.
3. Identify subpopulations of lymphocytes, and describe their functions.
4. Describe the process of cellular and humoral immunity.
5. Identify the external barriers, and describe their functions.
6. Describe the cellular components and their roles in the immune response.
7. Explain the activities and the processes involved in the complement cascade.
8. Differentiate specific from nonspecific immunity.
9. Describe the four types of specific immune responses.
10. Identify the four types of immune disorders, and describe the immune response of each.

ANATOMY

The immune system is a complex network of specialized cells and organs that protects the body from foreign substances, helps maintain homeostasis, and destroys mutant cells. The lymphoreticular (lymphoid/lymphatic) system is diffuse and houses the anatomic and cellular elements that make up the immune system (Fig. 47–1). Lymph is a transparent, slightly yellow fluid that circulates through body tissues and carries lymphocytes. Lymph drains into lymphatic vessels, a bodywide network of channels transporting lymph to immune organs and the bloodstream; then eventually the lymph drains into the regional lymph nodes.

The immune system includes the thymus, spleen, Peyer's patches, bone marrow, and lymph nodes (tonsils, adenoids, cervical, axillary, para-aortic, mesenteric, and inguinal). The overall functions of these organs include the storage, activation, proliferation, and differentiation of lymphocytes.

The spleen is a major site for the filtration of foreign

particles from the blood. It is composed of sinuses lined with macrophages, whose purpose is to remove antigens (substances capable of producing an immune response) or foreign invaders (see box on page 852 for definition of terms). The spleen contains lymphoid tissue, which is thought to play a role in the process of maturation of B lymphocytes into plasma cells.

Lymph nodes are small, bean-shaped structures distributed throughout the body. Each lymph node contains specialized compartments that house B lymphocytes, T lymphocytes, and other cells of the immune system. These nodes filter antigens from the blood and circulate lymphocytes throughout the body.

The bone marrow produces cells known as stem cells, which are undifferentiated, that is, they have no specific function except as precursors for white blood cells, red blood cells, or platelets. Stem cells are precursors for all cells of both the hematologic and immune systems. Those stem cells designated to become lymphocytes are known as pre–T lymphocytes (which undergo maturation in the thymus) and pre–

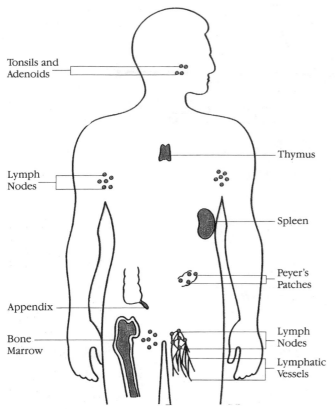

FIGURE 47–1. Organs of the immune system. (From Schindler, LW: Understanding the Immune System. NIH Publication No. 88-529, July 1988.)

TERMS ASSOCIATED WITH THE IMMUNE SYSTEM

Antigens: Substances that when introduced into the body cause an immune response.

Antigen-Presenting Cells: Macrophages that engulf and degrade antigens, presenting the antigens to the T cells in a form the T cells will recognize.

Chemical Mediator: Chemicals released by different cells of the immune system to communicate and direct other cells in the attack against antigens.

Complement: A complex series of circulating, enzymatic proteins that combine with antigen-antibody complexes to form a cascade. Complement destroys bacteria, regulates immune reactions, and produces inflammation (see Figure 47–4).

Leukocyte: Another term for a white blood cell.

Phagocytosis: The process by which white blood cells engulf antigens or cellular debris and destroy them through a series of degradative events.

B lymphocytes (which migrate to other areas in the bone marrow for maturation). When they mature, B lymphocytes produce plasma cells that secrete immunoglobulins (also known as antibodies).

CLASSIFICATION OF THE IMMUNE SYSTEM

The immune system is classified in two different ways: (1) specific or nonspecific and (2) humoral or cellular (Table 47–1). Nonspecific or specific immunity is determined by whether the immune resp

onse is directed toward a specific antigen. Nonspecific immunity is also called innate immunity because we are born with the chemical, mechanical, and physical factors involved in this type of immune response. In contrast, specific immunity is acquired as a result of the body's specific immune response triggered by invading organisms. Humoral immunity occurs when B lymphocytes stimulate the production of antibodies, and cellular immunity occurs when T lymphocytes secrete lymphokines.

Nonspecific/Innate Immunity

Barriers

External physical, mechanical, and chemical barriers are the first line of defense against antigens.

Physical barriers are structures such as intact skin and mucous membranes. Continuous shedding of dead epithelial cells rids the body surface of bacteria and denies the nutritional support necessary for replication of the antigen. Sebaceous glands of the skin secrete bactericidal and antifungal products, while dryness of the skin inhibits microbial growth. Intact mucous membranes protect the epithelial cells from viral and bacterial invasion.

Mechanical barriers include coughs and sneezes that help to expectorate particles. Eyelashes and eyelids protect eyes from invading particles. Ciliated epithelial cells along the respiratory tract constantly wave to move particles and organisms trapped in sticky mucus upward toward the oropharynx, where they are swallowed or expectorated. The intestines of the gastrointestinal tract undergo peristalsis, which propels food and associated bacteria out of the alimentary tract. In the genitourinary tract, urine flushes away microorganisms.

Chemical barriers include tears (lacrimation) that

TABLE 47–1
Classification of the Immune System

	Humoral Immunity	Cellular Immunity
Nonspecific (innate)	Complement	Granulocytes, mononuclear phagocytes
Specific (acquired)	Immunoglobulins	T lymphocytes

wash away microorganisms and particles. Lysozyme is a bactericidal component of tears, mucus, and saliva. The low pH in the stomach prohibits survival of most microbes, and digestive secretions in the small intestine deter bacterial growth. The acidic pH of urine and the production of bactericidal lysozyme by cells of the bladder also deter growth of microorganisms in the respiratory tract; mucous membranes secrete glycoproteins and lipoproteins that bind and neutralize viruses. These chemical barriers provide effective defenses for the body against antigens.

Cellular Components

The second line of defense is activated when antigens are able to pass through external barrier defenses (e.g., a staphylococcal infection from a central venous catheter). The cells making up the nonspecific immune system are known as phagocytes, which are large white blood cells that engulf and digest antigens. Phagocytes include monocytes, macrophages, granulocytes, and agranulocytes (box on page 854 and Fig. 47–2). Normal laboratory values for these cells are listed in Table 51–1.

Granulocytes. Granulocytes are phagocytes that envelop and destroy antigens. They contain granules filled with potent chemicals that contribute to inflammatory reactions. It is the granulocytes that produce symptomatology associated with allergies. Types of granulcocytes are neutrophils, eosinophils, and basophils.

Neutrophils are the most abundant and the most important phagocyte: they form the immune system's first response to bacterial invasions. Neutrophils release chemotoxins, which are substances that stimulate other cells of the immune system to migrate to the inflammatory site. The immune system has an intricate means of communicating and regulating itself through the release of chemical mediators such as the chemotoxins. Neutrophils spend about 12 hours in the blood and then enter tissues, where they complete their lifespan in a few days.

Eosinophils are granulocytes that contain granules filled with chemicals that damage parasites and have enzymes that diminish the inflammatory response. This type of granulocyte is important in allergic and immunologic reactions and against parasitic infections.

Basophils and mast cells are granulocytes that contribute to inflammatory reactions by releasing chemical mediators (e.g., histamine) that are responsible for the symptoms of allergies.

Nongranulocytes. Nongranulocytes are large cells that act as scavengers to engulf debris (e.g., phagocytosis) at the inflammatory site. Nongranulocytes include monocytes and macrophages. Monocytes are the nonspecific immune system's second internal line of defense after the granulocytes. They arrive at the site of antigen destruction 2 to 3 days after the granulocytes. Monocytes circulate in the bloodstream, while macrophages are seeded throughout body tissues, that is, in the walls of blood vessels and loose connective tissue. Monocytes transform into macrophages as they migrate from the intravascular to the interstitial space (Table 47–2). Macrophages not only phagocytize bacteria and other cellular debris but also remove dead neutrophils.

Monocytes secrete monokines, chemical mediators that help to direct and regulate the immune system. For example, interleukin-1 (IL-1) stimulates T and B lymphocytes. IL-1 also acts as an endogenous pyrogen, inducing prostaglandin production, which causes

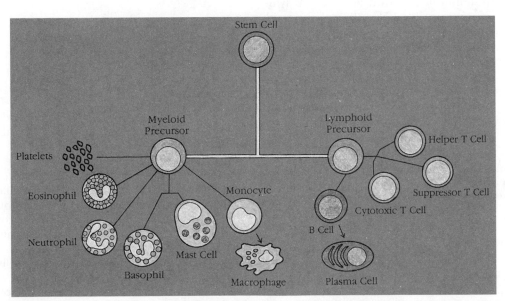

FIGURE 47–2. Cells of the immune system. (From Schindler, LW: Understanding the Immune System. NIH Publication No. 88-529, July 1988.)

CELLS OF THE IMMUNE SYSTEM

Stem Cells: Immature, undifferentiated white blood cells produced in the bone marrow.

GRANULOCYTES

Basophils: White blood cells that release histamine and heparin in response to tissue damage during inflammation. Basophils make up less than 0.5% of the total white blood cell count.

Eosinophils: White blood cells whose granules contain chemicals that are damaging to parasitic larvae, regulate inflammatory reactions, and release histamine in response to allergic reactions. Eosinophils make up 1%–2% of the total white blood cell count.

Neutrophils: Abundant white blood cells whose major function is the nonspecific ingestion and phagocytosis of antigens. Neutrophils make up 55%–70% of the total white blood cell count.

Mast Cells: A white blood cell located in tissue. Along with basophils, mast cells are responsible for the symptoms of allergies.

NONGRANULOCYTES

Monocytes: Large, phagocytic white blood cells when enter tissue, but develop into macrophages. Monocytes are capable of activating complement. They make up 2%–4% of the total white blood cell count.

Macrophages: Mature monocytes located in various body tissues. Macrophages act as phagocytes, as antigen-presenting cells, and they are an important source of the release of chemical mediators.

LYMPHOCYTES

Lymphocytes: White blood cells involved in cellular, specific immunity. Known as T and B lymphocytes, they account for 25%–30% of the total white blood cell count.

T Lymphocytes: A category of small white blood cells that coordinate and/or directly participate in the immune defenses. T lymphocytes are composed of helper, cytotoxic, suppressor, and memory cells.

Cytotoxic T Lymphocytes: A subset of T lymphocytes that carry the T8 marker. These cells are capable of killing cells either infected by viruses or transformed by cancer.

Helper T Lymphocytes: A subset of T lymphocytes that carry the T4 marker. They are essential for stimulating antibody production, activating cytotoxic T lymphocytes, and initiating other immune responses.

Suppressor T Lymphocytes: A subset of T lymphocytes that carry the T8 marker. They are responsible for stopping antibody production and other immune responses.

B Lymphocytes: A category of small white blood cells including plasma cells that secrete antibodies in response to particular antigens and memory cells.

Plasma Cells: Large antibody-producing cells that develop from B lymphocytes.

Antibody: One of five subsets of proteins that are secreted by plasma cells and are capable of neutralizing, eliminating, or destroying antigens. Antibodies are also known as **immunoglobulins.**

Memory Cells: T and B cells produced during the first encounter with a specific antigen. These cells circulate freely and respond quickly to antigens the next time of exposure.

Natural Killer Cells: Large granule-filled lymphocytes that attack antigens and aberrant cells. They are known as natural killers because they attack without first recognizing specific antigens.

fever and interferes with bacterial, viral, and tumor growth. Another mediator is interferon-α, which is activated in response to viral invasion. Interferon-α slows down viral replication and has an additional feature of inhibiting the proliferation of malignant cells.

TABLE 47–2
Monocytes and Macrophages of the Mononuclear Phagocyte System

Location	Name
Liver	Kupffer's cells
Connective tissue	Histiocyte
Bone	Osteoclast
Spleen	Dendritic cell
Nervous system	Microglial cell
Lung	Alveolar macrophage
Kidneys	Intraglomerular mesangial cell
Skin	Langerhans' cells

Phagocytosis

When an antigen enters the body, a chain of events called a phagocytic response is set in motion. First, a chemical is released either by the antigen or by the injured cell. This chemical (the chemotoxic factor) stimulates the body's initial efforts at search and destroy. Blood flow to the injured area is increased, causing the nonspecific local responses of erythema and heat production. Vasodilation follows, and the walls of the vessels become more permeable. This increased permeation allows neutrophils to leave

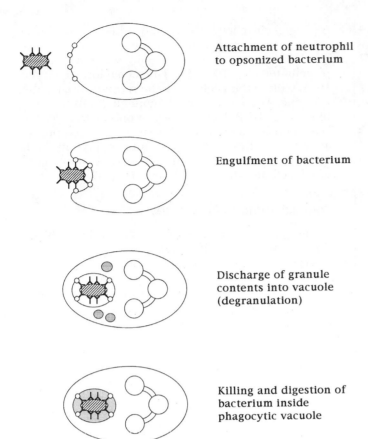

Attachment of neutrophil to opsonized bacterium

Engulfment of bacterium

Discharge of granule contents into vacuole (degranulation)

Killing and digestion of bacterium inside phagocytic vacuole

FIGURE 47–3. Phagocytosis.

blood vessels and migrate to the scene of the injury. Induration and swelling occur as a consequence of the arrival of a large number of white blood cells. Pus formation can occur from both the destruction of phagocytic cells and tissue injury.

The process of phagocytosis occurs when an antigen comes into contact with a granulocyte. Phagocytosis is the two-phase process by which antigens are engulfed by the phagocytic cells. In the attachment phase, the antigen and the phagocytic cell make contact. In the ingestion phase, the antigen is engulfed: it enters the cytoplasm and is enclosed within a pocket (vacuole); then the granules rupture, destroying the antigen (Fig. 47–3).

Complement System

The humoral arm of nonspecific immunity lies within the complement system. ''Complement'' is a collective term used to describe several different proteins that produce a series of events, or a cascade, that plays a role in the immune response. All of these proteins are given numbers that follow the letter ''C.'' Complement destroys bacteria, produces inflammation, and regulates immune reactions by the following actions: (1) lysis of cell membranes of the invading organism, (2) chemotaxis (the generation of peptide fragments that mediate the inflammatory and

immune responses), (3) opsonization (the process by which antigens are coated with a specific complement fragment to promote phagocytosis), and (4) release of mediators that increase vascular permeability (box on page 856).

The complement system is activated when the first complement molecule (C1) recognizes an antigen-antibody complex. This system activation occurs either in the classical complement activation pathway or the alternate pathway. The *classical complement system* cascade occurs when the protein C1 is activated by IgM or IgG coming into contact with an antigen (Fig. 47–4). When the complement cascade is completed, the result is a membrane attack complex. This complex resembles a trocar and pokes holes in the membranes of cells at the site of tissue destruction. Cytoplasm leaks out of these holes in the membrane walls of antigens, thus destroying the organism. Since the complement system is nonspecific, it can potentially destroy cells other than antigens involved in the immune response.

The complement cascade can also be activated through an *alternate pathway*. The alternate pathway starts at C3, bypasses C4, and then follows the classical complement pathway. It also differs from the classical pathway in that it is activated without the presence of IgG. Thus, antibody production is not necessary for this type of response.

MAJOR ANTIGEN-ANTIBODY REACTIONS

Agglutination: Antigens form a lattice with antibodies, resulting in clumping.

Complement Fixation: C1q binds to a site on the constant portion of immunoglobulin (Ig), activating the complement cascade and resulting in cell lysis.

Lysis: The cell membrane is destroyed by the late complement components.

Neutralization: The infectivity of an organism is neutralized by combining the toxins and preventing their attachment to cell membranes.

Opsonization: Antigens are coated to enhance phagocytosis.

Specific Immunity

Specific immunity presents the third line of defense. This system is activated when the defensive barriers and nonspecific immune responses are not effective in the destruction of antigens. The term "specific immunity" reflects the body's ability to manufacture antibodies that are selective for specific antigens.

To produce specific antibodies, the body has a complex means to distinguish self from nonself. Cells of the immune system are able to distinguish antigens (nonself) from themselves because of the characteristic shapes called epitopes that protrude from the surface of the antigens. Epitopes are unique shapes or markers carried on an antigen surface that trigger a corresponding antibody response. Most antigens carry several different types of epitopes. The immune system also recognizes self through a series of genes (human leukocyte antigen [HLA] genes) located on chromosome 6. When HLA antigens are transferred from the host (donor) to a recipient, they become foreign antigens to the recipient. This phenomenon is responsible for graft rejection with organ transplants.

The specific immune system is activated when mac-

rophage cells chemically modify antigens. The macrophage then again expresses the processed antigen on its surface along with a unique set of membrane proteins termed "DR." The DR gene is located on the HLA. Only certain cells have the receptor site for the DR gene. These cells include epithelial cells that line blood vessels, B lymphocytes, mononuclear phagocytes, and activated T lymphocytes. The macrophage, after chemically modifying the antigen, presents both the antigen and the DR molecule to the T lymphocyte, which activates the T lymphocyte (Fig. 47–5).

Specific Immune Responses

The specific immune system responds by proliferation (quantity) and differentiation (function) of lymphocytes, effector mechanisms, and memory.

Proliferation and Differentiation. Once the T lymphocyte is activated, it begins to undergo proliferation, reproducing multiple identical copies of itself in a process known as clonal expansion. During differentiation, the T lymphocyte produces four different subsets of lymphocytes: helper, suppressor, cytotoxic, and memory T lymphocytes. These cells are involved in discreet functions.

The T4 (CD4) lymphocyte is also known as the helper lymphocyte, helping orchestrate the specific immune response. T4 activates antibody production of B lymphocytes and cytotoxic lymphocytes and initiates many other immune responses.

Suppressor T8 lymphocytes help regulate the immune response by turning off antibody production and other immune responses. Once antigens are destroyed, the assault is inactivated by suppressor T lymphocytes that transmit chemical messages to B and T lymphocytes to shut down. B lymphocytes stop producing antibodies, and cytotoxic T lymphocytes stop their assault on the antigens.

Cytotoxic T lymphocytes (T8, CD8) are a subset of the T cells that carry the CD8 antigen receptor marker. These lymphocytes directly attack cell membranes, releasing toxic chemicals that cause the foreign particle to rupture and die. The CD8 cell is

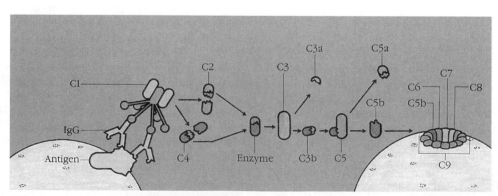

FIGURE 47–4. The complement cascade. (From Schindler, LW: Understanding the Immune System. NIH Publication No. 88-529, July 1988.)

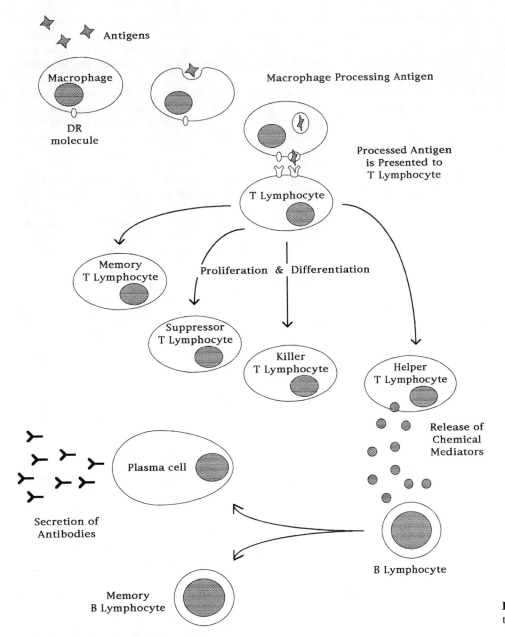

FIGURE 47-5. Activation of the specific immune system.

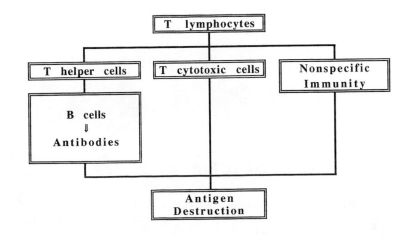

FIGURE 47-6. Effector mechanisms.

responsible for attacking cells that have been transformed into cancer cells, eliciting an immune response against engrafted tissues or organs and ridding the body of cells infected by bacteria or viruses.

Memory T lymphocytes are mobilized the next time the invading antigen enters the body. If the same antigen enters the body, these memory cells recognize the antigen and respond quickly.

Effector Mechanisms. Effector mechanisms inactivate or dispose of the remaining antigens. These functions are activated when antigens are presented to T lymphocytes, which then secrete lymphokines (chemical messengers that allow the T lymphocyte to communicate with other cells of the immune system). For example, the T lymphocyte can secrete a lymphokine called B cell growth factor (BCGF), whose function is to stimulate the proliferation of B lymphocytes. Another common lymphokine is interleukin-2 (IL-2), which acts as a stimulus for the proliferation of more T lymphocytes.

Once lymphokines are sent to the various cells, several events occur, as illustrated in Figure 47–6. T lymphocytes induce other T helper cells to stimulate B lymphocyte differentiation and antibody production. The T helper cells stimulate T cytotoxic cells. Next there is a release of a chemical mediator, which induces nonspecific immune cells to continue their activities against the antigen. What follows is a clonal

expansion of cytotoxic T lymphocytes capable of destroying antigens. Cytotoxic T lymphocytes bind to the surface of invading antigens, disrupt the cell membrane, and destroy the antigen by secreting lymphokines.

Stimulation of the B lymphocytes causes a proliferation of these cells, which mature into plasma cells. Antibodies (immunoglobulins) are produced by these plasma cells, which are specific for the particular invading antigen. There are five types of immunoglobulins, each serving different functions (box below).

Large granular lymphocytes known as natural killer (NK) cells are also stimulated by T lymphocytes. NK cells, also known as null cells, are not part of acquired immunity and respond as part of the nonspecific immune system. These cells are thought to be important in the detection and destruction of malignant cells.

Memory. The immune system also responds by memory, producing a proliferation of memory B and T lymphocytes. These memory cells remain viable and remember the foreign antigen from a previous exposure. Upon repeated exposure, these lymphocytes are then capable of responding more quickly to the antigen. Vaccinations help to elicit the memory function of lymphocytes. For example, when a vaccine (a substance that contains antigenic components from an infectious organism) is given to a host, it stimulates an

---

CLASSIFICATION OF IMMUNOGLOBULINS

IgG

- Major immunoglobulin class
- 85% of antibodies
- Found in the tissue and bloodstream
- Involved in opsonization, neutralization, and complement fixation
- Elevated with the chronic phase of an infection

IgA

- Composed of two IgA molecules, which can be secreted into mucus, intestinal juices, tears, and breast milk
- Protects the above areas from infection through neutralization
- Prevents surface attachment of antigens

IgM

- Composed of five immunoglobulin molecules
- Elevated with an acute phase of an infection
- Activates complement and causes agglutination of antigens

IgE

- Key role in allergic responses
- Attaches to a mast cell, causing the cell to lyse and release chemicals

IgD

- Possible role in regulating immune responses
- Located in the serum and on the surface of B lymphocytes

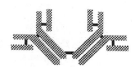

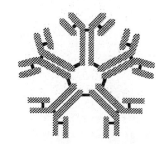

IgG, IgD, & IgE   *IgA*   *IgM*

TABLE 47–3
Immunodeficiency Disorders

Disorders	Immunity
Primary Disorders	
Cyclic neutropenia	Nonspecific immunity
Complement deficiencies	Nonspecific immunity
Transient hypogammaglobulinemia of infancy	Humoral immunity
Bruton's hypogammaglobulinemia	Humoral immunity
Selective IgA deficiency	Humoral immunity
DiGeorge's syndrome	Cell-mediated immunity
Severe combined immune deficiency (SCID)	Cell-mediated and humoral immunity
Secondary Disorders	
Acquired immunodeficiency syndrome (AIDS)	Cell-mediated immunity

TABLE 47–4
Type II: Autoimmune Disorders

Autoimmune Diseases	Disorders
Systemic lupus erythematous	Rheumatoid
Rheumatoid arthritis	Rheumatoid
Scleroderma	Rheumatoid
Sjögren's syndrome	Rheumatoid
Autoimmune hemolytic anemia	Hemopoietic
Idiopathic thrombocytopenia purpura	Hemopoietic
Pernicious anemia	Hemopoietic
Systemic necrotizing vasculitis	Vascular
Wegener's granulomatosis	Vascular
Goodpasture's syndrome	Renal
Immune complex glomerulonephritis	Renal
Hashimoto's disease	Endocrine
Grave's disease	Endocrine
Multiple sclerosis	Neurologic
Myasthenia gravis	Neurologic

immune response in which the lymphocytes remember being exposed to the infectious organism and are able to respond quickly to a subsequent exposure.

IMMUNOLOGIC DISORDERS

Immunologic disorders occur when the immune system is unable to defend the host against antigens either because of (1) a decreased ability to recognize antigens or (2) the inability to eliminate antigens. The disorders are classified as follows:

Type I: Immunodeficient
Type II: Autoimmune
Type III: Immunoproliferative
Type IV: Hypersensitive

Type I disorders can be either congenital (e.g., DiGeorge's syndrome) or acquired (e.g., AIDS), primary or secondary (Table 47–3). Primary deficiencies are generally very rare. The person usually has no underlying virus and no apparent underlying medical condition, nor has received immunosuppressive therapy. Secondary deficiencies are more common than primary deficiencies and may be due to underlying viral infections, other medical conditions, or medical treatments (e.g., chemotherapy).

Type II, autoimmune, disorders are the result of

mistaken attacks on the body's own tissue (Table 47–4). The immune system no longer recognizes self and activates immunologic mechanisms that react against self molecules. Rheumatoid arthritis, for example, is a type II disorder.

Type III, immunoproliferation, occurs when a component of the immune system proliferates without the appropriate signals to start and stop. Proliferation occurs when immunosurveillance is impaired and aberrant cells are allowed to proliferate. Leukemia is an example of this type of disorder.

Type IV, hypersensitivity, occurs when altered immune responses to specific antigens produce exaggerated or inappropriate immune responses. Hypersensitive reactions are categorized according to the speed of the reaction and the type of immune mechanism.

TYPE IV HYPERSENSITIVITY RESPONSES

1. Type I is the immediate hypersensitivity response (IgE mediated). When the host is exposed to an antigen, the T lymphocyte recognizes the antigen and sends a chemical message to B lymphocytes to produce IgE. The IgE binds to receptors on mast cells and then to antigens, causing the

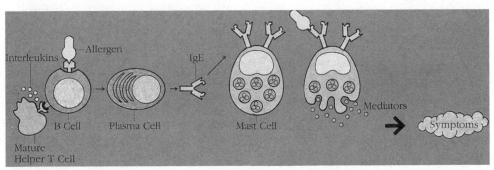

FIGURE 47–7. Type I hypersensitivity reaction. (From Schindler, LW: Understanding the Immune System. NIH Publication No. 88-529, July 1988.)

mast cells to degranulate. The release of chemical mediators, such as histamine, bradykinin, and prostaglandins, follows (Fig. 47–7). This release results in smooth muscle contraction, mucus production, vasodilation, puritis, capillary leakage, and bronchoconstriction. Type I reactions usually occur immediately or up to 12 hours after exposure. Type I hypersensitivity reactions include allergies, anaphylaxis, atopic eczema, and asthma.

2. Type II is the cytotoxic hypersensitivity reaction (antibody mediated). When the host's immune system begins to recognize self as foreign, B lymphocytes produce antibodies against the self cell. Macrophages, antibodies, and the complement cascade work in combination to destroy self cells. Examples of this type of reaction include immune hemolytic anemia, idiopathic thrombocytopenia purpura, Grave's disease, myasthenia gravis, rheumatoid arthritis, and systemic lupus erythematosus.

3. Type III is the immune complex–mediated reaction. Antigen-antibody complexes are formed and deposited into tissue, which results in increased vascular permeability and microthrombi formation. Platelets then aggregate at the site and release histamine, which causes further microthrombi development and capillary leakage. Components of the immune system respond to the injury, complement is activated, and phagocytes travel to the site. The granulo-

cytes are unable to phagocytize the immune complexes. Instead, lysosome from the phagocyte is released into the surrounding tissue, causing further damage. Examples of type III reactions include systemic lupus erythematosus and rheumatoid arthritis.

4. Type IV is the delayed hypersensitivity reaction. When antigens enter the host, T lymphocytes recognize the antigens and proliferate memory cells in response to them. The next time T lymphocytes encounter the antigens, they release lymphokines. These secretions cause a localized accumulation of lymphocytes and activated macrophages. Examples of type IV reactions include tuberculosis and contact dermatitis.

SUGGESTED READINGS

Huffer, TL, Kananpa, DJ, and Stevenson, GW: Introduction to Human Immunology. Jones and Bartlett, Boston, 1986.

Kirkwood, E, and Lewis, C: Understanding Medical Immunology, ed 2. John Wiley & Sons, Chichester, England, 1989.

Mudge-Grout, C: Immunologic Disorders. Mosby-Year Book, St. Louis, 1993.

Roitt, I, Brostoff, J, and Male, D: Immunology, ed 2. Gower Medical, London, 1989.

Schindler, LW: Understanding the Immune System. NIH publication no. 88–529, 1988.

Tribett, D: Immune system function: Implications for critical care nursing practice. Crit Care Nurs Clin North Am, 1(4):725–740, 1989.

Workman, ML, Ellerhorst-Ryan, J, and Hargrave-Koertge, V: Nursing Care of the Immunocompromised Patient. WB Saunders, Philadelphia, 1993.

CHAPTER 48

Assessment of Immunologic Function
Diane Ragsdale and Kristin Kane Ownby

CHAPTER OUTLINE

Health History
- Present Illness
- Past Medical History

Physical Examination

Laboratory Tests

Assessment Considerations for the Bone
   Marrow Transplant Patient

Quality of Life Considerations

Suggested Readings

LEARNING OBJECTIVES

After completing this chapter, you should be able to:

1. Complete a nursing assessment of the patient's immunologic function.
2. Correlate the clinical presentation with the type of immune response.
3. Identify the purposes of laboratory tests for nonspecific, humoral, and cell-mediated immunity.

As a result of the complexity of the immune system, a vast range of possibilities for defects and dysfunctions exist, and there are no standard signs and symptoms of immune disorders. Often, disorders of the immune system produce multiorgan and multisystemic effects. The focus of assessment should be on recognition of immune-related symptomatolgy.

An accurate assessment is crucial to the care of any patient who has a disorder of the immune system. Evaluation of immunologic status is based chiefly on laboratory findings; however, health history and physical examination provide important additional information. A nursing assessment for immunologic disorders begins with questions related to the present illness, past medical history, and family medical history. The SLIDT tool (Table 35–1) can be used to collect data related to the patient's complaints and problems. The next part of the assessment is a detailed, systematic physical examination. A variety of laboratory tests are then performed, based on clinical findings, to complete the assessment data.

HEALTH HISTORY

Present Illness

The clinical presentation of suspected immune dysfunction often suggests the type of immune response (Table 48–1).

Common signs of immune disorders are fatigue, fever, joint pain, lymphadenopathy, and bleeding (Table 48–2). Although these signs and symptoms are not always present, they are key indicators of immune system dysfunction. For example, spiking temperatures may indicate recurrent fevers and are often indicative of rapid cell proliferation; intermittent temperature elevations are characteristic of diseases such as Hodgkin's lymphoma. Joint pain often accompanies autoimmune disorders, such as rheumatoid arthritis (RA).

Past Medical History

Taking an immunologic history of the patient is the first step in identifying immune system dysfunctions. The components of the immunologic history include histories of infections, allergies, vaccinations, possible autoimmune symptoms, drugs, family illnesses, chronic illnesses, and sexual practices (box on page 862).

PHYSICAL EXAMINATION

The next step in identifying immune system dysfunctions is to make a thorough physical examination.

Skin. The skin is inspected for color, cyanosis, erythema, and petechiae. Because the skin is the first line

TABLE 48–1
Immune Dysfunction According to Clinical Presentation*

Type of Immunity	Clinical Presentation of Deficiency or Disorder
Cell-mediated	Fungal, viral, and protozoa infections
	Transplant/tissue rejection (graft versus host disease)
Humoral	Recurrent bacterial infections
Phagocytic	Recurrent skin and systemic (pyogenic bacterial) infections
Complement	Recurrent pyogenic infections

*This relationship is not present in all clinical cases.

TABLE 48–2
Indicators of Immune System Dysfunction

Signs and Symptoms	Nursing Assessment
Fatigue, weakness	Commonly present in many immune disorders; look for other signs and symptoms
Fever	Look for degree, characteristics (e.g., constant, intermittent, recurring, fluctuation)
Joint pain	Look for inflammation, limitation of movement; use SLIDT tool
Lymphadenopathy	Look for an inflammation/infection in the area drained by the involved lymph nodes
Bleeding	Look for hematuria, melena, ecchymosis, petechiae, anemia

of defense against infection, it should be assessed at portal sites (e.g., indwelling catheters, IVs, and vascular access devices) for signs of infection, such as redness, swelling, tenderness, or drainage. Allergic reactions may be manifested in rashes, dryness, itching, and scaling.

Eyes. The eyes are assessed for erythemia or pallor to the conjunctiva. Erythema may suggest conjunctivitis, which is seen in many allergies and immunodeficiency disorders. The lacrimal gland is palpated for enlargement, which may indicate Sjögren's syndrome. The six cardinal fields of gaze are checked for mus-

cular weakness because this condition can be seen in certain autoimmune disorders, such as multiple sclerosis (MS) or Grave's disease.

Oral Cavity. Ulcerations, lesions, white patches, or changes in color in the oral cavity may indicate an array of immunologic disorders. Oral ulcerations can indicate systemic lupus erythematosus or can result from treatment with antineoplastic agents. White exudate over the mucous membranes and tongue may be due to candidiasis, which may indicate an immunologic disorder, such as acquired immune deficiency

---

IMMUNOLOGIC HISTORY

INFECTIONS

Causative organism
Site of infection
Characteristics of infection
Recurrent
Chronic
Onset of infection—recent or childhood

ALLERGIES

Drug
Food
Environmental
Asthma
Hay fever
Urticaria

VACCINATIONS

Vaccination record
Unusually severe reaction to a vaccine
Resulted in desired immunity

POSSIBLE AUTOIMMUNE SYMPTOMS

Joint pain or limited range of motion
Anemia
Ulcerations of the oral cavity

Lymphadenopathy
Bleeding

DRUGS

Substance abuse:
Antineoplastic agents
Steroids
Chronic antibiotic therapy

FAMILY OR PERSONAL ILLNESSES

Autoimmune disease
Allergies
Immunodeficiency diseases
Diabetes
Cancer

SEXUAL PRACTICES

Multiple sexual partners
Homosexual
Heterosexual
Bisexual
Safer sex practices

syndrome (AIDS). Fine tremors of the tongue may indicate Grave's disease.

Lymph Nodes. The lymph nodes in the head and neck, axilla, inguinal, and popliteal areas should be assessed. Initially, nodes are inspected for edema, erythema, red streaks, or skin lesions. Inspection is followed by palpation, assessing for enlargement, temperature, tenderness, consistency, mobility, and shape. Lymph nodes that are large, fixed, matted, inflamed, or tender indicate some problem. Hard, discrete nodes are more indicative of malignancies. Enlarged lymph nodes related to an underlying malignancy are generally not tender. Particularly, a palpable left supraclavicular node indicates an underlying abdominal or thoracic malignancy. Tenderness tends to indicate an inflammatory process. With bacterial infections, nodes may become warm or tender, matted, and less discrete. In tuberculosis, the lymph nodes are usually at body temperature, soft, matted, and not tender.

Respiratory System. The respiratory system is assessed for signs of distress, such as dyspnea, persistent cough, wheezing, or cyanosis. Pneumonia can accompany many immune disorders, such as AIDS. The thoracic expansion is assessed for limitation in chest expansion, which may indicate pain, inflammation, or restriction. Restrictive chest expansion could indicate scleroderma. Auscultation of the chest is done to assess for adventitious breath sounds, such as hyperresonance and wheezes, which are often associated with asthma. Crackles and bronchial breath sounds are associated with pneumonia. Patients with systemic lupus erythematosus (SLE) or RA can develop pleural effusions.

Heart. The heart is auscultated for rate, rhythm, and abnormal heart sounds. Tachycardia may indicate Grave's disease, anemia, or an infection. Pericardial friction rubs, associated with endocarditis or pericarditis, can be seen in the patient with SLE, scleroderma, or RA.

Abdomen. The abdomen is assessed for bowel sounds. Hyperactive bowel sounds are frequently heard with diarrhea. Diarrhea is a common manifestation of immune disorders such as Crohn's disease or ulcerative colitis. Hypoactive bowel sounds secondary to constipation may be auscultated in the patient with scleroderma. The liver and spleen are palpated and percussed for enlargement. Hepatosplenomegaly is associated with immune disorders, such as idiopathic thrombocytopenic purpura (ITP) and hemolytic anemia, and with immunoproliferative disorders, such as lymphoma.

Neuromuscular. The neuromuscular system is also assessed for immunologic diseases. Gait, muscle strength, coordination, and range of joint motion should be assessed. Muscle weakness is associated with SLE, RA, myasthenia gravis (MG), and AIDS. Patients with MS or MG may have impaired coordination. Loss of balance is seen in patients with Grave's disease or progressive AIDS. Defects in sensory functions could indicate SLE, MS, or RA.

LABORATORY TESTS

Immunologic examination involves both in vivo and in vitro testing. The in vivo tests use three techniques: intradermal, prick, and patch skin testing.

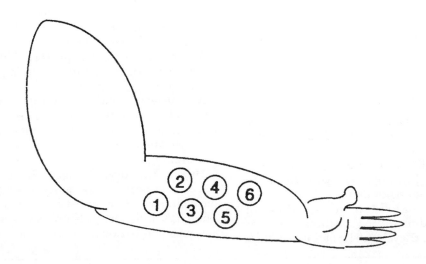

1 Candida	3 Purified protein derivative	5 Trichophyton
2 Mumps	4 Streptokinase	6 Control

FIGURE 48–1. Intradermal skin testing for anergy

IN VITRO IMMUNOLOGIC TESTS

TESTS OF NONSPECIFIC IMUNITY

Complete Blood Cell Count: Red blood cells (RBCs), hemoglobin, and hematocrit evaluate oxygen-carrying capacity and hydration. Platelets indicate the body's ability to clot. White blood cell (WBC) fluctuations may indicate infections or hematologic malignancies.

Erythrocyte Sedimentation Rate (SED rate) Test: In this nonspecific test for the inflammatory process, elevations of the SED rate may indicate RA, hemolytic anemia, thyroid disorders, nephritis, autoimmune disorders, and some malignancies.

Complement Activity Tests: C3 and C4 serum tests measure C3 and C4 levels. Elevation of C3, the most abundant component of the complement system, can occur in inflammatory disorders. C3 and C4 levels are decreased in diseases such as SLE, renal transplant rejection, glomerulonephritis, and MS. The CH50 assay evaluates the functioning of the whole classical complement pathway. Combined, these three tests are very effective in measuring the functioning of the complement system.

Neutrophil Function Tests: These tests evaluate the six stages of phagocytosis: motility, recognition, adhesion, ingestion, degranulation, and killing. The nitroblue tetrazolium (NBT) test is a rapid screening method to determine whether there are gross defects in the ability of neutrophils to phagocytize (kill) antigens. Another screening method to determine the neutrophils' ability to phagocytize is the chemiluminescence test.

C-Reactive Protein (CRP) Serum Test: The CRP level is generally not detectable in the healthy person; however, it is elevated 6 to 10 hours after an acute inflammatory process or tissue destruction. CRP is also elevated in diseases such as RA and SLE and in bacterial infections (however, not in viral infections).

TESTS OF HUMORAL IMMUNITY

Immunoglobulin Quantitation: This test measures the quantity of certain immunoglobulins: IgG, IgA, and IgM. The test is used especially in children who have repeated, severe infections. The infections may be related to impaired synthesis of one or more of the immunoglobulins.

IgE Estimation: This test is used for persons suffering from atopic diseases (e.g., asthma, hay fever, or food allergies). IgE levels will be elevated in these conditions. Based on the person's history, IgE antibody levels for specific antigens are measured.

Immunoelectrophoresis: This test detects antigen-antibody reactions by measuring precipitation. An example of this type of test is the Western blot for detecting antibodies for the human immunodeficiency virus.

Circulating Immune Complex Detection: This test assesses the formation of antigen-antibody with subsequent activation of the complement casade. Certain diseases, such as SLE, RA, lymphomas, and leukemias, are associated with the formation of immune complexes.

TESTS OF CELL-MEDIATED IMMUNITY

T and B Cell Quantitation: This test determines the actual number of T and B lymphocytes circulating in the blood.

Functional Lymphocyte Assays: These tests are used to measure the lymphocytes' ability to proliferate, recognize, and react to antigens.

Mixed Lymphocyte Cultures (MLC): This test is another means to measure proliferation of T and B lymphocytes. It is used primarily in organ and bone marrow transplants to determine donor/recipient compatibility.

MISCELLANEOUS TESTS

Coombs' Test: Direct Coombs' is used to detect antibodies on RBCs that induce agglutination of RBCs coated with these antibodies. Diseases associated with a positive direct Coombs' test include transfusion reactions and autoimmune hemolytic anemias. Indirect Coombs' test is used to detect antibodies in the serum. These antibodies bind with RBCs, inducing agglutination.

Rheumatoid (RA) Factor Test: This test detects the presence of an immunoglobulin present in the serum of patients with RA.

Antinuclear Antibody (ANA) Test: This test screens for connective tissue diseases, such as SLE. It detects the presence of an antibody by assessing for the affinity of the antibody to a nuclear preparation.

Human Leukocyte Antigen (HLA) Typing: This test is an important laboratory procedure when tissue-typing for bone marrow and organ transplants. The HLA antigens on lymphocytes are compared and matched between a donor and a recipient.

Intradermal skin testing to determine whether cell-mediated immunity is intact can be used to assess delayed hypersensitivity. Most people have been exposed to specific antigens: candida, mumps, purified protein derivative, trichophyton, and streptokinase. A 0.1 mL extraction of each of these antigens is injected intradermally into the forearm, which is observed for 48 hours (Fig. 48–1). A positive reaction is present when there is induration and erythema at the antigen sites. If there is no response, then the person is anergic (a state of cell-mediated unresponsiveness).

The prick test is used to assess immediate hypersensitivity by intradermally injecting antigens chosen based on the patient's history (e.g., house dust mites, grass pollen, and cat antigens). These skin tests are used to identify antigens that stimulate IgE antibody production.

Patch testing is used to diagnose contact dermatitis. A small amount of the suspected contact antigen is applied to the skin of the back. It is observed 48 hours later, and if a small patch of eczema is present, the test is positive.

In vitro testing is classified by the part of the immune system to be examined. The tests of the immune system are further classified as nonspecific, humoral, and cell-mediated immune system tests (box on page 864).

ASSESSMENT CONSIDERATIONS FOR THE BONE MARROW TRANSPLANT PATIENT

For the patient who has undergone an allogeneic bone marrow transplant, one of the most crucial immunologic processes that the nurse assesses for is graft versus host disease (GVHD). In the immunologic process of GVHD, the mature lymphocytes from the graft (the marrow) recognize the host (recipient) as being foreign. GVHD accounts for a mortality rate of about 45% after an allogeneic transplant. Acute GVHD may develop from 7 to 20 days after the transplant. The organ systems involved in GVHD are the skin, liver, and gastrointestinal tract. The signs and symptoms of GVHD are profuse diarrhea, elevation in the bilirubin, and a diffuse erythematous macular rash that can lead to desquamation of the skin. The rash typically begins on the soles, palms, and scalp and may spread to the trunk and extremities. Hyperbilirubinemia and jaundice occur as a result of inflammation of the small bile duct. Elevated laboratory values include serum alkaline phosphatase, alanine aminotranferase (ALT), and aspartate transferase (AST).

QUALITY OF LIFE CONSIDERATIONS

Immunodeficiency diseases (e.g., AIDS) and many of the autoimmune diseases (e.g., MS and MG) can have disastrous effects on patients and their families. Assess how the illness affects family members and how they are coping. Help the family identify effective coping mechanisms to enhance quality of life by decreasing stress, thus lessening the impact on the immune system.

SUGGESTED READINGS

Kee, JL: Handbook of Laboratory Diagnostic Tests with Nursing Implications, ed 2. Appleton & Lange, Norwalk, CT, 1994.
Kirkwood, E, and Lewis, C: Understanding Medical Immunology, ed 2. John Wiley & Sons, New York, 1989.
Mudge-Grout, CL: Immunologic Disorders. Mosby-Year Book, St. Louis, 1992.
Seidel, HM, Ball, JW, Dains, JE, and Benedict, GW: Mosby's Guide to Physical Examination, ed 2. Mosby-Year Book, St. Louis, 1991.

C H A P T E R 4 9

Clinical Application: Renal Transplantation

Wayne C. Waltzer

LEARNING OBJECTIVES

After completing this chapter, you should be able to:

1. Define "allotransplantation."
2. Discuss the significance of tissue matching in terms of tissue compatibility between donor and recipient and, thus, the best outlook for successful transplantation.
3. List key factors to be considered when evaluating a person/family as a potential recipient for organ transplantation.
4. Describe potential donor sources and key assessment considerations in donor selection.
5. List criteria for brain death in the clinical practice setting.
6. Describe major considerations in managing the patient after the transplant.
7. Discuss the impact of available immunosuppressive drug therapy on clinical transplantation and the special problems and concerns associated with specific immunosuppressive agents.
8. Examine classic presenting signs and symptoms and laboratory findings in kidney transplant rejection.

HISTORY

Over the past decades, kidney transplantation has evolved from an experimental procedure to a practical, everyday, and clinically accepted means for treating end-stage renal disease.

In 1912, Carrel[1] described the successful transplant of an autogenous kidney to the neck vessels of a dog by means of vascular suture. His experiments showed that while autogenous organs survived after vascular anastomosis and were able to function, unknown biologic factors caused failure in allogenic organ grafts.

Following decades of experimental work, it was discovered that the survival of grafted organs depended on similarities in the genetic constitution of the donor and recipient. With the discovery of the human leukocyte antigen (HLA) system in humans, the possibility of getting optimally compatible combinations between donors and recipients was enhanced. Dausset[2] first described the human leukocyte antigen, Mac, later known as HLA-2. This antigen was defined by the presence of antibody in the sera of multiply transfused patients, and later it was shown to be part of the major histocompatibility complex (MHC) in humans.

Advances in immunology, anesthesia, organ preservation, antibiotics, the use of heparin, and extracorporeal circulation for hemodialysis all made feasible a new phase of surgical activity and the rebirth of transplantation. In 1954, the first successful human kidney transplant was performed; the exchange of kidneys was between monozygotic twins.

After failure of nonimmunosuppressed allotransplants, the discovery of 6-mercaptopurine, steroids, and x-ray irradiation proved to be critical in controlling allograft rejection. The success of allotransplants improved, and in 1992, 7691 cadaveric kidney transplants were performed in the United States.[3] Unfortunately, about 24,000 patients were waiting for kidney transplants during the same period.

The introduction of cyclosporine, an even more effective means of suppressing host immune reactivity, has allowed the rapid clinical growth of transplantation of heart, liver, lungs, pancreas, bone marrow, and intestine. Other new immunosuppressive agents have further extended the immunosuppressive armamentarium (e.g., FK-506, rapamycin, mycophenolic acid, brequinar sodium.) Thus, most patients with irreversible organ damage are now potential candidates for transplantation.

HISTOCOMPATIBILITY

Histocompatibility testing determines the degree of tissue compatibility between donor and recipient. The discovery of the human MHC occurred in the 1950s when antibodies were found in the sera of multiply transfused patients and multiparous females. Subsequent research suggested that these antibodies could detect alloantigens (i.e., antigens present on the cells of individuals of a given species.)

The HLA is a single, complex genetic locus on the short arm of the C6 chromosome.[4] Based on results from family studies, the antigens have been grouped into two main divisions, or subloci: class I (HLA-A, B, and C) and class II (HLA-D, DR) antigens. The names assigned to antigens are uniform throughout the world to allow correlation of data and exchange of blood and tissue samples. These antigens are characteristic of an individual and stimulate rejection of foreign tissue allografts.

HLA tissue-typing is performed by exposing lymphocytes from both donor and recipient to antisera containing known HLA specificities.[4] Thus, it is possible to identify the antigens present on both donor and recipient tissue. HLA tissue-typing still remains important in the selection of renal allograft recipients, although the use of cyclosporine, transfusions, and OKT3 monoclonal antibody therapy have somewhat reduced the advantage gained by matching. Our policy is only to use tissues matched on either two antigens (A and B series antigens) or one DR locus.

The perfect match, or six antigens, or an HLA identical match, offers the best outlook for successful kidney transplantation.[5] The United Network for Organ Sharing (UNOS) requires that such kidneys be shared on a mandatory nationwide basis, with a kidney "payback" to the sharing institution.

Blood Group Matching: ABO System

ABO-typing is used for blood group determination (O, A, B, and AB) and is the first hurdle to successful transplantation.[5] The same rules apply to organ transplantation as to blood transfusion with regard to the ABO system. Red blood cell proteins cause an immune reaction if they are administered to a recipient of a different or incompatible blood group.

Thus, only organs from the same ABO groups are considered for transplantation; otherwise, incompatibility will result in immediate graft rejection. Recently, however, some progress has been made to alleviate this barrier. By performing pretransplant splenectomy and plasmapheresis to remove preformed antibodies, ABO-incompatible transplants have been performed.[6]

Crossmatching

Crossmatching is a histocompatibility technique that identifies the presence of preformed circulating antibodies in the recipient against antigens on the tissue of a potential donor. The presence of these antibodies is generally a contraindication to transplantation. Patients who have been presensitized by blood transfusion, pregnancy, or previous transplants are thus eliminated. The increasing sensitivity of crossmatching techniques, particularly flow cytometric crossmatching (FACS), can detect low levels of presensitization and readily distinguish between anti-T and anti-B lymphocyte antibodies.[7]

The test is done by mixing a sample of the recipient's serum with donor lymphocytes in the presence of complement. If cell agglutination or lysis occurs, this is considered a positive crossmatch, and transplantation generally cannot be performed, especially when this is a T-cell mediated event. A B-cell positive crossmatch does not automatically rule out transplantation.

Mixed Leukocyte Culture

Mixed leukocyte culture (MLC) measures the degree of compatibility between donor and recipient without defining the antigens responsible for these results, although this reaction is most likely controlled at the HLA-D locus.[8]

The MLC is performed by mixing lymphocytes from recipient and donor and culturing them for 5 days. Antigenic stimulation of T lymphocytes responding to foreign histocompatibility antigens on unrelated lymphocytes causes this reaction. DNA synthesis is then measured as a reflection of cellular response.

The MLC is useful in the selection of living, related

donors because it aids in predicting outcome of transplants between donor and recipient. By determining the MLC stimulation index (SI) those with a high (SI>8) versus low (SI<8) probability of success can be identified.[6] Unfortunately, it cannot be used for matching cadaver donors because organs cannot be preserved for the 5 to 6 days necessary to perform the test.

TYPES OF ORGAN TRANSPLANTATION

Renal Transplantation

Kidney transplantation has become a universally accepted form of therapy for patients with end-stage renal disease. For this reason, renal transplantation is presented in this chapter as a model for examining immunologic factors in transplantation.

Most people are eligible for transplantation if they meet the following criteria:

1. They are under the age of 70.
2. They have permanent, irreversible renal failure.
3. They have a functional lower urinary tract.
4. They are free from serious vascular, cardiac, or neurologic complications of uremia. Many high-risk patients who were previously excluded are now included in the growing lists of recipients awaiting renal allografts. Such high-risk patients include those with diabetes, abnormal lower urinary tract, prior malignancy, coronary artery disease, cystinosis, and collagen vascular disease.

Transplantation remains contraindicated for the management of renal failure secondary to oxalosis and for patients with active infections, uncontrolled or recently treated malignancies, or severe extrarenal disease, making the risks of surgery or anesthesia prohibitive. Patients less than age 1 or greater than age 70 are considered acceptable on an individualized basis.

Transplantation is usually not performed until the patient with end-stage renal disease has been stabilized on hemodialysis. Transplantation is recommended, however, as early as possible in patients with diabetic nephropathy, to prevent extrarenal manifestations, such as diabetic retinopathy and neuropathy. In young patients with chronic renal failure who are seen prior to the institution of dialysis and who have living related donors, transplantation may be scheduled for the same time when the patient would otherwise require the institution of dialysis. A general schema for the patient who develops end-stage renal disease is presented in the box at right.

Cardiac Transplantation

Selection of appropriate cardiac transplant recipients is crucial to the outcome of transplantation. These are patients with New York Heart Association class IV end-stage heart failure whose disease is not amenable to conventional medical or surgical therapy.

> ## RECIPIENT EVALUATION: A SCHEMA FOR THE PATIENT WITH END-STAGE RENAL DISEASE
>
> 1. Patient enters program.
>   a. Irreversible renal failure.
>   b. Biopsy.
>   c. Clinical course.
> 2. Medical, dietary management.
> 3. Vascular access for hemodialysis or peritoneal dialysis.
> 4. Dialysis.
> 5. Plans for transplantation.
>   a. Family psychological evaluation.
>   b. Tissue typing.
>   (1) ABO blood groups.
>   (2) HLA genotypes.
>   (3) Mixed lymphocyte culture.
>   c. Donor workup.
> 6. Urologic assessment of patient's status.
>   a. Voiding cystourethrogram.
>   b. Cystoscopy.*
>   c. Cystometrics.*
>   d. Urologic reconstruction.*
> 7. Surgical procedures.*
>   a. Parathyroidectomy.
>   b. Splenectomy.
>   c. Vagotomy/pyloroplasty.
>   d. Coronary artery bypass graft.
> 8. Living, related donor.
> 9. Transplantation.
>
> ---
>
> *If indicated.

Most patients have cardiomyopathy, usually idiopathic or of viral origin (50%). Another large group of patients consists of those with ischemic cardiomyopathy (40%).[9]

Transplant recipients must have no evidence of infection, cancer, or recent pulmonary infarction, because the infarcted area serves as an excellent locus for opportunistic pulmonary infection. Pulmonary hypertension manifested by significantly increased pulmonary vascular resistance contraindicates transplantation because acute failure of the normal donor right ventricle usually will occur. A relative contraindication for transplantation is age over 50 years, because older patients are less likely to tolerate such a major operation and the associated complications of infection and rejection.

Survival following heart transplantation has improved dramatically over the past years. At Stanford University, the 1-year survival rate is 80% to 85%, compared to 22% in 1963.[9] At least half of the patients are expected to be alive with good quality of life 5 years following transplantation. These improvements reflect better patient management, improved immunosuppressive therapy with cyclosporine, and the use of cardiac biopsy for the preclinical diagnosis of early acute graft rejection.

Liver Transplantation

Pioneering advances by Starzel[9] in liver transplantation have obtained >85% 1-year graft survival in this high-risk procedure. It is reserved for patients with irreversible chronic liver disease, most commonly in adults with nonalcoholic cirrhosis, including chronic active hepatitis. The indications include primary liver tumors and alcoholic cirrhosis. In children, biliary atresia and congenital metabolic abnormalities are the most common indications for hepatic transplantation.

Absolute contraindications to transplantation include ongoing alcoholism, poor cardiopulmonary or renal function, patient age over 55 years, portal vein thrombosis, and metastatic cancer. Hepatitis is a relative contraindication because not all such patients reinfect the donor liver. On the other hand, patients who are positive for hepatitis B both on the surface and in the core antigen inevitably reinfect the donor liver and must not receive a transplant.

Pancreatic Transplantation

Currently, methods of delivering exogenous insulin to diabetic patients have not proved effective in maintaining normal carbohydrate metabolism or in preventing microvascular disease. Thus, the aim of pancreas transplantation is to achieve perfect metabolic control and to stop the progression of these microvascular changes.[9] Pancreatic transplantation is unlikely to be of great value in persons with microvascular disease so far advanced that metabolic correction would not be expected to affect the course.

The first pancreas transplant was performed in 1966. Initially, the pancreas was transplanted with the duodenum, but, owing to complications related to the duodenum (i.e., leakage and fistula formation), pancreatoduodenal transplantation had largely been abandoned. However, it has recently had a resurgence of interest. Subsequent techniques have used (1) islet cells injected into the portal vein or small bowel mesentery (though this method never totally controlled diabetes); (2) segmental pancreas transplantation using half of the gland (body and tail), with vascular anastomosis between the donor splenic artery and splenic vein and the recipient iliac vessels; and (3) whole pancreas transplantation using the entire gland. The pancreatic duct can either be injected with a polymer or, alternatively, the duct can be anastomosed to be a defunctionalized limb of the small bowel or the urinary bladder. About two thirds of the grafts are functioning at 1 year; rejection and interstitial fibrosis

and vascular thrombosis account for the majority of failures.[9]

Blood Transfusions

Numerous studies have demonstrated improved cadaver allograft survival rates in patients receiving blood transfusions before the transplant.[6] Such transfusions, however, pose several risks to the recipient, including transmission of acquired immunodeficiency syndrome (AIDS), hepatitis, and cytomegalovirus (CMV). In addition, sensitization may occur and make less likely the chance of receiving a crossmatch negative kidney. Furthermore, with availability of recombinant human erythropoietin, the medical justification for such transfusions has decreased.[8] Fortunately, with the advent of improved immunosuppression, there remains little additional advantage in administering such transfusions.[6] If a transfusion must be given, frozen, washed red blood cells or leukocyte-depleted packed cells are preferred.

RECIPIENT EVALUATION

Before transplantation, the referring physician sends a complete medical history and physical examination and results of diagnostic studies and laboratory tests to the transplant center. Subsequent studies are done, depending on the patient's age, evaluation results, and the primary disease process. All adults undergo hepatitis studies, CMV titration, venereal disease research laboratory (VDRL) testing, and human immunodeficiency virus (HIV) testing.

Certain patients may require more extensive evaluation before operation. When indicated by history, an upper or lower gastrointestinal series is performed. If an ulcer is present, treatment is initiated with an intensive antacid and H_2 blocker program. Healing must be documented before transplantation. Patients older than 65, who constitute an increasingly large group with end-stage renal disease, require a more intensive evaluation of cardiovascular status. Diabetic patients have a high incidence of asymptomatic coronary artery disease; therefore, we currently perform stress thallium studies in all diabetic patients, and any significant lesions found are treated before transplantation. Similarly, patients with a significant history of peripheral vascular disease or aneurysmal disease are evaluated with noninvasive vascular imaging and, if indicated, an angiogram.

In children and select adults, a complete evaluation of the genitourinary tract is performed, including an ultrasound to evaluate for acquired cystic renal disease or for hydronephrosis and a voiding cystourethrogram to evaluate reflux; cystoscopy and cystometrics are used to evaluate neurogenic bladder disease and bladder outlet obstruction. Small children who undergo an intraperitoneal transplant can have simultaneous

INDICATIONS FOR NEPHRECTOMY BEFORE TRANSPLANT

Chronic renal infection
Infected calculi
Heavy proteinuria
Refractory hypertension
Polycystic kidney disease with infection or bleeding
Acquired renal cystic disease with malignancy
Infected reflux

TABLE 49–1

System Developed by UNOS to Allocate Cadaver Kidneys

Criteria	Assigned Points
1. Antigen mismatch (mm)	
a. 0 ABDR mm	10 points
b. 0 BDR mm	7 points
c. 0 AB mm	6 points
d. 1 BDR mm	3 points
e. 2 BDR mm	2 points
f. 3 BDR mm	1 point
2. Panel reactive antibody (PRA)	4 points for PRA >80%
3. Waiting time	0–1 point for <1 year
4. Medical urgency	Special request
5. Pediatric recipient	
a. ≤5 years	2 points
b. 6–10 years	1 point

bilateral nephrectomy and ureterectomy at the time of the surgery. Adults or children who require nephrectomy (e.g., those with congenital nephrotic syndrome, uncontrolled hypertension, reflux, pyelonephritis, or polycystic kidneys) undergo it as a separate procedure before transplant (box above).

Recently, living unrelated donors (usually a spouse, relative, or close friend) have been accepted for consideration. During the interview, they are informed about transplantation, the risks of the procedure, and possible complications.

After the interview, the recipient and all potential donors undergo histocompatibility studies. The patient without a compatible, related donor must wait for a kidney from a cadaveric donor source. To date, the system developed by UNOS to allocate cadaver kidneys has stressed mandatory sharing of six-antigen match kidneys and the use of blood type O kidneys for type O recipients. Transplant candidates are additionally assigned points, and the kidneys are assigned to those crossmatch-negative patients with the greatest number of points (Table 49–1).

DONOR SOURCES

The number of patients who can receive transplants is limited severely by the availability of donor organs. Because of this scarcity, in the United States in 1992, only about 7691 cadaveric kidney transplants were performed, while there are about 185,000 patients on maintenance hemodialysis.[10] As of August 1993, there were 23,948 patients waiting for kidney transplants in the United States.[11]

The paradox of this situation is that, while the number of potential donors far exceeds the number of organs needed for transplantation, most of the potential donors will never be considered. This situation is primarily due to insufficient efforts and awareness by physicians, nurses, and the public of the need for cadaveric organs. Because more than two thirds of patients with end-stage renal disease do not, by current criteria, have a suitable living, related donor, transplant programs increasingly depend on use of cadaveric organs. However, living donors confer the following significant advantages:

- Better short-term results (about a 95% 1-year graft survival).
- Better long-term results (about an 85% 5-year survival).
- Improved early graft function.
- Avoidance of wait for cadaveric transplant.
- Ability to time transplant.
- Less immunosuppression required.
- Emotional gain to donor.

To treat all patients with end-stage renal disease in a geographic area, an ongoing transplantation program must have an adequate supply of cadaveric organs in its own region.[12] Although sharing of cadaveric kidneys has received much attention, an active transplant center cannot depend primarily on the sharing of organs from other programs. Efforts to develop cadaveric donor sources have focused on increasing public awareness and encouraging physicians to participate in identifying potential donors and in efforts to enact legislation that would increase the number of organ donors. Some measures have been quite controversial, such as the use of tax credits to defer funeral expenses.[10]

DONOR SELECTION

Assessing the suitability of a donor begins when the referring hospital gives notification that a potential donor exists. At this time, the medical history of the donor, the circumstances and extent of the present injury, and the patient's immediate condition are evaluated. If a patient has not yet met the criteria for brain death, the patient should be managed without regard for his or her status as a potential donor, even if this management includes treatment with agents potentially detrimental to donor organ function. Specific questions on the suitability of such donors may be addressed at this time by the transplantation team. However, throughout the process of donor identification, members of the transplantation team do not play a role in the management of the patient, in certification of brain death, or in obtaining consent for organ donation. If brain death occurs and organ donation is feasible, a final decision regarding donor suitability is made.[12]

Kidneys from cadaveric donors older than 60 generally do not tolerate the insults of nephrectomy, preservation, and transplantation as well as kidneys from younger donors do. Therefore, cadaveric donors are usually less than 60 years old. Pediatric donors are also used and are generally older than 1 year; kidneys from these donors will sustain life even if transplanted as a single organ in an adult.

Careful evaluation of the medical history of the cadaveric donor is critical. Patients with malignant skin lesions or primary central nervous system lesions are not eliminated as potential donors, because there is a low tendency for dissemination and metastasis. However, the organs of donors with malignant lesions elsewhere in the body, despite the absence of documented metastasis, should not be used for transplantation. That the organ graft may serve as a source of malignant cells transferred from the donor to the immunosuppressed host has been reported.[12] The absence of neoplastic disease in the donor should not be assumed until there has been a thorough evaluation of the intra-abdominal cavity or a complete postmortem examination.

The cadaveric donor with injuries involving several organ systems frequently will have had a previous procedure, such as laparotomy, craniotomy, or orthopedic repair. These donors are acceptable unless the earlier operation showed bowel perforation, gangrenous changes of any intra-abdominal organs, or other conditions that may cause bacterial contamination of the kidneys, liver, or pancreas.

As an isolated finding, gross or microscopic hematuria does not contraindicate organ retrieval. These findings are often associated with pelvic fractures, urinary bladder contusions, or retroperitoneal hematomas, whereas the kidneys, ureters, and associated vascular structures remain normal. Occasionally, a single kidney can be used, despite a traumatized contralateral kidney. Significant elevations of the prothrombin time or partial thromboplastin time are no barrier to organ donation, provided the cause is not disseminated intravascular coagulation secondary to sepsis or carcinoma.

Organs from donors who have evidence of septicemia, an abscess, or viral or fungal disease are not used because the transfer of infection to the immunosuppressed host may have serious consequences. Positive CMV titers do not rule out a donor; however, positive HIV antibody status does. The presence of tracheobronchitis or bacteriuria does not contraindicate organ donation, because cadaveric donors with an endotracheal tube or urinary catheter often will have these findings without the kidneys being involved. An active pneumonia of any bacterial cause or an aspiration pneumonia associated with trauma does not entirely rule out organ donation. Many centers will

---

CONTRAINDICATIONS TO CADAVER ORGAN DONATION

Age >70
Chronic renal disease
Malignancy
Severe hypertension
Bacterial sepsis
Intravenous drug abuse
Positive HBsAg or anti-HCV
Positive HIV
Intestinal perforation
Prolonged warm ischemia

---

procure kidneys from these donors provided blood and urine cultures are negative. Of course, these donors would not be suitable for a heart or lung transplant. Thus, the basic rule in organ procurement is that any disease process that potentially could cause irreversible organ damage and could be transferred to the transplant recipient eliminates the possibility of organ donation (box above).

Brain Death

The concept of brain death, or irreversible coma, has been extensively reviewed, and generally accepted criteria are now present throughout the United States. The legal recognition that a patient can be declared dead although circulation is temporarily maintained by artificial means has been of great significance to organ transplantation. This development has allowed procurement of organs under accepted legal and ethical guidelines.

The diagnosis of brain death is a clinical diagnosis and can be made without ancillary investigation other than a detailed clinical examination. If the cause or extent of injury is unknown, it is essential that an electroencephalogram, brain scan, or arteriogram be performed.

When organs are to be removed for transplantation, two physicians must pronounce the donor brain dead. One of these physicians is usually a neurologist or neurosurgeon because the electroencephalogram commonly used in these circumstances is a specific diagnostic tool of these specialists and should be evaluated by them. The interval between two successive examinations (usually 6 to 24 hours) is determined by the examining physicians. The following criteria are generally agreed on as guidelines for brain death; however, these may differ from institution to institution.

BRAIN DEATH CRITERIA

1. Absence of induced hyperthermia and central nervous system depressant drugs.
2. Generalized flaccidity, no spontaneous muscle

movement, and no evidence of postural activity or shivering.

3. Absent cranial nerve reflexes.
   a. Pupils light-fixed and dilated.
   b. No corneal reflexes.
   c. No response to upper and lower airway stimulation.
   d. No ocular response to head turning and cold calorics.
   e. Absence of spontaneous breathing movements for 3 minutes.
   f. Isoelectric electroencephalogram.
   g. No blood flow seen on angiogram or brain scan.

ORGAN PROCUREMENT

The organ retrieval process should include the following orderly sequence of events:

- Identification of the potential donor.
- Notification of the transplant team by the referring hospital of a potential donor.
- Evaluation of donor's suitability.
- Discussion with the patient's family and physician.
- Consent obtained from the next of kin.
- Discussion with the medical examiner and district attorney, if necessary.
- Continued observation and maintenance of the donor.
- Pronouncement of donor death by two physicians according to protocol.
- Notification by the transplant coordinator of surgeon, operating room, and time for organ procurement.
- Notification of eye bank, skin bank, and other specialty areas.
- Surgery.
- Perfusion and preservation of organs.
- Transportation of organs.
- Tissue-typing of organs.
- Identification of recipients.
- Transplantation of organs.

Our preference is for heart-beating cadaveric donors, where kidneys are harvested en bloc with the aorta and vena cava to ensure preservation of multiple renal vessels and the ureteral blood supply. In a live donor, an anterior transperitoneal approach is preferred, which allows optimal exposure of the renal pedicle.

Legal Issues

Many physicians fear the consequences of pronouncing brain death and being involved with organ donation because of legal considerations. For example, questions can be raised about whether a physician is liable for taking a patient off a respirator, and if so, how the physician's liability could affect the question of who is responsible for the patient's initial injury.

The legal system, however, now recognizes that brain death criteria are legitimate, and the physician cannot be accused of taking the patient's life. Consultation with the medical examiner usually clarifies the issues involved and serves to protect the physician.

SURGICAL ASPECTS OF KIDNEY TRANSPLANTATION

A hockey stick–shaped incision is made either in the right or left lower quadrant and carried through the skin and subcutaneous tissue until a pocket is developed in the retroperitoneal space by mobilizing the peritoneum medially. The external iliac vein is dissected sharply, and either the internal iliac artery or external iliac artery is used for the arterial anastomosis. Subsequently, the renal allograft vein is anastomosed end-to-side to the external iliac vein, and the transplant renal artery is anastomosed either end-to-end to the internal iliac artery or end-to-side to the external iliac artery. After the completion of this procedure and the release of the vascular clamps, the kidney usually obtains a firm and pinkish appearance, indicating good vascular perfusion to the kidney. With multiple renal arteries and the absence of a Carrel patch, ex vivo arterial reconstruction is performed in the hypothermic flush solution.

The ureter is reimplanted by one of two general techniques: intravesical or extravesical. In the intravesical technique, the ureter is brought through the bladder and passed through a submucosal tunnel and anastomosed near the medial aspect of the ipsilateral ureter near the trigone; such is a traditional Ledbetter-Politano ureteroneocystostomy. In the extravesical technique, the ureter is anastomosed mucosa-to-mucosa on the dome of the bladder after a tunnel has been made in the seromuscular portion of the bladder. Each method has its own advocates, with the experience and comfort of the team governing results.

Complications of the transplant procedure may include infection, hematoma, ureteral obstruction, hematuria, arterial or venous thrombosis, ureteral necrosis, and hydrocele or lymphocele.

RENAL PRESERVATION

Organ preservation is a central part of any kidney transplantation program. The ultimate function of a transplant organ is highly dependent on the quality of procurement and preservation. The inadequate supply of cadaver organs in the United States and worldwide places further emphasis on these goals. Ischemic injury and deterioration during storage that leads to damage may severely impair the recovery of function and ultimately may lead to failure of procured kidneys.[13]

Causes of impaired graft functions include the following:

Donor factors
- Donor age >60
- Donor acute tubular necrosis
- Prolonged cold or warm ischemia time

Intraoperative factors
- Prolonged anastomosis time
- Intraoperative hypotension
- Negative intraoperative fluid balance

Recipient factors
- High plasma renin activity (PRA) level
- Postoperative hypotension or hypovolemia
- Cyclosporine toxicity.

Relevant features for effective donor procurement are support of blood pressure and fluid volumes to maintain adequate renal perfusion and diuresis and support of metabolic needs to avoid vasospasm and nephrotoxins.[14] Mannitol should be administered to promote an osmotic diuresis. Renal vasospasm is managed by giving phenoxybenzamine hydrochloride (Dibenzyline), an α-adrenergic blocker. Heparin is given for anticoagulation. Isoproterenol can be given for hypotension unresponsive to fluid challenge; however, kidneys obtained from such donors give inferior results.

Storage Methods

There are two methods of renal preservation. Simple cold storage has the advantages of simplicity, low cost, and ease of transportation. Hypothermic pulsatile perfusion has the advantages of extended preservation and the possibility of assessing the degree of ischemic damage to the kidney (viability testing). Both methods are currently in use in the United States and throughout the world. However, the recent discovery by Belzer and Southard of the University of Wisconsin (UW) solution has greatly extended the ability for simple cold storage to preserve organs for extended periods.[15] This development has resulted both in less postoperative acute tubular necrosis and in a rapid decline in serum creatinine to normal values. In addition, calcium channel blockers have been demonstrated to help achieve immediate graft function.[16] This has also resulted in a lower cost for those kidneys with immediate graft function than for those with delayed graft function (DGF).[17]

POST-TRANSPLANT COURSE

Fluid and Electrolyte Balance

The patient's early postoperative urinary output may be somewhat unpredictable and may range from complete anuria to polyuria. Fluid replacement must be adjusted accordingly. The general rule is to replace both the urine output volume per volume and the daily insensible loss. Diuretics should be considered only after a fluid challenge has failed to increase the urine output.

A difficult problem in clinical transplantation is anuria, which may occur in the absence of any other signs or symptoms during the early postoperative phase. The differential diagnosis of early anuria includes observation of the following: (1) acute tubular necrosis, (2) acute rejection, (3) urinary tract obstruction, (4) renal arterial or venous thrombosis, and (5) cyclosporine nephrotoxicity.

Anuria requires immediate attention because all drugs excreted by the kidney system are now recirculating in the recipient. As a consequence, the required therapeutic levels for antibiotics, for example, are significantly lower, and the continued administration of myelosuppressive agents, such as azathioprine (Imuran), can readily lead to marrow suppression and overwhelming infection. Recent evidence indicates that cyclosporine excretion is impaired in the presence of renal dysfunction.

When the anuria occurs, investigative procedures should include the following:

1. Technetium DTPA scan of the kidney, which provides evidence of the intactness of the renal vascular supply.
2. Ultrasound of the transplanted kidney, which may exhibit blurring of the corticomedullary junction characteristic of rejection or hydronephrosis indicative of urinary obstruction.
3. Cyclosporine levels by radioimmune assay (RIA).[18]
4. Transplant core needle biopsy or fine needle aspiration biopsy (FNAB).[19,20]

Immunosuppressive Therapy

Clinical transplantation would essentially cease if immunosuppressive drugs were removed from the therapeutic armamentarium. On the other hand, such drugs must be considered with the utmost care because of the potentially life-endangering side effects their use entails. The key agents in use today are prednisone, azathioprine (Imuran), cyclosporine, and OKT3. FK-506, anti-CD4 antibody, rapamycin, mycophenolic acid, and monoclonal antibody–bound immunotoxins now loom on the clinical horizon. Each transplant group, on the basis of preference, has its own variation of immunosuppressive regimens.

Prednisone

The drug shown to be of paramount importance in clinical transplantation is prednisone, a corticosteroid which is administered orally in doses of 2 to 2.5 mg/kg every 24 hours on the day of transplantation, with gradual tapering of this dosage to 1.5 mg/kg every 24 hours by the end of the first week. Under such circumstances, the eventual maintenance dosage upon discharge will be about 15 mg daily.

Recent evidence suggests that corticosteroids may exert their immunoregulatory function through several mechanisms. Corticosteroids impair cellular immune responses by inhibition of interleukin-1 (IL-1) production by monocytes (macrophages), with secondary inhibition of helper T-cell function by diminishing the production of interleukin-2 (IL-2).[21] Corticosteroids also impair cellular immune responses by reducing the migration of both T cells and monocytes into areas where they can interact with antigens. Within 6 hours of their administration in humans, they produce a significant lymphopenia, caused not by destruction of lymphocytes, but by redistribution of lymphocytes into extravascular sites and a change in their recirculation patterns. T cells are affected more than B cells, and the number of T-helper cells is diminished to a greater degree than the number of T-suppressor cells.

Azathioprine (Imuran)

Azathioprine (Imuran) is an antimetabolite, a thiopurine analogue of hypoxanthine that is converted to 6-thioinosine intracellularly, which competes with inosine as a substrate in the purine metabolic pathway.[21] It has a myelosuppressive effect, and excessive doses will result in hemopoietic ablation, associated with loss of the host's defenses against microorganisms. A specific program of therapy and close follow-up of key hematologic and physiologic indices is therefore required if this agent is to be used with a relative degree of safety.

Generally, azathioprine is first given to the recipient on the day before, or at the time of transplantation, with a total oral dosage of 2.5 to 3 mg/kg every 24 hours. The daily dosage is then reduced to 2 mg/kg every 24 hours. The maximal effect of a given dose of azathioprine may not be exerted until 48 hours after administration.

Because antimetabolites act primarily on cells during DNA synthesis, one would predict these agents would exert their effects mainly on actively proliferating cells. Experimental evidence supports this prediction, in that the best time to administer azathioprine is about 24 hours after antigen challenge. This is a time when resting lymphocytes have been activated and are beginning to synthesize new DNA. These agents have little effect on mature cells, like plasma cells or effector T cells, because these cells no longer have the capacity to replicate. Thus, it is not surprising that established immune responses are not affected as much as new responses.

For azathioprine, T cells seem to be the major target. In humans, phenomena related to T cells, like graft rejection and delayed hypersensitivity reactions, are sensitive to the effects of azathioprine at dosages of 3 to 5 mg/kg per day or less, but antibody production is not significantly altered until dosages of 5 to 6 mg/kg per day are given.

The increased sensitivity of T cells to azathioprine may not be entirely due to inhibition of DNA synthesis. Even in resting cells, azathioprine can inhibit the ability of T lymphocytes to form sheep rosettes, implying that it may directly interfere with T-cell surface receptors.

In addition to immunosuppressive effects, azathioprine has significant anti-inflammatory effects, which are due in part to the reduction in numbers of monocytes and neutrophils induced by this drug.

Cyclosporine

Cyclosporine, a fungal cyclic peptide, is a biologic product produced by the species *Tolyplocadium inflatum Gams*. It has a high degree of specificity for T lymphocytes and can prevent early T-cell activation in three ways: (1) by inhibiting T-cell help to accessory cells that normally produce IL-1; (2) by preventing T cells producing IL-2 from expressing receptors for IL-2, so that they cannot produce IL-2; and (3) by rendering cytoxic T cells unresponsive to IL-2. At the same time, cyclosporine has no significant effect on macrophage or monocyte function, resting T cells, T-cell counts, neutrophils, or hematopoiesis. It has no cytotoxic or antibiotic activity.[21]

Nephrotoxicity is the most important side effect. Unlike azathioprine, there is no simple laboratory test to detect toxicity, and patients taking cyclosporine must therefore have blood levels checked by RIA. A whole-blood level of 100 to 200 ng/mL is sought for renal transplantation recipients, and a level of 250 to 350 ng/mL for heart, liver, and pancreas transplant patients. Other side effects include hypertension, nephrotoxicity, hirsutism, gingival hypertrophy, hyperesthesia, tremor, gastrointestinal intolerance, and hepatic dysfunction.

Cyclosporine Nephrotoxicity. In clinical practice, there appear to be two forms of cyclosporine nephrotoxicity. One form is dose-dependent, and prompt recovery usually occurs when the dose is decreased before irreversible renal damage occurs. The other form of nephrotoxicity develops in susceptible patients despite normal levels of cyclosporine. These patients usually benefit from substitution of azathioprine for cyclosporine once rejection is excluded by renal biopsy. Low-dose cyclosporine combined with low-dose prednisone and azathioprine (triple drug therapy) is a promising approach to preventing rejection and may be associated with fewer drug-related side effects.

FK-506

FK-506 is a powerful new immunosuppressant that has proved to be an effective drug for the prevention and treatment of allograft rejection in humans and animals. While its mechanism of action is not entirely known, it has been shown to suppress T cell–mediated immunity by suppressing IL-2 synthesis in T cells. FK-506 inhibits the induction of T-lymphocyte proliferation at concentrations 10 to 100 times lower than the concentrations of cyclosporine required to achieve comparable inhibition in vitro.[18]

Rapamycin (RAPA)

Rapamycin (RAPA) is a potent immunosuppressant with structural similarity to FK-506. Recently, several groups reported that RAPA has 50 to 80 times higher therapeutic efficacy than cyclosporine in heart and kidney transplantation in rats and in large animals.[22] Furthermore, a short course of RAPA administration seems to induce a long-term allograft tolerance in the animal models. RAPA strongly suppresses the proliferation of T cells stimulated by mitogens.

It has also been demonstrated that RAPA strongly suppresses in vitro mitogen-stimulated immunoglobulin production by human lymphocytes and that such suppression is concomitant with the suppression of lymphocyte proliferation. This drug holds great promise for the future.

Allograft Rejection

Acceptance of renal allograft is the result of a delicate balance between the attempts of the host to reject the foreign tissues and the success of immunosuppressive drug therapy in inhibiting such a response. When the balance is tilted in the direction of the immunosuppressive drugs, the organ is tolerated and functions well, sustaining the life of the host. If, for a variety of reasons, the balance is tilted in the opposite direction, however, rejection ensues. Prompt recognition and management of rejection are essential in protecting the function and survival of the transplanted kidney. The classic presenting signs and symptoms include the following:

1. Fever
2. Hypertension
3. Tenderness at site of transplant
4. Decreased urinary output
5. Weight gain

The most common laboratory findings include the following:

1. Rise in serum blood, urea, nitrogen levels and in creatinine levels, and fall in creatinine clearance
2. Leukocytosis
3. Technetium DTPA scan showing decreased renal perfusion
4. Ultrasound demonstrating significant increase in the size of the transplanted kidney

As noted earlier, other situations may mimic rejection, including acute tubular necrosis (good vascular perfusion, but kidney is not enlarged and enzymes are not usually elevated), renal arterial or venous thrombosis (with typical nonperfusion of the transplanted renal cortex), urinary tract obstruction caused by extrinsic pressure (e.g., hematoma or lymphocele, which may be detectable by x-ray or by ultrasound scanning), and technical factors (ureteral obstruction), which may require cystoscopy and retrograde pyelogram. In addition, drug nephrotoxicity must be considered because cyclosporine, antibiotics, and H_2 antagonists[23] can all contribute to renal dysfunction.

Once the diagnosis has been established, rejection constitutes an emergency and should be managed immediately. A general approach includes methylprednisolone therapy, 1 g intravenously, daily for 3 to 5 days.

Polyclonal and Monoclonal Antibodies

Heterologous antilymphocyte globulin (ALG) and antithymocyte globulin (ATG) are potent immunosuppressive agents of value in preventing and reversing acute rejection.[24] Most often, ALG is used with azathioprine and prednisone. ALG causes lysis of circulating lymphocytes and depletion of T cells from the paracortical regions of the lymph nodes. The B cells in the medullary regions and germinal center of the nodes are less affected. The absolute T-cell count in the peripheral blood remains low up to 2 weeks after a course of ALG/ATG.

Recently, OKT3, a biochemically purified IgG2a immunoglobin that reacts with the T3 (CD3) antigen on the surface of all mature T lymphocytes has been developed.[25,26] OKT3 causes inhibition of signal transduction, essential for the T lymphocyte. It blocks the generation and function of cytoxic T cells, which is most probably the mechanism of reversing acute cellular allograft rejection. OKT3 has been successfully used in treating primary renal allograft rejection and as a second line of treatment in steroid-resistant allograft rejection. Such specific therapy holds great promise for the future of allotransplantation.

Remarkable advances have been made in numerous areas in renal transplantation over the past decade. The most serious problem facing the application of transplantation technology to patient care is the shortage of suitable organ donors. To bridge the gap between a readily adaptable clinical technique and a shortage of donor organs, bold advances will have to be forthcoming. These may include legislation to increase the number of cadaver or living donors, breakthroughs making possible xenotransplantation, enhanced allograft survival with better immunosuppression regimens, and finally, elimination of the need for transplantation by more effective means of treating those entities that lead to end-stage organ failure.

REFERENCES

1. Carrel, A: Techniques and remote results of vascular anastomosis. Surg Gynecol Obstet 14:246, 1912.
2. Hamilton, D: A history of transplantation. In Morris, PJ (ed): Tissue Transplantation. Grune & Stratton, New York, 1984, pp 1–13.
3. USRDS Annual Data Report 1991. Am J Kidney Dis 18 (suppl 2):38, 1991.
4. Schwartz, BD: The human major histocompatibility complex. In Stites, DP, et al (eds): Basic and Clinical Immunology, ed 6. Appleton & Lange, Norwalk, CT, 1987, pp. 55–68.
5. Mackintosh, P: ABO matching in kidney graft survival. Nature 250:351, July 1974.

6. Najarian, J and Matas, A: The present and future of kidney transplantation. Transplant Proc 23:2075–2082, 1991.
7. Bou-Habib, JC, et al: Impaired kidney graft survival in flow cytometric crossmatched positive donor-specific transfusion recipients. Transplant Proc 23:403, 1991.
8. Opelz, G, and Terasaki, PI: Significance of mixed leukocyte culture testing in cadaver kidney transplantation. Transplantation 23:375, 1977.
9. Simmons, RL, and So, SK: Clinical transplantation. In Stites, D, et al (eds): Basic and Clinical Immunology, ed 6. Appleton & Lange, Norwalk, CT, 1987, pp 491–499.
10. Rapaport, FT, and Anaise, D: Organ donation—1991. Transplant Proc 23:899, 1991.
11. UNOS Update, July/August 1993, 46.
12. Waltzer, WC: Procurement of cadaveric kidneys for transplantation. Ann Intern Med 98:536, 1983.
13. Miller, HC, Alexander, JW, and Nathan, P: Effects of warm ischemic damage on intrarenal distribution of flow in preserved kidneys. Surgery 72:193, 1972.
14. Lambert, R, et al: Glomerular damage after kidney preservation. Transplantation 42:125, 1986.
15. Southard, JH, et al: Important components of the UW solution. Transplantation 49:251, 1990.
16. Alcanaz, A, et al: Effect of Diltiazem in the prevention of acute tubular necrosis, acute rejection, and cyclosporine levels. Transplant Proc 23:2383, 1991.
17. Rosenthal, JT, et al: The high cost of delayed graft function in cadaveric renal transplantation. Transplantation 51:1115, 1991.
18. Rosano, TG, et al: Immunosuppressive metabolites of cyclosporine in the blood of renal allograft recipients. Transplantation 42:262, 1986.
19. Matas, AJ, et al: The value of needle renal allograft biopsy III: A prospective study. Surgery 98:922, 1985.
20. Hayry, P, and von Willebrand, F: Transplant aspiration cytology. Transplantation 38:7, 1984.
21. Webb, DR, and Winkelstein, A: Immunosuppression, immunopotentiation, and anti-inflammatory drugs. In Stites, DP, et al (eds): Basic and Clinical Immunology, ed 6. Appleton & Lange, Norwalk, CT, 1987, pp 55–68.
22. Luo, H, et al. Rapamycin suppresses in vitro immunoglobulin production by human lymphocytes. Transplant Proc 23:2236–2238, 1991.
23. Jarowenko, MV, et al: Ranitidine, cimetidine and the cyclosporine treated patient. Transplantation 42:311, 1986.
24. Matas, AJ, et al: Treatment of steroid resistant rejection in patients receiving cyclosporine. Transplantation 41:579, 1986.
25. Cosimi, AB, et al: A randomized clinical trial comparing OKT3 and steroids for treatment of hepatic allograft rejection. Transplantation 43:91, 1987.
26. Goldstein, G, et al: A randomized clinical trial of OKT3 monoclonal antibody for acute rejection in cadaveric renal transplants. N Engl J Med 3134:337, 1985.

CHAPTER 50

Immunodeficiency Disorders

Marc G. Golightly

LEARNING OBJECTIVES

After completing this chapter, you should be able to:

1. Differentiate between primary and secondary immunodeficiency disorders.
2. Describe clinical presentation of primary immunodeficiency diseases with possible pathophysiologic mechanisms underlying the immunologic dysfunction.
3. Explain why recurrent pyogenic infections in a child diagnosed to have a combined T- and B-cell immunodeficiency disorder generally do not manifest before 6 months of age.
4. Explain why strict T-cell immunodeficiencies in which the humoral immune system is not secondarily affected are very rare.
5. Examine the pathophysiologic mechanisms underlying the acquired immunodeficiency of AIDS, including the causative agent and its primary target.

The immune system is organized in a highly complex fashion with the cell-mediated, humoral, phagocytic, and complement components linked through complex interactions. Upon review of some of these interactions (see Chapter 47), it can be appreciated that the extreme complexity of the immune system, in turn, affords a tremendous number of possibilities for dysfunction and defects to occur.

When a defect does occur in one branch, it often affects another branch primarily or secondarily. The resultant clinical symptoms likewise depend on which of these branches and interactive relations are affected. As a result, the clinical presentation of suspected immunodeficient patients often suggests the type of immune dysfunction present. For example, patients with a defective *cell-mediated* immunity are more susceptible to infection by fungal, viral, and protozoan organisms (especially in the form of pneumo-

nia, chronic skin infection, and mucous membrane infections). A history of recurrent bacterial infections, particularly bacterial pneumonia and otitis media, suggests a *humoral* defect. *Phagocytic* dysfunctions are suggested by skin and systemic infections with pyogenic (pus-forming) bacteria. Often the systemic infection is by bacteria of normally low virulence. *Complement* deficiencies are also associated with recurrent pyogenic infections.

Although these associations generally do occur, it should be noted that they are not without exceptions. For example, a patient with humoral deficiency may have a fungal infection. Furthermore, the type of immunologic dysfunction present may range from no notable clinical symptoms to severe illness and even death. These associations will be examined with respect to the individual immunodeficiencies discussed later in this chapter.

877

IMMUNODEFICIENCIES: CLASSIFICATION

Immunodeficiencies are generally classified into two groups: *primary* immunodeficiencies and *secondary* immunodeficiencies. Primary immunodeficiencies are, as the name implies, inherent in the immune system itself as the primary cause of the immunologic dysfunction. These deficiencies are often congenital and may have a genetic component to them. They can occur at varying ages ranging from infancy to adulthood. While the cause of the defect(s) responsible for primary immunodeficiencies in many cases is known (e.g., embryologic abnormality or enzyme deficiencies), in many cases it is not. However, in most primary immunodeficiencies, the dysfunction can usually be identified (e.g., T-cell defect). Primary immunodeficiencies are known to occur in all four of the components of the immune system previously mentioned. These defects occur either alone or in combination with each other (Table 50–1). However, primary immunodeficiencies with relatively few exceptions (e.g., selective IgA deficiency) are uncommon (1 in 50,000 to 1 in 100,000).

In contrast, secondary immunodeficiencies are much more common and are often transient in nature. Secondary immunodeficiencies, as the name implies, may also occur secondary to a primary disease. They are associated with a variety of primary diseases or conditions, such as infection, malignancy, autoimmune diseases, protein-losing (wasting) states, immunosuppressive therapy, and a long list of other disorders (Table 50–2). Secondary immunodeficiencies often resolve when the primary disorder is successfully treated or corrected, and, like primary disorders, are also known to affect the cellular, humoral, phagocytic, or complement systems. While the underlying mechanisms of many of the secondary immunodeficiencies

TABLE 50–1
Primary Immunodeficiency Diseases

Combined B-Cell and T-Cell Immunodeficiencies
Severe combined immunodeficiency
Wiskott-Aldrich syndrome (WAS)
Hereditary ataxia-telangiectasia
Nezelof's syndrome
Others

B-Cell and Antibody Immunodeficiencies
X-linked infantile agammaglobulinemia
Transient hypogammaglobulinemia of infancy
Common, variable immunodeficiency
Selective immunoglobulin deficiencies
Others

T-Cell Immunodeficiencies
Thymic hypoplasia
Chronic mucocutaneous candidiasis
Others

Primary Phagocytic Deficiencies
Primary Complement Deficiencies

TABLE 50–2
Secondary Immunodeficiency Diseases*

Infection
Rubella
Measles
Leprosy
Tuberculosis
Human immunodeficiency virus (HIV)/AIDS
Coccidioidomycosis
Chronic infection
Acute viral infection
Multiple or repeated viral infections
Cytomegalovirus (CMV)

Neoplastic Disease
Hodgkin's disease
Acute leukemia
Chronic leukemia
Nonlymphoid malignancy
Myeloma

Autoimmune Disease
Systemic lupus erythematosus (SLE)
Rheumatoid arthritis

Protein-Losing States
Nephrotic syndrome
Protein-losing enteropathy

Other Disorders
Diabetes
Alcoholic cirrhosis
Chronic active hepatitis
Malnutrition
Burns
Sarcoidosis
Splenectomy
Sickle cell anemia
Uremia
Subacute sclerosing panencephalitis
Down syndrome
Premature infants

Immunosuppressive Treatment
Corticosteroids
Cytotoxic drugs
Antithymocyte globulin
Radiation
Cyclosporin A
Phenytoin, penicillamine

Anesthesia
Aging

*Adapted from Stites, DP, Stobo, JD, and Wells, JV (eds): Basic and Clinical Immunology, ed 6. Appleton & Lange, Norwalk, CT, 1987.

are also still in question, it is important to recognize the association of this group of immunologic dysfunctions with the various primary diseases and disorders for supportive and diagnostic purposes.

This chapter is devoted to the discussion of primary and secondary immunodeficiencies with respect to their basic defects, pathogenesis, and treatment. Although an examination of all of the immunodeficiencies is beyond the scope of this chapter, it is hoped that those presented will provide insight and the basis to understand most immunodeficiency diseases and the problems faced by patients with these diseases.

PRIMARY IMMUNODEFICIENCIES

Combined B- and T-Cell Immunodeficiencies

Combined B- and T-cell immunodeficiencies are variable in both their degree of severity and in their cause. The survival of patients with these disorders is likewise highly variable, ranging from less than a year of age in severe combined immunodeficiency to well into adulthood in partial combined immunodeficiency. The symptoms begin early in infancy in most of these patients. As might be expected, these patients are susceptible to a wide range of bacterial, fungal, viral, and protozoal infections. The basic defect of many of the combined immunodeficiencies is not known; however, there have been associations with enzyme deficiencies, genetic components, short-limbed dwarfism, and thymoma. These deficiencies require extensive immunologic laboratory workups.

Severe Combined Immunodeficiency

Severe combined immunodeficiency (SCID) is the most extreme of all immunodeficiency diseases. It is characterized by severe defects of both B-cell and T-cell immunity. This is evident by the scarcity of lymphoid tissue and the marked depressions in the numbers and/or functions of T and B cells. SCID should not be thought of as a single disease but rather a collection of disorders, all of which are manifested by a compromised cellular and humoral immunity. As such, SCID exhibits variable patterns of inheritance and different degrees of severity (albeit all are extremely serious and life-threatening). The forms of inheritance in SCID are autosomal recessive (the Swiss type lymphopenic agammaglobulinemia) and X-linked recessive type. Both of these forms are clinically similar.

SCID is basically a disorder of infants. The true incidence of SCID is difficult to determine because these patients usually die within the first 1 to 2 years of life, often before the diagnosis can be made. These patients fail to thrive, suffer from chronic diarrhea, and, as mentioned, are susceptible to a wide range of microbial infections. The infections are usually of skin and of respiratory and gastrointestinal tracts. However, during the first few months of life, they may be protected from bacterial infections and, to some extent, viral infections, by the maternal IgG transferred in utero.

Vaccination with live attenuated vaccines should never be attempted in these patients because death from progressive viremia is most likely. In addition, transfusions with nonirradiated blood should never be given to an infant suspected of SCID, or any other immunodeficiency for that matter. This is because of the graft-versus-host reactions that would occur in SCID patients and that may occur in other immunodeficient patients.

Pathogenesis. The pathogenesis of SCID has not been fully elucidated. This is most likely due to the fact that SCID is a heterogeneous group of disorders. In some forms of SCID, it appears that there is a defect in the pluripotential lymphoid stem cells' ability to differentiate into mature lymphocytes (see Fig. 51–1). In other forms, it may be a defect in the thymus that prevents proper maturation of regulatory T cells. In yet others, there is an association with a defective enzyme, adenosine deaminase, which may allow the buildup of a metabolite toxic to lymphocytes. A major histocompatibility complex class II deficiency has also been demonstrated as a cause of SCID.

Treatment. Treatment of SCID by bone marrow transplantation, fetal liver transplantation, and fetal thymus transplantation have all been tried with varying success. Following successful transplantation, survivals of 10 years and greater have been reported, depending on the procedure. Some of the treatment protocols are still too new to fully evaluate.

Wiskott-Aldrich syndrome (Immunodeficiency with Thrombocytopenia and Eczema)

Wiskott-Aldrich syndrome (WAS) is another disorder in which both the T- and the B-cell arms of the immune system are affected. It is characterized by severe thrombocytopenia, often with bleeding, recurrent infections with a wide range of microbial organisms, and eczema. B cells are present in normal numbers; however, they are unable to respond to polysaccharide antigens. Consequently, serum levels of IgM are usually decreased. On the other hand, serum IgA and IgE are frequently elevated.

The cellular responses are also abnormal (normal mitogen responsiveness, little or no antigen responsiveness). The T-cell immunity may deteriorate both quantitatively (T-cell numbers) and functionally with increasing age. WAS is inherited in an X-linked fashion.

The recurrent infections do not generally begin before 6 months of age; however, thrombocytopenia usually begins at birth. By the first year of life, eczema is evident and often becomes infected. Episodes of pneumonias, meningitis, and septicemia become more prevalent as time passes, and survival rarely exceeds the first decade of life. As with most immunodeficiencies, there is an increase in the frequency of lymphoreticular malignancies (as high as 30% in WAS patients).

Pathogenesis. The pathogenesis of WAS is largely unknown. However, increased Ig catabolism, regulatory cell failure, and a defective major glycoprotein in the T-cell membrane have all been implicated as having a role.

Treatment. Bone marrow transplantation has been performed to treat patients with WAS, with varying success. In addition, transfer factor has been used, but not enough data have been collected to evaluate this treatment adequately.

Hereditary Ataxia-Telangiectasia with Immunodeficiency

Hereditary ataxia-telangiectasia with immunodeficiency is primarily neurologic but also severely affects the immune, vascular, and endocrine systems. It is an autosomal recessive disorder characterized by ataxia (incoordination), telangiectasia of the eye (red lesions caused by dilated venules), and recurrent sinopulmonary infections. These infections dominate the clinical picture.

Both T and B cells are affected in a variable fashion. Although the B-cell numbers are relatively normal to slightly increased, these patients exhibit absent or decreased levels of serum and secretory IgA. IgE deficiencies have also been noted. T cells may be reduced in both absolute numbers, percentage, and functional ability.

Patients with this disorder are noted to have ataxia beginning in infancy, with the telangiectasia occurring later. The increased number of infections usually begins early in the first decade. If the recurrent infections begin before the ataxia and telangiectasia, it may be difficult to distinguish from other combined immunodeficiencies with abnormal Ig production and selective IgA deficiency (discussion following).

As the patient ages, the neurologic and immunologic functions progressively deteriorate, until about the second or third decade, when death from chronic respiratory infection or lymphoreticular malignancy is common. The pathogenesis of this disorder is still not clearly defined. DNA repair defects and defective germ-line tissue have been postulated.

Miscellaneous Combined Immunodeficiencies

The previously discussed immunodeficiencies are the major disorders that have been traditionally classified as primary combined immunodeficiencies. Others, such as Nezelof's syndrome (characterized by cellular immunodeficiency with abnormal immunoglobulin synthesis), seem to be a collection of disorders with T- and B-cell abnormalities to varying degrees that do not seem to be able to be classified into any of the groups discussed above.

It should be noted that, as our ability to elucidate the basic defects in immunodeficiency disorders increases, the distinction between combined T-cell and B-cell immunodeficiencies will also change. This will be evident in the later discussion of certain B-cell deficiencies that are now known to actually be the result of defective T-cell regulation.

B-Cell and Antibody Immunodeficiencies

Like the combined immunodeficiencies, the B-cell or antibody immunodeficiencies exhibit a wide range of extremes both in the defects and the resultant symptoms. The defects range from a complete lack of all immunoglobulin classes to a selective deficiency of an immunoglobulin subclass. The symptoms are closely linked to the type and extent of the immunoglobulin deficiency and range from severe recurrent infections to no apparent clinical symptoms.

The age at which symptoms appear depends on the severity of the antibody deficiency and the age of onset of disease. With prompt diagnosis and institution of proper therapy, usually gammaglobulin, many of these patients do extremely well. The defects have been attributed to inherent B-cell abnormalities at the various stages of B-cell maturation and to misregulation by T cells. Most of the laboratory workup for the detection of these B-cell deficiencies can be performed by the majority of hospital laboratories.

X-Linked Infantile Agammaglobulinemia (Bruton's Type Agammaglobulinemia)

X-linked infantile agammaglobulinemia (Bruton's disease) is the most severe of the B-cell deficiencies. It is, as the name implies, inherited in an X-linked recessive pattern and has an incidence of approximately 1 per 100,000. This disorder is characterized by a lack of circulating B cells and plasma cells. These patients do have pre-B cells in the bone marrow and in the circulation, but they do not secrete immunoglobulin.

As a result, the immunoglobulin levels are drastically reduced: IgG typically is less than 100 mg/dL, IgA and IgM less than 1% of normal. T-cell quantitations and functional analysis are normal. These patients are subject to recurrent pyogenic infections, but usually handle the common viral diseases of childhood without much sequelae.

Infants with Bruton's disease usually remain well during the first months of life because of the passive transfer of maternal antibodies. As these antibodies wane, however, an excessive susceptibility to infection becomes evident. These patients develop sinusitis, dermatitis, pneumonia, otitis media, sepsis, and meningitis. The most common infecting organisms are streptococci, staphylococci, and *Haemophilus influenzae*. These infections normally are easily controlled with appropriate antibiotic therapy.

The patient's quick response to treatment in these infections, however, may actually be unfortunate because it may delay the early diagnosis of Bruton's disease. Early diagnosis and institution of treatment are extremely important to the successful long-term maintenance of most immunodeficient patients. As mentioned previously, the therapy for most patients with B-cell immunodeficiencies is gammaglobulins, which can now be administered intravenously.

Pathogenesis. The pathogenesis of X-linked agammaglobulinemia was thought to be attributable to a lack of the stem cells that give rise to the B cells. However, pre-B cells have been found in the bone marrow and circulation of some of these patients, so the defect may be in the maturation of these pre-B cells into mature B cells.

Transient Hypogammaglobulinemia of Infancy

A normal infant begins to synthesize IgM at birth, IgA in about 3 weeks, and IgG by 6 to 8 weeks. At around age 5 to 6 months, the infant's serum concentration of IgG is at its lowest. This is because maternally transferred IgG has been almost completely catabolized at this point and the infant's own IgG has not yet offset the loss of maternal antibody. At this time, normal infants are more susceptible to those infections associated with lower IgG levels. Typically, this is soon corrected.

However, in infants with *transient hypogammaglobulinemia*, the production of IgG (occasionally IgM and IgA as well) is delayed by up to 2 years, and these individuals remain hypogammaglobulinemic. These infants do have circulating B cells, which distinguishes them from infants with congenital hypogammaglobulinemia, and the cellular immunity is intact.

Infants with transient hypogammaglobulinemia are prone to recurrent respiratory tract and skin infections. These eventually decrease as the patient's delayed immunoglobulin synthesis begins. Some patients may exhibit the same severity and type of infections as found in X-linked hypogammaglobulinemia and should be treated similarly.

Pathogenesis. Two different mechanisms for the pathogenesis of this disorder have been postulated: (1) the passive transfer of maternal anti-IgG antibody, which could, in turn, suppress the production of IgG in the infant; and (2) a transient deficiency in the number and/or function of the T-helper cells required for proper immunoglobulin production.

Common Variable Immunodeficiency (Primary Acquired Agammaglobulinemia)

Common variable immunodeficiency (CVI), like many of the deficiencies previously discussed, is a heterogeneous population disorder with similar features (in this case, *acquired* agammaglobulinemia). It is characterized by a clinical presentation similar to X-linked agammaglobulinemia except that the onset of the disorder may occur at any age, although usually between 15 and 35 years. There is no definitive inheritance pattern; however, there are familial cases reported, and there does seem to be a high incidence of immunologic abnormalities in the families of these patients.

The majority of CVI patients have circulating B cells. The immunoglobulin levels in these patients are slightly better than in those with the X-linked disorder; however, they are still extremely reduced.

The T-cell immunity in a large number of these patients does demonstrate some quantitative and functional abnormalities, which, in time, may actually worsen. These patients also have a higher-than-normal incidence of collagen vascular diseases and malignancy.

The clinical manifestations, as mentioned, are similar to the X-linked agammaglobulinemia and are essentially treated the same way. The long-term prognosis of treated patients is good.

Pathogenesis. Because this is a group of similar disorders, it might be expected that the pathogenesis would be variable. Indeed, this is the case. Intrinsic B cell defects, enzymatic abnormalities, increased activated suppressor T cells, and decreased helper T cells have all been demonstrated as causes of this disorder.

Selective Immunoglobulin Deficiencies

In contrast to all or many of the immunoglobulin classes being deficient, these disorders lack only one immunoglobulin class or subclass, with the rest being present in normal concentrations. *Selective IgA deficiency* is the most common of all immunodeficiencies, occurring in about 1 in 600 persons. The clinical presentations range from recurrent sinopulmonary infections and/or sepsis to being asymptomatic (most selective IgA deficients are asymptomatic). The treatments also vary from no gammaglobulin in IgA deficiencies to gammaglobulin in some of the other class and subclass deficiencies. The pathogenesis is not known but is speculated to be a defect in the terminal differentiation of the B cell.

T-Cell Immunodeficiencies

Strict T-cell immunodeficiencies in which the humoral immune system is not secondarily affected are very rare. This is because the humoral immune system depends on the regulatory T cells to mount a proper antibody response. There are, however, a few cases where T-cell deficiencies occur in the face of normal to near normal antibody production. These individuals suffer from severe recurrent infections with opportunistic fungal, viral, and protozoal organisms.

Thymic Hypoplasia (DiGeorge's Syndrome)

DiGeorge's syndrome is a congenital malformation that occurs early in gestation (in the third and fourth pharyngeal pouches). It is characterized at birth by multiple anomalies including abnormal facial structures, congenital heart defects, hypoparathyroidism, and a reduced or absent thymus. The cellular immune defect varies with the severity of the thymic defect. The lymphocyte counts are usually low. While the percentage of T cells and the responsiveness to the mitogens are reduced, the B-cell percentages may actually be increased with somewhat normal function. Immunoglobulin quantitations are of little value at birth because the majority of immunoglobulin will be of maternal origin when these infants present.

In these infants, it is not the cellular immune defect but rather the congenital heart defects and hypocalcemia that are the first manifestations of this syndrome requiring attention. These infants must first survive correction of these immediate life-threatening defects before the chronic recurrent infections become apparent. The cellular immunity has been known either to recover spontaneously or to deteriorate further, if left untreated. Fetal thymus transplants have been used successfully to reconstitute the T-cell immunity, resulting in long-term survival.

The cause of this congenital defect is not known, and it does not appear to occur generally in an inherited fashion. However, there appears to be an increased incidence of DiGeorge's syndrome in infants of alcoholic mothers.

Chronic Mucocutaneous Candidiasis

Chronic mucocutaneous candidiasis is a relatively restricted T-cell immunodeficiency. It is characterized by a selective inability to mount a cellular immune response against *Candida albicans* and related fungi. For the most part, the response against viral, protozoal, bacterial, and other fungal infections remains intact. There are varying forms of the disorder, including autosomal recessive inheritance, association with endocrine abnormalities, early onset, and late onset forms. The B-cell immunity and immunoglobulin levels are normal. The lymphocyte count is generally normal. Skin tests and blastogenesis assays are not responsive to candida; however, the response to other antigens and mitogens is, for the most part, normal.

The clinical manifestations of this disorder range from a very mild involvement of a single fingernail to a severe infection of the mucous membranes and skin. Life-threatening infections do not usually occur, and these patients do relatively well. Treatments, including antifungal agents and various *immunostimulatory* techniques, have had limited success.

Pathogenesis. Various models have been put forth to explain the pathogenesis of this disorder. These include genetic response restrictions, tolerance, specific suppressor cells, and monocyte/macrophage defects.

Phagocytic Deficiencies

A major proportion of primary phagocytic dysfunctions are related to the inability of the phagocytic cell to kill microorganisms. Usually this is the result of an enzymatic defect or deficiency. The clinical manifestations of these disorders, like many of the immunodeficiencies, vary widely. They range from recurrent mild bacterial infections to severe systemic fatal infections. Because T- and B-cell systems are intact in these patients, problems with viral and protozoal infections are not generally encountered.

Complement Deficiencies

Primary complement deficiencies are extremely rare, and, when they do occur, they are often associated with various autoimmune diseases. In addition, not all complement deficiencies are associated with an increased vulnerability to infections. This is surprising in light of what we know about complement's involvement in the microbial killing process, and it attests to the remarkable versatility of the immune system. A detailed treatment of these deficiencies is beyond the scope of the text (see Suggested Readings at the end of this chapter).

SECONDARY IMMUNODEFICIENCIES

As stated previously, secondary immunodeficiencies may be caused by an extremely wide range of primary disorders such as infection, malignancy, autoimmunity, protein-losing states, immunosuppressive therapy, and a long list of others (Table 50–2). The recognition of these associations is important because it often explains the increased susceptibility to infection seen in these disorders.

The immunologic abnormalities that occur in secondary immunodeficiencies are highly variable and range from being limited to very extensive. Because an exhaustive discussion of all of these disorders is beyond the scope of this chapter, a representative sampling of some of the more frequently encountered secondary immunodeficiency groups will be described: acquired immunodeficiency syndrome (AIDS), immunodeficiency in malignancy, and immunodeficiency associated with autoimmune disease.

Acquired Immunodeficiency Syndrome (AIDS)

AIDS is by far the most well-known immunodeficiency to both the health professional and the layperson. The incidence of AIDS among the *high-risk groups* ranges from 168–350/100,000 population in the United States.

AIDS has characteristics of both a primary and secondary immunodeficiency. The most severe manifestation of this disease is its profound effect on the immune system; however, this effect is *secondary* to and induced by infection with the *human immunodeficiency virus (HIV)*, formerly designated HTLVIII or LAV. Therefore, it is included here as a secondary immunodeficiency.

The effects of HIV infection on the immune system range from an asymptomatic immunodeficiency to the extreme immunodeficiency with its associated opportunistic infections and malignancies seen in classic AIDS. Virtually all arms of the immune system may be affected by HIV infection; however, the *primary* target is the T helper cell.

In clinical AIDS, there is usually a decrease in the lymphocyte count, with marked reductions in the percentage and absolute numbers of *T helper* cells. This results in the classic inversion of the T-helper to T-suppressor cell ratio, which is normally about 2 to 1.

Early in the disease, the number and percentage of T suppressor cells may actually increase. All of these lymphocyte values (including the T suppressor cells) eventually deteriorate as the disease progresses. Antigen proliferation responses are decreased, and, as the disease progresses further, the mitogen proliferation responses are affected as well. Immunoglobulin levels are frequently elevated by polyclonal B-cell activation.

Late in the disease course, these immunoglobulin (Ig) levels also deteriorate, most likely because of an obliteration of the lymphoid tissue germinal centers. Other cells of the immune system, such as macrophages and natural killer cells, are also adversely affected. The majority of these defects may be linked to the primary HIV-induced impairment and destruction of the T helper cells as well as the monocyte/macrophages also infected with the virus. Again, one only has to refer to the multitude of interactions and secreted regulatory factors involving the T helper cell to understand the majority of these defects (see Chapter 47 for a review of some of these interactions).

The clinical manifestations of HIV infection, like the immunologic abnormalities, vary considerably. One end of the spectrum is an asymptomatic carrier. This is followed by the AIDS-related complex (ARC), which includes abnormalities that may be predictive of AIDS. Finally, at the other end, is the full-blown AIDS. The first clinical symptoms in patients infected with HIV include fever, night sweats, lymphadenopathy, and fatigue. This may then be followed by extreme weight loss, diarrhea, opportunistic infections, and malignancies (Kaposi's sarcoma and lymphoma). The most common infection in AIDS is *Pneumocystis carinii* pneumonia. However, toxoplasmosis, cryptosporidiosis, fungal, bacterial, and concominant viral infections also occur. These infections are the prime cause of death in patients with AIDS. Treatment for HIV and the induced immunodeficiency is still experimental, with several clinical trials under way. The majority of these include the inhibitors of HIV replication (reverse transcriptase), such as azidothymidine (AZT), phosphonoformate, suramin, and HPA-23.

Pathogenesis

The pathogenesis is essentially related to the effects of HIV on the various cells that it infects. The main target for HIV is the T helper cell, in which rapid viral replication and cell death occur shortly after infection. Under certain conditions, a chronic viral infection may also be established. There are also reports that B cells and macrophages may become infected.

Nursing Care of the Patient with AIDS

Of utmost importance in caring for the immunosuppressed patient diagnosed as having either ARC (a condition attributed to HIV, in which the person tests positive for AIDS and demonstrates symptomatology, although less severe than in classic AIDS) or classic AIDS is to implement measures that prevent the transmission of HIV in the clinical setting and to focus on minimizing exposure of the immunosuppressed person to exogenous organisms. Toward this end, each

healthcare provider should be familiar with the "universal precautions" set forth by the Centers for Disease Control (CDC)* and should incorporate these recommendations into daily practice. Such precautions are essential in caring for *all* patients because HIV-infected patients are not always reliably diagnosed based on clinical history and physical examination.

Handwashing may provide the most important barrier to transmission of disease, and it should be performed meticulously using appropriate technique. Patients and family/significant others should be taught the need for and the appropriate technique in handwashing. Raising the consciousness and awareness of patient and visitors in this regard may help to influence their overall perceptions of health and how health is managed.

When exposure or contact with blood and body fluids is anticipated, *all such fluids should be considered to be infective.* Gloves should be worn, and articles in contact with such fluids should be disposed of in containers labeled "infectious waste." Handwashing before and after use of gloves and handling of such materials should be diligently performed. Care should be taken to avoid contaminating the outside of these receptacles.

For purposes of obtaining blood samples or administering parenteral medications, only disposable needles and syringes should be used and properly discarded in puncture-resistant containers. Recapping of needles after use should be *avoided* because of the risk of self-puncturing. Meticulous care of invasive lines should be provided. Acceptable practice is to use aseptic technique during insertion of lines and dressing changes. Sites of invasive lines should be assessed for any signs of infection (redness, swelling, pain, warmth). Use of indwelling urinary catheters should be avoided, if at all possible, because urinary tract infection is a major source of infection in hospitalized patients. If catheterization is necessary, scrupulous perineal care should be provided. Thorough mouth care and personal hygiene should be provided to prevent stomatitis. The skin should be assessed for signs of impairment, and special skin care should be provided to prevent breakdown of this first line of defense against opportunistic organisms.

In general, nurses caring for the immunosuppressed patient must adhere to high standards of practice in implementing personal hygiene, treatments, and procedures. It is essential to be thorough in assessing patients and to have a high degree of suspicion because these patients are at especially high risk of developing nosocomial infections. Nursing care considerations regarding the potential for infection are included in Table 56–5. See the case study at the end of this chapter for a depiction of a nursing approach, specifically psychological perspectives in the treatment of the patient with AIDS.

*Centers for Disease Control: Recommendations for prevention of HIV transmission in health care settings. HHS Pub. No. (CDC) 87-8017. MMWR CDC Surveill Summ 36(25): August 21, 1987.

Immunodeficiency Secondary to Malignant Disease

Immunodeficiency is very often associated with malignancy. In fact, this is such a common occurrence that excessive opportunistic infections are not only a risk to the diagnosed cancer patient but are also grounds to suspect an underlying malignancy. This is especially true of cancer involving the cells of the immune system.

B-cell malignancies, such as Burkitt's lymphoma, most chronic lymphocytic leukemia (CLL), multiple myeloma, and Waldenström's macroglobulinemia, often demonstrate hypogammaglobulinemia (excluding any monoclonal spikes) and a decreased in vivo antibody response to antigenic stimulation (e.g., vaccine, organisms). Often the cellular responses are also decreased. In CLL, the malignant B cells do not often secrete immunoglobulin and the defective humoral response seems to lie in a reduced immunoglobulin synthesis. In plasma cell malignancies such as multiple myeloma and Waldenström's macroglobulinemia, the malignant cells do produce immunoglobulin. In fact, the levels in the blood may become so high that the serum actually becomes viscous. However, the immunoglobulin is monoclonal (only one specificity), and these patients have very little polyclonal functional immunoglobulin. It has been suggested that this decrease in normal immunoglobulin may result from maturational block or inhibition of B cells by host suppressor monocytic cells.

The T-cell malignancies such as T-cell acute lymphocytic leukemia and Sézary syndrome (mostly a T-helper cell malignancy) have variable defects in both the humoral and cellular system. This often depends on whether the malignant cells are functional.

If the malignancy itself does not cause an immunodeficiency, very often the treatment will. This is because most cancer chemotherapy and radiation therapy are immunosuppressive.

Miscellaneous Secondary Immunodeficiencies

Although the secondary immunodeficiencies discussed in this chapter are among some of the more common ones encountered, the complete list is extremely large (Table 50–2) and cannot be discussed because of space limitations. Furthermore, equally as large as the number of secondary immunodeficiencies is the range of immune abnormalities that occur in them.

SUMMARY

Immunodeficiency disorders are by no means rare, and they are constantly being encountered by the health professional in one form or another, depending on the specific defect. It is hoped that this overview of the defects encountered in the immune system will enable the reader to appreciate the tremendous complexity and interactions of the immune system and the consequences of any errors or abnormalities that may occur.

CASE STUDY WITH SAMPLE CARE PLAN: PATIENT WITH AIDS: PSYCHOLOGICAL PERSPECTIVES*

WB is a 33-year-old white man, admitted to the medical unit with a chief complaint of increasing shortness of breath over a 1-week period. The patient states he is a lifelong homosexual whose ex-lover died last night of AIDS. Their last encounter was 3 years ago.

WB reported that the shortness of breath occurs while at rest, increasing significantly upon exertion. It is associated with a dry, unproductive cough and chest pain across the sternum. This pain is aggravated upon inspiration.

The patient also complains of dizziness at times but admits to not eating well over the past 2 weeks because he has had no appetite. WB denies fever, chills, night sweats, or any other associated complaints.

WB's past medical history includes hepatitis, 7 years before this admission; gonorrhea, 11 years before this admission, which was treated effectively with tetracycline; and herpes zoster, which developed about 4 months ago and was treated with acyclovir. A lesion attributed to the herpes infection is still evident on the patient's forehead.

WB's sexual history reveals that he has been exclusively a homosexual, active since age 14. He states that his last sexual contact was a year and a half ago. Before that, he had 5 partners; he estimated that he has had fewer than 50 partners over the last 19 years. He was active with his most recent lover about 3 years ago. The ex-lover was diagnosed as having AIDS about 2 years ago and has died.

Socially, WB has a history of cigarette smoking of about 18 pack years; he quit smoking altogether about 2 months before this admission. He describes himself as an occasional drinker. WB denies intravenous drug use; he admits to using recreational drugs, including cocaine, mescaline, and Quaalude.

WB reports that he was fired from his job as a manager of a store selling women's garments. He offered no explanation regarding the circumstances of his firing. He has no medical/health insurance and limited personal funds. He denies having had blood transfusions and has not traveled outside of the United States.

Significant family history reveals that the patient's father died at age 72 from heart disease; his mother is alive and well at age 71. There are five siblings, including three brothers and two sisters, all alive and well. Two of WB's brothers and one sister are homosexual.

On physical examination, the patient presents as a well-developed white man in no acute distress. A her-

*This case study and sample care plan were contributed by Kathleen Daley White and Margaret Connelly.

SAMPLE CARE PLAN FOR THE PATIENT WITH ACQUIRED IMMUNODEFICIENCY SYNDROME (AIDS): PSYCHOLOGICAL PERSPECTIVES

Nursing Diagnoses

Nursing Diagnosis #1

Fear of death and dying, related to AIDS diagnosis

Desired Patient Outcomes

Patient will be able to:
1. Verbalize fear regarding AIDS
2. Identify support systems to deal effectively with AIDS

Nursing Interventions

- Assess patient's perceived fear as expressed in own words.
- Help to identify factors the patient feels control over and those he or she does not.

- Use support persons and resources to help patient sort out and deal with fear.
  - Interview family members and identify those who are positive in their attitude and approach to the patient; encourage their participation in care.
  - Investigate patient's background to identify available support resources; contact these resources to help in creating a supportive environment in which the patient can verbalize fear.
- Document patient's questions and responses in progress notes, so as to communicate the patient's goals, progression, and regression in working toward goals.
- Document any key characteristic behavior exhibited by patient and reflective of underlying fear; use these to help the patient deal effectively with fear.
- Encourage family participation in patient care activities.

Rationales

- Separating those items that are able to be controlled from those that are not gives the patient an area on which to focus energies toward resolution of the fear.
- By working within the patient's own framework, support systems and resources can be used more effectively in assisting the patient to deal with fear.

- Documentation assists in providing continuity of care.

- Clarifying the status of AIDS, including what it is, what can be done to treat it, its prognosis, and expected course, for the patient and family members, ultimately will strengthen the effectiveness of the patient-family-health team and support system.
- It is essential to be honest and straightforward.

Nursing Diagnoses

Nursing Diagnosis #2

Body image, disturbance, related to actual bodily changes

Desired Patient Outcomes

Patient will:
1. Verbalize feelings regarding body changes
2. Demonstrate positive attitude regarding self:
   - Identify strengths
   - Express interest in self-care activities
   - Involve family in care

Nursing Interventions

- Assess thoughts and feelings regarding body changes.

- Ask patient to identify these changes.

- Help patient to become aware of the support systems that surround him or her and who accepts him or her as he or she is, regardless of body changes.

Rationales

- Underlying immune defect of cell-mediated immunity in AIDS places these patients at high risk of developing fungal and other opportunistic infections. Such infections can be physically unsightly and emotionally difficult for the patient to cope with.
- If patient can identify body changes that are particularly distressing, the nurse may help him or her to understand why the infections occur and what can be done to minimize the risk of infection—for example, frequent and meticulous oral hygiene, handwashing.
- By identifying a support system, the patient may begin to realize acceptance by those caring for him or her in spite of body changes; he or she may realize that body image in no way threatens their friendship, love, and support for him or her.

SAMPLE CARE PLAN FOR THE PATIENT WITH ACQUIRED IMMUNODEFICIENCY SYNDROME (AIDS): PSYCHOLOGICAL PERSPECTIVES (*Continued*)

Nursing Interventions

- Provide personalized nursing care: touch the patient and care for the patient in the manner you would care for any patient while implementing appropriate precautions.

- Work with family to help them be aware of patient's misgivings about body changes; help them to identify grooming habits important to patient and to implement a plan of care: haircut and shave; manicure; use of favorite cologne.
- Document patient's response to care and progress made toward accepting self; update and revise the care plan accordingly.

Rationales

- Nurses are able to demonstrate their acceptance of the patient by personalizing care; use of touch therapy is especially reassuring to the patient; furthermore, it sets an example for the family members and significant others to follow. Using this approach reassures the patient that he or she is accepted in spite of his or her own perceptions and self-doubts.
- Involving family in patient's care may enable them to feel positive about contributing in some way. By arranging for special grooming activities, the patient may be made to feel more positive about himself or herself and acceptance by others.
- Documentation assists in continuity of patient's care: efforts of all healthcare providers can be focused on identified goals and the achievement of desired patient outcomes.

Nursing Diagnoses

Nursing Diagnosis #3
Social isolation, related to:
1. Diagnosis of AIDS
2. Necessary isolation precautions

Desired Patient Outcomes

Patient will:
1. Explain the reasons for isolation precautions
2. Inform family and significant others of need for precautions
3. Demonstrate specific precautions in self-care

Nursing Interventions

- Explain need for and underlying rationales for instituting isolation precautions.

- Implement isolation techniques involving patient and family in performing specific procedures according to hospital protocol.
- Assess patient's previous social lifestyle and social interactions.

- Maintain socialization process on patient's behalf, and within the patient's activity tolerance.
  - After conferring with patient, encourage visitors when appropriate.
  - Keep door to patient room open except when the patient is sleeping.
  - Encourage timely use of television and radio to keep abreast of events.
  - Hang up pictures, cards, and other decorations with meaning to patient.
- Enlist family's help in determining important social situations in patient's life (e.g., birthday, holiday, and anniversary). Work with support system to bring a part of each of these to the patient.
- Encourage staff to carry out necessary isolation techniques, but caution not to overisolate.

Rationales

- Patient, family, and staff must understand what the disease AIDS entails and implications as to precautions to prevent its transmission to others. This is true not only within the hospital setting but also in daily activities of living.

- If patient has been active socially and enjoys people, this should not change because of AIDS. Patient's preferences should be respected and made known to all who interact with the patient. Maintaining some control over his or her life fosters self-confidence and self-esteem.
- Socially withdrawing could lead to a situational depression, or be reflective of depression already present. If patients see the staff as "overisolating," or perceive a "repugnance" on the part of the staff and/or visitors, they may become depressed and socially withdraw.

- For patients on isolation, special efforts should be made so that important events or interactions are not left unnoticed.

- Patients on isolation precautions sometimes feel they are missing something; such feelings as "being left out" can predispose to a depressive reaction and may delay progress in the patient's improvement.

SAMPLE CARE PLAN FOR THE PATIENT WITH ACQUIRED IMMUNODEFICIENCY SYNDROME (AIDS): PSYCHOLOGICAL PERSPECTIVES (*Continued*)

Nursing Diagnoses
Nursing Diagnosis #4

Verbal communication, impaired, related to:
1. CPAP mask
2. Constant tachypnea
3. Fatigue

Desired Patient Outcomes

Patient will be able to communicate with family, staff, and significant others to make needs known and to enjoy interacting with others

Nursing Interventions
- Assess the patient's ability to communicate.
  - Work with patient to identify the problem underlying inability to communicate.

- Work with patient to devise a communication tool to meet needs:
  - Use of chalk or alphabet board.
  - Use of "frequent words used" sheet.
  - Lip-reading.
  - Anticipate needs; remain accessible.
- Document key likes and dislikes so that the entire staff can anticipate patient's needs—for example, ice in water, call bell in left hand.

Rationales
- Patients who have had a terminal disease confirmed have a great deal of processing to go through intellectually, emotionally, and psychologically. If the patient needs to verbalize thoughts and feelings in this regard, an inability to communicate can cause the patient to feel isolated and alone.
- Inability to communicate can be extremely frustrating, particularly when it concerns the "small" needs that people in general take for granted. Aggravation associated with small concerns can become exaggerated and expand into major problems.

- If the patient who is already distressed and compromised must use remaining strength and energy requesting the same thing over and over again, or needs to continually make explanations regarding needs, then the therapeutic milieu provided for the patient needs to be reassessed, and a revised plan of care implemented accordingly.

---

pes lesion is evident on the forehead, and thrush is noted on the left lateral surface of the tongue. On auscultation, breath sounds are decreased bilaterally. Examination of lymph nodes reveals anterior cervical nodes about 1 to 2 cm in size and nontender; posterior cervical and inguinal nodes are also palpable and, likewise, 1 to 2 cm in size and nontender bilaterally.

Psychologically, the patient has experienced undue stress. He has had actual sexual contact with known AIDS victims; he has witnessed 10 close friends die of AIDS over the past 3 years.

Laboratory data of significance are as follows: Arterial blood gases on admission indicated pH 7.45, $PaCO_2$ 36, and PaO_2 62 mmHg (room air). A bronchoscopy performed on admission confirmed the diagnosis of *P. carinii* pneumonia associated with AIDS. Bactrim therapy was initiated.

On the second hospital day following admission, WB expressed a desire for his family to be informed regarding his status. The family was subsequently advised of his diagnosis in his presence, as he requested. On the third hospital day, the patient requested "no resuscitation," should this become an issue. The request was made based on his knowledge of AIDS and its prognosis. At this time, the patient was experiencing increasing dyspnea upon speaking, thus limiting his ability to communicate fully with family, nurses, social worker, priest, or other healthcare providers.

On day 5 of this admission, WB's arterial blood gas studies were as follows: pH 7.46, $PaCO_2$ 34, and PaO_2 46, HCO_3^- 24. He was transferred to the intensive care unit (ICU) and placed on continuous positive airway pressure (CPAP) at +5 cm/H_2O. The patient refused intubation. Subsequently, arterial blood gases were as follows: pH 7.41, $PaCO_2$ 36, PaO_2 107, HCO_3^- 28. The patient remained extremely tachypneic.

Over the next 24 hours, WB's condition remained unchanged. He confirmed: "I don't want to spend the rest of my life on a machine to breathe." Siblings were supportive of his decision and proud of his "bravery." The patient's mother was having a difficult time agreeing with her son's decision, but siblings were supportive to her.

On the eighth day after admission, the patient's body temperature rose to 103°F. Bactrim was discontinued, and pentamidine (Pentam) therapy was initiated. Patient reaffirmed, "no heroics." The entire family seemed at peace with this decision.

Twenty-four hours later, the patient became unresponsive, and apneic at times. The health team continued the treatment plan, hopeful that the patient could be supported until pentamidine would be effective. On consultation with an infectious disease expert, large doses of intravenous corticosteroids were recommended because there have been instances of abrupt reversal of fully fulminating *P. carinii* pneumonia with this approach.

The patient's mother and sister were upset with the steroidal therapy as they viewed this treatment as an "heroic" measure, one that was prolonging the patient's life in opposition to his request. When all siblings were called to the bedside, there was not full agreement by the family on the use of steroids. Following the administration of the first dose of intravenous steroidal therapy, the mother and one sister became so irate that further doses were discontinued. The patient appeared obtunded; body temperature remained at 103°F.

Over the next 18 hours following initial steroidal therapy, the patient became alert, oriented, and afebrile. He was agreeable to further steroidal therapy. Over the next 24 hours, WB had improved so that the CPAP was discontinued. The mother and one sister thought "a miracle had occurred."

On the 13th day following admission, the patient was able to celebrate his birthday with family and friends. He verbalized that his recovery and positive attitude were a result of the support from family, friends, and members of the health team.

Over the next 10 to 12 days, the patient continued to improve with a treatment regimen of pentamidine, steroids, and increased nutrition. He was subsequently transferred to an acute medical unit. During the ensuing 2 weeks, the patient established a new support system in religion, and he received his first holy communion as a Roman Catholic.

The patient continued to progress slowly and was discharged to his mother's home with referral to the AIDS Clinic, about 46 days following his admission.

Initial Nursing Diagnoses

1. Fear of death and dying, related to diagnosis of AIDS.
2. Body image, disturbance in, related to actual bodily changes, including herpetic lesion, *candida* infection (stomatitis), and cachexia (10-pound weight loss).
3. Social isolation, related to diagnosis of AIDS and necessary isolation precautions.
4. Verbal communication, impaired, related to CPAP mask and constant tachypnea and consequent fatigue.

Additional Nursing Diagnoses

1. Coping, ineffective, family (mother, sister), related to exhaustion of supportive capacity and questionable knowledge about AIDS.
2. Sleep pattern disturbance, related to dyspnea, febrile state, ICU setting.
3. Depression, reactive (situational), related to perceived powerlessness of future with AIDS.
4. Self-esteem, disturbance in, related to loss of job, loss of financial independence.
5. Anticipatory grief, related to prognosis of AIDS diagnosis.
6. Knowledge deficit.

SUGGESTED READINGS

Bellanti, JA: Immunology III. WB Saunders, Philadelphia, 1985.

Bellanti, JA: Immunology Basic Processes, ed 2. WB Saunders, Philadelphia, 1985.

Centers for Disease Control: Recommendations for prevention of HIV transmission in health care settings. HHS Pub. No. (CDC) 87-8017. MMWR CDC Surveill Summ 36(25):1987.

Lewandowski, AJ: The immunopathogenesis of AIDS. J Med Technol 3:145–149, 1986.

Mathewson, MK: Pharmacotherapeutics: A Nursing Process Approach. FA Davis, Philadelphia, 1986.

Nyamathi, A and van Servellen, G: Maladaptive coping in the critically ill population with acquired immunodeficiency syndrome: Nursing assessment and treatment. Heart Lung 18:113, March 1989.

Sigal, L and Ron, Y (eds): Immunology and Inflammation. McGraw-Hill, New York, 1994.

Stites, DP and Terr, A (eds): Basic Human Immunology, ed 1. Appleton & Lange, Norwalk, CT, 1991.

UNIT NINE

Hematologic System

UNIT OUTLINE

Anatomy and Physiology of the Hematologic System: Hematopoiesis and Hemostasis

Jan Foster

CHAPTER OUTLINE

Hematopoiesis
- □ Erythrocytes
- □ Leukocytes
- □ Platelets

Hemostasis
- □ Blood Vessels

- □ Platelets
- □ Coagulation Cascade
- □ Fibrinolysis

Integrated Reactions Among Hemostatic Components

References

LEARNING OBJECTIVES

After completing this chapter, you should be able to:

1. Define hemostasis in terms of the interaction among blood vessels, platelets, and the plasma systems of coagulation and fibrinolysis.
2. Describe the reaction of blood vessels to vascular injury.
3. Examine the role of platelets in the hemostatic process.
4. Distinguish the coagulation pathways and their clinical significance.
5. Explain the function of the fibrinolysis system.
6. Outline the major control mechanisms of hemostasis.
7. Describe the interrelationship among coagulation factors and the inflammatory process.

HEMATOPOIESIS

Hematopoiesis is the dynamic process of blood cell production and development. The hematopoietic system consists of the bone marrow, liver, spleen, lymph nodes, and thymus. These tissues and organs are involved in the production, maturation, and destruction of blood cells. All blood cells originate in the bone marrow as pluripotential stem cells that, when stimulated by a series of growth factors, colony-stimulating factors, and interleukins, proliferate and differentiate into erythrocytes, thrombocytes, and leukocytes. The stem cell pool is sustained by a process called self-renewal, which occurs through hematopoietic cells lodging in the stromal cell network of the bone marrow among energy-rich fat cells, adhering to reticular cells, and releasing growth factors by macrophages[1] (Fig. 51–1).

Erythrocytes

Mature erythrocytes, or red blood cells (RBCs), develop from erythroid progenitor cells through a series of mitotic divisions and maturation phases. Erythropoietin is the erythroid colony-stimulating factor responsible for the feedback regulation of erythropoiesis. Endothelial cells in the kidneys sense tissue hypoxia and secrete erythropoietin; erythroid precursor cells in the bone marrow are sensitive to erythropoietin and respond by proliferating and differentiating into fully mature RBCs.[2]

The primary role of RBCs is to transport oxygen and carbon dioxide between the lungs and the tissues. The normal mature RBC is a biconcave disk that is 7 to 8 μm in diameter. It is highly flexible and pliable, which facilitates its passage through tiny capillaries while affording optimal exposure of surface area for the

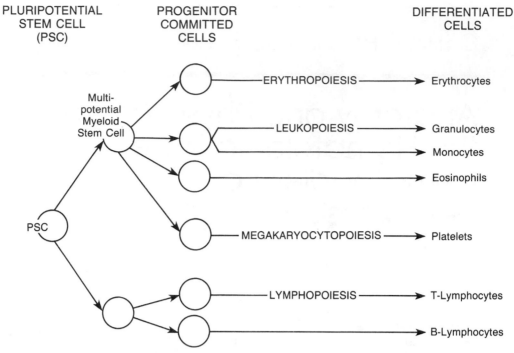

FIGURE 51–1. Hematopoiesis: differentiated cells.

exchange of oxygen and carbon dioxide. The hematocrit is the percentage of the total volume of blood occupied by RBCs.

The RBCs mature in the bone marrow over a period of 4 to 5 days. During this time there are successive morphologic alterations in the cells. The reticulocyte stage, which precedes the mature stage, is characterized by active hemoglobin synthesis, and it is at this stage that the reticulocyte is released into the circulation. Reticulocytes circulate in the blood for about 24 hours before maturing. The reticulocyte count is of particular clinical significance because it reflects the RBC production rate and is a good indicator of the erythropoietic response; an increase in the number of reticulocytes usually indicates an attempt by the bone marrow to respond to an increased need for RBCs. Table 51–1 lists the normal hematologic values.

Red blood cells have an average life span of about 120 days in the circulation and are then removed by the mononuclear phagocyte system. Circulating monocytes and tissue macrophages housed in the spleen, liver, bone marrow, and lymph nodes phagocytize senescent RBCs.[1]

Hemoglobin

The principal constituent of RBCs is hemoglobin, which transports oxygen from the lungs to the tissues and carbon dioxide from the tissues to the lungs. Hemoglobin also serves as a buffer in acid-base balance.

Hemoglobin consists of the protein globin (two pairs of polypeptide chains) and four heme groups,

each of which contains a protoporphyrin ring plus iron (Fe^{2+}). Oxygen specifically binds to the iron atom within each of the heme groups. One of the most important controls of hemoglobin affinity for oxygen is the RBC organic phosphate 2,3-diphosphoglycerate (2,3-DPG). When hemoglobin loads oxygen and becomes oxyhemoglobin, 2,3-DPG is expelled from the molecule. This relaxed form of hemoglobin has a higher affinity for oxygen. The hemoglobin molecule's multichain structure and its binding and expul-

TABLE 51–1
Normal Values in Hematology

Type	Percentage of Cell Count	Cell Count
Red Blood Cell (RBC)/Erythrocyte		4.5–6.0 K/μL (male)
		4.0–5.5 K/μL (female)
Reticulocyte	0.5%–1.5%	20–90 K/μL
Hematocrit	40%–54% (male)	
	37%–47% (female)	
Hemoglobin		14–18 g/dL (male)
		12–16 g/dL (female)
White Blood Cell (WBC)/Leukocyte		4–11 K/μL
Bands	3%–5%	1–6 K/μL
Neutrophils	42%–66%	1.7–3.7 K/μL
Lymphocytes	24%–44%	1.0–4.8 K/μL
Monocytes	2%–7%	0.08–0.07 K/μL
Eosinophils	1%–4%	0.04–4.0 K/μL
Basophils	0%–1%	0–0.1 K/μL
Platelet		140–440 K/μL

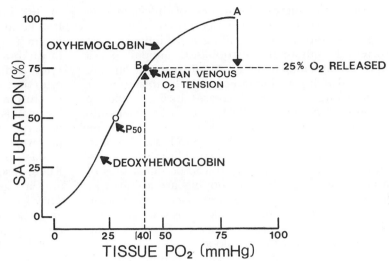

FIGURE 51–2. Normal hemoglobin-oxygen dissociation curve. (From Hillman, RF and Finch, CA: Red Cell Manual, ed 5. FA Davis, Philadelphia, 1985, with permission.)

sion of 2,3-DPG allow for movement that enables loading and unloading of oxygen.[3]

The amount of oxygen bound to hemoglobin is determined by the partial pressure (PO_2) of oxygen. When the partial pressure of oxygen is high, as at the alveolar-capillary membrane in the lungs, oxygen readily binds with hemoglobin; when the partial pressure of oxygen is low, as at the cellular-capillary membrane in the tissues, oxygen is readily released. The quantitative relationship between hemoglobin-bound oxygen and the partial pressure of oxygen is characterized by the oxyhemoglobin dissociation curve (Fig. 51–2). Conditions that reduce the affinity of hemoglobin for oxygen include acidemia, hyperthermia, and an increase in 2,3-DPG level. The result is increased oxygen release to the tissues. This is referred to as a "shift to the right" of the oxyhemoglobin dissociation curve (see Fig. 51–2). Conversely, alkalemia, hypothermia, and reduced levels of 2,3-DPG increase hemoglobin's affinity for oxygen, which reduces the amount of oxygen released to the tissues. This is a "shift to the left" of the oxyhemoglobin dissociation curve (see Fig. 51–2).

The patient suffering from anemia caused by loss of RBCs may be able to compensate if the oxyhemoglobin dissociation curve is shifted to the right, allowing delivery of adequate oxygen to the tissues. In this case, the RBCs, though fewer in number, are able to work more efficiently in tissue oxygenation.

Leukocytes

Leukocytes, or white blood cells (WBCs), include three different lineages: granulocytes, monocytes/macrophages, and lymphocytes. Granulocytes are subdivided into three groups: neutrophils, eosinophils, and basophils. Normal concentrations of the five types of WBCs are shown in Table 51–1.

Differentiation into the types of leukocytes occurs in response to colony-stimulating factors and interleu-

kins, which are produced by various types of hematopoietic cells. Colony-stimulating factors and interleukins act on myeloid colony–forming units, groups of immature cells arising from the pluripotential stem cell, and stimulate growth and proliferation into mature and functional neutrophils, eosinophils, basophils, monocytes, macrophages, and lymphocytes.

Neutrophils

Neutrophils arise from committed myeloid progenitor cells in the bone marrow. They are released from the bone marrow at the rate of 2.5 million cells per hour into the blood, where they carry out their functions. Because the neutrophil's life span is only about 7 to 10 hours, rapid proliferation is essential. Normally, the rate at which neutrophils enter the blood and the rate of egress from the blood are in equilibrium. Bands are an immature form of neutrophils. An increase in the number of bands together with an increase in the number of mature neutrophils usually reflects an acute infectious process.

Neutrophils serve as the primary defense against bacteria. In their host-defense function, neutrophils move to sites of injury, immobilize the invader, and kill the microbe. These functions are made possible because of the properties of chemical attraction to the injury (chemotaxis), adherence to the blood vessel endothelial wall to allow movement from the blood to the tissue (adhesion), ingestion of the organism (phagocytosis), and production of toxic oxygen substances (metabolic burst). Killing and digestion of the organism is the ultimate result.[4]

Eosinophils

Eosinophils have large, round secondary granules that have an affinity for the acid eosin stain. Mature eosinophils are stored in the bone marrow for several days before they migrate to the blood and then to the tissues, where they reside.

Eosinophils migrate into sites of infection and inflammation and are able to ingest bacteria, but their phagocytic and microbial killing capabilities are less efficient than those of neutrophils. Eosinophils play a key role in inflammatory and allergic reactions and are associated with parasitic infections. The total number of circulating eosinophils increases during an allergic response as these cells collect at sites of antigen-antibody reactions and remove the resulting immune complexes from the blood. Eosinophils are also present in large numbers in the mucosal lining of the gastrointestinal and respiratory tracts, potential sites of entry of antigens. When eosinophils are activated by antibodies, they attach to parasite larvae and release toxic substances that destroy the parasites.

Eosinophilia (i.e., the presence of increased numbers of eosinophils in the blood) occurs in allergic reactions (e.g., asthma), parasitic infections (e.g., trichinae), chronic skin diseases such as exfoliative dermatitis, Hodgkin's lymphoma, chronic myelocytic leukemia, pernicious anemia, tissue necrosis (e.g., after irradiation), sarcoid, vasculitis, and hypereosinophilic syndromes. Eosinophil counts are usually low during bacterial and viral infections, stress-induced increases, or exogenous administration of corticosteroids.

Basophils

Basophils contain granules that have a high content of histamine, serotonin, and heparin. Basophils have high-affinity receptors for IgE, which when bound to antigen triggers the release of these mediators. When released, the mediators can precipitate anaphylaxis (i.e., an allergic sensitivity reaction of the body to a foreign protein or drug).

Basophilic granules also contain eosinophil chemotactic factor, a substance that attracts eosinophils when released during immediate hypersensitivity reactions. The number of basophils is increased most often in chronic myelocytic leukemia and other myeloproliferative disorders. Basophilia also occurs in asthma, inflammatory bowel disease, splenectomy, and chronic inflammation.

Mast cells are structurally and functionally related to granulocytes, and like basophils, have granules that contain histamine. They are produced in the bone marrow but do not circulate in the blood; they are found in mucosal and connective tissues. Mast cells defend against certain parasites and fill a number of other roles in the regulation of lymphoid and granulocyte responses. When activated, they produce their primary effects through histamine release.[5]

Monocytes and Macrophages

Monocytes and macrophages are critical in cell-mediated immunity, which protects against infections caused by viruses, fungi, protozoa, and mycobacteria. Monocytes arise from the stem cell in the bone marrow, undergo several maturational stages, and are then released into the circulation. Circulating monocytes migrate to various tissues, where they further mature into macrophages. Tissue macrophages are housed in sinusoids of the liver and spleen, in alveoli in the lungs, in pleural and peritoneal serous cavities, in the brain as microglial cells, in the skin as histiocytes, and in the synovial membrane of joints. Monocytes and macrophages are more efficient than neutrophils in phagocytosis of very large molecules; their life span is also much longer. They ingest and destroy bacteria much less efficiently than neutrophils, however.

Macrophages play a key role in removing senescent RBCs, insoluble particles, activated clotting factors, and antigen-antibody complexes from circulation. They have the unique capacity to process and present antigens to T lymphocytes, and through this mechanism, play a central role in regulating T cell–mediated and B lymphocyte–mediated humoral immunity.[6] Macrophages release cytokines, substances that function in the immune response; interleukin-1 (IL-1) and tumor necrosis factor (TNF) are two of the cytokines. Cytokines have numerous functions in the immune response, including the production of fever and induction of proliferation of T lymphocytes.

Lymphocytes

Lymphocytes are primarily concerned with maintaining the body's immune defense system. Lymphocytes originate from lymphoid stem cells in the bone marrow and, when stimulated by interleukins and other cytokines, proliferate and differentiate into fully functional immune cells. There are two major types of lymphocytes, T cells and B cells. T lymphocytes mature in the thymus gland and have subpopulations called T helper cells, T suppressor cells, natural killer cells, and memory cells. B lymphocytes mature in the adult bone marrow and spleen and further differentiate into plasma cells that produce immunoglobulins (also called antibodies). T lymphocytes are responsible for cell-mediated immunity; protect against bacteria, viruses, cancer cells, and other foreign organisms; and orchestrate the immune response in general. B lymphocytes, through the actions of immunoglobulin, are responsible for humoral immunity and are particularly important in the immune responses to bacteria and allergic reactions.[2,7] For a detailed discussion of the role played by lymphocytes and plasma cells in the body's immune response, see Chapter 47.

Platelets

Platelets develop from the megakaryocytes in the bone marrow, which descend from the same multipotential stem cell as do the other myeloid cells. In the presence of the hormone thrombopoietin, megakaryocytes proliferate and fragment their cytoplasm into platelets. Their life span is about 10 days. Platelets have no nucleus and cannot synthesize protein. Their cytoplasm contains several substances, including enzymes and granules, that produce the clotting reaction. Platelets ordinarily circulate freely in the blood, but when tissues are injured, they adhere to damaged tissue and to each other to form hemostatic plugs or clots. Normally, 80% of platelets are in circulation in the blood, and 20% are pooled in the spleen. In the presence of splenomegaly, often associated with portal hypertension, however, up to 80% of platelets may be pooled in the spleen.

Thrombocytopenia results from diminished production or increased destruction of platelets. Conditions that diminish platelet production include administration of certain drugs (e.g., chloramphenicol and cancer chemotherapeutic agents) and aplastic anemia. Conditions that increase destruction of platelets include administration of certain drugs (e.g., quinidine), antibody formation (e.g., repeated blood transfusions), autoimmunity (e.g., idiopathic thrombocytopenia purpura), viral diseases, and disseminated intravascular coagulation.[4,7]

HEMOSTASIS

Hemostasis is initiated by local vascular injury and culminates in the formation of a platelet-fibrin plug that prevents blood loss through the damaged vessel.

Its purpose, quite simply, is to prevent bleeding. To promote blood flow, hemostasis is balanced by a finely tuned system of fibrinolysis. There are three major components to the hemostatic response: the blood vessel walls, the platelets, and the coagulation cascade, including the intrinsic and extrinsic pathways.

Blood Vessels

Endothelial cells line blood vessel walls and synthesize von Willebrand factor multimers. Following vessel injury and subendothelial exposure, platelets bind to von Willebrand multimers and collagen to initiate hemostasis. Direct insult to the vessel wall also stimulates sudden vasoconstriction, with a consequent reduction of blood loss and more effective contact of platelets and hemostatic processes (Fig. 51–3).

Platelets

When subendothelial structures are exposed to flowing blood, platelets adhere to collagen, bind von Willebrand multimers, change shape from disks to

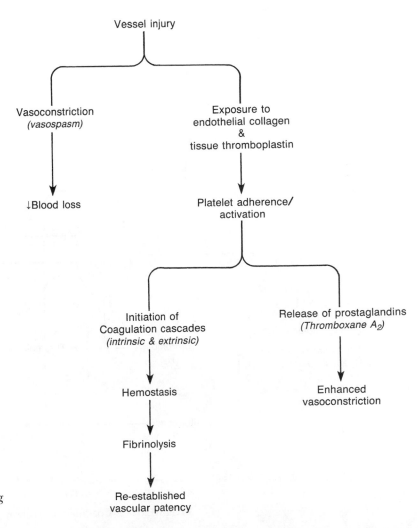

FIGURE 51–3. Vessel injury: triggering event.

spiny spheres, and release their granule contents. Adenosine diphosphate (ADP) is released from the platelet granules, which promotes platelet aggregation and alters the surface of the platelets. The altered surface binds fibrinogen from surrounding plasma and causes further aggregation of platelets to those already adhering to the endothelial lining and collagen of the blood vessel. Thrombin, generated from activation of the clotting cascade, amplifies platelet aggregation and release responses. Collagen and thrombin trigger the synthesis of multiple enzymes and prostaglandins, including thromboxane A_2, which potentiates the release of platelet granule contents. Thromboxane A_2 induces platelet aggregation and localized vasoconstriction.[8]

Coagulation Cascade

Because of common usage and international agreement, the coagulation factors are labeled by Roman numerals, which do not reflect the sequence in which they are activated in the coagulation process (Table

TABLE 51–2
Nomenclature of Coagulation Factors

Factor	Descriptive Name
Factor I	Fibrinogen
Factor II	Prothrombin
Factor III	Tissue thromboplastin (tissue factor)
Factor IV	Calcium
Factor V	Labile factor
Factor VI	Not assigned
Factor VII	Stable factor
Factor VIII	Antihemophilic factor (AHF)
Factor IX	Christmas factor
Factor X	Stuart-Power factor
Factor XI	Plasma thromboplastin antecedent
Factor XII	Hageman factor
Factor XIII	Fibrin stabilizing factor (FSF)

51–2). A small "a" next to the Roman numeral indicates that the factor is activated (Fig. 51–4). The coagulation factors are synthesized in the liver; factors II (prothrombin), IX, and X are vitamin K–dependent. In the final common pathway of the clotting cascade,

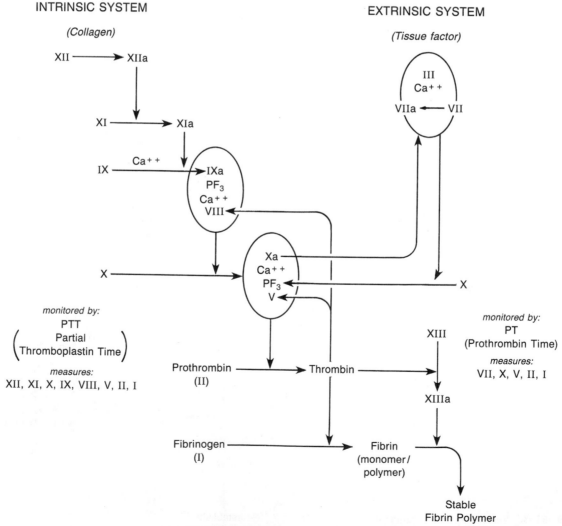

FIGURE 51–4. Coagulation pathways.

SUMMARY OF ACTIVITIES OF THE COAGULATION PATHWAYS

1. Initiation factors:
   a. Intrinsic pathway is initiated by injury to vessel wall or to blood itself; the injury occurs within the blood vessel.
   b. Extrinsic pathway is initiated by injury to tissues outside of the blood vessel or by blood coming into contact with injured tissues.
2. Major activators:
   a. Intrinsic pathway: collagen, antigen-antibody reaction, stasis, endotoxins.
   b. Extrinsic pathway: tissue factor III (thromboplastin).
3. Specific characteristics:
   a. Neither pathway involves the release of an enzyme from damaged tissue.
   b. Under normal conditions, the initiating factors are unavailable to flowing blood; phospholipid is essential to the initiation of both pathways.
   c. In both pathways, the initiators (e.g., collagen and tissue factor) are essential cofactors to the initial reactions of each respective pathway.
   d. Both pathways are essential for normal coagulation, although factors XII and XI are not essential.
   e. Initiation of the intrinsic pathway leading to the formation of fibrin occurs within *minutes;* initiation of the extrinsic pathway leading to the formation of fibrin occurs in *seconds.*
4. Mechanisms:
   a. Each pathway consists of a series of conversion reactions requiring cofactors wherein circulating proenzymes or precursor molecules are activated to proteolytic enzymes.
   b. The reactions of each pathway occur in a cascading fashion wherein each coagulation factor is activated by the preceding reaction, thus facilitating acceleration and amplification of the events of each pathway.
   c. All coagulation factors except for factors V, VIII, and IV (calcium) are proteins; factors V and VIII are cofactors that catalyze key reactions of the coagulation process.
   d. The acceleration phenomenon is caused by autocatalytic reactions whereby certain products formed in the coagulation process actually catalyze the reactions by which they themselves were formed. Thrombin is a principal autocatalyst.
   e. Vitamin K–dependent factors (VII, IX, X, and II) function in the tight binding of coagulation factors to calcium and phospholipid. This activity raises the localized concentrations of the reactants and increases the speed of reactions leading to the amplification effect.
   f. Thrombin is the pivotal molecule in these reactions, with the following key functions:
      1) Stimulates platelet aggregation, release reaction, and fusion into the secondary platelet plug that forms the basis for the interaction of coagulation factors.
      2) Enhances the activity of cofactors V and VIII, which accelerate the coagulation process.
      3) Converts fibrinogen to fibrin, which forms the basis for the clot.
      4) Activates factor XIII to XIIIa, which converts fibrin into a stable clot.
      5) Initiates the fibrinolysis system.

---

thrombin converts fibrinogen into fibrin, an insoluble meshwork that forms the plug that prevents bleeding.

The intrinsic pathway is triggered by factors circulating in the blood within the vascular compartment. The contact of Hageman factor (XII) with subendothelial structures at the site of vessel injury initiates the intrinsic pathway. Factor XI is activated to XIa, which cleaves XIIa to the subendothelium and produces a more effective proteolytic conversion of prekallikrein to kallikrein. Kallikrein is necessary for the activation of factor IX. Activation of factor IX to IXa in the presence of calcium triggers activation of factor X, which activates the common pathway.

The extrinsic pathway is initiated by exposure of plasma to tissue factor outside the circulating blood. Factor III (tissue thromboplastin) is released from the injured tissues and enters the vascular system; it provides the phospholipid component essential to the initiation of the extrinsic system. Factor VII is activated to VIIa in the presence of calcium, activating factor X, which in turn activates the common pathway. The extrinsic pathway generates thrombin; thrombin converts fibrinogen to fibrin. Factor XIII is converted to XIIIa, which covalently links fibrin monomers into fibrin polymers. A stable fibrin clot results (Fig. 51–4).[8] The activities of the coagulation pathways are summarized in the box above.

Fibrinolysis

Fibrin clots are sturdy and effective structures for stopping hemorrhage until endothelium-lined channels are reconstructed, but they are designed to be dissolved rapidly after vascular repair so blood flow can resume. Clot removal, fibrinolysis, is accomplished

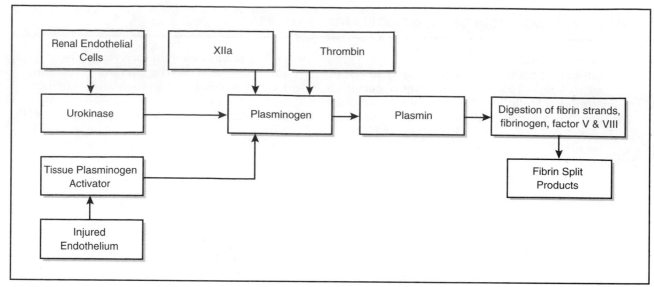

FIGURE 51–5. Fibrinolysis.

chiefly by a substance called plasmin. Plasmin is a proteolytic enzyme that digests the fibrin threads of the clot and other substances in the surrounding blood, including fibrinogen, factor V, factor VIII, prothrombin, and factor XII. Digestion of fibrinogen and other clotting factors prevents clot formation while fibrinolysis is in progress. Vascular repair begins under the stimulus of locally released platelet-derived growth factor (PDGF), which is released locally from platelet granules. Fibrin polymers are then slowly lysed. Plasmin is derived from its precursor, plasminogen. Plasminogen is activated by various substances, including factor XIIa, thrombin, tissue plasminogen activators released from injured endothelium, and urokinase, which is released by the renal glomerular endothelial and tubular cells. Plasmin remains bound to fibrin and splits it into fragments, called fibrin split products or fibrin degradation products (Fig. 51–5). The lysis of blood clots allows slow clearing of clotted blood in the tissues and reopens blood flow, including that through tiny peripheral vessels.

INTEGRATED REACTIONS AMONG HEMOSTATIC COMPONENTS

Because blood flow and hemostasis play key roles in the effectiveness of the inflammatory response to infection, tissue injury, and malignancy, several elements of the coagulation process also influence the inflammatory response. Hageman factor (XII), which triggers the intrinsic coagulation pathway, activates the precursor prekallikrein to kallikrein. Kallikrein, in turn, acts on plasmakinogens, converting them to kinin. Bradykinin is an example of a kinin that promotes dilation of blood vessels, increased vascular permeability, and smooth muscle contraction and causes the release of prostaglandins from tissue; all these functions facilitate the movement of neutrophils and macrophages to the source of injury or infection. Plasmin is another example of a clotting factor that affects the inflammatory process. Plasmin produces an interaction between the fibrinolysis and complement systems. The complement system is a series of 22 proteins that work together with antibodies that regulate the immune and allergic response.

REFERENCES

1. Jandl, JH: Blood: Pathophysiology. Blackwell Scientific Publications, Boston, 1991.
2. DiJulio, J: Hematopoiesis: An overview. In Baird SB (ed): New perspectives on the management of myelosuppression. Oncology Nursing Forum 18 (Suppl): 2, 1991.
3. Harmening, DM: The red blood cell: Structure and function. In Harmening, DM (ed): Clinical Hematology and Fundamentals of Hemostasis. FA Davis, Philadelphia, 1992, p 12.
4. Reich, PR, Kadin, ME, and Weller, PF: Leukocytes. In Robinson, SH and Reich, PR (eds): Hematology, Pathologic Basis for Clinical Practice. Little, Brown, Boston, 1993, pp 229–263.
5. Shoemaker, DL Hematopoiesis and the Impact of Cancer Therapy. Triclinica Communications Inc., New York, 1992.
6. Newcombe, D: Monocytes and macrophages. In Spivak, J and Eichner, ER (eds): The Fundamentals of Clinical Hematology. Johns Hopkins University Press, Baltimore, 1993, p 141.
7. Bell, A: Hematopoiesis: Morphology of human blood and marrow cells. In Harmening, DM (ed): Clinical Hematology and Fundamentals of Hemostasis. FA Davis, Philadelphia, 1992, p 21.
8. Bauer, KA: Hemotasis and Thrombosis, In Robinson, SH and Reich, PR (eds): Hematology, Pathologic Basis for Clinical Practice. Little, Brown, Boston, 1993, pp 391–441.

C H A P T E R 5 2

Assessment of Hematologic and Hemostatic Function

Jan Foster

CHAPTER OUTLINE

Clinical History
- ☐ Functional Health Patterns
- ☐ Medical History
- ☐ Family History

Physical Examination
- ☐ Integument
- ☐ Eyes
- ☐ Ears
- ☐ Mouth and Pharynx
- ☐ Head and Neck
- ☐ Systems

Laboratory Tests/Studies of Hematologic and Hemostatic Function
- ☐ Laboratory Tests of Hematopoietic Activity
- ☐ Laboratory Tests of Hematologic Function
- ☐ Laboratory Tests of Hemostasis

LEARNING OBJECTIVES

After completing this chapter, you should be able to:

1. Describe cardinal signs and symptoms of hematologic and hemostatic dysfunction.
2. Explain the clinical significance of ''shift to the left.''
3. Describe the manifestations of a bleeding disorder.
4. Describe the impact of hematologic and hemostatic dysfunction on a person's functional health patterns.
5. Discuss the significance of a thorough drug history in patients suspected of having a hematologic or hemostatic disorder.
6. Identify familial disorders of significance in hematologic and hemostatic dysfunction.
7. Outline key findings in the physical examination of patients with, or suspected of having, a hematologic or hemostatic disorder.
8. List tests of hematologic function and the normal ranges.
9. List tests of hemostatic function and the normal ranges.
10. Relate abnormalities in tests of hematologic and hemostatic function to the overall clinical presentation of the patient/family.

Disorders of hematologic function (i.e., the function of blood and blood-forming tissues) can be extremely complex. Hematologic problems frequently occur as a result of a disease of another organ system or as a consequence of treatment of another disease (e.g., chemotherapy).

Valid assessments are crucial to formulating nursing diagnoses, assisting with medical diagnoses, assessing response to treatment, and facilitating early recognition of complications. Symptoms reflective of hematologic dysfunction can be subtle, easily overlooked, or even misleading. As the healthcare provider who interacts most intimately with patient and family, the nurse must establish baseline assessment data, for-

mulate nursing diagnoses, and plan care accordingly. Ongoing assessment is necessary for evaluation of patient response to nursing and medical care. The diagnostic assessment and evaluation of hematologic function require a thorough history and physical examination of the patient and a variety of laboratory tests.

CLINICAL HISTORY

The clinical history affords the patient and family the opportunity to verbalize their problems and concerns about why they have chosen to seek healthcare assistance (subjective data); it also enables the nurse to observe closely for any overt or covert clues that may be helpful in diagnosing and planning care (objective data). The sequence and detail of the assessment process will vary according to the nurse's judgment about the patient's status. The extent and comprehensiveness of the initial interview and examination should be modified accordingly. Common hematologic diseases with which the patient may have been previously diagnosed that are pertinent to the clinical history include anemia, leukemia, lymphoma, myeloma, and other malignancies; and any bleeding disorder.

Functional Health Patterns

Patients who are experiencing alterations in hematologic and hemostatic function may present with changes in their functional health patterns. Assessment of these patterns is essential to nursing diagnosis, treatment, patient/family education, and discharge planning.

Health Perception and Health Maintenance. The nurse should ascertain the patient's perception of his or her overall health status. What levels of health and quality of life are desired, and how motivated are the patient and family to achieve them? What are their expectations of health care and healthcare providers? Decisions regarding health care rest with the patient and family, who must be well informed to make such decisions. Nurses support the patient and family through the crisis situation and plan for return to the community and resumption of role functions. The goal is to return to and maintain wellness and to adjust to changes in role, function, body image, and other areas when faced with chronic illness.

What is the patient's health status in general; are there other organ diseases with which he has to cope? Have family members observed changes in the patient's behavior or personality? Unexplained irritability, inability to concentrate, apathy, and depression often accompany hematologic disorders. What is the patient's occupation? Depression of bone marrow hematopoiesis is associated with exposure to toxic chemicals, radiation, and drugs.

Nutrition and Metabolic Status. Deficiencies in dietary intake over a period of time may place the patient at risk for developing hematologic dysfunction. Altered hematopoiesis may result from depleted iron stores or from vitamin B_{12} and folate deficiencies. Excessive alcohol consumption suppresses the appetite and predisposes to avitaminosis (vitamin deficiency), which may lead to various types of anemias. Alcohol may also impair platelet function, leading to coagulation defects and bleeding. The patient may present with a recent, unexplained weight loss, recurrent infection, or poor wound healing, all of which may occur in the presence of a hematologic disorder (e.g., erythrocyte deficiency or leukopenia).

Hemostasis is altered in the presence of vitamin K deficiency. Vitamin K deficiency may be associated with inadequate intake; ingestion of warfarin, a drug that blocks the action of vitamin K synthesis of clotting factors in the liver; or aggressive use of intravenous antibiotics, which obliterate the gastrointestinal bacterial flora essential to vitamin K synthesis and absorption. The end result is altered hemostasis as vitamin K–dependent coagulation factors (II, VII, IX, and X) become deficient.

Recent onset of anorexia, nausea, vomiting, food intolerance, or dysphagia may predispose to malnutrition and, in turn, compromise hematologic function.

Elimination. Recent changes in bowel habits (e.g., diarrhea or constipation) or in the characteristics of the stool (e.g., black or tarry) may contribute to a hematologic dysfunction, as in the case of anemia. Changes in bowel habits also may reflect an underlying hematologic dysfunction, as in the case of leukemia. Gastrointestinal bleeding may indicate a coagulation disorder. Severe diarrhea predisposes to malabsorption of essential nutrients. Malabsorption syndromes interfere with vitamin K absorption, predisposing to altered hemostasis. Hematuria may be an initial clue to the presence of a bleeding problem. Chronic renal failure may predispose to anemia, because erythropoietin, normally secreted by the kidneys and necessary for erythrocyte production in the bone marrow, is produced in insufficient quantities in this condition.

Activity and Exercise. Weakness, exercise intolerance, and inability to carry out activities of daily living commonly accompany hematologic dysfunction. Anemia, which causes a decrease in oxygen delivery to the tissues, may be a major contributing factor. Dyspnea on exertion may reflect an underlying anemia, or it may be associated with a thromboembolic disorder caused by altered hemostasis. It is important to establish the patient's usual exercise and rest patterns so that realistic goals for improvement may be set.

Coping with Stress. It is important to identify the psychosocial circumstances surrounding the occurrence of illness. How do the present circumstances differ from the usual lifestyle pattern? What changes in role function have been made in response to illness? Is the patient the family caretaker? Breadwinner? Decision maker? Stressors need to be identified.

It may be important to have the patient/family examine past coping strategies. Has a similar problem or illness been experienced previously? Under what circumstances? How was it handled? What can the patient/family do for themselves? What health- or illness–related education needs do they have? What community support systems are available? What changes in lifestyle are anticipated as a consequence of the illness? Malignant hematologic neoplasms, such as leukemia, multiple myeloma, and lymphoma, can have far-reaching effects on overall family dynamics and resources. The acuity and chronicity of such illnesses, many characterized by remissions and exacerbations, places a tremendous burden on family resources: physical, emotional, psychological, and financial. Bleeding and clotting disorders (e.g., hemophilias and von Willebrand disease) can similarly stress family resources. Patients who require blood replacement therapy have the additional risk of developing hepatitis and acquired immunodeficiency syndrome (AIDS).

Medical History

Pertinent medical history includes reports of any chronic or long-standing illness, recent acute illness, major trauma, and major surgery. Such pathophysiologic insults can predispose to hematopoietic disorders and hemostatic dysfunction. Disseminated intravascular coagulation (DIC), for example, an acute disorder of hemostasis, is a serious complication associated with a variety of pathophysiologic insults (see Chapter 53). Among others, these include shock states (e.g., anaphylactic, septic, hemorrhagic, or cardiogenic shock), crushing-type injuries, burns, major surgery, and childbirth. Tissue injury and/or disruption of the vascular system (i.e., the blood and blood vessels) place the patient at risk of developing such coagulopathy.

Major abdominal surgery (e.g., aortic aneurysm); cardiothoracic surgery (e.g., prosthetic heart valve replacement) and associated extracorporeal circulation; and splenectomy are examples of surgical procedures associated with hemostatic complications. The spleen, as part of the mononuclear phagocyte system, functions in the clearance of activated coagulation factors from the blood. Removal of the spleen alters this process, predisposing to higher concentrations of activated factors in the blood.

Certain types of gastrointestinal surgery, such as duodenal excision or total gastrectomy, predispose to hematologic disorders. Because iron absorption occurs largely within the duodenum, removal of the duodenum disrupts iron absorption and depletes iron stores, predisposing to anemia. A total gastrectomy results in loss of gastric parietal cells, which function to synthesize intrinsic factor, necessary for vitamin B_{12} absorption from the small intestine (ileum). Pernicious anemia results from vitamin B_{12} deficiency.

Replacement transfusions can suppress erythropoiesis and alter vitamin B_{12}, folate, and iron levels. Because such therapy can interfere with the interpretation of diagnostic tests, it is essential to elicit a history of recent blood transfusions.

Two of the functions of the liver are to synthesize many of the clotting factors and to clear activated factors from the blood. The presence of liver disease is significant to the hematopoietic history.

The patient's immunologic history should be ascertained. A history of immunodeficiency disease (e.g., AIDS), incompatible blood transfusion, bone marrow transplant, and transplant rejection may provide valuable clues to the patient's current status. Hematologic and immunologic functions are closely interrelated, and both affect overall body function.

Family History

Genetic factors are especially influential in certain hematologic disorders. Among these are a variety of hereditary hemolytic anemias, which are classified by whether the underlying defect is *intra*corpuscular (e.g., in the red blood cells [RBCs]) or extracorpuscular. Intracorpuscular defects include defects in the RBC membrane (e.g., hereditary spherocytosis), defects in enzymes (e.g., glucose-6-phosphate dehydrogenase), hemoglobinopathies (e.g., sickle cell anemia and methemoglobinemia), and thalassemia syndromes.

The following four extracorpuscular defects are major causes of hemolytic anemias.

1. Immune hemolytic anemias include alloimmune hemolytic anemia, wherein the individual develops antibodies upon stimulation by a foreign antigen, such as in a transfusion reaction, and autoimmune hemolytic anemia, wherein the ability for self-recognition of the individual's own RBCs is lost and the autoantibodies that are formed, in turn, destroy the individual's own RBCs.

2. Nonimmune hemolytic anemias include infection-induced anemia that occurs in malaria and aplastic anemia induced by certain chemicals (benzene), toxins, or physical agents.

3. Microangiopathic hemolytic anemias comprise anemias that result from fragmentation, shearing, or rupture of RBCs as they circulate; turbulent blood flow; or flow through blood vessels that are damaged or partially occluded by fibrin strands. Examples of microangiopathic anemias include thrombotic thrombocytopenia purpura, hemolytic uremic syndrome, DIC, malignant hypertension, and disseminated hematogenous carcinoma. Hemolytic anemias of this nature are known collectively as "red blood cell fragmentation syndromes."

4. Hypersplenism, which prolongs the transit time of RBCs through an enlarged spleen, results in decreased RBC survival and pooling within the spleen.

Anemias are associated with other diseases, such as infection, chronic renal disease (i.e., a decrease in erythropoietin), liver and endocrine disorders, and connective tissue disorders (e.g., rheumatoid arthritis and systemic lupus erythematosus), and with many types of malignancies.

Inquiry should be made about white blood cell (WBC) disorders during the patient/family interview. Certain types of leukemia are linked with chromosomal abnormalities. Lipid (lysosomal) storage diseases are largely inherited disorders. Gaucher's disease is caused by a genetic deficiency of an enzyme necessary for lipid degradation in macrophages; accumulation of lipids results in bone marrow encroachment by oversized macrophages and splenomegaly.

Hereditary disorders of platelet function include Bernard-Soulier syndrome and Glanzmann's thrombasthenia. Bernard-Soulier (giant platelet) syndrome is a rare disorder marked by very large platelets, mild thrombocytopenia, and defective platelet adhesion. Glanzmann's thrombasthenia is a rare genetic disorder characterized by severe mucous membrane and postoperative bleeding, prolonged bleeding time, absent clot retraction, and failure of platelets to aggregate in response to all physiologic agonists.

Von Willebrand disease is an inherited condition in which all elements of the factor VIII complex are decreased. Clinically, this disorder manifests as a mixed coagulopathy–qualitative platelet defect that results in abnormal bleeding. Hemophilia A, a hereditary disorder marked by a defect in factor VIII, is perhaps the most widely known of the bleeding disorders.

Other family history queries that pertain to hematologic disorders include the presence of jaundice, which is frequently associated with increased RBC hemolysis, and polycythemia vera, which is an excess of RBCs in peripheral blood.

PHYSICAL EXAMINATION

Components of the physical examination in assessing hematologic and hemostatic function include inspection, palpation, percussion, and auscultation. Meticulous techniques are required because physical findings of hematologic disorders can be very subtle, nonspecific, and easily overlooked. The presenting scenario often provides clues to the underlying problem and directs the physical exam.

Integument

Changes in skin coloration occur frequently in hematologic and hemostatic dysfunction. Pallor of skin, nailbeds, mucous membranes, and conjunctiva, may reflect an underlying anemia. Jaundice of the skin and sclera often reflects excessive RBC destruction with a consequent increase in serum bilirubin. Erythema or reddish discoloration is seen in fever; it may reflect an underlying polycythemia (excess in RBCs). Cyanotic, cold, mottled skin may reflect impaired tissue perfusion associated with coagulopathy that occurs, for example, in DIC.

Skin manifestations of bleeding problems commonly include purpura, petechiae, and ecchymoses. Gingival and mucosal bleeding and oozing from intravenous and intra-arterial puncture sites are highly indicative of bleeding disorders. Strict surveillance of all invasive tubes and lines (e.g., central lines; nasogastric, endotracheal, and tracheostomy tubes; and Foley catheter) is essential.

Eyes

The eyes should be examined for scleral icterus (jaundice), edema, and hemorrhage, and for retinal hemorrhages. Sunken orbits may reflect a dehydrated state. Periorbital edema may indicate renal failure.

Ears

The ears should be examined for evidence of bleeding from the external auditory canal; a bluish-colored tympanic membrane suggests the presence of blood in the middle ear.

Mouth and Pharynx

The mouth, tongue, and mucous membranes may be the most obvious indicators of an underlying hematologic disorder. Pallor, redness, and bleeding may indicate hematologic dysfunction. The lips and mucous membranes should be examined for cracks and fissures, herpetic lesions ("fever blisters" or "cold sores"), firm white plaques, ulcerations, and masses. White plaques often indicate candidiasis, a fungal infection; herpes and candidiasis are often associated with immunosuppression and neutropenia.

Head and Neck

Superficial lymph nodes should be assessed for lymphadenopathy. The location, size, texture, mobility, tenderness, and pain should be noted, because lymph nodes frequently reflect underlying pathophysiology. They may enlarge in acute infections. Changes in lymph nodes are evident in lymphoma, and often accompany leukemias and metastatic cancers. Changes include firmness or hardness on palpation, immobility, and irregular shape; unilateral changes may signify acute infection. Lymph nodes larger than 1 cm are often related to malignancy and warrant prompt medical attention.

Systems

Respiratory System

The respiratory rate, rhythm, and pattern should be assessed, noting tachypnea, dyspnea, orthopnea, and other signs. Dyspnea may be associated with an underlying anemia, with pulmonary embolus related to a thromboembolic disorder, or with a pulmonary infection. Hemoptysis should be noted, because it may indicate pulmonary hemorrhage. Symmetry of chest expansion, diaphragmatic excursion, and use of accessory muscles should be documented.

The lungs should be auscultated for normal and adventitious breath sounds. Patients with compromised hematologic function are at increased risk for pleural effusions, pulmonary hemorrhage and embolus, and pulmonary infections.

Cardiovascular System

The heart rate and rhythm and the quality of peripheral pulses should be assessed. Tachycardia is a common finding in anemias because the cardiac workload is increased to meet the oxygen demands of the cells. Peripheral pulses may feel full and bounding when associated with a high cardiac output; weak, thready pulses may indicate bleeding and volume depletion. The patient should be assessed for postural hypotension. Baseline hemodynamic parameters should be established and frequently monitored. Heart sounds should be auscultated for extra sounds, murmurs, and pericardial friction rub.

Gastrointestinal System

The abdomen should be inspected for skin texture, lesions, scars, discoloration, bruises, and distention. Bowel sounds should be auscultated in all four quadrants. If distention is present, the abdominal girth should be measured at regular intervals at the level indicated on the skin with a marking pencil. Abdominal distention may indicate the presence of ascites, usually associated with liver disease or malignancy; either may precipitate hematologic dysfunction. Abdominal distention also accompanies bowel obstruction secondary to infarction, which is associated with coagulopathy and vascular occlusion.

The abdomen should be percussed and palpated for masses, pulsations, hepatosplenomegaly, and tenderness. Splenomegaly is associated with a variety of hemolytic anemias and other hematologic disorders; the liver, as part of the mononuclear phagocyte system, may also become enlarged in hematologic disorders. The liver is also the site of bilirubin metabolism, and elevated bilirubin levels may reflect increased RBC hemolysis or altered liver function. The liver may be the source of altered hemostatic function because it is responsible for both the synthesis of most clotting factors and for the clearance and metabolism of activated factors from circulating blood. The stool should be examined for the presence of occult blood resulting from gastrointestinal bleeding, which may indicate a coagulation disorder.

Genitourinary System

Hematuria and back and flank pain may appear as presenting signs and symptoms of hematologic disorders; they may occur in the course of a hematologic or hemostatic problem, or they may result as a side effect of chemotherapy and radiotherapy for cancer. Oliguria may suggest renal failure. Menorrhagia (i.e., excessive menstrual bleeding) may be an indication of compromised hemostasis.

Musculoskeletal System

Bones and joints should be assessed for swelling, tenderness, pain, and range of motion. Hemarthrosis (i.e., bloody effusion into joints) can cause excruciating pain and is associated with hematologic disorders such as hemophilia, sickle cell anemia, and leukemia.

Nervous System

Changes in mental status, behavior, and neurologic function may signal increased intracranial pressure from intracranial bleeding, which is always a risk for patients with coagulopathy. Often the changes are subtle and recognized by family members more easily than by the healthcare practitioner. Patients may complain of headache or feelings of lightheadedness. They may experience visual disturbances from retinal hemorrhages, aphasia (absence or impaired speech), and paresthesias (numbness, tingling, altered proprioception, and vibratory sense).

Changes in the patient's mental status (memory loss, altered mood or affect) and level of consciousness may become apparent. The patient may become restless, irritable, lethargic, or comatose. Motor coordination may become impaired, and deep tendon reflexes may become hyperreflexic.

Vital signs and cranial nerve function should be monitored in patients with suspected intracranial hemorrhage. Neurologic findings may reflect intracranial bleeding or increased intracranial pressure caused by bleeding.

Immune System

Assessment of immunologic function includes inspection and palpation of lymph nodes, and examination for signs of infection, including fever, inflamed areas, and drainage. Patients who are neutropenic may have none of the usual signs of infection (e.g., swelling, redness, and pus) because they lack sufficient leukocytes to elicit the inflammatory response. Laboratory values assist the practitioner in assessment of immune function (see section that follows).

LABORATORY TESTS/STUDIES OF HEMATOLOGIC AND HEMOSTATIC FUNCTION

The laboratory assessment of hematologic function includes an examination of the cellular elements of blood: elevations and reductions, inadequate function, and abnormal ratios give clues to the patient's disease.

Laboratory Tests of Hematopoietic Activity

Hematopoiesis, the production and development of blood cells, occurs largely in the bone marrow. Hematopoietic activity can be evaluated by examining bone marrow tissue obtained by aspiration or biopsy. Cells normally present in bone marrow include granulocytes and erythrocytes in all stages of development and megakaryocytes, which give rise to platelets. Bone marrow examination is diagnostic for leukemias, multiple myeloma, lymphoma, and aplastic anemia. Before bone marrow can be removed, appropriate explanations should be made to the patient and family, and a consent form must be signed. Meticulous aseptic technique is necessary to avoid infection and potential septicemia. After the biopsy needle is withdrawn, application of firm pressure to the site, followed by a pressure dressing, is necessary to prevent bleeding.

Laboratory Tests of Hematologic Function

Complete Blood Count

Laboratory tests of hematologic function include an examination of whole blood for a complete blood count with differential and peripheral smear. The complete blood count (CBC) includes the RBC and WBC counts. The usual range for these and other tests are included in Appendix E. Specific blood tests are described here separately.

Red Blood Cells

RBC Count. Red blood cell count reflects the total number of circulating red blood cells per cubic millimeter of blood. In response to an increased need for oxygen, as in high altitudes, and with increased physical training, a physiologic increase in RBCs occurs.

Hemoglobin. The hemoglobin (Hb) laboratory test measures the hemoglobin attached to the RBC. This gives an indication of the oxygen-carrying capacity of the blood. It reflects the total amount of hemoglobin in peripheral blood.

Hematocrit. The hematocrit (Hct) laboratory test reflects the proportion of whole blood contributed by RBCs. Changes in plasma volume are reflected by changes in both the Hb and Hct. Overhydration produces a hemodilutional effect and decreases these parameters; dehydration causes these parameters to be fictitiously high.

RBC Indices

Mean Corpuscular Volume (MCV). This index reflects the relative size of the RBCs. An increase in the MCV reflects abnormally large RBCs (macrocytic), whereas a decrease in the MCV reflects microcytic or abnormally small RBCs, seen commonly in iron-deficiency anemia or thalassemias.

Mean Corpuscular Hemoglobin (MCH). This index reflects the average amount of hemoglobin in RBCs, calculated by dividing the hemoglobin concentration of whole blood by the number of RBCs present.

Mean Corpuscular Hemoglobin Concentration (MCHC). This index reflects the average concentration of hemoglobin in a single RBC and is derived by dividing the hemoglobin by the hematocrit.

Peripheral Smear. The peripheral smear test allows for a more exact evaluation of RBC size, shape, and composition. It is especially useful in diagnosing anemias.

Reticulocyte Count. Reticulocyte count reflects the number of immature RBCs circulating in the blood and provides a measure of bone marrow function. The number increases in response to acute hemorrhage.

Erythrocyte Sedimentation Rate (ESR). Erythrocyte sedimentation rate (ESR) reflects the composition and rate of "settling to the bottom" of red blood cells in plasma. It is a nonspecific test for disease, and merely indicates that an inflammatory response is in progress. A rise in the ESR accompanies most inflammatory disease, whether localized or systemic, acute or chronic. The ESR is helpful in monitoring response to therapy for chronic conditions, such as rheumatoid arthritis and tuberculosis.

White Blood Cells. White blood cells are distinguished from circulating RBCs by the presence of a nucleus. Fully mature circulating WBCs include granulocytes, lymphocytes, and monocytes.

WBC Count. WBC count reflects the total number of WBCs, or leukocytes, in circulating blood.

WBC Differential. WBC differential reflects the percentage of each type of WBC. These include neutrophils (polymorphonuclear cells, PMNs), eosinophils, basophils, lymphocytes, and monocytes. The absolute count of each specific type of WBC is important for differential diagnosis. An elevated neutrophil count is associated with infection. An increase in band neutrophils, immature neutrophils, is associated with acute bacterial infection.

The eosinophil count may be elevated in allergic reactions, parasitic infections, eczema, leukemia, and some autoimmune diseases. A decrease in eosinophils is associated with corticosteroid therapy.

The lymphocyte level may increase in some bacterial and viral infections, infectious mononucleosis, lymphocytic leukemia, and multiple myeloma. A decrease in lymphocytes occurs in immunodeficiency diseases (e.g., AIDS), sepsis, chemotherapy, radiotherapy, and certain leukemias.

Other Tests

Total Iron Binding Capacity Tests. The total iron binding capacity (TIBC) reflects a direct, quantitative measurement of transferrin, the globulin that binds iron and transports it in the blood. Reduced levels of iron and TIBC are frequently associated with iron-deficiency anemias.

Vitamin B_{12} Test. Vitamin B_{12} is necessary for RBC production. A low value may result from inadequate dietary intake, such as in vegetarianism. It may also be due to lack of absorption related to deficiency of intrinsic factor, which is secreted in gastric juices. People who have had a partial or complete gastrectomy require periodic injections of vitamin B_{12}.

Coombs' Tests. These tests differentiate types of hemolytic anemias and detect immune antibodies.

The direct Coombs' test measures antibodies (IgG) attached to RBCs. The indirect Coombs' test measures antibodies (IgG) in the serum. Both tests are read as normally negative.

Laboratory Tests of Hemostasis

Tests of Platelet Activity

Bleeding Time. A prolonged bleeding time is the single best indication of platelet function and is seen in thrombocytopenia of any etiology.

Platelet Count. The platelet count is the least accurate approach to assessing platelet function. In general, the bleeding time becomes prolonged when the platelet count falls below $100,000/mm^3$. Bleeding time is prolonged by aspirin therapy, because aspirin interferes with platelet aggregation.

Clot Retraction. Clot retraction reflects the process wherein platelets contract and serum is expressed from the clot, leaving only RBCs enmeshed in the fibrin mass. Platelet contraction is fundamentally necessary for the process of clot retraction. Patients with thrombocytopenia or abnormally functioning platelets will demonstrate altered clot retraction. Patients with polycythemia also demonstrate altered clot retraction.

Aggregation. Aggregation is a measure of platelet response to adenosine diphosphate (ADP), epinephrine, collagen, prostaglandin, thromboxane A_2, and serotonin. The release of these substances attracts more platelets to the site and plugs the vessel.

Platelet Factor 3. An unstable platelet plug causes exposure of platelet factor 3 on the platelet surface membrane, which attracts circulating clotting factors from the blood. Activation of the clotting factors continues the coagulation process and a more stable clot is formed. This laboratory test measures the time it takes for a measurable quantity of platelets to aggregate.

Coagulation Tests

Prothrombin Time. Prothrombin time (PT) is one of the most useful and commonly used tests to assess coagulation. PT evaluates the function of the extrinsic coagulation pathway (see Fig. 51–4). A firm fibrin clot normally forms in 11 to 13 seconds of injury. A PT exceeding 13 seconds represents excessive time needed for clot formation and may indicate a decrease in levels of fibrinogen or factors X, V, VII, and II.

Partial Thromboplastin Time. Partial thromboplastin time (PTT) evaluates the function of the intrinsic coagulation pathway. The normal range for clot formation is about 25 to 37 seconds. Factors XII, XI, and VIII must all be present at adequate levels to have a normal PTT. The presence of factors X and V, prothrombin, and fibrinogen is also reflected by normal PTT. This test does not reflect factor VII because that factor bypasses the extrinsic coagulation pathway.

Thrombin Clotting Time. Thrombin clotting time (TCT) reflects the conversion of fibrinogen to fibrin, the final phase of coagulation. TCT is prolonged in the presence of reduced levels of fibrinogen (<100 mg/100 mL) or if the fibrinogen is functionally abnormal.

Plasma Fibrinogen Levels. This test evaluates the level of fibrinogen in blood plasma. Elevation indicates that excessive clotting is in progress.

Fibrin Degradation Products. Fibrin degradation products (FDPs), sometimes referred to as fibrin split products (FSPs), result from products of fibrin cleavage or breakdown. Normally, when fibrin undergoes fibrinolysis, low levels of degradation products enter the circulation and are cleared by the liver. In the presence of excessive fibrinolysis, FDPs can be so elevated that blood flow becomes sludgy, and serious hemostatic complications can result. The FDPs interfere with the conversion of fibrinogen to fibrin and further compromise clotting by interfering with the formation of the hemostatic platelet plug. The presence of FDPs also reflects the activity of the fibrinolysis system, specifically the activity of plasmin, the principal fibrin-degrading factor. Levels of FDPs are elevated in DIC.

Euglobulin Clot Lysis Time. Results of this test reflect the presence of excessive fibrinolytic activity, thus providing a measure of the activity of the fibrinolytic system. Euglobulins are proteins found in the plasma and include fibrinogen, plasminogen, and plasminogen factor. Addition of thrombin to a euglobulin solution converts fibrinogen to fibrin and activates plasminogen. The time measured from clot formation to clot lysis is referred to as the euglobulin clot lysis time.

D-Dimer. D-dimers are fragments released in excess during extensive lysis of fibrin. They are specific markers for DIC, usually elevated to about 10 times normal levels in this condition.

Coagulation Factor Concentration Tests. These tests measure the concentration of specific clotting factors, including factors XI, IX, X, VIII, VII, and II (prothrombin).

CHAPTER 53

Nursing Management of the Patient with Disseminated Intravascular Coagulation

Susan D. Ruppert

CHAPTER OUTLINE

Disseminated Intravascular
   Coagulation: Defined
   □ DIC: Pathophysiology
   □ Etiologic Factors in DIC
Clinical Presentation
Diagnosis
   □ Laboratory Data: Interpretation and
   Analysis

Treatment and Management
   □ Nursing Care of the Patient with
   DIC
References
Suggested Readings

LEARNING OBJECTIVES

After completing this chapter, you should be able to:

1. Explain the pathophysiologic changes that occur in DIC.
2. Identify patients at risk of developing DIC.
3. Describe the clinical presentation of DIC.
4. Interpret common laboratory data reflective of the diagnosis of DIC.
5. Describe approaches to medical treatment and management of DIC.
6. Delineate the nursing process in the care of the patient with DIC, including the following: assessment, diagnosis, planning, and evaluation (desired patient outcomes and nursing interventions/rationales).

DISSEMINATED INTRAVASCULAR COAGULATION: DEFINED

Disseminated intravascular coagulation (DIC) is a pathophysiologic process caused by the presence of excess thrombin in the *systemic* circulation. Unlike normal clotting, which occurs as a *localized* reaction to vascular injury, the clotting of DIC occurs throughout the circulatory system and is characterized by widespread coagulation followed by excessive, diffuse fibrinolysis in an effort to bring about clot dissolution. DIC occurs *secondary* to an underlying pathologic process that initiates coagulation by either the intrinsic or extrinsic pathway.

Thrombin is the key factor triggering events. The action of this proteolytic enzyme results in the formation of fibrin, consumption of specific plasma proteins, irreversible platelet aggregation with a consequent depletion of platelets, and activation of fibrinolysis. The combination of these effects predis-

poses to the clinical manifestations of DIC, which include diffuse hemorrhage and fibrin thrombus formation. Bleeding is ultimately the major underlying clinical problem—not clotting. Therein lies the paradox, because it all begins as excessive clotting. Its onset may be insidious or rapid; its symptoms may be mild or severe. It may produce mild, occult bleeding, or widespread hemorrhage.

DIC: Pathophysiology

DIC is triggered by the presence of some unusual agent or substance in the bloodstream that initiates the clotting cascade (see Fig. 51–3, Fig. 51–4, and Table 51–2). The clotting mechanism can be initiated by the following:

1. Direct stimulation of the intrinsic pathway by injury to the endothelial cells
2. Stimulation of the extrinsic pathway by the

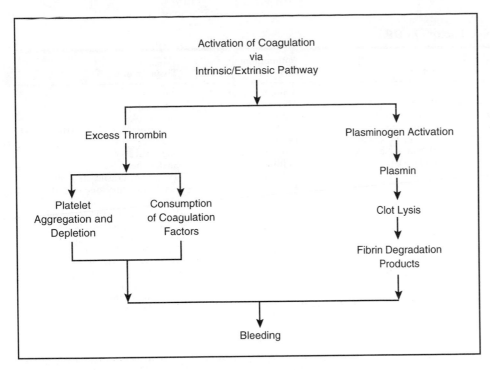

Activation of Coagulation
via
Intrinsic/Extrinsic Pathway

Excess Thrombin

Platelet Aggregation and Depletion

Consumption of Coagulation Factors

Plasminogen Activation

Plasmin

Clot Lysis

Fibrin Degradation Products

Bleeding

FIGURE 53–1. Pathophysiology of disseminated intravascular coagulation.

release of thromboplastin (i.e., tissue factor) into the circulation by procoagulants, such as bacterial toxins, cancer, tissue fragments, free hemoglobin, placental tissue fragments, hypoxia, and acidosis
3. Stasis or pooling of blood
4. Defective clearing of the activated clotting factors by the reticuloendothelial system
5. Defective fibrinolysis

Regardless of the initiating mechanism for clotting, the end result is the activation of thrombin. The excess thrombin, in turn, activates fibrinogen, causing fibrin to be deposited in the microcirculation. Platelet aggregation or adhesiveness is increased, thereby enabling fibrin clots to form. As the clots continue to form, red blood cells (RBCs) are trapped in the fibrin strands and destroyed. The resultant sluggish circulation of blood reduces the flow of nutrients and oxygen to the cells. This leads to tissue ischemia, injury, and necrosis, if untreated.

Concurrent with these events is the overuse of platelets, prothrombin, fibrinogen, and other clotting factors. As these factors are used up, a deficiency of these factors ensues, compromising coagulation and predisposing to bleeding. The excessive clotting at the microcirculatory level activates the fibrinolytic system, causing production of fibrin degradation products (FDP; i.e., fibrin split products). FDP has an anticoagulant effect with fibrinogen for thrombin, interfering with the formation of the stable fibrin clot and impairing platelet function, thereby perpetuating systemic bleeding.

To summarize, DIC is a condition characterized by a depletion of clotting factors, particularly fibrinogen

and factors V and VIII; the presence of FDP released by the activity of the fibrinolytic system; diffuse hemorrhage or bleeding; and fibrin thrombus formation with diffuse microthrombi causing ischemia, injury, and possible multiorgan dysfunction (Fig. 53–1).

Etiologic Factors in DIC

Etiologic factors can be examined according to the manner in which clotting is initiated (Table 53–1). Conditions that cause activation of the *intrinsic* coagulating pathway include hemolytic processes, such as transfusion of mismatched blood, or acute hemolysis from infection or immunologic disorders; endothelial tissue damage from extensive burns and trauma, transplant rejections, heat stroke, or surgery, particularly when extracorporeal circulation is used, because this results in destruction of RBCs; fat emboli, because this provides a source of lipid necessary to initiate clotting; circulatory crisis (e.g., shock state or septicemia); and acute pancreatitis. Conditions that cause the *extrinsic* coagulation pathway to become activated include obstetric and gynecologic conditions, such as abruptio placentae, amniotic fluid embolism, retained dead fetus, and septic abortion; neoplastic processes, such as prostatic cancer, acute leukemias, giant hemangiomas, and bronchogenic carcinoma; and chemotherapy.

Conditions in which the activating mechanism is not known include acute bacterial and viral infections (the effect of endotoxins may be to disrupt the endothelium); glomerulonephritis, purpura fulminans (large

TABLE 53-1
Common Predisposing Etiologic Factors in DIC

Obstetric Conditions	Cancer	Sepsis	Autoimmune Reactions	Tissue Injuries
Abortions	Leukemias	Viral	Acute pancreatitis	Burns
Abruptio placentae	Lymphomas	Bacterial, especially gram negative	Allograft rejection	Head injury
Amniotic fluid emboli	Solid tumors	Meningococcemia	Anaphylaxis	Heat stroke
Eclampsia	Metastasis	Mycotic histoplasmosis	Drug reaction or hypersensitivity	Hypovolemic or hemorrhagic shock
Placenta previa		Mycotic aspergillosis	Immune complex disease	Major surgery
Retained placental tissue		Rickettsial	Mismatched or massive transfusions	Snake bites
Stillbirths		Herpes		Trauma or crush syndrome
				Acute renal disease
				ARDS
				Vascular aneurysms, especially dissecting aortic aneurysms
				Liver disease
				Hypo/hyperthermia
				Prolonged cardiopulmonary bypass
				Giant hemangioma
				Acute hemolysis
				Pulmonary emboli

foci of skin necrosis), thrombotic thrombocytopenic purpura, cirrhosis, defects in the reticuloendothelial system, pulmonary embolism, adult respiratory distress syndrome (ARDS), and shock states.

Although there are many predisposing or etiologic factors, a common denominator occurring among patients with DIC is some type of circulatory crisis. Arterial hypotension, with its consequent systemic vasoconstriction and capillary dilatation, leads to stagnation of blood in the microvasculature. Such compromised circulation leads to hypoxemia and acidemia, because tissues, experiencing a reduction in the supply of oxygen and nutrients, must turn to anaerobic metabolism with a consequent increase in lactic acid production. Hypoxemia and acidemia, as procoagulants (i.e., precursors) initiate the onset of the clotting mechanism at the cellular level.

Etiologic factors of DIC share another common denominator—they all act by triggering mechanisms that eventually liberate free thrombin into the systemic circulation and subsequently lead to blood clotting.

Nurses must be aware of the patient's underlying condition and be able to identify patients at risk of developing DIC. Patients need to be assessed constantly for signs of its development, and appropriate measures must be implemented to prevent or control it.

Major areas of concern for nursing care include observing for pulmonary emboli, ARDS, renal failure, and gastrointestinal necrosis. Unrestrained clotting may predispose to neurologic deficits associated with cerebral emboli. The possibility of hemorrhage throughout the body is great, especially along the gastrointestinal tract and at the site of any open wounds, incisions, or abrasions. Patients need to be assessed for signs of decreased cardiac output, which may be

related to arrhythmias and myocardial infarction. These clinical phenomena may occur secondary to either clotting or hemorrhage.

CLINICAL PRESENTATION

Major signs and symptoms of DIC include bleeding, as reflected by the presence of purpura, petechiae, and ecchymoses; gastrointestinal bleeding (including hematemesis, melena, or tarry stools); genitourinary bleeding (e.g., hematuria, menorrhagia in women); wound bleeding, bleeding and oozing from puncture sites and around invasive catheters and lines; hematoma formation, pulmonary hemorrhage, purpura fulminans (i.e., large foci of skin necrosis resulting from tissue injury and necrosis associated with compromised circulation); and acrocyanosis (i.e., cyanosis of hands and feet associated with vasomotor and circulatory disturbances).

In addition to bleeding, the syndrome of acute multiorgan dysfunction may occur. This syndrome is characterized by hypotension, oliguria, dyspnea, confusion, convulsions, coma, abdominal pain, diarrhea, and other gastrointestinal symptoms.

The onset of symptoms may be slow or sudden. Through astute listening and observational skills, the nurse can assess the patient for changes early in the course of DIC. Table 53–2 lists subjective and objective symptoms of DIC. Usually the subjective signs are so vague that they may be overlooked by the patient, nurse, and other healthcare providers.

The nurse should be aware of early signs of impaired tissue perfusion. These include subtle mental changes, such as restlessness, confusion, and inappropriate behavior. Early physical signs include hypotension, especially orthostatic hypotension, dyspnea,

TABLE 53-2
Signs and Symptoms of DIC

Subjective	Objective
Angina	Anxiety/irritability
Dyspnea	Confusion
Fatigue	Convulsions
Headache	Coma
Malaise	Orthostatic hypotension
Nausea and vomiting	Pale yellow skin or sclera
Palpitations	Bleeding at venipuncture sites
Severe pain in the abdomen,	and surgical incisions
back, muscles, joints, and	Cutaneous petechiae,
bones	ecchymosis, hematomas
Sudden vision changes	Epistaxis
Vertigo	Hematuria
Weakness	Hemoptysis
	Peripheral thromboemboli
	Acrocyanosis
	Increasing abdominal girth
	Scleral or conjunctival
	hemorrhages
	Hyper/hypothermia

tachypnea, syncope, and decreased urinary output. The possibility of DIC may be overlooked because these signs are nonspecific alone. But in the presence of bleeding, whether overt or occult, they become substantiating data.

Overt bleeding may be reflected by oozing of blood from mucous membranes, needle puncture sites, or incisions. Hemorrhagic bullae, hematomas, ecchymosis, or petechiae may be observed. Occult bleeding can be suspected or documented by the presence of positive guaiac stools or emesis, abdominal distention, or hematuria. Jaundice of the skin and sclera, hemorrhages of the conjunctiva, air hunger, orthopnea, tachypnea, headache, and altered sensorium may all be reflective of an underlying bleeding problem.

DIAGNOSIS

Astute assessment and diagnosis of DIC requires (1) identifying the patient at risk of developing DIC, (2) implementing astute assessment skills and observation to detect subtle changes that may forewarn of the presence of DIC, and (3) interpreting and evaluating clinical and laboratory data to detect DIC and to follow its course and the patient's response to therapy.

The clinical history for a patient at risk of developing DIC should include any history of bleeding tendencies; coagulation disorders; intake of medications that may alter the coagulation mechanism (e.g., anticoagulants, aspirin, nonsteroidal anti-inflammatory drugs, or steroids); liver abnormalities; recent infections; bruising tendencies; hematuria; and menorrhagia. Also important is the history of any recent insult to the circulatory system, such as shock or vascular injury.

Laboratory Data: Interpretation and Analysis

Numerous bleeding disorders mimic DIC. Diagnosis may be difficult because bleeding is not always obvious. In general, when a patient has a disease known to be capable of eliciting or predisposing to DIC, DIC is probably present if bleeding appears suddenly.

Indications for specific laboratory tests include (1) bleeding in a patient with no history of bleeding; (2) the presence of acrocyanosis and generalized diaphoresis, with cold, mottled fingers and toes and petechiae or purpura; and (3) the patient who seems to be "going sour" for no obvious reason.

There is no one diagnostic test for DIC. Diagnosis requires a clinical suspicion elicited by thorough history, physical examination, and laboratory studies. The major screening tests for DIC include platelet count, prothrombin time and partial thromboplastin time, and fibrinogen level. Confirmatory tests include the concentration of fibrin degradation/split products (FDP/FSP), thrombin time, D-dimer, and antithrombin III (AT III).

A cardinal diagnostic finding in most patients with DIC is a significant decrease in the platelet count. Other findings include a decrease in fibrinogen levels, an increase in FDP/FSP and D-dimer, and a decrease in AT III. The D-dimer is more specific for DIC than FDP.[1] However, since the D-dimer is less sensitive, diagnosis of DIC should be made based on D-dimer and FDP results together. Diagnosis of DIC is frequently difficult if multiple transfusions have been given, because they may dilute clotting factors and platelets. Diagnosis may also be difficult in the presence of liver disease because the disease process causes a decrease in the synthesis of clotting factors, with a reduction in the clearance of activated clotting factors. Thrombocytopenia and activation of the fibrinolytic system may further complicate the clinical picture. See Table 53-3 for the common laboratory tests and findings in DIC.

TREATMENT AND MANAGEMENT

Successful treatment and management of patients with a disorder of the hemostatic mechanism depend on an accurate diagnosis and correction of the primary disorder. Other therapeutic approaches include (1) the use of heparin to inhibit the effects of thrombin, (2) replacement of deficient clotting factors, and (3) correction of other processes that may hinder the clotting mechanism, such as administration of vitamin K and folate.

The use of heparin in the treatment of DIC is controversial. While the drug does not have any effect on formed clots, it is thought to inhibit the formation of new clots, thereby slowing down the consumption of clotting factors. Heparin exerts its action through the molecule AT III, which inactivates thrombin. The

TABLE 53–3
Common Laboratory Findings in DIC

Test	Normal Values*	Values in DIC
Platelets	150,000–350,000 μL	<150,000 μL
Fibrinogen	200–400 mg/dL	<200 mg/dL
D-dimer	<0.5 μ/mL or <250 mg/mL	Increased
Prothrombin time (PT)	10–14 sec	Increased
Partial thromboplastin time (PTT)	30–45 sec	Increased
Activated partial thromboplastin time (aPTT)	16–25 sec	Increased
Thrombin time	10–15 sec ± 5 sec	Increased
Fibrin degradation products (FDP)	4 μg/mL	Increased
Antithrombin III (AT III)	18–40 mg/100 mL	<18 mg/100 mL
Euglobin lysis time factors assay	>2 h	<2 h
VIII	55%–145%	Low
XII	50%–150%	Low with sepsis
X	45%–155%	Low
VII and IX	60%–140%	Decreased
Paracoagulation tests:		
Fi test	Negative	Positive
Protamine sulfate test	Negative	Strongly positive

*Normal laboratory ranges may vary among institutions because of the technique used. Always check your facility's laboratory manual if in doubt.
Source: Fischbach, FT: A Manual of Laboratory Diagnostic Tests, ed 4. JB Lippincott, Philadelphia, 1992, and Swearingen, P and Keen, J: Manual of Critical Care: Applying Nursing Diagnoses to Adult Critical Illness, ed 3. Mosby, St. Louis, 1995.

drug causes increased amounts of thrombin to be *ad*sorbed by fibrin, which decreases the amount of thrombin available to convert fibrinogen to fibrin.

Heparin is thought to inhibit the action of thrombin on fibrinogen, thereby preventing conversion of fibrinogen to fibrin. It may prevent the formation of prothrombin activator by the intrinsic pathway. Specifically, it prevents the reaction between activated factor XI and factor IX, which is catalyzed by thrombin.

Heparin is most effective when given early in the course of DIC. The preferred route is by continuous intravenous drip, although it can be given in intermittent intravenous doses or subcutaneously. Heparin is frequently given in therapeutic doses, but the dose should be adjusted according to the patient's status, especially with the presence of both renal and hepatic impairment where the half-life of heparin is prolonged. Heparin is continued until the underlying cause of DIC has been corrected and the clinical and laboratory findings demonstrate a reversal of the abnormalities.

Blood products replacement therapy is also still controversial. When used, it should be given after heparin therapy has been initiated, otherwise the replacement components are consumed rapidly in the DIC process. Platelets and fresh frozen plasma may be given for severe depletion of platelets and coagulation factors. Cryoprecipitate is given for depletion of factors VIII and XIII, fibrinogen, and AT III.

Packed RBCs may be given to replace lost blood volume. A treatment still under investigation is the AT III concentrate. The purpose of this treatment is to replenish depleted stores of antithrombin. Although fibrinolytic inhibitors have no general value in the treatment of DIC, epsilon aminocaproic acid (Amicar) is sometimes used. Amicar slows bleeding by preventing lysis of microthrombi and stabilizing clots. Since this agent impedes clearance of microthrombi, Amicar should be given concurrently with heparin to prevent complications from acute thromboembolism.[2]

Effectiveness of treatment and management is monitored by serial fibrinogen levels and platelet counts. An increase in either parameter signals that clotting and depletion of clotting factors are normalizing.

Nursing Care of the Patient with DIC

Therapeutic Goals

Major goals of nursing care include detection of occult bleeding, prevention of further bleeding, correct measurement/estimate of blood loss, and support of the patient/family.

Nursing Diagnoses, Desired Patient Outcomes, and Nursing Interventions

Nursing diagnoses, desired patient outcomes, and nursing interventions/rationales in the care of the patient with DIC are presented in the care plan at the end of this chapter.

REFERENCES

1. Fischbach, FT: A Manual of Laboratory Diagnostic Tests, ed 4. JB Lippincott, Philadelphia, 1992.

2. Marder, VJ: Consumptive thrombohemorrhagic disorders. In Williams, WJ, Beutler, E, Erslev, AJ, and Lichtman, MA (eds): Hematology, ed 4. McGraw-Hill, New York, 1990.

SUGGESTED READINGS

Bell, T: Coagulation and disseminated intravascular coagulation. In Huddleston, V (ed): Multisystem Organ Failure: Pathophysiology and Clinical Implications. Mosby, St. Louis, 1992.

Bell, T: Disseminated intravascular coagulation and shock: Multisystem crisis in the critically ill. Crit Care Nurs Clin North Am 2(2):255–268, 1990.

Epstein, C and Bakanauskas, A: Clinical management of DIC: Early nursing interventions. Crit Care Nurse 11(10):42–53, 1991.

Griffin, JP: Hematology and Immunology: Concepts for Nursing. Appleton-Century-Crofts, Norwalk, CT, 1986.

Preston, FE: Plasma D-dimer levels and their relationship to serum fibrinogen/fibrin degradation products in hypercoagulable states. Br J Haematol 71:65–70, 1989.

Young, L: The insidious killer. Crit Care Nurse 10(9):26–33, 1990.

CARE PLAN FOR THE PATIENT WITH DISSEMINATED INTRAVASCULAR COAGULATION

Nursing Diagnoses

Nursing Diagnosis #1
Tissue Perfusion, alteration in: decreased cerebral, peripheral, pulmonary, renal, gastrointestinal, related to:
1. Intravascular coagulation with thrombosis in the microcirculation
2. Hypotension

Desired Patient Outcomes

Patient will:
1. Be alert and oriented to person, place, and date
2. Have peripheral pulses that are strong proximally and distally; skin normal pink in color, warm and dry to touch
3. Have urine output ≥30 mL/h
4. Have negative findings for occult blood in body secretions and drainage

Patient will:
1. Maintain respiratory rate <30 inspirations/min
2. Maintain adequate ventilation, as gauged by the work of breathing and arterial blood gases:
   - $PaO_2 > 60$ mmHg (room air)
   - $PaCO_2 \sim 35\text{--}45$ mmHg
   - pH 7.35–7.45
3. Maintain breath sounds clear to auscultation

Nursing Interventions

- Assess neurologic status.
  - General cerebral functions: mental status; level of consciousness; monitor for confusion, lethargy, obtundation, coma, seizures, behavioral changes, headache, dizziness.
  - Cranial nerve function:

    - Assess pupillary reaction to light and accommodation; drooping upper eyelid.
    - Assess for drooping lower eyelid and facial drooping.
    - Ability of patient to talk; presence of protective reflexes: cough, gag.
  - Sensorimotor function: assess movement and strength of all extremities.
    - Assess for the presence of paresthesias, numbness, tingling.
  - Monitor skin color and temperature of arms and legs. Monitor for signs of thromboemboli: Homans' sign.
- Assess pulmonary function.

  - Respiratory rate and breathing pattern.
  - Breath sounds.
  - Adventitious sounds: rales, rhonchi, stridor.
  - Chest pain: pleuritic causes.
  - Sputum production; hemoptysis.
  - Monitor arterial blood gases.

Rationales

- Ongoing assessment of neurologic status is essential because of risk of possible cerebral emboli/thrombi, intracranial bleeding, cerebral anoxia related to cerebral edema, hypoxemia.

  - Alterations in cranial nerve function reflect brainstem involvement.
    - Signals oculomotor nerve involvement.

    - Signals facial nerve involvement.
    - Reflect function of cranial nerves IX, X. Airway must be protected, especially in the compromised patient.
  - Peripheral thrombosis compromises systemic circulation.
    - Deep retroperitoneal bleed may cause pressure on lumbar nerve roots.
  - Presence of acrocyanosis reflects microthrombi within peripheral vasculature.
- Onset of respiratory distress suggests intravascular clotting and/or bleeding into pulmonary tissues.
  - Tachypnea, orthopnea, tachycardia reflect effort to maintain tissue oxygenation.

  - Hemoptysis suggests possible pulmonary emboli.
  - Altered pulmonary vascular dynamics predisposes to pulmonary shunting with compromised gas exchange and consequent hypoxemia.

CARE PLAN FOR THE PATIENT WITH DISSEMINATED INTRAVASCULAR COAGULATION
Continued)

Nursing Interventions

- Assess renal status.
  - Hydration: intake and output; urine specific gravity; body weight.
  - Hematuria.

  - Monitor renal function studies: BUN and creatinine.

Rationales

- Urine output less than 30 mL/h suggests dehydration, hypovolemic state, or possible microemboli within the kidneys.
  - Oliguria may be associated with renal insufficiency or acute tubular necrosis.
  - Massive fluid resuscitation may be necessary to maintain intravascular volume.
  - Altered renal function results in increases in BUN and creatinine.

Nursing Diagnoses

Nursing Diagnosis #2
Fluid volume deficit, related to bleeding/hemorrhaging

Desired Patient Outcomes

Patient will:
1. Be without signs of rebleeding:
   - Without hematemesis, melena
   - Without hematuria
   - Without oozing around invasive lines and wounds
2. Maintain balanced intake and output
   - Skin turgor elastic; warm to touch
3. Maintain stable laboratory parameters:
   - RBC and WBC counts within acceptable levels
   - Hb: 12–18 g/100 mL
   - Hct: 37–54%
   - BUN, creatinine, electrolytes, calcium, and glucose all within acceptable levels
4. Maintain normovolemia
   - Body weight within 5% of baseline
5. Achieve resolution of impaired coagulation
6. Achieve resolution of underlying cause
Patient will:
1. Remain without signs of intra-abdominal bleeding:
   - Without abdominal distention and pain
   - Stable abdominal girth
   - Without nausea and vomiting
   - Negative for occult blood in nasogastric drainage, emesis, stools
   - Bowel sounds appropriate
   - Vital signs stable

Nursing Interventions

- Initiate activities to detect the presence of occult bleeding.
  - Assess skin and mucosal membranes for pallor, cyanosis, jaundice, petechiae; observe sclera and conjunctiva; inspect for gingival bleeding, epistaxis, ecchymoses, purpura
  - Determine overall status: presence of fatigue, weakness, malaise.
    - Myalgia, hemarthrosis (i.e., bloody effusion into joint cavity).
    - Presence of visual disturbances.

  - Measurement of blood loss: all body fluids and secretions: stool (especially if diarrheal), hematochezia (i.e., stool containing red blood); urine; emesis, nasogastric drainage; sputum and/or hemoptysis; diaphoresis, wound drainage, drains.
    - Bandages and lines should be weighed and counted.
    - Sequential measurement of extremity circumference as well as abdominal girth.
    - Observe arterial and venipuncture sites for oozing of frank blood.
    - Hematest for occult blood: nasogastric secretions, stools, emesis.

Rationales

  - Acrocyanosis reflects microemboli in peripheral circulation; presence of jaundice suggests extensive hemolysis associated with underlying coagulopathy.

    - Bleeding into joint cavities may underlie joint/bone pain.
    - Retinal hemorrhages may underlie vision disturbances.
  - Multiorgan system involvement in some patients with DIC requires a delicate balance between hypovolemic shock on the one hand and overhydration from overly aggressive fluid/blood replacement therapy on the other. The key to therapy is accurate measure of all fluid and blood losses.
    - Persistent oozing or increase in bloody drainage may indicate a developing/increasing coagulopathy.

CARE PLAN FOR THE PATIENT WITH DISSEMINATED INTRAVASCULAR COAGULATION
(*Continued*)

Nursing Interventions

- ○ Monitor laboratory parameters: Hb and Hct.

- Administer prescribed fluid/blood replacement therapy.

  - ○ Administer lactated Ringer's/saline solutions, albumin, and other plasma expanders.

  - ○ Blood/blood products replacement therapy.
    - □ Packed RBCs, platelets, and fresh frozen plasma may be given for severe depletion of platelets and coagulation factors.
    - □ Cryoprecipitate is given for depletion of factor VIII and fibrinogen.
- Assess gastrointestinal function.
  - ○ Assess for signs of distention and increasing abdominal girth; abdominal cramps or pain; nausea/vomiting.
  - ○ Assess bowel sounds.
- Presence of paralytic ileus.

Rationales

- ○ These parameters are chief indicators of bleeding; however, the patient's hydration status must be considered when evaluating these values; blood administration may also alter these values.
- ○ Early identification of bleeding enables timely initiation of therapy to minimize and/or prevent bleeding.
- Adequate tissue perfusion requires an adequate intravascular blood volume.
- ○ Massive fluid resuscitation is frequently necessary to maintain intravascular volume at levels to maintain optimal cardiac output and blood pressure to meet the oxygen and nutrient needs of body tissues.
- ○ Blood replacement therapy remains controversial. When used, it should be initiated after heparin therapy has been administered, to prevent rapid consumption of blood products through the underlying disease process.

- ○ Bleeding into peritoneal cavity should be suspected in the presence of increasing abdominal girth.

- ○ Presence of microthromboemboli within splanchnic circulation may underlie mesenteric ischemia and/or necrosis.

Nursing Diagnoses

Nursing Diagnosis #3
Altered Protection, related to:
1. Decreased clotting factors
2. Increased anticoagulant effects of FDP

Nursing Interventions

- Initiate actions to prevent further bleeding.
  - ○ Gentleness is the rule of thumb when caring for the patient with DIC. Use an electric razor only.
  - ○ Gentle tooth brushing; cleansing of mouth with cotton or soft sponge.
  - ○ Skin protection through gentle handling; special attention to skin and mucous membranes, especially around catheters, endotracheal tubes, and other invasive lines and catheters. Avoid adhesive tape.
  - ○ Use pressure dressings over invasive line sites.
  - ○ Use only soft, loose restraints if needed; assess circulation frequently.
  - ○ Orotracheal suctioning should be performed only when absolutely essential, and with meticulous aseptic technique.
  - ○ Blood pressure cuffs should be used as infrequently as possible. Loosen cuff when not in use and inspect skin under cuff.

  - ○ Administer prescribed medications and monitor response: Oral medications should be given whenever possible; parenteral medications should be administered using the smallest-gauge needle and applying pressure to the puncture site for 5 to 10 min.
  - ○ Stool softeners should be given as prescribed.
  - ○ Avoid rectal temperatures.

Desired Patient Outcomes

Patient will:
1. Maintain intact skin and mucous membranes
2. Be without evidence of frank or occult bleeding

Rationales

- ○ Gentle care minimizes injury to fragile tissues, which may predispose to further bleeding.
- ○ Use of mild saline solution, bicarbonate, and peroxide as a rinse are recommended instead of a mouthwash; if a mouthwash is used, use alcohol-free mouthwash and dilute it 1:1. Avoid drying lemon swabs.

- ○ Careful and timely suctioning minimizes injury to mucosal lining, reducing the risk of bleeding and infection.
- ○ To avoid rupture of superficial capillaries with further bleeding. While an arterial line is invasive, it may be preferred to monitor vital signs and to obtain blood samples.

- ○ Help to prevent constipation with straining at stool.
- ○ May irritate friable tissues, resulting in bleeding.

CARE PLAN FOR THE PATIENT WITH DISSEMINATED INTRAVASCULAR COAGULATION
(*Continued*)

Nursing Interventions	Rationales

○ Heparin therapy via continuous infusion pump or intermittently (via minidose protocol).	○ Controversy regarding use of heparin in treatment of DIC.
	  □ Heparin is most effective when given early in the course of DIC.
	  □ Preferred route of administration is continuous intravenous drip. Doses are adjusted according to patient's overall status.
	  □ Heparin therapy is usually continued until clinical and laboratory data indicate patient's condition is stabilizing.

□ Vasopressors (e.g., dopamine).	□ Vasopressors may be indicated if blood pressure does not stabilize with full hydration.
• Monitor hematopoietic function. ○ Assess the following: bleeding—estimate loss; presence of petechiae, ecchymoses, purpura, hematomas—note size and location. ○ Monitor Hb, Hct, coagulation studies, especially platelets, prothrombin time, partial thromboplastin time, fibrin degradation products, D-dimer and bleeding time. ○ Monitor for exacerbation of bleeding.	• Changes in laboratory values are indicative of the patient's status and response to therapy; they afford the capability of following trends in the patient's condition that enable timely and appropriate therapy to be instituted. ○ Exacerbation of bleeding in patients receiving heparin therapy longer than 8 days may be indicative of antiplatelet antibody formation.
• Initiate precautionary/supportive therapy. ○ Teach patient to cough, sneeze, and blow nose gently. ○ Avoid sudden Valsalva's maneuver. ○ Avoid use of suppositories. ○ Avoid use of aspirin and steroids.	 ○ Reduces risk of dislodging clots and causing rebleeding. ○ May irritate friable rectal tissues, resulting in bleeding. ○ These drugs compromise hematologic and immunologic functions, leading to potential bleeding and infection.

• Institute precautionary measures:
 ○ Maintain proper body alignment.
 ○ Provide gentle passive range of motion.
 ○ Use extra assistance when moving patient; use draw sheet to *lift* patient.
 	
 ○ Use therapeutic beds; turn every 1 to 2 h
 ○ Keep skin well lubricated.
 	
    □ Provide meticulous skin and wound care.
    □ Be gentle with patients. Discourage scratching and removing scabs; keep nails trimmed.
	• Goal is to protect the patient from further trauma; minor injury/stress may potentiate bleeding.
	
	 ○ This avoids dragging the patient, as for example, when moving the patient up in bed; such action could cause skin abrasions and other trauma, increasing potential for bleeding.
	 ○ To avoid prolonged pressure areas
	 ○ To avoid dryness and cracking, which can predispose to skin breakdown and infection.
	    □ To prevent infection.
	    □ To avoid trauma.

Nursing Diagnoses	Desired Patient Outcomes
Nursing Diagnoses #4 Coping, ineffective: Individual/family	Patient/family will: 1. Verbalize feelings regarding underlying disease and prognosis 2. Identify strengths and coping mechanisms 3. Make decisions of importance to the patient/family 4. Identify familial and community resources

Nursing Interventions	Rationales
• Assess patient/family's prior coping methods. ○ Identify family/community resources.	• Identifying past coping capabilities may assist patient/family in dealing with current illness; familiarity breeds self-confidence.

CARE PLAN FOR THE PATIENT WITH DISSEMINATED INTRAVASCULAR COAGULATION
(*Continued*)

Nursing Interventions	Rationales
• Evaluate patient/family's understanding of illness: anticipate needs; be accessible; make necessary explanations.	• Knowledge of underlying problem may be especially helpful in coping with a bleeding disorder. The sight of even a little blood can be frightening.
• Provide emotional and psychological support.	• Support is important in assisting family members during the crisis of critical illness.

PaO_2 = partial arterial oxygen pressure; $PaCO_2$ = partial arterial pressure of carbon dioxide; BUN = blood urea nitrogen; WBC = white blood cell; Hb = hemoglobin; Hct = hematocrit.

UNIT TEN

Trauma, Emergencies, and Multisystem Disorders

UNIT OUTLINE

C H A P T E R   5 4

Nursing Management of the Patient with Thoracic, Abdominal, and Orthopedic Trauma

Karen Sue Hoyt and Peggy Hollingsworth-Fridlund

CHAPTER OUTLINE

LEARNING OBJECTIVES

After completing this chapter, you should be able to:

1. Identify patterns of trauma associated with thoracic, abdominal, and long bone trauma.
2. Describe the pathogenesis and pathophysiologic changes underlying trauma to the chest, abdomen, and long bones.
3. Describe the initial assessment considerations in patients with trauma of the chest, abdomen, and long bones.
4. Discuss therapeutic modalities indicated in specific types of trauma, including chest, abdominal, and long bone trauma.
5. Discuss why treatment is provided simultaneously with the diagnostic process in the management of the trauma victim.
6. Discuss implications for nursing management based on the nursing process: assessment, diagnoses, and planning (desired patient outcomes and nursing interventions/rationales).

INTRODUCTION TO TRAUMA SYSTEMS

Current Statistics

Traumatic injury has been termed the "neglected disease of modern society" and is viewed as the epidemic of the 1990s. Traumatic injury accounts for over 140,000 deaths per year in the United States, and one person in three suffers a nonfatal injury. Additionally, for every death, another two persons are permanently disabled. Trauma is the leading cause of death for individuals up to 44 years of age. It is the fourth overall cause of death for all individuals, exceeded only by cardiovascular disease, cancer, and stroke. Trauma affects predominantly young individuals, with its peak incidence in the 15- to 24-year-old age group. It is the leading killer of children. Research has shown that the injured die in three distinct time frames. The majority of patients die either at the accident scene or in the first several hours after injury. The third peak of deaths occurs days to weeks later when the patients succumb to sepsis or multiorgan failure. A knowledgeable critical care nurse functions as part of the trauma team in its efforts to decrease death and morbidity during this period.

Regionalization of Systems Approach

Regionalization of trauma care results in designated specialty centers working in concert with emergency medical services focusing upon the injured victims. The implementation of prehospital systems and trauma centers has been shown to decrease the mortality and morbidity related to accidental injury. A goal of trauma systems is to limit the number of facilities involved in the care of major trauma victims and to direct critically injured individuals to designated trauma centers. Institutions are designated as trauma centers if they consistently have the resources available to provide the services necessary to meet the special needs of victims of trauma. Trauma center designation may occur as a result of local, county, state, or federal processes.

Blunt Versus Penetrating Trauma

Trauma is an injury resulting from external forces. Injury occurs when energy is transferred to body tissues. The etiology may involve blunt or penetrating forces, with blunt trauma occurring more frequently. The most common causes of blunt trauma are motor vehicle crashes, falls, assaults, and sporting accidents. Penetrating trauma results largely from gunshot injuries and stabbings.

Triage/Initial Resuscitation Phase

The patient who sustains major trauma presents a special challenge to the healthcare team. Patients are identified as having sustained significant trauma by a process known as triage. Assessment of vital signs, identification of obvious wounds, and evaluation of the patient's mechanism of injury are all determinants of whether the patient may have major injuries. This process of triage occurs at the scene of the injury and also at the hospital admission area. During the initial assessment of the trauma patient, a systematic approach is used to identify the patient's status. Imme-

diate life-saving interventions are concerned with the ABCs (airway, breathing, and circulation) of trauma care. A patent airway is established and maintained, and supportive ventilation and oxygenation are provided. Cervical spine immobilization should be ensured at this time. Fluid volume replacement therapy is initiated to maintain effective cardiac output and tissue perfusion to vital organs. Once advanced life support is under way, a comprehensive assessment is performed simultaneously as diagnostic procedures and stabilization occur. At this time, decisions are made about the course of therapy, whether conservative medical management or surgical intervention should be undertaken. In some cases because of the need for rapid surgical therapy, not all of the patient's injuries will have been identified. The critical care nurse receiving the patient after resuscitation or operation must perform careful, thorough physical assessment serially and maintain skeletal or spinal immobilization as indicated.

Critical Care Phase

Even after the patient's initial condition has been stabilized, the critical care nurse must be especially vigilant for injuries not evident on the initial examinations. A knowledge of predictable patterns of trauma will assist the nurse to anticipate the occult injuries. Patterns of trauma as related to individual mechanisms of injury have been identified to assist the trauma team to anticipate specific injuries (Table 54–1). The details of the accident and knowledge of patterns of trauma help the trauma team accurately assess and plan the care for the trauma patient during the initial phase. An ongoing assessment of airway, breathing, and circulatory status must continue, and findings are documented accurately. Many patients are admitted to the critical care unit with additional diagnoses yet to be diagnosed. Particular attention must be directed toward assessing the patient's condition relative to these rule-out diagnoses. Therefore, frequent and accurate documentation is an essential element of patient care because it provides a most reliable method to communicate trends in the patient's condition and the response to therapies and to ascertain occult injuries.

Pathophysiology: Hypovolemic Shock

Patients with trauma to the torso, pelvis, or extremities frequently present in hypovolemic shock from hemorrhage. Shock is a profound alteration in tissue perfusion that results in a cellular oxygen demand that exceeds the supply. Without timely intervention, the shock state may become irreversible, leading to cellular or tissue death.

In response to the shock state, various bodily compensatory mechanisms are activated in an effort to

TABLE 54–1*
Patterns of Injury

Mechanism of Injury	Force	Associated Injury
1. Automobile Occupant		
a. Frontal impact		
1) Down and under pathway	Forward movement, knees strike dash; energy transferred along axis of femur	Patellar fracture; ligamentous injury; midshaft femur fracture; posterior dislocated hip
	If feet are braced on floor with legs trapped below dash	Femur fracture; ligamentous injury of knee—occult; ankle fracture
2) Up and over pathway	Body movement and energy transfer is up and over dash; head strikes windshield	Maxillofacial trauma (Le Fort fractures—with high-speed impact)
	Neck may be compressed, hyperextended or flexed;	Cervical spine injuries
	chest hits steering wheel or dash	Rib/sternal fractures; myocardial contusion; aortic tear; pneumothorax
b. Rear impact	Body pushed forward, excluding head	Cervical strain of anterior ligaments
c. Lateral impact	Impact by car door; moves body out from under head	Cervical strain of lateral ligaments
	Side chest impact	Rib fractures; pulmonary contusion; fractured humerus
	Femur head driven through acetabulum	Genitourinary system trauma; pelvic fracture
d. Rollovers and combination rotational impacts	Multiple forces	Constellation of injuries
2. Pedestrian	Victim turns sideways to avoid impact	Fractured femur, tibia, and fibula
a. Extremity triad	Lateral impact applied by hood and/or bumper	Ligamentous knee injury to opposite side (often missed)
b. Waddell's triad	Car impacts femur and chest and/or torso	Fractured femur, blunt chest, and/or abdominal trauma
	Victim thrown to ground by impact	Head injury
3. Falls/jumpers	Victim jumps or falls from great height	Bilateral wrist (Colles') fractures
a. Don Juan syndrome (triad)	Victim lands on heels	Bilateral calcaneal fractures
	Twisting motion during fall	Thoracic—lumbosacral fractures (L-1 and L-2)

*See also Tables 33–3 and 33–4 for vertebral and spinal cord injuries.

maintain perfusion to the vital organs, including the heart, brain, and liver. For a time, this is done at the expense of blood flow to the splanchnic circulation, kidneys, lungs, and skin.

Compensatory Mechanisms

The body responds to a traumatic insult by initiation of various compensatory mechanisms, including the sympathetic response, baroreceptor activity, fluid shifts, activation of the renin-angiotensin-aldosterone system, and enhanced secretion of antidiuretic hormone (ADH).

Sympathetic Response. An initial generalized response to the loss of circulating volume is stimulation of the sympathetic nervous system. Epinephrine and norepinephrine when released into the blood initiate arterial and venous vasoconstriction. This, in turn, increases systematic vascular resistance with a consequent increase in arterial blood pressure. Additionally, increased levels of circulating epinephrine enhance glycogenolysis.

Baroreceptor Response. Baroreceptors, located in the carotid sinus and aortic arch, respond to changes in arterial blood pressure. As blood pressure decreases, these pressure receptors respond by generating impulses that include an increase in heart rate and myocardial contractility and enhanced vasocon-

striction of the systemic vasculature, thereby further increasing the systemic vascular resistance.

Fluid Shifts. Fluid makes up about 60% of body weight, or about 40 liters in the average adult. In a state of hypovolemic shock, the body compensates for a depleted intravascular volume (i.e., the blood volume) by shifting fluid from the interstitial space into the blood vessels. The fluid in the interstitial compartment acts as a buffer, allowing fluid to move into the intravascular space when blood volume is depleted.

Renin-Angiotensin-Aldosterone System. Renin is an enzyme that is activated in response to hypoperfusion and ischemia of the kidneys, as in hypovolemic shock. The consequent diminished pulse pressure triggers the conversion of renin to angiotensin by a series of enzymatic reactions. The renin-angiotensin mechanism helps to maintain effective cardiac output in the presence of shock. Once formed, angiotensin stimulates secretion of aldosterone by the adrenal cortex. This hormone acts on cells of the distal tubules to increase the reabsorption of sodium and, thus, water. In this way, aldosterone functions to increase the circulating blood volume and cardiac output.

Secretion of ADH. ADH, also called vasopressin, secreted from the posterior pituitary gland in response to an increase in serum osmolality, acts on the epithelial cells of the distal tubules and collecting tubules to increase the reabsorption of water. The increase in serum osmolality is reflective of a relative increase in solutes that accompanies the loss of plasma. Receptors in the right atrium, stimulated in response to a decreased venous return to the heart associated with the hypovolemic state, also contribute to an increased secretion of ADH. The consequent reabsorption of water functions to expand the intravascular volume. Additionally, ADH exerts a potent vasopressor effect on the systemic vasculature, thereby increasing blood pressure and enhancing tissue perfusion.

In general, fluid resuscitation for the trauma patient includes administering crystalloid solutions at a ratio of 3 mL for every 1 mL of blood lost, which aids in restoration of the interstitial fluid space. Blood replacement is usually at a 1:1 ratio. In this way, the blood volume, essential for tissue perfusion, is maintained.

THORACIC TRAUMA

Anatomy and Physiology

The thoracic cavity extends from above the clavicles to the level of the diaphragm. It contains the left and right pleural spaces and the mediastinum. The mediastinal cavity is located between the pleural spaces and houses the heart, aortic arch, and other great vessels, including the pulmonary arteries and the superior and inferior vena cava. Other structures included are the esophagus, trachea, thymus, and vagus nerves. The lungs are contained in the pleural cavities.

Pathogenesis

Chest injuries can result in a variety of insults to cardiopulmonary function. They can be divided into five general categories (Table 54–2):

TABLE 54–2
Categories of Cardiothoracic Injury

Classification	Specific Trauma
1. Bony thoracic structure disruption	Rib and sternal fractures Flail chest
2. Parenchymal tissue disruption	Myocardial contusion Pulmonary contusion
3. Cardiothoracic dynamic disruption	Cardiac tamponade Tension pneumothorax Massive hemothoraces Sucking chest wounds (open pneumothorax) Simple pneumothorax Hemothorax
4. Conducting (upper and lower) airway disruption	Tracheobronchial injuries
5. Accessory structure disruption	Aortic rupture and other great vessel disruption

1. Bony thoracic structure disruption
2. Parenchymal tissue disruption
3. Cardiothoracic dynamic disruption
4. Conducting (upper and lower) airway disruption
5. Accessory structure disruption

These include airway impairment, derangement of chest wall mechanics, changes in intrathoracic pressures, and compromised cardiac function. These derangements, in turn, can result in impaired gas exchange with hypoxemia, alterations in cardiac output and tissue perfusion, and a depleted intravascular volume. In 85% of all chest trauma cases, however, the patient can be managed with a simple procedure, such as the insertion of a chest tube. Only about 15% of all thoracic trauma victims require immediate surgical intervention. These are the patients who require rapid assessment and quick intervention if death or permanent sequelae are to be prevented.

Clinical Presentation

Physical assessment of the patient with chest trauma includes inspection, auscultation, palpation, and percussion of the chest. The nurse should note the rate, rhythm, and depth of respirations as a key assessment parameter. The critical care nurse should listen to lung sounds, noting the presence or absence of breath sounds bilaterally. Patients with rib fractures, for example, will not breathe deeply since they are in pain. The absence of breath sounds can indicate a pneumothorax, and dullness to percussion may mean the patient has a hemothorax. In patients with rib fractures, crepitus can be heard when the bony fragments rub together. Patients with flail chest can exhibit severe respiratory distress with paradoxical movement of the chest at the location of the flail segment.

Chest trauma patients may develop hypovolemic or cardiogenic shock from hemorrhage, hemothorax, pneumothorax, pericardial tamponade, or injury to vascular structures or contusion of the heart. Life-threatening clinical signs and symptoms may include tracheal deviation (to the opposite side) and jugular venous distention as in tension pneumothorax. The heart should also be auscultated for the presence of muffled heart tones since this clinical manifestation is indicative of cardiac tamponade. Beck's triad of signs of pericardial tamponade also includes decrease in blood pressure and elevated jugular pressure. In the absence of breathing, the patient will require rapid intubation, ventilation, and other advanced cardiac life support (ACLS) measures.

Typically, the initial signs and symptoms experienced by the chest trauma patient will reflect anxiety; pain with associated dyspnea and tachypnea; tachycardia and signs reflective of a hypovolemic state with reduced tissue perfusion, including a decreased pulse pressure with declining arterial pressure, delayed capillary refill, and decreased urinary output; pale, cool, clammy skin with poor turgor; and dry mucous membranes. Arterial blood gases may reflect hypoxemia

(Pa_{O_2} < 80 mmHg) and hypocapnia (Pa_{CO_2} < 35 mmHg) initially; followed by hypercapnia (Pa_{CO_2} > 45 mmHg), with a consequent acidemia (pH < 7.35). Depending on the extent of injury, only a few or all of the above signs and symptoms may be present.

Diagnostic Considerations

The diagnosis of chest injury is based on clinical history, including mechanisms of injury, precipitating events, and assessment of pulmonary and cardiovascular status. The patient's clinical presentation and acuity status will determine the appropriateness of diagnostic studies. Worsening signs and symptoms resulting from the trauma may develop over time. Table 54–3 lists normal and abnormal values for commonly prescribed laboratory studies of significance in the chest trauma patient. Radiographic studies of diagnostic importance are listed in Table 54–4. Upright chest x-rays can be performed only after clearance of the cervical, thoracic, and lumbar spines for injuries. Since the majority of chest x-rays are done on patients still on spinal precautions, it is important for the nurse to realize that even large hemothoraces may not be easily seen on the supine film. Serial electrocardiographic (ECG) studies may be helpful in patients with blunt chest trauma, particularly in patients who sustain steering wheel impact. Significant ECG findings, depending upon the degree of myocardial injury, may vary from the presence of ischemic changes to life-threatening ventricular arrhythmia.

Nursing Care of the Patient with Thoracic Trauma

Effective treatment of chest trauma requires ongoing efforts to diagnose and treat the underlying injury while maintaining optimal respiratory and cardiovascular function. Of immediate concern is the stabilization of a patent airway to afford adequate alveolar ventilation. Arterial blood gases are serially monitored to determine the adequacy of ventilation. If the patient develops hypoxemia (Pa_{O_2} < 60 mmHg on room air), initiation of positive end-expiratory pressure (PEEP) with mechanical ventilation may be indicated. Such therapy helps to ensure adequate alveolar ventilation, maximize ventilation/perfusion matching, and minimize shunting. (For an in-depth discussion of ventilation/perfusion ratio and pulmonary shunting, see the appropriate sections in Chapter 22.) The critical care nurse should be aware that in the under fluid–resuscitated patient, initiation of positive pressure ventilation or PEEP may compromise venous return, cardiac output, and blood pressure. Hemodynamic monitoring using a pulmonary artery catheter affords ongoing assessment of pressures on the left side of the heart and hydration status. (Hemodynamic monitoring is discussed in detail in Chapter 16).

Aggressive fluid resuscitation may be initiated as

TABLE 54–3
Laboratory Values Associated with Shock

Laboratory Value	Normal Laboratory Value	Laboratory Value in Shock*
1. Hematocrit	37%–45%	30%
2. Arterial blood lactate level	5–20 mg/dL	>20 mg/dL
3. Arterial Pa_{O_2} (room air)	100 mmHg	<70 mmHg
4. Arterial pH	7.35–7.45	<7.30
5. Arterial Pa_{CO_2}	35–45 mmHg	Variable
6. Urine output	30–50 mL/h	<30 mL/h
7. Urine specific gravity	1.010–1.020	>1.025
8. Serum osmolality	285–295 mOsm/kg water	>300–310 mOsm/kg water

*This is a simplistic representation of laboratory values in shock. It should be appreciated that laboratory values may differ with the specific type of shock and/or the stage of shock.

TABLE 54–4
Common Radiologic Procedures Performed in Chest Trauma

Radiologic Procedure	Injury Suspected	Diagnostic Findings
Supine/upright chest (posteroanterior and lateral)	Any abnormality	Fractured ribs, flail chest, pneumothorax, hemothorax.
Chest x-ray	Ruptured diaphragm	Free air below the diaphragm.
	Aortic disruption	Widened mediastinum; fractures of 1st or 2nd ribs; obliteration of aortic knob; presence of pleural cap; obliteration of space between pulmonary artery and aorta; tracheal deviation to the right depression of left mainstream bronchus; elevation and shift of left bronchus to the right.
Aortogram	Aortic arch and great vessel injury	Aortic disruption/tear can be confirmed.
Serial chest x-rays	Pulmonary contusion; atelectasis	"White out"; infiltrates.
	Missed or developing pneumothorax or hemothorax	Partial or total lung collapse or fluid seen in the pleural space.

early therapy for hemothorax, hemomediastinum, and tension pneumothorax. The use of autotransfusion (autologous blood transfusions) has been used effectively in salvaging blood from life-threatening traumatic hemothorax. Cardiac output measurements and the response to fluid therapy may be helpful in the differential diagnosis of the etiology of the shock state.

Life-Threatening Chest Injuries

Life-threatening forms of chest trauma requiring immediate intervention include tension pneumothorax, massive hemothoraces, and cardiac tamponade. Their signs and symptoms may be present not only during the initial resuscitation but also in the critical care phase.

Tension Pneumothorax/Pneumothorax. A pneumothorax can result from both blunt or penetrating chest trauma. Air enters the pleural cavity and is trapped in the pleural space, causing partial or total lung collapse. As air accumulates in the pleural cavity, the lung continues to collapse. This is known as a *one-way valve effect.* Typical findings are shortness of breath, tachypnea, and respiratory distress. With a pneumothorax, there may be loss of auscultated breath sounds on the affected side and hyperresonance with percussion attributed to the air in the pleural cavity; with a hemothorax, there will be dullness with percussion. Confirmation of the diagnosis is by chest x-ray, and treatment is tube thoracostomy. Pneumothoraces are treated with a chest tube to underwater drainage (see Figs. 26–2 and 26–4 for landmarks).

Tension pneumothorax occurs when the trapped intrapleural air causes a degree of increased pressure that shifts the mediastinal structures toward the unaffected side. These dynamics impair venous return and result in a falling cardiac output. Signs and symptoms include severe dyspnea, hypotension, loss of breath sounds on the affected side, displacement of heart sounds, and tracheal deviation to the side opposite the pneumothorax. Patients on ventilators demonstrate a rise in peak inspiratory pressures and decreased ventilatory compliance. Distended neck veins and elevated central venous pressures are usually present unless severe hypovolemia exists. Cyanosis is a late, ominous sign. Treatment consists of needle thoracentesis at the 2nd intercostal space of the anterior axillary line of the affected side, which can be done rapidly (see Fig. 24–2 for landmarks). This life-saving intervention will temporarily relieve the pressure in the pleural space as the trapped air is allowed to exit. An insertion of a chest tube follows the needle thoracentesis. (For nursing care consideration related to thoracentesis and chest drainage, see Tables 26–2 and 26–3, respectively.) Patients who have sustained even moderate chest trauma are at risk for developing tension pneumothorax if they are placed on mechanical ventilation before the insertion of a chest tube. Patients with rib fractures or a small pneumothorax should be carefully monitored after initiation of positive pressure ventilation.

Hemothorax/Massive Hemothorax. A hemothorax is caused by either a blunt or penetrating injury that lacerates the lungs, mediastinal structures, diaphragm, or blood vessels. Hemothoraces are life-threatening when large amounts of blood accumulate in the pleural cavity, causing hemorrhagic shock and lung collapse. The massive hemothorax can also simulate the signs and symptoms of a tension pneumothorax. Venous return is impaired if a mediastinal shift occurs. The chest cavity can accumulate up to 4 liters of blood. Most hemothoraces are effectively treated with chest tube drainage and complete reinflation of the lung. A patient who drains excessive amounts of blood through a chest tube may require surgical intervention. The patient should have frequent monitoring of drainage until the amount has decreased. Chest tube output of greater than 1500 mL drainage at initial insertion or 300 mL/h for several hours suggests continuing hemorrhage and the need for immediate surgery. Clinical manifestations are those consistent with shock, namely, hypotension, tachycardia, and pale, cool skin.

Treatment of massive hemothoraces consists of rapid intravenous volume infusion with crystalloid solutions and replacement blood products. Autotransfusion of the patient's own blood is an alternative to rapid blood replacement. Chest tube placement should occur *simultaneously* with initiation of fluid resuscitation.

Cardiac Tamponade. Hemopericardium, accumulation of blood in the pericardial sac, may occur after blunt trauma but most commonly results from penetrating injury to the heart (see Fig. 59–1). This accumulation can result in cardiac tamponade, which impairs ventricular filling and decreases cardiac output. Clinical presentation may be that of Beck's triad of symptoms, including increased central venous pressure, muffled heart sounds, and decreased blood pressure with pulsus paradoxus (see Chapter 13). If the patient is hypovolemic, these classic symptoms may be obscured since blood pressure may already be decreased. There should be a high index of suspicion in patients with a poor cardiac performance if the other diagnosed injuries are known to be minor. Life-saving intervention requires draining the accumulated blood by pericardiocentesis or performing a surgical opening of the pericardium known as a pericardial window. Pericardiocentesis is the aspiration of the blood from the pericardial space by percutaneous needle insertion. An emergency thoracotomy may be done if the patient suffers a cardiopulmonary arrest. The patient will be taken to surgery to correct the underlying cardiac defect.

Other Potential Life-Threatening Chest Injuries

Other potential life-threatening chest injuries include aortic rupture or disruption of the integrity of other great vessels, myocardial contusion, pulmonary contusion, flail chest, tracheobronchial injuries, and thoracoabdominal trauma.

Aortic Rupture. Aortic ruptures are usually associated with blunt trauma, and they are fatal in about 90% of all cases. The most common cause of aortic rupture is a motor vehicle accident with rapid deceleration (e.g., steering wheel impact), resulting in the application of shearing and stress forces to intrathoracic structures. The aortic adventitia, mediastinum, and pleura may limit total rupture, and a false aneurysm is formed. Physical findings in patients with aortic rupture include asymmetric peripheral pulses, with a higher pulse amplitude and blood pressure in the upper extremities than in the lower extremities. A pressure difference between the right and left arm may also occur. If patients are conscious, they may complain of chest pain; they usually appear anxious, restless, and agitated. Fracture of the first rib and the presence of a left hemothorax raise the index of suspicion. The classic findings on x-ray are a widened mediastinum and loss of the normal shadow of the aortic knob. Definitive diagnosis is made on aortogram and at the time of surgery.

Treatment requires an emergency thoracotomy to correct the underlying pathology. The aorta may be clamped or the patient placed on cardiopulmonary bypass. If surgery is delayed, the patient should be kept as calm and comfortable as possible. The patient's urinary output and vital signs should be carefully monitored. Preoperative pharmacologic treatment may involve administration of agents to moderate elevated blood pressure. Moderation of blood pressure prevents hypertension and complete disruption of the involved vessel.

After operation, the patient requires careful assessment for residual effects of hypoperfusion to any organs or systems below the level of the aortic disruption. Decreased perfusion below this level can result from hypotension, decreased blood flow past the aneurysm, or intraoperative crossclamping of the aorta. Patients with known peripheral or primary vascular disease should be considered to be at particular risk. Common postoperative complications are bowel infarction, paraplegia, renal failure, and aortic graft infection or leak. Patients require serial monitoring for extreme variations in blood pressure, graft or anastamosis leak, or infection.

Myocardial Contusion. Myocardial contusion, a bruise to the muscular layer of the heart, occurs as the result of blunt trauma. It has often been identified in drivers who are not restrained with seat belts. This potentially lethal injury is difficult to diagnose because the clinical presentation varies from patient to patient. Evaluation for bruises to the anterior chest or seat belt ecchymosis, and for any chest pain should be done. Research has shown that the majority of arrhythmias associated with myocardial contusion occur early in the prehospital and hospital course. ECG findings observed usually within the first 48 hours range from ST- and T-wave changes to premature ventricular con-

tractions and atrioventricular blocks. The patient may even display signs of cardiogenic shock (see Table 19–9). A pericardial rub may be auscultated (see Chapters 13 and 24, respectively). Red blood cells are thought to extravasate around myocardial fibers and lead to increased serum levels of creatinine kinase MB (CK-MB). Serial levels of these isoenzymes are done to ascertain any elevations in CK-MB values. Echocardiography is also used to screen for contusions or abnormal cardiac wall motion. Treatment is generally supportive and similar to that of the patient with a myocardial infarction (see care plans in Chapter 18).

Pulmonary Contusion. Pulmonary contusion, a bruise of the lung parenchyma, occurs from a direct insult to the lungs or sudden compression of the thoracic cavity, which can be associated with fractured ribs or flail chest. The contusion results in leakage of blood and fluid into lung interstitium secondary to increased capillary permeability at the injury site. A contusion may occur more frequently in younger patients without rib fractures, who have a more compliant rib cage, or in patients with thinner chest walls. The patient is observed for dyspnea, tachypnea, hemoptysis, ineffective cough and copious secretions, tachycardia, and restlessness and anxiety in the conscious individual. Rales (crackles) may be heard on auscultation. Diagnosis is made based on the chest x-ray, although definitive findings may not be apparent on x-ray for the first 48 to 72 hours. Eventually, the bruised area is involved in the inflammatory response of interstitial and alveolar edema formation. These areas are then at risk for becoming atelectatic and infected. The accumulation of blood and mucus frequently produces upper and lower airway obstruction. The clinical picture may progress to that of adult respiratory distress syndrome (ARDS). (For nursing considerations in caring for the patient with pulmonary contusion complicated by ARDS, see Table 25–9.)

Meticulous attention should be given to pulmonary physiotherapy, postural drainage, and mobilization of secretions. Hemoptysis usually clears within 3 days. Efforts should be aimed at avoiding excessive fluid administration since it is felt to contribute to local pulmonary edema. Some patients receive diuretic therapy. Accurate intake and output information is a necessity. Intubation and institution of mechanical ventilation may be indicated in patients with large contusions and severe hypoxemia ($PaO_2 < 60$ mmHg on 40% fraction of inspired oxygen [FIO_2]) unresponsive to other supportive therapy. PEEP therapy in conjunction with mechanical ventilation may be implemented to improve hypoxemia. PEEP enhances functional residual capacity (FRC), prevents collapse of airways, enhances gas exchange and oxygen transport, and helps to reduce right to left shunting.

Flail Chest. A flail chest results from the fracture of multiple ribs in two or more places, causing instability of the bony thorax. Severe flail injuries can contribute to poor pulmonary ventilatory mechanics, as reflected by paradoxical respirations (i.e., collapse of flail segment of the chest wall on inspiration and expansion of the chest wall on expiration). It is most important to note that the flail segment is usually associated with an underlying pulmonary contusion. The patient may appear dyspneic and complain of severe pain with respiratory movement. Shallow respirations with poor tidal volume, increased work of breathing, and splinting are commonly observed, accompanied by varying degrees of hypoxia and hypercapnia. Many patients are able to use their chest muscles to prevent painful movement of the flail segment until the patient begins to fatigue. The chest wall may eventually demonstrate asymmetrical movement with the respiratory cycle, and crepitus may be palpated with movement of the rib ends. The amount of hypercapnia, hypoxia, and respiratory distress will vary depending upon the size of the parenchymal injury underlying the flail segment balanced by compensatory respiratory efforts made by the patient.

Mechanical ventilation with PEEP has been successful as an internal splinting of the rib cage and lung. With nonintubated patients in particular, the critical care nurse should serially monitor effectiveness of pain control therapies and pulmonary function, including tidal volume, maximum inspiratory pressures, oxygen therapy, and arterial blood gases. The goal is to maintain PaO_2 greater than 80 mmHg and $PaCO_2$ at normal levels. Management of the patient's pain is a very important part of therapy. The nurse should carefully evaluate the effectiveness of pain control therapies, based upon the patient's ability to move, deep-breathe, and participate in pulmonary toilet. One approach employed is to use thoracic epidural analgesic therapy. Another method is patient self-controlled administration of intravenous narcotics. On occasion, these techniques have eliminated the need for intubation because patients will breathe more efficiently and splint less if their pain is relieved. Intercostal nerve blocks have also been used with limited success.

Tracheobronchial Injuries. Tracheobronchial injuries are caused when shearing forces stretch and tear the tracheobronchial structures, usually involving the mainstem bronchi. Blunt trauma is the primary cause for this injury, although penetrating trauma is also a mechanism of injury. Although some patients may initially show no symptoms, several days after injury the symptoms of subcutaneous emphysema or pneumothorax may appear. Tension pneumothorax may be seen in conjunction with a tracheobronchial injury, further complicating the clinical picture and treatment options. Efforts to mechanically ventilate the patient are compromised by the large air leaks associated with the injuries. A portion of the tidal volume delivered by the ventilator is lost through the chest tube and can result in hypoventilation. Diagnosis is usually confirmed by bronchoscopy.

Treatment is directed toward establishing and maintaining an adequate airway and ventilation. The position of any artificial airway must be carefully protected from any movement. A patent airway may be maintained by positioning an endotracheal tube beyond the point of bronchial injury. Creation of a surgical opening by cricothyroidotomy or tracheotomy may be the only method available to establish a patent airway in patients who have sustained injury to the trachea, larynx, and bronchi (see Fig. 22–1). Definitive repair of the injury is performed in the operating room and is directed at correction of the underlying pathophysiology. After operation, care should be taken to avoid sharp increases in airway pressure, and the patient should be gently suctioned to avoid any stress of the sutured repair. Any change in the amount of chest tube air leak or decrease in the exhaled tidal volume should be carefully assessed.

Other Thoracic Injuries

Rib Fractures. Rib fractures are the most common chest injury. Such injuries can seriously compromise alveolar ventilation as a result of splinting of the rib cage secondary to pain. Puncture injury of the lung parenchyma may become potentially life-threatening. Patients usually complain of severe pain, and point tenderness over the fracture is frequently noted. Rib fractures can often be palpated. Patients will also be observed to splint the chest when they breathe, thereby compromising the ventilatory effort and predisposing to atelectasis. Diagnosis of the fracture and atelectasis may be confirmed on chest x-ray. Treatment usually involves adequate pain control to ease the work of breathing, depth of respirations, and pulmonary toilet.

Sternal Fractures. Sternal fractures are frequently the result of steering wheel injuries. A sternal fracture is also important because it is usually associated with significant blunt force and is associated with other potential serious injuries. The patient should be assessed carefully for cardiac rupture, myocardial contusion, cardiac tamponade, or pulmonary injury. Patients usually complain of point tenderness over the sternal area. Diagnosis is confirmed by chest x-ray.

Thoracoabdominal Trauma. Thoracoabdominal trauma is defined as trauma that involves both the thoracic and abdominal cavities. Injuries include esophageal trauma, diaphragmatic rupture, and other associated abdominal organ injuries. The clinical presentation varies, depending on the structures involved. The nurse must be cognizant of the fact that a chest injury also implies the presence of an abdominal injury, especially in penetrating trauma, for example, a stab wound. At exhalation, the diaphragm rises as high as the 5th intercostal space, and several abdominal organs lie beneath the lower rib cage. The liver and spleen are frequently involved in stab wounds to the lower thoracic areas. If the diaphragm is lacerated by blunt or penetrating trauma, bowel and other abdominal organs may herniate into the chest cavity. Esophageal trauma is usually due to penetrating injuries, but may also be caused by a severe blow to the abdomen.

Early diagnosis of the injury is very important because the surrounding tissue is damaged by spillage of the digestive juices and bacterial contamination.

Delays in diagnosis are usually associated with a high mortality rate. Initial signs and symptoms may be subtle until the patient develops mediastinitis, rupture into the pleural space with ensuing empyema, or signs of peritonitis appear. The patient may have particulate material draining from his chest tube after the blood has cleared. Treatment is usually surgical with good wound drainage and gastric decompression. Potential complications include intra-abdominal/thoracic abscess formation and esophageal fistula formation.

Complications in Thoracic Trauma

Patients who have sustained serious chest trauma are at high risk of complications involving other organ systems, in addition to cardiopulmonary function. Many of these patients are victims of multisystem trauma. Bleeding associated with a coagulopathy (i.e., a defect in blood clotting mechanism), induced by either the injury sustained or the dilution of clotting elements resulting from massive transfusion therapy, is a common occurrence. ARDS, pulmonary emboli, and respiratory failure often complicate the clinical picture. Sepsis, pneumonia, and renal and liver dysfunction are also common. The critical care nurse must be especially vigilant to detect subtle clues and to recognize trends that suggest underlying pathophysiology. Early recognition and timely institution of appropriate interventions may help to avert reversible pathophysiology from becoming *ir*reversible.

Therapeutic Goals

Nursing care in chest trauma is first directed toward use of an *anticipatory* approach to intervene in the immediate life-threatening types of chest trauma. Knowledge of the mechanism of injury, initial clinical status, typical injury sequelae, and patient history are helpful in providing appropriate and timely care. As diagnosis and stabilization occur, the nurse continues with comprehensive assessments to determine patient needs, emotional as well as physiologic, and to set priorities. Subtle changes in patient status may be significant in detecting complications or previously undetected injuries in these patients. Serial reassessments of the patient include airway and ventilatory status, vital signs, and neurologic status. Hemodynamic parameters are continuously monitored. The patient's fluid hydration status is monitored meticulously. Outputs, including nasogastric, urinary, and chest tube drainage, are documented carefully.

Overall management of the trauma patient begins with securing the ABCs (airway, breathing, and circulation) with stabilization of the cervical spine and control of external hemorrhage. Therapeutic goals for the patient with chest trauma involve the following:

1. Establish and maintain a patent airway.
2. Support alveolar ventilation and oxygenation to relieve hypoxemia.
3. Provide hemodynamic support to maintain adequate cardiac output and tissue perfusion.
4. Monitor/maintain fluid and electrolyte balance.
5. Monitor/maintain acid-base balance.
6. Recognize clues of underlying pathophysiology associated with ARDS, pulmonary embolism, hemorrhage.
7. Provide nutritional support.
8. Prevent infection.
9. Provide pain control and promote patient comfort.
10. Prevent impairment in skin integrity, related to immobility and stress.
11. Provide emotional and psychological support to patient and family.

Nursing Diagnoses, Desired Patient Outcomes, and Nursing Interventions

Implementation of the nursing process in the care of the patient with thoracic trauma centers around the therapeutic goals listed above. Nursing diagnoses, desired patient outcomes, and nursing interventions and their rationales are outlined in the care plan at the end of this chapter.

ABDOMINAL TRAUMA

Blunt Versus Penetrating Abdominal Trauma

Abdominal trauma is most frequently due to motor vehicle crashes and physical assault. Penetrating abdominal trauma is usually associated with violent acts, such as gunshot wounds and stabbings. Chest and pelvic trauma should be suspected in association with abdominal trauma.

The severity of blunt injury is directly related to the force of impact, the amount of time the force was applied, and the anatomic area where force was applied. The abdominal wall offers minimal protection from injury, as compared to the bony structures of the skull and thorax. Injuries from blunt trauma usually result from crushing or bursting of tissue.

Abdominal trauma may result in massive blood loss with hemorrhagic shock or peritoneal contamination with peritonitis. Abdominal injuries, therefore, may lead to fluid volume deficit, alteration in tissue perfusion, alteration in comfort, and alteration in bowel and urinary elimination.

Stab wounds result in low-velocity injuries (less wounding potential) that are confined to the instrument's tract. Gunshot wounds, however, also produce blast and concussive tissue injuries. Because this results in injury to more than just the area around the missile's tract, gunshot wounds usually require exploratory surgery.

The abdomen is the portion of the trunk located between the diaphragm and the pelvis. It consists of three sections: the intrathoracic abdomen, the pelvic or true abdomen, and the retroperitoneal space. The abdominal viscera contain both hollow and solid organs, with solid organs frequently injured by blunt force and hollow organ injuries resulting from penetrating trauma. The liver and spleen are the most frequently injured abdominal organs. The major abdominal vessels include the aorta and the inferior vena cava and the hepatic, renal, and iliac arteries and veins.

Clinical Presentation

The initial signs and symptoms exhibited by the abdominal trauma patient may be as severe as those indicative of profound hypovolemia or as subtle as no signs of injury or complaint of pain. The major life-threatening concern in abdominal injuries is severe blood loss and the resulting hemorrhagic shock (see Chapters 21 and 44). Clinical signs may include the so-called peritoneal signs: (1) abdominal ecchymosis, (2) decreased or absent bowel sounds, (3) pain with palpation, (4) muscular rigidity and involuntary guarding, and (5) rebound tenderness. Left shoulder pain, referred to as Kehr's sign, is a classic finding in patients with splenic rupture caused by blood below the diaphragm irritating the phrenic nerve. The critical care nurse should examine the patient carefully for bruising patterns and seat belt marks, which may indicate an occult injury. A central nervous system injury or the effects of drugs or alcohol may obscure the normal physical examination and make definitive workup for all the injuries difficult.

Diagnostic Considerations

Specific information regarding the mechanism of injury, events preceding the incident, location of the patient at the time of injury, and force of impact provide significant data for diagnosis of abdominal injury. Diagnostic studies must occur as part of the initial life-saving intervention. As with chest trauma, initial diagnostic efforts should address airway, breathing, and circulatory status. The most important decision in suspected abdominal trauma is whether the patient will require immediate surgical intervention to prevent death or significant morbidity/mortality.

Laboratory Studies

The patient with abdominal trauma requires many of the same laboratory studies as the chest trauma victim. Early determination of hemoglobin and hematocrit, electrolytes, urinalysis, and arterial blood gases is essential to direct resuscitative measures and to direct patient care in the critical care phase. Table 54–3 lists normal and abnormal values for commonly used laboratory data. Both actual or potential abdominal injury may require transfusion of blood products;

therefore, the number of units available in the blood bank should always be immediately ascertained by the critical care nurse. Guaiac of stool and gastric drainage may indicate injury and bleeding, particularly in penetrating trauma. Samples for baseline establishment of laboratory values include serum electrolytes, blood urea nitrogen (BUN), and creatinine done on admission to the critical care unit. Serial laboratory results may demonstrate development of complications. For example, an elevation in amylase can indicate post-traumatic pancreatitis, or rising creatinine and BUN may mean renal failure. A decrease in the hematocrit can signal coagulopathy and/or continuing hemorrhage. Increases in leukocytes can result from developing infection, abscess, or sepsis.

Radiographic Studies

Radiographic studies vary, depending on the severity of injury and institutional community attitudes, but the following radiographic studies may be indicated in abdominal trauma.

A simple anterior/posterior abdominal film may reveal (1) intra-abdominal free air, indicating disruption of a hollow organ; (2) abnormal densities associated with bleeding from solid organs (less than 800 mL of blood may not be visualized on x-ray); and (3) presence of foreign bodies, such as bullets or fragments.

A lateral decubitus film may reveal disruption of hollow organs through air along the lateral aspects of the abdomen. An intravenous pyelogram (IVP) may be used to determine extravasation of contrast media, indicating injury to the kidney or ureters. A cystogram may be done to evaluate bladder rupture. Computed tomography (CT) may be used to determine actual sites of hemorrhage. Unfortunately, the CT scan has limited ability to distinguish hollow organ injuries or pinpoint penetrating trauma.

Diagnostic Peritoneal Lavage (DPL)

Diagnostic peritoneal lavage is used to determine the presence of intra-abdominal bleeding in patients whose physical examination of the abdomen is unreliable or equivocal. It is most useful in assessment of blunt abdominal trauma and stab wounds of the flank or anterior abdomen. The accuracy of the peritoneal lavage is about 97% in identifying organ injury. Controversy exists regarding the efficiency and accuracy of peritoneal lavage versus the CT scan. Current modalities indicate a rise in popularity of the CT scan or ultrasound determination of abdominal injuries, but the peritoneal lavage continues to be the procedure of choice for most patients where time and resources are to be conserved.

Before the peritoneal lavage procedure, a nasogastric (NG) or orogastric tube and urinary catheter should be inserted. The NG tube is both diagnostic and therapeutic because it decompresses the stomach, prevents aspiration, and minimizes gastric content

TABLE 54–5
Positive Peritoneal Lavage Findings

Characteristic	Finding
Frank, nonclotting blood	Presence
Red blood cells	100,000 red blood cells/ mm^3 (blunt trauma)
	1000–100,000 red blood cells/mm^3 (penetrating trauma)
Hematocrit	>2%
White blood cells	>500 white blood cells/mm^3
Amylase	>200 somogyi units
Bile	Presence
Fecal material, bacteria, amniotic fluid, or urine	Presence

contamination of the abdominal cavity. A urinary catheter is inserted to empty the bladder, thereby decreasing the risk of puncturing the bladder during the procedure. It further allows monitoring of urine output and analysis of urine for gross or occult blood. If frank blood is not initially aspirated, 1000 mL saline solution or Ringer's lactate is rapidly infused into the abdominal cavity. The fluid is then drained out by gravity.

Laboratory analysis of peritoneal fluid is performed to determine the presence of blood cells, bile, amylase, urine, or feces, all indicative of intra-abdominal injury (Table 54–5).

Although DPL is a useful diagnostic tool, it does not assess all intra-abdominal structures. Retroperitoneal injuries to the kidneys, pancreas, and duodenum must be diagnosed by other means. It is important for the critical care nurse admitting a patient with the diagnosis of abdominal trauma to understand which methods have been used to work up the patient. If a DPL has been done, the patient still has the potential for intra-abdominal hemorrhage or chemical burn from the retroperitoneal organs and their vascular supply.

SELECTED ABDOMINAL TRAUMA

Lacerated Liver

The liver is one of the most frequently injured abdominal organs, occurring as a result of blunt trauma to the abdomen from motor vehicle crashes. Signs and symptoms specific to liver injury include right upper quadrant abdominal pain, abdominal wall musculature spasms, involuntary guarding, and signs of hypovolemic shock. Fracture of the lower right ribs and ecchymosis of the right upper quadrant are often associated with liver injury. A bleeding liver laceration requires immediate surgical control of blood loss. Because of the inability to intraoperatively control hemorrhage, the liver and abdomen may be packed with sponges and the patient returned to the intensive care unit for normalization of temperature and clotting factors. The patient is returned later to the oper-

ating room for completion of the repair and closure of the abdominal wall.

Splenic Injury

Blunt abdominal trauma most often results in injury to the spleen. Ecchymosis of the left upper quadrant and fractures of the lower left ribs are associated with splenic injuries. Pain radiating to the left shoulder, Kehr's sign, occurs when the intra-abdominal bleeding irritates the phrenic nerve. Additional signs and symptoms include point tenderness, involuntary guarding, and absent bowel sounds. The majority of traumatized spleens require surgical repair or resection (splenorrhaphy) or splenectomy. Unless contraindicated, splenectomized patients receive a pneumococcal vaccine because they are at higher risk for certain infections and sepsis, even later in life. Although some splenic injuries are managed nonoperatively, they require frequent CT scan assessment and continual monitoring of patient status and vital signs.

Kidney Injury

The kidney does not tolerate impact well, with multiple lacerations and fragmentation of the tissue. Trauma to the kidney frequently is a result of blunt trauma, and pedestrians struck by cars have a particularly high incidence. An IVP may be done to assess renal injury and the number of functioning kidneys. Ecchymosis over the involved flank area, tenderness on palpation, and gross hematuria are signs and symptoms associated with kidney trauma. Even in the most severe of renal injuries, however, hematuria is not necessarily present. The kidney is located retroperitoneally; therefore, the peritoneal lavage is not used to diagnose kidney injuries. Up to 85% of kidney injuries can be treated conservatively, including contusions and small lacerations. The patient is observed closely for infection of the hematoma or urinoma.

Trauma to the Hollow Viscus

The hollow organs (small bowel, colon, stomach, and bladder) frequently are injured in penetrating trauma to the abdomen but may also be damaged by blunt forces. Signs and symptoms include rebound tenderness, abdominal rigidity, involuntary guarding, and possibly hematuria, depending on the actual injury. The bladder is more likely to be injured by blunt forces when full because it rises up out of the protection of the pelvic cavity. Colon and small bowel pathology include contusions, seromuscular lacerations, perforations, and mesenteric injuries. Mesenteric blood supply to the bowel may be disrupted, requiring resection of the bowel before it becomes devitalized. Surgical intervention is often necessary to repair or resect the damaged tissue and to remove contaminants from the peritoneal cavity.

Nursing Care of the Patient with Abdominal Trauma

Critical intervention should include activities to support or reestablish vital physiologic functions. Airway patency requires continual assessment, optimal positioning with cervical spine stabilization, and suctioning as indicated. Volume replacement, initially with crystalloid solutions should begin immediately. Blood products should be transfused as indicated to maintain adequate perfusion and oxygenation of vital organs. Ongoing assessment by the nurse should continue as diagnostic procedures and stabilization occur. The critical care nurse should conduct a meticulous, head-to-toe admission assessment that gives particular attention to the patient's rule-out diagnoses. As diagnostic procedures and stabilization evolve, the critical care nurse should continue ongoing assessment and prepare for immediate transport to surgery if indicated. Insertion of the NG or orogastric tube and urinary catheter should be performed during stabilization of the patient.

Some patients who have known hepatic or splenic injuries are managed nonoperatively. The nurse should observe for subtle changes in level of consciousness, respiratory and circulatory status, and pain response to determine alterations indicating a need for immediate surgery. Throughout the care process, preparation for immediate transport and surgical intervention must be considered.

Abdominal injury resulting from penetrating trauma requires special attention. Impaled or foreign objects should be stabilized as they are and should not be removed until the patient is in the surgical suite. Removal of such objects may result in massive bleeding once the tamponading agent has been removed. Before operation, the patient usually receives antibiotics. Patients with stab wounds thought to be superficial may be admitted for close observation.

Tetanus immunization status and the need for antibiotics should be determined during the stabilization of the trauma victim. Antibiotics are indicated if intra-abdominal organs have been perforated and leakage of contents has occurred. The risk of peritonitis and sepsis is great in this event.

Important concerns for the patient with abdominal trauma are hemodynamic stability, recognition and identification of occult injuries, risk of sepsis, nutritional support, and psychosocial support for the patient and significant others. A high index of suspicion must be maintained for intra-abdominal injuries and other injuries commonly associated with a particular mechanism of injury or pattern of trauma.

Nutritional Support

Adequate nutrition is necessary to promote wound healing and prevent loss of body mass. This requires particular attention in the patient with gastrointestinal, pancreatic, gastric, and esophageal injuries. An assessment of the patient's nutritional requirements should be completed in the first 24 hours after admission to the critical care unit. Nutritional support is best attained through the use of a multidisciplinary approach, involving medical and surgical staffs, a nutritional support team, pharmacists, and above all, appropriately trained critical care nursing staff. (For a detailed discussion of nutritional support of the critically ill patient, see Chapter 9.)

Complications in Abdominal Trauma

Hemorrhage control and stabilization of hemodynamics is of great importance in the patient received from the resuscitation or operative phase of care. Long intraoperative procedures with large blood loss may make a patient prone to the development of symptoms of hypothermia, coagulopathy, and acidemia. Signs and symptoms of other complications are related to the specific organ system injured. Sepsis, peritonitis, and abscess formation is of major importance for any victim of abdominal trauma, particularly when injury results in perforation of a hollow organ. A perforation permits leakage of gastrointestinal contents into the peritoneum. This contamination of the abdominal cavity results in peritonitis and the potential for septic shock. (For a detailed discussion of septic shock, see Chapter 56.) Patients with pancreatic injuries may develop pancreatitis, glucose intolerance, pancreatic fistulas, and fluid and electrolyte imbalances. After surgical repair of the stomach, breakdown of the suture site resulting in gastric fistula or peritonitis can occur. Some patients develop acute cholecystitis after the stress of a traumatic episode. Tetanus immunization status should be determined because trauma results in contaminated wounds, which tend to be tetanus-prone.

Therapeutic Goals

Effective treatment of abdominal trauma requires immediate attention to airway, breathing, and circulatory status, and a high index of suspicion for severe injury. Therapeutic goals for the patient with abdominal trauma should include the following:

1. Establish a comprehensive database.
2. Establish and maintain a patent airway.
3. Provide necessary ventilatory support and oxygenation to relieve hypoxemia, hypercapnia, and consequent acidemia.
4. Provide hemodynamic support to ensure adequate cardiac output and tissue perfusion.
5. Maintain fluid, electrolyte, and acid-base balance (Chapter 23 and 36).
6. Prevent impairment to skin integrity.
7. Provide nutritional support (Chapter 9).
8. Prevent infection.
9. Provide emotional and psychological support to patient/family.
10. Provide pain relief.

Nursing Diagnosis, Desired Patient Outcomes, and Nursing Interventions

Implementation of the nursing process in the care of the patient with an abdominal injury revolves around the therapeutic goals listed above. Nursing diagnoses, desired patient outcomes, and nursing interventions and their rationales are outlined in the care plan at the end of this chapter.

ORTHOPEDIC TRAUMA

Extremity trauma is rarely life-threatening. There are, however, instances in which musculoskeletal trauma assumes a very high priority in the multisystem trauma patient. Severe pelvic fractures, complete neurovascular compromise, joint dislocation, and amputation can lead to significant morbidity and mortality. In the case of an amputation, which results in severe hemorrhagic shock, the loss of limb and life from circulatory collapse make this type of orthopedic trauma an immediate consideration. Joint dislocations and neurovascular injury or compromise can lead to permanent disability. Severe pelvic fractures can lead to heavy blood loss and transfusion requirements and hypotension.

Anatomy and Physiology

The musculoskeletal system is made up of muscles, bones, joints, tendons, and ligaments. The primary function of this system is to provide structure and form to the human body. Bones, the most dense connective tissue in the body, give the skeletal system a framework for leverage and protect the underlying organs from injury. They are composed of three tissue layers, the periosteum (outermost layer), the bone itself, and the cancellous of spongy bone (innermost layer). Bones act as a storehouse of calcium. Blood vessels and nerves are also part of the musculoskeletal system. The bone marrow, which forms the cancellous bone matrix, produces and stores red blood cells.

Pathogenesis

Musculoskeletal injuries frequently result from blunt forces. Motor vehicle and industrial accidents, falls, and sports injuries account for the majority of extremity trauma. Child and adult abuse, known as nonaccidental trauma (NAT), can also involve a form of blunt trauma. Statistics confirm the fact that NAT continues to be a major contributor to extremity trauma. Orthopedic trauma can also be caused by penetrating injury. These mechanisms include stab wounds, gunshot wounds, and missile and blast injuries.

Associated injuries often found in combination with

TABLE 54–6
Patterns of Associated Trauma for Extremity Injuries

Traumatic Injury	Associated Injury
Fractured humerus (distal ⅓)	Radial nerve palsy
Fractured humerus (supracondyle)	Compressed brachial artery; radial and/or median nerve injury
Anterior shoulder dislocation	Compressed auxiliary artery, nerve, vein
Wrist	Elbow or shoulder fracture
Calcaneal (heels)	L-1 or L-2 vertebrae fractures
Anterior knee fracture	Hip fracture/dislocation
Knee dislocation	Compression of popliteal vessel
Hip	Dislocated opposite hip
Posterior hip dislocation	Sciatic nerve compression; aseptic necrosis of femoral head
Fractured tibia (epiphysis) (proximal ⅓ tibia)	Popliteal artery laceration
	Anterior tibial artery and/or nerve compression; compartment syndrome
Fractures of femur (distal ⅓)	Dislocated hip
	Femoral artery laceration
Ankle dislocation	Compression of pedal artery

long bone trauma are listed in Table 54–6. Understanding these patterns of trauma based on the mechanism of injury provides the nurse with valuable information that can be used to anticipate orthopedic problems that may be present or may arise secondarily.

Certain types of extremity trauma, although single system, carry with them additional risks. The patient with a femur fracture, for example, may be in profound hypovolemic shock because the average femur fracture in an adult can result in a loss of up to 3 U of blood. Table 54–7 lists the approximate blood loss associated with each type of orthopedic trauma. (See Table 44–1 for signs and symptoms associated with approximate blood losses.)

Pathophysiology

In long bone trauma, the pathophysiology presents itself in the form of tissue deformity and ischemia. Fractures are categorized in a number of ways. One such classification system is presented in Table 54–8.

TABLE 54–7
Blood Loss Associated with Various Fractures

Fracture	Approximate Blood Loss
Fractured humerus	½–1 unit
Fractured tibia	1–2 units
Fractured femur	2–3 units
Pelvic fractures	1–2 units/fracture

TABLE 54–8
Classical Fracture Patterns

Type of Fracture	Definition/Description
Open	Skin integrity over or near fracture site disrupted
Closed	Skin integrity over or near fracture site intact
Complete	Total interruption of bony continuity
Incomplete	Incomplete interruption of bony continuity
Comminuted	Splintering of bone into fragments
Greenstick	Bone buckles, bends, but still securely hinged on one side
Impacted	Bone broken and wedged into other break
Overriding	Bone edges slip past one another out of alignment
Direction of Fracture	**Fracture Line Description**
Longitudinal	Parallel to bone axis
Transverse	Crosses bone at right angle to axis
Oblique	Crosses bone at a slanted angle to axis
Spiral	Runs through bone in a spiral direction

Orthopedic trauma can result in many kinds of disruptions. Bone can crack, bend, or break, and the skin surfaces may be bruised, abraised, or lacerated. Ligaments, the tissue that attaches bone to bone, may be sprained or torn from their attachments. Tendons, those structures that attach muscle to bone, may be pulled, stretched, or even sheared from their points of insertion. Nervous tissue disruption predisposes to inflammation and peripheral neuropathy (e.g., paresthesias). Such disruptions cause muscle strain and bony discontinuity leading to diminished sensory and motor function. Usually when a fracture occurs, a portion of the periosteum remains intact. This portion of the periosteum is responsible for helping in healing and reduction of the fracture. Extremity trauma can result in impaired mobility and severe pain.

In long bone trauma or joint dislocation, the blood supply may be disrupted by injury to blood vessels, altering circulation to the affected extremity. The extremity may become edematous from hematoma formation and tissue damage. The vascular status of the extremity, therefore, is disrupted, causing decreased blood flow, decreased tissue oxygenation, and, at times, cellular anoxia and death. The repair of these torn vessels, tendons, ligaments, skin, and nervous tissue occurs in a timely fashion in conjunction with bone realignment and results, eventually, in restoration of function.

Clinical Presentation

Complaints of pain and/or evidence of deformity indicate the possibility of a disrupted bone. Even if a closed fracture has occurred and a deformity is not readily apparent, a chief complaint of pain alerts the nurse to the possibility of an extremity injury. The six "P's" of fracture assessment are as follows:

Pain
Point tenderness
Pulses—distal to the fracture site
Pallor—skin color
Paresthesias—numbness or tingling
Paralysis—voluntary movement

Other factors to be assessed include the presence of muscle spasm, crepitus, swelling, discoloration, and associated wounds.

Diagnostic Considerations

Along with the history and physical examination, radiologic and laboratory assessment is undertaken. It is important to x-ray above and below all injured areas because other fractures may be missed. Angiography may be indicated for patients with compromised peripheral circulation, pelvic fractures with large blood loss, or fractures or dislocations. The overall goal is to limit hemorrhage, to prevent further injury or permanent disability, and to maintain the injured limb in a manner that will afford optimal function after healing and rehabilitation.

Nursing Care of the Patient with Orthopedic Trauma

The ABCs of care take precedence in the patient with a long bone injury. Management of the patient with orthopedic trauma includes ongoing monitoring of the patient's vital signs and hemodynamic status, laboratory data, and diagnostic studies performed and their results. It also requires the restoration of tissue perfusion and maintenance of skin integrity during the course of therapy. Fluid resuscitation is initiated with insertion of large-bore (14- to 16-gauge) angiocatheters. Ringer's lactate and normal saline are the crystalloids of choice. Blood is used when blood loss exceeds 20% of the patient's total blood volume. Appropriate amounts of typed blood should be kept available. The fluid/blood product should be warmed to prevent hypothermia. Attention to the affected limb and use of the six "P's" in assessment (see the preceding section on clinical presentation) will provide the critical care nurse with a complete database to evaluate comprehensively the patient and the response to therapy.

Complications

As is the case with chest and abdominal trauma (discussed previously), the nurse must be ever vigilant for complications. Complications seen in the care of the patient with long bone trauma include skin breakdown at pressure points, wound infections, compartment syndrome, fat emboli, and osteomyelitis.

Adequate fluid replacement during all phases of care is an essential treatment considered in the care of the patient with orthopedic trauma. Immediate measures to correct fluid and blood loss must be initiated to prevent hypoperfusion to the affected extremity (Table 54–7).

Wound infections are usually the result of a break in the skin noted at the time of injury. Wounds include severe degloving soft tissue injuries, lacerations, abrasions, avulsions, puncture wounds, and even wounds from foreign objects or missiles. Pin insertion or fixator sites may be observed for possible infection. Pin sites should be cared for per unit protocol. Vigilance by the critical care nurse who continually observes for signs of inflammation (heat, pain, redness, swelling, compromised function) or systemic infection is crucial in the care of the patient. Frequent assessment with adequate lighting; proper cleansing of the affected area with removal of debris; application of dry, sterile dressings as per unit protocol; and administration/ monitoring of prescribed antibiotic, both topically and systemically, will hasten wound healing. In particular, patients with open pelvic fractures are at high risk for sepsis and multiple organ failure.

Compartment syndrome, a state of excessive pressure within a muscle compartment caused by edema formation and bleeding, is seen in conjunction with arterial or venous vascular injuries or with massive swelling in the closed-space muscle compartment. The muscle contained in the fascial sheath becomes increasingly edematous and ischemic. Compartment pressures can be measured directly by the use of a slit or wick catheter device. Readings can easily be obtained by inserting an 18-gauge needle connected to a transducer into the suspected compartment. Normal pressure readings range from 9 to 15 mmHg in a relaxed muscle. Compartment pressure readings of greater than 30 mmHG are diagnostic of compartment syndrome. If the pressures are elevated, surgical incisions through the fascia are done to relieve the pressure. When the muscle has become necrotic, it will be surgically debrided. Usual sites for compartment syndrome development are the forearm, calf, and thigh. The role of the nurse in the care of the patient with compartment syndrome is *early* detection of this complication. The patient who continually complains of pain unrelieved by the use of narcotic analgesics is a classic example of a patient who may be developing compartment syndrome. The nurse should palpate compartment tension and compare it to the unaffected extremity. Other signs and symptoms include pain on passive stretching, loss of motor function, and throbbing pain. Paresthesias and diminished pulses in the affected extremity are later findings of the syndrome.

The etiology of fat embolization syndrome (FES) is still not well understood. There are two widely discussed theories based on the pathophysiology of FES. The *extra*vascular theory states that FES occurs from disruption of fat-containing tissues, resulting in the flow of fat globules into the microcirculation. The *intra*vascular theory states that fat, in some way, is altered in the bloodstream, forming large droplets and occluding small vessels. The result is the same and predisposes to ARDS and pulmonary embolism (see Chapters 25 and 26, respectively). Most orthopedic patients will develop symptoms within 48 hours after injury or after operative orthopedic procedure. Clinical manifestations include changes in mental status, dyspnea, tachycardia, restlessness, temperature spikes, and petechiae on the chest and in skinfolds. Laboratory diagnosis of FES includes elevated serum lipase, thrombocytopenia (platelet count <150,000), and a decreased PaO_2. Chest x-ray findings are consistent with ARDS; ECG findings may reflect ischemia (ST-segment and T-wave changes). Treatment is supportive. The critical care nurse must be cognizant of the fact that frequent manipulation of the involved extremity may increase the incidence of FES. Immediate immobilization, prompt stabilization of the fracture, adequate blood and fluid replacement, and prevention of hypotension are critical measures to be employed in the care of the patient with long bone trauma.

Osteomyelitis, a significant complication of long bone trauma, is infection of the bone. It is most common in patients who have an open fracture or who have undergone surgery for the repair of the fracture. Common symptoms include signs of local infection, pain, and temperature elevations. Therapy includes surgical debridement, immobilization, nutritional support, and even bone grafting for severely damaged sites. Nursing considerations include prevention of infection, pain control, administration of prescribed antibiotic therapy, and immobilization of the site. Careful monitoring of the wound drainage should be documented.

Therapeutic Goals

Nursing management considerations in caring for the patient with long bone trauma are focused on the following therapeutic goals:

1. Establish a thorough comprehensive database.
2. Establish and maintain a patent airway with adequate alveolar ventilation.
3. Provide necessary circulatory support to ensure adequate tissue perfusion.
4. Maintain fluid, electrolyte, and acid-base balance (Chapters 23 and 36).
5. Maintain skin integrity.
6. Provide nutritional support (Chapter 9).
7. Prevent complications of immobility, including thromboembolic and pulmonary embolic phenomena (Chapters 26 and 53).
8. Provide emotional and psychological support to patient and family (Chapters 5 and 6).
9. Monitor patient's expectation of therapy and concerns associated with body image and self-esteem.

Nursing Diagnoses, Desired Patient Outcomes, and Nursing Interventions

Implementation of the nursing process in the care of the patient with an extremity fracture centers around the previously mentioned therapeutic goals. Specific diagnoses, desired patient outcomes, nursing interventions and their rationales are presented in the care plan at the end of this chapter.

SUGGESTED READINGS

American College of Surgeons, Committee on Trauma. Shock. In Advanced Trauma Life Support (Provider) Manual, ed 5. Author, Chicago, 1993, pp 75–94.

Christensen, MA, and Sutton, KR: Myocardial contusion: New concepts in diagnosis and management. Am J Crit Care 2:28–34, 1993.

Demling, R and Pomfret, E: Blunt chest trauma. New Horiz 1:402–421, 1993.

Endersen, BL and Maull, KI: Missed injuries: The trauma surgeon's nemesis. Surg Clin North Am 71:399–418.

Freedland, M, Wilson, RF, Bender, JS, and Levison, MA: The management of flail chest injury: Factors affecting outcome. J Trauma 30:1460–1468, 1990.

Geiderman, JM: Orthopedic injuries: Management principles. In Rosen, P and Barkin, RM (eds): Emergency Medicine: Concepts and Clinical Practice, ed 3. Mosby Year Book, St Louis, 1992, pp 1, 522–544.

Injury Control in the 1990s: A National Action Plan: In the Report to the Second World Conference on Injury Control: Center for Disease Control and Prevention, National Center for Injury Prevention and Control. Waxweiller, RJ, Rosenberg, ML, Fenley, MA (Coordinators). Association for the Advancement of Automotive Medicine, 1993.

Johnson, KL: Trauma. In Thelan, LA, Davie, JK, Urden, LD, Lough, ME (eds): Critical Care Nursing. Mosby, St Louis, 1994, pp 729–765.

Landercasper, J, Cogbill, TH, and Strutt, PJ: Delayed diagnosis of flail chest. Crit Care Med 18:611–613, 1990.

Mackersie, RC, Karagianes, TG, Hoyt, DB, Davis, JW: Prospective evaluation of epidural and intravenous administration of fentanyl for pain control and restoration of ventilatory function following multiple rib fractures. J Trauma 31:443–451, 1990.

Mackersie, RC, Shackford, SR, Garfin, SR, and Hoyt, DB: Major skeletal injuries in the obtunded blunt trauma patient: A case for routine radiologic survey. J Trauma 28:1450–1455, 1988.

Mason, PJ: Abdominal trauma. In Cardona, V, Hurn, PD, Bastnegal-Mason, PJ, Scanlon, AM, and Veiss-Verry, SW (eds): Trauma Nursing: From Resuscitation Through Rehabilitation, ed 2. WB Saunders, Philadelphia, 1994, pp 512–547.

Proehl, JA: Compartment syndrome. J Emerg Nurs 14(5):283–292, 1988.

Rodriques, A: Injuries of the chest wall, lungs and the pleura. In Turney, SZ, Rodriquez, A, Cowley, RA (eds): Management of Cardiothoracic Trauma. Williams & Wilkins, Baltimore, 1990.

Ruth-Sahd, L: Pulmonary contusion: The hidden danger in blunt chest trauma. Crit Care Nurse 11(6):46–57, 1991.

Strange, JM and Kelly, PM: Musculoskeletal Injuries. In Cardonna, VD, Hurn, PD, Mason, PJ, Scanlon, AM, and Veise-Berry, SW (eds): Trauma Nursing. WB Saunders, Philadelphia, 1994, pp 549–586.

Vanek, VW, Gantt, N, and Spirtos, G: Review of the literature and recommendations for prophylaxis of deep vein thrombosis and pulmonary embolism in surgical and trauma patients. Curr Surg 44(4):539–553, 1991.

Wisner, DH, Reed, WH, and Riddick, R: Suspected myocardial contusion: Triage and indications for monitoring. Ann Surg 212:82–86, 1990.

CARE PLAN FOR THE PATIENT WITH MULTISYSTEMS TRAUMA: THORACIC, ABDOMINAL, AND LONG BONE (ORTHOPEDIC)

Nursing Diagnoses

Nursing Diagnosis #1
Alteration in tissue perfusion, related to:
1. Hypovolemia
2. Impaired blood supply
3. Vascular compromise from fracture

Nursing Interventions

- Perform patient assessment and monitoring (includes ABCs with C-spine and hemorrhage control).

- Perform mini neuro exam (Glasgow Coma scale and pupils).
- Note vital signs (including temperature) at frequent intervals (every 15 minutes unless patient condition dictates more frequent vitals, then every 1 to 5 minutes).
- Perform capillary refill checks with vital signs.
- Assess neurovascular function of immobilized extremity (pain, pulse, pallor, puffiness, paralysis, paresthesias).

Desired Patient Outcomes

Patient will maintain:
1. Skin temperature, color, and moisture—pink, warm, and dry
2. Normal neurovascular assessment of extremities: sensorimotor function intact
3. Urinary output of 30–50 mL/h

Rationales

- Complete patient assessment and monitoring aids the nurse in discovering overt/covert changes in patient status at frequent intervals in those with multisystem trauma.
- Early recognition of these changes results in timely care and the appropriate interventions to decrease trauma patient morbidity and mortality.

- Reflects status of tissue perfusion.

CARE PLAN FOR THE PATIENT WITH MULTISYSTEMS TRAUMA: THORACIC, ABDOMINAL, AND LONG BONE (ORTHOPEDIC) (*Continued*)

Nursing Diagnoses	Desired Patient Outcomes

Nursing Diagnoses

Nursing Diagnosis #2
Impaired gas exchange, related to:
1. Disruption of alveolar-capillary membrane
2. Decreased tissue perfusion
3. Other complication (e.g., fat emboli)

Desired Patient Outcomes

Patient will maintain:
1. Arterial blood gases:
   - PaO_2 > 80 mmHg (room air)
   - $PaCO_2$ 35–45 mmHg; pH 7.35–7.45
2. Minimum pulmonary function:
   - Tidal volume >7–10 mL/kg
   - Vital capacity >15 mL/kg
3. Cardiac output of 4–8 L/min
4. Respiratory rate of 12–20/min, eupneic
5. SvO_2 within normal limits

Nursing Interventions

- Ensure patent airway via appropriate route (chin lift, jaw thrust, without neck hyperextension).
- Provide high flow of oxygen at 6 to 10 L/min (use mask or cannula, or oral or nasal adjuncts).
- Give ventilatory support as needed FIO_2 of 100% (endotracheal or nasotracheal intubation; cricothyrotomy or tracheotomy, if indicated, for obstructed airway).
- Monitor serial arterial blood gases (ABGs) per physician.

- Obtain serial chest x-rays per physician.

- Cover sucking or open chest wounds.

- Observe for tension pneumothorax.

Rationales

- Establishing a patent airway provides the initial route for adequate intake of oxygen.
- Oxygen delivery in the proper amount by the appropriate method assists in the maintenance of adequate tissue oxygenation.

- Serial blood gas measurements accurately reflect gas exchange requirements in impaired patients with decreased tissue perfusion.
- Serial chest x-rays provide for ongoing monitoring of potential or missed lung injury (i.e., pulmonary contusion).
- Covering sucking or open wounds provides for more effective gas exchange until the defect can be repaired.

Nursing Diagnoses

Nursing Diagnosis #3
Fluid volume deficit, related to blood loss

Desired Patient Outcomes

Patient will maintain:
1. Wedge pressure (PCWP) of 8–12 mmHg
2. Systolic BP of >100 mmHg (including orthostatic BP)
3. Pulse pressure of >30 mmHg
4. Strong, palpable peripheral pulses of 2+ bilaterally
5. No external bleeding noted
6. Normal skin turgor
7. Level of consciousness: alert, awake, and oriented ×3
8. Absence of signs of internal bleeding (hematochezia, periumbilical ecchymoses)

Nursing Interventions

- Control external bleeding with direct pressure.

- Assess for signs of occult bleeding frequently (i.e., rigid abdomen, stools for guaiac).

- Start IVs with large-bore 14- to 16-gauge needles; crystalloids, colloids, and blood may be administered.
  - Fluid replacement therapy:
    - Crystalloids: 3 mL/1 mL blood loss
    - Blood: 1 mL/1 mL blood loss
- Assist with cutdowns or central lines as needed.

Rationales

- Controlling external bleeding prevents exsanguinating hemorrhage—direct pressure is the best method.
- Trendelenburg position aids in venous return to augment BP. Contraindicated in possible head injury—impedes blood flow from cranium.
- Assessment for occult bleeding is necessary to prevent missed injuries and to note the changing status of the patient.
- Large-bore IVs with crystalloids, colloids, and/or blood help replace fluid volume deficit.

- Cutdowns or central venous lines provide quick fluid access to central circulation.

CARE PLAN FOR THE PATIENT WITH MULTISYSTEMS TRAUMA: THORACIC, ABDOMINAL, AND LONG BONE (ORTHOPEDIC) (*Continued*)

Nursing Interventions	Rationales
• Prepare for autotransfusion if indicated with chest injuries.	• Autotransfusion provides an immediate autologous blood transfusion to the patient.
• Consider use of antishock garment in severe pelvic fractures. Monitor response: BP in hypotension; monitor ventilatory response as pressure over abdomen can compromise chest excursion.	• Antishock trousers enhance peripheral resistance, perform arterial tamponade, promote shunting of blood to vital organs, and splint fractures to decrease blood loss. (See Chapter 21 for discussion of antishock trousers.)
• Splint and immobilize fractured/dislocated extremities, prevent gross movement.	• Immobilization of fractures prevents further hemorrhage, reduces risk of fat emboli.
• Provide hemodynamic monitoring for critical patients.	• Hemodynamic pressure monitoring assists in determining fluid requirements in patients with fluid volume deficit.
• Monitor serial Hcts (as per physician).	• Serial Hcts determine the amount of packed red blood cells found in the blood.

Nursing Diagnoses	Desired Patient Outcomes
Nursing Diagnosis #4 Alteration in cardiac output (decreased), related to: 1. Hemorrhage shock 2. Tension pneumothorax 3. Cardiac injury	Patient will maintain: 1. Normal electrocardiogram 2. Heart sounds S_1 and S_2 normal without extra sounds 3. Cardiac output of 4–8 L/min 4. Normal skin temperature, color, and moisture (as noted previously) 5. Pulse rate of 60–100 beats/min 6. Signs of adequate tissue perfusion (e.g., brisk capillary refill)

Nursing Interventions	Rationales
• Obtain 12-lead ECG (per physician). • Perform continuous ECG monitoring.	• 12-lead ECG provides baseline electrocardiographic data. • Continuous ECG monitoring is performed to note potential cardiac arrhythmias, a complication of impaired gas exchange and alteration in cardiac output.
• Consider antishock garment (controversial).	• Antishock garment enhances peripheral resistance (see Nursing Diagnosis #3, preceding)
• Monitor hemodynamic status to titrate fluids (see Nursing Diagnosis #3, preceding).	• Hemodynamic monitoring detects status of cardiopulmonary function and measures cardiac output.
• Obtain serial labwork (Hb, Hct, chemistries, and cardiac enzymes).	• Maintaining Hct in normal range ensures tissue oxygenation.

Nursing Diagnoses	Desired Patient Outcomes
Nursing Diagnosis #5 Impaired skin integrity, related to: 1. Open wounds from fractures 2. Penetrating trauma 3. Abrasions, contusions, lacerations, edema 4. Neurovascular compromise	Patient will maintain: 1. Absence of bacterial infection and secondary infections 2. Intact skin surfaces 3. Proper wound healing and reduced inflammatory response 4. Absence of sepsis or other systemic reactions 5. Body temperature at baseline: 98.6°F (37°C)

Nursing Interventions	Rationales
• Stabilize all impaled objects before operative removal.	• Stabilization of impaled objects prevents further injury.
• Cleanse and irrigate all open wounds with solution of choice.	• Cleansing and irrigation of open wounds removes debris and decreases bacteria, which cause infection.
• Cover all open wounds with sterile dressings. Perform sterile dressing changes as needed. Note amount, color, and consistency of drainage from wounds.	• Covering wounds maintains sterile environment.
• Cover "sucking" wounds with impregnated (petroleum jelly) gauze.	• Covering sucking wounds with impregnated gauze temporarily restores skin integrity and may reduce chest wall defect.

CARE PLAN FOR THE PATIENT WITH MULTISYSTEMS TRAUMA: THORACIC, ABDOMINAL, AND LONG BONE (ORTHOPEDIC) (*Continued*)

Nursing Interventions

- Provide antibiotic therapy as ordered (IV, intramuscular, or oral).
  - Obtain specimens for culture and sensitivity (as appropriate).
- Give tetanus toxoid or tetanus immunoglobulin (per physician).
- Turn and position every 2 h; range-of-motion exercises (as indicated).

Rationales

- Antibiotic therapy inhibits and/or kills microorganisms and the growth of anaerobic gram-positive and gram-negative organisms.

- Tetanus toxoid and tetanus immune globulin prevent tetanus.
- Maximizes perfusion, reduces risk of thrombophlebitis and pressure ulcer in immobilized patient.

Nursing Diagnoses

Nursing Diagnosis #6
Impaired physical mobility, related to chest, abdominal, and/or long bone trauma

Desired Patient Outcomes

Patient will: demonstrate mobility to pre-injury capacity, or to optimal level of restored function

Nursing Interventions

- Remove all constrictive clothing and jewelry.

- Splint and immobilize all extremities above and below joints.
- Provide gait training and crutches during limited mobility.

- Assist with cast, traction, pin, and/or fixator application if indicated.

- Encourage early ambulation in multisystem trauma patients.

Rationales

- Removing constrictive clothing and jewelry provides for enhanced mobility and increased circulation to promote healing.
- Immobilization and splinting allow for increased mobility and the prevention of further injury.
- Proper gait training prevents injury, and crutch walking provides a method of early ambulation in patients with long bone trauma.
- Casting, pin insertion, external and/or internal fixators, and/or traction promote alignment of bone, restore tissue function, and increase circulation to the affected area to promote healing.
- Early ambulation prevents other complications (e.g., pulmonary).

Nursing Diagnoses

Nursing Diagnosis #7
Pain, related to tissue, nerve, or vessel disruption from penetrating, blunt, or extremity trauma

Desired Patient Outcomes

Patient will:
1. Verbalize that pain is diminished or that pain relief has occurred (if conscious)
2. Display relaxed musculature, no facial grimace, and minimal signs of combativeness

Nursing Interventions

- Provide position of comfort for patient as permitted by patient's clinical status.
- Provide pain medication by proper route and monitor response.
- Use other pain reduction techniques if alternative therapy indicated (biofeedback, transcutaneous electrical nerve stimulation, distraction, guided imagery).
- Splint and immobilize all fractured/dislocated extremities.

- Cover all wounds.

Rationales

- Providing position of comfort for patients in pain may alleviate or reduce discomfort.
- Pain medication binds to receptor sites, which function to reduce perception of pain.
- Pain reduction techniques alter pain perception and/or sensation.

- Splinting of fractured/dislocated extremities brings about immobilization, which reduces edema and restores circulation and, therefore, tissue perfusion, to reduce or eliminate pain.
- Dressings to wounds decrease pain to the injured site and reduce risk of infection.

CARE PLAN FOR THE PATIENT WITH MULTISYSTEMS TRAUMA: THORACIC, ABDOMINAL, AND LONG BONE (ORTHOPEDIC) (*Continued*)

Nursing Diagnoses

Nursing Diagnosis #8

Alteration in elimination (bowel or urinary), related to:
1. Decreased circulating volume
2. Associated hypoperfusion from multisystem organ failure, gastrointestinal injury, or renal trauma

Desired Patient Outcomes

Patient will maintain:
1. Urinary output of 30–50 mL/h (mL/kg)
2. Urine specific gravity of 1.010–1.025
3. Normal color, amount, consistency of urine
4. Decreased gastric distention
5. Expected NG drainage (if NG tube is in place)
6. Abdomen soft and not tender
7. Normal bowel sounds; bowel movement if appropriate

Nursing Interventions

- Insert continuous urinary drainage catheter. Monitor urinary output. Note color, amount, consistency, and specific gravity.
- Insert NG or orogastric tube.
- Monitor gastric drainage (to suction if indicated).
- Note color, amount, and consistency of gastric drainage.

Rationales

- Continuous urinary drainage allows for monitoring of potential alterations in urinary and/or renal function.

- Continuous gastric drainage allows for monitoring of gastrointestinal function and potential bleeding; decompressed stomach allows for full chest excursion and lung expansion; minimizes risk of aspiration in patients with an altered level of consciousness.

Nursing Diagnoses

Nursing Diagnosis #9

Knowledge deficit, related to lack of information regarding injury or illness

Desired Patient Outcomes

Patient/family comprehends treatment regimen through verbalization and resultant compliance in self-care.

Nursing Interventions

- Assess for readiness of the learner(s).

- Provide for patient and family education.

- Give one-to-one teaching about specific aspects of care.

- Teach to level of patient/family.

Rationales

- Assessing for learner readiness provides information as to the patient/family level of comprehension.
- Patient/family education may promote an understanding of the injury and therefore greater acceptance and compliance with treatment regimens.
- One-to-one teaching may result in enhancing absorption of information and reinforcement.
- Teaching to the level of the patient allows for greater retention and understanding.

Nursing Diagnoses

Nursing Diagnosis #10

Ineffective coping patterns (patient and/or family or significant others) to stress of trauma

Desired Patient Outcomes

Patient/family will:
1. Exhibit effective coping mechanisms.
2. Verbalize feelings.
3. Identify/access support systems (persons, institutions, associations).
4. Identify past coping mechanisms that have been successful.
5. Be able to set short-term goals and objectives.
6. Eventually be able to set long-term goals, and a plan of action for the future. Anxiety reaction, if present, will be appropriate to crisis or event.

CARE PLAN FOR THE PATIENT WITH MULTISYSTEMS TRAUMA: THORACIC, ABDOMINAL, AND LONG BONE (ORTHOPEDIC) (*Continued*)

Nursing Interventions

- Assess for life-threatening injury or illness and/or patient and family perceptions of such illness.

- Communicate and develop trusting relationship with patient/family.

- Act as patient/family advocate.

- Encourage patient/family to verbalize feelings.

- Assist patient/family to identify past coping mechanisms.

- Help patient/family define immediate areas where decision making is involved.
- Provide emotional and verbal support during crisis.

- Involve patient/family in as many decisions as possible (includes care activities, short- and long-term decisions).

- Encourage the development of new coping mechanisms where past mechanisms have proven ineffective for problem-solving.
- Initiate referral system as needed.

Rationales

- Assessing for life-threatening injuries may assist in relating patient prognosis information to patient/family and clarifying patient's overall clinical status.
- Development of a trusting relationship increases communication, thereby giving clear messages to the client.
- Acting as patient/family advocate may assist in patient support.
- Verbalization of feelings encourages dealing with perceptions about the injury and known/unknown fears.
- Identifying past coping mechanisms may help in knowing which techniques were helpful.
- Patient/family participation is imperative for future well-being and overall healthcare management.
- Provide emotional support during crisis may decrease anxiety.
- Involving patient/family in decisions about care allow them to assume responsibility for actions and promotes dignity and patient self-esteem.
- Encouraging the use of new coping methods may strengthen patient/family and assist them in identifying effective coping mechanisms.
- Use of a referral system (social service, pastoral care, psychological counseling) will be significant in planning total, comprehensive, holistic patient care during acute phase and rehabilitation.

Nursing Diagnoses

Nursing Diagnosis #11
Alteration in nutritional status, decreased from multisystem trauma. (See appropriate tables in Chapter 9, Nutritional Support of the Critically Ill Patient.)

Desired Patient Outcomes

Patient will maintain:
1. Adequate nutritional intake via oral, IV, and/or parenteral or enteral route (regular diet or diet to tolerance)
2. Positive nitrogen balance will be achieved
3. Normal serum electrolytes:
   - Potassium 3.5–5.0 mEq/L
   - Sodium 135–145 mEq/L
   - Chloride 100–106 mEq/L
   - CO_2 content 24–30 mEq/L
   - Glucose 70–110 mg/100 mL
   - Creatinine 0.6–1.5 mg/100 mL
   - BUN 8–25 mg/100 mL
4. Normal skin turgor present

Nursing Interventions

- Provide nutritional support by appropriate route (oral, parenteral, or enteral route, as indicated).
- Obtain serial electrolytes per physician.

- Assess skin turgor and mucous membranes during complete patient assessment.
- Monitor nitrogen balance in critically injured patients.

Rationales

- Nutritional support is necessary for the repair of injured tissue and the promotion of health.
- Serial electrolytes provide baseline data for the monitoring of the patient's nutritional and overall status.
- Skin turgor assessment detects dehydration or overhydration status of the patient.
- Positive nitrogen balance is imperative for the multisystems trauma patient in a compromised, catabolic state caused by injury.

CARE PLAN FOR THE PATIENT WITH MULTISYSTEMS TRAUMA: THORACIC, ABDOMINAL, AND LONG BONE (ORTHOPEDIC) (*Continued*)

Nursing Diagnoses

Nursing Diagnosis #12
Alteration in body image, related to:
1. Traumatic incident
2. Disfigurement
3. Perceived body image disturbance

Desired Patient Outcomes

Patient will:
1. Be able to discuss body image disturbance if present and verbalize feelings about self, including positive comments
2. Demonstrate signs of acceptance of self in actions like dress and performance of the activities of daily living

Nursing Interventions

• Assess patient coping style.

• Discuss with patient body image perceptions.

• Offer praise and accomplishment when appropriate.

• Establish open lines of communication.

• Make appropriate referrals as needed.

Rationales

• Assessment of patient coping styles assists in discovering successful methods of dealing with body image crises.
• Verbalizing feelings regarding body perceptions may reduce anxiety and fears and help patients overcome disturbances.
• Offering praise and support when appropriate creates feelings of enhanced human dignity, self-worth, and self-esteem.
• Open lines of communication allows for verbalization of body image concerns.
• Making appropriate referrals will assist in patient well-being.

PaO_2 = arterial oxygen pressure; $PaCO_2$ = arterial carbon dioxide pressure; SvO_2 = mixed venous blood oxygen tension (saturation); BP = blood pressure; IV = intravenous; Hct = hematocrit; Hb = hemoglobin; and NG = nasogastric.

C H A P T E R 5 5

Nursing Management of the Patient with Burns

Rita Bolek Trofino

LEARNING OBJECTIVES

After completing this chapter, you should be able to:

1. Discuss pathophysiology underlying burn injury and its impact on total body function.
2. Identify key assessment factors in establishing the severity of burn injury.
3. Examine the major complications of a major burn injury and implications for nursing care.
4. Delineate therapeutic goals in the management of burn injury during the emergency and acute phases.
5. Describe the major considerations underlying effective wound management and the implications for nursing care.
6. Describe therapeutic modalities used to enhance wound healing.
7. Discuss the nursing process in caring for the patient with a major burn injury, including assessment, nursing diagnoses, desired patient outcomes, and nursing interventions.

BURN (THERMAL) INJURY

Description

An energy transfer from a heat source to the body, heating the tissue enough to cause damage, will result in a burn injury. Major causes of this energy transfer are listed in Table 55-1. The amount of heat transfer can be altered by the thickness of the skin; the surface pigmentation; the presence of hair, dirt, and natural skin oils; surface cellular water content; peripheral circulation in the area of contact; and the temperature of and duration of exposure to the burning agent.

Pathophysiology

Local Skin Response

Heat transfer denatures cellular protein, inactivates or blocks thermolabile enzymes, and interrupts vas-

cular supply. Three zones of injury, or dimensions to the burn wound, have been identified (Fig. 55–1).

The extent of integumentary alterations is determined by the burning agent, temperature of the burning agent, conductivity of the tissues, duration of exposure, and thickness of the integumentary structures involved. The major alterations in normal skin functioning that can occur from thermal injury are as follows:[1]

Loss of protection
Impaired thermoregulation
Impaired defense against infection
Decreased or absent sensory function
Loss of fluids
Decreased vitamin D production
Impaired skin regeneration
Impaired secretory function
Impaired excretory function
Loss of hair growth
Alteration in appearance

TABLE 55–1
Causes of Injury

Thermal Injuries	Description
Dry Heat	
Flame	→ Most common injury.
Flash	→ Sudden ignition or explosion of short duration.
Contact	
Tar	→ Splatter-type injuries; temperature >400°F.
Metals	→ Industrial injuries; temperature usually >200°F.
Grease	→ Household injury; temperature >200°F.
Moist Heat	
Steam	→ Under pressure, trauma is greater.
Scald	→ Third-degree burns occur in 1 second if the temperature is 156°F.
Chemicals	→ 25,000 products capable of producing burns are used in industry, agriculture, and the home.
Electrical	→ Low-voltage direct current creates less damage than low-voltage alternating current. High-voltage direct current creates more hazard than high-voltage alternating current.
Lightning	→ Uncommon injury with extremely variable trauma.

Systemic Response

Altered functional capacity of the skin affects all body systems either directly or indirectly because of the interdependence of all body systems.

Hemodynamics. After a major burn injury occurs, increased capillary permeability leads to the extravasation of water, electrolytes, albumin, and protein into the interstitial and intracellular compartments, leading to the formation of edema. Beginning immediately after the burn occurs, this process can lead to a 60% loss of intravascular volume because the capillary response extends to unburned tissues if the burn injury is greater than 30% of body surface area (BSA). An increase in the body's metabolic rate will lead to further water loss through the respiratory system. Insensible water loss through burn wounds can range from 90 to 350 mL/h. Impaired circulation and decreased peripheral perfusion lead to metabolic acidosis.

Burn shock (hypovolemic) causes a decrease in blood pressure, blood flow, and polycythemia because of hemoconcentration. Blood viscosity leads to sludging in the vasculature. This vascular volume depletion can continue up to 36 hours after injury, although capillary integrity is generally restored after 24 hours.

Cellular Response

Similar to the action in an inflammatory response, neutrophils converge in the area of injury, and phagocytosis of bacteria occurs. An increase of monocytes, which convert to macrophages in tissues, continues to

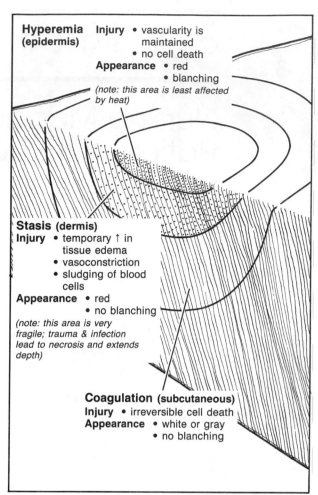

FIGURE 55–1. Three zones of tissue damage. *Hyperemia* (epidermis): This area is least affected by heat. Vascularity is maintained with no cellular death. Skin is red and blanches. *Stasis* (dermis): Damage to this layer is due to temporary lack of good blood supply. Vasoconstriction occurs, leading to sludging of the blood cells and an increase in tissue edema. Appearance is red with no blanching. This area is very fragile as trauma and infection lead to necrosis and extend depth. *Coagulation* (subcutaneous): Innermost area. Cellular death is an irreversible process. Appearance is white or gray, with no blanching. Size will increase with heat intensity and exposure time.

act on residual wound debris. Interference with cellular enzyme processes leads to red blood cell destruction in the area of injury and partial destruction of those red blood cells on the periphery of the wound. Progressive anemia occurs for the first 2 weeks after the burn. Disseminated intravascular coagulopathy (DIC) may occur because of a decrease in platelet and fibrinogen levels; these levels return to normal in 24 to 36 hours. (DIC is discussed in detail in Chapter 53.)

Cardiac Function

The occurrence of myocardial depressant factor in burn victims with greater than 50% BSA injury may decrease cardiac output by 30% during the first 30 minutes after injury. Cardiac output may also decrease to 20% of normal because of further compromise by the circulating plasma volume loss. Cardiac function at this time is supported with aggressive fluid therapy.

Renal Function

The renal stress response—hypovolemia and the release of antidiuretic hormone—alters renal function. Inadequate fluid resuscitation can lead to acute tubular necrosis. Hemoglobin, released in large amounts because of red blood cell destruction, and myoglobin, freed by muscle destruction when the depth of injury involves the muscle compartment, also lead to tubular necrosis. Adequate fluid and electrolyte replacement can help either to reverse this process or to decrease the incidence of renal dysfunction.

Gastrointestinal Tract Function

Hypovolemia produces splanchic vasoconstriction with a reflex ileus. Abdominal distention, regurgitation, malabsorption, ulcerations, and hyperacidity are all in response to the burn injury. Common gastrointestinal problems that can develop following a major burn include gastric dilatation, Curling's ulcer (acute gastroduodenal ulcer), superior mesenteric artery syndrome, and paralytic ileus.

Stress Response

The release of catecholamines triggered by the stress response increases the release of norepinephrine out of proportion to other traumas. A blood sugar increase is secondary to adrenal hormone release with a decrease in insulin effectiveness. Acceleration of the metabolic rate is directly proportional to the size and depth of the burn injury, evaporative water loss through burned tissue, and increased protein losses. Hypoglycemia, unique in the pediatric age group, is due to inadequate glycogen stores in the liver.

Immune Response

With the loss of the first line of defense, the skin, the burn wound offers the ideal entry and medium for bacterial growth. Severe burns cause an immediate depression of the immunoglobins IgA, IgG, and IgM. With host defenses depressed, bacterial invasion at the site of injury can quickly lead to a septic episode. (The immune response is discussed in detail in Chapter 47.)

Assessment: Severity of Injury

The following factors influence the severity of burn injury:
1. Depth of injury
2. Size of the burn
3. Age of the patient
4. Past medical history
5. Location of burn injury
6. Associated trauma

Depth of Injury

Depth of injury is classified as partial-thickness injury, which affects the epidermal layer and from one half to seven eighths of the dermal layer of skin; and full-thickness injury, which can involve all epidermis and dermis, subcutaneous tissue, and in many cases, muscle and bone (Table 55–2).

TABLE 55–2
Classification of Burn Depth

Classification	Formerly	Areas Involved	Appearance	Sensitivity	Healing Time
Partial-thickness (superficial)	1°–2°	Epidermis Papillae of dermis	Bright red to pink. Blanches to touch. Serum-filled blisters. Glistening, moist.	Sensitive to air, temperature, and touch.	7–10 days
Partial-thickness (deep)	2°	Epidermis, ½ ⅞ of dermis Appendage usually present	Blisters may be present. Pink to light red to white. Soft and pliable. Blanching present.	Pressure may be painful from exposed nerve endings.	14–21 days. May need grafting to decrease scarring.
Full-thickness	3°–4°	Epidermis Dermis Tissue Muscle Bone	Snowy white, gray, or brown. Texture is firm and leathery. Inelastic.	No pain as nerve endings are destroyed, unless surrounded by areas of partial-thickness burns.	Needs grafting to complete healing.

Partial-thickness injuries can easily convert to full-thickness injuries when ice is used initially to cool the wound, which leads to vasoconstriction in the zone of stasis. Other factors that can convert a partial-thickness injury to a deeper injury include drying effects of air; infection; and inadequate hydration, nutrients, and oxygen.

Size of the Burn

The size of the wound must be determined correctly to accurately calculate fluid requirements during resuscitation. There are three methods to determine the extent of the injury. The *palmer* method is a quick assessment that uses the palms of the hand to represent 1% of the BSA. This method is inaccurate and is used to assess smaller wounds. The *rule of nines* method, most commonly used in emergency departments, is the simplest calculation. In this method, the total body is divided into nine sections or multiples of nine (with the perineum counted as 1%), as indicated in Figure 55–2. This method is quick and convenient but not the most accurate, especially in children, because of the head size and the size of the lower extremities. The *Lund and Browder* method is the most accurate way to assess the size of a burn wound because it allows for age-related differences (Fig. 55–3). Many emergency departments provide convenient charts for this purpose.

Age of the Patient

Children less than 2 years old and adults older than 65 are the populations at risk for burn injury. Poor antibody response in the very young results in early infection leading to septicemia. Pre-existing illness and the inability of the aged body to handle stress leads to increased mortality in elderly persons.

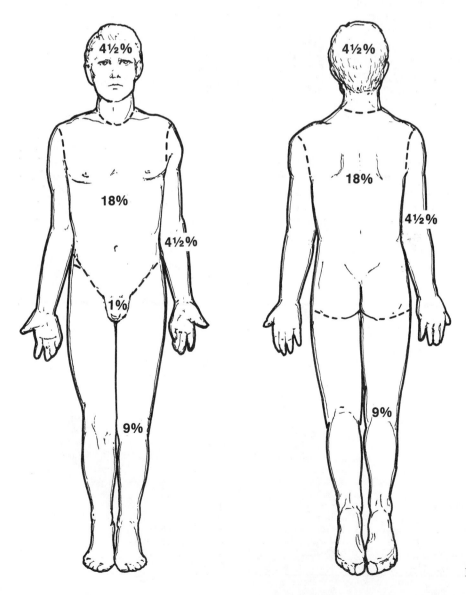

FIGURE 55–2. Rule of nines.

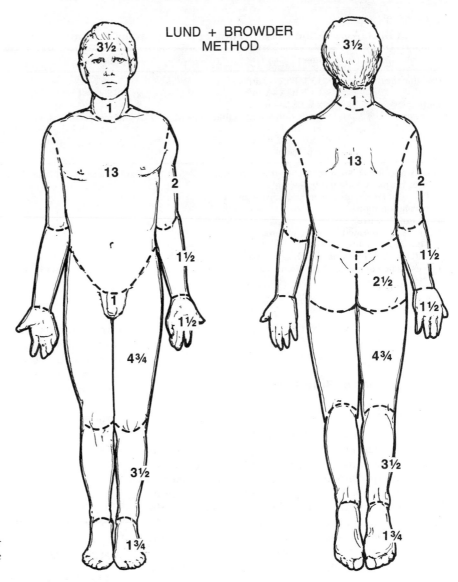

LUND + BROWDER
METHOD

FIGURE 55–3. Lund and Browder method of estimation of percentage of burn injury.

Past Medical History

Major burns can aggravate degenerative disease processes and exacerbate pre-existing illnesses. These pre-existing conditions can also complicate wound management and healing. In addition, certain medications that the patient has been taking for other conditions can also alter the body's response to the burn injury. To decrease mortality and morbidity, any medical condition and medications must be identified early in the course of therapy and must be appropriately managed.

Location of the Injury

Pulmonary complications are increased with burns of the head, neck, and chest. The incidence of functional or cosmetic alterations increases with burns in critical body areas, such as face, hands, feet, or joints.

Perineal burns increase the risk of infection. Circumferential burns can decrease circulation in limbs or decrease respiratory excursion of the trunk. Loss of mobility can occur, especially in hands if the joints are involved.

Associated Trauma

Trauma other than burns can further complicate the burn victim's course of therapy. A thorough assessment for associated injuries must be completed as quickly as possible. Because burn wounds do not bleed, frank bleeding indicates other injury. Intra-abdominal trauma, head trauma, long bone fractures, and spinal cord injuries can occur as a result of impact injuries that occur frequently with burn trauma.

The American Burn Association classification of the severity of injury is presented in Table 55–3. Severity

TABLE 55–3
American Burn Association Classification Severity Grading System*

	Minor†	Moderate	Major
Partial-thickness	<15% BSA—Adults <10% BSA—Child	15–25%—Adults 10–20%—Child	>25% BSA—Adults >20% BSA—Child
Full-thickness	<2% BSA—Adult	2–10% BSA—Adults	>10% of BSA
Treatment	Usually outpatients, children, and elderly Possibly 1–2 days hospital admission	Admission to hospital, preferably one with expertise in burn care (e.g., burn unit)	Admission to burn center

*In Trofino, RBT: Nursing Care of the Burn-Injured Patient, FA Davis Company, Philadelphia, 1991, p 143, with permission.
†Minor burns exclude the following:
1. Burns of face, hands, feet, and perineum.
2. Inhalation injury.
3. Electrical burns.
4. Burns complicated by other trauma.
5. Poor-risk patients.
6. Patients with improper psychosocial facilities.
The existence of any of these circumstances would further classify the patient as a moderate or major burn.

of injury is determined by the depth of injury and total BSA involved.

Complications of Burn Injury

Pulmonary Injury

The most immediate threat to life associated with burns is inhalation injury. Carbon monoxide poisoning and smoke inhalation are the greatest killers at the scene of the fire and are the leading cause of death in admitted patients. Of the 50,000 fire victims admitted to hospitals per year, smoke or thermal damage to the respiratory tract may occur in about 30%. Smoke inhalation influences survivability of fire victims by doubling the mortality for a burn of any size. The four types of pulmonary injury are presented in the box on page 947.

Sepsis

The burn wound is an excellent culture medium for bacterial growth. The incidence of serious infection in burn patients increases with the size of the burn wound. The burn wound flora must be monitored carefully for signs of colonization and infection. Bacterial growth greater than 10^5 colonies/gram of tissue can predict a septic episode. The use of topical agents on the burn wound can control the number of bacteria sufficiently to prevent invasive infection. Types of infection are presented in Table 55–4.

When sepsis is suspected, prompt identification of the offending organisms is essential, and antibiotic therapy should be instituted. Wound care must be meticulous and constant with evaluation of topical antimicrobials for their effectiveness against the offending organisms.

Neurovascular Compromise

Full-thickness burns form as inelastic, thick, tight eschar over the wounds. With edema formation caused by the capillary leak, this eschar forms tight constricting bands on injured limbs, creating pressure on underlying structures and decreasing blood flow to areas distal to the burned area.

TABLE 55–4
Types of Infection

	Noninvasive	Invasive Without Bacteremia	Invasive with Bacteremia
Signs and symptoms	Stays on the surface of the wound, can grow and divide.	Granulation area of burn wound that was healing deteriorates as organisms invade viable tissue.	Both colonizing and invading bacteria may enter the lymphatic system and systemic circulation.
	Bacterial count is 10^3–10^5. Low-grade but spiking fever. Mild leukocytosis. Patient is awake and alert.	Invaded tissue is edematous, pale, and progresses to dry, crusty, and necrotic. Persistent temperature elevation. Bacterial count is 10^6–10^8. Leukocytosis. Patient becomes less responsive, may progress to coma.	Same as invasive without bacteremia. Bacterial count is 10^9–10^{12}. If caused by gram-negative organisms, the temperature may fall and white blood cells may be depressed. Septicemia is followed by septic shock and death.

TYPES OF PULMONARY INJURY

CARBON MONOXIDE POISONING

Carbon monoxide (CO) is a colorless, odorless, tasteless, nonirritating gas given off by nearly everything that burns. The biologic effects are due to tissue hypoxia as the CO molecule replaces the oxygen molecule on the hemoglobin sites.

The victim is usually trapped in an enclosed or poorly ventilated smoke-filled area.

Signs and Symptoms

Toxicity depends on the concentration of CO in the inspired air, the length of exposure, and the individual victim's response. Carboxyhemoglobin (CO + Hb) produces the following symptoms:

<10%	Does not cause symptoms.
10%–20%	Complaints of headaches, nausea, vomiting, loss of manual dexterity.
21%–40%	Confusion, lethargy, may show depressed ST segment on ECG. This level can be lethal because the victim loses both the interest and the ability to flee the smoke.
41%–60%	Ataxia, convulsions, coma with respiratory failure.
>60%	Usually fatal.

Treatment

Restoration of adequate oxygenation is the primary goal. Since there is a 50% reduction in the CO + Hb level in the first 20 minutes in the presence of 100% oxygen, this therapy must be initiated as quickly as possible with an established airway.

SMOKE OR CHEMICAL INHALATION INJURY

Injury to lung mucosa from the inhalation of smoke is primarily a chemical injury.

The chemical composition of smoke depends on the type of materials being burned, as follows:

Cyanide→nylon carpets, polyurethane carpets, chair cushions.

Hydrochloric acid→burning or smoldering vinyl. When inhaled, this very strong acid corrodes lung and throat tissue.

Aldehydes→acrylics such as curtains and drapes.

Two hundred-eighty separate toxic products have been found in wood smoke.

Fire history is very important. Suspect this injury if the victim was in a closed space, if it was a smoky fire, or if the smell of smoke is on the victim's clothes. Question the rescuers or the victim on the type of items burning, the length of time the victim was exposed to smoke, and the condition of the victim on rescue.

Signs and Symptoms

Initial Response:

1. Immediate loss of bronchial cilia. (See Chapter 22 for discussion of anatomy and physiology of respiratory tract and lungs.)
2. Decrease in alveolar surfactant.
3. Atelectasis.
4. Mucosal edema in small airways.
5. Wheezing and air hunger.

12–24 Hours' Response:

1. Tracheal and bronchial epithelium begins to slough and hemorrhagic tracheobronchitis develops.
2. Patients may expectorate mucosa and bronchial casts.

24–48 Hours' Response:

1. Interstitial edema becomes prominent, resulting in a typical adult respiratory distress syndrome pattern.
2. Pulmonary macrophages are destroyed, leading to bacterial pneumonia.

Suspect this injury if the following are present:

1. Facial burns
2. Intraoral burns
3. Singed nasal hair
4. Soot in the oropharynx
5. Carbonaceous sputum
6. Hoarseness and wheezing
7. Hypoxemia with an elevated CO_2 level and CO present on blood gas analysis
8. Positive bronchoscopy that shows mucosal erythema, hemorrhage, ulceration, edema, and carbonaceous particles in the lower airways

Treatment

In the presence of increasing laryngeal edema, establishment of a patent airway is indicated; usually endotracheal intubation is required.

Mechanical ventilation or humidified O_2.

Vigorous pulmonary toilet.

Bronchodilators as needed.

Sputum cultures.

Management of IV fluids to decrease the incidence of pulmonary edema and to maintain hemodynamic stability without compromising pulmonary function.

Treatments completed aseptically to prevent pneumonia, a lethal complication of burns.

TYPES OF PULMONARY INJURY (Continued)

UPPER AIRWAY INJURY

Direct exposure to superheated air at temperatures >150°F can cause burns of the face, nose, oropharynx, and larynx above the trachea.

Reflex closure of the glottis prevents further injury to the lower airway.

Superheated steam is capable of burning the respiratory tract to the bronchioles because it has a greater heat-carrying capacity (4000 times greater) than air.

Signs and Symptoms

Heat injury to the mucosa results in erythema, ulcerations, and edema. When associated with face and neck burns, airway obstruction increases from increased edema.

Suspect this injury if physical examination shows the following:

1. Burns of the face and neck.
2. Carbon deposits in mouth and throat; singed nasal hairs and nares.
3. Inflammation of nasal and buccal mucosa with posterior pharyngeal swelling.
4. Tachypnea, respiratory distress, hoarseness, cough, anxiety, stridor, disorientation, combative behavior, sore throat, and dysphagia.

Treatment

Early endotracheal intubation is indicated. Airway edema forms in the first hour after injury, leading to difficulty in intubation as signs of tracheal edema worsen.

RESTRICTIVE DEFECT

This defect is caused by third-degree or circumferential burns of the chest and/or neck, inhalation of smoke, and aggressive fluid therapy.

The inelastic quality of the eschar and splinting effect of the edema in the burn area prohibit lung expansion.

Noncardiogenic pulmonary edema can occur and can decrease lung compliance.

Signs and Symptoms

Abdominal respirations	Decreased tidal volume
Severely restricted respiratory excursion	Increased respirations
Inability to ventilate with an endotracheal tube in place	Decreased PaO_2

Treatment

Escharotomies may have to be performed to allow for proper respiratory excursion and adequate ventilation.

Signs and symptoms of diminished blood flow begin 1 hour after burn injury. Assess pulses hourly using an ultrasonic Doppler. Elevate the affected limb. In the absence of pulses and with positive symptoms of decreased perfusion, an escharotomy must be performed to release the constriction and increase blood flow to compromised limbs. An escharotomy is a linear excision that extends through the eschar down to the superficial fat.

NURSING MANAGEMENT OF THE PATIENT WITH BURNS: EMERGENT, ACUTE, AND REHABILITATION

The management of burn care is usually divided into three overlapping stages: emergent, acute, and rehabilitation (Table 55–5).

Emergent Stage

Critical management of the wound is essential at the time of injury. The burning process must be halted;

clothes must be removed; and the wound must be cooled with tepid water or normal sterile saline to decrease depth and extent of the injury. These steps are followed by the ABCs (airway, breathing, circulation) of trauma resuscitation (see Chapter 54). Every attempt must be made to stabilize the patient; to control any hemorrhage, fractures, or suspected injuries;

TABLE 55–5
Stages of Burn Care

Stage	Duration
I (emergent)	From onset of injury to completion of fluid resuscitation
II (acute)	From start of diuresis to near completion of wound closure
III (rehabilitation)	From wound closure to return of optimal level of physical and psychosocial function

TABLE 55–6
Fluid Resuscitation Formulas

	Crystalloids	Colloid	5% Dextrose/Water	Urine Output
First 24 Hours				
Evans	Normal saline 1 mL/kg wt per % burn	1 mL/kg wt per % burn	2000 mL	30–50 mL/h (adult)
Brooke	Lactated Ringer's 1.5 mL/kg wt per % burn	0.5 mL/kg wt per % burn	2000 mL	30–50 mL/h (adult)
Parkland (Baxter)	Lactated Ringer's 4 mL/kg wt per % burn	None	None	50–70 mL/h (adult)
	Rate of infusion for all formulas listed is as follows: ½ of the total in the first 8 hours ¼ of the total in the second 8 hours ¼ of the total in the third 8 hours			
Second 24 Hours				
Evans	Lactated Ringer's 0.5 mL/kg wt per % burn	0.5 mL/kg wt per % burn	1500–2000 mL	30–50 mL/h (adult)
Brooke	Lactated Ringer's 0.75 mL/kg wt per % burn	0.25 mL/kg wt per % burn	1500–2000 mL	30–50 mL/h (adult)
Parkland	None	700 to 2000 mL (adult)	Sufficient to maintain urine output	30–50 mL/h (adult)

and to maintain cervical spine control. Inhalation injury is suspected if the fire occurred in a closed space, if the face and neck are burned, if the nares or buccal mucosa are singed, if vocal changes are present, and if the patient is coughing carbonaceous particles. Treatment for hypovolemic shock is begun using one of the formulas in Table 55–6. The burn wound should not be treated at this time. The wound should be covered with clean blankets in an attempt to decrease the amount of contamination of the wound. Body temperature should be maintained.

As soon as possible, an accurate history should be obtained of how the injury occurred, what the burning agent was, and what occurred at the scene. This accurate account can aid in determining the severity of injury and any associated trauma. An accurate medical history at this time must also include allergies, current medications, past and present illnesses, and substance abuse. Crisis intervention and emotional support for the patient/family begins as the victim arrives in the emergency care facility. Burn care treatment modalities are explained, and the need for admission to a burn care facility is discussed.

Acute Stage

The acute phase of burn care begins with the start of diuresis and the stabilization of the burn victim after injury, usually 48 to 72 hours, and continues until wound healing is complete. A multidisciplinary approach to care begins, and complex care is provided. Major energies of the burn team are directed at managing the burn wound. Therapeutic goals include (1) providing pain relief; (2) providing adequate nutritional support; (3) maintaining fluid, electrolyte, and acid-base balance; (4) providing ongoing monitoring for complications; (5) providing emotional support to the patient and family; and (6) planning for rehabilitation and discharges.

Wound Management

Regardless of the etiology or extent of burn wound injury, the principles of wound care remain the same. Immediately stopping the burning process is the first priority in emergency care. Specific wound care is never initiated before stabilization of the burn-injured patient. Upon stabilization of the patient's condition, wound care begins. The four goals of wound care are (1) contain bacterial growth, (2) provide comfort, (3) facilitate the healing process, and (4) promote restoration and function.

Stages of Repair

Inflammatory Phase. Inflammation begins immediately and lasts about 72 hours after injury. The immediate response is vasoconstriction with fibrin clot formation. Damaged cells release histamine, serotonin, and intracellular enzymes, which disrupt endothelial membranes and increase capillary permeability. As a result, fluid and hydrophilic protein molecules leak into the interstitial space, leading to edema formation and intravascular volume depletion. Polymorphonuclear leukocytes (PMNs) move into the interstitial space. Monocytes convert to macrophages. PMNs and macrophages begin the repair process by attacking the foreign material, digesting this debris, and transporting it from the wound site.

Destructive Phase. The destructive phase lasts from day 1 to day 6. The PMNs and macrophages clear the wound of debris. Macrophages attract more macrophages to the wound site, which facilitates the healing process. These macrophages stimulate formation and multiplication of fibroblasts. With increased cellular activity, more enzymes are released to debride unwanted fibrin and necrotic material. Edema increases as protein is released from digested cells.

Proliferative Phase. In the proliferative phase, from day 3 to day 24, healing is evident. Fibroblasts, stimu-

RESEARCH APPLICATION: PAIN ASSESSMENT FROM PATIENTS WITH BURNS AND THEIR NURSES
Everett, JJ, et al. J Burn Care Rehabil 15:194, 1994.

Purpose: The purpose of this study was to investigate pain assessment ratings by both patients and nurses during burn wound debridement, to identify the relations among nurse and patient pain ratings, and to show how different patient and nurse variables are related to pain reports.

Methods: *Patients:* The total number of adult patients was 49: 11 women and 38 men, with a mean age of 38.3 years. The percentage of burn area ranged from 1% to 69%, with a mean of 14%. Each patient had wound care once or twice daily.

Nurses: A total of 27 registered nurses participated: 24 women and 3 men. Nursing experience was as follows: a mean of 4.1 years and a median of 5.0 years. Years of experience working in a burn unit were as follows: a mean of 7.5 years and a median of 2 years. Fifteen nurses had AD degrees, 3 had BS degrees, and 9 had BSN degrees.

Measures: Both patients and nurses used the Visual Analog Scales (VAS) to estimate pain during wound care.

Procedures: Shortly after wound care was completed, VAS measures were obtained on a daily basis at a regional university-based burn center. The total number of pairs of nurse/patient ratings were 123.

Results: The nurses' and patients' mean VAS overall ratings were essentially equal. The mean absolute difference between paired nurse and patient VAS overall scores was 1.27 cm. There were no differences in low and high worst pain groups for age, total BSA, or sex. Nurses were able to accurately assess patients' pain 53.7% of the time. The accuracy of pain estimation was not found to be related to either nursing experience, burn nursing experience, or educational level. Nurses' VAS ratings for overall pain were highly correlated with both patients' worst pain and overall pain.

Practice Implications: Even though the correlation between nurse and patient ratings was strong, many of the nurse ratings failed to be within the 1.0-cm accuracy range. Therefore, there is a lack of agreement between the nurse and patient pain ratings despite a high correlation. Nurses do, however, have some ability to correctly estimate pain from burns. Providing appropriate forms or guidelines to assist nurses in identifying pain behavior may help to increase the nurses' accuracy.

lated by an acidic environment, begin synthesis of collagen, the principal component of connective tissue, and mucopolysaccharides. Early collagen synthesis is disorganized, and the quality of the synthesis will depend on tissue vascularity and perfusion. The increased cellular and chemical activity results in the formation of granulation tissue along fragile capillary loops supported by collagen fibers. Granulation tissue will remain highly vascular, fragile, and dusky red in color.

Maturation Phase. The maturation phase begins on day 24 and lasts for years. Progressively, vascularity of the scar decreases. Fibroblasts exit the wound, and collagen fibers strengthen and reorient. The wound changes from a dusky red of vascular granulation to a pale white avascular scar. Gradually, the skin softens and tissues flatten. During this plase, hypertrophic scar or keloid formation becomes evident and may require surgical intervention or preventive measures to control the scar formation.

Other Healing Processes

Contracture. Wound healing by contracture is especially important when there is a great deal of tissue loss. Healing occurs from wound edges converging at the center of the wound. Myofibroblasts are necessary for this type of wound closure, which begins on the fourth day. Cell viability at the edge of the wound con-tributes to the ability of contractures to heal the wound.

Epithelialization. Epithelialization occurs by the migratory effort of new cells over live epithelial cells in the wound, usually around the skin appendages not totally destroyed in the injury. Epithelial cells usually form under eschar as the healing progresses. In large wounds, eschar or a dressing can protect these fragile cells from trauma.

Other factors that influence the healing process are (1) hemostasis, (2) hypovolemia, (3) infection, (4) inadequate nutrition, and (5) dressing type.

Definitive Wound Care

Cleansing and debridement of the burn wound must be a daily procedure to promote healing and decrease the risk of infection. The wound is inspected for suspect areas, and wound cultures are obtained. Confirmed invasive burn wound sepsis mandates aggressive therapies with the use of topical antimicrobials and systemic antibiotics.

Wound cleansing can be accomplished by tubbing, using a Hubbard tank; by showering, using a shower trolley or shower chair; and by bedside dressing changes.

Debridement. Debridement of eschar, or nonviable tissue, from the burn wound helps to control infection and prepares the wound for skin grafting. Mechanical debridement involves cutting away dead tissue from viable granulation bed. Chemical debridement, with the use of proteolytic enzymes, aids in the initial debridement before a patient can tolerate surgery. Easily applied, these agents selectively digest necrotic soft tissue without harming viable tissue. These agents are not bactericidal, may cause bleeding, and may be irritating to the wound or surrounding tissues; therefore, dressings need to be changed more frequently, at least every 8 hours. Surgical debridement is the excision of burn wounds. This is indicated in the treatment of full-thickness and deep partial-thickness burns of special areas and for early closure of the wound.

Selection of Burn Dressing. Selection of a burn dressing includes selection of a method of treatment, a topical agent, and design of the dressing. Many topical agents are used in burn wound care (Table 55–7). Dressing types are influenced by area, extent, and depth of injury (Table 55–8).

Dressing design depends on the status of the wound. Protective dressings are used on clean healing wounds. If mechanical debridement is needed, dressings can be used to cleanse the surface of the wound. Bulky dressings can be based on the need for absorption of fluids from the wound. Some principles of burn wound dressings are as follows:

1. Wound surfaces must not be wrapped together.
2. Limit the bulk of dressing to facilitate maximum mobility.
3. Individualize dressing based on the need for absorption, debridement, or protection.
4. Wrap extremities distal to proximal to promote venous return.
5. Ace-wrap dependent areas to limit edema formation and bleeding and to facilitate graft take.

Wound Healing: Therapeutic Modalities

The overall goal of wound care in burn therapy is wound closure with minimal scarring. This is accomplished with autografting, beginning 48 to 72 hours after injury when stabilization of the patient is complete. An autograft is a skin graft from an unburned area on the burn victim to be placed on a clean excised wound. The grafts used for burn wound closure are split-thickness skin grafts (STSGs), which are a partial thickness of epidermis and dermis; or full-thickness skin grafts (FTSGs), which include the entire thickness of the dermal layer.

STSG may be applied as a meshed graft, which can be expanded 1½ to 9 times its original size to cover a large wound, or as a sheet graft for cosmetic effect. The STSG is nourished by an osmotic exchange of tissue nutrients until healing is complete. Graft take is complete in 3 to 5 days when collagen strands have attached the graft to the base supporting tissues and an effective blood supply develops.

FTSGs are used over areas of muscle mass or soft tissue loss. A type of FTSG is a pedicle graft, or flap,

TABLE 55–7
Topical Antibiotic Agents

Agent	Dressings	Advantages	Disadvantages
Silver sulfadiazine 1% cream	Buttered on. With light dressings once or twice a day.	Broad spectrum. Low toxicity. Painless, easy to apply and remove. Can be used with or without dressings.	Intermediate penetration of eschar; leukopenia.
Mafenide acetate (Sulfamylon)	Buttered on. Open exposure method. Applied 3–4 times daily.	Broad spectrum. Rapid, deep penetration of eschar. Rapid excretion.	Pain on application. Pulmonary toxicity. Metabolic acidosis. Inhibits wound healing. Hypersensitivity.
Silver nitrate solution 0.5%	Wet dressings. Change bid. Resoak every 2 h.	Broad spectrum. Nonallergenic. Low toxicity. Inexpensive. Does not interfere with healing.	Poor penetration of eschar. Ineffective on established wound infections. Can cause an electrolyte imbalance. Discoloration of wound and environment makes assessment difficult.
Povidone-iodine	Buttered on. Used with or without dressing 1–2 times daily.	Broad spectrum. Antifungal. Low toxicity. Eases debriding by tanning of eschar.	Poor penetration of eschar. Pain on application. Iodine sensitivity. Metabolic acidosis. Absorption of iodine.
Bacitracin	Buttered on. Reapply every 4–6 h.	No pain. Clear, odorless. Useful for face burns. Softens eschar.	Poor penetration of eschar. Not effective in reducing sepsis in large burns. Occasional allergic sensitivity.
Gentamicin	Apply gently 3–4 times daily.	Broad spectrum. May be covered or left open to air.	Ototoxic. Nephrotoxic. Pain on application.
Nitrofurazone	Apply thin layer directly to wounds or impregnate into gauze. Change dressings twice daily.	Bactericidal. Broad spectrum.	Painful application. May lead to overgrowth of fungus and pseudomonas.

TABLE 55–8
Dressing Types

Method	Advantage	Disadvantage
Open exposure (no topical dressings)	Wound is always visible for inspection. Bacterial growth is suppressed by the drying effect of air. Facilitates physical therapy. Especially used for burns of face, neck, ear, and perineum.	Increases heat loss. Requires strict isolation. Requires frequent linen changes. Open to both direct and indirect transmission of contamination. Cannot be effective with uncooperative children and adults. Increases discomfort from exposure of wounds.
Semi-open exposure (light dressings)	Patient is more mobile. Frequent observation of the wound. Patient can be treated on an outpatient basis.	On an outpatient basis, dressings must be changed at least three times a week. Requires skilled personnel.
Closed-occlusive (inner layer of fine mesh gauze or coarse mesh gauze; after layer of roll gauze)	Decreases pain. Decreases exposure to bacterial contamination. Can be treated on an outpatient basis with minimal dressing changes. Increases absorption of fluid and exudate into dressing. Aids in immobilizing injured areas. Decreases evaporative fluid losses. Facilitates debridement.	Decreases effectiveness of topical agents. Limitation of mobility. Decreased wound observation may delay diagnosis of wound infection. Partial-thickness injury may convert to full-thickness injury.

in which the flap includes not only skin and subcutaneous tissue but also an artery and vein. However, FTSGs are not used for extensive full-thickness wounds because the donor sites also require an STSG to heal.

Cadaver skin; synthetics, such as Op Site; semisynthetics, such as Biobrane or artificial skin; and biologic dressings, such as pigskin, may be used as temporary wound coverings over clean partial- and full-thickness injuries. These dressings can decrease pain, evaporative water loss, bacterial proliferation, and dessication of a viable wound surface. These skin substitutes can be used to maintain a wound surface until healing occurs or the wound is in condition for autografting as donor skin becomes available.

Rehabilitation Stage

Survival in any burn victim is the immediate goal after injury. The scarring process and the potential for severe deformity, however, cannot be overlooked or accepted on the basis of burn severity. Rather, aggressive treatment of burns should begin during the acute stage, once the patient's condition is stabilized, and such therapy should continue throughout the rehabilitation stage.

During the rehabilitation stage, two conditions of the burn wound must be recognized: (1) the position of comfort is the position of contracture, and (2) the burn wound will shorten until it meets an opposing force. Contractures can be avoided by starting patients on an active exercise program 24 to 48 hours after burn injury. Gentle sustained stretching with the use of splinting devices can be used to maintain a range of motion. Effective therapeutic positioning requires

a full team effort and support. These critically ill immobile patients require frequent repositioning to achieve rehabilitation.

Rehabilitation is often a long process, not only encompassing physical injuries but also the psychosocial care of the patient and family. Changes in self-image and lifestyle may be required. Reconstructive surgery may be necessary to address functional and cosmetic problems. Counseling for the patient and family is a necessary component of care. This phase of care provides many challenges for the patient, family, and healthcare providers.

NURSING DIAGNOSES, DESIRED PATIENT OUTCOMES, AND NURSING INTERVENTIONS

Nursing diagnoses, desired patient outcomes, nursing interventions, and rationales for the management of the patient with major burns through the phases of care are presented in the care plan at the end of this chapter.

CASE STUDY: PATIENT WITH BURNS

A 43-year-old woman is admitted to the emergency room. Her history was significant for sustaining thermal burns in an enclosed space during a house fire. The patient required intubation at the scene and was transported about 1½ hours after injury. Third-degree burns totaling 35% BSA included her posterior torso, buttocks, and patchy areas of her lower and upper extremeties. The patient was lethargic and confused. Her carboxyhemoglobin level at the time of admission was 30%, with sooty sputum, rales, and a respiratory rate of 24. She has a history of hypertension and smokes one pack per day.

REFERENCE

1. Trofino, RBT: Nursing Care of the Burn-Injured Patient. FA Davis, Philadelphia, 1991, p 16.

SUGGESTED READINGS

Achaer, BM and Martinez, SE: Burn wound pathophysiology and care. Crit Care Clin 1:47, March 1985.
Aggarwal, SJ, et al: Burn induced alterations in vasoactive function of the peripheral cutaneous microcirculation. J Burn Care Rehabil 15:1–12, 1994.
Arturson, MG: The pathophysiology of severe thermal injury. J Burn Care Rehabil 6:129, 1985.
Artz, CP, Moncrief, JA, and Pruitt, BA: Burns: A Team Approach. WB Saunders, Philadelphia, 1979.
Baxter, C and Waeckerle, J: Emergency treatment of burn injury. Ann Emerg Med 17:1305–1314, 1988.
Bayley, EW and Smith, GA: The three degrees of burn care. Nursing 17(3):34, March 1987.
Boswick, JA: The Art and Science of Burn Care. Aspen Publishers, Rockville, Maryland, 1987.
Constable, JD: The state of burn care: past, present and future. Burns 20(4):316, August 1994.
Dressler, DP, Hozid, JL, and Nathan, P: Thermal Injury. CV Mosby, St. Louis, 1988.
Geisser, ME, et al: Pain and anxiety during burn dressing changes: Concordance between patients' and nurses' ratings and relation to medication administration and patient variables. J Burn Care Rehabil 16:165–172, 1995.
Kuehn, C, Ahrenholz, D, and Solem, L: Care of the burn wound. Trauma 5(4):34–35, 1989.
Mikhail, JN: Acute burn care: An update. J Emerg Nurs 14:9, 1988.
Ogle, CK, et al: A long term study and correlation of lymphocyte and neutrophil function in the patient with burns. J Burn Care Rehabil 11:105, 1990.
Powers, PS, et al: Safety and efficacy of debridement under anesthesia in patients with burns. J Burn Care Rehabil 14:176–80, 1993.
Trofino, RBT: Nursing Care of the Burn-Injured Patient. FA Davis, Philadelphia, 1991.
Wagner, M: Care of the Burn-Injured Patient: A Multidisciplinary Approach. Publishing Sciences Group, Littleton, MA, 1980.

CARE PLAN FOR THE PATIENT WITH THERMAL INJURY

Nursing Diagnoses

Nursing Diagnosis #1
Impairment of skin integrity, related to thermal injury: dry/moist heat, chemical or electrical

Desired Patient Outcomes

The patient will:
1. Have the burning process halted
2. Maintain a skin pH near normal
3. Have no complaints of burning on the wound
4. Maintain a decrease in the degree of corneal ulcerations and eye infection
5. Have burned areas healed with no infection present
6. Maintain adequate body temperature and perfusion

Nursing Interventions

- Assess burning process. If fire or scald injury and heat are evident on the wound, cool the area with tap water.
- Remove clothing and jewelry

- Do not apply ice.

- Cover patient with clean sheet or blanket.

- Obtain history of the burning agent.

- Initiate extensive lavage with tepid-to-cool water for all chemical burns along with simultaneous removal of contaminated clothing. Brush off dry chemicals before lavage.

- If eyes are affected, lavage with a minimum of 2 to 3 L of normal sterile saline. If blepharospasm occurs during irrigation, apply topical ophthalmic anesthetic agent as prescribed.

Rationales

- Depth of injury increases from length of exposure to the burning agent.
- Clothing, jewelry, belts, etc., retain heat and can increase depth of injury.
- Vasoconstriction occurs, damaging the surrounding tissues. Core temperature decreases.
- Prevents excessive heat loss. Body heat is lost through the burned area.
- Decreases pain from exposure to air.
- Protects from emergency room contamination.
- Provides information on agent as extent and depth of injury are directly related to the concentration, activity, and penetrability of the chemical; also, duration of contact and the resistance of tissues affect severity of injury.
- Dilution of the chemical and removal of the chemical from the injured tissues will halt the burning process. Although some chemicals create heat when united with water, copious lavage can dissipate that heat away from the body. (Healthcare workers must protect themselves from exposure to chemicals.)
- Important to remove all chemicals from the eyes to preserve sight. (Blepharospasm refers to a twitching or spasm of orbicularis oculi muscle.)

CARE PLAN FOR THE PATIENT WITH THERMAL INJURY (*Continued*)

Nursing Diagnoses

Nursing Diagnosis #2
Impaired gas exchange, related to:
1. Upper airway edema
2. Carbon monoxide poisoning
3. Smoke inhalation injury
4. Disruption of alveolar-capillary membrane
5. Heat-damaged tracheal-bronchial tissue

Desired Patient Outcomes

The patient will:
1. Have a CO level less than 10%
2. Maintain a patent airway
3. Maintain acceptable blood gas parameters:
   - pH ~ 7.35–7.45
4. Maintain clear lung sounds
5. Maintain respiratory pattern regular and unlabored
6. Maintain PaO_2 80–100 mm Hg
7. Maintain $PaCO_2$ 35–45 mmHg
8. Have effective mobilization of secretions
9. Be responsive, awake, and cognizant of the surroundings

Nursing Interventions

- Assess for signs or symptoms of tracheal obstruction and respiratory distress, as indicated in Table 55–5.

- Establish an airway. Administer humidified oxygen at 100%.
- Monitor arterial blood gases and CO level.

- Elevate head of bed.
- Monitor intake and output.

- Obtain sputum cultures. Note color, amount, and consistency of pulmonary secretions. Note carbonaceous sputum.

- Assess arterial pH.

- Assess chest x-ray.

- Prepare for endotracheal intubation and mechanical ventilation with positive signs and symptoms of inhalation injury.
- Assess breath sounds for abnormalities: wheezing.

  ○ Rales
- Prepare for bronchoscopy.
- Administer prescribed bronchodilators as indicated.

- Begin vigorous pulmonary toilet.
  ○ Suction frequently.
  ○ Use incentive spirometer every 2–4 h.
  ○ Turn, cough, and deep-breathe every 2–4 h.

- Assess chest wall excursion and the use of accessory muscles for breathing.

Rationales

- Upper airway edema with smoke inhalation can cause a rapid, progressive airway obstruction leading to respiratory arrest.
- Promotes oxygenation to maintain adequate PaO_2.

- CO and acute airway obstruction are the greatest threats to life immediately after burn injury. CO level of more than 10% to 20% is indicative of CO poisoning.
- Decreases swelling of face and neck.
- Assists in modification of fluid therapy. Adequate hydration aids in liquefying secretions. Overhydration leads to pulmonary edema.
- Infectious agents will change color, consistency, and amount of sputum. Carbonaceous sputum is diagnostic for smoke inhalation.
- Monitors microbial growth and assists in selection of appropriate antibiotic therapy.
- Patient will demonstrate a metabolic acidosis from decreased tissue perfusion.
- This may initially be negative but may demonstrate inflammation or pulmonary edema in 12–24 h after burn injury.
- Early intubation before the development of airway obstruction is preferred over tracheostomy because of the increased chance of infection from tracheostomy.
- Wheezing is heard across all lung fields because of edema and inflammation caused by carbon deposits and damage to the airways.
  ○ Rales can occur 12–24 h after injury.
- Bronchoscopy will be diagnostic for inhalation injury.
- Respiratory pharmacologic agents decrease bronchospasms and mucosal edema.
- Frequent suctioning of smoke inhalation victims is necessary to clear the airway of copious secretions and carbon deposits.
  ○ This must be completed aseptically to prevent the lethal complication of pneumonia.
  ○ Mobilizes secretions and promotes lung expansion.
- For severe burns of the neck and chest, eschar and edema formation create a splinting effect that prohibits lung expansion.

CARE PLAN FOR THE PATIENT WITH THERMAL INJURY (*Continued*)

Nursing Interventions

- With positive signs of restrictive defect, prepare for escharotomy.

Rationales

- Eschar is released by cutting the eschar on both sides of the chest and from the zyphoid process and/or sternal notch to the outer chest wall.

Nursing Diagnoses

Nursing Diagnosis #3
Fluid volume deficit, related to:
1. Capillary leak—loss of plasma proteins
2. Insensible water loss
3. Decreased fluid intake

Desired Patient Outcomes

The patient will be maintained with adequate circulating volume and cardiac output, as evidenced by:
1. Urine output of 50 mL/h. If hemochromogens* are in the urine, an output of 100 mL/h is maintained.
2. Adequate blood pressure, as evidenced by an arterial systolic pressure of about 100 mmHg and urine output maintained as above.
3. Heart rate: ~ 100 beats/min.
4. Hemoglobin and hematocrit within normal range.
5. Stabilized body weight.

Nursing Interventions

- Obtain admission weight and monitor weight daily.

- Monitor for signs and symptoms of hypovolemia, including hypotension, tachycardia, tachypnea, extreme thirst, restlessness, disorientation.

- Administer IV fluids according to fluid resuscitation formulas in Table 55–6. Insert large-bore IV catheter.

  ○ Prepare for the insertion of subclavian catheters and arterial lines.

  ○ Send blood specimens for determination of hematocrit and hemoglobin, electrolytes, prothrombin/partial thromboplastin times, blood sugar, BUN, and creatinine.

- Insert indwelling urinary catheter.

  ○ Monitor urine for amount, specific gravity, and the presence of hemochromogens.

  ○ Administer osmotic diuretics as ordered, and monitor response to diuretic therapy.

- Monitor serum pH. Administer prescribed sodium bicarbonate.
- Continue to monitor hourly for the effectiveness of fluid resuscitation.
- Assess gastrointestinal function: absence of bowel sounds.

  ○ Insert a nasogastric tube and attach to suction.

Rationales

- Assesses weight gains and losses common to fluid shifting. Measures fluid loss.
- Fluid volume is lost through increased capillary permeability, which begins at the time of injury. Insensible fluid loss through the burn wound contributes to decreasing circulation volume.
- Fluid resuscitation begins immediately. IV placement should be in large vessels for the rapid delivery of fluid.
  ○ Difficulty of peripheral IV insertion is caused by vasoconstriction and volume depletion.
  ○ With the insertion of subclavian catheters, hemodynamics can be more accurately assessed and monitored.
  ○ Hemodynamic status is also assessed through the laboratory data.
  ○ Increased potassium (K^+) is due to cellular trauma, which releases K^+ into extracellular fluid.
  ○ Sodium is lost from the circulation as edema forms.
  ○ Metabolic acidosis results from the loss of bicarbonate ions with the sodium.
- Most effective measurement of volume replacement at this time is a urine output of 50–100 mL/h.
  ○ Specific gravity can predict the volume replacement.
  ○ Myoglobin is released in the bloodstream from muscle damage, especially in electrical injuries. Hemoglobin is released through the destruction of red blood cells. These hemochromogens can cause renal-tubular obstruction. Osmotic diuretics can aid in reversing this process.
  ○ Decreased urinary output can be a result of decreased renal blood flow, increased secretion of antidiuretic hormone, increased adrenocortical activity.
- Correct the metabolic acidosis that results from vasoconstriction and tissue ischemia.
- Hypervolemia will lead to increased edema and pulmonary congestion.
- Splanchnic constriction as a result of hypovolemia leads to paralytic ileus.
  ○ Paralytic ileus occurs in burn victims with a > 20%– 25% total body surface burn.

CARE PLAN FOR THE PATIENT WITH THERMAL INJURY (*Continued*)

Nursing Interventions

- ○ Monitor gastric pH every 1–2 h. Administer antacids via nasogastric tube as prescribed to maintain a gastric pH > 5.
- Record all intake and output hourly. Record hourly specific gravity.

Rationales

- ○ Antacids help neutralize gastric secretions. Antacids decrease the risk of Curling's ulcer related to stress.
- Serves as a guide to fluid loss and replacement.

Nursing Diagnoses

Nursing Diagnosis #4
Pain, related to:
1. Exposure of nerve endings in partial-thickness burns
2. Donor site area

Desired Patient Outcomes

The patient will:
1. Receive assistance in controlling the pain
2. Verbalize that the pain is tolerable
3. Receive validation that the pain exists

Nursing Interventions

- Assess level of pain through verbalization, facial expression, and body positioning. Rate pain or have patient rate pain on a visual analogue scale.
- Assess the degree and duration of pain during painful procedures, such as wound care and exercise.
- Observe for varied responses to pain:
  - ○ Increases in blood pressure, pulse, and respiratory rate
  - ○ Facial grimaces
  - ○ Guarding
  - ○ Increased irritability and restlessness
  - ○ Increased muscle tension
- Decrease the anxiety of the patient through the use of relaxation, distraction, or music.

- Acknowledge the presence of pain. Explain the causes of pain in burn injury.

- Provide privacy for painful therapies.
- Decrease the fear associated with pain and the use of narcotics.
- Motivate the patient to participate in noninvasive methods to reduce the intensity of pain.

- Administer narcotic analgesics as prescribed to provide optimal relief:
  - ○ Administer IV narcotics during the emergent phase.

  - ○ Administer narcotics as often as necessary during the acute phase, especially before dressing change and exercise.

  - ○ Assess adequate doses of drugs. Assess the patient's response to the medication. Recommend increasing prescribed doses as necessary.
- Decrease the amount of narcotic analgesia as the burn wound heals.

Rationales

- Monitors individual responses to therapy, pain, and changes in pain response. Monitors subjective sensations. Changes in pain may indicate developing complications.

- Responses to pain are variable. These parameters change in response to pain.

- Relaxation can reduce intensity.
  - ○ Acute anxiety can be related to anger or guilt about the accident and the chance of survival.
- In partial-thickness injury, the presence of prostaglandins and histamines in and around the injured area stimulates peripheral pain receptors and intensifies central perceptions of discomfort. Full-thickness burns initially are painless, but as the nerve endings regenerate, pain occurs from exposure to air.
- Patients feel a loss of control during painful modalities.
- Patients frequently will not ask for medication for fear of becoming addicted to a drug.
- Patients exhibit wide variability in both pain perception and response to pain, attributed to sociological background and previous pain threshold.
  - ○ How the injury occurred also contributes to the patient's response.

  - ○ Because of the capillary leak, intramuscular medications are not absorbed adequately to provide acute pain relief.
  - ○ Inadequate narcotic doses are frequently prescribed because of the fear by the medical professionals of producing respiratory depression or addiction to a narcotic.
  - ○ Careful titration of narcotic doses can provide adequate pain relief.
- At the time of discharge, the patient's pain should be adequately controlled with oral agents.

CARE PLAN FOR THE PATIENT WITH THERMAL INJURY (*Continued*)

Nursing Interventions
- Maintain comfortable environment:
  - Bed cradle
  - Quiet environment
  - Environmental temperature 86°–91.4°F

Rationales
- Pressure from bed linens may cause discomfort. With loss of integument, body is unable to self-regulate environmental changes in temperature.

Nursing Diagnoses

Nursing Diagnosis #5
Alteration in peripheral perfusion, related to:
1. Circumferential eschar
2. Compartment syndrome
3. Release of myocardial depressant factor

Desired Patient Outcomes

The patient will have:
1. Pulses present and of good quality distal to burn area on limbs
2. Extremities warm to touch
3. Edema minimized to prevent vascular compromise

Nursing Interventions
- Assess pulses on burned extremities every 15 min. Use the ultrasonic Doppler as necessary. Assess capillary refill, color, swelling, and motion.

- Assess for numbness, tingling, and increased pain in the burned extremity.
- Elevate burned extremities above the level of the heart.

- Apply burn dressing loosely.
- Assess muscle compartment pressure.

  - If signs and symptoms of circulatory impairment and inadequate deep tissue perfusion are present, prepare the patient for escharotomy and/or fasciotomy.
- Measure circumference of burned extremity.
  - Monitor cardiac output if pulmonary catheter is in place.
  - Monitor urine output

Rationales
- As edema forms on circumferential burns, eschar forms a tight constricting band, decreasing the circulation to the limb distal to the circumferential site. Assess peripheral perfusion.
- Increasing pain in extremities can be predictive of increasing pressure from tight bands.
- Elevation of the limb promotes venous return and decreases edema.
- To allow for expansion as edema forms.
- Increasing pressure readings from muscle compartments are indicative of decreased tissue perfusion.
  - These surgical procedures will release constricting eschar bands and improve deep tissue perfusion.

- Assists in identifying edema formation.
  - Indicator of fluid volume deficit and cardiac function to determine replacement needs.
  - Assesses adequacy of circulation and maintenance of renal perfusion.

Nursing Diagnoses

Nursing Diagnosis #6
Potential for sepsis, related to wound infection. (Refer to Table 56–1 and the care plan at the end of Chapter 56.)

Desired Patient Outcomes

The patient will have:
1. Healthy granulation tissue on unhealed areas with < 10^5 colonies of bacteria as demonstrated on wound culture
2. Absence of clinical manifestation of infection (body temperature, white blood cell count)
3. Skin graft sites that have taken
4. Donor sites that are free of infection

Nursing Interventions
- Use sterile technique when caring for the burn wound.
- Maintain protective isolation with good handwashing technique.
- Administer immunosupportive medications as prescribed: tetanus, gamma globulin.
- Perform wound care as prescribed:
  - Inspect and debride wounds daily; culture wounds three times a week or at any sign of infection; shave all burned areas, especially the scalp and invasive line site for inflammation, especially if the line is through a burn area.

Rationales
- Burn wound is a culture medium for bacterial growth.
- Prevent the spread of bacteria from patient to patient.

- Immunoglobulins are depressed at the time of severe burn injury.
- Provides quick identification of bacterial wound invasion and decreases the incidence of septic episodes.

CARE PLAN FOR THE PATIENT WITH THERMAL INJURY (*Continued*)

Nursing Interventions
- Monitor the patient constantly for signs and symptoms of sepsis: temperature, sensorium, vital signs, increase/ decrease in bowel sounds, decreased output, fluid translocation; positive blood/wound cultures.
- Administer systemic antibiotics as prescribed and monitor response to therapy.

Rationales
- The burn patient will experience several septic episodes during hospitalization until the burn wound is healed.

- Judicious use of antibiotics can decrease the incidence of drug-resistant organism development.

Nursing Diagnoses
Nursing Diagnosis #7
Alteration in nutrition, related to:
1. Inadequate intake caused by inability to eat, therapeutic regimen, or multiple surgeries
2. Increased metabolic demands

Desired Patient Outcomes

The patient is:
1. Maintained within 10% of preburn weight
2. Healing burn wound
3. In a positive nitrogen balance

Nursing Interventions
- Institute enteral feedings as soon as bowel sounds are present.
- Ensure required caloric and protein intake by:
  ○ Having a dietitian calculate caloric needs.
  ○ Accurate calorie counts; accurate intake and output; daily weights.
- If tube feedings are needed to supplement caloric needs, insert a feeding tube, assess patency and placement every 4 h, place patient in a semi-Fowler's position:
  ○ Assess for gastric residuals at least every 4 h.
  ○ Assess bowel sounds every 2 to 4 h.
  ○ Increase feeding regimen as prescribed.
  ○ Monitor for adverse side effects, such as diarrhea or gastric distention.
  ○ Accurately document amount of feeding administered.
- Avoid painful procedures during feeding times.

Rationales
- The burn patient may require up to 4000 calories per day.
- Formulas have been developed to assess necessary caloric needs using total BSA burn (see Chapter 9).
  ○ Maintenance of protein mass is critical to survival.

- Burn victims frequently require more calories than they are able to eat.
- Frequent treatment modalities and surgeries interrupt feeding schedules.
  ○ Absence of bowel sounds is frequently the first sign of impending sepsis.
  ○ If the patient is unable to tolerate enteral feedings, hyperalimentation may need to be considered.

- Severe pain decreases desire to eat.

Nursing Diagnoses
Nursing Diagnosis #8
Impairment of activity, related to:
1. Re-formation of collagen
2. Excisional wound therapy
3. Auto-grafting

Desired Patient Outcomes

The patient will:
1. Maintain positioning as prescribed during multiple surgeries
2. Be able to perform activities of daily living
3. Be ambulatory with no assistive devices
4. Retain full range of motion of all affected joints

Nursing Interventions
- Assess the need for positioning and/or splinting.
  ○ Consult occupational therapy.

  ○ Apply splints and check frequently for fit or areas of pressure.
  ○ Clean splints at least every shift. Evaluate the need for continuous splinting or night-time use only.
  ○ Encourage patient to exercise burned limbs and to actively participate in as many activities of daily living as possible.
- Observe the burn wound closely for any exposed tendons, unresolved edema, peripheral neuropathies, or points of pressure.
- Assess problem areas:

Rationales
- Attempt to maintain neutral positioning of burned areas.
- Maintain a stretch of skin to decrease the pull of contracture.
  ○ As edema subsides, splints might need revision.

  ○ Decrease contamination of the burn wounds.

- Rapid identification of problem areas helps to decrease additional injury to burned areas.

CARE PLAN FOR THE PATIENT WITH THERMAL INJURY (*Continued*)

Nursing Interventions

- ○ Position patient with neck burns in extension. Use no pillow.
- ○ Inspect ears frequently.
- ○ Position patient with axilla burns in 90-degree shoulder abduction and 10-degree elbow flexion.
- ○ Use special skin care and topical agent of choice after each voiding or defecation.
- ○ For facial injuries elevate head of the bed. Lubricate lips every 4 h.
- • Inspect the burn wound for early signs of webbing, contracture, banding, or keloid formation.

Rationales

- ○ Prevent the development of neck contractures.
- ○ Pressure can cause necrosis, and bending can cause chondritis.
- ○ Prevent the formation of scar bands in the axilla.
- ○ Prevent infection or contamination of the burn wound.
- ○ Decrease edema formation. Avoid lips that crack and bleed.
- • Quick identification of defects can lead to reversal through the use of splints or pressure.

Nursing Diagnoses

Nursing Diagnosis #9

Ineffective coping of individual/significant others, related to:

1. Trauma of burns
2. Family loss
3. Lack of knowledge of the disease process
4. Surgical procedures
5. Expected outcomes
6. Role changes caused by hospitalization
7. Prolonged hospitalization

Desired Patient Outcomes

The patient/significant other will:

1. Demonstrate acceptance of the accident with a decreased level of anxiety
2. Verbalize fears, grief, and acceptance of an altered body image
3. Verbalize treatment modalities, process of skin healing, and scar/contracture formation
4. Develop supportive behaviors

Nursing Interventions

- • Assess patient/significant other for level of understanding of burn treatment.
- • Describe the pathophysiology of the burn process and what the patient will experience.
- • Explain the precautionary isolation of the victim.
- • Assist and identify the coping mechanisms of both patient/significant other. Provide time for questions and discussion of feelings and fears.
- • Be honest. Do not protect the patient/significant other from necessary emotional experiences.

- • Keep patient and significant others informed of the progress of the patient.
- • Explain all procedures and enlist the patient's cooperation.
- • Develop a contract with the patient/significant other and set realistic short-term goals. Allow the patient to make decisions and choices when possible.
- • Approach and administer care in a consistent, positive manner. Carry out your part of the contract regardless of the patient's behavior.
- • Administer sedatives and analgesics as needed.
- • Provide adequate rest time.
- • Encourage discussion of feelings, family, and future plans.
- • Support and encourage the patient to participate in self-care. Provide assistive devices.
- • Recommend a psychiatric consult if the patient/significant other needs help in coping.
- • Refer the patient/significant other to appropriate resources for aid: burn support groups; social services; rehabilitation centers; financial services.

Rationales

- • At high-stress times, repetition is necessary for understanding.
- • Attempt to enlist the support of the family in helping the patient cope with pain and disfigurement.

- • This event is disruptive to patient/significant other lifestyles, relationships, careers, and finances.

- ○ Frequently there are other injuries or deaths at the scene. Burn victims will ask about the outcome of loved ones. These concerns must be dealt with to enable the patient to cope with his/her injury.
- • If the burn is severe, the death and dying process needs to be instituted.
- • Painful procedures preclude patient cooperation.

- • Allows the patient to have some control over his/her environment. (Contracting is discussed in Chapter 3.)

- • The patient will be cognizant of the inability to manipulate staff. Burn patients frequently become combative, argumentative, and resistant to therapeutic modalities because of the pain.

- • Patients will experience a positive self-image as activities of daily living increase.
- • Patient/significant others frequently need help in dealing with body disfigurement and the long-term care needs.

PaO₂ = arterial oxygen pressure; PaCO₂ = arterial carbon dioxide pressure; IV = intravenous; BUN = blood urea nitrogen.
*Hemochromogens—compounds containing heme and a nitrogen-containing substance such as a protein.

CHAPTER 56

Nursing Management of the Patient with Septic Shock

Carol F. Evans

CHAPTER OUTLINE

LEARNING OBJECTIVES

After completing this chapter, you should be able to:

1. Define septic shock.
2. Identify causative microorganisms and their portal of entry.
3. List patients at high risk of developing septic shock.
4. Examine the pathophysiology underlying septic shock.
5. Differentiate between early and late signs and symptoms of septic shock based on the underlying pathophysiology.
6. Discuss approach to treatment of septic shock and its prevention.
7. Delineate the nursing process in caring for the patient with septic shock, including assessment, nursing diagnoses, and planning desired patient outcomes and nursing interventions/rationales.

Septic shock, like other forms of shock, is a syndrome which produces inadequate tissue oxygenation and impaired cellular function. It is a clinical problem posing a continuous challenge to physicians and nurses in the critical care setting. Multiple organ dysfunction or failure is a frequent consequence of septic shock and is a primary contributor to the high mortality rate. Despite advances in the treatment of infections and the management of shock, septic shock continues to be a major cause of death in intensive care units.[1–3]

DEFINITIONS

Table 56–1 lists the accepted definitions for septic shock and other terms discussed in this chapter. *Sepsis* is the body's response to overwhelming infection. In sepsis, the usually protective inflammatory response is intensified, leading to tissue and organ damage. *Septic* *shock* is a form of severe sepsis characterized by refractory hypotension and altered tissue perfusion. It frequently occurs with the failure of early interventions to improve hemodynamic status and tissue perfusion in the septic patient.

The sepsis response can be seen in clinical situations in which no infectious process is evident. The variety of clinical situations that produce a sepsis-like response has led to the naming of a new clinical syndrome: *systemic inflammatory response syndrome (SIRS)*.[3] *SIRS* differs from sepsis in that it can occur in the absence of infection. Noninfectious causes of SIRS include pancreatitis, multiple trauma, hemorrhagic shock, and autoimmune organ injury. "Sepsis" is the term used when a confirmed infection is present in the patient with SIRS.[3]

Multiple organ dysfunction syndrome (MODS) may occur in both sepsis and SIRS. MODS is the presence of altered organ function in acutely ill patients that requires medical intervention to maintain function.[3]

TABLE 56–1
Definitions

Term	Definition
Infection	Local inflammatory response to microorganisms, such as bacteria, viruses, fungi, or parasites, or the invasion of normal sterile tissue by these organisms.
Bacteremia	Presence of live bacteria in the blood.
Systemic inflammatory response syndrome (SIRS)	Systemic inflammatory response to a variety of clinical problems. Two or more conditions exist: • Temperature >100.4°F or <96.8°F • Heart rate >90 beats/min • Respiratory rate >20 inspirations/min or P_{CO_2} <32 mmHg • White blood cell count >12,000/mm^3, <4000/mm^3, or >10% bands
Sepsis	Systemic response to infection. Two or more of the following conditions exist as a result of infection: • Temperature >100.4°F or <96.8°F • Heart rate >90 beats/min • Respiratory rate >20 inspirations/min or P_{CO_2} <32 mmHg • White blood cell count >12,000/mm^3, <4000 mm^3, or >10% bands
Severe sepsis	Sepsis associated with organ dysfunction, hypoperfusion, or hypotension. Perfusion abnormalities may include lactic acidosis, oliguria, or acute altered mental status.
Septic shock	A form of severe sepsis with hypotension (systolic BP <90 mmHg), despite fluid resuscitation, and perfusion abnormalities, including lactic acidosis, oliguria, or acute altered mental status. Patients on vasoactive drugs may not be hypotensive when perfusion alterations are measured.
Multiple organ dysfunction syndrome (MODS)	Presence of altered organ function in acutely ill patient that requires medical intervention to maintain function.

Source: Adapted with permission from ACCP-SCCM Consensus Conference Committee, Bone, RC, et al: Definitions for sepsis and organ failure and guidelines for the use of innovative therapies in sepsis. Chest 101:6, 1992.

Although multiple organ failure can be initiated by noninfectious causes of inflammatory response, 50% of MODS is initiated by infection or sepsis.[4]

ETIOLOGY OF SEPSIS

Sepsis is caused by the effects of toxins, produced by pathogenic microorganisms, on the vascular, coag-

ulation, immune, and metabolic systems. It is usually precipitated by bacteremia, defined as the presence of pathogens in the circulating blood.

Although gram-negative bacilli are most frequently associated with sepsis, gram-positive cocci and bacilli also have been implicated. Moreover, sepsis may develop secondary to systemic infections caused by fungi and viruses.[5]

Pathogens may be a part of the patient's normal body flora or may be endemic to the hospital environment. Critically ill patients are prone to bacterial invasion, especially after surgery or other invasive procedures. The risk of sepsis is increased in the very young or very old and in patients with a compromised immune system, such as cancer patients, transplant patients, and patients with acquired immunodeficiency syndrome (AIDS). The risk factors and predisposing causes of infection and sepsis are as follows:[1,2,5–7]

Invasive Devices
Venous catheters
Arterial lines
Pulmonary artery catheters
Endotracheal tubes
Tracheostomy tubes
Intracranial monitoring catheters
Urinary catheters

Invasive Procedures
Cystoscopic examination
Surgery

Age
Neonates/young infants <1 year old
Elderly adults >65 years old

Underlying Conditions
Poor state of health
Malnutrition
Chronic alcoholism
Pregnancy
Diabetes mellitus
Cancer
Major organ disease—cardiac, hepatic, or renal dysfunction

Medications/Therapeutic Regimens
Radiation therapy
Corticosteroids
Oncologic chemotherapy
Immunosuppressive drugs
Extensive antibiotic use

PATHOPHYSIOLOGY

The pathophysiology of sepsis is complex. Effects on hemodynamics, coagulation factors, immune response, and metabolic processes are attributed to a series of biochemical reactions triggered by the body's own chemicals (endogenous mediators). The production of endogenous mediators is stimulated by endotoxin, a lipopolysaccharide that is part of the cell wall of gram-negative bacilli.

Endotoxin is released and begins its activity after the bacteria have been destroyed by the host's immune system or by antibiotic therapy. Therefore, sepsis can occur even if live, viable bacteria are no longer in circulation.[1,6]

Gram-positive bacteria do not produce endotoxin. However, the endogenous chemical mediators of the sepsis response are activated in gram-positive sepsis.[5] Gram-positive bacteria, fungi, and viruses can produce a systemic inflammatory response similar to gram-negative sepsis, although usually not as severe.

As mentioned previously, a sepsislike SIRS can develop without the presence of infection. Endogenous mediator responses are triggered in multiple trauma, burn trauma, and acute pancreatitis, with or without evidence of infection.[3]

Despite the absence of endotoxin in some forms of sepsis, the effects of endotoxin can be used as a model to explain the physiologic changes seen in SIRS, sepsis, and septic shock.

Effects of Endotoxin

The biochemical processes initiated by endotoxin and subsequent physiologic effects are presented in Table 56–2 and Figure 56–1. Endotoxin activates the classic and alternative complement pathways. C3a and C5a are the primary complement protein products produced. These mediators produce vasodilation through histamine release and increase capillary permeability, leading to interstitial fluid shifts.[8]

Interstitial fluid shifts caused by vasodilation and permeability changes are promoted by other endotoxin/mediator reactions. Examples of these are bradykinin, β-endorphin, prostaglandin, and leukotriene metabolism (see Table 56–2). Shifting of fluid from the intravascular to the interstitial space leads to distributional hypovolemia, decreased tissue perfusion, and tissue hypoxia.

Tissue perfusion also is reduced through the formation of emboli in the microcirculation. Coagulation is triggered by endotoxin, which activates the intrinsic coagulation pathway, through the Hageman factor (see Chapter 51). Coagulation is further promoted by complement/prostaglandin–enhanced platelet aggregation and the release of platelet activating factor. Platelet activating factor production is stimulated by

TABLE 56–2
Biochemical Processes Triggered by Endotoxin in Sepsis/SIRS

Process	Mediator(s)	Effects
Activation of classic and alternative complement pathway	C3a C5a	Vasodilation Increased capillary permeability Histamine release Chemotaxis of leukocytes Platelet aggregation
Activation of intrinsic coagulation pathway	Hageman factor (factor XII)	Intravascular coagulation
Activation of kallikrein-bradykinin system through factor XII (Hageman factor)	Bradykinin	Vasodilation Increased capillary permeability
Activation of arachidonic acid metabolism	Prostaglandins Leukotrienes	Vasodilation Platelet aggregation Increased capillary permeability Bronchoconstruction Myocardial depression
Macrophage production of cytokines	Tumor necrosis factor (TNF) Interleukin-1	Intravascular coagulation (platelet activating factor) Neutrophil aggregation Damage of endothelial cells through phagocytosis and adhesion of PMNs Release of proteolytic enzymes Decreased lipase activity Fever Amplification of other mediator reactions
Release of pituitary hormones	β-Endorphin, ACTH	Vasodilation Hypotension Hyperglycemia

Source: Data from Bone, RC: Gram-negative sepsis: Background, clinical features and interventions. Chest 100:3, 1991; Waage, A, Brandtzaeg, P, Espevik, T, and Halstensen, A: Current understanding of the pathogenesis of gram negative shock. In Young, LS and Glauser, MP (eds): Infect Dis Clin North Am 5:4, 1991; and Brown, KA and Sheagren, JN: Recognition and emergent treatments of septic shock/multiple organ systems failure syndrome. Intern Med 11(2):3, 1990.

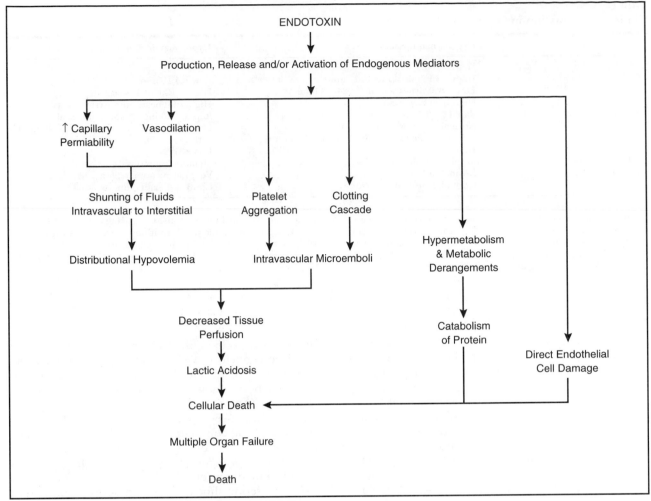

FIGURE 56-1. Summary of pathophysiologic effects of endotoxin.

yet another endogenous mediator—tumor necrosis factor (TNF, cachectin).[8,9]

Tumor Necrosis Factor

TNF is considered a major mediator in sepsis and SIRS. Endotoxin stimulates the macrophage to produce TNF and other cytokines, such as interleukin-1, interferon, and interleukin-6. TNF has direct effects and also amplifies other mediator reactions, such as the coagulation cascade and leukotriene production.[6,7]

TNF is directly toxic to endothelial cells. Moreover, cell destruction is enhanced through TNF activation of polymorphonuclear cells (PMNs), which adhere to and phagocytize endothelial cells, and through TNF-promoted release of proteolytic enzymes. TNF also has been implicated in metabolic derangements observed in sepsis. This is thought to be related to a TNF-induced decrease in lipase activity that prevents the absorption and storage of triglycerides.[5]

METABOLIC EFFECTS

Several metabolic aberrations are seen during the septic response. A hypermetabolic, hyperglycemic, catabolic state occurs as a result of the stress response (catecholamine release), endotoxin-induced adrenocorticotropic hormone (ACTH) release, and TNF-induced decreased lipase activity.[4,5] Glucose, fat, and protein metabolism are altered. Serum glucose is elevated related to increased hepatic glucose production and peripheral insulin resistance. Lipolysis and protein catabolism are increased.[5] The catabolic state, coupled with impaired perfusion and tissue hypoxia, contributes to cell and organ destruction.

CLINICAL PRESENTATION

The clinical presentation of sepsis and septic shock may best be viewed as a continuum of signs and symptoms as the patient develops sepsis, responds to chemical mediator effects, and responds to medical inter-

TABLE 56–3
Clinical Presentation in Septic Shock

	Hyperdynamic Shock	Hypodynamic Shock
Core temperature	High >100.4°F or low <96.8°F	Same
CO*	**High >8 L/min up to 15 L/min***	Low <4 L/min
SVR*	**Low <800 dynes sec cm^{-5} (24–48 hours)***	High >1200 dynes sec cm^{-5}
Heart rate	High >90 beats/min	High >90 beats/min Arrhythmias
Respiratory rate and depth	Rapid >20 inspirations/min Deep	Rapid >20 inspirations/min Shallow
Blood pressure (BP)	Normal or low with change of position (orthostatic hypotension) or low <90 mmHg	Low <90 mmHg or decrease of ≥40 mmHg from baseline
SvO$_2$	High >80%	Low <60%
Acid-base balance	Respiratory alkalosis	Metabolic acidosis
Urine output	Normal or low	Very low or none <30 mL/h
Mental status	Normal, confused, or anxious	Confusion, agitation, or coma

*****Bold** = hallmark signs of septic shock.
Source: Data from Bone, RC: Gram-negative sepsis: Background, clinical features and interventions. Chest 100:3, 1991; ACCP-SCCM Consensus Conference Committee: American College Physicians/Society of Critical Care Medicine: Definitions of sepsis and organ failure and guidelines for the use of innovative therapies in sepsis. Chest 101:6, 1992; Hazinki, MF, et al: Epidemiology, pathophysiology and clinical presentation of gram-negative sepsis. Am J Crit Care 2:3, 1993; and Brown, KA and Sheagren, JN: Recognition and emergent treatments of septic shock/multiple organ systems failure syndrome. Intern Med 11(2):3, 1990.

ventions. Moreover, there is a continuum of hemodynamic changes from hyperdynamic to hypodynamic (Table 56–3). Hallmarks of hyperdynamic sepsis and septic shock are decreased systemic vascular resistance (SVR) and increased cardiac output (CO). Decreased SVR is a result of profound vasodilation triggered by endogenous mediator reactions. Increased CO is a compensatory response to decreased SVR and increased catecholamine levels.[10]

Change in core body temperature is an early sign of the response to infection. Either hyperthermia or hypothermia may be present. TNF and interleukin-1 contribute to the febrile reaction. However, elderly, immunocompromised, or debilitated patients may become hypothermic, not hyperthermic.[1]

Vasodilation and hyperthermia produce warm, flushed skin, which may be misinterpreted as adequate tissue perfusion, when in fact organ/tissue perfusion is poor and tissue hypoxia is present. High blood flow rates from decreased SVR and decreased tissue perfusion from mediator effects lead to decreased oxygen extraction by the cells from the blood. Increased SvO$_2$ (venous oxygen saturation) is an early manifestation of this effect.[6]

Other early signs of sepsis and septic shock include hyperventilation, respiratory alkalosis, tachycardia, and orthostatic hypotension.[1,10] Hyperventilation is related to effects of chemical mediators on the respiratory center and to the stress response. Respiratory alkalosis is secondary to hyperventilation. Tachycardia is a compensatory response to maintain CO. Orthostatic hypotension, when present, reveals the true fluid state of distributional hypovolemia.

Hypotension and severe altered tissue perfusion (septic shock) may occur later in the continuum of response, usually when the patient is unresponsive to fluid replacement and other interventions to treat hemodynamic changes.[1] In refractory septic shock, a small percentage (10%) of patients develop a hypodynamic state in which CO falls below normal and SVR increases because of catecholamine-induced vasoconstriction. CO also may decrease because of myocardial failure. The causes of myocardial failure in late septic shock are not completely understood. Contractility and ejection fraction may decrease because of the effects of a *myocardial depression factor* (MDF) and other chemical mediator effects on cardiac cells.[6,7]

In late septic shock, MODS may occur. The most common organs to fail, in order, are the lungs (adult respiratory distress syndrome [ARDS]), liver, intestines, and kidneys.[4] (For signs and symptoms of ARDS, hepatic failure, and renal failure see Chapters 25, 45, and 37). Intestinal dysfunctions may include paralytic ileus, inability to absorb/tolerate enteral feedings, and stress ulcer formation. Hematologic system failure, in the form of disseminated intravascular coagulation (DIC), also may occur. The sequence of organ failure may be altered in the presence of underlying pre-existing pathology. However, prognosis appears to be related to the number of organ failures, not to the sequence.

LABORATORY FINDINGS

Alterations in laboratory tests are related to immune response, metabolic dysfunction, and organ damage. Early laboratory findings may include hyperglycemia, leukocytosis with a left shift, thrombocytopenia, and increased serum cortisol.[1,10] Respiratory alkalosis is evident during the early phase because of compensatory hyperventilation. In septic shock, after tissue perfusion is severely reduced, metabolic acidosis develops.

Cultures of blood, urine, and sputum may be obtained to identify the potential causative agent and to direct antibiotic therapy. Because the presence of viable bacteria in the blood may be transient, negative blood cultures do not necessarily rule out the possibility of bacteremia or sepsis.

TREATMENT

Early recognition of sepsis is important because prompt intervention may prevent septic shock and multiple organ failure. Nurses should observe for hallmark signs of evolving septic shock in patients at risk: hyperthermia (>100.4°F) or hypothermia, decreased SVR (<800 dynes/cm^5), and increased CO (>8 L/min).

Other signs and symptoms to monitor are tachycardia, hyperventilation, and orthostatic hypotension. The nurse should also monitor for signs of organ failure and decreased perfusion. Decreased urine output may be an early sign of renal dysfunction, and altered mental status suggests decreased cerebral perfusion.

Treatments are directed at preventing complications of SIRS and/or blocking the effects of endotoxin and endogenous chemical mediators (Table 56–4).

Initial interventions include fluid volume replacement, antibiotic therapy, and identification and removal (if necessary) of the focus of the infection.[1] Fluid replacement with crystalloids and/or colloids is essential in correcting hypovolemia and improving tissue perfusion. Colloids may be needed to increase osmotic pressure, thus promoting the retention of fluids in the intravascular space.

Colloid replacement with packed red blood cells, if indicated, has the added benefit of improving oxygen transport to the tissues. Initial volume replacement will usually be substantial, with up to 6 liters of crystalloid or 2 liters of colloid. Actual amounts of fluid given will be titrated according to pulmonary capillary wedge pressure (PCWP) and other hemodynamic measures obtained through pulmonary artery pressure monitoring.[5]

Antibiotic therapy is based on the results of positive cultures that indicate the sensitivities of the invading organism. Usually the physician will order two antibiotic agents, one of which is an aminoglycoside. The second antibiotic may be an antipseudomonal penicillin or third-generation cephalosporin.[10] Using two antibiotics broadens the spectrum of antibacterial action.

Identification and removal of the focus of entry of infection is important to prevent the recurrence of sepsis. If a surgical wound or abscess is at fault, it must be drained or excised. Suspect venous or arterial catheters must be removed and replaced in another site. If the urinary tract is the focus of infection, the decision to remove or avoid a urinary catheter must be weighed against the need to monitor urinary output.

Some treatments listed in Table 56–4 are directed toward the prevention and treatment of complications, such as hypotension, acidosis, respiratory failure, and cardiac failure. Inotropic agents such as dopamine and dobutamine may be needed if fluid resuscitation is not fully effective in improving perfusion. Dopamine is the preferred inotropic agent because at midrange (5 to 10 μg/kg per minute) it improves contractility and renal perfusion. Higher-dose dopamine (>10 μg/kg per minute) produces vasoconstriction to aid in correcting hypotension.

In hypodynamic septic shock, fluid resuscitation and initial vasoactive drug therapy are ineffective in maintaining blood pressure and tissue perfusion. Vasoactive drugs that have α-adrenergic effects, such as epinephrine, norepinephrine, and phenylephrine, may be needed. Phenylephrine is indicated for patients with cardiac arrhythmias because it is less arrhythmogenic than the other drugs. Norepinephrine has been shown to be safe and effective in treating refractory hypotension and may be combined with dopamine to improve renal perfusion. Epinephrine should be the last choice because it may cause tachycardia and ventricular arrhythmias.[7]

The potential for respiratory failure is increased in septic shock, because decreased pulmonary tissue perfusion may damage pulmonary capillary membranes, resulting in ARDS. Early oxygenation and ventilatory support, in the form of intubation and mechanical ventilation, will help to decrease the work of breathing, prevent respiratory muscle fatigue, and improve tissue oxygenation.[5]

TABLE 56–4
Treatments for Sepsis and Septic Shock (SIRS)

Treatment	Purpose
Fluid volume replacement	Correct hypovolemia
• Crystalloid	Improve tissue perfusion
• Colloid	
• Blood products	
Antibiotic therapy (two-drug combination)	Prevent/treat infection
Identification/removal of infection source	Prevent/treat infection
• Arterial/venous catheters	
• Urinary catheters	
Inotropic agents	Increase BP
• Dopamine	Increase CO
• Dobutamine	Increase renal perfusion
Respiratory support	Improve tissue oxygenation
• Oxygen therapy	Prevent/treat respiratory failure
• Mechanical ventilation	Decrease work of breathing

Source: Data from Bone, RC: Gram-negative sepsis: Background, clinical features and interventions. Chest 100:3, 1991; Deitch, EA: Multiple organ failure: Pathophysiology and potential future therapy. Ann Surg 216:2, 1992; Rackow, EC and Astiz, ME: Pathophysiology and treatment of septic shock. JAMA 266:4, 1991; and Brown, KA and Sheagren, JN: Recognition and emergent treatments of septic shock/multiple organ systems failure syndrome. Intern Med 11(2):3, 1990.

TABLE 56–5
Potential for Infection: Nursing Care Considerations

Nursing Actions	Rationales
• Define major risk factors for hospital-acquired infections in intensive care units: ○ Invasive devices: pressure monitoring devices, intravascular (IV) catheters, urinary catheters, respiratory therapy equipment, continuous ambulatory peritoneal dialysis (CAPD), hemodialysis ○ Resistant microorganisms ○ Altered immune response ○ Antimicrobial therapy ○ Underlying chronic or debilitating disease	• Most frequently involved organisms (some with highly resistant strains) include members of the following: *Serratia, Pseudomonas, Enterobacter, Proteus, Klebsiella, Enterococcus, Staphylococcus aureus,* and *Streptococcus* (these latter two strains are frequently implicated in bacterial pneumonias). *Candida* infections proliferate in hyperalimentation solutions.
• Monitor for urinary tract infection (UTI): ○ Avoid inserting catheter when alternative techniques for urinary drainage can be used. ○ Remove catheter as soon as possible. ○ Assess for signs/symptoms of UTI: urgency, frequency, dysuria, fever, chills, sweats; septic shock may be associated with a secondary bacteremia. ○ Insert catheter using aseptic technique: ○ Use smallest size possible. ○ Secure catheter, leaving enough slack to prevent pull on bladder neck and urinary meatus. ○ Maintain closed sterile drainage system.	○ The incidence of UTI is directly related to the length of time a urinary catheter is in the bladder. ○ Major complications of UTI include gram-negative sepsis and acute/chronic pyelonephritis. ○ To minimize trauma to urinary tract.
• Monitor for intravascular infection: ○ Identify risk factors for IV-catheter related infections: patient's health status and susceptibility (e.g., immunosuppressed). ○ Method of insertion: percutaneous approach; centrally placed catheters (subclavian, central venous pressure). ○ Duration of cannulation. ○ Degree of manipulation of infusion system: replacement of infusion solution container upon infusion completion; piggyback infusions. ○ Stopcocks—hemodynamic monitoring equipment. ○ Contaminated infusion solutions.	○ Percutaneous approach has lower infection rate than cutdown or centrally placed catheters. ○ Infection rate markedly increases after 72 h of insertion. ○ Bacteremias are most commonly associated with hemodynamic pressure monitoring.
• Assess for signs and symptoms of intravascular cannula-related infection: ○ Swelling, pain, tenderness, warmth, and erythema at insertion site, or over an indurated vessel, suggests phlebitis. ○ Elevation of body temperature.	○ Phlebitis is highly implicated in intravascular infections and bacteremia. ○ When cause of elevated body temperature cannot be determined, suspect the IV-catheter site.
• Note precautions for the insertion and maintenance of IV line: wash hands carefully prior to insertion; use antiseptic to prepare insertion site: ○ Anchor line securely. ○ Follow unit protocols for IV tubing, IV fluid, and dressing changes (technique/time interval).	○ Securing line reduces risk of injury to cannulated vessel.
• Note precautions for the insertion and maintenance of pressure-monitoring system: ○ Avoid inappropriate use of hemodynamic pressure-monitoring lines. ○ Use strict aseptic technique (masks, gloves, gowns). ○ Use closed flush system to maintain patency of line. □ Use saline solutions.	□ Glucose solutions support bacterial colonization.
• Monitor for respiratory tract infection (RTI): ○ Risk factors for RTI include: □ Compromised pulmonary defense mechanisms (e.g., intubation, tracheostomy, suctioning); aspiration of oropharyngeal and/or gastric secretions. □ Antibiotic therapy □ Hematogenic spread of infection to the lungs from distant foci (e.g., UTI). □ Debilitating disease multiorgan system failure. ○ Assess for signs and symptoms of RTI: fever (spiking), dyspnea, tachypnea. □ Dullness to percussion. □ Abnormal breath sounds (bronchial in place of vesicular), and adventitious sounds (crackles, wheezes) on auscultation.	□ Occasionally predisposes to gram-negative infection of mouth and oropharynx. □ Suggests lung consolidation in this clinical setting.
• Review laboratory data and other studies: ○ Increase in white blood cells. ○ Chest x-ray may indicate pulmonary consolidation. ○ Sputum production.	○ In immunosuppressed patients, white blood cells may decrease. ○ Purulent sputum production, in conjunction with other clinical findings, is highly suggestive of pneumonia.

TABLE 56–5
Potential for Infection: Nursing Care Considerations (*Continued*)

Nursing Actions	Rationales

• Implement care considerations:
  ○ Rigorous handwashing.
  ○ Institution of timely and aggressive chest physiotherapy and bronchial hygiene; coughing; deep breathing; incentive spirometry.
  ○ Minimize risk of aspiration:
    □ Confirm placement of nasogastric tube before tube feeding.
    □ Maintain in semi-Fowler's position.
 	
  ○ Monitor use and handling of respiratory therapy equipment.
  ○ Follow unit protocols in maintenance of artificial airways (endotracheal and tracheostomy tubes).
	○ Common source of cross-contamination.
	  ○ Facilitates secretion mobilization and removal.
	
	    □ Reduces risk of aspiration; allows for maximum respiratory excursion.
	  ○ Highly implicated in hospital-acquired infections.
	  ○ See Tables 25–3 and 25–4 for complications of endotracheal intubation and for procedure for endotracheal suctioning, respectively.

• Appreciate significance of widespread antimicrobial use as a contributing factor in the selection of resistant strains of microorganisms:
  ○ Mechanisms underlying microbial resistance include: enzymatic inactivation of antibiotic, alterations in biochemical pathways, alterations in drug-receptor sites, changes in cell-wall binding sites, alterations in genetic coding.
• Nursing care considerations:
  ○ Administer prescribed antibiotics as directed: avoid too rapid IV infusion; avoid infusion of two different antibiotics via the same line because the drug interaction may alter the desired effects of each drug (e.g., penicillins and aminoglycosides).
• Appreciate infection control actions by healthcare providers:
  ○ Elements of the infectious process include causative agent, reservoir, portal of exit, transmission, portal of entry, susceptible host.
	• Selection of resistant strains occurs when sensitive microflora are suppressed by an antibiotic, enabling colonization and/or superinfection by resistant bacteria.
	  ○ *Candida* is an example of an infectious process, or superinfection, which becomes clinically evident after the antibiotic has eliminated the normal flora.
	
	• It is essential for nurses to appreciate potential adverse drug interactions:
	  ○ Excessively high levels of some drugs may predispose to drug toxicity.
	
	• Healthcare providers have a responsibility to implement steps necessary to control the spread of infection in the patient population, environment, and in themselves and fellow healthcare professionals.
	• Viral hepatitis B is a commonly occurring infectious disease.
	• Disease-specific precautions have been established for most known infectious diseases (refer to hospital's infection control manual).

New and Experimental Treatments

New and experimental treatments for sepsis and septic shock include ibuprofen, naloxone, and monoclonal antibodies to endotoxin. Ibuprofen, a nonsteroidal anti-inflammatory agent, has been effective in blocking the cardiovascular effects of TNF and interleukin-1 in clinical studies.[5] Studies are ongoing to determine the effectiveness of ibuprofen in treating septic shock. Naloxone, an opiate antagonist, is being studied for use in septic shock because it blocks the effect of β-endorphin.[5] HA-1A and E5, two monoclonal antibodies to endotoxin, have shown varying degrees of effectiveness in treating septic shock. These drugs block the effects of endotoxin in initiating mediator effects but appear to be effective primarily in gram-negative sepsis.[11,12]

NURSING CARE

Nurses have an important role in the prevention, recognition, and management of sepsis. Prevention of infection is a primary goal in the care of all patients, and, as previously mentioned, early recognition and intervention may prevent the progression to septic shock and organ failure. Early recognition of septic shock is enhanced through careful patient assessment coupled with the knowledge of the signs and symptoms of septic shock and infection. Nursing care considerations for the patient with potential for infection are described in Table 56–5.

Baseline assessment data assist the nurse to identify and interpret subtle changes, which may indicate decreased cerebral or peripheral perfusion. Part of the nursing care involves monitoring for symptoms of potential complications. Potential complications include cardiac failure, arrhythmias, renal failure, ARDS, paralytic ileus, gastrointestinal hemorrhage, and DIC. Additional nursing care considerations, nursing diagnoses, patient outcomes, and nursing interventions/rationales are presented in the care plan at the end of this chapter.

REFERENCES

1. Bone, RC: Gram-negative sepsis: Background, clinical features and interventions. Chest 100:3, 1991.
2. Hoyt, NJ: Preventing septic shock: Infection control in the intensive care unit. Crit Care Nurs Clin North Am 2:2, 1990.

3. ACCP-SCCM Consensus Conference Committee: American College Physicians/Society of Critical Care Medicine: Definitions of sepsis and organ failure and guidelines for the use of innovative therapies in sepsis. Chest 101:6, 1992.

4. Deitch, EA: Multiple organ failure: Pathophysiology and potential future therapy. Ann Surg 216:2, 1992.

5. Rackow, EC and Astiz, ME: Pathophysiology and treatment of septic shock. JAMA 266:4, 1991.

6. Hazinski, MF, et al: Epidemiology, pathophysiology and clinical presentation of gram-negative sepsis. Am J Crit Care 2:3, 1993.

7. Quesado, ZMN and Natanson, C: Systemic hemodynamic abnormalities and vasopressor therapy in sepsis and septic shock. Am J Kidney Dis 20:3, 1992.

8. Sable, CA and Wispelwey, B: Pharmacologic interventions aimed at preventing the biologic effects of endotoxin. In Young, LS and Glauser, MP (eds). Infect Dis Clin North Am 5:4, 1991.

9. Waage, A, Brandtzaeg, P, Espevik, T, and Halstensen, A: Current understanding of the pathogenesis of gram negative shock. In Young, LS and Glauser, MP (eds): Infect Dis Clin North Am 5:4, 1991.

10. Brown, KA and Sheagren, JN: Recognition and emergent treatments of septic shock/multiple organ systems failure syndrome. Intern Med 11(2), 1990.

11. Ziegler, EJ, Fisher, CJ, Sprung, CL, et al: Treatment of gram-negative bacteremia and septic shock with HA-1A human monoclonal antibody against endotoxin. New Engl J Med, 324:7, 1991.

12. Gorelick, KJ and Chmel, H: The role of monoclonal antibodies in the management of gram negative sepsis: Experience with E5 antibody. In Young, LS and Glauser, MP (eds): Infect Dis Clin North Am 5:4, 1991.

SUGGESTED READINGS

Brown, KK: Septic shock: How to stop the deadly cascade, part I. Am J Nurs 94:9, 1994.

Brown, KK: Clinical interventions in septic shock: Part II. Am J Nurs 94:10, 1994.

Rice, V: Shock, A clinical syndrome: An update, part 1: An overview of shock. Crit Care Nurse 11:4, 1991.

Rietschel, ET and Brade, H: Bacterial endotoxins. Sci Am 267: 54–61, 1992.

Russell, S: Septic shock: Can you recognize the clues? *Nursing 94* 24:4, 1994.

CARE PLAN FOR THE PATIENT WITH SEPSIS/SEPTIC SHOCK

Nursing Diagnoses

Nursing Diagnosis #1
Fluid volume deficit, related to:
1. Distributional volume loss; shift to interstitial space
2. Increased insensible loss with high fever

Desired Patient Outcomes

Patient will:
1. Maintain adequate circulating blood volume and stable hemodynamic variables:
   • Heart rate 60–100 beats/min when resting
   • Systemic arterial BP adequate for tissue perfusion; BP > 90 mmHg systolic
   • PCWP 8–12 mmHg
   • CO > 4 L/min
   • SVR 800–1400 dynes sec cm^{-5}
   • Normal central venous pressure 0–8 mmHg
2. Maintain normal body temperature
3. Maintain adequate urine output > 30 mL/h
4. Maintain baseline and/or optimal neurologic status
5. Maintain fluid and electrolyte balance as demonstrated by laboratory data in normal limits:
   • Electrolytes
   • Hemoglobin and hematocrit
   • Blood urea nitrogen and creatinine
6. Demonstrate adequate peripheral tissue perfusion:
   • Warm, dry skin
   • Absence of cyanosis
   • Absence of skin breakdown

Nursing Interventions

• Assess for signs and symptoms of sepsis:

Rationales

• Early recognition of sepsis is important for instituting prompt measures to prevent shock and/or multiple organ failure:

CARE PLAN FOR THE PATIENT WITH SEPSIS/SEPTIC SHOCK (*Continued*)

Nursing Interventions	Rationales
○ Assess for early signs of bacteremia: hyperthermia, warm, dry, flushed skin; chills; weakness; nausea, vomiting, diarrhea. ○ Obtain baseline cultures: urine, sputum, blood, wound (if applicable). □ Bacteremia may be transient. Blood cultures should not be obtained through indwelling venous or arterial catheters, because they may be colonized with bacteria not responsible for the sepsis response. ○ Obtain and monitor: serum glucose, electrolytes, prothrombin time, partial thromboplastin time, platelet count, fibrin split products, hemoglobin and hematocrit, white blood cell count with differential.	○ Determination of the portal of entry and focus of infection is crucial to successful treatment. ○ Laboratory data will be helpful in monitoring fluid replacement therapy and in identifying complications, such as DIC. ○ Serum glucose may be elevated in sepsis. ○ Elevated leukocyte count with a left shift is frequently observed in sepsis; indicative of acute infection.
• Assess hemodynamic status: ○ CO ○ PCWP ○ SVR ○ Arterial BP ○ Heart rate • Observe for ventricular arrhythmias. • Assess neurologic status: ○ Altered level of consciousness ○ Anxiety • Assess renal function; urine output, urine specific gravity, urinary sodium.	• Increased CO and decreased SVR are observed early in the continuum of the sepsis response; however, if septic shock develops, CO is reduced and SVR may increase. ○ Monitoring these variables will determine effectiveness of therapeutic interventions, including fluid replacement and inotropic medications. • Arrhythmias may indicate decreased coronary perfusion. • Changes in neurologic status may indicate decreased cerebral perfusion. • Reduced renal perfusion will reduce glomerular filtration, causing a decrease in urine output. A decrease in urinary sodium is indicative of hypovolemia secondary to aldosterone release.
• Assess peripheral pulses and condition of the skin.	• In early sepsis, skin may be warm and flushed from vasodilation. Pulses may be normal or increased. If hypodynamic septic shock develops, skin may become cool and pale because of decreased peripheral perfusion. Pulses may be normal or decreased.

• Administer and monitor prescribed fluid replacement therapy:
○ Monitor hemodynamic variables (as mentioned previously).
 	
○ Monitor hourly urinary output.
 	
○ Assess respiratory status: respiratory rate; rhythm of breathing; presence of adventitious breath sounds: crackles and wheezes.
• Institute measures to control body temperature:
 	
○ Monitor body temperature every 2 h if the patient is febrile.
○ Administer antipyretic drugs as ordered; evaluate response to therapy.
○ Apply hypo/hyperthermia blanket as prescribed:
  □ Automatic cooling mode using rectal probe.
  □ Monitor temperature continuously.
  □ Protect skin during cooling.
  □ Avoid shivering.
	○ Higher-than-normal central venous pressure, pulmonary artery pressure, and PCWP may indicate a too rapid infusion of fluids and impending fluid overload.
	○ Urine output of greater than 30 mL/h indicates adequate renal perfusion.
	○ Tachypnea and crackles may indicate fluid overload.
	
	• Insensible fluid loss may increase when the patient is febrile.
	○ High body temperature increases the metabolic rate of the tissues and may exacerbate tissue ischemia and hypoxia:
	
	○ Continuous measurement of temperature while the patient is on a cooling blanket will prevent excessive cooling and chills.

CARE PLAN FOR THE PATIENT WITH SEPSIS/SEPTIC SHOCK (*Continued*)

Nursing Diagnoses

Nursing Diagnosis #2
Potential for impaired gas exchange, related to:
1. Hypovolemia resulting in reduced pulmonary perfusion (ventilation/perfusion mismatch)
2. Altered alveolar/capillary membrane
3. Compensatory tachypnea/hyperventilation

Desired Patient Outcomes

Patient will:
1. Maintain acceptable blood gas parameters:
   - pH 7.35–7.45
   - Po_2 >60 mmHg
   - Pco_2 ~35–45 mmHg
2. Maintain an effective breathing pattern and respiratory rate
3. Maintain acceptable Svo_2 between 60%–80%
4. Verbalize ease of breathing
5. Maintain baseline and/or optimal neurologic status

Nursing Interventions

- Assess respiratory status:

  - Respiratory rate and rhythm

  - Breath sounds

  - Arterial blood gases and pH

  - Observe for increased peak inspiratory pressures in mechanically ventilated patient.

  - Svo_2

- Implement measures to decrease the work of breathing:
  - Place patient in semi-Fowler's or semiprone position.
  - Maintain patent airway: suction if necessary.
  - Teach breathing techniques (see Chapter 25 care plan, nursing diagnosis #2).
- Administer and monitor oxygen therapy.
- Assess neurologic status:
  - Level of consciousness
  - Cognitive ability
  - Orientation

Rationales

- Respiratory distress syndrome may occur in sepsis secondary to decreased perfusion and endotoxin damage to the pulmonary vasculature (see Chapter 25).
  - Altered respiratory patterns, such as hyperventilation and tachypnea, occur secondary to fever and sympathetic nervous system stimulation.
  - Development of abnormal breath sounds, such as crackles, indicates fluid overload and pulmonary edema.
  - Decreased Pao_2 <60 mmHg, and increased $Paco_2$ >50 mmHg (room air) are signs of impending respiratory failure.
  - Patients with septic shock may require endotracheal intubation and mechanical ventilation. In the patient requiring mechanical ventilation, increased inspiratory pressures indicate decreased lung compliance observed in respiratory distress syndrome.
  - Svo_2 increases in early septic shock because of decreased O_2 extraction. Decreased Svo_2 may occur later as hypoxic tissues extract greater amounts of O_2.

  - Allows for greater lung expansion and improves ventilation.
  - See Chapter 25 care plan, nursing diagnosis #2.

  - May improve tissue oxygenation.
- Changes in mental status may indicate cerebral hypoxia.

Nursing Diagnoses

Nursing Diagnosis #3
Potential impairment of skin integrity, related to:
1. Immobility
2. Decreased tissue perfusion

Desired Patient Outcomes

Patient will demonstrate skin integrity as evidenced by the absence of skin breakdown and pressure ulcers

Nursing Interventions

- Assess skin condition frequently.
- Perform passive range-of-motion exercises.
- Provide pressure relief device.
- Teach the patient to shift position frequently.
- Establish a turning schedule of every 1–2 h depending on the patient's condition.

Rationales

- To improve peripheral circulation.

- Pressure ulcers may be prevented by reducing the amount and duration of pressure to a given area.

C H A P T E R   5 7

Nursing Management of the Patient with Anaphylactic Shock

Lorraine Fallon and Jeannette Waterman

CHAPTER OUTLINE

Anaphylactic Shock
- Pathophysiology
- Diagnosis
- Clinical Presentation
- Therapeutic Management

- Nursing Diagnoses, Patient Outcomes, and Nursing Interventions

Case Study with Sample Care Plan: Patient with Anaphylactic Shock

References

LEARNING OBJECTIVES

After completing this chapter, you should be able to:

1. Define anaphylaxis.
2. Identify etiologic factors and patients at risk for anaphylactic shock.
3. Examine pathophysiology underlying anaphylactic shock, including the actions of chemical mediators released in this immune response.
4. Identify key factors of importance to assessment and diagnosis of anaphylactic shock, including the patient's past history and the clinical presentation.
5. Outline key considerations in the emergent care of the patient with anaphylactic shock.
6. Delineate the nursing process in caring for the patient with anaphylactic shock, including assessment, nursing diagnoses, and planning (desired patient outcomes and nursing interventions/rationales).

ANAPHYLACTIC SHOCK

Anaphylaxis (type I, atopy) is one of four basic immune mechanisms underlying host responses to foreign substances (i.e., antigens). The other mechanisms are cytotoxic responses (type II), circulating immune complexes or antigen-antibody complexes (type III), and delayed hypersensitivity or cell-mediated responses (type IV) (Table 57–1).

Anaphylactic shock is an immediate, systemic, normovolemic vasogenic reaction that occurs when an antigen interacts with the preformed antibody (immunoglobulin IgE) found on the surface of mast cells and basophils. The interaction between the antigen and the antibody causes the release of chemical mediators from mast cell granules. These mediators trigger the life-threatening clinical manifestations that we call anaphylactic shock. Unless treatment is immediately given, the results of this shock can be fatal.

Pathophysiology

Anaphylactic shock is a two-phase reaction. The first phase occurs when persons are exposed to a foreign substance (an antigen) and their body produces specific IgE antibodies against this antigen. These IgE antibodies bind with mast cells found in the connective tissue of the lungs, uterus, spleen, liver, omentum, kidneys, heart, and skin, as well as in the connective tissues that surround the blood vessels. IgE also binds with basophils, the counterparts of mast cells found in blood plasma. Once the person's immune system has become sensitized to that specific antigen (i.e., antigen-specific IgE antibodies are on the surface of mast cells), phase one is completed. The person is now at risk for anaphylactic shock.

Phase two occurs when the person is again exposed to the same or similar antigen. The antigen now reacts with the preformed IgE antibodies that are attached

TABLE 57–1
Effector Mechanisms Underlying Immune Responses/Reactions*

Type	Name	Response/Reaction	Examples
I	Anaphylaxis (atopy), immediate	Specific antigen attaches to IgE antibody bound to mast cells and basophils. Rapid release of chemical mediators. A strong hereditary component is evident.	Anaphylaxis (food, drugs, preservatives)
II	Cytotoxic response	Antibody attacks/binds with a cell or tissue antigen, resulting in humoral (complement activation) or antibody-dependent, cell-mediated cytotoxicity; cell lysis, pH inactivation, or phagocytosis occur.	ABO transfusion reactions Rh incompatability Erythroblastosis fetalis Drug-related hemolytic anemias, leukopenias
III	Antigen-antibody complexes (immune complex–mediated)	Insoluble antigen-antibody complexes are too small for liver/spleen to remove, and they become deposited in small arteries and capillaries of the kidney, nervous system, and skin. The result is an inflammatory response.	Acute glomerulonephritis Rheumatoid arthritis Lupus Serum sickness
IV	Cell-mediated reactions (delayed hypersensitivity)	Specific, sensitized T lymphocytes react with an antigen, causing lysosomal enzyme release and inflammation.	Contact dermatitis Poison ivy Organ transplant rejection Herpes Tuberculosis

*See Chapter 47 for a more detailed discussion of these immune mechanisms.
Source: Mathewson Kuhn, MA: Anaphylaxis versus anaphylactoid reactions: Nursing interventions. Crit Care Nurse 10(5):126, 1990.

to the mast cells and basophils. The consequent reaction causes cellular integrity to become disrupted, degranulation occurs, and the mast cell surface ruptures. Chemical mediators are released from the intracellular granules and catalyze the sequence of reactions that underlie anaphylactic shock.

An anaphylactoid syndrome, having clinical manifestations nearly identical to those of anaphylactic shock, has been recognized.[1] In this anaphylactoid reaction, however, there is no prior sensitization, and preformed IgE antibodies are not involved. There is no immune mechanism involved. The chemical agent itself causes a direct mediator release, triggering the anaphylactoid reaction. Agents that have been identified with these reactions include radiographic contrast materials; nonsteroidal anti-inflammatory drugs, such as acetylsalicylic acid (aspirin), ibuprofen, and opiates; and antibiotics, such as vancomycin. These reactions have been found to be dose-related.

Another anaphylactoid reaction has been associated with vigorous exercise, and three patterns have been identified.[2] The first pattern is an exercise-induced reaction that does not correlate with recent ingestion of foods. The second pattern is an exercise-induced reaction that occurs during exercise and shortly after eating specific foods, such as shellfish, nuts, and celery. The third pattern occurs in people who exercise within 2 hours of having eaten any foods. There is speculation that changes in blood volume distribution during the digestive/absorption phase may be a possible explanation for the three patterns of reactions. Perhaps some unexplained deaths of runners

and swimmers are related to exercise-induced anaphylaxis.

Antigens

Many different antigens (allergens) have been implicated as possible causes of anaphylactic shock. They are classified by how they enter the body, falling predominantly into three categories: injections, ingestions, and bites and stings (Table 57–2).

Because of the unpredictable pathogenesis, morbidity, and mortality associated with anaphylactic shock, attempts to identify persons at increased risk of experiencing anaphylaxis have been unsuccessful. For example, it has been discovered that persons who suffer with ragweed hay fever will also frequently have a local anaphylactic reaction to melons and bananas. This local reaction is manifested by acute swelling, burning, and itching of the mouth. This reaction is IgE-mediated but is not to be confused with systemic anaphylactic shock. An allergy to fish products or iodine may predispose individuals to reaction when contrast media are used in diagnostic testing. Yet individuals with general allergies and or asthma are not necessarily at a greater risk for anaphylactic shock.

While prevention of anaphylaxis would be the best defense, it is difficult to recognize high-risk groups. After surviving one reaction, the individual must create an environment with limited or no exposure to that allergen. Health histories are beneficial in identifying persons who have had previous reactions, but they will not help to distinguish the remaining high-

TABLE 57–2
Antigens Causing Anaphylactic Shock

Mode of Entrance	Antigen
Injection or Ingestion	
1. Drugs*	• Antibiotics (e.g., penicillin, sulfonamides)
a. Sera	• Foreign proteins (e.g., vaccines or medications made from animal serum, including insulin, tetanus antitoxin, rabies antitoxin, snakebite antitoxin)
	• Local anesthetics (e.g., procaine hydrochloride [Novocain])
	• Salicylates (e.g., aspirin compounds)
	• Diagnostic contrast media
	• Plasma expanders, blood, and blood products
	• Barbiturates and narcotics(e.g., codeine, meperidine hydrochloride [Demerol])
	• Muscle relaxants (e.g., methocarbamol [Robaxin])
2. Foods	• Legumes (soybeans, peanuts)
	• Nuts and seeds
	• Shellfish (lobster, shrimp, clams, crabs)
	• Egg albumin
	• Cereals (wheat, corn)
	• Fish (salmon, cod)
	• Milk products
	• Chocolate
	• Fruits (berries, bananas, oranges)
a. Additives	• Food coloring agents
	• Preservatives (e.g., sodium bisulfite, monosodium glutamate, tartrazine, and sodium benzoate)
Stings and Bites	• Honey bee, wasp, hornet, yellow jacket, fire ant, and deer fly
	• Snake venom—pit vipers (e.g., rattlesnakes, cottonmouths, and copperheads)
Environmental Factors	• Sunlight, cold, exercise, heat, pollens, molds, and spores.
Miscellaneous	• Latex products (gloves, catheters)
	• Vitamin K

*Drugs administered by the parenteral route rank highest as the cause of anaphylactic shock. Anaphylaxis to penicillin is a well-known phenomenon, but fatal reactions to oral penicillin are rare. Beta blockage can apparently potentiate anaphylactic reactions to penicillin and unusually aggressive treatment may be necessary to reverse the shock state. From Beta blockers and penicillin anaphylaxis. Nurses' Drug Alert 10(5):38, 1986.

risk persons in our general population. For patients who have had a reaction to radiocontrast media, a pretreatment regimen has been developed in the event another radiocontrast study is necessary. An example of one such pretreatment regimen is to administer diphenhydramine hydrochloride (Benadryl) 50 mg intramuscularly (IM) 1 hour before procedure, prednisone 50 mg orally (PO) at 13, 7, and 1 hour before the procedure, and ephedrine 25 mg PO 1 hour before the procedure.[3]

Chemical Mediators

The degranulation of mast cells releases chemical mediators into the tissues and circulation (Table 57–3). The major mediator is histamine, which is released in large doses. Histamine causes smooth muscles to contract, blood capillaries to dilate, and capillary permeability to increase. The resulting fluid shift and vascular dilation progress to a sudden and severe drop in blood pressure and cardiac output. The contraction of smooth muscle results in constriction of the bladder, uterus, intestines, and bronchioles of the lungs. Respiratory distress, bronchospasm and laryngospasm, and severe abdominal cramps ensue. The increased capillary permeability leads to a shift of fluid, blood, plasma proteins, and leukocytes from the vascular system into the interstitial space. Although this change in permeability is beneficial to promote healing in tissue injuries, the degree seen in anaphylactic shock causes so great a response that it becomes a threat to life itself.

Serotonin is another mediator released from mast cells. It also increases capillary permeability, particularly in the lungs. As plasma leaks into the alveoli, the integrity of the alveolar-capillary membrane (see Figs. 22–5, and 22–11) becomes disrupted, impairing gas exchange. Unless the process can be reversed quickly, hypoxemia and hypercapnia will ensue. Leakage of plasma into the alveoli also precipitates pulmonary edema (see Fig. 25–1), which can quickly become fatal if not arrested.

Other substances released from mast cells include bradykinins, platelet-activating factor, eosinophil chemotactic factor, and prostaglandins (see Table 57–3).

The slow-reacting substance of anaphylaxis (SRS-A) has similar effects on the body as does histamine, except that it is slower and more prolonged. This slower response follows the more rapid histamine response and must be considered when treating patients in anaphylactic shock (a relapse can result if the patient is discharged prematurely). Thus, patients not only require adequate treatment but extended observation.

Diagnosis

A carefully elicited history is essential to the diagnosis and treatment of the patient with anaphylactic shock. An attempt should be made to identify the following: (1) the specific allergen; (2) the patient's initial exposure to the allergen; (3) the type of reaction triggered by the allergen, including signs and symptoms and the initial symptoms; and (4) what was done to treat the problem.

Typically, the patient with atopy relates a history of a previous reaction to a specific antigen. A family history of allergies is common, although the clinical presentation in each member may vary.

Characteristically, most cases of anaphylaxis have a

TABLE 57–3
Chemical Mediators: Actions and Physiologic Effects

Mediator	Actions/Physiologic Effects
1. Histamine	• Increased vascular permeability, causing fluid shifts from the circulation to the interstitial space • Decreased cardiac output associated with diminished circulating blood volume, decreased venous return, and altered cardiac contractility • Hypotension caused by fluid shifts and vasodilation • Arrhythmias associated with decreased coronary artery perfusion and hypoxia • Smooth muscle contraction, resulting in bronchospasm • Pulmonary edema • Urticaria and pruritus
2. Slow-reacting substance of anaphylaxis (SRS-A) (leukotriene)	• Increased vascular permeability that predisposes to fluid shifts from the intravascular to interstitial space, resulting in hypotension, decreased venous return, and decreased cardiac output • Smooth muscle contraction, resulting in bronchospasm
3. Platelet-activating factor	• Platelet aggregation triggered, with release of histamine and serotonin
4. Eosinophil chemotactic factor of anaphylaxis (ECF-A)	• Unidirectional migration of eosinophils to the tissue sites involved in allergic inflammation • Exact role of ECF-A remains unclear
5. Prostaglandins (D and F)	• Smooth muscle contraction and vasodilation, resulting in bronchospasm and hypotension
6. Serotonin (5-hydroxytryptamine)	• Increased capillary permeability, especially in the lungs; predisposes to noncardiogenic pulmonary edema
7. Bradykinin	• Smooth muscle contraction and increased capillary permeability

rapid onset occurring within minutes of exposure to an allergen. Occasionally, the response may not develop for as long as 1 hour after exposure. It is imperative that nurses monitor anyone who has been in contact with a potential allergen, for at least 1 hour. Since patients experience side effects of medications almost routinely, the nurse must assess all patients and be aware of the many different reactions that may occur. The nurse must be able to differentiate between an anaphylactic reaction and a cutaneous or flush reaction, which may or may not portend more serious sequela. Certain drugs such as vancomycin, opiates, plasma expanders, and radioactive contrast media are known for causing a flush reaction. This reaction may be related to the dosage or to the infusion rate and not a true drug reaction. A few patients, however, may go on to develop a true anaphylactic reaction. Victims of insect stings or those who have ingested a food allergen must likewise be closely assessed to differentiate a local histamine release from anaphylaxis. For patients with life-threatening food allergies, avoidance may be difficult. Many food offenders, such as peanuts and fish, are used as food extenders, thickeners, and taste enhancers. For these potential victims, anaphylaxis may begin as the food allergen passes into the intestinal mucosal surface. The reaction may also be biphasic (i.e., the initial symptoms are immediate, and, as the food is digested, the symptoms reappear 6 to 8 hours later).[4]

A reaction may occur after the first contact with the allergen, although the individual will sometimes relate a slight reaction from a previous exposure. A thorough nursing history is mandatory before administering any medication or other suspected allergens. See Table 57–4 for specific symptomatology.

TABLE 57–4
Symptomatology of Anaphylactic Shock

System Affected	Symptoms
H1 and H2 Receptor-Stimulated	
1. Integumentary	Flushing Erythema Pruritus Urticaria Angioedema
2. Respiratory	Dypsnea Hoarseness Pharyngeal edema Wheezing Stridor
3. Cardiovascular	Arrhythmia Tachycardia Hypotension Ischemia
4. Gastrointestinal	Nausea Vomiting Cramps Diarrhea Mucus secretion
H1 Receptors—Immunologic Reaction	Nonvascular smooth muscle contraction, such as bronchoconstriction; increased peristalsis Capillary permeability, resulting in third spacing Coronary artery vasoconstriction
H2 Receptors—Nonimmunologic Reaction	Increased gastric secretion Increased mucus production Cardiac stimulation, resulting in ischemic changes from inotropy Coronary vasodilation

Clinical Presentation

Early Phase

Initially, the patient may be observed to be restless, apprehensive, uneasy, or fearful. Minor complaints may include lightheadedness and/or paresthesias (e.g., abnormal sensations of burning or tingling). Pruritus may develop with local or generalized urticaria. As fluid shifts occur between intravascular and interstitial spaces, angioedema may become evident. Edema may be observed particularly in the face (lips and eyelids), tongue, hands, feet and possibly the genitalia.

Intermediate Phase

With progression to the intermediate phase, patients experiencing laryngospasm and bronchospasm display increasing dyspnea and wheezing. They may appear exhausted from the increased work of breathing. As fluid shifts progress, pulmonary edema develops, along with abdominal cramps, diarrhea, and vomiting. Smooth muscle contraction may lead to incontinence of urine and, in women, uterine bleeding.

Advanced Phase

As fluid shifts continue, the circulatory system experiences a marked decrease in blood volume. Hypotension, tachycardia, and ECG changes that mimic myocardial infarction may occur. These changes include ST-segment elevation and T-wave flattening (see Chapter 18). Respiratory distress occurs as laryngeal edema obstructs the airway and pulmonary edema prevents adequate gas exchange. The respiratory complications and circulatory collapse contribute to the high death rate associated with anaphylaxis.

Therapeutic Management

The best treatment for anaphylactic shock is prevention. The initial emergent treatment is to halt the spread of the antigenic agent. In the case of an insect sting, scraping off the stinger from the epidermis will diminish absorption of the antigen. Never try to pinch or pull out the stinger with the fingertips or tweezers because this may only inject more venom or toxin into the wound.[5] If the bite or stinger is on an extremity, obstructing the venous and lymph circulation with a tourniquet will reduce the allergen's entry into the systemic circulation. The tourniquet must be removed at 3-minute intervals for 1 minute until definitive treatment (e.g., medications and intravenous fluids) is available. Careful removal of the stinger can then be followed by local injection of subcutaneous epinephrine to further retard antigen absorption. A 1:1000 epinephrine dilution is given 0.1 to 0.2 mL directly into the wound. The application of ice to the site will decrease pain and slow toxin activation.

The patient may show only early clinical manifestations of shock if the initial interventions have been successful. Should the shock state progress, maintaining a patent airway becomes the priority. The leading cause of death from anaphylaxis is laryngeal edema with airway obstruction. For patients experiencing upper airway (laryngeal edema) and/or lower airway (bronchospasm) obstruction, epinephrine administered subcutaneously or intravenously is the drug of choice. Epinephrine counteracts the adverse effects of histamine. If there is a delay in establishing an intravenous access, this medication can be instilled directly into the tracheobronchial tree by the endotracheal route. Table 57–5 may be used as a reference guide for epinephrine dosages, but it should be understood that it is only a guide.

Other interventions helpful in eliminating anaphylaxis are possible at several stages in the pathway of the reaction. For example, H1 and H2 histamine antagonists such as diphenhydramine (Benadryl) and ranitidine hydrochloride (Zantac) are administered as part of the initial treatment. Used concurrently, antihistamines block immunologic reactions and cutaneous symptomatology (see Table 57–4). However, they are not the primary drugs for the treatment of major reactions. An H1 blocker may relieve mild bronchospasm, but an H2 blocker will complete the antihistamine effect. This is because both H1 and H2 mediators contribute to peripheral vasodilation. Antihistamines cannot be used solely in anaphylactic treatment since they do not deactivate the effects of leukotrienes, which are more potent bronchoconstrictor agents than histamine[6] (Table 57–3).

Supplemental medications are used in conjunction with epinephrine to complete the armamentarium for patients whose condition is refractory to treatment. Before the advent of β-adrenergic drugs (Proventil, Alupent, Brethaire) that were inhaled, intravenous aminophylline or theophylline was employed to relieve bronchospasm. Intravenous aminophylline may still be used, but the β-adrenergic drugs by inhalation are preferred, since large amounts of medication can be delivered to airway tissue before systemic effects occur. Corticosteroids may also be prescribed, but their effect is not beneficial immediately. They are administered to stabilize lysosomal membranes, maintain intravascular volume, and preclude fluid imbalance. Respiratory support with mechanical ventilation and oxygenation may become necessary.

The patient who develops unstable hemodynamics and vascular collapse will need intravenous fluid resuscitation and vasopressor continuous therapy. Fluids are administered aggressively to restore circulating blood volume and perfuse vital organs. Fluids may not reverse the vasogenic hypovolemia, and vasopressor treatment may be initiated. Infusion therapy with 1 mg of a 1:1000 epinephrine dose in 250 mL of normal saline provides a concentration of 4 μg/mL, infused

TABLE 57–5
Drugs Used to Treat Anaphylaxis

Drugs	Dosage	Nursing Interventions
*Epinephrine** Clinical manifestations Early (mild to moderate)	0.1–0.5 mL of 1:1000 subcutaneous (SQ) or IM. SQ doses may be repeated at 10- to 15-min intervals as necessary.	The site should be massaged vigorously to increase absorption. The SQ route may be safer because the medication is absorbed more slowly. The intravenous (IV) route may cause fatal cardiac arrhythmias, especially in the elderly. If the patient is experiencing a cutaneous reaction (hives) or mild bronchospasm, but can still maintain a patent airway, SQ or IM doses can be continued. If the patient's condition deteriorates or if the blood pressure falls, the IV route is indicated. Asthmatic patients may be less sensitive to β-adrenergic stimulation and need to receive a higher dose of epinephrine. Patients receiving β-blocker medications will not respond to β-agonist drug effects unless given larger concentrations. The vasopressor effect of epinephrine may be reversed and hypotension may occur in patients receiving α-adrenergic blocking drugs, such as phentolamine.
Severe	0.1–0.25 mL of 1:1000 or 1.0–2.5 mL of a 1:10,000 IV. Any patient who is unconscious should be treated by this route.	The IV route is necessary for shock states since other routes offer poor absorption from impaired circulation. An IV injection given slowly is recommended because β-receptor sites respond to low and slow dosages at 10 μg/min. Epinephrine has a rapid antagonistic effect on histamine. Patients need close monitoring for the α- and β-agonist properties of this drug. Too much alpha stimulation can elevate blood pressure and cause cerebral hemorrhage, while too much beta stimulation can lead to myocardial ischemia, angina, and arrhythmias.
β-Adrenergic Bronchodilators Albuterol (Proventil) Terbutaline (Brethine) Metaproterenol (Alupent)	Dose depends on individual response. Given via handheld nebulizer or intermittent positive pressure breathing device. May be the only treatment needed if bronchospasm is the only symptom.	
Supplemental Drugs and Drugs Used to Treat Refractory Anaphylaxis H1 receptor blockers Diphenhydramine hydrochloride (Benadryl)	25–50 mg, PO, IM, IV.	May help relieve bronchospasm, but has little effect on major reactions. Should not be used in place of epinephrine. Will compete with histamine at the receptor-binding sites and block further absorption, but will not prevent histamine release. Is contraindicated in acute asthma and narrow-angle glaucoma. Help control symptoms of cutaneous reactions, such as pruritus and urticaria. May help reverse hypotension, but use cautiously as blood pressure may decrease.
Hydroxyzine (Vistaril)	25–100 mg, PO, IM.	Reverses cutaneous reactions.
H2 receptor blockers Cimetidine (Tagamet) Ranitidine hydrochloride (Zantac)	300 mg diluted in normal saline, given IV over 5, 10, or 15 min. 50 mg, administered slowly, diluted in 10–20 mL of normal saline.	Unopposed H1 stimulation causes coronary vasoconstriction. To negate this effect, H1 and H2 blockers are now combined for their synergistic effects. May help to reverse hypotension.
Aminophylline	Loading dose: 6 mg/kg administered over 30 min; not to exceed 25 mg/min. Maintenance dose: 0.5–0.7 mg/kg per h.	Desired effect is to reduce bronchospasm. Adverse effect may include hypotension tachyarrhythmias. Maintain serum levels at 10–20 μg/mL.
Hydrocortisone	100–1000 mg IV initially, then 100 mg every 6 hours, or continued as an IV drip 500 mg in 250 mL at 60 mL/h.	Controversy remains as to its benefits. Inhibits the formation of preformed mediators. Decreases the severity of symptoms. Increases the number of receptor sites available for sympathomime interaction. Dosages must be tapered.

TABLE 57–5
Drugs Used to Treat Anaphylaxis (*Continued*)

Drugs	Dosage	Nursing Interventions
Dopamine	2–5 μg kg^{-1} min^{-1} IV; may be increased gradually up to 20–50 μg kg^{-1} min^{-1}.	Clinical effects include α/β stimulation to support blood pressure.
Norepinephrine bitartrate (Levophed)	4–8 μg kg^{-1} min^{-1} IV; dose is individualized, based on the patient's response.	Used when dopamine is not effectual. A potent, direct-acting sympathomimetic. Adverse effects are many for sympathomimetic drugs, such as hypertension, arrhythmia, angina, dyspnea, and extravasation necrosis at IV site.

*The recommended dose of epinephrine is individualized and in cardiac arrest states is 1 mg IV push every 3–5 minutes as the starting dose. If this dose fails, other regimens can be considered: intermediate, escalating, and high-dose epinephrine. (Currents in Emergency Cardiac Care) 12, 1992.
Source of data: Hopfer Deglin, J and Hazard Vallerand, A: Davis's Drug Guide for Nurses, ed 3. FA Davis, Philadelphia, 1993.

at 1 to 4 μg/min. The sympathomimetic effects of epinephrine will increase peripheral vascular resistance, heart rate, and stroke volume to augment blood pressure.

In patients who are already intubated, a simple measure to treat hypotension is to place the patient supine and elevate the legs. This increases venous return to the heart, thus increasing cardiac output, mean arterial pressure, and tissue perfusion. If hypotension continues to be problematic, other vasopressors (dopamine and norepinephrine bitartrate) may be necessary (Table 57–5).

Discharge Planning

Once ventilation and circulation are restored, comfort measures and education can be employed. The patient and family/significant others must be taught preventive strategies and emergency interventions before discharge. After anaphylactic shock, patients need teaching instructions to eliminate the allergen from their surroundings. If this is impossible because of the patient's lifestyle, immunotherapy (hyposensitization) is initiated. Cutaneous tests are used to evaluate the immune system's ability to respond to known allergens.

Follow-Up Care: Hyposensitization. The basic problem in most atopic or allergic patients is that they produce too many IgE antibodies. The goal of hyposensitization or desensitization therapy is to reduce the number of IgE antibodies produced in the body in response to a specific allergen (antigen). This is accomplished by administering a long series of injections of the allergen, beginning initially with a low dosage, and gradually increasing it until the patient can tolerate an environmentally induced dosage. The mechanism underlying this form of immunotherapy is thought to involve a proliferation of the population of T suppressor cells specific for the allergen in question. Unfortunately, this is not always effective. Injections may be given throughout the year or beginning 3 to 6 months before the season starts. Treatment may continue for years or until the patient is free of allergic symptomatology. (For a discussion of T suppressor cells, see Chapter 47.)

Follow-Up Care: Medical Notification Bracelet or Tag. Patients with a known history of hypersensitivity should be instructed to wear a medical notification (Medic Alert) bracelet or necklace. Any individual who experiences a severe systemic reaction from a bee sting, a bite, or other various causes needs an allergy referral for further evaluation and care. Patients who have had or who are presently undergoing hyposensitization therapy should be reminded that immunotherapy is not a cure, but can provide protection against further exposure to the particular allergen(s).

Instruction regarding continuity of care after anaphylactic shock should be individualized according to each patient's allergy history and may include some of the discharge instructions and follow-up recommendations listed in the box on page 978. The patient and at least one family member should be able to state the emergency first aid measures that should be performed if the patient develops anaphylaxis. Commercial kits, available for this purpose, can readily be purchased with a physician's prescription. The patient and family member will need guidance and instruction in its appropriate use. If the patient is apprehensive about self-injection, pocket pressure nebulizers are available.

Effective immunotherapy for insect sting prophylaxis is specific venom therapy. However, the patient's history may not reveal what the causative insect was that precipitated the attack. If the patient can bring the dead vector to the treatment center, absolute identification and treatment with the appropriate antidote may be possible. If the causative vector is unknown, a mixture of venoms may be administered.

Upon discharge following an anaphylactic episode, the patient must be instructed to avoid any medication or activity that induces a state of vasodilation. Therefore, after anaphylaxis treatment, patients must avoid vasodilator drugs and alcoholic beverages. They should also avoid strenuous exercise and hot showers or baths for at least 24 to 36 hours.

PATIENT TEACHING: PROPHYLAXIS

The following are key nursing considerations for patient/family instruction regarding follow-up and preventative care:

1. The patient must be responsible for informing all healthcare personnel of specific medications, foods, etc., that elicit a hypersensitivity response. It is highly recommended that the patient wear a medical notification bracelet or tag.
2. As an outpatient, the patient can expect to wait 30–60 minutes after any injection so that direct observation can guarantee the patient is allergy-free.
3. At least one member of the family should be versed in emergency first aid measures in the event the patient develops anaphylaxis.
4. Patient/family must be aware of high-risk situations and have access to information regarding insect-breeding areas and characteristics of vectors.

Insect Anaphylaxis: Self-Protective Measures

1. Caution is needed when near insect habitats, such as flowering and fruit shrubbery or fields. Realize that warm weather increases insect numbers.
2. Clothing can be sprayed with repellent, and long-sleeved shirts, long pants, and shoes should be worn whenever possible for outings.
3. Because insects are attracted to dark and bright clothing, as well as shiny jewelry, avoid these items.
4. Avoid aromatics, such as fragrances and scented cosmetics.
5. Remain calm and still if insects swarm.
6. Avoid stings around the face and neck because these areas are vascular and the sting more threatening. Lie on the ground and/or cover the face with arms and hands.
7. Keep windows up in cars and use air-conditioning whenever possible.

Household Preventative Measures

1. Limit shrubs and plants in and around the house. Keep screens and doors in good repair.
2. Consider hiring a professional gardener, or assign another family member to perform the garden chores.
3. Exterminate all nests and hives in the vicinity.
4. Wear garden gloves for all outdoor work.
5. Keep trash cans clean and sprayed with insecticide.

Nursing Diagnoses, Desired Patient Outcomes, and Nursing Interventions

The case study that follows provides the assessment data used as the basis for care planning. See the sample care plan for the patient with anaphylactic shock, for specific nursing diagnoses, desired patient outcomes, and nursing interventions.

CASE STUDY WITH SAMPLE CARE PLAN: PATIENT WITH ANAPHYLACTIC SHOCK

JP is a 25-year-old housewife and dental hygienist who has a history of sulfonamide allergy and allergies to dust, pollen, molds, and mildew. Her medical history reveals a diagnosis of rheumatoid arthritis within the last 3 months. Tonight, 10 minutes after eating dried apricots, she developed warmth, flushing, and a maculopapular rash that quickly became generalized. She read the container label and discovered the apricots were preserved with a sulfur preparation.

Her husband drove her to the emergency department about 20 miles away, although another hospital was within 5 miles from their home. On arrival, she presented with shortness of breath, diaphoresis, no fever, pulse 110/min, regular respirations 28/min, and blood pressure 150/86. JP is anxious, and between breaths blurts out that she thought that she would never make it to the hospital. "I cannot catch my breath; my throat feels tight." Angioedema is seen on her lips and hands. Five minutes later, she becomes hypotensive.

INITIAL NURSING DIAGNOSES

1. Airway clearance, ineffective, related to:
   a. Bronchospasm, laryngospasm
   b. Increased pulmonary secretions
2. Fluid volume deficit, related to:
   a. Vasodilation
   b. Increased capillary permeability
3. Anxiety, related to:
   a. Respiratory distress
   b. Hypotensive state
4. Skin integrity, impairment of, related to severe urticaria
5. Knowledge deficit, related to:
   a. Inability to identify allergen
   b. Delay in receiving treatment

REFERENCES

1. Dickerson, M: Anaphylaxis and anaphylactic shock. Crit Care Nurs Q 11(1):68, 1988.
2. Corren, J and Schocket, AL: PGM Symposium. Anaphylaxis: A preventable emergency. Postgraduate Medicine 87(5):171, 1990.
3. Lieberman, P: Anaphylactoid reactions to radiocontrast material. Ann Allergy 67:95, 1991.
4. Sampson, HA: Peanut anaphylaxis. J Allergy Clin Immunol 86:2, 1990.
5. Settipane, GA and Boyd, GK: Anaphylaxis from insect stings. Postgrad Med 86:278, 1989.
6. Bush, WH: Treatment of systemic reactions to contrast media. Urology 35:148, 1990.

SAMPLE CARE PLAN FOR THE PATIENT WITH ANAPHYLACTIC SHOCK*

Nursing Diagnoses

Nursing Diagnosis #1

Airway clearance, ineffective: actual or risk of, related to
1. Bronchospasm, laryngospasm
2. Increased pulmonary secretions in response to release of chemical mediators from degranulated mast cells

Desired Outcomes

Patient will:
1. Maintain adequate alveolar ventilation and oxygenation:
   - Pulse oxymetry >95%
   - $PaCO_2$ 35–45 mmHg room air
   - PaO_2 > 60 mmHg
   - pH 7.35–7.45
2. Verbalize ease of breathing; breath sounds clear on auscultation; absence of adventitious breath sounds
3. Verbalize reduced anxiety; perform relaxation exercises; demonstrate a relaxed demeanor

Nursing Interventions

- Assess respiratory function:
  - Respiratory parameters: respiratory rate, rhythm; diaphragmatic excursion; use of accessory muscles.
  - Presence of abnormal or adventitious breath sounds on auscultation.

  - Neurologic parameters: mental status: orientation to person, place, and date.
  - Cardiovascular parameters: vital signs
  - Arterial blood gas parameters.
- Implement measures to assure a patent airway:
  - Maintain upright position.

  - Place suction and intubation equipment at the bedside.

  - Initiate oxygen therapy as prescribed (e.g., nasal cannula at 2 L/min).
  - Obtain baseline arterial blood gases (room air) before initiating oxygen therapy.
  - Monitor serial arterial blood gas parameters.

- Administer medication regimen as prescribed:
  - Anticipate injection of epinephrine.

  - Implement bronchodilator treatments in conjunction with the respiratory therapy department as per unit protocol and physician orders.

- Provide restful and calm environment to reduce tensions and anxiety.
  - Spend time at the patient's bedside.
  - Keep abreast of progress.
  - Instruct about relaxation exercises.
  - Provide periods of uninterrupted rest and/or sleep.

Rationales

- It is essential to establish presenting symptomatology to facilitate the ongoing evaluation of the patient's response to treatment measures.
  - Adventitious sounds are noted, with special emphasis placed on the presence of stridor and wheezing. Inspiratory wheezes and stridor are ominous signs.
  - A deterioration in the level of consciousness may be the first warning sign of inadequate oxygenation and tissue perfusion.

  - Upright position allows for chest wall expansion and diaphragmatic excursion; accessory muscles can be used to the fullest.
  - Suction equipment, etc., is needed for prophylactic readiness in case laryngospasm or edema compromises the airway.
  - Oxygen prevents hypoxia and consequent respiratory acidemia.
  - Monitoring of arterial blood gases provides a direct indication of the effectiveness of therapeutic measures in assisting the patient to maintain adequate gas exchange.

  - Subcutaneous route may be safer because it is more slowly absorbed. There are fewer adrenergic side effects. Epinephrine will help to control bronchospasm and improve ventilation.
  - Metaproterenol sulfate (Alupent), a frequently used adrenergic agent, stimulates β receptors and thus exerts the following effects: bronchodilation, positive inotropic and chronotropic cardiac activity, and decreased synthesis and release of chemical mediators by mast cells.

Nursing Diagnoses

Nursing Diagnosis #2

Fluid volume deficit: actual or risk of, related to:
1. Vasodilation
2. Increased capillary permeability with increased third spacing (angioedema)

Desired Outcomes

Patient will:
1. Maintain stable vital signs:
   - Blood pressure within 10 mmHg of baseline
   - Heart rate <100 beats/min
2. Remain without evidence of third spacing (e.g., no angioedema or pitting edema)

SAMPLE CARE PLAN FOR THE PATIENT WITH ANAPHYLACTIC SHOCK* (*Continued*)

Nursing Interventions	Rationales
• Monitor vital signs, particularly blood pressure and heart rate.	• An increase in blood pressure and decrease in heart rate may be indicative of restoring circulatory volume and cardiac output.
• Monitor intake and output hourly.	• Renal function parallels normal cardiac output and normovolemia. Urine output should be maintained at >30 mL/h.
• Implement prescribed fluid regimen.	• Initial fluid challenges must be monitored in relation to patient's clinical status.
○ Initiate intravenous therapy with lactated Ringer's solution (fluids may need to be infused wide open).	○ Ringer's lactate is the most compatible physiologic (isotonic) solution and can be infused at a rapid rate in an attempt to stabilize intravascular volume.
○ Anticipate repeated doses of SQ epinephrine, followed by IV administration if there is no clinical improvement.	○ Epinephrine is an endogenous catecholamine that stimulates both α and β receptors. It will increase the heart rate and myocardial contractility; it will increase systemic vascular resistance and thereby increase arterial blood pressure. It may be necessary to give epinephrine intravenously since peripheral perfusion may be inadequate for SQ or IM injection if the shock state progresses. The IV route is fast and efficacious, but when this route is unavailable, epinephrine may be instilled directly into the endotracheal tube after intubation (as prescribed).

Nursing Diagnoses	Desired Outcomes
Nursing Diagnosis #3 Anxiety, related to: 1. Respiratory distress (hypoxia and dyspnea stimulate flight/fight responses and emotional distress) 2. Hypotensive state	Patient will: 1. Verbalize ways to reduce stress and avoid panicking 2. Assume a relaxed demeanor

Nursing Interventions	Rationales
• Implement measures to assist patient/family to maintain control and react appropriately in the event of an emergency.	
○ Assist patient to assume a position of comfort—may try orthopnea.	○ Facilitates ease of breathing and may relieve respiratory distress.
○ Allow patient decision-making alternatives.	○ Anxiety may be decreased when patients are permitted decision-making power. ○ Choices facilitate autonomy and self-control.
○ Speak in a calm, soothing voice. ○ Offer optimistic reassurances.	○ There are positive psychological benefits derived from reassurances.
○ Do not leave patient unattended.	○ Fear is perpetuated when patient is left alone. The patient's condition may deteriorate rapidly.
○ Keep patient/family informed of treatments and progress.	○ Fear of the unknown is alleviated.
○ Consider the sedative effects of drugs such as diphenhydramine hydrochloride (Benadryl) to assist in managing anxiety.	○ Diphenhydramine can be used as an adjunct epinephrine therapy, after the acute symptoms are controlled.

Nursing Diagnoses	Desired Outcomes
Nursing Diagnosis #4 Skin integrity, impairment of, related to severe urticaria with pruritus	Patient will: 1. Avoid scratching 2. Demonstrate ways to avoid scratching (e.g., massaging with prescribed lotion) 3. Maintain intact skin, with absence of angioedema

SAMPLE CARE PLAN FOR THE PATIENT WITH ANAPHYLACTIC SHOCK* (*Continued*)

Nursing Interventions

- Implement measures to relieve itching and maintain skin integrity:
  - Apply cool compresses to affected areas, as needed.

  - Remove all unnecessary clothing/bedding.

  - Instruct patient to avoid scratching; if all else fails, instruct patient to use fingertips rather than nails and to use a massaging motion.
  - Administer diphenhydramine as prescribed.

  - A prescription may be given upon discharge that includes oral diphenhydramine and/or a topical cream.

Rationales

- Cool temperatures reduce the discomfort that coincides with pruritus and angioedema.
- Removal of clothing sometimes relieves itching and feelings of constriction.
- Scratching disrupts skin integrity, the first line of defense against infection.

- Diphenhydramine competes with histamine for the histamine receptor sites. It effectively controls localized itching.
- Since some chemical mediators (e.g., SRS-A) have slower and more prolonged action, an antihistamine and local, topical agents may be prescribed to counteract the annoying skin eruptions (urticaria).

Nursing Diagnoses

Nursing Diagnosis #5
Knowledge deficit, related to:
1. Inability to identify allergen (allergen was disguised as a preservative)
2. Delay in receiving treatment (driving to distant hospital rather than the one nearby; this may have exacerbated the shock state)

Desired Outcomes

Patient will:
1. Review sources of sulfur preparations
2. Discuss cross-reactivity with allergens
3. Verbalize need to expedite emergency treatment upon exposure to allergen(s)

Nursing Interventions

- Assess patient/family knowledge regarding allergic status: known allergens; precautions taken to avoid exposure to allergen(s); emergency care with onset of allergic reaction.

- Assess readiness to learn.
  - Identify support system in family.

- Implement patient/family education program:
  - Teach the importance of reading all labels.

  - Reinforce responsibility to notify all health professionals of specific allergies.
  - Encourage patient to wear a medical notification tag or bracelet.

  - Recommend an allergy referral.

  - Inform patient/family that treatment must be sought immediately because subsequent reactions may be more severe.

Rationales

- Assessing patient/family knowledge base regarding anaphylaxis assists in determining essential information to include in patient/family instruction; it may also help to discern misunderstandings that might complicate the patient's care.
- It is imperative that one or more family members be versed in emergency first aid measures in case the patient develops anaphylactic shock.

- Sulfiting agents (e.g., sulfur, sodium, or potassium bisulfate or sodium sulfite) are commonly used as antioxidants and food preservatives. Potatoes, shellfish, and wines are just a few items that contain sulfites.*
- Patients are active participants as well as recipients of interdisciplinary health care.
- Identification of the allergen or anaphylactoid reaction may be lifesaving, especially if only minutes can be spared.
- Clients who experience severe systemic reactions need a referral for further evaluation and care.
- Phase two reactions cause chemical mediators to be released into the blood, since the patient is already sensitized (i.e., has preformed IgE antibody from initial exposure). Treatment must be solicited at *nearest* hospital, via ambulance if necessary.

$PaCO_2$ = arterial carbon dioxide pressure; PaO_2 = arterial oxygen pressure.
*Effective August 1987, the Food and Drug Administration has banned the use of sulfite agents on fruits and vegetables intended for raw consumption. Also, effective January 1987, foods and nonalcoholic beverages must be labeled when sulfites are present in detectable amounts. Individuals can now test for sulfites right at the table just by dipping a test strip into the suspect food or drink. A simple color change indicates the presence of sulfites. From A continuing education service for physicians and nutritionists. Nutrition and the M.D. 12(10):1, 1986.

CHAPTER 58

Nursing Management of the Patient with Acute Poisoning/Substance Abuse

Cynthia J. Abel

CHAPTER OUTLINE

Epidemiology of Acute Poisoning
- Substance Abuse
- Prevention of Acute Poisoning
- Regional Poison Control Centers

Pathophysiology of Poisonings

Assessment of the Poison Victim
- History
- Physical Examination and Initial Management
- Laboratory Studies
- X-Ray Examination

Treatment
- Antidotes and Antagonists
- Prevention of Absorption
- Elimination of Substance
- Enhancement of Elimination

Specific Poisons

References

Suggested Readings

LEARNING OBJECTIVES

After completing this chapter, you should be able to:

1. Discuss the incidence of acute poisoning and substance abuse.
2. Define poisoning exposure, routes of exposure, and adverse reactions.
3. List common substances involved in acute poisoning or substance abuse.
4. Identify strategies for prevention of acute poisoning.
5. Identify the regional poison control center as the major resource available for the prevention, identification, and treatment of poisonings.
6. Examine the pathophysiology of common poisonings.
7. Describe the key components of assessment of the poison victim.
8. Differentiate therapeutic approaches and implications for nursing care in the treatment of a variety of acute poisoning exposures.
9. Delineate the nursing process in the care of a patient with acute poisoning or substance abuse.

Acute poisoning is a result of exposure to any substance that may damage the structure of the body or disturb the function of living tissues. Exposure may occur through ingestion, inhalation, absorption, or injection (Table 58–1). The number and type of agents potentially toxic to the human body are endless. New potentially toxic drugs and chemicals are continuously being reformulated or developed. Almost any substance can be toxic if the dose is high enough or the exposure is long enough. Care of the patient with acute poisoning from toxic exposure requires knowledge of a variety of toxic substances and a multidisciplinary team approach. Critical care nurses play an integral role in the care of the poisoned

patient. This chapter focuses on the epidemiology, pathophysiology, assessment, diagnosis, treatment, and nursing care of the patient with acute poisoning in the critical care setting.

EPIDEMIOLOGY OF ACUTE POISONING

In 1992, the American Association of Poison Control Centers (AAPCC) estimated 2.4 million human poison exposures to toxic substances occurred. Children under 6 years old accounted for 59% of all poisonings, but adults and adolescents accounted for

982

TABLE 58–1
Routes of Exposure for Human Poisonings as Reported by the American Association of Poison Control Centers (AAPCC) 1992

Route*	All Cases	Fatal Cases
Ingestion	75.4%	78.3%
Dermal	7.7%	0.5%
Ophthalmic	6.3%	0%
Inhalation	6.1%	13.1%
Bites and stings	3.6%	0.5%
Parenteral	0.3%	4.6%
Other	0.7%	2.9%

*Multiple routes of exposure were observed in many poison victims.

Source: Adapted from Litovitz, TL, et al: 1992 Annual Report of the American Association of Poison Control Centers Toxic Exposure Surveillance System. Am J Emerg Med 11:494, Sep 1993.

TABLE 58–2
Common Categories of Substances Involved in Poisonings

Substance	Ranking: % of Total Number of Poisonings Reported for 1992 (n = 1,864,188 reported)
Pharmaceuticals Prescription and nonprescription (over-the-counter) drugs (e.g., aspirin, acetaminophen)	31.8%
Cleaning Substances Household bleach, ammonia, cleansers, washing and laundry detergents	10.5%
Cosmetics and Personal Care Products Mouthwashes, aftershaves, colognes, perfumes, shampoos, nail polish	8.2%
Plants In the home, in the yard, or in the wild	5.7%
Bites and Envenomations Snakes, spiders, and stinging insects	4.0%
Pesticides and Rodenticides Agents to kill rodents and insects in the home environment; highly concentrated industrial agents used by professional exterminators	3.8%

Source: Adapted from Litovitz, TL, et al: 1992 Annual Report of the American Association of Poison Control Centers Toxic Exposure Surveillance System. Am J Emerg Med 11:494, 1993.

95% of all deaths from toxic exposure. Of poisoning fatalities, 56% occurred in 20- to 49-year-olds.[1]

In 1992, 92% of toxic exposures occurred in the home and involved ingestion. Over-the-counter analgesics, such as aspirin and acetaminophen, made up a major category of substances involved in poisonings. Tricyclic antidepressants (TCA) and central nervous system (CNS) depressants in combination with alcohol accounted for a high proportion of hospital and critical care admissions and were the most common causes of death following acute poisoning.[1] Other substances commonly involved in acute poisoning include cleaning products, plants, cosmetics, insect bites, envenomations, and pesticides (Table 58–2).

Although most poison victims are children, all age groups and socioeconomic levels are affected. Recently, the problem of geriatric poisoning has grown significantly and will probably continue to do so as the population ages.[2,3]

Exposure to a toxic substance or poisoning may be intentional or unintentional (accidental) (see box on poisoning terminolgy on page 984). Intentional exposure occurs as a result of a suicide attempt, substance abuse, or intentional misuse of a substance. Intentional exposure to a toxic substance may be referred to as an "overdose." Unintentional exposure to a toxic substance may occur as a result of misreading a label, workplace exposure, environmental exposure, or a hazardous material spill. The AAPCC reported that 87.1% of human poison exposures in 1992 were unintentional; suicidal intent was present in 7.2% of cases; 1.6% were food or drug reactions; and 0.2% were not classified.[1] Of the 705 human poisoning fatalities reported in 1991, 80% of adult deaths were intentional.[1]

Substance Abuse

Substance abuse is a form of intentional poisoning often leading to overdose, which may require critical care admission. Substance abuse episodes include any nonmedical use of a substance for recreational or psy-

chic effects, for dependence, or for suicide attempt or gesture.[4] Groups of substances commonly involved in this type of acute poisoning include narcotics/opioids, CNS depressants, CNS stimulants, hallucinogens, inhalants, and alcohol.[4]

Drugs most frequently identified in substance abuse episodes leading to acute poisoning and requiring hospital care include alcohol, cocaine, and heroin/morphine. Table 58–3 lists the top nine drugs responsible for substance abuse poisonings. The boxes on pages 984 and 985 define the nonmedical use of a substance and list some commonly abused substances.

It is important to make the distinction between intentional and unintentional poisoning. If the patient was involved in an intentional poisoning or episode of intentional substance abuse, psychosocial support for both patient and family is necessary. A nonjudgmental, supportive attitude from healthcare providers can enhance the therapeutic environment even in the critical care setting. Patients who routinely abuse chemical substances are a varied and complicated group. No particular personality traits or style can describe all of these patients. Some have additional psychiatric problems or other compulsive or addictive behaviors. These patients may appear hopeless, frightened, selfish, aggressive, and disheveled.

POISONING TERMINOLOGY

Acute: A single exposure occurring over a relatively short time, usually within 8 hours.

Chronic: A repeated exposure to the same substance, or a single exposure lasting longer than 8 hours.

Unintentional: An unintended poisoning exposure; commonly involves situations where children gain access to a toxic substance in the home, where it is obvious that they did not realize the potential danger of their actions.

Intentional: Implies a purposeful action with an exposure that results from an inappropriate use of a substance for self-destructive, or manipulative reasons, such as a suicide gesture, or the improper use of a substance in an attempt to gain a psychotropic effect.

Adverse Reaction: An unexpected reaction to a drug, food, or other agent; or the patient experiences an unwanted effect, which is usually caused by either an allergic, hypersensitive, or idiosyncratic response at a normal dose or with normal use of a substance.

Substance Abuse: The nonmedical use of a substance for psychic effect, dependence, or suicide attempt or gesture.

Both patients and family members may express a wide range of emotions from anger and hostility to guilt, shame, and denial.

There are a few red flags that may alert the critical care nurse to a patient with a potential substance abuse problem. A patient who cannot be made comfortable even with maximum doses of analgesics or who seems to have a high tolerance for various analgesics may require closer observation. A patient with multiple complaints of symptoms not generally associated with the primary complaint, such as nausea, headache, and abdominal pain, and requiring additional medications may be exhibiting signs of drug-seeking behavior.

Patients who have taken an overdose or who have a history of substance abuse may be harmful to themselves or others. It is necessary to identify this risk and consult a psychiatric nurse or mental health professional to assess the patient and significant others before discharge. Suicide precautions should be initiated for any patient who has intentionally overdosed or for whom suicide is suspected.

The Centers for Disease Control estimates that 300,000 high school students make a serious suicide attempt each year, that 6% to 50% will make another suicide attempt, and that up to 11% will eventually be successful. Many of these adolescents will require intensive care.[5,6] It is important that the critical care nurse caring for survivors of a suicide attempt be aware of risk factors for repeat attempts (see box on risk factors for adolescent suicide on page 985).

Patients with a history of substance abuse are more likely to have a variety of other medical problems. These commonly include hepatitis, human immunodeficiency virus, bacterial endocarditis, poor nutrition, poor hygiene, anorexia, weight loss, mental deterioration, and depression. Long-term abuse of substances such as alcohol may also cause hepatic dysfunction and coagulopathies.[7]

Interruption of a regular cycle of substance abuse may result in symptoms of withdrawal (Table 58–4). The time period the patient is in the critical care unit may be critical. Signs, symptoms, and time of onset are dependent on the substance, usual dose, and time of last dose.

Prevention of Acute Poisoning

Reference to unintentional poisoning as "accidental" should be avoided. The use of the term "acci-

TABLE 58–3
Drugs Most Frequently Identified in Substance Abuse Episodes

Substance	Rank
Alcohol in combination	1
Cocaine	2
Heroin/morphine	3
Acetaminophen	4
Aspirin	5
Marijuana/hashish	6
Alprazolam	7
Ibuprofen	8
Diazepam	9

Source: Adapted from National Institute on Drug Abuse. Annual Emergency Room Data 1991. Statistical Series. Series 1, No. 11-A. Rockville, MD, US Department of Health and Human Services.

NONMEDICAL USE OF A SUBSTANCE

- Use of prescription drugs in a manner inconsistent with accepted medical practice
- Use of over-the-counter drugs contrary to approved labeling
- Use of any substance (heroin, cocaine, marijuana, glue, aerosols) for psychic effect, dependence, or suicide (Drug Abuse Warning Network [DAWN], 1991)

Source: Adapted from National Institute on Drug Abuse: Annual Emergency Room Data, 1991. Statistical Series. Series 1, No. 11-A. Rockville, MD, US Department of Health and Human Services.

COMMONLY ABUSED SUBSTANCES

Narcotics:
- Opium
- Morphine
- Codeine
- Heroin
- Hydromorphone (Dilaudid)
- Oxycodone (Percodan)
- Meperidine (Demerol)
- Methadone (Dolophine)
- Pentazocine (Talwin)

CNS Depressants:
Barbiturates
- Pentobarbital (Nembutal)
- Amobarbital (Amytal)
- Secobarbital (Seconal)
Nonbarbiturates
- Chloral hydrate
- Paraldehyde
- Ethchlorvynol (Placidyl)
- Glutethimide (Doriden)
- Methaqualone (Quaalude)
Antianxiety agents
- Meprobamate (Miltown)
- Chlordiazepoxide (Librium)
- Diazepam (Valium)

CNS Stimulants:
Amphetamines
- Benzedrine
- Dextroamphetamine (Dexedrine)
- Methamphetamine (Desoxyn, Methampex)
Phenmetrazine (Preludin)
Methylphenidate (Ritalin)
Cocaine

Hallucinogens:
Indole group
- Lysergic acid diethylamide (LSD)
- Psilocybin
- Dimethyltryptamine (DMT)
Phenylethylamine group
- Peyote, mescaline
- Methylenedioxyamphetamine (MDA)
Miscellaneous
- Phencyclidine hydrochloride (PCP)
- Nutmeg
- Cannabis, tetrahydrocannabinol (THC)

Inhalants:
Anesthetics
- Nitrous oxide
- Ethylene
- Halothane
- Cyclopropane
- Diethyl ether
- Chloroform
Solvents
- Gasoline
- Kerosene
- Toluene
- Benzene
- Carbon tetrachloride
Miscellaneous
- Freon
- Amylnitrate
- White correction fluid

Alcohol

Source: Adapted from Levine, DG, et al: Drug abuse. In Schwartz, GR (ed): Principles and Practice of Emergency Medicine, ed 2. WB Saunders, Philadelphia, 1986.

RISK FACTORS FOR ADOLESCENT SUICIDE

- Previous suicide attempts
- Early sexual behavior
- Substance abuse
- Trouble at school and with the law
- Depression

Source: Adapted from Piacentini, J: 1993 pediatric update. Evaluating adolescent suicide attempters: What emergency nurses need to know. JEN 19(5):465, 1993.

dent'' implies that the event was not preventable. On the contrary, most poisonings are preventable. Use of an epidemiological framework related to prevention could assist in the development of strategies aimed at the prevention of poisonings and the education of clients to prevent reexposure.[8]

The Haddon matrix for prevention of injury can be applied to acute poisonings. This framework examines the acute poisoning event by dividing it into phases composed of pre-event, event, and post-event occurrences (see box on poison prevention model on page 987). For each phase, contributing factors to the event related to the host, toxic agent, and environment may be evaluated. Haddon's 10 strategies for prevention can be adapted and applied to the event[9] (Table 58–5).

TABLE 58–4
Signs and Symptoms of Withdrawal

Substance	Onset	Symptoms
Alcohol	8 hours after last drink, or a rapid 25% drop in ethanol alcohol (ETOH) level	*Stage 1* Tremors, tachycardia, hypertension, perspiration, anorexia, insomnia, hyperthermia *Stage 2* Intensification of stage 1 and hallucinations *Stage 3* Delusions, disorientation, delirium, amnesia *Stage 4* Seizure activity
Cocaine	Rapid Up to 9–12 months	Fatigue Depression Dysphoria Intense craving for drug
Opiates	6 hours after last dose	*6 Hours* Anxiety, drug craving *14 Hours* Rhinorrhea, lacrimation, perspiration, yawning *16 Hours* Dilated pupils, piloerection, tremors, anorexia, muscle, bone aching *24–36 Hours* Insomnia, hypertension, elevated temperature, tachycardia, nausea *36–48 Hours* Vomiting, diarrhea, hyperglycemia

Regional Poison Control Centers

Regional poison control centers should be regarded as the best source of current information concerning toxic or poisonous substances. In the United States there are currently 38 AAPCC-designated regional poison control centers. Regional poison control centers may be staffed with nurses, pharmacists, and physicians certified as specialists in poison information by the AAPCC, the American Board of Medical Toxicology, or the American Board of Applied Toxicology.

Each regional poison control center offers 24-hour telephone access to a population base of at least 1 million people. The poison control center is often the first facility contacted to determine the potential for toxicity of exposure and to recommend treatment.

In addition to telephone assessment of risk and advice on treatment, regional poison control centers provide education programs for the public on the use of the center, what to do in case of poisoning, and how to prevent poisoning. They also provide education for healthcare providers involved in the treatment of poisoned patients, interface with all healthcare facilities and emergency transport systems in the region served, and interface with local, state, and federal agencies in identifying and dealing with hazards to the community. Actions may include product

TABLE 58–5
Ten Strategies and Countermeasures to Prevent Poisoning

Strategy/Countermeasure	Example
1. Prevent creation of the poison.	Eliminate iron from children's vitamins.
2. Reduce the amount of poison brought into being.	Decrease lead content in paint. Give disulfiram (Antabuse) for alcohol abuse. Establish drug abuse prevention campaign in schools. Reduce quantity of drugs kept in home.
3. Prevent the release of the poison that already exists.	Control narcotic substances. Store hazardous products out of reach of children.
4. Modify the rate or spatial distribution of the poison from its source.	Limit prescriptions and refills for emotionally disturbed clients. Provide automatic shut-off valves for hazardous materials. Use medication containers that separate each day's medications for the elderly.
5. Separate in time or in space, the poison and that which is to be protected.	Use air packs or respiratory filters around toxic fumes.
6. Separate the poison by material barrier.	Use childproof poison containers.
7. Modify the basic qualities of the poison.	Modify drug dose for elderly. Alter chemical agents to reduce poison content. Use antidotes.
8. Increase resistance to damage from poison.	Improve nutrition, self-esteem, family dynamics.
9. Counter damage already done by poison.	Assess and treat: decontaminate, eliminate. Support vital functions.
10. Repair and rehabilitate poisoned individual.	Provide substance abuse treatment programs.

Source: Adapted from Robertson, LS: Injury epidemiology and the reduction of harm. In Mechanic, D: Handbook of Health, Health Care, and the Health Professions. The Free Press, New York, 1984.

recalls, contaminated food investigation, chemical spill treatment, and recognition of a threat to the community by the appearance of new or more lethal strains of street drugs.[10]

PATHOPHYSIOLOGY OF POISONINGS

Any substance is potentially toxic if exposure is at a high enough dosage or a long enough duration. Death and tissue damage from poisons may be due to the direct mechanism of drug action or to secondary complications from the substance or the substance's actions. An example of a direct action of a toxic substance on tissue would be the burn that results from skin exposure to cleaning substances. An example of secondary complications from a poisoning might be

POISON PREVENTION MODEL

Phase	Human Factors	Toxic Substance	Environmen-tal Factors
Pre-Exposure Phase			
Acute Exposure Phase			
Post-Exposure Phase			

Pre-Exposure: Includes events and factors that are present before the poisoning. The interaction of these elements leads to the poisoning.

Acute Exposure: The actual poisoning. This includes the physical response, the duration of the exposure, and the dose or strength of the poison.

Post-Exposure: Follows the acute exposure. Includes factors related to the body's response to the poison, the final dose, and care provided.

Human Factors: Includes all biologic and physiologic factors, such as age, health, comorbids, and emotional state.

Toxic Substance: Includes all characteristics and properties of the drug, such as how the drug acts on the body and toxic dose.

Environmental Factors: Includes all physical and sociocultural factors surrounding the poisoning, such as easily opened drug containers and family stress.

Source: Adapted from Robertson, LS: Injury epidemiology and the reduction of harm. In Mechanic, D: Handbook of Health, Health Care, and the Health Professions. The Free Press, New York, 1984.

TABLE 58–6
Common Mechanisms of Action for Toxic Substances

Mechanism of Action	Toxin Example
1. Direct surface/cellular injury[14]	Caustic acids, alkalis
a. Enzyme degradation	Snake venom
b. Tissue digestion	Hymenoptera venom
2. Enzyme inhibitors[15]	Heavy metals: arsenic, lead, mercury; Cyanide
3. Neurotransmitter potentiation/inhibition	
a. Increased neurotransmitter release[16]	Black widow spider
b. Inhibition of neurotransmitter breakdown[17]	Organophosphates
c. Mimics neurotransmitter[18]	Nicotine
d. Sensitization of effector tissue to neurotransmitter[19]	Freon
e. Blockade of postsynaptic receptors[20]	Atropine
f. Blocked re-uptake of neurotransmitter[21,22]	Cocaine; Cyclic antidepressant
g. Impaired production of neurotransmitter[23]	Isoniazid
h. Inhibited release of neurotransmitter[24]	*Clostridium botulinum*
4. Derangement of metabolic/respiratory processes[25–27]	Carbon monoxide; Acetylsalicylic acid
5. Target organ specifically[28]	Acetaminophen—liver; Paraquat—lungs
6. Alteration of cellular function[29]	Methemoglobin producers
7. Inhibition of anabolic processes[30–32]	Cyclopeptide mushrooms; Caster bean; Rosary pea

respiratory arrest caused by the CNS depression from narcotic ingestion.

Some poisons may cause immediate effects or damage, such as alkaline corrosives, exposure to which results in a liquefaction necrosis of tissue within seconds of contact.[11] Other substances may be delayed in their effects, such as paraquat, an herbicide, exposure to which can result in pulmonary fibrosis 1 to 2 weeks following contact.[12]

Duration of exposure also has a bearing on the toxic potential of many agents in the overall outcome of the poisoning. Generally, the longer the duration of exposure, the more toxic the outcome. This is exemplified by chronic salicylism poisoning, which is due to repeated intake of high doses of aspirin over a period of days, versus acute salicylism, which is due to a one-time ingestion.[13] Chronic salicylism is associated with a higher incidence of severe symptoms and death.

Table 58–6 lists seven mechanisms of action with their corresponding toxins. It should be noted that this is not an all-inclusive list and that certain substances may mediate their effects by multiple mechanisms.

ASSESSMENT OF THE POISON VICTIM

The assessment of the poison victim entails the solicitation of a poisoning history, the physical examination of the poison patient, the observation of response to pharmacologic antagonists, and the analysis of gastric contents, blood, and urine from the poison victim. It should be noted, especially with intentional exposures (substance abuse or suicide gestures), the agent involved in the poisoning is frequently unknown, so that all four components of the assessment must be considered collectively.

History

Following any necessary initial stabilization of the poisoning victim, securing a detailed history of the poisoning event is essential. Information about the substance and its toxic ingredient is necessary (1) to assess the immediacy of the situation, (2) to assess the toxic potential of the exposure, and (3) to identify the medical treatment needed to support the patient's vital system functions and to minimize the effects of the exposure. It is vital to gather information about the following: substance, amount ingested, route, time since exposure, drug allergies, age, weight, symptoms, past medical history, routine medicine taken, history of chemical dependency, and how and why the poisoning occurred (see box on elements of a poison history on page 989).

Obtaining an accurate history from a patient with known or suspected poisoning is very difficult. The patient may be too lethargic or confused to describe events accurately. A suicidal patient may give false information or may be uncooperative. A patient who has been poisoned unintentionally may not be fully cognizant of the drug or amount. Patients intoxicated with street or recreational drugs may give inaccurate information about the involved substances because they fear retribution and embarrassment or because they simply never knew what was actually mixed with, or cut into, the drug they used.

In-depth questioning of the patient's psychiatric history may be better obtained from family, friends, or a private physician. An objective and professional attitude toward the patient should prevail. Feelings of disapproval or disgust for the patient will limit the patient's cooperation and ability to trust providers. Patients may show anger, hostility, or reluctance to talk. It is more productive to begin communication with questions such as "How are you feeling?" or "What happened?" than to ask "Why did you do it?"

Physical Examination and Initial Management

The initial priorities in physical assessment of the poisoned patient are assessment of airway, breathing, and circulation (the ABCs) and assessment of neurologic status, as follows:

1. Assess and establish a patent airway and adequate ventilation. If the patient is unable to protect his own airway from secretions or emesis or if the poisoned patient is not breathing adequately, assisted ventilation and endotracheal intubation is essential. Suctioning may be required frequently.
2. Assess for other trauma, and control bleeding if present. Hypotension may be treated cautiously with fluid and blood if indicated by the underlying pathology. Do not overhydrate to the point of pulmonary edema. Hypotension may also require treatment with vasopressor agents.
3. Assess cardiac status. Blood pressure, pulse, peripheral skin color, and cardiac rhythm must be evaluated and treated if necessary. Cardiac monitoring is essential for any comatose patient. Many toxic substances may result in cardiac arrhythmias.
4. Assess neurologic status based on Glasgow Coma Scale, pupillary size and reactivity, sensory and

motor function, and patient's behavior. Restraint of a violent patient may be necessary to protect the patient from harming himself. Naloxone hydrochloride (Narcan) may be administered to the comatose patient. It is a pure narcotic antagonist and will reverse narcotic effects if present. Intravenous 50% dextrose may also be given to comatose patients without adverse effects.

A head-to-toe assessment should follow the initial assessment and emergency intervention. Many clues to the cause of the poisoning may be gathered from data obtained during careful examination. Needle marks, signs of trauma, pill fragments, or certain odors may be helpful. In addition, many physical signs can be associated with characteristics reflective of a particular toxic substance or group of substances (Table 58–7).

Ongoing patient assessment includes observation and maintenance of airway, and continuous monitoring of the cardiac rhythm, vital signs, urinary output, response to treatment, level of consciousness, and thermoregulation. Critically ill patients may require invasive monitoring with devices such as a Swan-Ganz catheter and arterial line.

Laboratory Studies

Blood, urine, emesis, or gastric specimens should be obtained in the early phase of care. Qualitative screening tests to identify drugs and other substances are routinely run on urine samples. Analysis of gastric contents may determine what was acutely ingested or may confirm exposure to a drug or chemical before significant systemic absorption has occurred. Quantitative serum analysis for substances such as methanol, ethylene glycol, acetaminophen, salicylates, iron, lead, arsenic, mercury, lithium, or TCA may be done to determine if the substance is at a toxic or lethal level. Most times a toxicology analysis is necessary only as confirmatory evidence of the substance ingested.

Severe poisoning or overdose victims may require monitoring of other laboratory values, including complete blood cell count (CBC), serum electrolytes, blood urea nitrogen (BUN), glucose, ethanol alcohol (ETOH), and arterial blood gases (ABG). Data may reveal acute drug-related changes in acid-base balance, electrolyte shift, hypo/hyperglycemia, carbon dioxide (CO_2) retention from respiratory depression, or hypoxia from aspiration or pulmonary edema. An ETOH level should be documented in any patient suspected of poisoning because it is a commonly associated factor.

Drugs such as acetaminophen and aspirin require baseline quantitative serum levels, with repeat levels 3 to 6 hours after ingestion. Serum levels of these drugs may be monitored for several days until the drug is completely eliminated. Serum levels may also be monitored for drugs that have a lethal dose or an amount per kilogram that is considered lethal or life-threatening.

ELEMENTS OF A POISON HISTORY

The following include basic questions and elements of a poison history:

1. What was involved in the poisoning?

This information may be difficult to ascertain because the substance involved in the poisoning may not be in the original container, products are frequently reformulated, and many poisonings are unsupervised. If possible, information about the substance should be obtained from the label on the container from which the substance was taken. Any patient transported to a hospital should be accompanied by the container with the substance involved in the poison incident.

At the site of exposure, it should be noted whether other substances could have been available to the poisoning victim, if there is any evidence of open medicine containers and household products, or if there were any characteristic smells or odors.

2. Who was involved in the poisoning?

Characteristics of the poisoning victims, such as age, weight, and past medical history, are important components of the poisoning history. Poisonings involving older children, teenagers, and adults are more likely to be the result of an intentional exposure than those involving a victim under 5 years old. Weight can also be helpful, because for many toxins the dose of the toxin in relation to the weight of the patient can be calculated to provide an expected range of toxicity.

3. When did the poisoning occur?

Knowing when the poisoning occurred helps to establish a causal relationship between the poison exposure and the symptoms the patient is manifesting, and helps to predict upcoming symptomatology.

4. Where did the poisoning occur?

Knowing where the poisoning occurred is especially important for children, to assist with the determination of what product was involved. For instance, a child found in the bathroom may have access to the set of substances normally found in that area of the home, such as toilet bowl cleaners, bleaches, and medications in the medicine cabinet, versus a poisoning occurring in the yard, or the garage, where substances such as automotive products, pesticides, or garden care products are available.

5. How much of the substance was involved in the poisoning?

This question is important, especially when a substance has been ingested. This information can provide an estimate of the dose of a toxin that a victim was exposed to, which will allow an estimation of the toxic potential of the poisoning incident.

6. What was the route or routes of exposure?

In addition to being ingested, poisons may also be inhaled, may come in direct contact with the eye, may be splashed on the skin, or may be rejected. There are a significant number of poisons that do involve multiple routes of exposure. Each route of exposure requires a specialized decontamination procedure. Also, for each route, those tissues exposed to a toxin may incur direct injury or may become a route of administration for systemic absorption.

7. What symptoms has the patient had?

Is the patient conscious? Is the patient breathing? Does the patient have a pulse? Are the symptoms likely to be related to the exposure?

8. What was the reason for exposure?

It is important to distinguish an unintentional from an intentional exposure. Many intentional exposures involve multiple drugs, have worse outcomes in terms of morbidity and mortality, and are often accompanied by inaccurate or incomplete histories. Therefore, they may require more aggressive therapy and monitoring.

9. What first aid has been performed?

It is important to determine whether the patient has had an adequate decontamination procedure performed. Many first aid procedures can complicate the poisoning, such as using salt water as an emetic in children, which has resulted in fatalities from hypernatremia.[33]

10. What current medication is the patient on?

The substances involved in a poisoning may interact with another medication that a patient is chronically administered for a therapeutic purpose. For example, a patient taking a monoamine oxidase inhibitor who ingests a therapeutic dose of a sympathomimetic or decongestant, such as phenylpropanolamine, could develop a life-threatening hypertensive crisis.[34]

11. What allergies does the patient have?

Some patients are at risk for hypersensitivity reactions to medications, chemicals, and venoms. A patient who has previously been exposed and sensitized to hymenoptera venom may be at greater risk for an acute anaphylactic reaction when stung by a honey bee, wasp, or hornet (see Chapter 57).

12. What other chronic disease states does the patient have?

Many times, patients with chronic disease states will be at higher risk for severe toxicity to exposures of certain substances. For instance, elderly patients with cardiovascular disease are more sensitive to the effects of, and respond poorly to, exposures to carbon monoxide.[35,36]

13. What is the race of the poison victim?

A poison victim with an enzyme deficiency, such as glucose-6-phosphate dehydrogenase deficiency, will be at greater risk for an acute hemolytic episode after ingestion of a mothball containing naphthalene than a patient without this enzyme deficiency.[37] It has been determined that certain populations, such as blacks or those of Mediterranean origin, have a higher incidence of this enzyme deficiency.[38]

TABLE 58–7
Physical Findings and Laboratory Clues to Poisonous Substances

Finding	Substance
Blood Pressure	
Hypotension	Sedative hypnotics (barbiturates, glutethimide), theophylline, iron, TCA, antihypertensives (methyldopa [Aldomet], clonidine hydrochloride).
Hypertension	Amphetamines, cocaine, PCP, anticholinergics (atropine), black widow spider venom
Bronchospasm	Organophosphates, toxic fumes, β-blockers
Respirations	
Slowed rate, apnea	Opiates, alcohols, sedative hypnotics
Hyperpnea, tachypnea	Salicylates, theophylline, dinitrophenol, CNS stimulants
Electrocardiogram (ECG)	
Bradyarrhythmias	β-blockers, clonidine, organophosphate insecticides, calcium channel blockers (verapamil hydrochloride)
Tachyarrhythmias	Amphetamines, cocaine, caffeine, theophylline, anticholinergics (atropine), TCA, nicotine
Conduction defects (PR, QRS, QT prolongation)	TCA, quinidine, arsenic, mercury, propoxyphene, propranolol
Temperature	
Hyperthermia	Salicylates, amphetamine, cocaine, anticholinergics, dinitrophenol, PCP
Hypothermia	Opiates, ethanol, sedative hypnotics, phenothiazines
Pupils	
Miosis (pinpoint)	Organophosphate insecticides, phenothiazines, chloral hydrate, clonidine, sedative hypnotics, opiates
Mydriasis (dilated)	Anticholinergics, TCA, cocaine, LSD, amphetamine
Nystagmus	Phenytoin, barbiturates, PCP
Bowel Sounds	
Increased	Organophosphate insecticides, sympathomimetics
Decreased	Anticholinergics (atropine, TCA), sedative hypnotics
Guaiac test (Hemoccult)—stool	Iron, nonsteroidal/anti-inflammatory
Muscular System	
Muscle tremor	Amphetamines, cocaine, caffeine, theophylline, lithium, alcohol, and sedative hypnotic withdrawal
Muscle flaccid/paralysis	Opiates, clonidine, sedative hypnotics, botulism
Muscle rigidity	Strychnine, tetanus, PCP, haloperidol, methaqualone, phenothiazines
Fasciculations	Organophosphate insecticides, nicotine, lithium, PCP
Myoclonus	TCA, carbamazepine, phenytoin, methaqualone
Integumentary System	
Dry skin	Anticholinergics, vitamin A
Sweaty skin (diaphoresis)	Organophosphate insecticides, nicotine, sympathomimetics
Cyanosis (slate-blue discolorations)	Methemoglobin producers (nitrates, phenazopyridines, aniline)
Alopecia	Thallium, antineoplastic agents
Fingernails (Aldrich-Mees lines; transverse leukonychia)	Arsenic, thallium
Needle tracks, pitted scars	Subcutaneous injections
Blackened needle tracks	Matches used to sterilize needle, leaving carbon on skin
Large cutaneous blisters	Barbiturates, carbon monoxide exposure
Oral mucosal burns	Acids, alkalis
Pseudomembrane or white film posterior on pharynx	Paraquat
Acid-Base Disorders	
Respiratory acidosis	Sedative hypnotics, opiates
Metabolic acidosis	Salicylates, methanol, paraldehyde, iron, isoniazid, ibuprofen, ethanol, ethylene glycol, carbon monoxide, cyanide
Respiratory alkalosis	Salicylates
Metabolic alkalosis	Sodium bicarbonate
Breath odors	
Pungent, volatile	Hydrocarbons, gasoline, kerosene, toluene, carbon tetrachloride
Bitter almond	Cyanide
Garlic	Arsenic

X-Ray Examination

A chest radiograph may reveal pulmonary edema or aspiration pneumonia. An abdominal radiograph may show a drug-induced ileus, but its main use is to determine the presence of any radiopaque substances in the gastrointestinal tract. The acronym CHIPE (chloral hydrate, heavy metals, iron, phenothiazines, and enteric-coated tablets) may be a useful adjunct for recalling drugs visible on x-ray.[39]

Any patient with suspected toxic ingestion should be continuously observed on a cardiac monitor. If there is a suspicion of drug-related cardiac toxicity, a 12-lead ECG should be obtained. Conduction or rhythm abnormalities with potential substances are noted in Table 58–7.

TREATMENT

Once initial stabilization has been achieved, other therapeutic options aimed at the identification of the substance, reversal with antidote, prevention of absorption, elimination of a specified drug, or disruption of the toxin can be instituted. The method of choice for removal or interruption of the poison and its effects depends on the method of exposure and the toxin.

Antidotes and Antagonists

Few poisons have specific antidotes, but there are some commonly used antidotes and antagonists (Table 58–8).[40] Although the mechanisms of action of various antidotes differ from agent to agent, the principal means by which antidotes work include direct binding of antidote to poison, drug receptor-site competition or receptor modification, alteration in poison metabolism, and direct counteraction of physiologic effects.

Administration of a certain antidote may be a useful diagnostic tool in a poisoned patient. If a patient's condition improves after the administration of a particular antidote, this may become a key diagnostic element. For example, it is common to administer parenteral naloxone (Narcan) in a comatose patient. If the patient has been poisoned by narcotics he may waken or demonstrate improved levels of consciousness after the administration of the naloxone.

Recently, the benzodiazepine antagonist flumazenil has become a valuable adjunct in the diagnosis and treatment of benzodiazepine poisonings. Patients who respond to this antagonist regain consciousness immediately, verifying the diagnosis and making a brief history possible. The effect of flumazenil deteriorates after 1 to 2 hours and leads to deterioration of the patient's level of consciousness.

TABLE 58–8
Pharmacologic Antagonists and Antidotes

Antagonists and Antidotes	Toxic Substance
Antivenin	Pit viper (Crotalidae) snake bites (rattlesnakes, water moccasins, copperheads)
	Black widow (*Latrodectus mactans*) spider bites
	Coral snake (*Micrurus fulvius*) bites
Atropine	Organophosphate and carbamate insecticide poisonings
Calcium gluconate	Calcium channel blocker (verapamil), hydrofluoric acid burns
Oxygen	Carbon monoxide
Cyanide antidote kit (amyl nitrite, sodium nitrite, sodium thiosulfate)	Cyanide
Deferoxamine	Iron
Dimercaprol (BAL)	Arsenic, gold, lead, and mercury
Diphenhydramine	Phenothiazine and butyrophenone-induced dystonias
Edetate calcium disodium	Lead
Ethanol	Ethylene glycol and methanol
Fab fragments (Digibind)	Digoxin and digitoxin
Flumazenil (Romazicon)	Benzodiazepines
Glucagon	β-blocker (propranolol)
Methylene blue	Drug- and chemical-induced methemoglobinemias
Acetylcysteine	Acetaminophen
Naloxone	Opiates
Physostigmine	Anticholinergic substances (antihistamines, atropine, antispasmodics, phenothiazines, TCA)
Pralidoxime	Organophosphate insecticide
Pyridoxine	Isoniazid, hydrazine-containing mushrooms

Prevention of Absorption

The general premise for decontamination is to remove the substance involved in the poisoning from the victim to decrease the amount of local tissue damage and to limit the amount of the substance absorbed into the body. The decontamination procedure chosen should be based on the amount of substance involved, its potential for local and systemic toxicity, the routes of exposure, and the patient's physical condition.

Dermal Exposures

Many toxins can cause direct irritation or burns to the skin, as well as be absorbed systemically into the body by this route, which is known as *percutaneous absorption*. For example, a primary route of exposure through the skin is observed with the organophosphate insecticides. Therefore, it is important to decontaminate exposed skin immediately on exposure to one of these agents to prevent severe systemic toxicity.

In addition, during the decontamination procedure, it is important to protect the decontaminator. Often the persons performing the decontamination may, themselves, become contaminated with the poisonous substance. So, the decontaminator, if using liquid, should wear gloves, an apron, and a mask if necessary when fumes have evolved.

The exposed patient should be washed from head to toe, including the hair and under the nails. Because some agents, such as the organophosphate insecticides, are fat-soluble, they may require special washing solutions, such as tincture of green soap (alcohol-based soap solution), to decontaminate the victim. The patient should be first rinsed with cold water, then with warm water, and finally with hot water. The reason to commence with cold water is to avoid causing peripheral vasodilation, thereby minimizing systemic absorption. It is extremely important to decontaminate a poisoned patient at the site of exposure, rather than "scoop and run." In addition, it is important to remove all clothing from the victim. Certain clothing articles, such as leather products, absorb pesticides and are difficult to decontaminate.

Ocular Exposures

Following ocular exposures to substances, it is important to irrigate the substance from the eye as soon as possible.[41] This should be done, preferably, at the site of exposure. Proper irrigation of the eye or of the affected eye or eyes should consist of a continuous irrigation for at least 15 to 20 minutes. The irrigation solution may include tap water if at home, or sterile saline in an emergency department.

Eyedroppers and irrigating syringes are worthless. In the home, the irrigation may be performed on a patient by holding his or her head back over a sink and pouring tap water from a large pitcher, liter bottle, or running faucet at low pressure about 6 inches from the eye. To avoid cross-contamination of the eyes, the irrigant should be poured from the bridge of the nose to the outward portion of the eye. Always avoid direct high-pressure irrigation. The irrigant can be just poured on the eye, even with children, because the eyes will usually open and close.

Prolonged irrigation may be necessary in cases of exposure to caustic substances. Neutralizing substances should not be administered. An ophthalmologist should be consulted. A device called a Morgan lens is available for hospital use for the purpose of ocular irrigation. This device attaches to intravenous (IV) tubing and fits over the eye like a contact lens. A continuous flush of normal saline can then be initiated. It is helpful to first instill anesthetic eye drops before placing the Morgan lens.

Inhalation

Frequently, victims exposed to fumes or gases will also require measures to decrease the amount of exposure and alleviate local irritation. With exposures involving the respiratory tract, measures, such as having the victim breathe fresh air or, in many cases, humidified air or oxygen, will alleviate local irritation of the mucous membranes and upper airway. If the patient is cyanotic due to asphyxiation or to an impairment of gas exchange or delivery of oxygen through the pulmonary system, then oxygen administration to the patient is required. It should be noted that patients exposed to fumes or gases may incur injury to the eyes as well as the upper and lower airways; therefore, it is always important to consider the possibility of multiple routes of exposure and to target the decontamination procedure toward each route.

Ingestion

The most common route of exposure for poisonings is by ingestion. The approach taken by the clinician to decontaminate the gastrointestinal tract of the poisoned victim has been an issue of ongoing controversy. The premise for gastrointestinal decontamination is to prevent absorption of a toxin that has a potential for systemic effects. There are many options in the area of gastrointestinal decontamination, such as the induction of emesis, gastric lavage, use of activated charcoal, use of cathartics, and even in some circumstances, endoscopy and surgery.

Gastrointestinal dilution with water or milk has long been touted as a first aid procedure for poisonings. This maneuver, if done inappropriately, can complicate a poisoning. For instance, milk used as the dilution fluid may delay the ability to induce emesis with ipecac syrup, or if a drug has been ingested, oral administration of water may enhance the dissolution of the tablets or capsules,[42,43,44] thereby facilitating systemic absorption and possibly resulting in faster onset of toxic effects from the drug. Administration of water is appropriate for a toxic ingestion that produces local tissue irritation or is a caustic. This results in decreasing the contact time between the toxin and the exposed tissue, as well as decreasing the concentration of the caustic agent, thereby decreasing the amount or degree of irritation and injury.[11,42]

The use of neutralizers after acid or alkaline caustic ingestion is not recommended because of the production of heat during the neutralization process. This first aid measure is still recommended on the labels of commercially packaged products and first aid charts. A policy statement regarding the gastrointestinal dilution with water as a first aid procedure in poisoning has been issued by the AAPCC.[42] Their recommendations include the following:

1. Oral dilution with water should *not* be used as a general first aid measure to treat ingestions of medications.
2. Following the ingestion of a caustic or corrosive substance, the immediate oral administration of water or milk is recommended.
3. Water is the appropriate fluid to administer in conjunction with ipecac syrup.

It has been demonstrated that the first aid recommendations on labels of commercial products are often hazardous, inappropriate, and inaccurate.[43] There are reported cases of patients developing severe toxicity, not from a substance initially involved in the poisoning, but from the first aid procedure.[33] If in doubt regarding the appropriate treatment of an ingestion, contact the regional poison control center.

Elimination of Substance

Part of decontamination includes gastric emptying. Two primary options to accomplish gastric emptying are to induce vomiting or emesis or to perform gastric lavage with the use of a large-bore orogastric tube. It should be noted that studies assessing the outcome of poisonings have not clearly demonstrated the beneficial effect on patients who are provided gastric-emptying procedures. In fact, many ongoing studies have failed to show a beneficial effect of gastric emptying on the outcome of the poisoned victim.[44] However, it is commonly observed that during these procedures the substance that was ingested is retrieved, as evidenced by pill fragments or retrieval of a colored fluid.

Ipecac Syrup

Ipecac syrup, because of its safety, efficacy, and oral route of administration, is considered by most to be the emetic of choice in poisonings. Ipecac is derived from a plant, *Cephaelis ipecacuanha,* and contains a mixture of alkaloids, such as emetine, psychotrine, and cephaeline.[45] Ipecac has both local and central emetic properties. Cardiotoxicity, resulting in fatalities, has been attributed to the use of fluid extract of ipecac, which is 14 times more concentrated than ipecac syrup, and to chronic abuse (of ipecac syrup) by bulimics.[46,47,48] Ipecac syrup is shown to induce emesis in about 96% of the patients to whom it was administered, and the onset of emesis will usually occur in 20 to 30 minutes.[49]

Contraindications to the induction of emesis include those situations in which the risk of pulmonary aspiration in the poisoned patient is high, such as in the comatose or seizing patient or after the loss of gag reflex; those situations in which the induction of emesis could precipitate severe gastrointestinal injury, such as with the patient who has ingested a strong acid or base, or solid objects, such as razor blades or nails; or in patients predisposed to hemorrhagic diathesis, such as patients with cirrhosis and esophageal varices or thrombocytopenia. As previously noted, removal of the ingested toxin from the gastrointestinal tract is based on the assertion that there is a significant risk for systemic absorption with significant toxicity once absorbed.

Certain hydrocarbons, such as gasoline, kerosene, or mineral oil, may mediate their toxicity primarily through direct aspiration into the lungs (rather than by absorption from the stomach). Therefore, it is not advisable to induce vomiting because of the increased risk of aspiration during the procedure. If the hydrocarbon is aromatic, such as benzene, or halogenated, such as carbon tetrachloride, or is contaminated by another toxic substance, such as a pesticide, the potential for systemic absorption and toxicity is greater and may require emesis. Because of the delayed onset of emesis with ipecac syrup, an assumption must be made that the clinical status of the patient will not change sufficiently to contraindicate the induction of emesis during that time period. Ingestion of substances such as TCA, camphor, or strychnine may also produce a rapid unpredictable onset of seizures and coma, and, therefore, the induction of emesis in that situation may be hazardous and not recommended.

Gastric Lavage

Gastric lavage is another procedure used to empty the stomach. This requires the use of a large-bore orogastric tube. Lavage should be performed in those situations where induction of emesis with ipecac syrup is contraindicated, such as in the patient who is seizing or comatose. The patient must be placed in the left lateral decubitus position, and, if severely obtunded or comatose or if the patient has a loss of the gag reflex, the airway should be protected with a cuffed endotracheal tube before the lavage procedure. Then a lavage solution, usually saline, in 200-mL aliquots in adults or 10 mL/kg in a child, is instilled into a lavage tube and then removed by aspiration or gravity suction. This should be continued until several liters of lavage fluid have been used or until the lavage fluid is clear. The tube can then be used for the instillation of activated charcoal and a cathartic.

There are limitations with gastric lavage. Large pill fragments may be unable to travel through the tube, especially those used for children, because of the size of the bore.

Gastric emptying is most effective if performed soon after the poisoning. However, the rate at which a substance is absorbed is quite variable and depends on a variety of patient-related and toxin-related parameters: the presence of food, the patient's intrinsic gastrointestinal motility, the amount of substance ingested, the effect of a substance on gastric-emptying time, the time since ingestion, and the physical properties of the substance. Ingestion of substances with anticholinergic properties, which decrease gastric motility and increase gastric-emptying time, may be amenable to gastric-emptying procedures even a day after ingestion.

Activated Charcoal

Activated charcoal is another useful adjunct to the treatment of poisoning and has been identified as the primary line of therapy.[50,51] Activated charcoal is made from the destructive distillation or burning of organic materials, such as wood, coconut, bones, and rice starch. It is activated by treatment with oxidizing gases, such as steam. Activated charcoal, itself, is a fine, black, odorless, and tasteless powder comprised of extremely small and porous particles. This porosity provides a large surface area to adsorb a large quantity of a substance. One gram of activated charcoal has a surface area ranging from 1000 to 3000 m^2. Substances that are adsorbed by charcoal include most medications, as well as a wide variety of other chemicals and natural toxins. Substances poorly adsorbed by activated charcoal include small ionic compounds, such as cyanide and caustic acids or alkalis, or small organic molecules, such as methanol. Recent research suggests that the use of charcoal alone without forced emesis may offer a better method of absorbing and removing poisons that were orally ingested.[50,51]

Enhancement of Elimination

Cathartics

Cathartics, such as magnesium sulfate and citrate, sorbitol, and sodium sulfate, have all been used in the treatment of poisonings.[52] It is important that activated charcoal, in most cases, be accompanied by the use of a cathartic to facilitate transport of the charcoal-drug complex. It should also be noted that there is no scientific basis to substantiate the use of cathartics alone. In addition, cathartics are contraindicated and may cause problems in the following situations: small children, in whom it may result in fluid and electrolyte imbalances; very old patients; patients with pre-existing renal disease, following the ingestion of nephrotoxic substances and caustics; and patients with recent bowel surgery, absent bowel sounds, hypertension, or congestive heart failure.

Other Methods

Another method used to decrease absorption of a compound from the gastrointestinal tract is to administer agents that chemically react with a toxin to result in an insoluble, nonabsorbable complex. Examples include the administration of a calcium-containing compound to the patient who has ingested fluoride,[53] which results in an insoluble, neutralized calcium-fluoride complex, and the use of bicarbonate for an iron poisoning,[54] where a bicarbonate solution is either administered orally or instilled through a lavage tube following an iron ingestion, which results in the production of insoluble iron salts, such as ferrous carbonate.

Forced diuresis may also be used to enhance the elimination of specific substances. In particular, acidification of the urine with ascorbic acid or ammonium chloride has been found useful in PCP and amphetamine poisonings.

Another less frequent mode of removal of a toxic product from the gastrointestinal tract is by endoscopy and/or surgery. Certain products when ingested may either lodge in parts of the gastrointestinal tract or form tenaciously adhering concretions. These are difficult to remove by either lavage or emesis or other

methods for gastrointestinal decontamination and, if left in contact with the gastrointestinal mucosa, may result not only in systemic absorption but also in severe damage to the lining of the gastrointestinal tract. Examples of such substances are iron, especially perinatal ferrous sulfate tablets, and disk batteries, both of which can be removed by either endoscopy or surgery.[55,56]

It is beyond the scope of this text to describe the best treatment modalities for all potential poisoning events. It is most important for the nurse to identify the potential poisoning, to assess and intervene in maintaining the ABCs and supportive therapy, and to contact a regional poison control center or specialized resource in order to determine the most appropriate treatment for the particular poisoning.

SPECIFIC POISONS

The following is a discussion of selected poisonings commonly treated in the critical care setting.

Ethanol Alcohol (ETOH). ETOH is a relatively weak poison and is most commonly treated in the critical care setting as part of a poisoning involving more than one substance. Alcohol abuse/use may have a cumulative toxic effect on all major systems because its metabolism interferes with vital functions.

ETOH poisoning kills by depressing respiratory effort, inducing hypoglycemia and potentiating hypothermia. In addition, alcoholics are prone to chronic malnutrition, gastrointestinal bleeding, hepatic dysfunction, pancreatitis, Wernicke's encephalopathy, and Korsakov's psychosis.[7]

Clinical findings of ETOH poisoning include slurred speech, ataxia, dehydration, hypotension, and hyponatremia. A blood concentration greater than 1.0 g/L is considered legal drunkenness and more than 5.0 g/L induces coma.

Treatment of ETOH poisoning includes airway maintenance, oxygen administration, gastric lavage, and fluid hydration. Intravenous 50% dextrose and 100 mg of thiamine intramuscularly (IM) may be administered to prevent the complications of alcohol abuse.

Alcohol abstinence syndrome or withdrawal symptoms may occur at any time after the serum ETOH level begins to decrease and up to 96 hours after the last drink. The most severe symptoms usually occur in 12 to 48 hours after the last drink. There are four stages to alcohol abstinence syndrome (Table 58–9). The stages are unpredictable and may overlap. Treatment is aimed at minimizing or decreasing the hyperirritability and managing medical complications of fluid and electrolyte imbalances, hypoglycemia, and other underlying problems.[57] Patient safety and injury prevention must be a major nursing consideration.

Acetaminophen. Acetaminophen is found in more than 70 over-the-counter products. It is used as an antipyretic and analgesic. Poisoning may occur as the result of unknown cumulative dosing with combination medications, such as cough syrups or cold medi-

TABLE 58–9
Four Stages of Alcohol Abstinence Syndrome

Stage	Characteristics	Nursing Considerations
I	Psychomotor agitation, autonomic hyperactivity, tachycardia, hypertension, diaphoresis, anorexia, insomnia, auditory and visual illusions	Hydroxyzine (Vistaril) 50–100 mg orally/ IM every 2–3 h or diazepam 10–20 mg IM or IV every 2–4 h. Assessment, close observation, patient safety
II	Hallucinations, amnesia	Haloperidol 2.5–5 mg IM every 2–4 h
III	Delusions, disorientation, delirium	Phenobarbital IV or diazepam IV
IV	Seizures	Diazepam IV

Source: Adapted from Knott, DH: Intoxication and the alcohol abstinence syndrome. In Schwartz, GR (ed): Principles and Practice of Emergency Medicine, ed 2. WB Saunders, Philadelphia, 1986.

cations. A single dose of 10 to 15 g or chronic use of 3 to 6 g daily may be fatal to adults; 150 mg/kg is considered potentially toxic.

Clinical findings occur 4 to 7 hours following ingestion and can be identified in four phases:

Phase I (up to 24 hours): Anorexia, nausea, vomiting, malaise, pallor, diaphoresis.

Phase II (24 to 48 hours): Right upper quadrant pain, increased liver enzymes, oliguria.

Phase III (72 to 96 hours): Peak liver function abnormalities, anorexia, nausea, vomiting, malaise, jaundice, hepatic necrosis, death.

Phase IV (96 hours to 2 weeks): Liver functions return to baseline.

Treatment includes monitoring acetaminophen levels 4 hours after ingestion, administering antidote acetylcysteine 140 mg/kg × 1 and 709 mg/kg every 4 hours for 17 doses, and administering activated charcoal to reduce absorption.[58]

Tricyclic Antidepressants (TCA). TCA poisoning is the most common cause of death after overdose, and it is very often encountered in the critical care unit. Cardiac arrest occurs in 12% of cases. Death has been reported after ingestion of as little as 500 mg. TCA inhibits the re-uptake of norepinephrine, which produces an anticholinergic effect on the body.

TCAs are used to treat depression. The most frequently reported TCAs associated with poisoning include amitriptyline hydrochloride (Elavil, Endep, and Emitrip), imipramine hydrochloride (Tofranil and Janimine), trimipramine maleate (Surmontil), and nortriptyline hydrochloride (Aventyl, Pamelor).

Clinical findings include mydriasis (dilated pupils), tachycardia, dry mucous membranes, urinary retention, decreased peristalsis, confusion, agitation, hallucinations, seizures, coma, and respiratory depression. Myocardial depression with conduction abnormalities may be seen. Sinus tachycardia, QRS-segment widening, right bundle branch block, and

first degree heart block may be identified on the monitor.

Treatment includes gastric lavage followed by multiple dose charcoal. Induction of emesis is not recommended because of the possibility of rapid deterioration of level of consciousness. Physostigmine (Antilirium) may be administered as an antidote. Hypotension should be treated initially with normal saline and followed by vasoactive drugs if necessary.

Continuous cardiac monitoring is recommended for a minimum of 24 to 48 hours following TCA poisoning. Diazepam (Valium) is the drug of choice for seizure activity. Ongoing nursing care includes airway maintenance, cardiac monitoring, frequent neurologic assessment, and measurement of urine output.[59]

Recently, hypertonic sodium bicarbonate has been found to be effective in the treatment of moderate to severe TCA overdose. Serum alkalinization with hypertonic sodium bicarbonate appeared to reverse toxic effects, such as hypotension, QRS-segment prolongation, and depressed level of consciousness.[60]

A care plan for TCA overdose is presented at the end of this chapter.

Cocaine. Cocaine is an alkaloid anesthetic. Cocaine-related deaths have increased more than 200% in the last decade. Cocaine may be taken intramuscularly, intranasally (snorting), orally, or intravenously. "Body packing," or swallowing pure cocaine in sacks to prevent detection, is particularly lethal if the bags burst. Typically 3 to 5 g of pure cocaine is released into the gut.

Crack is a very potent, inexpensive smokeable form of cocaine, which has increased in availability and popularity. Smoking crack results in more immediate absorption, quicker and greater euphoria, and an increase in addiction potential and toxic reactions. Chest pain, tachycardia, and ventricular fibrillation are more likely with this route of administration.

Clinical findings associated with cocaine toxicity include the following: CNS stimulation manifested by excitement, excessive talking, anxiety, mydriasis, diaphoresis tremors, vertigal nystagmus, hallucinations, and hyperthermia. Death is related to cardiovascular collapse and ventricular arrhythmias. Seizure and metabolic acidosis may also occur.

Treatment includes support of vital function and close monitoring of ABCs. Intravenous propranolol hydrochloride (Inderal) may be administered to alleviate cardiac toxicity. Sodium nitroprusside (Nipride) may be used to treat hypertension. Diazepam (Valium) may be used to suppress seizure activity. Hyperthermia may be managed with a cooling blanket or ice packs.[61]

Volatile Inhalants. Volatile inhalants are a diverse group of chemicals that produce vapors that cause an alteration in the state of consciousness and perception. They are used for recreational purposes. Abuse of these substances has been documented since 1962 and has been increasing steadily among adolescents. Multiple substances make up this category of poisoning, including solvents, glues, gasoline, lighter fuel, paints, antifreeze, and aerosol sprays. Generally, inhaled solvents are CNS depressants and may produce euphoria and hallucinations.

Clinical findings may include hallucinations, euphoria, excitement, blurred vision, tinnitus, slurred speech, headache, abdominal pain, chest pain, or bronchospasm. Patients may appear drunk, and their clothing, breath, and hair may smell of the solvent. Late findings may include decreased level of consciousness, convulsions, status epilepticus, and coma. A characteristic rash may be noted around the nose and mouth if the method of inhalation was from a bag or aerosol can—"bagging" or "huffing."

Long-term effects of solvent abuse are due to damage to the liver, kidneys, nervous system, and bone marrow. These effects may include peripheral neuropathies, bone marrow depression and aplastic anemia, cerebellar degeneration, disorders of equilibrium, marked moodiness, and encephalopathy.

Treatment is supportive and may include decontamination, oxygen, and treatment of arrhythmia or seizures. Patients may require intubation and mechanical ventilation, dialysis, or treatment of hepatic failure.[62]

Salicylates. Salicylates (aspirin) are used as antipyretics and analgesics. Salicylates are a common substance in unintentional and intentional adult poisonings.

Clinical findings may be divided into three phases:

Initial: Tachypnea, hyperventilation, and respiratory alkalosis.

Mild intoxication: Headache, vertigo, tinnitus, confusion, sweating, thirst, nausea, vomiting, and drowsiness.

Severe intoxication: Electrolyte imbalance, agitation, restlessness, seizures, coma, pulmonary edema.

Treatment includes gastric decontamination and administration of activated charcoal and cathartics. Alkalinization of urine to pH of 7 to 8 is recommended. One liter of dextrose 5% in water with 44 to 132 mg sodium bicarbonate and 20 to 40 mEq of potassium chloride should run 2 to 3 mL/kg per minute to produce urine flow of 3 to 6 mL/kg per hour. Treatment is dose-related. In general, if ingestion is 100 mg/kg or less, no treatment may be necessary. If ingestion is greater than 100 mg/kg, induction of emesis or lavage, activated charcoal, and cathartics should be part of patient management. For ingestions greater than 300 mg/kg, measuring salicylate levels every 6 hours is recommended. Additional lab work may include ABG, electrolytes, CBC, prothrombin time (PT), and partial thromboplastin time (PTT). Supportive nursing care and the maintenance of vital functions are also important.

Benzodiazepines. Benzodiazepines are sedative hypnotics commonly prescribed as antianxiety agents and may appear in acute poisonings as a single substance or in combination with alcohol or other drugs. Their general action is CNS depression.

Clinical findings include drowsiness, hypotension, tachycardia, depressed respirations, dilated pupils, slurred speech, coma, and respiratory arrest.

Treatment includes gastric decontamination and activated charcoal with cathartic. Recent research has demonstrated that administration of intravenous flumazenil may lighten the CNS depression. Continuous assessment and maintenance of ABCs is essential. In general, hypotension may be successfully managed with fluids.[40,63]

Phencyclidine (PCP). PCP is a hallucinogen that can be ingested, smoked, or snorted.

Clinical findings include wild and bizarre behavior. Patients often exhibit periods of lethargy with intermittent episodes of extreme hostility, belligerence, and destructive behavior. Coma may also be observed.[7]

Treatment may include care in a confident, deliberate manner, decreasing external stimuli and sedation with minor tranquilizers and sedatives. The patient may require physical or chemical restraint in intensive care. Care should be given to protect the patient from injury while meeting basic physiologic needs.

Iron. Iron is a mineral supplement found in a variety of preparations. Iron has a direct effect on gastric mucosa when ingested and may cause severe hemorrhagic necrosis in less than 2 hours.

Clinical findings occur in four phases:

Phase 1: Lethargy, restlessness, hematemesis, abdominal pain, bloody diarrhea.

Phase 2: Apparent recovery.

Phase 3: Shock, acidosis, cyanosis, and fever.

Phase 4: Hepatic necrosis.

Treatment includes support of the ABCs, prevention of absorption with gastric lavage and activated charcoal, and correction of shock by administration of fluids and blood. Deferoxamine may be administered for severe symptoms or if serum iron is greater than 350 mg/dL.

Organophosphates. Organophosphates are insecticides such as chlorpyriphos (Dursban), diazinon, malathion, and those used in pesticide strips. These substances prevent the breakdown of neurotransmitter acetylcholine, which creates a cholinergic crisis.

Clinical findings include increased secretions, salivation, lacrimation, urination, diarrhea, vomiting, muscle weakness, respiratory paralysis, psychotic behavior, and coma.

Treatment includes support of vital functions (the ABCs), prevention of absorption, and rigorous decontamination for dermal exposure. Atropine 1 to 2 mg IV repeated every 2 to 3 minutes until secretions are dry is the drug of choice. Pralidoxine (Protopam or 2-PAM) 1 to 2 g IV at 0.5 g/min or infused in 250 mL/ns over 30 minutes may also be used for the respiratory and muscular manifestations.[64]

Narcotics. Narcotics include drugs such as opium, morphine, codeine, heroin, oxycodone hydrochloride, meperidine hydrochloride, pentazocine. These drugs are used as analgesics and have CNS effects that include analgesia, sedation, mental clouding, and suppression of cough reflex and gastrointestinal motility.

In addition, a dose-related, centrally mediated respiratory depression is produced.

Clinical findings include pinpoint pupils, respiratory depression, lethargy, coma, and hypotension.

Treatment should include support of vital functions (the ABCs) and gastric decontamination. Oxygen and ventilatory support should be anticipated. Naloxone should be administered intravenously as antidote. Close observation and supportive care may be required for 24 to 48 hours.[7]

Carbon Monoxide. Carbon monoxide is an odorless, tasteless gas that results from incomplete combustion of carbon-containing fuels. It has a 200 times stronger affinity to hemoglobin than oxygen and will bind more quickly than oxygen to produce carboxyhemoglobin (CO-HB). This results in hypoxia, with primary effects on the brain and heart, which can be fatal.

Clinical findings can be divided into four levels of toxicity:

Level 1: Tightness across forehead, slight headache, dilation of cutaneous vessels. CO-HB level up to 20%.

Level 2: Nausea, abdominal discomfort, throbbing headache. CO-HB level up to 30%.

Level 3: Weakness, dizziness, nausea, vomiting, severe headache, dim vision, dyspnea, syncope, tachycardia, and collapse. CO-HB up to 50%.

Level 4: Syncope, ataxia, tachypnea, tachycardia, confusion, coma, convulsions, depressed respirations, depressed cardiac activity, and death. CO-HB up to 80%. Permanent neurologic damage and death is likely with CO-HB 60% or greater.

Treatment includes supportive care and maintenance of vital functions (the ABCs). Cardiac monitoring should be continuous. CO-HB levels should be measured every 2 to 4 hours until below 15%. Supplemental oxygen should be delivered as close to 100% FIO_2 as possible. In some cases this will require endotracheal intubation and mechanical ventilation. Hyperbaric oxygen therapy may be considered for the most severe cases.

Dexamethasone and fluid restriction can be used to treat cerebral edema. Patients with neurologic symptoms, abnormal ECG, metabolic acidosis, or CO-HB levels greater than 30% will require hospital admission.[65]

REFERENCES

1. Litovitz, TL, et al: 1992 Annual Report of the American Association of Poison Control Centers Toxic Exposure Surveillance System. Am J Emerg Med 11:494, 1993.
2. Klein-Schmartz, W and Oderda, GM: Poisoning in the elderly. J Am Geriatr Soc 31:195, 1983.
3. Oderda, GM and Klein-Schwartz, W: Poison prevention in the elderly. Drug Intell Clin Pharm 18:183, 1984.
4. National Institute on Drug Abuse. Annual Emergency Room Data 1991. Statistical Series. Series 1, No. 11-A. Rockville, MD, US Department of Health and Human Services.
5. Centers for Disease Control (CDC). Attempted suicide among high school students. United States, 1990. MMWR 40:633, 1991.
6. Spirito, A, et al: Attempted suicide in adolescence: A review and critique of the literature. Clin Psych Review 9:935, 1989.
7. Levine, DG, Schwartz, GR, and Ungar, JR: Drug abuse. In Schwartz, GR (ed): Principles and Practice of Emergency Medicine, ed 2. WB Saunders, Philadelphia, 1986.
8. Temple, AR: Poison prevention education. Pediatrics 74(suppl):964, 1984.
9. Robertson, LS: Injury epidemiology and the reduction of harm. In Mechanic, D: Handbook of Health, Health Care and the Health Professions. The Free Press, New York, 1984.
10. Manoguerra, AS and Temple, AR: Observations on the current status of poison control centers in the United States. Emerg Med Clin North Am 2:185, 1984.
11. Rothstein, FC: Caustic injuries to the esophagus in children. Pediatr Clin North Am 33:665, 1986.
12. Mofenson, HC, et al: Paraquat intoxication: Report of a fatal case. Discussion of pathophysiology and rational treatment. J Toxicol Clin Toxicol 19:821, 1982–1983.
13. Gaudreault, P, Temple, AR, and Lovejoy, FH, Jr: The relative severity of acute versus chronic salicylate poisoning in children. Pediatrics 70:566, 1982.
14. Kunkel, DB, et al: Reptile envenomations. J Toxicol Clin Toxicol 21:503, 1983–1984.
15. Chisolm, JJ: Poisoning from heavy metals (mercury, lead, and cadmium). Pediatr Ann 9:28, 1980.
16. Rauber, H: Black widow spider bites. J Toxicol Clin Toxicol 21:473, 1983–1984.
17. Mortensen, ML: Management of acute childhood poisonings caused by selected insecticides and herbicides. Pediatr Clin North Am 33:421, 1986.
18. Oberst, B and McIntyre, R: Acute nicotine poisoning. Pediatrics 11:338, 1953.
19. Baselt, RC and Cravey, RH: A fatal case involving trichloromonofluoromethane and dichlorodifluoromethane. J Forensic Sci 13:407, 1968.
20. Weiner, N: Atropine, scopolamine, and related antimuscarinic drugs. In Gilman, AG, et al (eds): Goodman and Gilman's The Pharmacological Basis of Therapeutics, ed 7. Macmillan, New York, 1985, p 132.
21. Gay, GR: Clinical management of acute and chronic cocaine poisoning. Ann Emerg Med 11:562, 1982.
22. Pentel, PR and Benowitz, NL: Tricyclic antidepressant poisoning. Med Toxicol 1:101, 1986.
23. Messing, RO, Closson, RG, and Simon, RP: Drug-induced seizures: A 10-year experience. Neurology 34:1582, 1984.
24. Dowell, VR: Botulism and tetanus: Selected epidemiologic and microbiologic aspects. Rev Infect Dis 6(suppl 1):S202, 1984.
25. Zimmerman, SS and Traxal, B: Carbon monoxide poisoning. Pediatrics 68:215, 1981.
26. Temple, AR: Acute and chronic effects of aspirin toxicity and their treatment. Arch Intern Med 141:364, 1981.
27. Gosselin, R, Smith, R, and Hodge, H: Clinical Toxicology of Commercial Products (Section III, Therapeutics Index), ed 5. Williams & Wilkins, Baltimore, 1984, pp 111–156.
28. Rumack, BH: Acetaminophen overdose in children and adolescents. Pediatr Clin North Am 33:691, 1986.
29. Smith, RP and Olson, MV: Drug-induced methemoglobinemia. Semin Hematol 10:253, 1973.
30. Davis, JH: Abrus precatorius (rosary pea): The most common lethal plant poison. J Fla Med Assoc 65:189, 1978.
31. Wedin, GP, et al: Castor bean poisoning. Am J Emerg Med 4:259, 1986.
32. Olson, KR, et al: Amanita phalloides-type mushroom poisoning. West J Med 137:282, 1982.
33. Barer, J, et al: Fatal poisoning from salt used as an emetic. Am J Dis Child 125:889, 1973.
34. Smookler, S: Hypertensive crisis resulting from an MAO inhibitor and an OTC appetite suppressant. Ann Emerg Med 11:482, 1982.
35. Aronom, WS and Isbell, MW: Carbon monoxide effect on exercise-induced angina pectoris. Ann Intern Med 79:392, 1973.
36. Grace, TW and Platt, FW: Subacute carbon monoxide poisoning: Another great imitator. JAMA 246:1698, 1981.
37. Shannon, K and Buchanan, GR: Severe hemolytic anemia in black children with glucose-6-phosphate dehydrogenase deficiency. Pediatrics 70:364, 1982.
38. Piomelli, S and Vora, S: G6PD Deficiency and Related Disorders

of the Pentose Pathway. In Nathan, DG, and Oski, FA (eds): Hematology of Infancy and Childhood, ed 2. WB Saunders, Philadelphia, 1981, p 608.

39. O'Brien, RP, et al: Detectability of drug tablets and capsules by plan radiography. Am J Emerg Med 4:302, 1986.
40. Kulka, PJ and Lauven, PM: Benzodiazepine antagonists: An update of their role in the emergency care of overdose patients. Drug Saf 7:381, 1992.
41. Rost, KM, Jaeger, RW, and deCastro, FJ: Eye contamination: A poison center protocol for management. Clinical Toxicology 14:295, 1979.
42. American Association of Poison Control Centers: Policy statement: Gastrointestinal dilution with water as a first-aid procedure in poisoning. Vet Hum Toxicol 25:55, 1983.
43. Alderman, D, Burke, M, and Cohan, B: How adequate are warnings and first-aid instructions on consumer product labels? An investigation. Vet Hum Toxicol 24:8, 1982.
44. Kulig, K, et al: Management of acutely poisoned patients without gastric emptying. Ann Emerg Med 14:562, 1985.
45. Manno, BR and Manno, JE: Toxicology of ipecac: A review. Clinical Toxicology 10(2):221, 1977.
46. Miser, JS and Robertson, WO: Ipecac poisoning. West J Med 128:440, 1978.
47. Smith, RP and Smith, DM: Acute ipecac poisoning. N Engl J Med 265:523, 1961.
48. Brotman, MC, et al: Myopathy due to ipecac syrup poisoning in a patient with anorexia nervosa. Can Med Assoc J 125:453, 1981.
49. Manoguerra, AS and Krenzelok, EP: Rapid emesis from high-dose ipecac syrup in adults and children intoxicated with antiemetics or other drugs. Am J Hosp Pharm 35:1360, 1978.
50. Derlet, RW and Albertson, TE: Activated charcoal: Past, present and future. West J Med 145:493, 1986.
51. Park, GD, et al: Expanded role of charcoal therapy in the poisoned and overdosed patient. Arch Intern Med 146:969, 1986.
52. Reigel, JM: Use of cathartics in toxic ingestions. Ann Emerg Med 10:254, 1981.
53. Monsour, PA, et al: Acute fluoride poisoning after ingestion of sodium fluoride tablets. Med J Aust 13:503, 1984.
54. Czajka, PA, Konrad, JD, and Duffy, JP: Iron poisoning: An in-vitro comparison of bicarbonate and phosphate lavage solutions. J Pediatr 98:491, 1981.
55. Venturelli, J, et al: Gastrotomy in the management of acute iron poisoning. J Pediatr 100:768, 1982.
56. Litovitz, TL: Button battery ingestions: A review of 56 cases. JAMA 249:2495, 1983.
57. Knott, DH: Intoxication and the alcohol abstinence syndrome. In Schwartz, GR (ed): Principles and Practice of Emergency Medicine, ed 2. WB Saunders, Philadelphia, 1986.
58. Riggs, B: Acetaminophen. In Noji, E and Kelen, G: Handbook of Toxicologic Emergencies. Year Book, Chicago, 1989.
59. Keough, V. Case review: A 27-year-old with a tricyclic overdose. J Emerg Nurs 19(5):382, 1993.
60. Hoffman, JR, et al: Effect of hypertonic sodium bicarbonate in the treatment of moderate-to-severe cyclic antidepressant overdose. Am J Emerg Med 11:336, 1993.
61. Higgins, R: Cocaine abuse: What every nurse should know. JEN 15:318, 1989.
62. Graham, DR: Solvent abuse. In Haddad, L and Winchester, J (eds): Clinical Management of Poisoning and Drug Overdose, ed 2. WB Saunders, Philadelphia, 1990.
63. Karb, V, Queener, S, and Freeman, J: Handbook of Drugs for Nursing Practices. CV Mosby, St. Louis, 1989.
64. Arena, J: Management of specific poisonings. In Schwartz, GR (ed): Principles and Practice of Emergency Medicine, ed 2. WB Saunders, Philadelphia, 1986.
65. Talbert, SR: Case review. Inhalation injuries: Review and two case studies. J Emerg Nurs 19(6):482, 1993.

SUGGESTED READINGS

SUBSTANCE ABUSE

Alderman, D, Burke, M, and Cohan, B: How adequate are warnings and first-aid instructions on consumer product labels? An investigation. Vet Hum Toxicol 24:8, 1982.

Alspach, JAG: American Association of Critical Care Nurses (AACN) Core Curriculum for Critical Care Nursing. WB Saunders, Philadelphia, 1991.

American Association of Poison Control Centers: Policy statement: Gastrointestinal dilution with water as a first-aid procedure in poisoning. Vet Hum Toxicol 25:55, 1983.

Aronom, WS and Isbell, MW: Carbon monoxide effect on exercise-induced angina pectoris. Ann Intern Med 79:392, 1973.

Barer, J, et al: Fatal poisoning from salt used as an emetic. Am J Dis Child 125:889, 1973.

Bertino, JS and Reed, MD: Barbiturate and nonbarbiturate sedative hypnotic intoxication in children. Pediatr Clin North Am 33:703, 1986.

Chin, L: Induced emesis: A questionable procedure for the treatment of acute poisoning. Am J Hosp Pharm 29:877, 1972.

Davis, JH: Abrus precatorius (rosary pea): The most common lethal plant poison. J Fla Med Assoc 65:189, 1978.

Derlet, RW and Albertson, TE: Activated charcoal: Past, present and future. West J Med 145:493, 1986.

Dowell, VR: Botulism and tetanus: Selected epidemiologic and microbiologic aspects. Rev Infect Dis 6(suppl 1):S202, 1984.

Gay, GR: Clinical management of acute and chronic cocaine poisoning. Am J Emerg Med 11(10):562, 1982.

Grace, TW and Platt, FW: Subacute carbon monoxide poisoning: Another great imitator. JAMA 246:1698, 1981.

Klein-Schwartz, W and Oderda, GM: Poisoning in the elderly. J Am Geriatr Soc 31:195, 1983.

Knukel, DB, et al: Reptile envenomations. J Toxicol Clin Toxicol 21:503, 1983–1984.

Kulig, K, et al: Management of acutely poisoned patients without gastric emptying. Ann Emerg Med 14:562, 1985.

Litovitz, TL, Normal, SA, and Veltri, JC: Annual Report of the American Association of Poison Control Centers National Data Collection System. Am J Emerg Med 4:427, 1986.

Manno, BR and Manno, JE: Toxicology of ipecac: A review. Clinical Toxicology 10:221, 1977.

Manoguerra, AS and Temple, AR: Observations on the current status of poison control centers in the United States. Emerg Med Clin North Am 2:185, 1984.

Messing, RO, Closson, RG, and Simon, RP: Drug-induced seizures: A 10-year experience. Neurology 34:1582, 1984.

Miser, JS and Robertson, WO: Ipecac poisoning. West J Med 128:440, 1978.

Mofenson, HC, et al: Paraquat intoxication: Report of a fatal case. Discussion of pathophysiology and rational treatment. J Toxicol Clin Toxicol 19:821, 1982–1983.

O'Brien, RP, et al: Detectability of drug tablets and capsules by plan radiography. Am J Emerg Med 4:302, 1986.

Park, GD, et al: Expanded role of charcoal therapy in the poisoned and overdosed patient. Arch Intern Med 146:969, 1986.

Pentel, PR and Benowitz, NL: Tricyclic antidepressant poisoning. Med Toxicol 1:101, 1986.

Reigel, JM: Use of cathartics in toxic ingestions. Ann Emerg Med 10:254, 1981.

Rost, KM, Jaeger, RW and deCastro, FJ: Eye contamination: A poison center protocol for management. Clinical Toxicology 14(3):295, 1982.

Rumack, BH: Acetaminophen overdose in children and adolescents. Pediatr Clin North Am 33:691, 1986.

Shannon, K and Buchanan, GR: Severe hemolytic anemia in black children with glucose-6-phosphate dehydrogenase deficiency. Pediatrics 70:364, 1982.

Smith, RP and Olson, MV: Drug-induced methemoglobulinemia. Semin Hematol 10:253, 1973.

Smookler, S: Hypertensive crisis resulting from an MAO inhibitor and an OTC appetite suppressant. Ann Emerg Med 11:482, 1982.

Temple, AR: Poison prevention education. Pediatrics 74(suppl):964, 1984.

Temple, AR: Acute and chronic effects of aspirin toxicity and their treatment. Arch Intern Med 141:364, 1981.

Vogel, SN and Sultan, TR: Cyanide poisoning. Clinical Toxicology 18(3):367, 1981.

CARE PLAN FOR THE PATIENT WITH TRICYCLIC ANTIDEPRESSANT (TCA) OVERDOSE

Nursing Diagnoses

Nursing Diagnosis #1
Ineffective breathing pattern (shallow, slow, or apneic), related to:
1. Altered state of consciousness (CNS depression)
2. Blunted hypoxic drive

Nursing Interventions

- Perform overall assessment.
- Assess respiratory function:
  - Respiratory rate, rhythm, depth; chest excursion; tone of respiratory musculature.
  - Breath sounds/presence of adventitious sounds and air exchange.
  - Oxygen saturation monitoring.

  - Supplemental oxygen if respiratory depression evident.
  - Assist ventilation if necessary.
  - Administer the following:
    - Naloxone hydrochloride (Narcan)
    - Thiamine
    - Glucose

Desired Patient Outcomes

Patient will maintain:
1. Respiratory rate >12 inspirations/min; regular rhythm and depth
2. Adequate chest excursion
3. Tidal volume >5–7 mL/kg with spontaneous breathing
4. Mental status: alert, oriented to name

Rationales

- Establishes a baseline with which to evaluate the response to therapy.
  - Respiratory depression or apnea are commonly and quickly associated with tricyclic drugs.
  - CNS depression results in decreased depth of respiratory effort.
  - Decreased respiratory effort will manifest by decreased oxygen saturation.
  - Improves oxygenation of vital organs.

  - May improve level of consciousness.

Nursing Diagnoses

Nursing Diagnosis #2
Ineffective airway clearance, related to CNS depression, loss of gag reflex

Nursing Interventions

- Assess serial ABG.

- Assess neurologic function: mental status, level of consciousness; sensorimotor function; and deep tendon reflexes.
- Avoid use of emetics.
- Gastric emptying per orogastric tube and instillation of activated charcoal after placement of cuffed endotracheal tube.

Desired Patient Outcomes

Patient will demonstrate ability to cough and expectorate secretions to protect own airway

Rationales

- CNS depression predisposes to aspiration.
  - Disruption of CNS function can be an ominous sign in acute poisoning.
- Acute TCA overdose predisposes to rapid neurologic deterioration.

Nursing Diagnoses

Nursing Diagnosis #3
Altered perfusion, related to myocardial depression and arrhythmia

Nursing Interventions

- Assess cardiac function: blood pressure, heart rate and rhythm, peripheral pulses, 12-lead ECG.
  - Fluid challenge
  - Serum alkalinization
  - Monitor ECG.
  - Treat arrhythmia per advanced cardiac life support (ACLS) protocol
  - Swan-Ganz catheter to monitor central venous pressure and pulmonary capillary wedge pressure
- Alkalinization with bicarbonate drip.

Desired Patient Outcomes

Patient will:
1. Demonstrate ability to maintain systolic blood pressure above 100 mmHg, regular heart rate above 60 beats/min and less than 100 beats/min
2. Demonstrate normal sinus rhythm with normal QRS segment and conduction
3. Demonstrate cardiac output in acceptable range

Rationales

- Establishes baseline.

  - TCAs cause negative inotropic effects.
  - Treats hypotension.
  - TCAs cause decreased conduction and decreased automaticity.

  - Decreased cardiac output possible.

- Enhances drug binding and decreases toxicity.

CARE PLAN FOR THE PATIENT WITH TRICYCLIC ANTIDEPRESSANT (TCA) OVERDOSE
(*Continued*)

Nursing Diagnoses

Nursing Diagnosis #4
Potential for poisoning, related to intentional ingestion of TCA

Desired Patient Outcomes

Patient will recuperate from poisoning episode without any obvious sequelae; patient will maintain:
1. Mental status: alert; states name
2. Usual personality
3. Respiratory function within acceptable parameters: breathing easy, breath sounds clear to auscultation.
4. Cardiac function within acceptable parameters: normal sinus rhythm, systolic blood pressure BP above 100 mmHg.

Nursing Interventions

- Assess potential/actual poisoning:
  ○ What/who was involved in the poisoning?
  ○ What was the route of exposure, and how much of the agent was taken?
  ○ What were the signs and symptoms?
  ○ What medications or other emergent actions were taken?
- Implement antagonistic treatment as prescribed.
  ○ Initiate gastric lavage.

  ○ Ensure that E/T tube cuff is inflated.

  ○ Administer activated charcoal as prescribed and monitor response to therapy.

    □ Auscultate for bowel sounds prior to administration.

    □ Monitor gastric pH.
    □ Administer prescribed dosage of activated charcoal: 50–100 g/adult.

  ○ Administer cathartic therapy: sorbitol 1 g/kg.

  ○ Administer sodium bicarbonate drip to alkalinize blood pH to 7.5.

Rationales

- Thorough assessment, including history, physical examination, and laboratory testing are essential to timely diagnosis and treatment (Table 58–4).
- Timely treatment is essential to reverse the effects of the poisoning agent before irreversible pathophysiologic changes occur.

  ○ Controversy exists as to the clinical efficacy of this modality. The decision to initiate lavage therapy is based on the time of exposure; the more recent the occurrence (30 to 60 min), the more effective the outcome.
  ○ An inflated cuff will help to prevent aspiration in the comatose patient.
  ○ Activated charcoal decreases toxicity by adsorbing chemical to its surface. Efficacy depends on timing of administration (most effective in 30 to 60 min, but may be effective up to 24 h).
    □ Activated charcoal is not given if bowel sounds are absent.
    □ Food in stomach may decrease effect of charcoal.
    □ Inadequate dose may induce *desorption:* a reversible process in which an adsorbed chemical is removed from the charcoal, causing free chemical to again be available to exert its untoward effects.
  ○ Cathartic maintains bowel motility to hasten elimination of drug/chemical/charcoal complex.
  ○ Alkalinization of blood increases protein binding and decreases free drug availability and resultant toxicity.

Nursing Diagnoses

Nursing Diagnosis #5
Potential for injury, related to CNS effects of ataxia, confusion, hallucinations, seizures

Desired Patient Outcomes

Patient will demonstrate:
1. Glasgow Coma Scale ≥ 14
2. Calm, appropriate behavior
3. Absence of ataxia, confusion, hallucinations, seizure activity

Nursing Interventions

- Perform neurologic assessment on arrival and at frequent intervals.
- Do not leave patient unattended.

- Provide quiet environment.
- Pharmacologic intervention as appropriate.
- Pad side rails.
- Explain all procedures.

Rationales

- Establish baseline.

- Tricyclic overdoses may have rapid neurologic deteriorization.
- Decreases stimulation.
- Decreases drug toxicity.
- Prevents injury if seizure occurs.
- Gains cooperation.

CARE PLAN FOR THE PATIENT WITH TRICYCLIC ANTIDEPRESSANT (TCA) OVERDOSE
(*Continued*)

Nursing Diagnoses

Nursing Diagnosis #6
Ineffective family coping, related to feelings of guilt

Desired Patient Outcomes

Family will:
1. Verbalize feelings about poisoning episode and the circumstances under which it occurred
2. Verbalize actions to be taken to prevent a recurrence

Nursing Interventions

- Assess the circumstances of the poisoning exposure.

- Allow the family the opportunity to verbalize their feelings.
- Have family verbalize the telephone number of the local branch of the poison control center.
- Have family verbalize emergency measures to be taken if such an episode would recur.

Rationales

- It is essential to evaluate how the poisoning occurred so that measures may be taken to prevent a recurrence.
- Verbalizing their feelings may help them to cope with this family crisis.
- It is essential for all households to have the telephone number of the poison control center.
- In the event of an emergency, it is essential that the family not panic, but follow the necessary steps to get help immediately. Minutes can mean the difference between life and death.

Nursing Diagnoses

Nursing Diagnosis #7
Ineffective individual coping, related to perceived lack of alternatives

Desired Patient Outcomes

Patient will demonstrate:
1. Appropriate knowledge as indicated by verbalizations of
   a. Medical complications
   b. Dangers of abuse
2. Acceptance of referral for care

Nursing Interventions

- Assist patient to identify feelings.
- Help patient to identify current and past successful coping strategies.
- Assess risk for repeat suicide attempt.
  - Provide referral for counseling when stable.
- Use nonjudgmental approach.
- Assess family support system.

Rationales

- May be successful when applied to this crisis

  - Serious intent demonstrated
- Establishes trust
- Resource for patient

UNIT ELEVEN

Oncologic Critical Care Nursing

UNIT OUTLINE

C H A P T E R   5 9

Nursing Management of Patients with Neoplastic-Related Medical Emergencies

Merri D. Walkenstein and
Deborah Rodzwic Pennypacker

CHAPTER OUTLINE

LEARNING OBJECTIVES

After completing this chapter, you should be able to:

1. Identify patients at risk for developing neoplastic emergencies, including:
   a. Cardiac tamponade
   b. Septic shock
   c. Spinal cord compression
   d. Syndrome of inappropriate antidiuretic hormone (SIADH)
   e. Superior vena cava syndrome (SVCS)
   f. Hypercalcemia
   g. Pain

2. List tentative etiologies for each of these oncologic emergencies.
3. Discuss pathophysiology underlying these oncologic emergencies.
4. Recognize the clinical presentation of these oncologic emergencies.
5. Discuss the clinical diagnosis and treatment of these oncologic emergencies.
6. Identify pertinent aspects in the nursing care of the patient with an oncologic emergency, including assessment, diagnosis, planning (desired patient outcome), and nursing interventions/rationales.

NEOPLASTIC CARDIAC TAMPONADE

Etiology and Pathophysiology

Cardiac tamponade is a life-threatening condition caused by an accumulation of fluid in the inelastic parietal pericardial space. This fluid accumulation, referred to as a "pericardial effusion," may result from a variety of syndromes and can result in a decrease in cardiac output (CO) with subsequent shocklike symptoms. *Neoplastic* cardiac tamponade implies that the cause of this fluid accumulation is cancer-related, which accounts for the majority of pericardial effusions.[1] For some patients, symptoms of cardiac tamponade are the initial presentation of their cancer.[2]

The accumulation of fluid causes an increase in the pressure around the heart, thereby preventing the ventricles from completely filling during diastole (Fig. 59–1). As a result, CO is markedly impaired. This rise in pericardial pressure may be rapid or gradual with fluid accumulation between 200 to 1200 mL.[3] If the fluid accumulation is gradual, the patient is often able to tolerate several hundred milliliters of fluid before symptoms occur.[4] If the fluid accumulation is rapid, acute symptoms of decreased CO are apparent.

Oncology-related conditions most likely associated with tamponade include the following:
- Malignant tumors that invade the mediastinum, blocking the normal resorption of pericardial fluid
- Malignant tumors that metastasize to the heart
- Constrictive pericarditis that results from the effects of radiotherapy on the pericardium or mediastinum

Patients at Risk

About 20% of patients with cancer will have metastases involving the pericardium and, to a lesser extent, the myocardium.[5] Patients at the highest risk for developing neoplastic tamponade include those diagnosed with melanoma, leukemia, lymphoma, and metastatic tumors of the lung and breast. Cancers of the lung and breast have the highest incidence of tamponade,[5] related, in part, to the lymphatic drainage of the heart, lungs, and breast. These patients are often treated with large doses of radiotherapy to the chest and may develop tamponade because of radiation pericarditis.[6]

Diagnosis

Although the clinical symptoms of cardiac tamponade may appear gradually, the signs and symptoms must be recognized immediately, or death will ensue rapidly. Diagnosis of cardiac tamponade is made by evaluating the patient's clinical signs and symptoms and by evaluating the x-rays, the electrocardiogram (ECG), and the hemodynamic invasive-monitoring values, using a pulmonary artery (PA), flow-directed, balloon-tipped catheter.

Common signs and symptoms of cardiac tamponade include the following:
- Hypotension
- Tachycardia
- Muffled heart sounds
- Narrow pulse pressure
- Kussmaul's breathing

Hypotension with classic shocklike symptoms occurs related to the decreased CO. A weak, tachycardic pulse is a compensatory mechanism resulting from the decreased CO. Auscultation of heart sounds is muffled because the heart is now surrounded by fluid. A narrowing pulse pressure indicates a decreased stroke volume with arterial constriction. One of the classic signs of tamponade is distended neck veins, or Kussmaul's sign. This sign is present if the neck veins distend during inspiration while the patient is lying with the head of the bed at a 60-degree angle, indicating an increase in right atrial pressure. Normally, the neck veins collapse during inspiration, decreasing the right atrial pressure and allowing the ventricles to fill.

Other signs and symptoms of tamponade include a pulsus paradoxus $\geq$ 10 mmHg. This paradox is characterized by a decline in systolic arterial pressure with normal inspiration and is usually absent if the patient's pressure is below 50 mmHg. Additional manifestations of cardiac tamponade are apprehension and restlessness (often the first sign indicating impaired cerebral oxygenation); cool, pale, and diaphoretic skin; shortness of breath; coughing; and decreased urine output. The following three classic signs of cardiac tamponade are often referred to as "Beck's triad": distention of neck veins, hypotension, and muffled heart sounds.

More definitive clinical signs that the nurse should

look for include values obtained by using a PA catheter. These values include the following:

Increased central venous pressures

Increased PA systolic and diastolic pressures

Increased pulmonary capillary wedge pressures (PCWP)

Decreased CO

An echocardiogram, computed tomography (CT) scan, and chest x-ray often show an enlarged heart with fluid accumulation. Continuous cardiac monitoring is essential because the ECG may demonstrate ST-T wave changes and/or electrical alternans (alternating large and small QRS complexes or altered direction of the complexes). This may indicate a diseased pericardium and is not commonly seen in other conditions.

A pericardiocentesis (aspiration or removal of blood or fluid from the pericardial sac) confirms the diagnosis of cardiac tamponade. This procedure is performed by a physician inserting a large-bore needle into the pericardial space to withdraw the fluid (Fig. 59–1). The fluid is tested for cytologic identification of malignant cells. Complications of this diagnostic procedure include the following:

- Irritated or perforated ventricles
- Lacerated coronary arteries
- Air embolism
- Pneumothorax

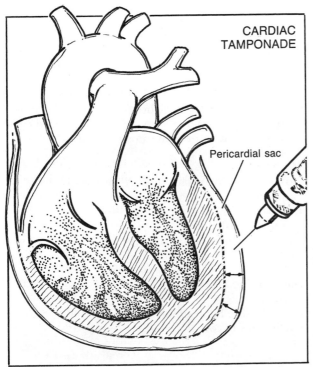

FIGURE 59–1. Cardiac tamponade. A pericardiocentesis, performed by introducing a needle into the pericardial sac, confirms the diagnosis of cardiac tamponade in addition to relieving the symptoms of decreased cardiac output.

- Infection
- Cardiac arrest

The nurse must anticipate these problems and be prepared to employ emergency measures.

Treatment

The patient and significant others need to be aware that the treatment for cardiac tamponade is often palliative, depending on the ability to control the underlying malignancy.[7] Therapy is aimed at restoring fluid volume and CO, relieving pressure around the heart, and enhancing oxygen perfusion of tissues. Fluid volume and CO are improved with administration of saline solution, alone or in combination with an inotropic agent such as dobutamine. This combination therapy increases the arterial pressure, CO, and stroke volume, while decreasing the systemic vascular resistance.[8] The pressure around the heart is decreased by performing a pericardiocentesis, in which case removal of fluid will usually return the patient's blood pressure to normal in 15 minutes.[4] A pericardial catheter may be inserted for repeated drainage of fluid and for instillation of chemotherapy or sclerosing agents into the pericardial sac. In addition, a pericardiectomy may be surgically performed to allow subsequent fluid accumulation to drain from the pericardial space.[9] Tissue perfusion, maintenance of cardiopulmonary function, and comfort are achieved by the administration of supplemental oxygen, fluid replacement, inotropic agents, vasopressors, and rest.

Nursing Diagnoses, Desired Patient Outcomes, and Nursing Interventions

For nursing diagnoses, desired patient outcomes, and nursing interventions in the care of the patient with neoplastic cardiac tamponade, refer to the care plan at the end of this chapter.

CASE STUDY: PATIENT WITH NEOPLASTIC CARDIAC TAMPONADE

The following case study illustrates the classic signs and symptoms, diagnostic studies, and therapy related to neoplastic cardiac tamponade. Although not all patients present with every symptom mentioned in this particular case, clinical manifestations such as dyspnea on exertion, tachycardia, ECG changes, Beck's triad, and pulsus paradoxus are almost universally present.[5]

Ms. C is a 55-year-old woman with metastatic adenocarcinoma of the lung. She is admitted to the hospital complaining of shortness of breath, dyspnea on exertion, and right lateral chest pain. Ms. C is restless and apprehensive, and assessment findings include cool, moist, and pale skin; hypotension with a narrowing pulse pressure; and a pulsus paradoxus of 15 mmHg. Neck veins are engorged with Kussmaul's breathing; heart sounds are muffled; and tachycardia with weak peripheral pulses is present.

Shortly after admission to the intensive care unit, a PA catheter is inserted to provide continuous hemodynamic monitoring. Hemodynamic readings include an elevated right atrial pressure, elevated PA systolic and diastolic pressures during expiration, an increased PCWP, and a decreased CO. The ECG reveals electrical alternans of the P waves and QRS complexes and ST-T wave changes. An echocardiogram reveals a collapsed right ventricle and confirms the suspected diagnosis of cardiac tamponade. Ms. C's low CO is treated with volume expanders and inotropic agents in preparation for a pericardiocentesis.

The pericardiocentesis is performed for two reasons: (1) it relieves the pressure around the heart, allowing for increased ventricular filling, and (2) it confirms the diagnosis of cardiac tamponade. During the procedure, 850 mL of grossly bloody pericardial fluid is obtained. A specimen for cytologic identification is analyzed and reveals the presence of malignant cells consistent with adenocarcinoma of the lung. This confirms a neoplastic etiology, allowing for appropriate therapy to be initiated. A pericardial window is performed, at which time a portion of the fifth rib is removed. This procedure allows for a decrease in pressure around the heart. A pericardial catheter is inserted for instillation of thiotepa (used as a sclerosing agent and a cytotoxic drug) and for continued drainage of pericardial fluid.

The nurse assessed this patient quickly, allowing appropriate measures to be taken. Ms. C's vital signs returned to normal within minutes, and her complaints subsided almost immediately. Although the therapy instituted did not change the overall prognosis of the disease process, it allowed Ms. C to continue to receive further palliative therapy.

SEPTIC SHOCK

Etiology and Pathophysiology

Septic shock is an oncologic emergency that must be recognized and treated in the early stages to improve the patient's outcome. Neoplasms, immunosuppressive therapy, and invasive procedures increase an oncology patient's risk for developing septic shock. Sepsis often begins with a gram-negative or gram-positive bacterial invasion; however, viral and fungal infections have also been identified as causative organisms.[10,11]

Septic shock is associated with systemic vasodilation leading to a decreased CO and tissue perfusion. The end result is cellular hypoxia, acidosis, and the potential for death. The patient initially responds to this process with mild hypotension, increased CO, hyper- or hypothermia, chills, mental confusion, tachycardia, and tachypnea. As the process progresses, capillary leakage and vasoconstriction occur, leaving the patient with cool skin, peripheral edema, and oliguria.

Without treatment, the condition worsens, causing further hypovolemia and the formation of microthrombi. At this point, the patient appears cold and clammy, has severe hypotension, and may develop multiple organ failure exhibited by adult respiratory distress syndrome (ARDS), renal failure, and disseminated intravascular coagulation (DIC). For more information, refer to Chapter 56.

Patients at Risk

Any patient who succumbs to an overwhelming infection is at risk for developing septic shock. However, patients with cancer are especially prone because of a variety of factors compromising immune function. These include such factors as altered mucous membranes and skin integrity secondary to invasive lines, chemotherapy, radiation therapy, malnutrition, and surgical intervention. Fistula formation can potentially occur in patients who have had abdominal or head and neck surgery because of poor healing, tumor invasion, or a past history of radiotherapy to the operative area. In addition, alterations in total white blood cell counts predispose patients with cancer to infection. Likely causes of myelosuppression in cancer patients include malignant tumor invasion of the bone marrow and bone marrow suppression. Tumor invasion of the bone marrow is frequently seen in patients with leukemias, lymphomas, and certain solid tumors. Bone marrow suppression may occur secondarily to systemic chemotherapy or radiation therapy to the bone reserves in the iliac crest, spine, or sternum. The absolute neutrophil count is an important determinant in assessing the risk of infection. (See Chapter 56 for other risk factors and laboratory data related to sepsis.)

Cancers commonly treated by chemotherapy and radiotherapy include lung, breast, and colon cancer. The following are some commonly administered cytotoxic agents that cause immunosuppression:

Busulfan
Methotrexate
Doxorubicin hydrochloride (Adriamycin)
Cisplatin
Etoposide (VP-16)
5-Fluorouracil (5-FU)
Cyclophosphamide (Cytoxan)
Vinblastine sulfate (Velban)
Mitomycin
Dacarbazine (DTIC)
Ifosfamide
Procarbazine hydrochloride
Paclitaxel (Taxol)

Diagnosis

Once it is determined that a shock state exists (decreased blood pressure and CO, tachycardia, and poor peripheral tissue perfusion), the type of shock must be identified (cardiogenic, neurogenic, anaphylactic, hypovolemic, or septic). The differential diagnosis of septic shock is based on a careful history and physical assessment. Certain factors, such as diagnosis, surgery, age, or treatment modalities, are essential to consider. These factors may constitute a significant risk for the occurrence of septic shock. Other data to evaluate are the absolute neutrophil count, coagulation studies, body temperature, and blood culture results.

Vital signs; hemodynamic measurements, including CO and PCWP; and urine output are monitored frequently, along with assessment of capillary refill and tissue perfusion. The patient's oxygenation status is assessed, including mental status and arterial blood gases (ABGs). The patient is continuously monitored for signs of respiratory failure (see Chapter 25).

Treatment

Therapy is directed at supporting the vital body systems while identifying and eliminating the source of infection. Antibiotic therapy must be started immediately after cultures are obtained. Efforts are made to conserve the patient's energy, so vital functions are maintained despite the anaerobic metabolic state resulting from cellular hypoxia. Limiting activity, promoting rest, and reducing environmental stimuli may be helpful. Ventilation support may warrant mechanical ventilation to conserve the patient's energy or to improve oxygenation status.[12]

Intravascular fluid volume is replaced based on the PCWP and urine output. Blood pressure may be maintained by administering traditional drugs such as dopamine, dobutamine, or isoproterenol, or an experimental agent such as naloxone hydrochloride, a narcotic antagonist.[13] Administering antiserum to endotoxins has been limited because the organism causing the septic shock syndrome cannot be identified at the onset of the clinical symptoms, a time when the drug must be given.[14] Temperature regulation is managed by using a warming or cooling blanket, iced saline gastric lavages, or ice packs to the groin. If complications, such as ARDS, DIC, or acidosis, appear, they are treated accordingly.

The best way of dealing with septic shock is prevention and recognition of the signs and symptoms as early as possible. Preventative measures may include the following:

- Observing strict handwashing technique
- Observing meticulous aseptic technique
- Identifying patients at risk
- Assessing baseline mental and physical status for subtle changes
- Recognizing signs and symptoms of impending shock so that treatment can be instituted early
- Teaching patients and families how to care for wounds and tubes and the importance of handwashing

Nursing Diagnoses, Desired Patient Outcomes, and Nursing Interventions

For nursing diagnoses, desired patient outcomes, and nursing interventions in the care of the patient in septic shock, refer to the care plan at the end of this chapter. For a detailed discussion of septic shock the reader is referred to Chapter 56. For additional nursing diagnoses, desired patient outcomes, and nursing interventions, see also the care plan at the end of that chapter.

The following case study includes some of the classic signs and symptoms, diagnostic studies, and therapy related to septic shock.

CASE STUDY: PATIENT WITH SEPTIC SHOCK

Mrs. G is a 78-year-old woman with adenocarcinoma of the colon with metastasis to the liver. Several months ago she was hospitalized with malignant ascites, at which time a paracentesis was done. A sigmoidectomy with a resulting colostomy was performed, and treatment with 5-fluorouracil by a newly implanted port was instituted. Mrs. G has a high risk for developing an infection that could lead to septic shock from compromised immune function, related to the malignancy, antineoplastic drug therapy, and the invasive procedures.

Today, Mrs. G is admitted to the hospital 2 years after diagnosis with a persistent cough, chills, and urinary frequency. Assessment findings include decreased breath sounds, a systolic pressure of 70 mmHg, a pulse of 135 beats per minute, 30 respirations per minute, a temperature of 98.4°F, 3+ bilateral pretibial pitting edema, and barely palpable peripheral pulses. Laboratory values are as follows: an absolute neutrophil count of 900 mm^3; hemoglobin of 12 g/100 mL; platelets of 60,000 per mm; prothrombin time of 31 seconds; partial thromboplastin time of 56 seconds; pH of 7.47; carbon dioxide pressure (PCO_2) of 22 mmHg; and an oxygen pressure (PO_2) of 82 mmHg.

Mrs. G's primary nurse notes a change in her mental status since the last admission. To compensate for Mrs. G's falling blood pressure and platelet count, fluid therapy is begun with normal saline and fresh frozen plasma, and platelets are transfused. A dopamine infusion is started to increase CO and a Foley catheter is inserted to provide accurate urine measurements. Although a positive culture has not yet been obtained, broad spectrum antibiotic therapy is begun.

A flow-directed PA balloon-tipped catheter is inserted to continuously monitor hemodynamic status. CO and PCWP are below normal from the massive vasodilation that occurs in the later stage of septic shock. Mrs. G becomes increasingly lethargic because of decreased organ and tissue perfusion. Assessment findings include cyanotic nail beds, oliguria, and hypotension. To maintain a PO_2 of 60 mmHg, Mrs. G is placed on mechanical ventilation set at a fraction of inspired oxygen (FIO$_2$) of 70% and 10 cm of positive end expiratory pressure (PEEP). Rapid assessment and implementation of nursing and physician orders led to Mrs. G's stabilization and recovery from septic shock. (See the care plan for septic shock at the end of this chapter. See also the care plan at the end of Chapter 56.)

SPINAL CORD COMPRESSION

Etiology and Pathophysiology

Compression of the spinal cord from a neoplasm is classified as an oncologic emergency because a successful patient outcome depends on *accurate* and *rapid* assessment, diagnosis, and treatment. The nurse has an important role in recognizing the symptoms of a cord compression and in advocating emergent follow-up care.

Spinal cord compression can occur when a tumor reaches the extradural space by direct extension from vertebral bony metastases, by growth through the intravertebral foramina, or by hematogenous spread. The neurologic symptoms associated with the compression may be related to the following:[15]

- Venous occlusion
- Vascular congestion
- Edema
- Arterial ischemia
- Hemorrhage

Any portion of the spinal cord may be invaded; however, the most common sites are in the lower thoracic region.[16] The location of spinal metastases can be summarized as 4% in the cervical spine, 71% in the thoracic spine, 22% in the lumbosacral region, and 3% in multiple sites.[16]

Patients at Risk

Spinal cord compression is one of the most common neurologic complications of metastatic cancer. It occurs in about 20,000 patients a year in the United States[17] (or 5% of the patients who die of cancer). The cancers most commonly associated with spinal cord compression are lung, prostate, breast, and kidney cancer.[16] In two large studies, lung cancer accounted for 20% of all cases.[16,18] In women, spinal cord compression is most commonly associated with metastatic breast cancer, with an incidence of 70% documented in advanced disease.[19] Table 59–1 lists the incidence of spinal cord compression by primary tumor.[16,20]

The *clinical* presentation depends on the level at which the spinal cord is compressed, rather than the location of the primary tumor. Neurologic symptoms may be what initially brings the patient into the hospital for evaluation, especially in the case of rapidly growing metastatic tumors.[21] The most common symptoms associated with spinal cord compression are as follows:

TABLE 59–1

Incidence of Spinal Cord Compression by Site of Primary Tumor

Site	Percent Range
Lung	12–19
Breast	13–24
Prostate	18–27
Kidney	5–10
Lymphoma	6–9
Myeloma	5
Unknown	5–11

Back pain
Weakness
Sensory loss
Autonomic dysfunction

Back pain is the presenting symptom in the majority of patients. It is initially local, with the potential to radiate weeks to months later.[22] The pain may be described as persistent, intense, and aggravated by movement, coughing, Valsalva's maneuver, sneezing, and neck flexion.[17,23] The pain may be worse while in the supine position; therefore, the patient may find it more comfortable to sleep sitting up.

Other symptoms commonly encountered include weakness, sensory loss, and autonomic dysfunctions. The location and extent of weakness depends on the level and degree of spinal cord compression. An initial complaint of a neurologic deficit may progress to paraplegia within hours to days.[17] Sensory dysfunctions may include loss of light touch, pain, and thermal sensation. There may also be loss of proprioception and deep pressure. Autonomic dysfunctions include urinary retention or hesitancy, bowel and bladder incontinence, constipation, and sexual impotence (see Tables 33–10 and 33–11). (See Chapter 28 for details about the neurologic assessment.)

Diagnosis

Early detection and treatment of spinal cord compression is instrumental in maintaining the patient's current neurologic status and in preventing further nerve damage. Patients with known or suspected malignancies complaining of back pain or unexplained weakness should have spinal cord compression ruled out. Diagnosis is confirmed with CT scan, myelogram, or with magnetic resonance imagery (MRI).

Prognosis

The most important factor in determining a patient's ability to maintain motor function is the degree of neurologic deficit the patient is experiencing before the initiation of treatment.[16,24] For example, if the patient is ambulatory when first diagnosed with spinal cord compression, the chance of maintaining an ambulatory status after therapy is 79% and only 18% for patients unable to walk before treatment.[16] Ambulation also has significance in terms of survival time. Of patients who walked before therapy, 47% survive for 1 year after treatment versus only 7% of non-ambulatory patients who live after 1 year.[24] Another prognostic indicator is the radiosensitivity of the primary tumor.[16] For example, patients with breast cancer respond to radiotherapy better than patients with lung cancer. The median survival time for patients with spinal cord compression is 3 to 6 months.[16,22,24]

Treatment

The choice of treatment for spinal cord compression consists of corticosteroid administration, laminectomy, radiotherapy, or a combination of therapies. Therapy is aimed at either preventing neurologic complications or treating symptoms already present. The type of therapy selected depends on the type, radiosensitivity, and location of the tumor. Early treatment is essential to regain neurologic function, to prevent further neurologic damage, and to relieve pain, all important to an individual's quality of life.

Nursing Diagnoses, Desired Patient Outcomes, and Nursing Interventions

Nursing diagnoses, desired patient outcomes, and nursing interventions in the care of the patient with spinal cord compression are presented in the care plan at the end of this chapter. The care plan at the end of Chapter 33 also presents essential information related to nursing care of the patient with spinal cord injury.

CASE STUDY: PATIENT WITH SPINAL CORD COMPRESSION

The following case illustrates how a patient with a spinal cord compression may present, be diagnosed, and be treated.

Mr. B is a well-nourished 61-year-old man with cancer of the lung admitted for a thoracotomy. He is ambulatory after surgery, but several days later complains of rapidly increasing numbness and leg weakness to the point where he collapses when getting out of bed. He has severe back pain managed with oral narcotics. Over the next 24 hours Mr. B develops marked weakness of his lower extremities, has a moderate decrease in pain sensation around the middle of his back, and has become incontinent of stool and urine.

An emergency myelogram reveals a complete block at T-3. A radiotherapy consult is obtained, and radiotherapy is started immediately, along with high-dose steroids to decrease the inflammation around the spi-

nal cord. Mr. B's neurologic and pain status are evaluated frequently for any changes.

Several days later Mr. B's condition remains stable; however, there is no return of motor and sensory function. He is discharged to a long-term facility and is confined to chair and bed rest. This case emphasizes the importance of early recognition and prompt treatment of symptoms in oncology patients with back pain and leg weakness. The nurse, as patient advocate, must be alert for symptoms of spinal cord compression so that treatment is instituted early.

SYNDROME OF INAPPROPRIATE ANTIDIURETIC HORMONE

Etiology and Pathology

In syndrome of inappropriate antidiuretic hormone (SIADH) there is a continuous release of antidiuretic hormone (ADH) that cannot be explained by normal stimuli. Normal, or appropriate, stimuli for secretion of ADH include the following:[25]

- Increased serum osmolality that may occur when a person becomes dehydrated or is given large volumes of hyperosmolar solutions
- Decreased plasma volume related to hemorrhage or capillary leakage
- Reduced central blood pressure (hypotension) seen in patients in cardiogenic or septic shock

Failure of the negative feedback system that regulates ADH secretion results in continued reabsorption of solute-free water, which expands the extracellular fluid volume. The system fails to respond to decreased osmolality or increased extracellular (intravascular and interstitial) fluid volume, resulting in the continued inappropriate secretion of ADH. The end result of SIADH is excessive water retention, decreased serum osmolality, hyponatremia, and increased urine sodium and urine osmolality.[26]

If SIADH is not discovered and treated early, the complications of hyponatremia and water intoxication may lead to severe neurologic complications that may ultimately end in coma and death. There are many diseases and medications associated with the development of SIADH. *Cancer-related* causes are as follows:[25,27]

- Carcinomas: bronchogenic, duodenum, pancreas, colon, prostate, thymoma, Hodgkin's lymphoma
- Cytotoxic drugs: vincristine sulfate, vinblastine sulfate, cyclophosphamide, cisplatin
- Miscellaneous: nausea, pain, stress, analgesics, trauma

Some neoplasms synthesize, store, and release ADH that is identical to the ADH produced in the hypothalamus.[27] The mechanism by which drugs produce SIADH is not known. Some drugs may increase hypothalamic ADH production and release. Others may act on the renal tubules, increasing their sensitivity to circulating ADH. Some cytotoxic agents, listed in the previous paragraph, may produce SIADH either by acting directly on the osmoreceptors in the supraoptic nucleus of the hypothalamus (Fig. 59–2) or by acting indirectly by causing nausea, which stimulates ADH secretion.[26,27]

Regardless of the underlying cause of SIADH, patients experience defects in the normal feedback mechanism of ADH. Therefore, patients become hypervolemic, with resulting dilutional hyponatremia and hypo-osmolality. As the kidneys conserve water, there is an increase in the urine sodium and urine osmolality. The plasma volume expands increasing blood pressure. As water retention progresses, patients demonstrate the signs and symptoms of water intoxication:[25,26,28] anorexia, nausea, vomiting pattern, diarrhea, confusion, hypothermia, alteration in respiratory pattern, and coma. Serum sodium drops from the hemodilution, and there is increased renal excretion of sodium, resulting in signs and symptoms of hyponatremia:[25,28,29] headache, lethargy, mental confusion, anorexia, muscle cramps, weight gain, weakness, nausea, vomiting, seizures, coma, and death. In both cases, the symptoms are related to how low the serum sodium is and how quickly it is lowered.[28]

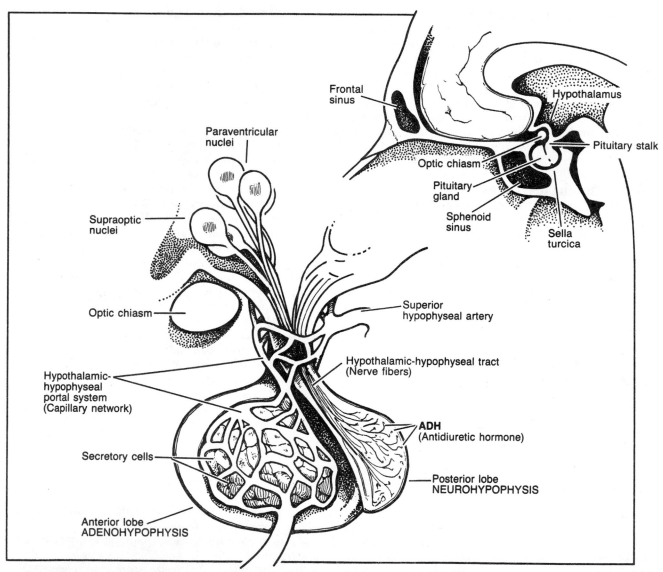

FIGURE 59–2. The pituitary gland, or hypophysis, lies within the bony sella turcica at the base of the skull. It is connected to the hypothalamus by the hypophyseal stalk. Anterior and superior to the pituitary as it sits in the sella turcica is the optic chiasm; anterior and inferior to the pituitary is the sphenoidal sinus. These structural relationships account for the visual field deficits experienced by individuals with a pituitary tumor. During pituitary-related surgery, access to the pituitary is achieved through a trans-sphenoidal approach (i.e., through the sphenoid sinus into the sella turcica). Continuity between the hypothalamus and neurohypophysis occurs via hypothalamic-neurohypophyseal nerve tracts; continuity between the hypothalamus and adenohypophysis is non-neural; rather, it occurs via the hypothalamic-hypophyseal portal system.

Patients at Risk

Cancer-related factors responsible for SIADH are listed in the preceding discussion. Indirect cancer-related causes of SIADH include severe pain, emotional stress, nausea, and narcotic administration. Other related factors seen in the oncology patient that can cause SIADH are central nervous system disorders, such as infection or seizures, and pulmonary disorders, such as pneumonia.

Clinical Presentation

Clinically, manifestations of SIADH occur secondary to the two primary pathophysiologic states: water intoxication and hyponatremia. There may be an initial gradual onset of neurologic symptoms—headache, confusion, disorientation, and weakness—together with the nausea, vomiting, diarrhea, and anorexia associated with the hyponatremia. Subsequently, muscle cramps, twitching, and seizures may ensue. Since the signs and symptoms are nonspecific, a high index of suspicion is necessary in assessing the patient. Therefore, a thorough history is critical to help distinguish etiologic from contributory factors.

Critically ill oncology patients are frequently ventilator-dependent. Positive pressure breathing may predispose the patient to an increase in ADH secretion. The underlying mechanism is associated with the reduction in venous return and CO, resulting from positive pressures generated in the thorax during the inspiratory phase. The consequent reflex reduction in CO (e.g., by baroreceptors) triggers the release of ADH. Nurses caring for the ventilated patient should therefore be vigilant for signs and symptoms of SIADH.

Diagnosis

Diagnosis of SIADH depends on several criteria being present:[25,28]
  Hyponatremia
  Decreased serum osmolality
  Inappropriately increased urine osmolality
  Increased urine sodium
  Normal renal, cardiac, and adrenal function
  No known defect in circulating volume or free water generation
The syndrome should be suspected in patients who are hyponatremic and have urine that is hypertonic in relation to plasma osmolality.

A *water-loading* test may be used to diagnose SIADH. The water-loading test is initiated by giving the patient 20 to 25 mL of water per kilogram of body weight over a 15- to 20-minute period every 4 hours. Urine is collected and measured over the same 4-hour period. Patients with SIADH have concentrated urine versus the normal individual who excretes 80% of the fluid given in the 4 hours.[25]

Another diagnostic test measures serum ADH levels with radioassay.

Treatment

Before treatment is begun, one should consider the cause of SIADH, the degree of water intoxication, and subsequently, the extent of hyponatremia. Treatment of SIADH begins with free water restriction of about 500 to 1000 mL of fluid per day. In mild cases, water restriction may be all that is required. In more severe cases of water intoxication—when confusion, seizure, or coma is present—hypertonic (3%) saline solution may be given at a rate of 1 to 2 mL/kg per hour for 2 to 3 hours to restore plasma osmolality and serum sodium.[25,29] If fluid overload is excessive, the patient is monitored closely for symptoms of congestive heart failure, and loop diuretics are administered. The goal for correcting hyponatremia should be attained in 48 hours.[28]

When SIADH is the result of a neoplasm, attempts are made to surgically remove the tumor or to treat it with radiation or chemotherapy. This treatment may not necessarily cure the cancer, but may alleviate the life-threatening symptoms of SIADH. If SIADH occurs as a result of chemotherapy, therapy may be discontinued or other chemotherapeutic agents may be administered. When SIADH is chronic, as may be the case with oncology patients, in addition to a water restriction, drugs that inhibit ADH may be instituted, such as demeclocycline, an antibiotic that inhibits the response of the renal tubules to ADH.[25]

Nursing Diagnoses, Desired Patient Outcomes, and Nursing Interventions

Nursing diagnoses, desired patient outcomes, and nursing interventions in the care of the patient with inappropriate secretion of ADH are presented in the care plan at the end of this chapter.

CASE STUDY: PATIENT WITH SYNDROME OF INAPPROPRIATE ANTIDIURETIC HORMONE

Mr. J is a 64-year-old man with small cell cancer of the lung. While Mr. J is being treated with vincristine, he notices both feet and ankles are swollen. He contacts the nurse, reporting symptoms of fatigue, restlessness, and slight confusion. Mr. J is admitted to the hospital with a blood pressure of 188/106 mmHg and a pulse of 94 to 140 beats per minute with occasional premature atrial contractions. A serum sodium is drawn, and a level of 128 mEq/L is reported. Careful urine output reveals an average of 18 mL/h, with a specific gravity of 1.030. Mr. J's hematocrit is 32%.

Within hours, his sodium levels fall to 116 mEq/L. The nurse immediately places Mr. J on seizure precautions and explains to his family the importance of maintaining strict fluid restriction. Mr. J becomes more confused, begins hallucinating, and experiences a hyponatremic seizure. SIADH is diagnosed. Intravenous (IV) demeclocycline, sodium replacement, and IV furosemide are started immediately, and the chemotherapy regimen is revised to eliminate vincristine. This therapy will be continued with close observation of additional signs and symptoms of SIADH.

With continued therapy, sodium levels return to 130 mEq/L, and the symptoms of SIADH are temporarily relieved. Before discharge, Mr. J and family members are instructed about the importance of the prescribed therapy, the relationship between the tumor and SIADH, and the signs and symptoms of hyponatremia and water intoxication that must be reported.

SUPERIOR VENA CAVA SYNDROME

Etiology and Pathophysiology

Superior vena cava syndrome (SVCS) is a clinical diagnosis that refers to either an external or an intraluminal compression of the superior vena cava, resulting in impaired venous drainage. This condition is observed most frequently in patients with bronchogenic carcinoma and malignant lymphomas. The syndrome has also been increasingly reported as a complication of the use of central venous catheters. Therefore, knowledge of the signs and symptoms, patients at risk, and therapeutic interventions is necessary to prevent serious consequences.

The superior vena cava is the principal vein draining the upper portion of the body, which includes the head, neck, arms, and upper trunk. This vein empties into the right atrium and is surrounded by lymph nodes, pericardium, and the right lung. As a thin-walled, low-pressure vessel, the superior vena cava is particularly vulnerable to compression.

Obstruction to venous return in the superior vena cava causes a selective increase in upper body venous pressure. The pressure forces blood to return from this region to the right atrium by collateral vascular channels. The resulting venous hypertension and all its complications constitute the signs and symptoms of SVCS.

The clinical manifestations of SVCS include dyspnea, coughing, and chest pain. Shortness of breath, facial edema, and arm and trunk swelling are commonly observed. Other complaints are facial swelling, headache, and visual disturbances. These symptoms worsen when the patient is recumbent. Thoracic vein distention may be present but is not universally observed. Left untreated, SVCS can progress into laryngeal edema, severe upper airway obstruction, cyanosis, and altered consciousness, including coma.

Diagnosis

Because up to 90% of all SVCS cases are associated with a malignant disease, diagnostic proceedings usu-

ally focus on obtaining a tissue biopsy specimen. In addition to tissue diagnosis, a chest x-ray may be performed to confirm SVCS. After an accurate tissue diagnosis has been made, appropriate treatment for the underlying disease may begin.

Treatment

Radiation therapy is the standard treatment for SVCS. Most patients will feel subjective relief from their symptoms after 72 hours. A decrease in edema is noted after about 7 days of therapy. Chemotherapy is a useful treatment for SVCS if the underlying disease is small cell carcinoma of the lung or lymphoma. These malignancies are responsive to the effects of chemotherapy, and the patient will experience relief of symptoms. The patient with lung cancer is more prone to experience the emergency again. Recurrence of the symptoms after treatment for patients with lymphoma is rare.

Nursing Management

The major nursing interventions are to identify patients at risk for SVCS, to manage symptoms, and to prevent acute complications. Patient positioning is very important. An upright position to promote drainage by gravity and prevent fluid accumulation in the upper body is essential. Administration of oxygen for dyspnea may be indicated. Cautious use of diuretics and steroids is also appropriate. The provision of emotional support in what is a frightening scenario for the patient is of utmost importance. The patient and family must be taught to recognize impending signs and symptoms of recurrence.

HYPERCALCEMIA

Hypercalcemia, defined as an elevated serum calcium greater than 11 mg/dL, occurs in at least 20% of all cancer patients. Because an increase in calcium causes many potentially life-threatening effects, prompt diagnosis and treatment are necessary.

Etiology and Pathophysiology

The serum calcium level is regulated by three major factors. The equilibrium between calcium intake, turnover, and loss of calcium is a result of a sensitive regulatory mechanism involving parathyroid hormone (PTH), calcitonin, and vitamin D. A disturbance in the absorption of calcium from the gastrointestinal tract, renal excretion of calcium, or resorption of calcium in the bones may all result in a hypercalcemic episode.

Oncology patients are commonly at risk for developing hypercalcemia. Cancers of the lung and breast, multiple myeloma, hypernephroma, and head and neck tumors are the most frequent etiologies. Over half of the patients will develop hypercalcemia as a result of bone metastasis.

Clinical Presentation

Calcium is crucial to muscle contraction and nerve impulse transmission. It is also essential to maintain teeth, bones, and normal clotting mechanisms. Symptoms of hypercalcemia may be observed in the central nervous, renal, gastrointestinal, cardiovascular, and ocular systems. Central nervous system symptoms include fatigue, weakness, hyporeflexia, lethargy, apathy, stupor, and coma. Renal complaints may range from polyuria, polydipsia, and renal insufficiency to renal calculi and failure. Patients with gastrointestinal symptoms experience anorexia, nausea, vomiting, constipation, and abdominal cramping. Cardiovascular problems include arrhythmias, ECG changes (increased PR interval and shortened QT interval [see Fig. 15–41]), and a risk of digoxin toxicity. Conjunctivitis and corneal calcifications result from the effect of calcium deposition in the ocular system.

Treatment

Reduction of the tumor burden is the only way to cure hypercalcemia. The treatment for hypercalcemia depends on the signs and symptoms and degree of calcium elevation. The goals of treatment are reducing bone resorption of calcium and enhancing the excretion of calcium from the body.

Hydration with large volumes of saline is indicated. The usual rate is 4 to 6 liters every 24 hours. When large volumes of saline are administered, the patient is monitored for fluid overload and electrolyte imbalances. Nursing measures are to take daily weights, intake and output, and central venous pressure measurements, if applicable, and to monitor electrolytes.

Newer drug therapy includes intravenous etidronate and gallium nitrate. Oral phosphates are occasionally used for long-term management of hypercalcemia but may cause severe nausea and diarrhea. Nonthiazide diuretics may be used to increase calcium excretion. Caution is required in maintaining hydration to prevent hypovolemia.

Depending on the acuity of the situation, glucocorticoids, mithramycin, and calcitonin may be administered. Glucocorticoids are used in treating hypercalcemia associated with breast cancer and malignant melanoma. The efficacy of glucocorticoroids may be explained by the direct effect of these drugs on the tumor or by the increase in bone resorption of calcium. Mithramycin, an antineoplastic agent, is used in very symptomatic cases of hypercalcemia. Myelosuppression may result with prolonged use. Hypocalcemia is also associated with the use of mithramycin. Therefore, patients are also monitored for low serum calcium levels. Calcitonin, a polypeptide hormone secreted by the thyroid gland, lowers calcium by inhib-

iting bone resorption. It is usually not effective by itself.

Nursing Diagnoses, Desired Patient Outcomes, and Nursing Interventions

Nursing interventions are directed toward preventing fluid overload, electrolyte imbalances, and cardiac abnormalities.

PAIN

Pain related to cancer is said by some professionals to be the newest of the oncologic emergencies. Prolonged, unrelieved pain is a pathologic state, which often limits one's ability to perform everyday tasks of daily living, severely compromising the person's quality of life. The cancer pain experience not only involves physiologic processes, but also has psychological, intellectual, interactional, and spiritual components. It is a multidimensional and highly subjective experience. Therefore, pain is defined in terms of the patient's description of it. Health professionals must uphold the notion that the patients are the authority on their pain.

Even though not all patients with cancer experience pain, about two thirds do. It is believed that 25% of all patients with cancer die with severe, unrelieved pain.

The Nature of Cancer Pain

Recognition of the complex nature of cancer pain is imperative. The first and most common cause of pain in cancer patients is the tumor itself. The second type of pain is associated with the therapy, such as surgery, radiotherapy, or chemotherapy. The physiologic mechanisms of common cancer pain syndromes are not well understood. A series of neuropharmacologic and neurophysiologic changes are most likely responsible.

Pain Management

The goals of pain management are to identify the cause, prevent the pain, maintain an unclouded sensorium, and minimize side effects. Pain assessment is crucial, and the healthcare team, together with the patient, must choose and then use an appropriate tool for measuring pain.

The first goal is to identify the cause of the pain. If the cause is treatable, such as local infection or hemorrhoids, efforts to manage the source of pain become a priority. If the pain is related to the primary cancer, antitumor therapy is initiated. When neither the tumor nor other source of pain can be managed, therapy aimed at alleviating the pain through analgesic interventions is tried.

A second important aim is to prevent the pain. Medications are given in adequate amounts and at appropriate intervals to prevent recurrences or worsening of the pain. Pain medicine is administered around the clock and not "as needed."

The maintenance of an unclouded sensorium is another aim. Sedation usually occurs on initiation or on an increase in narcotics but dissipates after 48 to 72 hours. In most instances, as the pain worsens and narcotics are safely escalated, sedation is rarely a long-term problem. Of utmost importance in any pain management regimen is to promote maximum participation in activities of daily living and to allow the patient to remain as alert as possible.

A last goal of any pain management program is to prevent physical side effects from the medication. Side effects are anticipated and prevented or minimized. Relief of one symptom should not be traded for the presence of another. The nurse who is knowledgeable about the pharmacology and clinical use of analgesics can have significant impact on the analgesic plan.

A variety of drugs are currently available for pain management. For mild pain, aspirin or acetaminophen can be used. For moderate pain, oxycodone hydrochloride and oxycodone terephthalate, or acetaminophen with codeine are effective drugs. Morphine, hydromorphone hydrochloride, levorphanol tartrate, methadone hydrochloride, and fentanyl citrate in various dosages and methods of administration can be given to patients who complain of severe to very severe pain. Meperidine hydrochloride should be avoided. Its short duration of action (2 to 3 hours) and decreased analgesic potency when given by mouth deem it unsuitable for patients with cancer pain. In addition, safe dosage escalations beyond normal dosages are virtually impossible because of the accumulation of meperidine's toxic metabolite, normeperidine.

Patients with cancer pain may be on extremely high doses of medication. Many clinicians remain afraid of the risk of addiction in these patients. Because addiction is a behavior pattern of abusing a narcotic for its psychic effects rather than medical reasons, it is not a problem for the overwhelming majority of patients with cancer.

In addition to administering medication, nurses should also consider nonpharmacologic approaches to pain management. Distraction is the use of activity or other measures to move a patient's focus from the pain onto something else. Simple conversation, music, television, and reading are examples of this technique. Progressive muscle relaxation is another useful tool. Although learning how to relax the body takes practice by both the nurse and the patient, it is very therapeutic for episodic, acute pain. For example, a patient about to undergo a bone marrow biopsy would benefit from muscle relaxation. Guided imagery is also helpful for patients with both acute and chronic pain. This technique involves either a nurse "leading" a patient "somewhere else" by the use of dialogue or by the patient doing it alone. Guided imagery has undergone scrutiny for its therapeutic effectiveness as well as psychological benefits. Therapeutic touch has also been investigated for use in other areas in addition to pain control. In its simplest form, it involves the transfer of energy between practitioner and patient. All other nonpharmacologic measures of pain management are useful tools; however, they should be used in conjunction with medication, not in place of it.

Nursing Diagnoses, Desired Patient Outcomes, and Nursing Interventions

Nursing diagnoses, desired patient outcomes, and nursing interventions in the care of the patient with pain attributed to neoplastic disease are presented in the care plan at the end of this chapter.

REFERENCES

1. Kirkland, L and Taylor, R: Pericardiocentesis. Crit Care Clin 8:699–712, 1992.
2. Aggarwal, P and Sharma, S: Cardiac tamponade as the initial presentation of malignance. Int J Cardiol 22:157–159, 1989.
3. Okamoto, H, et al: Cardiac tamponade caused by primary lung cancer and the management of pericardial effusion. Cancer 71:93–98, 1993.
4. Brown, J, et al: Elevated arterial blood pressure in cardiac tamponade. N Engl J Med 327:463–466, 1992.
5. Gilbert, I and Henning, R: Adenocarcinoma of the lung presenting with pericardial tamponade: Report of a case and review of the literature. Heart Lung 14:83, 1985.
6. Joiner G and Kolodychuk, G: Neoplastic cardiac tamponade. Crit Care Nurse 11(2):50–55, 57–58, 1991.
7. Levitan, Z and Kaplan, A: Survival after malignant pericardial effusion and cardiac tamponade in advanced ovarian cancer. South Med J 82:241–242, 1990.
8. Hoit, B, Gabel, M, and Fowler, N: Hemodynamic efficacy of rapid saline infusion and dobutamine versus saline infusion alone in a model of cardiac rupture. J Am Coll Cardiol 16:1745–1749, 1990.
9. Wall, T, et al: Diagnosis and management (by subxiphoid pericardiotomy) of large pericardial effusions causing cardiac tamponade. Am J Cardiol 69:1075–1078, 1992.
10. Rostad, M: Management of myelosuppression in the patient with cancer. Oncol Nurs Forum 17(suppl):4–8, 1990.
11. Francis, P and Walsh, T: Current approaches to the management of fungal infections in cancer patients. Oncology 6:81–90, 1992.
12. Hartnett, S: Septic shock in the oncology patient. Cancer Nurs 12:191–201, 1989.
13. Shumann, L and Remington, M: The use of naloxone in treating endotoxic shock. Crit Care Nurse 10(2):63–73, 1990.
14. Parrillo, J: Management of septic shock: Present and future. Ann Intern Med 115:491–493, 1991.
15. Arguello, F, et al: Pathogenesis of vertebral metastasis and epidural spinal cord compression. Cancer 65:98–106, 1990.
16. Sørensen, P, et al: Metastatic epidural spinal cord compression. Cancer 65:1502–1508, 1990.
17. Byrne, T: Spinal cord compression from epidural metastases. N Engl J Med 327:614–619, 1992.
18. Pedersen, A, Bach, F, and Melgaard, B: Frequency, diagnosis, and prognosis of spinal cord compression in small cell bronchogenic carcinoma: A review of 817 consecutive patients. Cancer 55:1818, 1985.
19. Harrison, K, Muss, H, Ball, M, et al: Spinal cord compression in breast cancer. Cancer 55:2839, 1985.
20. Landman, C, Hunig, R, and Gratzl, O: The role of laminectomy in the combined treatment of metastatic spinal cord compression. Int J Radiat Oncol Biol Phys 24:627–631, 1992.

21. Klein, P: Neurologic emergencies in oncology. Semin Oncol Nurs 1:278, 1985.
22. Gilbert, R, Kim, J, and Posner, J: Epidural spinal cord compression from metastatic tumor: Diagnosis and treatment. Ann Neurol 3:40–51, 1978.
23. Choucair, A: Myelopathies in the cancer patient: Incidence, presentation, diagnosis and management. Oncology 5:71–80, 1991.
24. Maranzano, E, et al: Radiation therapy in metastic spinal cord compression. Cancer 67:1311–1317, 1991.
25. Poe, C and Taylor, L: Syndrome of inappropriate antidiuretic hormone: Assessment and nursing implications. Oncol Nurs Forum 16:378–381, 1989.
26. Lindaman, C: S.I.A.D.H. Is your patient at risk? Nursing 22(6):60–63, 1992.
27. Shimizu, K, et al: Ectopic atrial natriuretic peptide production in small cell lung cancer with the syndrome of inappropriate antidiuretic hormone secretion. Cancer 68:2284–2288, 1991.
28. Ayus, J and Arieff, A: Symptomatic hyponatremia: Correcting sodium deficits safely. J Crit Illn 5(9):905–918, 1990.
29. Sterns, R: The management of hyponatremic emergencies. Crit Care Clin 7:127–142, 1991.

SUGGESTED READINGS

SUPERIOR VENA CAVA SYNDROME

Morse, L, Heery, M, and Flynn, K: Early detection to avert the crisis of superior vena cava syndrome. Cancer Nurs 8:228, 1985.

HYPERCALCEMIA

Doogan, R: Hypercalcemia of malignancy. Cancer Nurs 4:299, 1981.
Elbaum, N: With cancer patients, be alert for hypercalcemia. Nursing '84 14(8):58, 1984.
Mahon, S: Signs and symptoms associated with malignancy-induced hypercalcemia. Cancer Nurs 12:153–160, 1989.
Meriney, D: Application of Orem's conceptual framework to patients with hypercalcemia related to breast cancer. Cancer Nurs 13:316–323, 1990.
Poe, C and Radford, A: The challenge of hypercalcemia in cancer. Oncol Nurs Forum 12:29, 1985.
Valentine, A and Stewart, J: Oncologic emergencies. Am J Nurs 83(9):1283, 1983.

PAIN MANAGEMENT

Anderson, J: Nursing management of the cancer patient in pain: A review of the literature. Cancer Nurs 5:33, 1982.
Foley, K: The treatment of cancer pain. N Engl J Med 313:84, 1983.
Hauck, S: Pain: Problem for the person with cancer. Cancer Nurs 9:66, 1986.
Johnson, L and Gross, J (eds): Handbook of Oncology Nursing. Wiley, New York, 1985, 145–147.
Levine, J: Pain and analgesia: The outlook for more rational treatment. Ann Intern Med 100:269, 1984.
McCaffrey, M and Beebe, A: Pain: A clinical manual for nursing practice. CV Mosby, St. Louis, 1989.
Paice, J: Unraveling the mystery of pain. Oncol Nurs Forum 18(5):843–849, 1991.
Spross, J: Cancer pain relief: An international perspective. Oncol Nurs Forum 19:5–11, 1992.

CARE PLAN FOR THE PATIENT WITH NEOPLASTIC CARDIAC TAMPONADE

Nursing Diagnoses

Nursing Diagnosis #1
Decreased CO, related to elevated intrapericardial pressure

Desired Patient Outcomes

Patient will maintain hemodynamic stability:
- Heart rate: <100 beats/min
- Central venous pressure: 0–8 mmHg
- Pulmonary artery pressure: <25 mmHg
- PCWP: 8–12 mmHg
- CO: 4–8 L/min

Nursing Interventions

- Assess heart rate and blood pressure every 15 min until stable. Note pulse pressure difference.
- Assess for pulsus paradoxus with each blood pressure.
- Assess for neck vein distention with the head of bed elevated 60° every 2 h.
- Assess dependent areas for edema every 4 h.
- Assess hemodynamic pressure measurements every 1 h (CO and PCWP every 4 h).
- Administer inotropic agents as prescribed and monitor response.
- Administer fluid volume replacements as prescribed and monitor response.
- Assess heart and breath sounds every 1 h.

- Measure urine output every 1 h.

- Palpate peripheral pulses for presence and strength every 4 h.
- Maintain patient in low Fowler's position.
- Assist with pericardiocentesis.
- Assess hemodynamic changes after pericardiocentesis.

- Monitor for cardiac irregularities related to needle placement.

Rationales

- CO can become significantly compromised as fluid accumulates in the pericardium.
- Present with variations of the filling pressures on the right side of the heart.

- May increase CO.

- Significant volume replacement may help restore the volume in the left ventricle.
- As fluid accumulates in the pericardium, heart sounds become distant on auscultation.
- Reduced CO compromises renal perfusion, reducing glomerular filtration.
- Peripheral pulses reflect perfusion of extremities.

- Removal of fluid will often improve blood pressure and CO.
- The needle may irritate the ventricles.

CARE PLAN FOR THE PATIENT WITH NEOPLASTIC CARDIAC TAMPONADE (*Continued*)

Nursing Diagnoses

Nursing Diagnosis #2
Impaired gas exchange, related to decreased
cardiopulmonary perfusion

Desired Patient Outcomes

Patient will:
1. Maintain effective cardiopulmonary function—stable
   ABGs:
   • pH 7.35–7.45
   • $Paco_2$ 35–45 mmHg
   • Arterial oxygen pressure (Pao_2) > 60 mmHg
2. Remain oriented to person, place, and date

Nursing Interventions

• Administer oxygen as prescribed.
• Assess blood pressure and heart rate every 15 min until
  stable.
• Assess for evidence of respiratory distress.

• Perform neurologic assessment as it relates to mental
  status and level of consciousness.
• Assess ABG results.

Rationales

• Mediastinal fluid accumulation can compromise lung
  expansion and respiratory mechanics.
• Changes in mental status and orientation may reflect
  decreased cerebral perfusion.

Nursing Diagnoses

Nursing Diagnosis #3
Fluid volume deficit, related to decreased CO

Desired Patient Outcomes

Patient will:
1. Have a balanced fluid intake and output
2. Maintain serum electrolytes, blood urea nitrogen,
   creatinine, and total protein within the physiologically
   normal range

Nursing Interventions

• Measure intake, output, and specific gravity every 1 h.

• Assess skin turgor every shift.
• Palpate for peripheral edema every 4 h.
• Assess for Kussmaul's breathing every 2 h.
• Auscultate breath sounds every 1 h.

• Take daily weights.
• Assess related laboratory work every 4 h, or as reported.

Rationales

• Fluid overload may enhance fluid accumulation within
  the pericardium, further complicating the patient's
  clinical status.

• Crackles on auscultation may reflect pulmonary
  congestion.
• Daily weight is best measure of fluid status.

Nursing Diagnoses

Nursing Diagnosis #4
Fear, related to severity of illness

Desired Patient Outcomes

Patient/significant others will verbalize fears and concerns

Nursing Interventions

• Assess knowledge regarding condition and treatments.

• Encourage verbalization of fears.
• Help patient/significant others identify resources.
• Refer to chaplain, social service, for additional support.

Rationales

• Patient/significant others may have preconceived
  perceptions of cancer.
• Patient may experience a "feeling of impending doom."
• Treatments are often palliative versus curative.

Nursing Diagnoses

Nursing Diagnosis #5
Anxiety, related to:
1. Decreased cerebral oxygenation
2. Underlying diagnosis of cancer

Desired Patient Outcomes

Patient will demonstrate ability to use effective relaxation
measures

Nursing Interventions

• Assess for signs and symptoms of anxiety.

Rationales

• Anxiety can further compromise respiratory status;
  tachypnea associated with anxiety can significantly
  compromise alveolar ventilation.

CARE PLAN FOR THE PATIENT WITH NEOPLASTIC CARDIAC TAMPONADE (*Continued*)

Nursing Interventions
- Monitor pulse oximeter for effectiveness of oxygen therapy.
- Orient patient to relaxation techniques.
- Remain with patient during stressful periods; provide a "listening ear."
- Medicate as prescribed, and monitor response.

Rationales

Nursing Diagnoses

Nursing Diagnosis #6
Pain, related to physical and psychological changes

Desired Patient Outcomes

Patient will:
1. Verbalize feeling pain-free
2. Exhibit eupneic pattern of breathing

Nursing Interventions
- Administer pain medications as prescribed, and monitor response.
- Monitor output from pericardiocentesis and evaluate effect on symptoms.
- Monitor output from pericardial catheter.
- Administer oxygen as prescribed.
- Position patient in low Fowler's position.

Rationales
- Goal is to prevent pain. Analgesics should be given in adequate amounts and at appropriate intervals to prevent recurrence or worsening of pain and to control respiratory rate.
- Acknowledge that patients are the authority on their pain.

Nursing Diagnoses

Nursing Diagnosis #7
Knowledge deficit, related to emergency procedures

Desired Patient Outcomes

Patient and/or significant other will verbalize understanding of procedures such as pericardiocentesis, pericardial window, and/or pericardial catheter

Nursing Interventions
- Clarify/reinforce explanations of procedures for patient/significant other.
- Assess patient's/significant other's understanding of procedure.

Rationales
- Patients/significant others may tolerate procedures better when they are given instruction.

CARE PLAN FOR THE PATIENT WITH SEPTIC SHOCK

Nursing Diagnoses

Nursing Diagnosis #1
Decreased CO, related to systemic arterial hypotension associated with vasodilation of vasculature

Desired Patient Outcomes

Patient will:
1. Maintain hemodynamic stability
   • Heart rate 60–80 beats/min; rhythm regular sinus
   • Blood pressure within 10 mmHg of baseline
   • Central venous pressure 0–8 mmHg
   • PCWP 8–12 mmHg
2. Maintain hourly urine output greater than 1 mL/kg per hour
3. Maintain intact neurologic function:
   • Mental status alert; oriented to person, place, and date

Nursing Interventions

• Assess heart rate and blood pressure every 15 min until stable.

• Assess dependent areas for edema every 4 h.
• Assess hemodynamic pressure measurements every 1 h (CO, PCWP, every 4 h).
• Administer inotropic and/or vasopressor agents as prescribed, and monitor response to therapy.
• Administer fluid volume replacements as prescribed.
• Measure urine output every 1 h.

• Palpate peripheral pulses for presence and strength every 4 h.

Rationales

• Signs/symptoms of early septic shock reflect the body's compensatory response to reduce perfusion: there is an increase in heart rate and peripheral vascular resistance.

• Monitoring CO and PCWP is essential to evaluate fluid needs and the patient's response to therapy.

• Monitoring urine output hourly is essential to determine status of renal perfusion.

Nursing Diagnoses

Nursing Diagnosis #2
Impaired gas exchange, related to hypoxic respiratory failure

Desired Patient Outcomes

Patient will maintain a $PaO_2 > 60$ mmHg

Nursing Interventions

• Assess mental status and level of consciousness.

• Assess ABGs as prescribed.

• Provide frequent rest periods.
• Follow appropriate procedure for endothacheal suctioning as needed.
• Administer oxygen therapy as prescribed.
• Monitor patient for acute respiratory failure.

Rationales

• Changes in mental status and neurologic function may reflect decreased cerebral perfusion related to reduced CO. This may be the first manifestation of infection.
• Respiratory alkalosis or metabolic acidoses may be present.
• Patients have little energy reserve because they are in an anaerobic metabolic state.

Nursing Diagnoses

Nursing Diagnosis #3
Alteration in peripheral tissue perfusion, related to capillary leakage and vasoconstriction

Desired Patient Outcomes

Patient will maintain a viable peripheral circulatory status:
• Easily palpable pulses
• Brisk capillary refill
• Usual skin color, absence of mottling and cyanosis

Nursing Interventions

• Assess peripheral pulses every 4 h.
• Assess for peripheral edema every 4 h.

• Assess skin for color and warmth.
• Instruct patient to avoid positions that compromise blood flow to extremities.

Rationales

• Altered endothelial permeability allows blood albumin to leak into the interstitium, reducing the capillary oncotic pressure and predisposing to peripheral edema.

CARE PLAN FOR THE PATIENT WITH SEPTIC SHOCK (*Continued*)

Nursing Diagnoses

Nursing Diagnosis #4

Activity intolerance, related to oxygen supply/demand imbalance

Desired Patient Outcomes

Patient will conserve energy for vital functions:
- Verbalize feeling rested
- Demonstrate relaxation techniques

Nursing Interventions

- Assess patient's vital signs related to activity.
- Assist patient with all activities to conserve energy.
- Explain importance of energy conservation to patient/ significant others.

Rationales

Nursing Diagnoses

Nursing Diagnosis #5

Knowledge deficit, related to infection control

Desired Patient Outcomes

Patient/significant others will state measures effective in reducing the risk of infection

Nursing Interventions

- Instruct patient/significant others on proper infection control measures.

- Follow procedures for patient on white blood cell count precautions.

Rationales

- For detailed information on infection control, refer to Chapter 56, Table 56–5, for the nursing diagnosis: potential for infection.

Nursing Diagnoses

Nursing Diagnosis #6

Ineffective thermoregulation, related to infectious process

Desired Patient Outcomes

Patient will maintain a core body temperature within normal limits

Nursing Interventions

- Assess for hypothermia/hyperthermia every 1 h
- Alter the environment to control temperature.
- Administer antipyretics as prescribed and monitor response.
- Administer antibiotics as prescribed.

Rationales

- Patients may be warm to touch in the early stages of shock.

- Timely antibiotic administration may decrease the number of organisms and their toxins.

CARE PLAN FOR THE PATIENT WITH SPINAL CORD COMPRESSION

Nursing Diagnoses

Nursing Diagnosis #1
High risk for injury, related to sensory deficits

Desired Patient Outcomes

Patient will remain free from injury while hospitalized

Nursing Interventions

- Keep side rails up at all times.

- Have call light and personal items within patient's reach.
- Instruct patient to call for assistance if desiring to get out of bed.
- Assess level of consciousness as indicated.
- Assess sensory level every shift.

Rationales

- Patients have an altered sensorium and may not have a clear sense of where they are in bed.

- Loss of sensation places patient at increased risk of injury.

Nursing Diagnoses

Nursing Diagnosis #2
Pain related to damaged spinal cord

Desired Patient Outcomes

Patient will:
1. Use measures effective in managing pain
2. Verbalize relief from pain
3. Present relaxed facies and overall demeanor

Nursing Interventions

- Assess patient for intensity, radiation, and character of pain.
- Inform patient and/or significant others of available methods of pain relief.
- Administer pain medication on a round-the-clock basis as appropriate. Assess for effect in 10–20 min using a standardized scale.
- Explain importance of pain medication in patient's progress.
- Collaborate with physician and patient in altering pain medication as needed.
- Suggest alternate positions.
- Log roll when needed.
- Position on pressure relief mattress.

Rationales

- Pain associated with spinal cord compression may be especially severe.

- Patient should be encouraged to request pain medication early on instead of waiting until the pain becomes unbearable.

- Log roll to prevent further damage to spinal cord.

Nursing Diagnoses

Nursing Diagnosis #3
Bowel and urinary incontinence, related to nerve disruption

Desired Patient Outcomes

Patient will:
1. Maintain regular bowel elimination
2. Adhere to a bladder and bowel control program

Nursing Interventions

- Explain need for scheduled bowel elimination program.
- Support patients psychosocial needs related to change in voluntary bowel habits.

- Monitor intake and output every shift.
- Offer fluids to patient every 2 h.
- Offer bedpan or assist patient to bathroom every 2 h.
- Palpate bladder for distention.
- Explain importance of bladder program.
- Catheterize patient if necessary.

Rationales

- It is essential for the patient to establish and maintain regular bowel elimination. The patient's usual bowel habits should be assessed and incorporated into daily schedule.

- Urinary retention can predispose to infection.
- Patient/significant others should be able to check for urinary retention of which the patient may not be aware.

Nursing Diagnoses

Nursing Diagnosis #4
Constipation, related to:
1. Immobility
2. Narcotic administration

Desired Patient Outcomes

Patient will maintain regular bowel elimination.

CARE PLAN FOR THE PATIENT WITH SPINAL CORD COMPRESSION (*Continued*)

Nursing Interventions	Rationales
• Instruct patient on need for good hydration. • Force fluids as necessary unless contraindicated.	• Patient/family should be able to explain the importance of hydration and diet high in fiber, in terms of overall bowel function. • Patient/family should be aware of signs and symptoms suggestive of constipation: abdominal fullness or distention, loss of appetite, nausea, headache, feeling of fullness in rectum. • Appearance of diarrheal stool may suggest the presence of fecal impaction.
• Administer stool softeners/laxatives as needed and prescribed. • Consult dietician to increase fiber in foods.	

Nursing Diagnoses	Desired Patient Outcomes
Nursing Diagnosis #5 High risk for impaired skin integrity, related to decreased mobility	Patient will be free from skin breakdown

Nursing Interventions	Rationales
• Inspect patient's skin integrity every shift.	• Loss of mobility and sensation, immunosuppressed state, and altered nutrition place patient at greater risk of skin breakdown. • Meticulous surveillance of pressure areas is essential to maintain skin integrity.
• Encourage/assist patient to turn every 2 h while in bed. • Apply lotion to dry skin every shift. • Apply pressure relief mattress to bed. • Force fluids as necessary unless contraindicated.	

Nursing Diagnoses	Desired Patient Outcomes
Nursing Diagnosis #6 Impaired physical mobility, related to motor neuron damage	Patient will maintain muscle tone and coordination: • Demonstrate active range of motion of all extremities • Verbalize importance of exercise and avoidance of fatigue

Nursing Interventions	Rationales
• Inspect muscles of arms and legs for atrophy and involuntary movements. • Assess for muscle coordination. • Perform active and/or passive range-of-motion exercises to all extremities four times a day. • Encourage activity as prescribed/tolerated. • Collaborate with physical therapists about mobility and an individualized exercise plan.	• A baseline assessment should be performed to establish the patient's physical capabilities. • Actions should be performed to maintain muscle strength and mobility. • Team participation in exercise regimen should be encouraged.

Nursing Diagnoses	Desired Patient Outcomes
Nursing Diagnosis #7 Self-esteem disturbance, related to incontinence and immobility	Patient and/or significant other will begin accepting the change in usual functions: • Verbalize feelings • Initiate discussion of disease and impact on lifestyle

Nursing Interventions	Rationales
• Explain to patient and/or significant others reasons for changes in muscle control. • Assess patient's/significant other's usual coping mechanisms, encouraging positive ones. • Encourage patient and/or significant other to discuss their feelings about these changes.	• Recognizing one's feelings and emotions is the first step in dealing with them. • Observing patient/family/significant other interactions may assist in determining strengths and effective coping capability.

CARE PLAN FOR THE PATIENT WITH SYNDROME OF INAPPROPRIATE ANTIDIURETIC HORMONE SECRETION

Nursing Diagnoses

Nursing Diagnosis #1
Fluid volume excess, related to overproduction of ADH (Note: see Table 36–3).

Desired Patient Outcomes

Patient will be free from signs and symptoms of water intoxication:
• Serum sodium 135–145 mEq/L
• Serum osmolality 285–295 mOsm/kg water

Nursing Interventions
• Maintain water restriction as indicated.

• Divide the fluid allowed into an AM and PM allotment.
• Take daily weights.
• Monitor for and teach patient to report anorexia, nausea, vomiting, or diarrhea.
• Assess patient for confusion, hypothermia, and aberrant respirations.
• Assess for changes in blood pressure and respiratory status.
• Administer diuretics and ADH-inhibiting drugs as prescribed, and monitor response to therapy.

Rationales
• Water intake is severely restricted to prevent aggravating state of water intoxication and hyponatremia.
• Provides the patient with some control over therapy.

• Altered neurologic function reflects severe hyponatremia and water intoxication.

• Diuretics enhance water excretion and help prevent congestive heart failure.

Nursing Diagnoses

Nursing Diagnosis #2
High risk for injury, related to hyponatremia

Desired Patient Outcomes

Patient will be free from hyponatremic-related injury:
• Serum sodium: 135–145 mEq/L
• Serum osmolality: 285–295 mOsm/kg water
• Urine osmolality: 50–1400 mOsm/kg water
• Urine sodium: 80–180 mEq/L per 24 h
• Urine specific gravity: 1.010–1.025

Nursing Interventions
• Assess laboratory values for sodium level.

• Monitor for and teach patient to report headache, anorexia, muscle cramps, nausea, vomiting, or weakness.
• Assess for lethargy, confusion, and seizures.
• Administer hypertonic saline solution, as prescribed, and monitor response.

• Encourage intake of fluids high in sodium: milk, broth, tomato juice.
• Maintain patient on seizure precautions.

Rationales
• Serial electrolytes, serum, and urine osmolality should guide therapy.
• Signs of hyponatremia and water intoxication should be treated quickly.

• Hypertonic saline increases serum sodium rapidly and assists to relieve seizures and other neurologic dysfunction.
• A decreased sodium may cause patient to develop seizure activity.

Nursing Diagnoses

Nursing Diagnosis #3
Knowledge deficit regarding SIADH and its treatment

Desired Patient Outcomes

Patient and/or significant others will verbalize an understanding of SIADH and its treatment

Nursing Interventions
• Assess patient's/significant other's knowledge of SIADH.

• Explain the relationship between cancer and this syndrome.

• Explain the importance of water restrictions.

• Teach patient/significant other to report any of the symptoms of SIADH to a health professional.
• Explain the importance of taking ADH-inhibiting drugs.

Rationales
• Patient/significant other should be able to explain the relationship between underlying pathophysiology and occurrence of SIADH.
• Patient/significant other should be able to describe symptoms reflective of hyponatremia and actions to take to relieve the problem.
• Patient/significant other should understand the significance of strict intake/output measurements and daily weights.
• Efforts should be made to help patient/significant other to remain responsible for self-care.

CARE PLAN FOR THE PATIENT WITH NEOPLASTIC-RELATED PAIN

Nursing Diagnoses	Desired Patient Outcomes
Nursing Diagnosis #1 Pain (See the care plan in Chapter 60, nursing diagnosis #6.)	Patient will be free from pain: • Verbalizes pain relief • Demonstrates relaxed facies and overall demeanor

Nursing Interventions	Rationales
• Acknowledge that patient has pain. • Administer pain medication around the clock. • Be alert for possible side effects of narcotics: constipation, nausea, and drowsiness. Promote measures that prevent and control them. • Suggest nonpharmacologic methods of pain control, such as relaxation and distraction. • Evaluate and document effectiveness of pain relief measures. • Encourage verbalization about the pain experience. • Include family members and significant others in teaching.	• Recognize that patients are the authority on their own pain. • This will prevent pain and erase the pain memory. • These can be used in addition to medications.

Nursing Diagnoses	Desired Patient Outcomes
Nursing Diagnosis #2 High risk for alteration in sensorium (drowsiness), related to narcotics	Patient will: 1. Not knowingly become injured as a result of taking pain medication 2. Verbalize potential side effects of pain medication

Nursing Interventions	Rationales

• Inform patient/significant others that drowsiness is transient and should dissipate in 36 to 72 h.
• Promote safety measures:
  ○ Assistance with ambulation
  ○ Night lights
  ○ Side rails
  ○ Call bell in reach
	• This reassurance will encourage patients to continue taking their medication without fear of somnolence.

Nursing Diagnoses	Desired Patient Outcomes
Nursing Diagnosis #3 High risk for constipation, related to narcotic-induced constipation	Patient will: 1. Not become constipated 2. Resume usual bowel routine

Nursing Interventions	Rationales

• Be alert for the possibility of constipation with administration of narcotics.
  ○ Encourage a preventive mode.
  ○ Administer stool softeners and laxatives at the onset of administration of narcotics.
  ○ Encourage patient to eat bulky foods and to increase fluid intake (when feasible).
  ○ Record all stools.
  ○ Check for impaction if no stool for 3 days.
	• Preventing constipation is simpler than remedying it once it has occurred.

Nursing Management of Patients With Neoplastic-Related Surgery

Janet Donnard White and
Deborah Rodzwic Pennypacker

CHAPTER OUTLINE

Therapeutic Modalities in the Treatment
of Cancer
Esophageal Carcinoma
□ Incidence and Etiology
□ Staging
□ Adjuvant Therapy
□ Surgical Procedure:
Esophagogastrectomy

□ Postoperative Care: Nursing
Management
Nursing Diagnoses, Desired Patient
Outcomes, and Nursing Interventions
References

LEARNING OBJECTIVES

After completing this chapter, you should be able to:

1. Identify key nursing care considerations for patients with surgery for cancer of the head and neck.
2. Discuss symptomatology closely associated with esophageal carcinoma.
3. Describe surgical procedure for esophagogastrectomy and implications for nursing care.
4. Identify major complications of esophagogastrectomy surgery and pertinent preventive and therapeutic interventions.
5. Examine implications for nursing care based on implementation of nursing process: assessment, specific nursing diagnoses, planning (patient outcomes and nursing interventions/rationales).

THERAPEUTIC MODALITIES IN THE TREATMENT OF CANCER

Cancer is a prevalent disease in our society. Public awareness of cancer has increased over the years, which has led to early detection, prompt treatment, and improved survival. Today, the seven warning signals of cancer (box on page 1027) are widely publicized. Comprehensive cancer treatment centers are now available to those seeking diagnosis and treatment.

The three most common modalities in the treatment of cancer are surgery, radiation therapy, and chemotherapy. Tumor staging and cell type determine which methods are used. The box on page 1027 lists the principles of surgery. Surgery is the most common initial therapy used either to diagnose a malig-

nant tumor or to remove it for purposes of cure or palliation. However, surgical recovery is likely to be complicated by the addition of radiation or chemotherapy. The latter two forms of treatment are used to eradicate residual tumor cells by either focusing on the primary malignant tumor site or treating it systematically. Both radiation therapy and chemotherapy may impair wound healing, cause fistula formation, or alter immunologic functioning necessary to guard against infection.

Patients with head and neck carcinoma and esophageal carcinoma face the possibilities of receiving a combination of cancer therapies, experiencing a variety of complications, and requiring intensive nursing care. In this chapter, we highlight these sites as representatives of the radical surgical techniques often necessary in the treatment of patients with cancer and of the sophisticated nursing care required. This chapter provides information about the use of myocutaneous flaps in head and neck surgery and about the chest and abdominal surgery required in the treatment of esophageal neoplasms. Both topics include nursing care plans, which provide the nurse with desired patient outcomes, specific nursing interventions, and associated rationales.

ESOPHAGEAL CARCINOMA

Incidence and Etiology

Tumors of the esophagus account for 1% of new cases and 10,200 deaths each year.[1] The most frequently found forms include squamous cell carcinoma and adenocarcinoma. The majority of cases are found in men, the median age being 60.

Risk factors include chronic cigarette smoking and excessive alcohol consumption.[2] Poor nutrition has been cited when there are deficiencies in vitamins A and B, iron, and zinc. Diets high in nitrites and foods contaminated by fungal toxins have been shown to be carcinogenic. Genetics has also been implicated. A correlation has been found between esophageal cancer and a genetic syndrome known as tylosis, a condition in which there is an overgrowth of epidermis on the soles of the feet and palms of the hands.[3]

Staging

Symptoms in the early stages are often vague complaints of gastrointestinal fullness and indigestion (box below). Unfortunately, the cancer is usually not diagnosed until 50% of the esophagus has occluded. The chance tumor cells may have spread to lymph nodes or by direct invasion through the muscle wall is increased by this late finding.

Diagnosis is based on findings from a number of different sources. Included is a thorough physical examination, esophagogastroscopy with biopsy and brush cytology, barium swallow, and computed tomography (CT) scan.

Once identified, the staging of the tumor is determined. There are four outcomes from this process.[4] First, a description of the tumor is made. This includes tumor size, location, lymph node involvement, and distant metastasis. The universal tool adopted by the American Joint Committee on Cancer (AJCC) is known as the TNM system (box on page 1028). This tool facilitates the second purpose of communication among all disciplines involved in the patient's care.

The remaining outcomes of staging provide a guide to therapy and a prognosis of the disease. At present there are multiple therapies to choose from at each stage, many under clinical trial. Depending on the TNM classification, surgery, radiation therapy, and chemotherapy may all play a part.

**THE TNM CLINICAL CLASSIFICATION
SYSTEM**

    T: Identifies the primary tumor and the
       extent of invasion into surrounding
       structures
    N: Identifies the degree of lymph node
       involvement
    M: Identifies the presence or absence of dis-
       tant metastasis.

Adjuvant Therapy

As with all oncology cases, early detection is important if there are hopes of achieving a cure. As stated
previously, esophageal tumors are usually diagnosed
late, when spread to the lymphatic system has already
occurred. In an effort to improve patient survival, studies have been conducted of the use of radiation therapy before operation and concurrent with chemotherapy.[2] The goal is to decrease the tumor burden
before surgery and to treat possible systemic metastasis. Studies also evaluate the use of drugs such as 5-
fluorouracil, cisplatin, and mitomycin-c along with
external beam radiation. It is postulated that in combination, the chemotherapy will enhance the effects
of radiation.[5]

Both radiation and chemotherapy carry risk to the
patient.[6] Bone marrow suppression, a common side
effect, can lead to anemia, neutropenia, and thrombocytopenia. Patients will require blood and blood
product transfusions to offset the abnormalities. They
will also need to be monitored closely for opportunistic infections and sepsis.

A second side effect of treatment is anorexia. Nausea and vomiting caused by the chemotherapy regimen and radiation-induced esophagitis contribute to
the already poor nutritional state of someone with
esophageal cancer. Preoperative enteral or parenteral
nutrition may be necessary. Serum albumin and transferrin levels are used as guides in determining the
patient's nutritional status.[7]

Surgical Procedure:
Esophagogastrectomy

An understanding of the surgical procedure is
needed to use the nursing process and successfully
accomplish patients' goals. There are several
approaches to the surgical treatment of esophageal
neoplasms. The type of procedure chosen depends in
part on tumor location, the presence or absence of
metastasis, and the surgeon's preference. For the purposes of this chapter, the esophagogastrectomy

approach will be discussed. The goal of such extensive
surgery is curative.

The procedure is as follows (Fig. 60–1). A midline
abdominal incision is carried out from the xiphoid to
the umbilicus. The abdominal cavity is examined for
any metastatic disease. If the examination is benign
for tumor, the stomach and esophagus are freed up
from accessible organs by releasing the major blood
vessels that feed them. This allows the stomach to be
pulled up into the thoracic cavity. A pyloroplasty or
stretching of the pyloric sphincter is performed.
Lymph nodes from this area will be sent to pathology
for frozen section determination.

Attention is then turned to the jejunum. A feeding
jejunostomy tube is placed about one and a half feet
distal to the ligament of Treitz. A drainage tube is
placed through a separate stab wound in the left upper
quadrant. The abdominal incision is closed.

The patient is then turned on the side, and a thoracotomy is performed through the 5th or 6th intercostal space. The ribs are gently spread with a rib
retractor, although rib resections are occasionally
required. The parietal pleura overlying the esophagus
is divided. An incision is made in the diaphragm for
placement of the stomach in the chest. The esophagus
is freed from its posterior mediastinal bed; the neoplasm is located and transected completely. The specimen is sent to pathology to ensure that the margins
are free of tumor. Once established, the two ends are
anastomosed by either hand sewing or use of the end-
to-end circumferential anastomotic stapler. A nasogastric tube is inserted into the remaining esophagus,
through the anastomosis, and into the remaining
stomach. Two chest tubes are placed through separate
stab wounds, one laterally at the anastomosis and the
second midway up the thorax. The chest is then
closed.[8]

Postoperative Care: Nursing Management

The nursing management of the surgical oncology
patient is very challenging. The patient's preoperative
physical status is often compromised by side effects of
the disease, treatment of the disease, or both.

Complications of Respiratory Function

Because of the nature of the surgical procedure,
potential complications involving the pulmonary system often exist. It is therefore important for the nurse
to be mindful of pre-existing health problems identified in the nursing history. For example, the combination of smoking or pulmonary disease along with
the manipulation of the lungs at the time of surgery
potentiates postoperative complications. In a study
done by Galandiuk and associates at the Cleveland
Clinic, the most common complication was atelactasis
followed by pneumonia.[9]

The nurse can provide support to the patient by

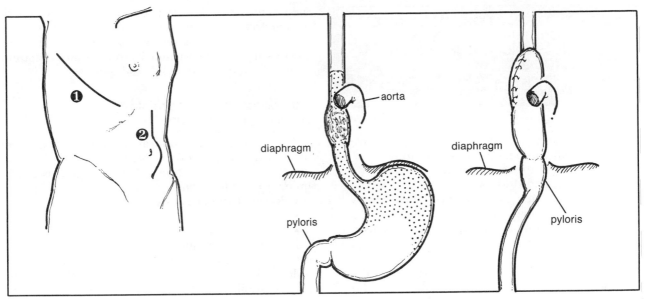

FIGURE 60–1. Esophagogastrectomy; a surgical approach for the treatment of esophageal carcinoma is a two-step approach involving (2) an initial abdominal incision, followed by (1) thoracotomy.

evaluating the effectiveness of pain control and instructing the patient to splint incisions while coughing and deep breathing. Movements that place tension on the abdominal and thoracic incisions tend to increase pain and inhibit lung expansion.[10] This results in the following:

- Decreased vital capacity (VC)
- Ventilation:perfusion (V:Q) ratio abnormalities
- Hypoxia

Advances in pain control and subsequent reduction of pulmonary complications have been related to the use of intraspinal narcotics.[11] A catheter is placed by an anesthesiologist at the time of surgery into either the epidural or intrathecal space of the spinal column. The narcotic is then injected once a day or administered continually by infusion pump.

Other measures implemented to maintain an adequate respiratory status include placing the patient in a semi-Fowler's position and turning every 2 hours. The necessity for oxygen therapy is determined by arterial blood gas and/or pulse oximetry, which monitors the oxygen saturation of available hemoglobin. Lung expansion is enhanced by two chest tubes, and progress is checked daily by chest film. Lungs are auscultated every 4 hours during the acute period, and the quality/quantity of sputum production is noted. (For additional details related to assessment of respiratory function, see Chapter 24.)

Complications of Cardiovascular Function

Closely involved with the pulmonary system is the cardiovascular system. The patient's cardiac history is noted so baseline data can be used as a form of comparison. The patient undergoing chest surgery is at greater risk for the development of arrhythmias, most commonly atrial fibrillation. Etiology is unknown, although studies suggest an increased incidence with an increase in the patient's age. If the patient develops this arrhythmia after the operation, the nurse should be aware of potential complications, such as the following:

- Increased oxygen demands
- Decreased cardiac output
- Emboli formation

Increased oxygen demands may tax or stress an already compromised cardiopulmonary system, causing cardiac ischemia/arrhythmias. The nurse notes the ventricular rate and the regularity of the apical pulse. An increased rate is associated with increased oxygen consumption. In a nonacute setting, the nurse promotes rest and administers antianxiety agents or pain medication as prescribed and monitors the patient's response to therapy.

The second complication, a 20% to 30% decrease in cardiac output, occurs when the atria do not function properly, as with atrial fibrillation. This directly affects coronary, cerebral, and renal perfusion. The nurse performs an ongoing cardiovascular assessment with continuous cardiac and hemodynamic monitoring. (For details related to cardiovascular assessment and hemodynamic monitoring, see Chapters 13 and 16.) The lungs are auscultated for the presence of rales (crackles), a sign of fluid overload. Neck vein distention and pedal edema also indicate heart failure. An altered level of consciousness may be suggestive of cerebral hypoxia. Serum electrolytes, blood urea nitrogen (BUN), creatinine, and hourly urine output are monitored to observe for abnormalities of renal perfusion.

RESEARCH APPLICATION: PATTERNS OF NAUSEA, VOMITING, AND DISTRESS IN PATIENTS RECEIVING ANTI-NEOPLASTIC DRUG PROTOCOLS
Rhodes, VA, Watson, PM, Johnson, MH, Madsen, RW and Beck, NC Oncol Nurs Forum 14, 35–44, 1987.

Purpose:
1. To identify patterns of symptom occurence after chemotherapy administration.
2. To analyze the relationship of duration, frequency, and distress of nausea and vomiting associated with specific chemotherapy drug combinations.
3. To determine if the experience of nausea and vomiting is altered with repeated cycles.

Methods: The authors chose a time series–designed study with a sample of 309 adults who had cancer. The sample was divided into groups according to antineoplastic drug protocols. Participation in this study was from 25 hospitals and 15 physician practices in 2 midwestern states. Subjects were 20 to 84 years old and selected from both urban and rural areas. Requirements for subject selection included the following:
1. First-time recipients of chemotherapy.
2. Receiving specific drug combinations.
3. Receiving treatment for at least six cycles without interruption.

Results:
1. The majority of patients experienced minimal nausea and vomiting, indicating a good response to antiemetic drug therapy.
2. Symptoms differed from patient to drug protocol.
3. There appears to be an increase in nausea and vomiting with each cycle of chemotherapy.

Implications for Nursing Practice: Instruct patients to expect little or no nausea and vomiting before chemotherapy administration. This will potentially limit the symptom experience.

Finally, 30% of all patients who develop atrial fibrillation experience systemic or pulmonary emboli. An increase in patient activity will decrease venous stasis, a precurser to emboli formation. Such activity includes sitting in a chair within the first 24 hours after surgery and performing range-of-motion exercises to extremities. (See Chapter 26 for the signs, symptoms, and medical and nursing management of pulmonary embolisms.)

Treatment of atrial fibrillation will depend on the clinical status of the patient. Therapy for one experiencing cardiac decompensation consists of synchronized cardioversion. A conservative approach with

medications may be used for those patients experiencing arrythmias without major sequelae. This form of treatment includes the use of conventional drugs such as digoxin, verapamil hydrochloride, diltiazem hydrochloride, propranolol, and quinidine.

Complications of Gastrointestinal Function and Nutrition

The most serious complication of esophagogastrectomy is dehiscence of the anastomotic site. Factors linked to the separation of the esophagus-gastric union are the following:
- Poor nutritional status
- Radiation therapy before operation
- Tumor present at the margins of resection

Nursing care requires prudent attention to the drainage catheters. If the nasogastric tube becomes dislodged from its original placement, the surgeon may be hesitant to replace it.[12] Reinsertion has the potential to disrupt the anastomosis. Observation of the color and amount of drainage is equally important. If the chest tube or sump begins to drain either bile or "coffee-grounds" drainage, the physician should be notified and specimens sent for analysis.

Once a leak occurs, gastric contents are emptied into the mediastinum, causing thoracic empyema, mediastinitis, cardiopulmonary dysfunction, and general sepsis. The patient may have chest pain, arrhythmia, an elevated white blood cell count, and fever. Diagnosis is often made by meglumine diatrizoate (Gastrograffin) esophogram and analysis of the drainage from the chest tubes or sump. Treatment is aimed both at draining the site of the leakage to promote healing and at managing related symptoms.

Nutrition plays an important role in coping with this problem. The patient with a negative nitrogen balance before operation is placed on total parenteral nutrition (TPN). TPN is a hypertonic solution consisting of dextrose, fat emulsions, and L-amino acids. Attempts to restore an adequate nutritional state enhance the patient's immunologic capabilities.

The nurse who is monitoring a patient receiving TPN should be cognizant of the potential for infection. The high glucose concentration is a good medium for bacterial growth. The central line catheter provides access for systemic sepsis. Special attention to vital signs and white blood cell counts is prudent. Care of the central venous line site is performed according to the institution's policy. A transparent dressing allows the nurse to assess the site for signs of redness, swelling, pain, or drainage. (For additional nursing care related to a patient on TPN, see Chapter 9.)

During the operative procedure, the patient will have a feeding tube placed in the jejunum (J-tube). If the gastrointestinal tract is able to absorb nutrients, it is the preferred route for nutrition. Gastrointestinal motility is evidenced by auscultated bowel sounds or the presence of flatulence. Feedings are initiated and gradually increased according to the patient's tolerance. The nutritional support service will determine caloric intake and will gradually wean the patient off TPN. Intolerance may be evidenced by residual feeding that is not emptying from the gastrointestinal tract or the development of diarrhea. Medications such as metroclopramide hydrochloride (Reglan), which stimulates gastric and intestinal motility, or paregoric, which decreases gastrointestinal motility, are often used.

In summary, a person with a malignancy requiring surgical intervention who has been previously treated with chemotherapy and radiation therapy has the potential for poor wound healing. When such complications do not respond to conservative medical management, the patient may require surgical repair with an associated poor prognosis. Therefore, it is vital that the nurse understand the surgical procedure, the potential complications, and the essential role of the nurse.

NURSING DIAGNOSES, DESIRED PATIENT OUTCOMES, AND NURSING INTERVENTIONS

A comprehensive nursing care plan for the patient with cancer of the esophagus treated by surgery is presented at the end of this chapter. Included in the table are pertinent nursing diagnoses, desired patient outcomes, and nursing interventions/rationales.

REFERENCES

1. American Cancer Society. Cancer facts and figures, 1993.
2. Held, JL and Peahota, A: Nursing care of patients with esophageal cancer. Oncol Nurs Forum 19:627–633, 1992.
3. Leichman, L and Israel, V: Neoplasms of the esophagus. In Calabrisi, P and Schein, PS (eds): Medical Oncology, rev ed. McGraw-Hill, New York, 1993, pp 650–666.
4. Grunberg, SM and Groshen, S: Concepts of cancer staging. In Calabrisi, P and Schein, PS (eds): Medical Oncology rev ed. McGraw-Hill, New York, 1993, pp 229–230.
5. Kelsen, DP, Barns, M, and Burt, M: Neoadjuvant chemotherapy and surgery of cancer of the esophagus. Semin Surg Oncol 6:268–273, 1990.
6. Orringer, MB, et al.: Chemotherapy and radiation therapy before transhiatal esophagectomy for esophageal carcinoma. Ann Thorac Surg 49:348–353, 1990.
7. Burnett, CM, Rosemary, AS, and Pheiffer, EA: Life-threatening acute posterior mediastinitis due to esophageal perforation. Ann Thorac Surg 49:979–982, 1990.
8. Data compiled from patient records at the Fox Chase Cancer Center, Philadelphia.
9. Galandiuk, S, et al: Cancer of the esophagus: The Cleveland Clinic experience. Ann Surg 203:101, 1986.
10. Bonica, JJ: Postoperative pain. In Bonica, JJ (ed): The Management of Pain, rev ed. Lea & Febiger, Philadelphia, 1990.
11. Ready, LB: Acute postoperative pain. In Cucchiara, RF, et al (eds): Anesthesia, ed 3. Churchill Livingstone, New York, 1990.
12. Hoebler, L and Irwin, MM: Gastrointestinal tract cancer: Current knowledge, medical treatment, and nursing management. Oncol Nurs Forum 19:1403–1407, 1992.

CARE PLAN FOR THE PATIENT WITH CANCER OF THE ESOPHAGUS TREATED BY SURGERY

Nursing Diagnoses

Nursing Diagnosis #1
Decreased cardiac output, related to altered hemodynamics associated with thoracic/abdominal surgery.

Nursing Diagnosis #2
Alteration in tissue perfusion: cardiopulmonary, cerebral, renal

Desired Patient Outcomes

Patient will:
1. Maintain presurgical cardiovascular function, as manifested by:
   - Stable hemodynamics
     - Blood pressure within 10 mmHg of baseline
     - Heart rate: <100 beats/min
     - Cardiac output: ~5 L/min
     - Central venous pressure: 0–8 mmHg
     - Pulmonary capillary wedge pressure: 8–12 mmHg
   - Absence of extreme weakness or fatigue, peripheral edema, neck vein distention, or chest pain
   - Absence of cardiac arrhythmias
2. Maintain intact neurologic status:
   - Mental status: alert and oriented
3. Maintain fluid and electrolyte balance
   - Stable body weight
   - Balanced intake and output
   - Hourly urine output >30 mL/h

Nursing Interventions
- Perform ongoing cardiovascular assessment:
  - Continuous cardiac monitoring. Establish baseline rate, rhythm, and ectopy.
  - Continuous hemodynamic monitoring when indicated. Establish baseline central venous pressure and pulmonary capillary wedge pressure measurements.

Rationales
- Chest surgery may cause cardiac irritability. Many patients develop atrial fibrillation. This arrhythmia may decrease cardiac output by 20%–30%.

CARE PLAN FOR THE PATIENT WITH CANCER OF THE ESOPHAGUS TREATED BY SURGERY (*Continued*)

Nursing Interventions
- ○ Auscultate lungs every 4 h.
- ○ Auscultate heart sounds—presence of S_3
- ○ Assess for fatigue, neck vein distention, sacral edema.
- • Perform neurologic assessment.
  - ○ Level of consciousness.
  - ○ Behavior.
- • Assess fluid and electrolyte status.

  - ○ Daily weight.
  - ○ Intake and output with hourly urine outputs.
  - ○ Serum electrolytes, BUN, creatinine.

Rationales
- ○ Rales (crackles) are an indication of fluid overload.
- ○ Diagnostic sign for congestive heart failure.

- • Compromised hemodynamics and hypoxemia predispose to cerebral hypoxia with altered cerebral function.

- • Reduced blood volume will further compromise venous return and cardiac output; blood volume may need to be expanded with use of colloids or fluids.
  - ○ Reduced cardiac output may diminish renal perfusion, placing patient at risk of developing acute renal failure.

Nursing Diagnoses

Nursing Diagnosis #3
Impaired gas exchange, related to:
1. Pulmonary congestion associated with surgical manipulation of intrathoracic structures.
2. Atelectasis

Desired Patient Outcomes

Patient will maintain effective respiratory function:
- • Rate <25/min
- • Rhythm eupneic
- • Breath sounds clear on auscultation
- • Mental status: alert and oriented
- • Usual skin color
- • Arterial blood gases at baseline

Nursing Interventions
- • Monitor and report signs and symptoms of altered respiratory function:
  - ○ Presence of rapid, shallow, or irregular respirations; dyspnea, orthopnea; use of accessory muscles.
  - ○ Presence of adventitious breath sounds on auscultation.
  - ○ Presence of restlessness, irritability, confusion, or somnolence.
  - ○ Presence of mottled or cyanotic skin color.
- • Note amount and color of sputum production.
- • Monitor arterial blood gas values, and report abnormal results.
- • Monitor pulse oximetry. Obtain arterial blood gas measurements for desaturation.
- • Monitor hemoglobin and hematocrit.
- • Implement measures to maintain adequate respiratory function:
  - ○ Maintain semi-Fowler's position.
  - ○ Maintain prescribed O_2 therapy and monitor response.
  - ○ Encourage coughing and deep breathing every 1–2 h.
  - ○ Assist in turning every 2 h.
  - ○ Instruct to splint incision when coughing.
  - ○ Encourage use of pain medication as prescribed and monitor response.

Rationales

- • Monitors the oxygen saturation of available hemoglobin.

- • Anemia provokes tissue hypoxia.

  - ○ Because of extent of surgery, patient will "guard" incision, which leads to decreased lung expansion, atelectasis, and poor gas exchange.

Nursing Diagnoses

Nursing Diagnosis #4
Alteration in bowel elimination, related to surgical trauma, stress, and enteral tube feedings

Nursing Interventions
- • Maintain nasogastric tube to low suction. Irrigate with 30 mL normal saline solution every 4 h, or as prescribed.

Desired Patient Outcomes

Patient will:
1. Regain peristaltic activity and presurgical bowel function

Rationales
- • Maintains patency and prevents gastric distention, which may cause stress to suture line and lead to an anastomotic leak.

CARE PLAN FOR THE PATIENT WITH CANCER OF THE ESOPHAGUS TREATED BY SURGERY (*Continued*)

Nursing Interventions
○ **Do not reposition or reinsert.**

- Assess for presence of abdominal distention and auscultate for bowel sounds every shift.

- Inquire as to the presence or absence of flatulence.
  ○ Encourage ambulation when indicated.
- Monitor daily intake and output, weight, and electrolyte balance.

- Assess character and frequency of stool.

Rationales
○ The tube is placed during surgery. Care must be taken to avoid harm to the anastomosis. Physician will determine benefit, risk, and method of replacement.
- Distention may indicate malfunctioning nasogastric tube and stress to the anastomosis.
- Bowel sounds indicate that the intestines have regained peristaltic activity.

- Fluid loss after gastrointestinal surgery may approach 2 liters or more. Fluid and electrolyte replacement may be required with the loss of large amounts of fluids.
- Diarrhea may result in wasting of Mg^{2+} and Ca^{2+}. Observe for muscle weakness or tetany.

Nursing Diagnoses

Nursing Diagnosis #5
Impairment of skin integrity, related to:
1. Surgical incision with potential for impaired wound healing, resulting from:
   - Preoperative radiation therapy
   - Poor nutrition
   - Infection
2. Irritation or breakdown, related to:
   - Contact of skin with wound drainage
   - Stress from drainage tubes
   - Use of tape

Desired Patient Outcomes

Patient will experience normal healing of surgical wounds

Nursing Interventions
- Position patient to reduce stress on suture lines.
- Maintain nasogastric tube patency.
- Splint wounds while coughing.

- Change dressings frequently and perform aseptic wound care.
- Note type and amount of drainage. Obtain culture if indicated and monitor results.
- Note drainage tube sites. Provide anchoring tape to prevent tensions or pulling at insertion sites.
  ○ Consider use of Montgomery straps.
- Monitor laboratory values for signs of anemia, decreased albumin levels, or an increased leukocyte count.

Rationales

- Prevents gastric distention.
- Equalizes pressure to the wounds. Reduces the possibility of dehiscence.
- Minimizes skin irritation from drainage and prevents nosocomial infections.

  ○ Prevents skin abrasions from frequent tape changes.
- Anemia will result in decreased oxygenation to the tissues. Low albumin level indicates a decrease in the colloidal osmotic pressure, which will lead to edema and interference with healing. A leukocytosis may indicate an infectious process.

Nursing Diagnoses

Nursing Diagnosis #6
Alteration in comfort level: pain, related to surgical procedure

Desired Patient Outcomes

Patient will:
1. Use measures effective in managing pain
2. Verbalize pain relief
3. Exhibit relaxed demeanor:
   - Relaxed facial expression and body posturing
   - Ease of breathing

CARE PLAN FOR THE PATIENT WITH CANCER OF THE ESOPHAGUS TREATED BY SURGERY (*Continued*)

Nursing Interventions

- Determine pain "tolerance." Assess patient's willingness to use pain medication versus stoic behavior.
- Assess for physical manifestations of pain.
  - Restlessness, reluctance to move, guarding incision, clenched fist.
  - Diaphoresis, rapid shallow breathing, tachycardia, hypertension.
- Assess complaints of pain, including severity, location/radiation, duration, and quality (i.e., sharp, dull, knifelike).
- Collaborate with physician and patient in titrating pain medication as needed.
- Suggest alternate position changes.

Rationales

- Many people fear they will become addicted to narcotics.

Nursing Diagnoses

Nursing Diagnosis #7

Alteration in nutrition: less than body requirements, related to presence of a neoplasm in the gastrointestinal tract before operation and NPO status after operation (See Chapter 9, Nutritional Support of the Critically Ill Patient.)

Desired Patient Outcomes

Patient will:
1. Meet the estimated nutrients:
   - Calories per day
   - Grams of protein per day as established by the nutritional support service
2. Maintain body weight within 5% of baseline
3. Maintain laboratory data within acceptable range: BUN, creatinine, electrolytes, glucose, albumin, and transferrin levels

Nursing Interventions

Parenteral nutrition

- Monitor daily intake and output, calorie count, and weight. Notify physician for weight gain greater than 2 lb in 24 h.
- Monitor blood glucose levels and ketone levels in urine every 6 h.

- Monitor lab values (while on TPN):
  - Hematology profile.
  - Serum glucose and electrolytes, calcium, phosphorus.
  - BUN and creatinine.
  - Liver profile.
  - Serum cholesterol, triglycerides.
  - Total protein and serum albumin, transferrin.
  - Coagulation profile.
  - 24-h urine for BUN
- Maintain a constant IV infusion via infusion pump. Should therapy be interrupted, run dextrose 10W at the TPN rate.
- Administer vitamin K 20 mg IM once per week as prescribed.
- Infuse lipids (10% or 20%) and amino acids daily as prescribed.
- Consider physical therapy consult for resistance and endurance training.

Enteral tube feedings

- Monitor daily intake and output, caloric counts.
  - Weigh patient 3 times per week.
  - Monitor serum glucose and ketone levels in urine every 6 h.
- Monitor laboratory values: complete blood cell count with differential, albumin, and total iron-binding capacity, electrolytes, BUN, and glucose.
- Place continuous tube feeding on infusion pump. Keep head of bed elevated 45°. Check residual volume of feeding every 4 h. If >100 mL, discontinue feeding for 1 h. If feeding held for more than 2 h, notify physician.

Rationales

- Monitors effectiveness of therapy.

- The increased glucose load may overtax the pancreas and its ability to produce insulin. Patient may require regular insulin coverage.
- Obtain full complement of blood work before initiation of TPN for baseline values. Repeat weekly.
  - Monitors adequacy of replacement therapy.

- Allows pancreas to adjust to a high glucose level.

- Provides nutritional supplement.

- Monitors effectiveness of therapy.

- Obtain full complement weekly.

CARE PLAN FOR THE PATIENT WITH CANCER OF THE ESOPHAGUS
TREATED BY SURGERY (*Continued*)

Nursing Interventions
- ○ Irrigate feeding tube with at least 20 mL water every 4 h.

- Notify physician if patient develops diarrhea. (See Research Application box.)

- Administer formula at room temperature. Discard unused feeding every 4 h.
- Provide frequent mouth care.
- Consider physical therapy consult for resistance and endurance training.

Rationales
- ○ Patients receiving enteral nutrition in high osmolar concentrations require free water to prevent dehydration.
- Indicates patient's intolerance to glucose and/or osmolar concentration. May require either a decrease in rate or concentration. Patient may require antidiarrheal medication to prevent fluid and electrolyte imbalance.

- Aesthetically pleasing to patient. Keeps mucous membranes moist and intact.

Nursing Diagnoses

Nursing Diagnosis #8
Potential for infection, related to central line and TPN infusion

Nursing Interventions
- Monitor for symptoms of infection: fever, tachycardia, increased white blood cell count.
- Perform central venous line site care as per unit protocol. The area is cleansed with acetone and betadine and redressed with a transparent, occlusive dressing.
- Assess dressing integrity and catheter site every shift for redness, swelling, pain, or drainage. Obtain cultures as needed. Tubing changes are done daily. TPN bottles are discontinued after 24 h.
- Note: Once a central line is dedicated for TPN use, it *should not* be used for additional medication, infusions, central venous pressure readings, or blood aspiration.

Desired Patient Outcomes

Patient will be free from catheter- and infusion-related infections

Rationales
- Patients receiving TPN are susceptible to infection from high glucose concentration.
- TPN solution is a media for bacterial growth. The central line allows for systemic access into the patient.

- Allows for additional entry of bacteria into system.

Nursing Diagnoses

Nursing Diagnosis #9
Social isolation, related to prolonged hospital stay.

Nursing Interventions
- Encourage verbalization about social contacts.

- Consult social service when indicated.
- Promote privacy for patients and visitors.

Desired Patient Outcomes

Patient will maintain social contacts developed before surgery

Rationales
- Identifies contacts that the nursing staff may make on behalf of the patient while in intensive care.

North American Nursing Diagnosis Association (NANDA) Taxonomy of Nursing Diagnoses

This list represents the NANDA-approved nursing diagnoses for clinical use and testing (1994).

PATTERN 1: EXCHANGING

Altered nutrition: more than body requirements
Altered nutrition: less than body requirements
Altered nutrition: potential for more than body requirements
Risk for infection
Risk for altered body temperature
Hypothermia
Hyperthermia
Ineffective thermoregulation
Dysreflexia
Constipation
Perceived constipation
Colonic constipation
Diarrhea
Bowel incontinence
Altered urinary elimination
Stress incontinence
Reflex incontinence
Urge incontinence
Functional incontinence
Total incontinence
Urinary retention
Altered tissue perfusion (specify type: renal, cerebral, cardiopulmonary, gastrointestinal, peripheral)
Fluid volume excess
Fluid volume deficit
Risk for fluid volume deficit
Decreased cardiac output
Impaired gas exchange
Ineffective airway clearance
Ineffective breathing pattern
Inability to sustain spontaneous ventilation
Dysfunctional ventilatory weaning response (DVWR)

Risk for injury
Risk for suffocation
Risk for poisoning
Risk for trauma
Risk for aspiration
Risk for disuse syndrome
Altered protection
Impaired tissue integrity
Altered oral mucous membrane
Impaired skin integrity
Risk for impaired skin integrity
Decreased adaptive capacity: intracranial
Energy field disturbance

PATTERN 2: COMMUNICATING

Impaired verbal communication

PATTERN 3: RELATING

Impaired social interaction
Social isolation
Risk for loneliness
Altered role performance
Altered parenting
Risk for altered parenting
Risk for altered parent-infant-child attachment
Sexual dysfunction
Altered family process
Caregiver role strain
Risk for caregiver role strain
Altered family process: alcoholism
Parental role conflict
Altered sexuality patterns

PATTERN 4: VALUING

Spiritual distress (distress of the human spirit)
Potential for enhanced spiritual well-being

PATTERN 5: CHOOSING

Ineffective individual coping
Impaired adjustment
Defensive coping
Ineffective denial
Ineffective family coping: disabling
Ineffective family coping: compromised
Family coping: potential for growth
Potential for enhanced community coping
Ineffective community coping
Ineffective management of therapeutic regimen: individuals
Noncompliance (specify)
Ineffective management of therapeutic regimen: family
Ineffective management of therapeutic regimen: community
Effective management of therapeutic regimen: individual

Decisional conflict (specify)
Health-seeking behaviors (specify)

PATTERN 6: MOVING

Impaired physical mobility
Risk for peripheral neurovascular dysfunction
Risk for perioperative positioning injury
Activity intolerance
Fatigue
Risk for activity intolerance
Sleep pattern disturbance
Diversional activity deficit
Impaired home maintenance management
Altered health maintenance
Feeding self-care deficit
Impaired swallowing
Ineffective breastfeeding
Interrupted breastfeeding
Effective breastfeeding
Ineffective infant feeding pattern
Bathing/hygiene self-care deficit
Dressing/grooming self-care deficit
Toileting self-care deficit
Altered growth and development
Relocation stress syndrome
Risk for disorganized infant behavior
Disorganized infant behavior
Potential for enhanced organized infant behavior

PATTERN 7: PERCEIVING

Body image disturbance
Self-esteem disturbance
Chronic low self-esteem
Situational low self-esteem
Personal identity disturbance
Sensory-perceptual alterations (specify: visual, auditory, kinesthetic, gustatory, tactile,
    olfactory)
Unilateral neglect
Hopelessness
Powerlessness

PATTERN 8: KNOWING

Knowledge deficit (specify)
Impaired environmental interpretation syndrome
Acute confusion
Chronic confusion
Altered thought processes
Impaired memory

PATTERN 9: FEELING

Pain
Chronic pain

Dysfunctional grieving
Anticipatory grieving
Risk for violence: self-directed or directed at others
Risk for self-mutilation
Post-trauma response
Rape-trauma syndrome
Rape-trauma syndrome: compound reaction
Rape-trauma syndrome: silent reaction
Anxiety
Fear

APPENDIX B

NANDA-Approved Nursing Diagnoses: Definitions*

Altered Nutrition: More Than Body Requirements

The state in which an individual is experiencing an intake of nutrients exceeding metabolic needs.

Altered Nutrition: Less Than Body Requirements

The state in which an individual experiences an intake of nutrients insufficient to meet metabolic needs.

Altered Nutrition: Potential for More Than Body Requirements

The state in which an individual is at risk of experiencing an intake of nutrients exceeding metabolic needs.

Risk for Infection

The state in which an individual is at risk for being invaded by pathogenic organisms.

Risk for Altered Body Temperature

The state in which the individual is at risk for failure to maintain body temperature within normal range.

Hypothermia

The state in which an individual's body temperature is reduced below normal range.

Hyperthermia

A state in which an individual's body temperature is elevated above his or her normal range.

Ineffective Thermoregulation

The state in which an individual's temperature fluctuates between hypothermia and hyperthermia.

Dysreflexia

The state in which an individual with a spinal cord injury at T-7 or above experiences a life-threatening, uninhibited sympathetic response of the nervous system to a noxious stimulus.

Constipation

A state in which an individual experiences a change in normal bowel habits characterized by a decrease in frequency and/or passage of hard, dry stools.

Perceived Constipation

The state in which an individual makes a self-diagnosis of constipation and ensures a daily bowel movement through abuse of laxatives, enemas, and suppositories.

Colonic Constipation

The state in which an individual's pattern of elimination is characterized by a hard, dry stool resulting from a delay in passage of food residue.

Diarrhea

A state in which an individual experiences a change in normal bowel habits characterized by the frequent passage of loose, fluid, unformed stools.

---

*Adapted from North American Nursing Diagnosis Association: Definitions and Classification 1995–1996. NANDA, Philadelphia, 1994.

Bowel Incontinence

A state in which an individual experiences a change in normal bowel habits characterized by involuntary passage of stool.

Altered Urinary Elimination

The state in which the individual experiences a disturbance in urine elimination.

Stress Incontinence

The state in which an individual experiences a loss of urine of less than 50 mL, occurring with increased abdominal pressure.

Reflex Incontinence

The state in which an individual experiences an involuntary loss of urine, occurring at somewhat predictable intervals when a specific bladder volume is reached.

Urge Incontinence

The state in which an individual experiences involuntary passage of urine soon after a strong sense of urgency to void.

Functional Incontinence

The state in which an individual experiences an involuntary, unpredictable passage of urine.

Total Incontinence

The state in which an individual experiences a continuous and unpredictable loss of urine.

Urinary Retention

The state in which the individual experiences incomplete emptying of the bladder.

Altered Tissue Perfusion (Specify Type: Renal, Cerebral, Cardiopulmonary, Gastrointestinal, Peripheral)

The state in which an individual experiences a decrease in nutrition and oxygenation at the cellular level because of a deficit in capillary blood supply.

Fluid Volume Excess

The state in which an individual experiences increased fluid retention and edema.

Fluid Volume Deficit

The state in which an individual experiences vascular, cellular, or intracellular dehydration.

Risk for Fluid Volume Deficit

The state in which an individual is at risk of experiencing vascular, cellular, or intracellular dehydration.

Decreased Cardiac Output

A state in which the blood pumped by an individual's heart is sufficiently reduced that it is inadequate to meet the needs of the body's tissues.

Impaired Gas Exchange

The state in which an individual experiences a decreased passage of oxygen and/or carbon dioxide between the alveoli of the lungs and the vascular system.

Ineffective Airway Clearance

The state in which an individual is unable to clear secretions or obstructions from the respiratory tract to maintain airway patency.

Ineffective Breathing Pattern

The state in which an individual's inhalation and/or exhalation pattern does not enable adequate pulmonary inflation or emptying.

Inability to Sustain Spontaneous Ventilation

A state in which the response pattern of decreased energy reserves results in an individual's inability to maintain breathing adequate to support life.

Dysfunctional Ventilatory Weaning Response (DVWR)

A state in which a patient cannot adjust to lowered levels of mechanical ventilator support, which interrupts and prolongs the weaning process.

Risk for Injury

A state in which the individual is at risk of injury as a result of environmental conditions interacting with the individual's adaptive and defensive resources.

Risk for Suffocation

Accentuated risk of accidental suffocation (inadequate air available for inhalation).

Risk for Poisoning

Accentuated risk of accidental exposure to, or ingestion of, drugs or dangerous products in doses sufficient to cause poisoning.

Risk for Trauma

Accentuated risk of accidental tissue injury, such as wound, burn, fracture.

Risk for Aspiration

The state in which an individual is at risk for entry of gastrointestinal secretions, oropharyngeal secretions, or solids or fluids into tracheobronchial passages.

Risk for Disuse Syndrome

A state in which an individual is at risk for deterioration of body systems as the result of prescribed or unavoidable musculoskeletal activity.

Altered Protection

The state in which an individual experiences a decreased ability to guard the self from internal or external threats such as illness or injury.

Impaired Tissue Integrity

A state in which an individual experiences damage to mucous membrane, corneal, integumentary, or subcutaneous tissue.

Altered Oral Mucous Membrane

The state in which an individual experiences disruptions in the tissue layers of the oral cavity.

Impaired Skin Integrity

A state in which the individual's skin is adversely altered.

Risk for Impaired Skin Integrity

A state in which the individual's skin is at risk of being adversely altered.

Decreased Adaptive Capacity: Intracranial

A clinical state in which intercranial fluid dynamic mechanisms that normally compensate for increased intracranial volumes are compromised, resulting in repeated disproportionate increases in intracranial pressure (ICP) in response to a variety of noxious and non-noxious stimuli.

Energy Field Disturbance

A disruption of the flow of energy surrounding a person's being that results in a disharmony of the body, mind, and/or spirit.

Impaired Verbal Communication

The state in which an individual experiences a decreased or absent ability to use or understand language in human interaction.

Impaired Social Interaction

The state in which an individual participates in an insufficient or excessive quantity or ineffective quality of social exchange.

Social Isolation

Aloneness experienced by the individual and perceived as imposed by others and as a negative or threatened state.

Risk for Loneliness

A subjective state in which an individual is at risk of experiencing vague dysphoria.

Altered Role Performance

Disruption in the way one perceives one's role performance.

Altered Parenting

The state in which a nurturing figure experiences an inability to create an environment that promotes the optimum growth and development of another human being.

Risk for Altered Parenting

The state in which a nurturing figure is at risk of experiencing an inability to create an environment that promotes the optimum growth and development of another human being.

Risk for Altered Parent-Infant-Child Attachment

Disruption of the interactive process between parent/significant other and infant that fosters the development of a protective and nurturing reciprocal relationship.

Sexual Dysfunction

The state in which an individual experiences a change in sexual function that is viewed as unsatisfying, unrewarding, inadequate.

Altered Family Process

The state in which a family that normally functions effectively experiences a dysfunction.

Caregiver Role Strain

A caregiver's felt difficulty in performing the family caregiving role.

Risk for Caregiver Role Strain

A caregiver is vulnerable for felt difficulty in performing the family caregiving role.

Altered Family Process: Alcoholism

The state in which the psychosocial, spiritual, and physiologic functions of the family unit are chronically disorganized, leading to conflict, denial of problems, resistance to change, ineffective problem-solving, and a series of self-perpetuating crises.

Parental Role Conflict

The state in which a parent experiences role confusion and conflict in response to crisis.

Altered Sexuality Patterns

The state in which an individual expresses concern regarding his or her sexuality.

Spiritual Distress (Distress of the Human Spirit)

Disruption in the life principle that pervades a person's entire being and integrates and transcends one's biologic and psychosocial nature.

Potential for Enhanced Spiritual Well-Being

Spiritual well-being is the process of an individual's developing and unfolding of mystery through harmonious interconnectedness that springs from inner strengths.

Ineffective Individual Coping

Impairment of adaptive behaviors and problem-solving abilities of a person in meeting life's demands and roles.

Impaired Adjustment

The state in which the individual is unable to modify his or her lifestyle and behavior in a manner consistent with a change in health status.

Defensive Coping

The state in which an individual repeatedly projects falsely positive self-evaluation based on a self-protective pattern that defends against underlying perceived threats to positive self-regard.

Ineffective Denial

The state of conscious or unconscious attempts to disavow the knowledge or meaning of an event to reduce anxiety and fear to the detriment of health.

Ineffective Family Coping: Disabling

Behavior of significant person (family member or other primary person) that disables his or her own capacities and the client's capacity to effectively address tasks essential to either person's adaptation to the health challenge.

Ineffective Family Coping: Compromised

A usually supportive primary person (family member or close friend) provides insufficient, ineffective, or compromised support, comfort, assistance, or encouragement that may be needed by the client to manage or master adaptation tasks related to his or her health challenge.

Family Coping: Potential for Growth

Effective managing of adaptive tasks by family member involved with the health challenge, who now is exhibiting desire and readiness for enhanced health and growth in regard to self and in relation to the client.

Potential for Enhanced Community Coping

A pattern of community activities for adaptation and problem-solving that is satisfactory for meeting the demands or needs of the community but can be improved for management of current and future problems or stressors.

Ineffective Community Coping

A pattern of community activities for adaptation and problem-solving that is unsatisfactory for meeting the demands or needs of the community.

Ineffective Management of Therapeutic Regimen: Individuals

A pattern of regulating and integrating into daily living a program for treatment of illness and the sequelae of illness that is unsatisfactory for meeting specific health goals.

Noncompliance (Specify)

A person's informed decision not to adhere to a therapeutic recommendation.

Ineffective Management of Therapeutic Regimen: Family

A pattern of regulating and integrating into family processes a program for treatment of illness and the sequelae of illness that is unsatisfactory for meeting specific health goals.

Ineffective Management of Therapeutic Regimen: Community

A pattern of regulating and integrating into community processes programs for treatment of illness and the sequelae of illness that is unsatisfactory for meeting specific health-related goals.

Effective Management of Therapeutic Regimen: Individual

A pattern of regulating and integrating into daily living a program for treatment of illness and its sequelae that is satisfactory for meeting specific health goals.

Decisional Conflict (Specify)

The state of uncertainty about course of action to be taken when choice among competing actions involves risk, loss, or challenge to personal life values.

Health-Seeking Behaviors (Specify)

A state in which an individual in stable health is actively seeking ways to alter personal health habits and/or the environment to move toward a higher level of health.

Impaired Physical Mobility

A state in which the individual experiences a limitation of ability for independent physical movement.

Risk for Peripheral Neurovascular Dysfunction

A state in which the individual is at risk of experiencing a disruption in circulation, sensation, or motion of an extremity.

Risk for Perioperative Positioning Injury

A state in which the client is at risk for injury as a result of the environmental conditions found in the perioperative setting.

Activity Intolerance

A state in which an individual has insufficient physiologic or psychological energy to endure or complete required or desired daily activities.

Fatigue

An overwhelming sustained sense of exhaustion and decreased capacity for physical and mental work.

Risk for Activity Intolerance

A state in which an individual is at risk of experiencing insufficient physiologic or psychological energy to endure or complete required or desired daily activities.

Sleep Pattern Disturbance

Disruption of sleep time causes discomfort or interferes with desired lifestyle.

Diversional Activity Deficit

A state in which an individual experiences a decreased stimulation from (or interest or engagement in) recreational or leisure activities.

Impaired Home Maintenance Management

Inability to independently maintain a safe, growth-promoting immediate environment.

Altered Health Maintenance

Inability to identify, manage, or seek out help to maintain health.

Feeding Self-Care Deficit

A state in which one experiences an impaired ability to perform or complete feeding activities for oneself.

Impaired Swallowing

A state in which an individual has decreased ability to voluntarily pass fluids and/or solids from the mouth to the stomach.

Ineffective Breastfeeding

The state in which a mother, infant, or child experiences dissatisfaction or difficulty with the breastfeeding process.

Interrupted Breastfeeding

A break in the continuity of the breastfeeding process as a result of inability or inadvisability to put baby to breast for feeding.

Effective Breastfeeding

The state in which a mother-infant dyad/family exhibits adequate proficiency and satisfaction with breastfeeding process.

Ineffective Infant Feeding Pattern

A state in which an infant demonstrates an impaired ability to suck or coordinate the suck-swallow response.

Bathing/Hygiene Self-Care Deficit

A state in which one experiences an impaired ability to perform or complete bathing/hygiene activities for oneself.

Dressing/Grooming Self-Care Deficit

A state in which one experiences an impaired ability to perform or complete dressing and grooming activities for oneself.

Toileting Self-Care Deficit

A state in which one experiences an impaired ability to perform or complete toileting activities for oneself.

Altered Growth and Development

A state in which an individual demonstrates deviations in norms from his or her age group.

Relocation Stress Syndrome

Physiologic and/or psychological disturbances as a result of transfer from one environment to another.

Risk for Disorganized Infant Behavior

Risk for alteration in integration and modulation of the physiologic and behavioral systems of functioning (i.e., automatic, motor, state, organizational, self-regulatory, and attentional-interactional systems).

Disorganized Infant Behavior

Alteration in integration and modulation of the physiologic and behavioral systems of functioning (i.e., automatic, motor, state, organizational, self-regulatory, and attentional-interactional systems).

Potential for Enhanced Organized Infant Behavior

A pattern of modulation of the physiologic and behavioral systems of functioning of an infant (i.e., automatic, motor, state, organizational, self-regulatory, and attentional-interactional systems) that is satisfactory but can be improved, resulting in higher levels of integration in response to environmental stimuli.

Body Image Disturbance

Disruption in the way one perceives one's body image.

Self-Esteem Disturbance

Negative self-evaluation and feelings about self or self-capabilities, which may be directly or indirectly expressed.

Chronic Low Self-Esteem

Long-standing negative self-evaluation and feelings about self or self-capabilities.

Situational Low Self-Esteem

Negative self-evaluation and feelings about self that develop in response to a loss or change in an individual who previously had a positive self-evaluation.

Personal Identity Disturbance

Inability to distinguish between self and nonself.

Sensory-Perceptual Alterations (Specify: Visual, Auditory, Kinesthetic, Gustatory, Tactile, Olfactory)

A state in which an individual experiences a change in the amount or patterning of oncoming stimuli accompanied by a diminished, exaggerated, distorted, or impaired response to such stimuli.

Unilateral Neglect

A state in which an individual is perceptually unaware of, and inattentive to, one side of the body.

Hopelessness

A subjective state in which an individual sees limited or no alternatives or personal choices available and is unable to mobilize energy on own behalf.

Powerlessness

Perception that one's own actions will not significantly affect an outcome; a perceived lack of control over a current situation or immediate happening.

Knowledge Deficit (Specify)

Absence or deficiency of cognitive information related to specific topic.

Impaired Environmental Interpretation Syndrome

Consistent lack of orientation to person, place, time, or circumstances over more than 3 to 6 months, necessitating a protective environment.

Acute Confusion

The abrupt onset of a cluster of global, transient changes and disturbances in attention, cognition, psychomotor activity, level of consciousness, and/or sleep-wake cycle.

Chronic Confusion

An irreversible, longstanding, and/or progressive deterioration of intellect and personality characterized by decreased ability to interpret environmental stimuli and decreased capacity for intellectual thought processes, and manifested by disturbances of memory, orientation, and behavior.

Altered Thought Processes

A state in which an individual experiences a disruption in cognitive operations and activities.

Impaired Memory

The state in which an individual experiences the inability to remember or recall bits of information or behavioral skills. Impaired memory may be attributed to pathophysiologic or situational causes that are either temporary or permanent.

Pain

A state in which an individual experiences and reports the presence of severe discomfort or an uncomfortable sensation.

Chronic Pain

A state in which the individual experiences pain that continues for more than 6 months in duration.

Dysfunctional Grieving

Extended, unsuccessful use of intellectual and emotional responses by which individuals attempt to work through the process of modifying self-concept based upon the perception of loss.

Anticipatory Grieving

Intellectual and emotional responses and behaviors by which individuals work through the process of modifying self-concept based on the perception of potential loss.

Risk for Violence: Self-Directed or Directed at Others

A state in which an individual experiences behaviors that can be physically harmful to either the self or others.

Risk for Self-Mutilation

A state in which an individual is at risk of performing an act upon the self to injure, not kill, which produces tissue damage and tension relief.

Post-Trauma Response

The state of an individual experiencing a sustained painful response to an overwhelming traumatic event.

Rape-Trauma Syndrome

Forced, violent sexual penetration against the victim's will and consent. The trauma syndrome that develops from this attack or attempted attack includes an acute phase of disorganization of the victim's lifestyle and a long-term process of reorganization of lifestyle.

Rape-Trauma Syndrome: Compound Reaction

Forced, violent sexual penetration against the victim's will and consent. The trauma syndrome that develops from this attack or attempted attack includes an acute phase of disorganization of the victim's lifestyle and a long-term process of reorganization of lifestyle.

Rape-Trauma Syndrome: Silent Reaction

Forced, violent sexual penetration against the victim's will and consent. The trauma syndrome that develops from this attack or attempted attack includes an acute phase of disorganization of the victim's lifestyle and a long-term process of reorganization of lifestyle.

Anxiety

A vague, uneasy feeling whose source is often nonspecific or unknown to the individual.

Fear

Feeling of dread related to an identifiable source that the person validates.

APPENDIX C

Functional Health Patterns: Definitions

Health Perception–Health Management

Describes the client's perceived pattern of health and well-being and how his or her health is managed. Includes the individual's perception of health status and its relevance to current activities and future planning. Also included is the individual's general level of healthcare behavior, such as adherence to mental and physical prevention health practices, medical or nursing prescriptions, and follow-up care.

Nutritional-Metabolic

Describes patterns of food and fluid consumption relative to metabolic need and pattern indicators of local nutrient supply. Includes the individual's patterns of food and fluid consumption, daily eating times, the types and quantity of food and fluids consumed, particular food preferences, and the use of nutrient or vitamin supplements. Reports of any skin lesions and general ability to heal are included. The condition of skin, hair, nails, mucous membranes, and teeth and measures of body temperature, height, and weight are included.

Elimination

Describes patterns of excretory function (bowel, bladder, and skin) of individuals. Includes the individual's perceived regularity of excretory function, use of routines or laxatives for bowel elimination, and any changes or disturbances in time pattern, mode of excretion, quality, or quantity. Also included are any devices employed to control excretion. Includes family or community waste disposal pattern when appropriate.

Activity-Exercise

Describes pattern of exercise, activity, leisure, and recreation. Includes activities of daily living requiring energy expenditure, such as hygiene, cooking, shopping, eating, working, and home maintenance. Also included are the type, quantity, and quality of exercise, including sports, which describe the typical pattern. (Factors that interfere with the desired or expected pattern for the *individual*, such as neuromuscular deficits and compensations, dyspnea, angina, or muscle cramping on exertion, and, if appropriate, his or her cardiac-pulmonary classification, are included.) Leisure patterns are included and describe the recreational activities undertaken with others or alone. Emphasis is on activities of major importance to the client.

Sleep-Rest

Describes patterns of sleep, rest, and relaxation. Includes the patterns of sleep and rest/relaxation periods during the 24-hour day. Includes the perception of the quality and quantity of sleep and rest, and perception of energy level. Included also are aids to sleep, such as medications or night-time routines that are employed.

Cognitive-Perceptual

Describes sensory-perceptual and cognitive pattern. Includes the adequacy of sensory modes, such as vision, hearing, taste, touch, or smell, and the compensation or prostheses used for disturbances. Reports of pain perception and how pain is managed are also included when appropriate. Also included are the cognitive functional abilities, such as language, memory, and decision-making.

Self-Perception–Self-Concept

Describes self-concept pattern and perceptions of self. Includes the attitudes about self, perception of abilities (cognitive, affective, or physical), image, identity, general sense of worth, and general emotional pattern. Patterns of body posture and movement, eye contact, voice, and speech patterns are included.

Role-Relationship

Describes pattern of role engagements and relationships. Includes perception of the major roles and responsibilities in current life situation. Satisfaction or disturbances in family work, social relationships, and responsibilities related to these roles are included.

Sexuality-Reproductive

Describes patterns of satisfaction or dissatisfaction with sexuality; describes reproductive pattern. Includes the perceived satisfaction or disturbances in sexuality or sexual relationships. Included also is the female's reproductive stage, before or after menopause, and any perceived problems.

Coping–Stress Tolerance

Describes general coping pattern and effectiveness of the pattern of stress tolerance. Includes the reserve or capacity to resist challenges to self-integrity, modes of handling stress, family or other support systems, and perceived ability to control and manage situations.

Value-Belief

Describes patterns of values, goals, or beliefs (including spiritual) that guide choices or decisions. Includes what is perceived as important in life and any perceived conflicts in values, beliefs, or expectations that are health-related.

Nursing Diagnoses Grouped Under Functional Health Patterns*

Health Perception–Health Management

Energy field disturbance
Altered growth and development
Altered health maintenance
Health-seeking behaviors
Effective management of therapeutic regimen: individual
Ineffective management of therapeutic regimen: individual
Ineffective management of therapeutic regimen: community
Ineffective management of therapeutic regimen: family

Noncompliance: (specify)
Risk for injury
   Risk for suffocation
   Risk for poisoning
   Risk for trauma
Risk for perioperative positioning injury

Nutritional-Metabolic

Decreased adaptive capacity: intracranial
Risk for altered body temperature
   Hypothermia
   Hyperthermia
   Ineffective thermoregulation
Fluid volume deficit
Fluid volume excess
Risk for infection
Altered nutrition: more than body requirements
Altered nutrition: potential for more than body requirements

Altered nutrition: less than body requirements
   Effective breastfeeding
   Ineffective breastfeeding
   Interrupted breastfeeding
   Ineffective infant feeding pattern
   Impaired swallowing
Altered protection
   Impaired tissue integrity
      Altered oral mucous membrane
      Impaired skin integrity

---

*The Functional Health Patterns were identified in Gordon, M: Nursing Diagnosis: Process and Application, ed 3. McGraw-Hill, New York, 1994, with minor changes by the author.

Elimination

Constipation
Colonic constipation
Perceived constipation
Diarrhea
Bowel incontinence
Altered urinary elimination

Urinary retention
Total incontinence
Functional incontinence
Reflex incontinence
Urge incontinence
Stress incontinence

Activity-Exercise

Activity intolerance
Decreased cardiac output
Risk for disuse syndrome
Diversional activity deficit
Impaired home maintenance
  management
Disorganized infant behavior
Risk for disorganized infant behavior
Potential for enhanced organized infant
  behavior
Impaired physical mobility
Risk for peripheral neurovascular
  dysfunction
Dysfunctional ventilatory weaning
  response

Ineffective airway clearance
Ineffective breathing pattern
Impaired gas exchange
Inability to sustain spontaneous
  ventilation
Self-care deficit: (specify)
Altered tissue perfusion
  (specify: cerebral,
  cardiopulmonary, renal,
  gastrointestinal, peripheral)

Sleep-Rest

Sleep pattern disturbance

Cognitive-Perceptual

Altered comfort
  Pain
  Chronic pain
  Acute confusion
  Chronic confusion
Decisional conflict (specify)
Dysreflexia
Impaired environmental interpretation
  syndrome
Knowledge deficit: (specify)
Risk for aspiration

Sensory-perceptual alteration: (specify:
  visual, auditory, kinesthetic, gustatory,
  tactile, olfactory)
Altered thought processes
Impaired memory
Unilateral neglect

Self-Perception–Self-Concept

Anxiety
Fatigue
Powerlessness
  Body image disturbance
  Personal identity disturbance

Fear
Hopelessness
  Self-esteem disturbance
    Chronic low self-esteem
    Situational low self-esteem

Role-Relationship

Impaired communication
Impaired communication: verbal
Altered family process
Altered family process: alcoholism
Anticipatory grieving
Dysfunctional grieving
Risk for loneliness

Risk for altered parent-infant-child
  attachment
Risk for altered parenting
Parental role conflict
Altered role performance
Impaired social interaction
Social isolation

Sexuality-Reproductive

Altered sexuality patterns

Coping-Stress Tolerance

Impaired adjustment
Caregiver role strain
Risk for caregiver role strain
Ineffective individual coping
  Defensive coping
  Ineffective denial
Ineffective family coping: disabling
Ineffective family coping: compromised

Family coping: potential for growth
Ineffective community coping
Potential for enhanced community
  coping
Post-trauma response
  Rape-trauma syndrome
Relocation stress syndrome
Risk for self-mutilation
Risk for violence

Value-Belief

Spiritual distress
Potential for enhanced spiritual well-
  being

Normal Reference Laboratory Values*

BLOOD VALUES

Ammonia	12–55 μmol/L
Amylase	4–25 U/mL
Bilirubin	Direct: up to 0.4 mg/100 mL
	Total: up to 1.0 mg/100 mL
Calcium	8.5–10.5 mg/100 mL
Carbon dioxide content	24–30 mEq/L
Carcinoembryonic antigen (CEA)	0–2.5 ng/mL
Chloride	100–106 mEq/L
Creatine kinase isoenzymes	CK-MM: 100%
	CK-MB: 0%–5%
	CK-BB: 0%
Creatinine	0.6–1.5 mg/100 mL
Digoxin	0.8–2.0 ng/mL
Glucose	70–110 mg/100 mL (fasting)
Iron	50–150 μg/100 mL
Iron-binding capacity	250–410 μg/100 mL
Lacticdehydrogenase (LDH)	45–90 U/L
LDH-1	17%–27%
LDH-2	27%–37%
LDH-3	18%–25%
LDH-4	3%–8%
LDH-5	0%–5%
Lipase	2 U/mL or less
Lipids:	
Cholesterol	120–220 mg/dL
	HDL: male > 45 mg/dL
	female > 55 mg/dL
	LDL: 60–180 mg/dL
	VLDL: 25%–50%
Triglycerides	Male: 40–160 mg/dL
	Female: 35–135 mg/dL
Magnesium	1.5–2.0 mEq/L
Osmolality	280–296 mOsm/kg water
Oxygen saturation (arterial)	95%–100%
P_{CO_2}	35–45 mmHg

*Adapted from Scully, RE (ed): Case records of the Massachusetts General Hospital. N Engl J Med, 314:39–49, January 2, 1986, with permission. Normal laboratory ranges may vary among institutions because of techniques used. Always check your facility's laboratory manual if in doubt.

pH	7.35–7.45
PO$_2$	80–100 mmHg
Phenobarbital	15–50 µg/mL
Phenytoin	10–20 µg/mL
Phosphatase (Acid)	Male: total: 0.13–0.63 sigma U/mL
	Female: total: 0.01–0.56 sigma U/mL
Phosphatase (Alkaline)	13–39 U/L
Phosphorus (Organic)	3.0–4.5 mg/100 mL
Potassium	3.5–5.5 mEq/L
Protein: Total	6.0–8.4 g/100 mL
Albumin	3.5–5.5 g/100 mL
Globulin	2.3–3.5 g/100 mL
Sodium	135–145 mEq/L
Theophylline	10–20 µg
Transaminases, serum glutamic-oxaloacetic transaminase (SGOT) (Aspartate aminotransferase—AST)	7–27 U/L
Transaminases, serum glutamate pyruvate transaminase (SGPT) (Alanine aminotransferase—ALT)	1–21 U/L
Urea nitrogen (BUN)	8–25 mg/100 mL
Uric acid	3.0–7.0 mg/100 mL
Vitamin A	0.15–0.6 µg/mL

Special Endocrine Tests

Adrenocorticotropin (ACTH)	15–70 pg/mL
Aldosterone	Excretion: 5–19 µg/24 h
Calcitonin	Male: 0–14 pg/mL
	Female: 0–28 pg/mL
Cortisol:	
8 AM	5–15 µg/100 mL
8 PM	<10 µg/100 mL
4-h ACTH test	30–45 µg/100 mL
Overnight suppression test	<5 µg/100 mL
Parathyroid hormone	<25 pg/mL
Thyroid-stimulating hormone (TSH)	0.5–5.0 uU/mL
Thyroxine-binding globulin capacity	15–25 µg T$_4$/100 mL
Total triiodothyronine (T$_3$)	75–195 ng/100 mL
Total thyroxine by radioiodine uptake (RAIU) (T$_4$)	4–12 µg/100 mL
T$_3$ resin uptake	25%–35%
Free thyroxine index (FT$_4$I)	1–4
Vitamin D derivatives:	
1,25-Dihydroxyvitamin D	26–65 pg/mL
25-Hydroxyvitamin D	8–56 ng/mL

URINE VALUES

Acetone plus acetoacetate (quantitative)	0
Amylase	24–76 units/mL
Calcium	300 mg/day or less
Catecholamines:	
Epinephrine	Under 20 µg/day
Norepinephrine	Under 100 µg/day
Copper	0–100 µg/day

Creatine	Under 100 mg/day or less than 6% of creatinine
Creatinine	15–25 mg/kg of body weight/day
Hemoglobin (myoglobin)	0
pH	5–7
Phosphorus (inorganic)	Varies with intake; average = 1 g/day
Protein:	
Quantitative	<150 mg/24 h
Steroids:	
17-Ketosteroids	

Age	Male	Female
10	1–4 mg	1–4 mg
20	6–21	4–16
30	8–26	4–14
50	5–18	3–9
70	2–10	1–7

17-Hydroxysteroids	3–8 mg/day (women lower than men)
Glucose	0
Urobilinogen	Up to 1.0 Ehrlich U
Vanillylmandelic acid (VMA)	Up to 9 mg/24 h

HEMATOLOGIC VALUES

Coagulation factors:	
Factor I (Fibrinogen)	200–400 mg/dL
Factor II (Prothrombin)	60%–140%
Factor VII	70%–130%
Factor X (Stuart factor)	70%–130%
Factor VIII (antihemophilic globulin)	50%–200%
Factor IX (Plasma thromboplastic cofactor)	6%–140%
Factor IX (Plasma thromboplastic antecedent)	60%–140%
Factor XII (Hageman factor)	60%–140%
Coagulation screening tests:	
Bleeding time	3–9.5 min
Prothrombin time	Less than 2-sec deviation from control
Partial thromboplastin time (Activated)	30–45 sec
Whole blood clot lysis	No clot lysis in 24 h
D-dimer	$\leq$0.5 μg/mL or 250 mg/mL
Fibrinolytic studies:	
Euglobin lysis	No lysis in 2 h
Fibrinogen split products	< 10 μg/mL or dilution < 1:20
Thrombin time	Control $\pm$5 sec
Complete blood count:	
Hematocrit	Male: 45%–52%
	Female: 37%–48%
Hemoglobin	Male: 13–18 g/100 mL
	Female: 12–16 g/100 mL
White blood cell count	4300–10,800/mm^3
Differential count:	
Neutrophils	55%–70%
Lymphocytes	20%–40%
Monocytes	2%–8%
Eosinophils	1%–4%
Basophils	0.5%–1.0%
Erythrocyte count	4.2–5.9 million/mm^3
Mean corpuscular volume (MCV)	86–98 μm^3/cell

Mean corpuscular hemoglobin (MCH)	27–32 pg/red blood cell
Mean corpuscular hemoglobin concentration (MCHC)	32–36 percent
Erythrocyte sedimentation rate	Male: 1–13 mm/h
	Female: 1–20 mm/h
Platelet count	150,000–350,000/mm^3
Platelet function tests:	
Clot retraction	50%–100%/2 h
Platelet aggregation	Full response to adenosine diphosphate, epinephrine, and collagen
Platelet factor 3	33–57 sec
Reticulocyte count	0.5%–2.5% red blood cells

CEREBROSPINAL FLUID VALUES

Bilirubin	0
Cell count	0–5 mononuclear cells
Chloride	120–130 mEq/L
Albumin	Mean: 29.5 mg/100 mL
Immunoglobulin G (IgG)	Mean: 4.3 mg/100 mL
Glucose	50–75 mg/100 mL
Pressure (initial)	70–180 mm of water
Protein:	
Lumbar	15–45 mg/100 mL

IMMUNOLOGIC TESTS

α-Fetoprotein	Undetectable in normal adult
α-Antitrypsin	83–213 mg/100 mL
Rheumatoid factor	<60 IU/mL
Anti-DNA antibodies	Negative at a 1:8 dilution of serum
Autoantibodies to:	
Thyroid colloid and microsomal antigens	Negative at a 1:10 dilution of serum
Gastric parietal cells	Negative at a 1:20 dilution of serum
Adrenal gland	Negative at a 1:10 dilution of serum
Bence Jones protein	No Bence Jones protein detected in a 50-fold concentrate of urine
Complement, total hemolytic	150–250 U/mL
Cryoprecipitate proteins	None detected
Hemoglobin A$_{1C}$	3.8%–6.4%
Immunoglobulins:	
IgG	639–1349 mg/100 mL
IgA	70–312 mg/100 mL
IgM	86–352 mg/100 mL

APPENDIX F

Hemodynamic Formulas/Parameters*

Parameter	Formula	Normal Values
Arterial O_2 content (CaO_2)	$(Hb \times 1.39 \times SaO_2) + (PaO_2 \times 0.003)$	16–22 mL/dL
Arteriovenous oxygen difference (A-VDO$_2$)	CaO_2 − Venous O_2 content	4–8 L/min
Cardiac index (CI)	$\dfrac{CO}{BSA}$	2.5–4 L/min
Cardiac output (CO)	Heart rate × Stroke volume	4–8 L/min
Central venous pressure (CVP)	$Cm\ H_2O = mmHg \times 1.34$	2–6 mmHg or 5–12 cm H_2O
Cerebral perfusion pressure (CPP)	MAP − ICP	80–100 mmHg
Coronary artery perfusion pressure (CAPP)	DBP − PAWP	60–80 mmHg
Ejection fraction	% Ventricular end-diastolic volume ejected in one beat	55%–70%
Left atrial pressure (LAP)		8–12 mmHg
Left ventricular stroke work index (LSWI)	SVI (MAP − PCWP) × 0.0136	38–85 g/m^2/beat
Mean arterial pressure (MAP)	$SBP + \dfrac{(DBP \times 2)}{3}$	70–105 mmHg
Oxygen consumption (VO_2)	$(SaO_2 - SvO_2)\ (CO \times Hb \times 1.39)$	3.5 mL/kg/min
Oxygen delivery (DO_2)	$CO \times CaO_2 \times 10$	1000 mL/min
Partial pressure of inspired O_2 (PIO$_2$)	$PIO_2 = (PB - PH_2O)\ FIO_2$	149.73 mmHg room air
Pulmonary artery pressure (PAP)		$\dfrac{20–30}{8–12}$ mmHg
Pulmonary artery wedge pressure (PAWP)		8–12 mmHg
Pulmonary vascular resistance (PVR)	$\dfrac{Mean\ PAP - PCWP}{CO} \times 80$	100–250 dynes/sec/cm^{-5}
Right atrial pressure (RAP)		2–6 mmHg
Right ventricular stroke work index	$(MAP - CVP) \times SI \times 0.0136$	7–12 g/m^2/beat
Stroke index (SI)	$\dfrac{CI \times 1000}{HR}$	30–650 mL/beat/m^2
Stroke volume (SV)	$\dfrac{CO}{HR} \times 1000$	60–120 mL/beat
Saturation of mixed venous blood oxygen (SvO$_2$)		60%–80%
Systemic vascular resistance	$\dfrac{MAP - RAP}{CO} \times 80$	800–1200 dynes/sec/cm^{-5}

*BSA = body surface area; DBP = diastolic blood pressure; FIO$_2$ = fraction of inspired oxygen; Hb = hemoglobin; HR = heart rate; ICP = intracranial pressure; PaO$_2$ = partial oxygen pressure; PB = barometric pressure; PCWP = pulmonary capillary wedge pressure; PH$_2$O = water pressure; SaO$_2$ = saturation with oxygen, arterial blood; SBP = systolic blood pressure; SVI = stroke volume index.

Use a straightedge to connect the patient's height in the left-hand column to weight in the right-hand column. The intersection of this line with the center scale estimates the body surface area.

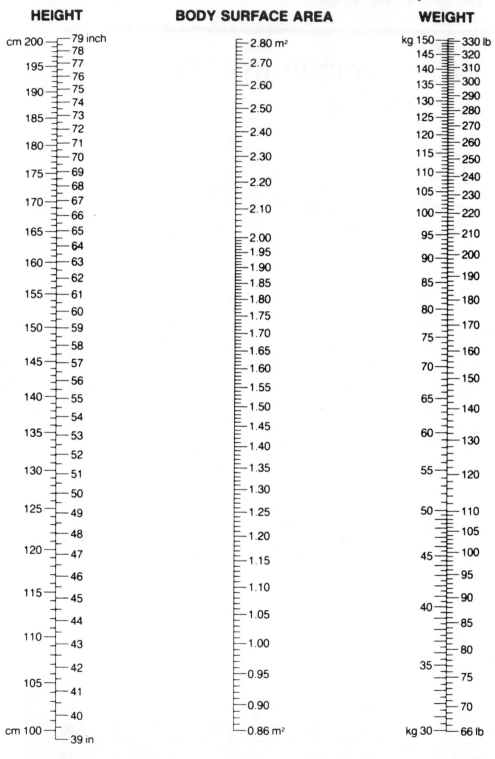

FIGURE F–1. Body surface area nomogram. [From Lenter, C (ed): Geigy Scientific Tables, ed 8, courtesy CIBA-GEIGY, Basel, Switzerland.]

Drug Calculation Formulas for Critical Care

1. Calculate micrograms per milliliter.
   Example: A drip sent from the pharmacy has 800 mg dopamine in 250 mL D_5 W. How many micrograms of dopamine per milliliter does the solution contain?

   $$800 \text{ mg}/250 \text{ mL} \times 1000 \text{ μg}/1 \text{ mg} = 3.2 \times 1000 = 3200 \text{ μg/mL}$$

2. Calculate μg/kg/min of drug infusing.

   $$\text{FORMULA: } \frac{(\text{μg/mL}) \times (\text{mL/h})}{(60 \text{ min/h}) \times (\text{kg body weight})} = \text{μg/kg/min}$$

   Example: The patient weighs 93 kg, and a sodium nitroprusside (Nipride) drip is infused at the rate of 26 mL/h. There are 100 mg/500 mL of nitroprusside in D_5 W. How many μg/kg/min is the patient getting?

   $$100 \text{ mg}/500 \text{ mL} \times 1000 \text{ μg}/1 \text{ mg} = 0.2 \times 1000$$
   $$= 200 \text{ μg/mL} \quad \frac{(200 \text{ μg/mL}) \times (26 \text{ mL/h})}{(60 \text{ min/h}) \times (93 \text{ kg})} = 0.93 \text{ μg/kg/min}$$

3. Calculate mL/h to infuse for prescribed dose in μg/kg/min.

   $$\text{FORMULA: } \frac{(\text{Prescribed dose in μg/kg/min}) \times (60 \text{ min/h}) \times (\text{kg})}{(\text{μg/mL of the solution})} = \text{mL/h}$$

   Example: An order is written to begin nitroprusside at 1 μg/kg/min. The patient weighs 84 kg, and there is 200 μg/mL in the solution.

   $$\frac{(1 \text{ μg/kg/min}) \times (60 \text{ min/h}) \times (84 \text{ kg})}{200 \text{ μg/mL}} = 25.2 \text{ or } 25 \text{ mL/h}$$

   Note: To calculate μg/mL if your additive is in mg, you must:

   $$\frac{\text{mg} \times 1000}{\text{mL of solution}} = \text{μg/mL}$$

4. Calculate mg/min of drug infusing.

   $$\text{FORMULA: } \frac{(\text{mg/mL}) \times (\text{mL/h})}{(60 \text{ min/h})} = \text{mg/min}$$

   Example: A lidocaine (Xylocaine) drip is infused at 15 mL/h, and there is 4 mg lidocaine per milliliter of D_5 W. How many mg/min is the patient receiving?

   $$\frac{(4 \text{ mg/mL}) \times (15 \text{ mL/h})}{(60 \text{ min/h})} = 1 \text{ mg/min}$$

5. Calculate mL/h to infuse prescribed dose of mg/min.

FORMULA: $\dfrac{(\text{Prescribed dose in mg/min}) \times (60 \text{ min/h})}{(\text{mg/mL})} = \text{mL/h}$

Example: The physician prescribes procainamide hydrochloride (Pronestyl) at 3 mg/min, and the solution contains 4 mg/mL. What is the needed rate of infusion in mL/h?

$\dfrac{(3 \text{ mg/mL}) \times (60 \text{ min/h})}{(4 \text{ mg/mL})} = 45 \text{ mL/h}$

Infusion Rate Tables*

ALTEPLASE (ACTIVASE)

Dilution: 20-mg vial with 20-mL diluent or 50-mg vial with 50-mL diluent = 1 mg/mL.

Alteplase 1 mg/mL Patient wt > 65 kg	*Dose (vol)* *First H** 60 mg (60 mL)	*Dose (vol)* *Second H* 20 mg (20 mL)	*Dose (vol)* *Third H* 20 mg (20 mL)
Alteplase 1 mg/mL Patient wt < 65 kg	*Dose (mg/kg)* *First H†* 0.75 mg/kg	*Dose (mg/kg)* *Second H* 0.25 mg/kg	*Dose (mg/kg)* *Third H* 0.25 mg/kg

*Give 6–10 mg (6–10 mL) as a bolus over first 1–2 min.
†0.075–0.125 mg/kg of this given as a bolus over the first 1–2 min.

AMINOPHYLLINE

Dilution: 250 mg in 250 mL or 500 mg in 500 mL or 1000 mg in 1000 mL = 1 mg/mL.
Loading dose in patients who have not received aminophylline in preceding 24 h = 5.6 mg/kg (5.6 mL/kg) of above dilution administered over 20 min.

Aminophylline Infusion Rates (mL/h)
Concentration = 1 mg/mL

Patient Weight

Dose	50 kg	60 kg	70 kg	80 kg	90 kg	100 kg
Loading dose (mg)*	280 mg	336 mg	392 mg	448 mg	504 mg	560 mg
0.9 mg/kg/h	45 mL/h	54 mL/h	63 mL/h	72 mL/h	81 mL/h	90 mL/h
0.8 mg/kg/h	40 mL/h	48 mL/h	56 mL/h	64 mL/h	72 mL/h	80 mL/h
0.7 mg/kg/h	35 mL/h	42 mL/h	49 mL/h	56 mL/h	63 mL/h	70 mL/h
0.6 mg/kg/h	30 mL/h	36 mL/h	42 mL/h	48 mL/h	54 mL/h	60 mL/h
0.5 mg/kg/h	25 mL/h	30 mL/h	35 mL/h	40 mL/h	45 mL/h	50 mL/h
0.4 mg/kg/h	20 mL/h	24 mL/h	28 mL/h	32 mL/h	36 mL/h	40 mL/h
0.3 mg/kg/h	15 mL/h	18 mL/h	21 mL/h	24 mL/h	27 mL/h	30 mL/h
0.2 mg/kg/h	10 mL/h	12 mL/h	14 mL/h	16 mL/h	18 mL/h	20 mL/h
0.1 mg/kg/h	5 mL/h	6 mL/h	7 mL/h	8 mL/h	9 mL/h	10 mL/h

*Loading dose administered over 20 min

AMRINONE (INOCOR)

Dilution: 100 mg/100 mL = 1 mg/mL.
Dilute with 0.45% or 0.9% sodium chloride.
Loading dose: 0.75 mg/kg (0.75 mL/kg) over 2–3 min.
To calculate infusion rate (mL/min), multiply patient's weight (kg) by dose in mL/kg/min.
To calculate infusion rate (mL/h), multiply patient's weight (kg) by dose in mg/kg/min × 60.

Amrinone Infusion Rates (mL/h)
Concentration = 1 mg/mL

Patient Weight

Dose	50 kg	60 kg	70 kg	80 kg	90 kg	100 kg
Loading dose (mg)*	37.5 mg	45 mg	52.5 mg	60 mg	67.5 mg	75 mg
5 μg/kg/min	15 mL/h	18 mL/h	21 mL/h	24 mL/h	27 mL/h	30 mL/h
6 μg/kg/min	18 mL/h	21.6 mL/h	25.5 mL/h	28.8 mL/h	32.4 mL/h	36 mL/h

---

*Reprinted from Deglin, JH and Vallerand, AH: Davis's Drug Guide for Nurses, ed. 4. FA Davis, Philadelphia, 1995, with permission.

Amrinone Infusion Rates (mL/h)
Concentration = 1 mg/mL

Patient Weight

Dose	50 kg	60 kg	70 kg	80 kg	90 kg	100 kg
7 μg/kg/min	21 mL/h	25.2 mL/h	29.4 mL/h	33.6 mL/h	37.8 mL/h	42 mL/h
8 μg/kg/min	24 mL/h	28.8 mL/h	33.6 mL/h	38.4 mL/h	43.2 mL/h	48 mL/h
9 μg/kg/min	27 mL/h	32.4 mL/h	37.8 mL/h	43.2 mL/h	48.6 mL/h	54 mL/h
10 μg/kg/min	30 mL/h	36 mL/h	42 mL/h	48 mL/h	54 mL/h	60 mL/h

*Given over 2–3 min.

BRETYLIUM TOSYLATE (BRETYLOL)

A. For life-threatening ventricular arrhythmias (ventricular fibrillations or hemodynamically unstable ventricular tachycardia): Administer 5 mg/kg (0.1 mL/kg) of *undiluted* drug by rapid intravenous (IV) injection. *Undiluted* drug concentration = 50 mg/1 mL.

Rapid IV Injection of Undiluted Bretylium
Doses given in volume of undiluted bretylium injection
50 mg/1 mL

Patient Weight

Dose	50 kg	60 kg	70 kg	80 kg	90 kg	100 kg
5 mg/kg	5 mL	6 mL	7 mL	8 mL	9 mL	10 mL

B. For other ventricular arrhythmias: Dilution: 2 g/500 mL = 4 mg/mL. Administer as 5–10 mg/kg (1.25–2.5 mL/kg) IV over 10–30 min, may be repeated every 6 h or administered as a continuous infusion at 1–2 mg/min.

Bretylium Intermittent Infusion Rates
Volume of diluted bretylium to infuse over 10–30 min
Concentration = 4 mg/mL

Patient Weight

Dose	50 kg	60 kg	70 kg	80 kg	90 kg	100 kg
5 mg/kg	62.5 mL	75 mL	87.5 mL	100 mL	112.5 mL	125 mL
6 mg/kg	75 mL	90 mL	105 mL	120 mL	135 mL	150 mL
7 mg/kg	87.5 mL	105 mL	122.5 mL	140 mL	157.5 mL	175 mL
8 mg/kg	100 mL	120 mL	140 mL	160 mL	180 mL	200 mL
9 mg/kg	112.5 mL	135 mL	157.5 mL	180 mL	202.5 mL	225 mL
10 mg/kg	125 mL	150 mL	175 mL	200 mL	225 mL	250 mL

Bretylium Continuous Infusion Rates
Concentration = 4 mg/mL

Dose mg/min	Dose mL/h
1.0 mg/min	15 mL/h
1.5 mg/min	23 mL/h
2.0 mg/min	30 mL/h

DOBUTAMINE (DOBUTREX)

Dilution: May be prepared as 250 mg/1000 mL = 250 μg/mL.
500 mg/1000 mL = 500 μg/mL.
1000 mg/1000 mL = 1000 μg/mL.
To calculate infusion rate (mL/min), multiply patient's weight (kg) by dose in mL/kg/min.
To calculate infusion rate (mL/h), multiply patient's weight (kg) by dose in mL/kg/min × 60.

Dobutamine Infusion Rates (mL/h)
Concentration = 250 μg/mL

Patient Weight

Dose	50 kg	60 kg	70 kg	80 kg	90 kg	100 kg
2.5 μg/kg/min	30 mL/h	36 mL/h	42 mL/h	48 mL/h	54 mL/h	60 mL/h
5 μg/kg/min	60 mL/h	72 mL/h	84 mL/h	96 mL/h	108 mL/h	120 mL/h
7.5 μg/kg/min	90 mL/h	108 mL/h	126 mL/h	144 mL/h	162 mL/h	180 mL/h
10 μg/kg/min	120 mL/h	144 mL/h	168 mL/h	192 mL/h	216 mL/h	240 mL/h

Dobutamine Infusion Rates (mL/h)
Concentration = 500 μg/mL

Patient Weight

Dose	50 kg	60 kg	70 kg	80 kg	90 kg	100 kg
2.5 μg/kg/min	15 mL/h	18 mL/h	21 mL/h	24 mL/h	22.5 mL/h	30 mL/h
5 μg/kg/min	30 mL/h	36 mL/h	42 mL/h	48 mL/h	54 mL/h	60 mL/h
7.5 μg/kg/min	45 mL/h	54 mL/h	63 mL/h	72 mL/h	81 mL/h	90 mL/h
10 μg/kg/min	60 mL/h	72 mL/h	84 mL/h	96 mL/h	108 mL/h	120 mL/h

Dobutamine Infusion Rates (mL/h)
Concentration = 1000 μg/mL

Patient Weight

Dose	50 kg	60 kg	70 kg	80 kg	90 kg	100 kg
2.5 μg/kg/min	7.5 mL/h	9 mL/h	10.5 mL/h	12 mL/h	11.3 mL/h	15 mL/h
5 μg/kg/min	15 mL/h	18 mL/h	21 mL/h	24 mL/h	27 mL/h	30 mL/h
7.5 μg/kg/min	22.3 mL/h	27 mL/h	31.5 mL/h	36 mL/h	40.5 mL/h	45 mL/h
10 μg/kg/min	30 mL/h	36 mL/h	41 mL/h	48 mL/h	54 mL/h	60 mL/h

DOPAMINE HYDROCHLORIDE (INTROPIN)

Dilution: May be prepared as 200 mg/500 mL = 400 μg/mL.
400 mg/500 mL = 800 μg/mL.
800 mg/500 mL = 1600 μg/mL.
To calculate infusion rate (mL/min), multiply patient's weight (kg) by dose in mL/kg/min.
To calculate infusion rate (mL/h), multiply patient's weight (kg) by dose in mL/kg/min × 60.

Dopamine Infusion Rates (mL/h)
400 μg/mL Concentration

Patient Weight

Dose	50 kg	60 kg	70 kg	80 kg	90 kg	100 kg
2 μg/kg/min	15 mL/h	18 mL/h	21 mL/h	24 mL/h	27 mL/h	30 mL/h
5 μg/kg/min	37.5 mL/h	45 mL/h	52.5 mL/h	60 mL/h	67.5 mL/h	75 mL/h
10 μg/kg/min	75 mL/h	90 mL/h	105 mL/h	120 mL/h	135 mL/h	150 mL/h
20 μg/kg/min	150 mL/h	180 mL/h	210 mL/h	240 mL/h	270 mL/h	300 mL/h
30 μg/kg/min	225 mL/h	270 mL/h	315 mL/h	360 mL/h	405 mL/h	450 mL/h
40 μg/kg/min	300 mL/h	360 mL/h	420 mL/h	480 mL/h	540 mL/h	600 mL/h
50 μg/kg/min	375 mL/h	450 mL/h	525 mL/h	600 mL/h	675 mL/h	750 mL/h

Dopamine Infusion Rates (mL/h)
800 μg/mL Concentration

Patient Weight

Dose	50 kg	60 kg	70 kg	80 kg	90 kg	100 kg
2 μg/kg/min	7.5 mL/h	9 mL/h	10.5 mL/h	12 mL/h	13.5 mL/h	15 mL/h
5 μg/kg/min	18.8 mL/h	22.5 mL/h	26.3 mL/h	30 mL/h	33.8 mL/h	37.5 mL/h
10 μg/kg/min	37.5 mL/h	45 mL/h	52.5 mL/h	60 mL/h	67.5 mL/h	75 mL/h
20 μg/kg/min	75 mL/h	90 mL/h	105 mL/h	120 mL/h	135 mL/h	150 mL/h
30 μg/kg/min	112.5 mL/h	135 mL/h	157.5 mL/h	180 mL/h	202.5 mL/h	225 mL/h
40 μg/kg/min	150 mL/h	180 mL/h	210 mL/h	240 mL/h	270 mL/h	300 mL/h
50 μg/kg/min	187.5 mL/h	225 mL/h	262.5 mL/h	300 mL/h	337.5 mL/h	375 mL/h

Dopamine Infusion Rates (mL/h)
1600 μg/mL Concentration*

Patient Weight

Dose	50 kg	60 kg	70 kg	80 kg	90 kg	100 kg
2 μg/kg/min	3.8 mL/h	4.5 mL/h	5.3 mL/h	6 mL/h	6.8 mL/h	7.5 mL/h
5 μg/kg/min	9.4 mL/h	11.2 mL/h	13.1 mL/h	15.0 mL/h	16.9 mL/h	18.7 mL/h
10 μg/kg/min	18.8 mL/h	22.5 mL/h	26.3 mL/h	30 mL/h	33.8 mL/h	37.5 mL/h
20 μg/kg/min	37.5 mL/h	45 mL/h	52.5 mL/h	60 mL/h	67.5 mL/h	75 mL/h
30 μg/kg/min	56.3 mL/h	67.5 mL/h	78.8 mL/h	90 mL/h	101.3 mL/h	112.5 mL/h
40 μg/kg/min	75 mL/h	90 mL/h	105 mL/h	120 mL/h	135 mL/h	150 mL/h
50 μg/kg/min	93.8 mL/h	112.5 mL/h	131.3 mL/h	150 mL/h	168.8 mL/h	187.5 mL/h

*Appropriate concentration for patients with fluid restriction.

EPINEPHRINE

Dilution: 1 mg/250 mL = 4 μg/mL.

Epinephrine Infusion Rates (mL/h)
Concentration = 4 μg/mL

Dose (μg/mL)	Dose (mL/h)
1 μg/min	15 mL/h
2 μg/min	30 mL/h
3 μg/min	45 mL/h
4 μg/min	60 mL/h

ESMOLOL HYDROCHLORIDE (BREVIBLOC)

Dilution: 5 g/500 mL = 10 mg/mL.

Loading regimen = 500 µg/kg (0.05 mL/kg) loading dose over 1 min, followed by 50 µg/kg/min (0.005 mL/kg/min) infusion over 4 min. If no response, repeat loading dose over 1 min and increase infusion rate to 100 µg/kg/min for 4–10 min. If no response, loading dose may be repeated before increasing infusion rates in 50 µg/kg/min increments.

Esmolol Hydrochloride Infusion Rates
Concentration = 10 mg/mL

Patient Weight

Dose	50 kg	60 kg	70 kg	80 kg	90 kg	100 kg
Loading dose (mL)*	2.5 mL	3 mL	3.5 mL	4 mL	4.5 mL	5 mL
50 µg/kg/min	15 mL/h	18 mL/h	21 mL/h	24 mL/h	27 mL/h	30 mL/h
75 µg/kg/min	22.5 mL/h	27 mL/h	31.5 mL/h	36 mL/h	40.5 mL/h	45 mL/h
100 µg/kg/min	30 mL/h	36 mL/h	42 mL/h	48 mL/h	54 mL/h	60 mL/h
125 µg/kg/min	37.5 mL/h	45 mL/h	52.5 mL/h	60 mL/h	67.5 mL/h	75 mL/h
150 µg/kg/min	38 mL/h	54 mL/h	63 mL/h	72 mL/h	81 mL/h	90 mL/h
175 µg/kg/min	52.5 mL/h	63 mL/h	73.5 mL/h	84 mL/h	94.5 mL/h	105 mL/h
200 µg/kg/min	60 mL/h	72 mL/h	84 mL/h	96 mL/h	108 mL/h	120 mL/h

*Loading dose given over 1 min.

HEPARIN

Dilution: 20,000 U/1000 mL = 20 U/mL.
Loading dose: 1000–2000 units as a bolus.

Heparin Infusion Rates (mL/h)
Concentration = 20 U/mL

*Dose (U/h)	Dose (mL/h)
500 U/h	25 mL/h
750 U/h	37.5 mL/h
1000 U/h	50 mL/h
1250 U/h	62.5 mL/h
1500 U/h	75 mL/h
1750 U/h	87.5 mL/h
2000 U/h	100 mL/h

ISOPROTERENOL (ISUPREL)

Dilution: 2 mg/500 mL.

Isoproterenol Infusion Rates (mL/h)
Concentration = 4 µg/mL

Dose (µg/min)	Dose (mL/h)
2 µg/min	30 mL/h
5 µg/min	75 mL/h
10 µg/min	150 mL/h
15 µg/min	225 mL/h
20 µg/min	300 mL/h

LIDOCAINE (XYLOCAINE)

Dilution: May be prepared as 1 g/1000 mL = 1 mg/mL.
2 g/1000 mL = 2 mg/mL.
4 g/1000 mL = 4 mg/mL.
8 g/1000 mL = 8 mg/mL.
Loading dose: 50–100 mg at 25–50 mg/min.

Lidocaine Infusion Rates (mL/h)

Dose (mg/min)	1 mg/mL Concentration	2 mg/mL Concentration	4 mg/mL Concentration	8 mg/mL Concentration
1 mg/min	60 mL/h	30 mL/h	15 mL/h	7.5 mL/h
2 mg/min	120 mL/h	60 mL/h	30 mL/h	15 mL/h
3 mg/min	180 mL/h	90 mL/h	45 mL/h	22.5 mL/h
4 mg/min	240 mL/h	120 mL/h	60 mL/h	30 mL/h

MILRINONE

Loading dose: 50 µg/kg given over 10 min.

Milrinone Infusion Rates (mL/h)

Patient Weight

Dose	50 kg	60 kg	70 kg	80 kg	90 kg	100 kg
Loading dose (mg)	2.5 mg	3.0 mg	3.5 mg	4.0 mg	4.5 mg	5.0 mg

Milrinone Infusion Rates (mL/h)
Concentration = 100 µg/mL

Patient Weight

Dose	50 kg	60 kg	70 kg	80 kg	90 kg	100 kg
0.375 µg/kg/min	11 mL/h	13.2 mL/h	15.4 mL/h	17.6 mL/h	19.8 mL/h	22.0 mL/h
0.400 µg/kg/min	12 mL/h	14.4 mL/h	16.8 mL/h	19.2 mL/h	21.6 mL/h	24.0 mL/h
0.500 µg/kg/min	15.0 mL/h	18.0 mL/h	21.0 mL/h	24.0 mL/h	27.0 mL/h	30.0 mL/h
0.600 µg/kg/min	18.0 mL/h	21.6 mL/h	25.2 mL/h	28.8 mL/h	32.4 mL/h	36.0 mL/h
0.700 µg/kg/min	21.0 mL/h	25.2 mL/h	29.4 mL/h	33.6 mL/h	37.8 mL/h	42.0 mL/h
0.750 µg/kg/min	22.5 mL/h	27.0 mL/h	31.5 mL/h	36.0 mL/h	40.5 mL/h	45.0 mL/h

Concentration = 150 µg/mL

Patient Weight

Dose	50 kg	60 kg	70 kg	80 kg	90 kg	100 kg
0.375 µg/kg/min	7.5 mL/h	9.0 mL/h	10.5 mL/h	12.0 mL/h	13.4 mL/h	15.0 mL/h
0.400 µg/kg/min	8.0 mL/h	9.6 mL/h	11.2 mL/h	12.8 mL/h	14.4 mL/h	16.0 mL/h
0.500 µg/kg/min	10.0 mL/h	12.0 mL/h	14.0 mL/h	16.0 mL/h	18.0 mL/h	20.0 mL/h
0.600 µg/kg/min	12.0 mL/h	14.4 mL/h	16.8 mL/h	19.2 mL/h	21.6 mL/h	24.0 mL/h
0.700 µg/kg/min	14.0 mL/h	16.8 mL/h	19.6 mL/h	22.4 mL/h	25.2 mL/h	28.0 mL/h
0.750 µg/kg/min	15.0 mL/h	18.0 mL/h	21.0 mL/h	24.0 mL/h	27.0 mL/h	30.0 mL/h

Concentration = 200 µg/mL

Patient Weight

Dose	50 kg	60 kg	70 kg	80 kg	90 kg	100 kg
0.375 µg/kg/min	5.5 mL/h	6.6 mL/h	7.7 mL/h	8.8 mL/h	9.9 mL/h	11.1 mL/h
0.400 µg/kg/min	6.0 mL/h	7.2 mL/h	8.4 mL/h	9.6 mL/h	10.8 mL/h	12.0 mL/h
0.500 µg/kg/min	7.5 mL/h	9.0 mL/h	10.5 mL/h	12.0 mL/h	13.5 mL/h	15.0 mL/h
0.600 µg/kg/min	9.0 mL/h	10.8 mL/h	12.6 mL/h	14.4 mL/h	16.2 mL/h	18.0 mL/h
0.700 µg/kg/min	10.5 mL/h	12.6 mL/h	14.7 mL/h	16.8 mL/h	18.9 mL/h	21.0 mL/h
0.750 µg/kg/min	11.0 mL/h	13.5 mL/h	15.4 mL/h	17.6 mL/h	19.8 mL/h	22.0 mL/h

NITROGLYCERIN (NITRO-BID, NITROL, NITROSTAT, TRIDIL)

Dilution: May be prepared as 5 mg/100 mL (25 mg/500 mL, 50 mg/1000 mL) = 50 µg/mL.
            25 mg/250 mL (50 mg/500 mL, 100 mg/1000 mL) = 100 µg/mL.
            50 mg/250 mL (100 mg/500 mL, 200 mg/1000 mL) = 200 µg/mL.
Note that different products are available in different concentrated solutions and should be used with appropriate infusion tubing. Changes in tubing may result in altered response to a given dose.

Nitroglycerin Infusion Rates (mL/h)

Dose (µg/min)	50 µg/mL Concentration	100 µg/mL Concentration	200 µg/mL Concentration
2.5 µg/min	3 mL/h	1.5 mL/h	0.75 mL/h
5 µg/min	6 mL/h	3 mL/h	1.5 mL/h
10 µg/min	12 mL/h	6 mL/h	3 mL/h
15 µg/min	18 mL/h	9 mL/h	4.5 mL/h
20 µg/min	24 mL/h	12 mL/h	6 mL/h
30 µg/min	36 mL/h	18 mL/h	9 mL/h
40 µg/min	48 mL/h	24 mL/h	12 mL/h
50 µg/min	60 mL/h	30 mL/h	15 mL/h
60 µg/min	72 mL/h	36 mL/h	18 mL/h

NITROPRUSSIDE (NIPRIDE, NITROPRESS)

Dilution: May be prepared as 50 mg/1000 mL = 50 µg/mL.
100 mg/1000 mL = 100 µg/mL.
200 mg/1000 mL = 200 µg/mL.
To calculate infusion rate (mL/min), multiply patient's weight (kg) by dose in mL/kg/min.
To calculate infusion rate (mL/h), multiply patient's weight (kg) by dose in mL/kg/min × 60.
Dosing range: 0.3 µg/kg/min–10 µg/kg/min.

Nitroprusside Infusion Rates (mL/kg/min)

Dose (µg/kg/min)	50 µg/mL Concentration	100 µg/mL Concentration	200 µg/mL Concentration
0.3 µg/kg/min	0.006 mL/kg/min	—	—
0.5 µg/kg/min	0.01 mL/kg/min	—	—
1 µg/kg/min	0.02 mL/kg/min	0.01 mL/kg/min	—
2 µg/kg/min	0.04 mL/kg/min	0.02 mL/kg/min	0.01 mL/kg/min
3 µg/kg/min	0.06 mL/kg/min	0.03 mL/kg/min	0.015 mL/kg/min
4 µg/kg/min	0.08 mL/kg/min	0.04 mL/kg/min	0.02 mL/kg/min
5 µg/kg/min	0.1 mL/kg/min	0.05 mL/kg/min	0.025 mL/kg/min
6 µg/kg/min	0.12 mL/kg/min	0.06 mL/kg/min	0.03 mL/kg/min
7 µg/kg/min	0.14 mL/kg/min	0.07 mL/kg/min	0.035 mL/kg/min
8 µg/kg/min	0.16 mL/kg/min	0.08 mL/kg/min	0.04 mL/kg/min
9 µg/kg/min	0.18 mL/kg/min	0.09 mL/kg/min	0.045 mL/kg/min
10 µg/kg/min	0.2 mL/kg/min	0.1 mL/kg/min	0.05 mL/kg/min

Nitroprusside Infusion Rates (mL/h)
50 µg/mL Concentration

Patient Weight

Dose	50 kg	60 kg	70 kg	80 kg	90 kg	100 kg
0.3 µg/kg/min	18 mL/h	22 mL/h	25 mL/h	29 mL/h	32 mL/h	36 mL/h
0.5 µg/kg/min	30 mL/h	36 mL/h	42 mL/h	48 mL/h	54 mL/h	60 mL/h
1 µg/kg/min	60 mL/h	72 mL/h	84 mL/h	96 mL/h	108 mL/h	120 mL/h
2 µg/kg/min	120 mL/h	144 mL/h	168 mL/h	192 mL/h	216 mL/h	240 mL/h
3 µg/kg/min	180 mL/h	216 mL/h	252 mL/h	288 mL/h	324 mL/h	360 mL/h
4 µg/kg/min	240 mL/h	288 mL/h	336 mL/h	384 mL/h	432 mL/h	480 mL/h
5 µg/kg/min	300 mL/h	360 mL/h	420 mL/h	480 mL/h	540 mL/h	600 mL/h
6 µg/kg/min	360 mL/h	432 mL/h	504 mL/h	576 mL/h	648 mL/h	720 mL/h
7 µg/kg/min	420 mL/h	504 mL/h	588 mL/h	672 mL/h	756 mL/h	840 mL/h
8 µg/kg/min	480 mL/h	576 mL/h	672 mL/h	768 mL/h	864 mL/h	960 mL/h
9 µg/kg/min	540 mL/h	648 mL/h	756 mL/h	864 mL/h	972 mL/h	1080 mL/h
10 µg/kg/min	600 mL/h	720 mL/h	840 mL/h	960 mL/h	1080 mL/h	1200 mL/h

Nitroprusside Infusion Rates (mL/h)
100 µg/mL Concentration

Patient Weight

Dose	50 kg	60 kg	70 kg	80 kg	90 kg	100 kg
0.3 µg/kg/min	9 mL/h	11 mL/h	13 mL/h	14 mL/h	16 mL/h	18 mL/h
0.5 µg/kg/min	15 mL/h	18 mL/h	21 mL/h	24 mL/h	27 mL/h	30 mL/h
1 µg/kg/min	30 mL/h	36 mL/h	42 mL/h	48 mL/h	54 mL/h	60 mL/h
2 µg/kg/min	60 mL/h	72 mL/h	84 mL/h	96 mL/h	108 mL/h	120 mL/h
3 µg/kg/min	90 mL/h	108 mL/h	126 mL/h	144 mL/h	162 mL/h	180 mL/h
4 µg/kg/min	120 mL/h	144 mL/h	168 mL/h	192 mL/h	216 mL/h	240 mL/h
5 µg/kg/min	150 mL/h	180 mL/h	210 mL/h	240 mL/h	270 mL/h	300 mL/h
6 µg/kg/min	180 mL/h	216 mL/h	252 mL/h	288 mL/h	324 mL/h	360 mL/h
7 µg/kg/min	210 mL/h	252 mL/h	294 mL/h	336 mL/h	378 mL/h	420 mL/h
8 µg/kg/min	240 mL/h	288 mL/h	336 mL/h	384 mL/h	432 mL/h	480 mL/h
9 µg/kg/min	270 mL/h	324 mL/h	378 mL/h	432 mL/h	486 mL/h	540 mL/h
10 µg/kg/min	300 mL/h	360 mL/h	420 mL/h	480 mL/h	540 mL/h	600 mL/h

Nitroprusside Infusion Rates (mL/h)
200 µg/mL Concentration

Patient Weight

Dose	50 kg	60 kg	70 kg	80 kg	90 kg	100 kg
0.3 µg/kg/min	5 mL/h	5 mL/h	6 mL/h	7 mL/h	8 mL/h	9 mL/h
0.5 µg/kg/min	7.5 mL/h	9 mL/h	10.5 mL/h	12 mL/h	13.5 mL/h	15 mL/h
1 µg/kg/min	15 mL/h	18 mL/h	21 mL/h	24 mL/h	27 mL/h	30 mL/h
2 µg/kg/min	30 mL/h	36 mL/h	42 mL/h	48 mL/h	54 mL/h	60 mL/h

Nitroprusside Infusion Rates (mL/h)
200 μg/mL Concentration

Patient Weight

Dose	50 kg	60 kg	70 kg	80 kg	90 kg	100 kg
3 μg/kg/min	45 mL/h	54 mL/h	63 mL/h	72 mL/h	81 mL/h	90 mL/h
4 μg/kg/min	60 mL/h	72 mL/h	84 mL/h	96 mL/h	108 mL/h	120 mL/h
5 μg/kg/min	75 mL/h	90 mL/h	105 mL/h	120 mL/h	135 mL/h	150 mL/h
6 μg/kg/min	90 mL/h	108 mL/h	126 mL/h	144 mL/h	162 mL/h	180 mL/h
7 μg/kg/min	105 mL/h	126 mL/h	147 mL/h	168 mL/h	189 mL/h	210 mL/h
8 μg/kg/min	120 mL/h	144 mL/h	168 mL/h	192 mL/h	216 mL/h	240 mL/h
9 μg/kg/min	135 mL/h	162 mL/h	189 mL/h	216 mL/h	243 mL/h	270 mL/h
10 μg/kg/min	150 mL/h	180 mL/h	210 mL/h	240 mL/h	270 mL/h	300 mL/h

NOREPINEPHRINE (LEVOPHED)

Dilution: May be prepared as 1 mg/250 mL = 4 μg/mL.
To calculate infusion rate (mL/h), multiply infusion rate in mL/min × 60.

Norepinephrine Infusion Rates (mL/h)
Concentration = 4 μg/mL

Dose (μg/min)	Dose (mL/h)
8 μg/min	120 mL/h
9 μg/min	135 mL/h
10 μg/min	150 mL/h
11 μg/min	165 mL/h
12 μg/min	180 mL/h

PHENYLEPHRINE HYDROCHLORIDE (NEO-SYNEPHRINE)

Dilution: 10 mg/500 mL = 20 μg/mL.

Phenylephrine Infusion Rates (mL/h)
Concentration = 20 μg/mL

Dose (mg/min)	Dose (mL/h)
0.04 mg/min	120 mL/h
0.06 mg/min	180 mL/h
0.08 mg/min	240 mL/h
0.10 mg/min	300 mL/h
0.12 mg/min	360 mL/h
0.14 mg/min	420 mL/h
0.16 mg/min	480 mL/h
0.18 mg/min	540 mL/h

PROCAINAMIDE HYDROCHLORIDE (PRONESTYL)

Dilution: May be prepared as 1000 mg/500 mL = 2 mg/mL.
Loading dose: 50–100 mg every 5 min until arrhythmia is controlled, adverse reaction occurs, or 500 mg has been given; or 500–600 mg as a loading infusion over 25–30 min.

Procainamide Infusion Rates (mL/h)
Concentration = 2 mg/mL

Dose (mg/min)	Dose (mL/h)
1 mg/min	30 mL/h
2 mg/min	60 mL/h
3 mg/min	90 mL/h
4 mg/min	120 mL/h
5 mg/min	150 mL/h
6 mg/min	180 mL/h

APPENDIX I

Advanced Cardiac Life Support (ACLS) Guidelines*

These guidelines use algorithms as an educational tool. They are an illustrative method to summarize information. Providers of emergency care should view algorithms as a summary and a memory aid. They provide a way to treat a broad range of patients. Algorithms, by nature, oversimplify. The effective teacher and care provider will use them wisely, not blindly. Some patients may require care not specified in the algorithms. When clinically appropriate, flexibility is accepted and encouraged. Many interventions and actions are listed as "considerations" to help providers think. These lists should not be considered endorsements or requirements or "standard of care" in a legal sense. Algorithms do not replace clinical understanding. Although the algorithms provide a good "cookbook," the patient always requires a "thinking cook."

The following clinical recommendations apply to all treatment algorithms:

1. First, treat the patient, not the monitor.
2. Algorithms for cardiac arrest presume that the condition under discussion continually persists, that the patient remains in cardiac arrest, and that cardiopulmonary resuscitation (CPR) is always performed.
3. Apply different interventions whenever appropriate indications exist.
4. The flow diagrams present mostly Class I (acceptable, definitely effective) recommendations. The footnotes present Class IIa (acceptable, probably effective), Class IIb (acceptable, possibly effective), and Class III (not indicated, may be harmful) recommendations.
5. Adequate airway, ventilation, oxygenation, chest compressions, and defibrillation are more important than administration of medications and take precedence over initiating an intravenous (IV) line or injecting pharmacologic agents.
6. Several medications (epinephrine, lidocaine, and atropine) can be administered through the endotracheal tube, but clinicians must use an endotracheal dose 2 to 2.5 times the IV dose.
7. With a few exceptions, IV medications should always be administered rapidly, in bolus method.
8. After each IV medication, give a 20- to 30-mL bolus of IV fluid and immediately elevate the extremity. This will enhance delivery of drugs to the central circulation, which may take 1 to 2 minutes.
9. Last, treat the patient, not the monitor.

---

*CPR issue of JAMA, October 28, 1992, copyright American Heart Association, with permission.

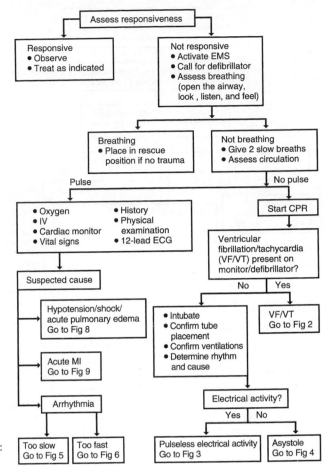

FIGURE I–1. Universal algorithm for adult: emergency cardiac care.

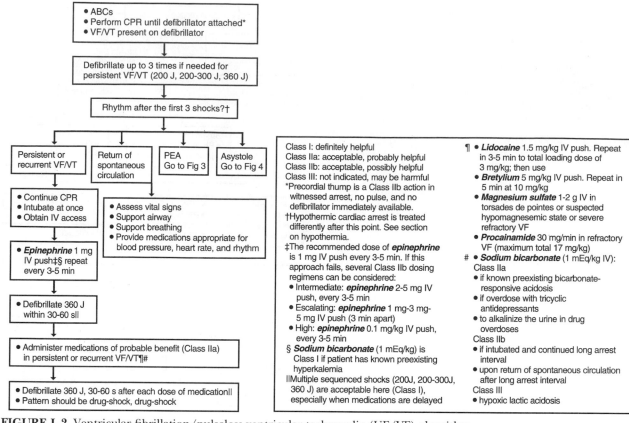

FIGURE I–2. Ventricular fibrillation/pulseless ventricular tachycardia (UF/VF) algorithm.

PEA includes
- Electromechanical dissociation (EMD)
- Pseudo-EMD
- Idioventricular rhythms
- Ventricular escape rhythms
- Bradyasystolic rhythms
- Postdefibrillation idioventricular rhythms

- Continue CPR
- Intubate at once
- Obtain IV access
- Assess blood flow using Doppler ultrasound

↓

Consider possible causes
(Parentheses=possible therapies and treatments)
- Hypovolemia (volume infusion)
- Hypoxia (ventilation)
- Cardiac tamponade (pericardiocentesis)
- Tension pneumothorax (needle decompression)
- Hypothermia (see hypothermia algorithm, Section IV)
- Massive pulmonary embolism (surgery, *thrombolytics*)
- Drug overdoses such as tricyclics, digitalis, β-blockers, calcium channel blockers
- Hyperkalemia*
- Acidosis†
- Massive acute myocardial infarction (go to Fig 9)

↓

- *Epinephrine* 1 mg IV push, *‡ repeat every 3-5 min

↓

- If absolute bradycardia (<60 beats/min) or relative bradycardia, give *atropine* 1 mg IV
- Repeat every 3-5 min up to a total of 0.04 mg/kg§

Class I: definitely helpful
Class IIa: acceptable, probably helpful
Class IIb: acceptable, possibly helpful
Class III: not indicated, may be harmful
Sodium bicarbonate 1 mEq/kg is Class I if patient has known preexisting hyperkalemia.
†*Sodium bicarbonate* 1 mEq/kg:
   Class IIa
- if known preexisting bicarbonate-responsive acidosis
- if overdose with tricyclic antidepressants
- to alkalinize the urine in drug overdoses
   Class IIb
- if intubated and long arrest interval
- upon return of spontaneous circulation after long arrest interval
   Class III
- hypoxic lactic acidosis
‡The recommended dose of *epinephrine* is 1 mg IV push every 3-5 min. If this approach fails, several Class IIb dosing regimens can be considered.
- Intermediate: *epinephrine* 2-5 mg IV push, every 3-5 min
- Escalating: *epinephrine* 1 mg-3 mg-5 mg IV push (3 min apart)
- High: *epinephrine* 0.1 mg/kg IV push, every 3-5 min
§ Shorter *atropine* dosing intervals are possibly helpful in cardiac arrest (Class IIb).

FIGURE I–3. Pulseless electrical activity (PEA) algorithm (electromechanical dissociation [EMD]).

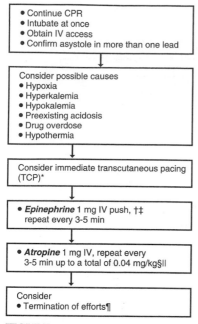

- Continue CPR
- Intubate at once
- Obtain IV access
- Confirm asystole in more than one lead

↓

Consider possible causes
- Hypoxia
- Hyperkalemia
- Hypokalemia
- Preexisting acidosis
- Drug overdose
- Hypothermia

↓

Consider immediate transcutaneous pacing (TCP)*

↓

- **Epinephrine** 1 mg IV push, †‡ repeat every 3-5 min

↓

- **Atropine** 1 mg IV, repeat every 3-5 min up to a total of 0.04 mg/kg§‖

↓

Consider
- Termination of efforts¶

Class I: definitely helpful
Class IIa: acceptable, probably helpful
Class IIb: acceptable, possibly helpful
Class III: not indicated, may be harmful

*TCP is a Class IIb intervention. Lack of success may be due to delays in pacing. To be effective TCP must be performed early, simultaneously with drugs. Evidence does not support routine use of TCP for asystole.

†The recommended dose of **epinephrine** is 1 mg IV push every 3-5 min. If this approach fails, several Class IIb dosing regimens can be considered:
- Intermediate: **epinephrine** 2-5 mg IV push, every 3-5 min
- Escalating: **epinephrine** 1 mg-3 mg-5 mg IV push (3 min apart)
- High: **epinephrine** 0.1 mg/kg IV push, every 3-5 min

‡**Sodium bicarbonate** 1 mEq/kg is Class I if patient has known preexisting hyperkalemia.

§Shorter **atropine** dosing intervals are Class IIb in asystolic arrest.

‖**Sodium bicarbonate** 1 mEq/kg:
Class IIa
- if known preexisting bicarbonate-responsive acidosis
- if overdose with tricyclic antidepressants
- to alkalinize the urine in drug overdoses
Class IIb
- if intubated and continued long arrest interval
- upon return of spontaneous circulation after long arrest interval
Class III
- hypoxic lactic acidosis

¶If patient remains in asystole or other agonal rhythms after successful intubation and initial medications and no reversible causes are identified, consider termination of resuscitative efforts by a physician. Consider interval since arrest.

FIGURE I–4. Asystole treatment algorithm.

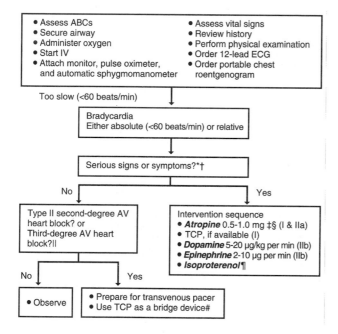

- Assess ABCs
- Secure airway
- Administer oxygen
- Start IV
- Attach monitor, pulse oximeter, and automatic sphygmomanometer

- Assess vital signs
- Review history
- Perform physical examination
- Order 12-lead ECG
- Order portable chest roentgenogram

↓

Too slow (<60 beats/min)

Bradycardia
Either absolute (<60 beats/min) or relative

↓

Serious signs or symptoms?*†

No ← → Yes

No:
Type II second-degree AV heart block? or
Third-degree AV heart block?‖

Yes:
Intervention sequence
- **Atropine** 0.5-1.0 mg ‡§ (I & IIa)
- TCP, if available (I)
- **Dopamine** 5-20 μg/kg per min (IIb)
- **Epinephrine** 2-10 μg per min (IIb)
- **Isoproterenol**¶

No ↓   ↓ Yes

- Observe

- Prepare for transvenous pacer
- Use TCP as a bridge device#

*Serious signs or symptoms must be related to the slow rate. Clinical manifestations include:
  symptoms (chest pain, shortness of breath, decreased level of conciousness) and
  signs (low BP, shock, pulmonary congestion, CHF, acute MI).
†Do not delay TCP while awaiting IV access or for **atropine** to take effect if patient is symptomatic.
‡Denervated transplanted hearts will not respond to **atropine**. Go at once to pacing, **catecholamine** infusion, or both.
§**Atropine** should be given in repeat doses in 3-5 min up to total of 0.04 mg/kg. Consider shorter dosing intervals in severe clinical conditions. It has been suggested that atropine should be used with caution in atrioventricular (AV) block at the His-Purkinje level (type II AV block and new third-degree block with wide QRS complexes) (Class IIb).
‖Never treat third-degree heart block plus ventricular escape beats with **lidocaine**.
¶**Isoproterenol** should be used, if at all, with exteme caution. At low doses it is Class IIb (possibly helpful); at higher doses it is Class III (harmful).
#Verify patient tolerance and mechanical capture. Use analgesia and sedation as needed.

FIGURE I–5 Bradycardia algorithm (patient is not in cardiac arrest).

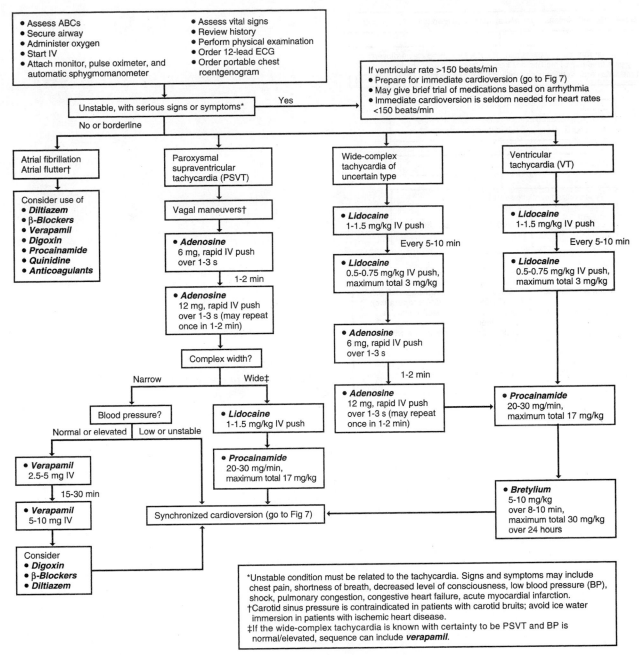

FIGURE I–6. Tachycardia algorithm.

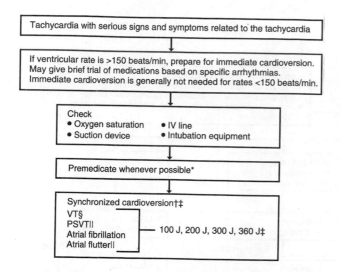

Tachycardia with serious signs and symptoms related to the tachycardia

↓

If ventricular rate is >150 beats/min, prepare for immediate cardioversion. May give brief trial of medications based on specific arrhythmias. Immediate cardioversion is generally not needed for rates <150 beats/min.

↓

Check
- Oxygen saturation
- Suction device
- IV line
- Intubation equipment

↓

Premedicate whenever possible*

↓

Synchronized cardioversion†‡

VT§
PSVT‖
Atrial fibrillation
Atrial flutter‖
— 100 J, 200 J, 300 J, 360 J‡

*Effective regimens have included a sedative (eg, *diazepam, midazolam, barbiturates, etomidate, ketamine, methohexital*) with or without an analgesic agent (eg, *fentanyl, morphine, meperidine*). Many experts recommend anesthesia if service is readily available.
†Note possible need to resynchronize after each cardioversion.
‡If delays in synchronization occur and clinical conditions are critical, go to immediate unsynchronized shocks.
§Treat polymorphic VT (irregular form and rate) like VF: 200 J, 200-300 J, 360 J.
‖PSVT and atrial flutter often respond to lower energy levels (start with 50 J).

FIGURE I–7. Electrical cardioversion algorithm (patient is not in cardiac arrest).

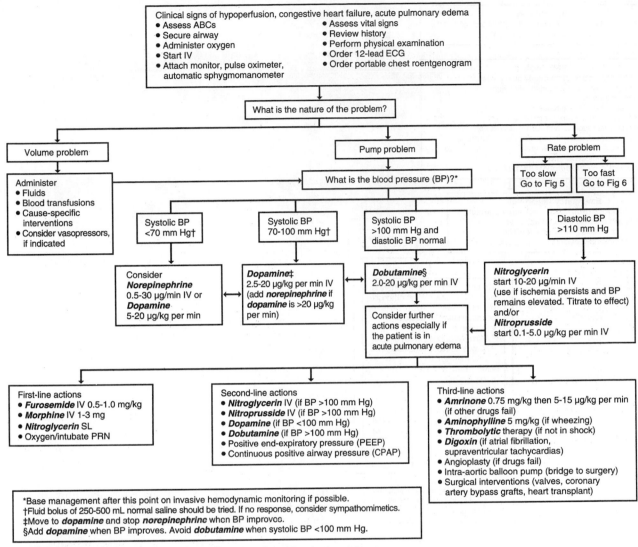

Clinical signs of hypoperfusion, congestive heart failure, acute pulmonary edema
- Assess ABCs
- Secure airway
- Administer oxygen
- Start IV
- Attach monitor, pulse oximeter, automatic sphygmomanometer

- Assess vital signs
- Review history
- Perform physical examination
- Order 12-lead ECG
- Order portable chest roentgenogram

What is the nature of the problem?

Volume problem

Administer
- Fluids
- Blood transfusions
- Cause-specific interventions
- Consider vasopressors, if indicated

Pump problem

What is the blood pressure (BP)?*

Rate problem

Too slow
Go to Fig 5

Too fast
Go to Fig 6

Systolic BP
<70 mm Hg†

Systolic BP
70-100 mm Hg†

Systolic BP
>100 mm Hg and
diastolic BP normal

Diastolic BP
>110 mm Hg

Consider
Norepinephrine
0.5-30 µg/min IV or
Dopamine
5-20 µg/kg per min

Dopamine‡
2.5-20 µg/kg per min IV
(add ***norepinephrine*** if
dopamine is >20 µg/kg
per min)

Dobutamine§
2.0-20 µg/kg per min IV

Consider further
actions especially if
the patient is in
acute pulmonary edema

Nitroglycerin
start 10-20 µg/min IV
(use if ischemia persists and BP
remains elevated. Titrate to effect)
and/or
Nitroprusside
start 0.1-5.0 µg/kg per min IV

First-line actions
- ***Furosemide*** IV 0.5-1.0 mg/kg
- ***Morphine*** IV 1-3 mg
- ***Nitroglycerin*** SL
- Oxygen/intubate PRN

Second-line actions
- ***Nitroglycerin*** IV (if BP >100 mm Hg)
- ***Nitroprusside*** IV (if BP >100 mm Hg)
- ***Dopamine*** (if BP <100 mm Hg)
- ***Dobutamine*** (if BP >100 mm Hg)
- Positive end-expiratory pressure (PEEP)
- Continuous positive airway pressure (CPAP)

Third-line actions
- ***Amrinone*** 0.75 mg/kg then 5-15 µg/kg per min (if other drugs fail)
- ***Aminophylline*** 5 mg/kg (if wheezing)
- ***Thrombolytic*** therapy (if not in shock)
- ***Digoxin*** (if atrial fibrillation, supraventricular tachycardias)
- Angioplasty (if drugs fail)
- Intra-aortic balloon pump (bridge to surgery)
- Surgical interventions (valves, coronary artery bypass grafts, heart transplant)

*Base management after this point on invasive hemodynamic monitoring if possible.
†Fluid bolus of 250-500 mL normal saline should be tried. If no response, consider sympathomimetics.
‡Move to ***dopamine*** and stop ***norepinephrine*** when BP improves.
§Add ***dopamine*** when BP improves. Avoid ***dobutamine*** when systolic BP <100 mm Hg.

FIGURE I–8. Acute pulmonary edema/hypotension/shock algorithm.

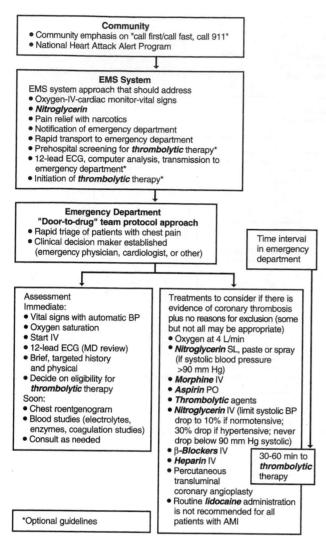

Community
- Community emphasis on "call first/call fast, call 911"
- National Heart Attack Alert Program

EMS System
EMS system approach that should address
- Oxygen-IV-cardiac monitor-vital signs
- *Nitroglycerin*
- Pain relief with narcotics
- Notification of emergency department
- Rapid transport to emergency department
- Prehospital screening for *thrombolytic* therapy*
- 12-lead ECG, computer analysis, transmission to emergency department*
- Initiation of *thrombolytic* therapy*

Emergency Department
"Door-to-drug" team protocol approach
- Rapid triage of patients with chest pain
- Clinical decision maker established (emergency physician, cardiologist, or other)

Time interval in emergency department

Assessment
Immediate:
- Vital signs with automatic BP
- Oxygen saturation
- Start IV
- 12-lead ECG (MD review)
- Brief, targeted history and physical
- Decide on eligibility for *thrombolytic* therapy
Soon:
- Chest roentgenogram
- Blood studies (electrolytes, enzymes, coagulation studies)
- Consult as needed

Treatments to consider if there is evidence of coronary thrombosis plus no reasons for exclusion (some but not all may be appropriate)
- Oxygen at 4 L/min
- *Nitroglycerin* SL, paste or spray (if systolic blood pressure >90 mm Hg)
- *Morphine* IV
- *Aspirin* PO
- *Thrombolytic* agents
- *Nitroglycerin* IV (limit systolic BP drop to 10% if normotensive; 30% drop if hypertensive; never drop below 90 mm Hg systolic)
- β-*Blockers* IV
- *Heparin* IV
- Percutaneous transluminal coronary angioplasty
- Routine *lidocaine* administration is not recommended for all patients with AMI

30-60 min to *thrombolytic* therapy

*Optional guidelines

FIGURE I–9. Acute myocardial infarction algorithm (recommendations for early management of patients with chest pain and possible acute myocardial infarction).

Glossary

Absorption: Movement of particles across a cellular membrane from a body compartment toward the blood or intravascular compartment.

Absorptive State: Period during which nutrients are being absorbed from the gastrointestinal tract into the bloodstream.

Abulia: Lack of spontaneity; inability to make a decision.

Accommodation: Adjustments in the eye for viewing distances by changes in the shape of the lens, pupillary constriction, and convergence of eyeballs.

Acetone: Ketone body produced from metabolism of acetyl coenzyme A (CoA) during prolonged fasting or in diabetic ketoacidosis.

Acetylcholine: Neurotransmitter released at neuromuscular junctions, preganglionic synapses, and cholinergic synapses of parasympathetic nervous system.

Acetylcholinesterase: Enzyme that degrades acetylcholine.

Acid: Substance capable of releasing hydrogen ions (H^+) in a solution; a solution having an H^+ concentration greater than that of water (i.e., pH < 7.0).

Acidemia: Reflects an increase in the concentration of H^+ in the blood, resulting in a pH < 7.35.

Acidosis: Any circumstances in which the H^+ concentration in blood is in the process of becoming increased, thereby lowering the pH to < 7.35.

Acquired Immunodeficiency Syndrome (AIDS): Caused by the human immunodeficiency virus (HIV). The immunologic defect is due to the effect the virus has in making T4 lymphocytes ineffective.

ACTH: Adrenocorticotropic hormone secreted by the anterior pituitary gland.

Action Potential: Reversal in the polarity of the membrane potential, in which the inside of the cell momentarily becomes positive with respect to the outside; the electrical signal conducted over nerve and muscle cells.

Active Hyperemia: Increased blood flow through tissues in response to metabolic activity.

Active Transport: An energy-requiring, carrier-mediated transport system, in which molecules can be moved across a membrane against an electrochemical gradient.

Primary Active Transport: Chemical energy is transferred directly from ATP to carrier proteins.

Secondary Active Transport: The energy released during the transmembrane movement of one substance from a higher to lower concentration is transferred to the simultaneous movement of another substance from lower to higher concentrations (coupled, facilitated diffusion).

Adenosine Diphosphate (ADP): Two-phosphate product from the breakdown of ATP.

Adenosine Monophosphate (AMP): Monophosphate derivative from the breakdown of ATP.

Adenosine Triphosphate (ATP): Major molecule that accepts energy from the breakdown of fuel molecules during formation from ADP and phosphatidylinositol.

Adenylcyclase: Enzyme that catalyzes the transformation of ATP to cyclic AMP.

Adrenal Cortex: Endocrine gland that forms the outer perimeter of each adrenal gland; secretes glucocorticoids (cortisol), mineralocorticoids (aldosterone), and androgens.

Adrenal Medulla: Endocrine gland that forms the inner core of each adrenal gland and secretes mainly epinephrine and, to a lesser extent, norepinephrine.

Adrenergic: Term applied to nerve fibers that when stimulated release epinephrine at their axon endings; sympathetic nervous system response.

Adrenocorticotropic Hormone (ACTH): Hormone secreted by the anterior pituitary, essential to the growth, development, and continued function of the adrenal cortex.

Aerobic: Living only in the presence of oxygen.

Affect: Emotional reactions associated with an experience.

Afferent Neuron: Neuron that transmits impulses from receptors in the periphery to the central nervous system (brain and spinal cord).

Afferent Pathway: Series of afferent (sensory) neurons that transmit impulses from receptors in the periphery to the integrating centers and primary sensory centers in the brain.

Affinity: Attraction between molecules.

Afterload: Load against which the heart muscle must exert its contractile force.

Agonist: Molecule that binds to a receptor site and triggers the same response as the true chemical messenger.

1077

Aldosterone: Mineralocorticoid hormone secreted by adrenal cortex that stimulates reabsorption of sodium by distal tubule cells.

Alkalemia: Decrease in H^+ concentration of the blood (pH > 7.45).

Alkaline: Having an H^+ concentration lower than that of water (pH > 7).

Alkalosis: Any state in which the H^+ concentration of arterial blood is reduced (pH > 7.45).

All or None: Event that occurs maximally or not at all.

Allergy: Acquired hypersensitivity to a substance (antigen, allergen) that does not normally evoke an immune response.

α-Adrenergic Receptor: A site in autonomic nerve pathways wherein excitatory responses occur when adrenergic agents, such as norepinephrine and epinephrine, are released. α-Adrenergic and β-adrenergic receptors are distinguished from one another by the type of response elicited.

Alpha Cells: Glucagon-secreting cells of the pancreatic islets of Langerhans.

Alternate Complement Pathway: Sequence for complement activation that is initiated nonspecifically and is not antibody dependent.

Alveolar-Arterial Oxygen Difference (A-a Gradient): Difference between alveolar and arterial oxygen tensions.

Alveolar Ventilation: Volume of inspired gas that reaches the alveoli and participates in gas exchange.

Ammonia: Produced by breakdown of amino acids; converted to urea in the liver.

Amphipathic Molecule: Molecule containing a polar or ionized group at one end and a nonpolar group at the other.

Amylase: Enzyme that breaks down starch into disaccharides.

Anabolism: Constructive phase of metabolism wherein cells take nutrients from the blood for the growth and repair of tissue.

Anaerobic: In the absence of oxygen.

Analgesia: Pain relieving.

Anaphylaxis: Sudden, acute allergic hypersensitivity reaction to an antigen or drug.

Anatomic Dead Space: Volume of inspired gas that occupies the space in the upper airways and tracheobronchial tree (i.e., the conducting zone) that does not participate in gas exchange.

Alveolar Dead Space: Alveoli that are fully ventilated but do not receive adequate perfusion to facilitate gas exchange.

Physiologic Dead Space: Dead space ventilation equal to the anatomic dead space plus the alveolar dead space.

Anemia: Condition characterized by a reduction in the number of circulating red blood cells (RBCs) and total hemoglobin in the blood.

Anemic Hypoxia: State in which the arterial partial pressure of oxygen (PaO_2) is normal, but the total oxygen content of the blood is reduced because of reduction in total blood hemoglobin.

Aneurysm: Abnormal localized dilatation of a blood vessel usually associated with the weakening of the vessel wall.

Angiotensin I: Vasopressor substance formed in the blood by the interaction of renin and angiotensinogen (a plasma precursor).

Angiotensin II: Potent vasopressor substance formed from angiotensin I by the action of converting enzyme; stimulates secretion of aldosterone from adrenal cortex.

Anion: Negatively charged ion (e.g., chloride [Cl^-], bicarbonate [HCO_3^-]).

Anosognosia: Lack of awareness of the presence of neurologic deficits.

Anoxia: Absence of oxygen.

Antagonist: Molecule that binds to a receptor site and triggers a response opposed to that elicited by the true chemical messenger.

Antibody: Protein substance synthesized and secreted by plasma cells in response to, and interacting specifically with, an antigen.

Antibody-Mediated Immunity: Specific immune response in which circulating antibodies play a central role (see *humoral immunity*).

Antidiuretic Hormone (ADH): Hormone synthesized in the hypothalamus and released from the posterior pituitary; increases the permeability of cells of the distal renal tubules and collecting ducts to water; also called vasopressin.

Antigen: Foreign molecule, usually a protein, that stimulates a specific immune response when introduced into the body.

Antihistamine: Chemical that blocks the action of histamine.

Antrum (Gastric): Lower portion of the stomach (i.e., the region closest to the pyloric sphincter).

Aphasia (Dysphasia): Absence or impairment of the ability to communicate by formulating or understanding oral or written language; receptive (sensory) reflects the inability to understand spoken or written word; expressive (motor) reflects inability to speak one's thoughts.

Apnea: Cessation of respiration.

Apraxia: Disturbance in the execution of learned movements or the manipulation of objects in space.

Arachidonic Acid: Fatty acid that is the major precursor of prostaglandins.

Arrhythmia (Dysrhythmia): Any variation from the usual rhythm of the heartbeat.

Arteriolar Resistance: Resistance to the flow of blood offered by the arterioles.

Asterixis: See *tremor*.

Asthenia: Debilitated, loss of strength, extreme weakness.

Astigmatism: Defect in vision from irregularities in the curvature of the cornea and/or lens of the eye.

Atelectasis: Collapse of alveoli; failure of expansion or resorption of gas (resorptive atelectasis).

Atherosclerosis: Pathologic process characterized by a thickening of the arterial wall associated with accumulation of lipids, cholesterol, platelets, and calcium deposits, and by infiltration of abnormal smooth muscle and connective tissue cells.

Athrombia: Impairment in blood clotting from thrombin deficiency.

Atmospheric Pressure: The air pressure of the environment at sea level (760 mmHg).

Atom: Smallest unit of matter that has unique chemical characteristics.

ATPase: Enzyme that breaks down ATP to ADP and inorganic phosphate.

Autoimmune Disease: Disease produced by antibodies or T cells acting against the body's own cells, resulting in alteration of cellular function.

Automaticity: Capable of self-excitation.

Autonomic Dysreflexia: Clinical emergency characterized by an exaggerated sympathetic response occurring below the level of the spinal cord lesion and resulting in uncontrolled paroxysmal hypertension.

Autonomic Nervous System: Component of the efferent division of the peripheral nervous system that innervates cardiac muscle, smooth muscle, and glands; consists of the parasympathetic and sympathetic subdivisions.

Autoregulation: Ability of individual organs and tissues to alter their vascular resistance to maintain a relatively constant blood flow to meet their oxygen and nutrient needs.

Axon Terminals (Synaptic Knob): Network of fine branches at the end of each axon, each branch ending at a synapse or neuromuscular junction.

Azotemia: Renal dysfunction characterized by a progressive accumulation and retention of nitrogenous waste.

B Cells: Immune system: lymphocytes that upon activation proliferate and differentiate into antibody-secreting plasma cells. Endocrine system: insulin-secreting cells in the islets of Langerhans of the pancreas.

Baroreceptor: Sensory nerve endings located in the carotid sinus, *vena cava,* and aortic arch, and sensitive to pressure or the degree of stretch.

Basal Ganglia: Nuclei deep in the cerebral hemispheres that relay information associated with the control of body movements.

Base: Any molecule that can combine with H^+.

Basement Membrane: Thin proteinaceous layer of extracellular material associated with the plasma membranes of many cells.

β-Adrenergic Receptor: Receptor in the sympathetic nervous system to which epinephrine and norepinephrine bind, thereby triggering a sympathetic response. α-Adrenergic and β-adrenergic receptors are distinguished from one another by the type of response elicited.

Bile: Fluid secreted by the liver, containing bile salts, cholesterol, lecithin, bile pigment, and other endproducts of organic metabolism.

Bile Canaliculi: Tiny, intercellular, biliary vessels that channel bile into bile ducts.

Bile Duct: Conveys bile from the liver to the hepatic duct, which joins the cystic duct, carrying bile from the gallbladder, to form the common bile duct. The common bile duct conveys bile to the duodenum.

Bile Pigments: Colored substances derived from the breakdown of the heme group of hemoglobin and secreted in the bile.

Bile Salts: Steroid molecules secreted by the liver in the bile that promote solubilization and digestion of fat in the small intestine.

Bilirubin: Yellow substance resulting from the breakdown of heme excreted in the bile as a bile pigment.
Direct: Bilirubin conjugated by the liver cells to form water-soluble bilirubin diglucuronide.
Indirect: Fat-soluble unconjugated bilirubin present in blood.

Biliverdin: Greenish pigment formed in bile by the oxidation of bilirubin.

Binding Site: A region on the surface of a protein that has a chemical group/conformation with which molecules interact and specifically bind.

Blood-Brain Barrier: Barrier membrane between circulating blood and the brain interstitium, which closely controls the kinds of substances allowed to enter the brain's substance (and the rate at which they enter).

Blood Types: Classification of the blood determined by the presence of antigens of the A, B, C, or AB types on the plasma membranes of erythrocytes, and by the presence in the plasma of anti-A or anti-B antibodies (or both, or neither).

Bone Marrow: Highly vascular cellular substance of the central cavity of some bones; site of synthesis of RBCs, white blood cells (WBCs), and platelets.

Bradykinin: Molecule formed by the action of the enzyme, kallikrein, on a protein precursor; a potent vasodilator that increases capillary permeability.

Bruit: Adventitious sound of venous or arterial origin heard on auscultation.

Buffering: Reversible binding of H^+ by various compounds; these reversible reactions tend to minimize changes in acidity of a buffered solution when acid is added or removed.

Bulk Flow: Movement of fluids or gases from a region of higher pressure to one of lower pressure.

Calcitonin: Hormone secreted by parafollicular cells of the thyroid gland; involved in calcium regulation.

Calcium Antagonist: Calcium-blocking agents that inhibit transmembrane flow of Ca^+.

Calmodulin: Intracellular protein that binds calcium and mediates many of calcium's second messenger functions.

Calorie (cal): Unit in which heat energy is measured; the amount of heat needed to raise the temperature of 1 g of water 33.8°F.

Carbon Monoxide (CO): Gas that reacts with the same iron-binding sites on hemoglobin as does oxygen but with a much greater affinity than oxygen; decreases the oxygen-carrying capacity of blood.

Carbonic Anhydrase: Enzyme that catalyzes the reaction in which carbon dioxide (CO_2) and water (H_2O) combine to form carbonic acid (H_2CO_3).

Carcinogen: Any of a number of agents (radiation, viruses, certain chemicals) that can induce the cancerous transformation of cells.

Cardiac Cycle: One episode of contraction–relaxation of the heart muscle.

Cardiac Output: Volume of blood pumped by each ventricle each minute.

Carotid Sinus: Dilated area at the bifurcation of the common carotid that is richly supplied with sensory nerve endings sensitive to pressure and degree of stretch (baroreceptors).

Carrier: Integral membrane protein capable of combining with specific molecules and facilitating their passage through a membrane.

Catabolism: Degradative phase of metabolism wherein cells break down complex substances into their simpler parts, usually with the release of energy.

Catalyst: Substance that accelerates chemical reactions but does not itself undergo any net chemical change during the reaction.

Catechol O-Methyltransferase: Enzyme that breaks down catecholamine neurotransmitters.

Catecholamines: Neurotransmitters that have a similar chemical structure, including dopamine, epinephrine, and norepinephrine; they have marked effects, especially on the nervous and cardiovascular systems, smooth muscle, cardiac muscle, and glands.

Cation: Ion having a net positive charge.

Cell-Mediated Immunity: Type of immune response mediated largely by cytotoxic T lymphocytes.

Central Venous Pressure: Blood pressure in large veins of the thorax (superior, inferior vena cavae) and right atrium.

Cephalic Phase (Gastrointestinal Control): Initiation of the neural and hormonal reflexes regulating gastrointestinal functions by stimulation of the receptors in the head—sight, smell, taste.

Cerebral Edema: Increase in water content of brain parenchyma.

Cerebral Perfusion Pressure: Driving force underlying cerebral blood flow; determinants include mean arterial blood pressure minus intracranial pressure.

Cerebrospinal Fluid (CSF): Fluid that fills the cerebral ventricles and subarachnoid space surrounding the brain and spinal cord.

Chemical Equilibrium: System in which the rates of the forward and reverse components of a chemical reaction are equal (i.e., no net change in the concentrations of the reactants or products occurs).

Chemical Specificity: Property of a protein-binding site such that only certain molecules or ions can bind with it.

Chemoreceptor: *Peripheral:* Sensory receptors or sensory nerve endings stimulated by and reacting to concentrations of certain chemicals (outside of the central nervous system); chemoreceptors in the carotid body and aortic arch are sensitive to changes in serum oxygen, CO_2, and H^+ concentration. *Cen-*

tral: Sensory receptors in the brain stem that respond to changes in H^+ concentration in the brain extracellular fluid.

Chemotaxis: Orientation and movement of cells in a specific direction in response to a chemical stimulus (i.e., movement of neutrophils to area of inflammation).

Cholecystokinin (CCK): Hormone secreted by cells in the upper small intestine that regulates several gastrointestinal activities, including motility of and secretion by the stomach, gallbladder contraction, and enzyme secretion by the pancreas.

Cholesterol: Steroid molecule that is the precursor of the steroid hormones and bile salts; a component of plasma membranes.

Cholinergic: Substance that acts like acetylcholine.

Chylomicron: Lipid droplet composed of phospholipid, cholesterol, triacylglycerol, free fatty acids, and proteins, which is released from the intestinal epithelial cells and enters the lacteals during fat absorption.

Cilia: Hairlike projections from the surface of specialized epithelial cells; they sweep back and forth in a synchronized manner to propel material along the cell surface.

Classical Complement Pathway: Antibody-dependent system for activating complement.

Coagulation: Process of clotting.

Coagulopathy: Disturbance in blood-clotting mechanisms.

Collagen: Fibrous protein that has great strength; functions as a structural element in the interstitium of various types of connective tissues (i.e., tendons and ligaments).

Collateral Circulation: Circulation of small anastomosing blood vessels connecting branches of the same vessels and other blood vessels.

Collateral Ventilation: Movement of air between alveoli through pores in the walls separating the alveoli.

Colloid: Large molecule to which the capillaries are relatively impermeable (i.e., a plasma protein).

Compensatory Mechanisms: Activities that function to make up for a deficiency or defect and to restore/maintain a central function; compensatory mechanisms usually have limitations beyond which they are no longer effective.

Complement: A group of plasma proteins that upon activation kill microbes directly and facilitate the inflammatory process. (See *alternate complement pathway* and *classical complement pathway*.)

Compliance: Measure of the ease with which a structure or substance may be deformed (e.g., compressed, expanded, distended).

Concentration Gradient: Gradation in concentration that occurs between two regions having different concentrations.

Conjugate Gaze: Both eyes move together so that one image is perceived.

Contralateral: Originating in or affecting the opposite side of the body.

Control System: Collection of interconnected components that function to keep a physical or chemical parameter within a predetermined range of values.

Converting Enzyme: Enzyme that catalyzes the reaction in which angiotensin I is changed to angiotensin II.

Corpus Callosum: Large wide band of myelinated nerve fibers that connects the two cerebral hemispheres.

Corticotropin-Releasing Hormone (CRH): Hypothalamic hormone that stimulates ACTH secretion by the anterior pituitary.

Cortisol: Glucocorticoid steroid hormone secreted by the adrenal cortex that regulates various aspects of cellular metabolism and has many other actions.

Countercurrent Multiplier System: Mechanism associated with the loop of Henle that creates a high fluid osmolality in the medullary interstitium.

Creatine Phosphate: Molecule that transfers phosphate and energy to ADP to generate ATP.

Creatinine: Waste product derived from muscle creatine.

Cross-Bridge: Projection extending from a thick filament in muscle; a portion of the myosin molecule capable of exerting force on the thin filament and causing it to slide past the thick one.

Crystalloid: Low-molecular-weight solute (e.g., sodium [Na^+], glucose, or urea).

Current: Movement of electrical charge achieved by the movement of ions.

Cyclic AMP (cAMP): Cyclic $3',5'$-adenosine monophosphate; a cyclic nucleotide that serves as a second messenger for many hormones and neurotransmitters.

Cytotoxic T Cells: Class of T lymphocytes that, on activation by specific antigens, directly attack the cell bearing that type of antigen.

D Cells: Somatostatin-secreting cells of the islets of Langerhans of the pancreas.

Deamination: Removal of an amino ($^-NH_2$) group from a molecule such as amino acid.

Decerebrate: Pattern of abnormal posturing/rigidity in which an abnormal extensor response occurs in both upper and lower extremities.

Decorticate: Pattern of abnormal posturing/rigidity in which an abnormal flexor response occurs in the upper extremities and an abnormal extensor response occurs in the lower extremities.

Decussation: Crossing over of nerve tracts to the side opposite their origin.

Deoxyhemoglobin: Hemoglobin (Hb) not combined with oxygen; reduced Hb.

Deoxyribonucleic Acid (DNA): Nucleic acid that stores and transmits genetic information; consists of a double strand (double helix) of nucleotide subunits that contain the sugar deoxyribose.

Depolarization: Change in the value of the membrane potential toward zero because of an increase in membrane permeability to sodium.

Dermatomes: Segments of skin innervated by the various spinal cord segments.

Desmosome: Type of cell junction whose function is to hold cells together.

Diastole: Period of the cardiac cycle when ventricular muscle fibers are not contracting; ventricular relaxation.

Diastolic Pressure: Minimum blood pressure during the cardiac cycle; ventricular end–diastolic pressure is the pressure in the ventricles just before ventricular systole, ventricular contraction.

Diffusion: Movement of molecules from a region of higher concentration to one of lower concentration because of random molecular motion.

Diffusion Equilibrium: State during which the diffusion fluxes in opposite directions are equal.

2,3-Diphosphoglycerate (DPG): Substance produced by RBCs that binds reversibly with Hb, decreasing Hb's affinity for oxygen, thereby allowing oxygen to be released to the tissues.

Diplopia: Double vision.

Diuretic: Any substance that inhibits fluid reabsorption in the renal tubule, causing an increase in the volume of urine excreted.

Dominant Hemisphere: Cerebral hemisphere that controls the hand used most frequently for intricate tasks (i.e., left hemisphere in a right-handed person).

Dopamine: Catecholamine neurotransmitter; a precursor of epinephrine and norepinephrine.

Dorsal: Posterior, toward the back.

Dual Innervation: Innervation of an organ or gland by both sympathetic and parasympathetic nerve fibers.

Dysarthria: Speech impairment from a disruption of the muscles of the tongue and other muscles essential to speech.

Dyskinesia: Alteration in movement; loss of functional integrity related to movement.

Ectopic Focus: Region of the heart other than the sinoatrial (SA) node that assumes the role of the cardiac pacemaker.

Edema: Accumulation of excess fluid in the interstitial space.
  Vasogenic: Fluid accumulation in interstitial space (extracellular edema).
  Cytotoxic: Fluid accumulation in the cells (intracellular edema).

Effector: Structures, including nerves, muscles, and glands, through which the response of the central nervous system to sensory input is actualized; results in response or altered activity.

Efferent Neuron (Motor): Neuron that carries information away from the central nervous system to muscle cells, glands, and other neurons.

Efferent Pathway: Motor neurons that transmit impulses from the receptive/integrating unit in the brain and spinal cord to the periphery, where the response to the central nervous system is evoked by muscles and glands.

Elastance: Measure of the tendency of a structure to return to its original form after removal of a deforming force.

Electric Force: Force that causes the movement of charge particles toward regions having an opposite charge and away from regions having a similar charge.

Electrochemical Gradient: Force determining the magnitude of the net movement of charge particles; a combination of the electrical gradient (as determined by the voltage difference between two points) and the chemical gradient (as determined by the concentration differences between the same two points).

Electrode: A probe to which electrical charges can be added (or from which they can be removed) to cause changes in the electrical current flow to a recorder.

Electrolyte: Substance that dissociates into ions when in solution.

Embolus: Foreign body, such as a fragment of a blood clot or an air bubble, circulating in the blood.

Emulsification: Fat-solubilizing process in which large, lipid droplets are broken into smaller droplets.

End-Diastolic Volume (EDV): Amount of blood in a ventricle of the heart just before systole.

End-Systolic Volume (ESV): Amount of blood remaining in the heart after ejection.

Endocytosis: Method of cellular digestion of a foreign body; a process in which the plasma membrane invaginates and the invaginations become pinched off, forming small, intracellular, membrane-bound vesicles that enclose a volume of material.

Endogenous Pyrogen: Protein secreted by monocytes and macrophages, which acts in the brain to cause fever.

Endorphins: Chemical substances synthesized in the brain that act as opiates and produce analgesia by binding to opiate receptor sites; β-endorphins are highly active endorphins with morphinelike effect.

Endothelium: Thin layer of cells that lines the cavities of the heart and the vasculature.

Enkephalin: Peptide that functions as a neurotransmitter at synapses activated by opiate drugs.

Enterohepatic Circulation: Recycling pathway for bile salts and other substances by reabsorption from the intestines, passage to the liver by way of the hepatic portal vein, and passage back to the intestines by way of the bile duct.

Enzyme: Protein that accelerates specific chemical reactions but does not itself undergo any net change during the reaction; a biochemical catalyst.

Eosinophil: Granulocyte leukocyte whose granules stain readily with red dye eosin; involved in allergic responses and destruction of parasitic worms.

Epinephrine: Hormone secreted by the adrenal medulla and involved mainly in the regulation of metabolism; a catecholamine neurotransmitter.

Equilibrium Potential: Voltage difference at which there is zero net flux of an ion between two compartments.

Erythropoietin: Hormone that stimulates RBC production in bone marrow.

Essential Amino Acid: Amino acid that cannot be formed by the body at all and, therefore, must be obtained from the diet.

Excitability: Ability to produce action potentials.

Excitation-Contraction Coupling: Mechanisms in muscle fibers linking depolarization of the plasma membrane with generation of force by the cross-bridges.

Excitatory Synapse: Response of the postsynaptic membrane to the chemical neurotransmitter released by the presynaptic neuron is depolarization (i.e., moving the resting membrane potential toward threshold potential).

Exocytosis: Process in which the membrane of an intracellular vesicle fuses with the plasma membrane, the vesicle opens, and the vesicle contents are liberated into the extracellular fluid (e.g., release of chemical neurotransmitter at cholinergic and adrenergic synapses).

Expiratory Reserve Volume (ERV): Volume of air that can be exhaled by maximal active contraction of the expiratory muscles at the end of a normal expiration.

Extracellular Fluid: Fluid surrounding cells; includes interstitial fluid and intravascular blood volume.

Extrasystole: Heartbeat that occurs before the normal time in a cardiac cycle.

Extrinsic Clotting Pathway: Formation of fibrin clots by a pathway using tissue thromboplastin.

Facilitated Diffusion: Simple: Carrier-mediated transport system that moves molecules from high to low concentration across a membrane; energy is not required, and equilibrium is reached when the concentrations on the two sides of the membrane become equal. Coupled facilitated diffusion.

Fasciculations: Involuntary contraction or muscle twitching.

Fat-Soluble Vitamins: Vitamins that are soluble in nonpolar solvents and insoluble in water; vitamins A, D, E, and K.

Feedback Control System: Type of control system in which the output of the system (response) influences the input.

Ferritin: Iron-binding protein that is the storage form for iron.

Fibrillation: Extremely rapid contraction of myocardial fibers in an unsynchronized repetitive manner, which compromises the pumping action of the heart, thereby reducing cardiac output.

Fibrinolysis: Dissolution of fibrin by plasmin (fibrinolysin).

Fight-or-Flight Response: Overall activation of the sympathetic nervous system in response to stress.

Filtration: Movement of essentially protein-free plasma across the walls of a capillary out of its lumen as a result of a pressure gradient across the capillary wall.

Fluid Mosaic Model: Molecular structure of cell membranes consists of proteins embedded in a bimolecular layer of phospholipids; the phospholipid layer has the physical properties of a fluid, allowing the membrane protein to move laterally in the lipid layer.

Flux: An excessive flow or discharge from an organ or cavity of the body.

Functional Residual Capacity (FRC): Equal to the sum of the expiratory reserve volume plus the residual volume. The FRC is the volume of gas that remains in the lungs at end-expiration during quiet breathing to ensure gas exchange continues uninterrupted.

Functional Unit: Subunit of which an organ is composed; all subunits have similar structural and functional properties.

Gammaglobulin: Immunoglobulin G (IgG), the most abundant class of plasma antibodies.

Ganglion (Ganglia): Cluster of neuronal cell bodies; generally restricted to neuronal clusters located outside the central nervous system.

Gap Junction: Type of cell junction allowing ions and small molecules to flow between the cytoplasm of adjacent cells by way of small channels or gaps.

Gastric Phase (Gastrointestinal Control): Initiation of neural and hormonal reflexes controlling gastrointestinal function by stimulation of the wall of the stomach.

Gastrin: Hormone secreted by the antral region of the stomach that stimulates gastric acid secretion.

Gastroileal Reflex: Physiologic relaxation of the ileocecal valve resulting from food in the stomach.

Globulin: One of the types of protein found in blood plasma.

Glomerular Filtration: Movement of an essentially protein-free plasma through the capillaries of the renal glomeruli into Bowman's capsule.

Glomerular Filtration Rate (GFR): Volume of fluid filtered through the renal glomerular capillaries into Bowman's capsule per unit time.

Glucagon: Hormone secreted by the A cells of the islets of Langerhans of the pancreas; its action on target cells leads to a rise in plasma glucose.

Glucocorticoid: One of several steroid hormones produced by the adrenal cortex and having major effects on glucose metabolism.

Gluconeogenesis: Formation of glucose from noncarbohydrate sources, including amino acids, fatty acids, pyruvate, and lactate.

Glycogen: Major form of carbohydrate storage in the body, composed of thousands of glucose subunits.

Glycogenolysis: Breakdown of glycogen.

Glycolysis: Metabolic pathway that breaks down glucose to form two molecules of pyruvate (in the presence of oxygen) or two molecules of lactate (in the absence of oxygen).

Granuloma: Mass or growth consisting of numerous layers of lymphoid or epithelial cells at the center of which may be a microbe or potentially harmful nonmicrobial substance, all enclosed in a fibrous capsule, which isolates the substance from healthy tissue.

Growth Hormone (GH): Hormone secreted by the anterior pituitary; stimulates the release of somatomedins; stimulates body growth by means of its action on carbohydrate and protein metabolism; somatotropin.

Growth Hormone-Releasing Hormone (GH-RH): Hypothalamic hormone that stimulates the secretion of growth hormone by the anterior pituitary.

Halo Sign: Presence of dark or bloody drainage encircled by a yellow stain on dressing or linen. Highly suggestive of CSF leak. Presence of glucose detected by testing drainage with a reagent strip (Dextrostix) confirms the presence of CSF; CSF contains glucose, while mucus is glucose-free.

Hapten: Small molecule that does not itself elicit an immune response but can attach to an existing antigen and thereby acquire the ability to trigger an immune response.

Heat Exhaustion: Acute reaction to heat exposure, characterized by a state of hypotension precipitated by a depletion of intravascular volume associated with extreme diaphoresis and by extreme vasodilation of cutaneous blood vessels; thermoregulatory centers are still intact.

Heat Stroke: Condition characterized by impairment of thermoregulatory centers caused by a positive feedback state wherein the heat gain is greater than the heat loss, causing body temperature to become extremely elevated.

Helper T Cells: Class of T cells that enhance antibody production and cytotoxic T-cell function.

Hematemesis: Vomiting of blood.

Hematochezia: Passage of stools containing red blood rather than tarry stools.

Hematocrit: Percentage of total blood volume occupied by blood cells.

Hematoma: Collection or mass of blood confined to an organ, tissue, or space and associated with injury to a blood vessel (e.g., epidural, subdural, and subarachnoid hematomas).

Hematomyelia: Bleeding into spinal cord parenchyma.

Hematopoiesis: Production and growth of RBCs in bone marrow.

Heme: Iron-containing organic molecule bound to each of the four polypetide chains of a hemoglobin molecule.

Hemianesthesia: Loss of sensation of one side of the body.

Hemianopia (Hemianopsia): Loss of one half of the field of vision in one or both eyes.

   Homonymous Hemianopia: Loss of sight in corresponding halves of both eyes.

   Bitemporal Hemianopia: Loss of temporal half of visual field in each eye.

Hemiparesis: Weakness to slight paralysis affecting only one side of the body.

Hemiplegia: Paralysis of one side of the body.

Hemoglobin: Red protein located in erythrocytes; transmits most of the oxygen in the blood.

Hemostasis: Cessation of bleeding from damaged vessel.

Hepatic Portal Vein: Vein that conveys blood from the capillary beds in the intestines to the capillary beds in the liver.

Herniation: Protrusion of an organ, or part of any organ, through the wall of the cavity that normally compartmentalizes it (i.e., brain herniation, protrusion of uncal portion of temporal lobe into tentorial notch).

Histamine: Inflammatory mediator released mainly by mast cells; exerts a vasodilatory effect on blood vessels, resulting in flushing of skin and reduction in blood pressure; stimulates gastric secretion.

Histamine$_2$ Antagonist: Drug that blocks the effect of histamine on its receptors.

Histocompatibility (HLA) Antigens: Tissue antigens present on the surface of all nucleated cells. They are controlled by genes at several loci termed the major histocompatibility complex (MHC).

Histotoxic Hypoxia: Hypoxia in which the quantity of oxygen reaching the tissues is normal, but the cell is unable to use the oxygen because a toxic agent has interfered with its metabolism (e.g., cyanide poisoning).

Homeostasis: State of dynamic equilibrium of the internal environment, maintained by various feedback and regulatory mechanisms.

Hormone: Chemical messenger synthesized by a specific endocrine gland in response to certain stimuli and secreted into the blood, which carries it to the other cells in the body, where its actions are exerted.

Humoral Immunity: Type of specific immune response in which circulating antibodies play a central role.

Hydrogen Ion (H$^+$): Single free proton; the concentration of H$^+$ in a solution determines the pH of the solution.

Hydrolysis: The breaking of a chemical bond with the addition of water to the products formed; a hydrolytic reaction.

Hydrostatic Pressure: Pressure exerted by a fluid (e.g., blood).

Hypercapnia: Increased CO_2 concentration in the blood (>45 mmHg); hypercarbia.

Hyperemia: Increased blood flow.

Hyperesthesia: Increase in sensitivity to sensory stimuli such as touch, pain, vibration.

Hyperglycemia: Plasma glucose concentrations increased above normal levels (serum glucose > 110 mg/100 mL).

Hyperplasia: Excessive proliferation of normal cells in a tissue or organ whereby the bulk of the part or the organ is increased.

Hyperpolarization: Change in the membrane potential so that the inside of the cell becomes more negative than its resting state; associated with efflux of potassium ions (K$^+$) from the cell.

Hypersensitivity: An acquired reactivity to an antigen that can result in bodily damage on subsequent exposure to that particular antigen.

Hyperthermia: Body temperature above normal; hyperpyrexia; fever.

Hypertonic: Having a higher concentration and thus a higher osmotic pressure than a compared solution (e.g., blood).

Hypertrophy: Increase in size; enlargement of tissue or organ that results from an increase in cell size rather than in cell number.

Hyperventilation: Ventilation greater than that needed to maintain normal plasma arterial partial pressure of CO_2 (PaCO_2).

Hypervolemia: Abnormally increased blood volume.

Hypocalcemic Tetany: Skeletal muscle spasms caused by a low extracellular calcium concentration.

Hypoesthesia: Reduced sensitivity to touch, tactile stimuli.

Hypoglycemia: Low blood sugar (glucose concentration). Serum glucose <70 mg/100 mL.

Hypothalamic-Releasing Hormones: Hormones released from hypothalamic neurons into the hypothalamo-pituitary portal vessels to control the release of anterior pituitary hormones.

Hypothermia: Body temperature below normal.

Hypotonic Solution: Having a lesser concentration and thus a lower osmotic pressure than a compared solution (e.g., blood).

Hypoventilation: Ventilation insufficient to maintain normal plasma PaCO_2.

Hypoxemia: Insufficient oxygenation of the blood.

Hypoxia: Reduction in tissue oxygen concentration (see also *anemic hypoxia, histotoxic hypoxia,* and *ischemic hypoxia*).

Hypoxic Hypoxia: Hypoxia caused by decreased PaO_2.

Idiopathic: Of undetermined cause.

Ileogastric Reflex: Reflex reduction in gastric motility in response to a distention of the ileum.

Immunity: Physiologic mechanisms that allow the body to recognize foreign or abnormal substances (i.e., antigens) and to neutralize and/or eliminate them; allows the body to recognize and protect/maintain what is "self."

Immunoglobulin: Antibody, includes five classes: IgG, IgM, IgA, IgE, IgD.

Immunologic Tolerance: Ability of the body to recognize those molecules that are foreign; to distinguish self from nonself.

Infarction: Area of necrotic tissue resulting from localized ischemia caused by diminished blood supply.

Inflammation: Local response to tissue injury characterized by swelling, heat, redness, and pain.

Inhibitory Synapse: Response of the postsynaptic neuron to the chemical neurotransmitter released by the presynaptic neurons causes the membrane potential to become more negative, that is, moving away from threshold potential.

Inotropic: Pertaining to the heart's contractile state; factor influencing force of myocardial contractility.

Insensible Loss: Imperceptible loss of water (e.g., by evaporation from cells of the skin or respiratory tract).

Inspiratory Reserve Volume: Maximum volume of air

that can be inspired over and above the resting tidal volume.

Insulin: Hormone secreted by B cells of islets of Langerhans of the pancreas, which facilitates uptake of glucose and amino acids by most cells.

Intercalated Disks: Low resistance pathways between adjacent cardiac muscle cells.

Interferon: Protein or proteins formed when cells are exposed to viral or other foreign nucleic acids; important to immune function and have antitumor activity (especially in hairy cell leukemia).

Interleukin-1 (IL-1): Substance secreted from macrophages that stimulates the activated B cells to proliferate and the T cells to secrete interleukin-2.

Interleukin-2 (IL-2): Protein (lymphokine) secreted by helper T cells that causes activated T cells to proliferate (secretion of interleukin-2 is stimulated by interleukin-1).

Internal Environment: Includes interstitial fluid that bathes each cell and the blood plasma.

Interstitial Fluid: Extracellular fluid surrounding cells.

Interstitium: Space between cells containing extracellular (interstitial) fluid.

Intestinal Phase (Gastrointestinal Control): Initiation of neural and hormonal reflexes controlling gastrointestinal functions by stimulation of the walls of the gastrointestinal tract.

Intrapleural Pressure: Pressure in the pleural space generated by the tendency of the lungs and chest wall to pull away from each other.

Intrinsic Clotting Pathway: Intravascular sequence of fibrin formation initiated by Hageman factor (factor XII).

Intrinsic Factor: Substance normally secreted by cells of the stomach and essential for the absorption of vitamin B_{12} in the ileum.

Ion: Particle or small molecule carrying an electrical charge in solution.

Ipsilateral: Pertains to the same side; affecting the same side of the body.

Ischemia: Reduced blood supply to a tissue or organ.

Ischemic Hypoxia: Hypoxia in which the underlying defect is too little blood flow to tissues to ensure adequate oxygen supply.

Isometric Contraction: Contraction of muscles under conditions in which they develop tension but do not change length.

Isotonic Contraction: Contraction of a muscle under conditions in which a load on the muscle remains constant but the muscle length shortens.

Isotonic Solution: Solution in which the concentration and, thus, the osmotic pressure are equivalent to the solution to which it is being compared (e.g., blood).

Isovolumetric Ventricular Contraction: Early phase of systole when myocardial tension increases but both the atrioventricular and semilunar valves remain closed.

Isovolumetric Ventricular Relaxation: Early phase of diastole when myocardial tension is decreasing but both the atrioventricular and semilunar valves remain closed.

Ketone Bodies: Certain products of fatty acid metabolism, including acetoacetic acid, acetone, and β-hydroxybutyric acid, that accumulate in the blood and contribute to the metabolic acidosis of diabetic ketoacidosis (DKA).

Kinesthesia: Ability to sense the extent, direction, and weight of movement.

Kinins: Group of peptides derived from kininogens that have considerable biologic activity; that facilitate vascular changes associated with inflammation, including an increase in blood flow and capillary permeability; and that stimulate pain receptors.

Laryngospasm: Spasm of laryngeal muscles; major concern is closing off of airway.

Lecithin: Phospholipid.

Leukotrienes: Group of chemical mediators of inflammation; stimulate contraction of bronchiolar smooth muscle (related to prostaglandins).

Lipoproteins: Protein molecules that combine with lipids (including cholesterol, phospholipids, and triglycerides) and transport lipids in the blood. Lipoproteins are classified as high-density (HDL), low-density (LDL), and very-low-density (VLDL) lipoproteins.

Local Current Flow: Movement of positive ions from a membrane region with a high positive charge directly through the cytoplasm or extracellular fluid toward a membrane region of more negative charge; and the simultaneous movement of negative ions in the opposite direction; in this way, adjacent segments of membrane become depolarized.

Lung Compliance: Change in lung volume caused by a given change in pressure difference across the lung wall (i.e., the greater the lung compliance, the more easily the lungs can be expanded).

Lymphokines: Substances (nonantibody) released by sensitive lymphocytes when in contact with specific antigens that contribute to cellular immunity by stimulating macrophages and monocytes.

Lysosome: Cell organelle containing digestive enzymes and surrounded by a limiting membrane. These enzymes are capable of breaking down proteins and some carbohydrates; if released into the cytoplasm, they can digest components of the cell itself.

Macrophage: Cell of the reticuloendothelial system that functions as a phagocyte in many tissues, processes and presents antigen to lymphocytes, and secretes chemicals involved in the proliferation of activated lymphocytes in the inflammatory processes and in the body's overall response to infection.

Major Histocompatibility Complex (MHC): Group of genes that code for many proteins important for immune responses, including HLA, or histocompatibility antigens, present on the surface of all nucleated cells.

Mast Cells: Connective tissue cells that release histamine and other chemicals in response to local tissue injury.

Maximum Tubular Capacity (Tm): Maximum rate of mediated transport of a substance (e.g., glucose) across the membrane of renal tubule cells.

Mean Arterial Blood Pressure: Average blood pressure during the cardiac cycle; equal to diastolic pressure plus one third the pulse pressure.

Mediated Transport: Movement of molecules across membranes by binding to protein carrier molecules located in the membrane (see *active transport* and *facilitated diffusion*).

Melanosis: Disorder of pigment metabolism resulting in abnormal dark brown or brown/black pigmentation of various tissues or organs.

Membrane Potential: Voltage difference between the inside and outside of the cell caused by the separation of charge across the membrane.

Memory Cells: B and T lymphocytes produced after initial exposure to an antigen that respond expeditiously during a subsequent exposure to the same antigen.

Metabolic Acidosis: Associated with an accumulation of acid by-products of metabolism other than CO_2 (lactate production during exercise; ketone formation in DKA).

Metabolic Alkalosis: Reduction in the H^+ concentration in the body associated with mechanisms other than the respiratory removal of CO_2 (loss of H^+ from stomach caused by vomiting or continuous nasogastric suctioning).

Metabolic Rate: Reflects total energy expenditure in the body per unit time.

Micelle: Soluble cluster of amphipathic molecules in which the polar regions of the molecules line the surface of the micelle; the nonpolar regions are oriented toward the middle of the micelle. Formed during digestion of fats in the small intestine.

Microvilli: Small hairlike projections from the surface of some epithelial cells, which greatly increase the absorptive surface area of the cell.

Micturition: Urination.

Mineralocorticoids: Steroid hormones synthesized and secreted by the adrenal cortex, having their major effect on sodium and potassium balance (e.g., aldosterone).

Mitochondria: Intracellular organelles that produce ATP.

Mixed Venous Blood: Status of the oxygen and CO_2 tensions of blood in the pulmonary artery, as a reflection of the total extraction of oxygen from circulating blood by all tissues in the body.

Monoclonal Antibodies: Identical immunoglobulins secreted by a clone of hybrid cells.

Muscarinic Receptors: Acetylcholine receptors that can be stimulated by the drug muscarine; occur primarily at postganglionic synapses in the parasympathetic branches of the autonomic nervous system.

Myelin: Insulating substance containing lipid and protein that forms a sheath around axons of certain nerves; presence of nodes of Ranvier facilitates rapid impulse transmission by saltatory conduction.

Myenteric Plexus: Network of nerve cells lying between muscle layers in the gastrointestinal tract.

NA^+, K^+-ATPase: Primary active transport carrier protein present in all plasma membranes, which releases energy used to pump Na^+ out of the cell in exchange for K^+.

Natriuretic Factor: A hormonelike substance secreted by cells, especially in the right atrium, that enhances renal excretion of sodium. Concomitant with sodium loss, both extracellular fluid volume and intravascular blood volume decrease slightly.

Natural Killer (NK) Cells: Cells, probably lymphocytes, that bind relatively nonspecifically to cells exhibiting foreign surface antigens and kill them directly; no prior exposure to the antigen is required.

Negative Balance: State wherein the loss of a substance from the body is greater than that gained, and the total concentration of that substance in the body is decreased.

Negative Feedback: System wherein a series of changes are initiated to return a factor that has become excessive or depleted back toward a certain mean value; type of feedback wherein an increase in the output of the system results in a decrease in the input.

Neuroglycopenia: Presence of adrenergic and central nervous system alterations in the presence of serum glucose levels <55 mg/100 mL.

Neurotransmitter: Chemical messenger released at chemical synapses through which the electrical activity of the presynaptic neuron influences the activity of the postsynaptic neuron (e.g., norepinephrine, acetylcholine).

Nicotinic Receptors: Acetylcholine receptors that respond to nicotine; primarily occurs at neuromuscular junctions and ganglia in the autonomic nervous system.

Nystagmus: Continuous involuntary movement of the eyeball in any direction.

Oncogene: Gene in a virus that appears to be able to induce a cell to become malignant. Oncogenes have been identified in human tumors.

Onycholysis: Loosening of nails, usually beginning at the free border with detachment from the nailbed.

Ophthalmoplegia: Paralysis of ocular muscles.

Opisthotonos: Tetanic spasm causing the head and heels to bend backwards and the trunk to bow forward.

Osmolality: Osmotic concentration, the characteristic of a solution determined by the ionic concentration of dissolved particles per unit of solvent, expressed as osmoles per kilogram of water.

Osmolarity: Concentration of osmotically active particles in solution.

Osmole: The amount of substance that dissociates in solution to form one mole of osmotically active particles.

Osmosis: Net diffusion of water from a region of high water concentration to one of low water concentration across a membrane; water moves from regions of low solute concentration (high water concentration) to a region of high solute concentration (low water concentration).

Osmotic Pressure: Pressure that develops when two solutions of different concentrations are separated by a semipermeable membrane; or pressure that must be applied to a solution on one side of a membrane to prevent osmotic flow of water into the solution from a source of pure water on the opposite side of the membrane.

Otorrhea: Drainage or discharge from the ear; suspect CSF leakage in the scenario of head injury.

Oxidative Phosphorylation: Process by which energy derived from the reaction between hydrogen and oxygen (to form water) is transferred to ATP during its formation from ADP and inorganic phosphate; this reaction occurs in mitochondria.

Oxyhemoglobin: Hb combined with oxygen.

Oxyhemoglobin Dissociation Curve: Reflects that the amount of oxygen bound to Hb is a function of the partial pressure of oxygen.

Paralytic Ileus: State of complete atony of the small bowel with an absence of peristalsis; associated with abdominal surgery/trauma.

Parasympathetic Nervous System: Division of the autonomic nervous system whose preganglionic fibers leave the brain and sacral region of the spinal cord; most of its postganglionic fibers release the neurotransmitter acetylcholine.

Parasympathomimetic: Drug that produces effects similar to those of the parasympathetic nervous system.

Parenchyma: Essential substance or components of an organ concerned with its function.

Paresthesia: Heightened sensitivity; sensations of prickling, tingling, numbness.

Parietal Cells: Gastric gland cells that secrete hydrochloric acid and intrinsic factor (oxyntic cell).

Partial Pressure: Pressure exerted by the molecules of one specific gas (e.g., PO_2, the partial pressure of oxygen, is that part of total atmospheric pressure attributed to oxygen molecules).

Permissiveness: Situation whereby a small quantity of one hormone is required for a second hormone to exert its effect.

pH: Measure of the acidity or concentration of H^+ of a solution; as acidity increases, pH decreases.

Phagocytosis: Form of endocytosis or pinocytosis, involving the engulfment and digestion of bacteria and particles by phagocytic cells (e.g., leukocytes, macrophages).

Phospholipid: Lipid molecules containing phosphorus, fatty acids, and a nitrogenous base (e.g., lecithin).

Phosphorylation: Addition of a phosphate group to an organic molecule.

Pinocytosis: Cellular process of engulfing liquid.

Plasma: Fluid, noncellular portion of the blood, making up about 3% of total extracellular fluid.

Plasma Cells: Cells derived from activated B lymphocytes that secrete antibodies.

Plasma Proteins: Include albumin, globulins, and fibrinogens present in blood plasma.

Plasmapheresis: Process of plasma exchange wherein blood is removed from the body and centrifuged to separate the cellular components from the plasma. Undesired components (e.g., autoantibodies) can be removed and the remainder of the blood can be returned to the patient.

Plasmin: Fibrinolytic enzyme derived from its precursor, plasminogen; functions to decompose fibrin and, thereby, to dissolve blood clots.

Plethora: Hypervolemia: excess of any body fluid; expanded blood volume.

Polarized: Having two electric poles: one positive, the other negative.

Polydipsia: Excessive thirst.

Polyunsaturated Fatty Acid: Fatty acid that contains more than one double bond.

Portal Vessels: Blood vessels that link two separate capillary networks (e.g., hypothalamic-hypophyseal portal system).

Postabsorptive State: Period between meals during which nutrients are not being absorbed by the gastrointestinal tract and energy must be supplied by the body's endogenous stores.

Postganglionic Neuron: Neuron of the autonomic nervous system whose cell body lies in a ganglion and whose axon endings terminate in effector organs (i.e., neuromuscular junction, glands).

Postsynaptic Neuron: Neuron that conducts impulses away from a synapse.

Postural (Orthostatic) Hypotension: Reduction in blood pressure upon assuming an erect position or upon standing.

Postural Reflexes: Those reflexes that maintain or restore upright, stable posture.

Potential (Potential Difference): Voltage differences between two points.

Precapillary Sphincter: Ring of smooth muscle around a capillary at the point at which it exits from an arteriole.

Preganglionic Neuron: Neuron of the autonomic nervous system whose cell body lies in the central nervous system and whose axon terminals lie in a ganglion; conducts impulses from the central nervous system toward a ganglion.

Preload: Distending force stretching the ventricular muscle fibers just before contraction.

Presynaptic Neuron: Neuron that conducts impulses toward a synapse.

Proprioception: Awareness of posture and the knowledge of position and weight in relation to the body.

Prostaglandins: Large group of biologically active, unsaturated fatty acids derived from arachidonic acid. Biologic effects are short-lived and are not mediated by the blood. They exert their effects locally, in the tissues in which they are formed. Physiologic activities influenced by prostaglandins include platelet aggregation, local blood flow, fluid balance, lypolysis, and neurotransmission, among others.

Proteolysis: Breakdown of proteins into simpler substances; amino acid components.

Pulse Pressure: Difference between systolic and diastolic arterial blood pressures.

Raynaud's Phenomenon: Intermittent attacks of pallor followed by cyanosis, then redness of digits, before return to normal.

Reactive Hyperemia: Transient increase in blood flow following the release of occlusion of the blood supply to a tissue or organ; attributed to the vasodilatory effects of chemical mediators released by ischemic tissues.

Receptor: Specialized peripheral ending of an afferent (sensory) neuron, or distinct cell intimately related to it, that detects changes in the environment; receives stimulus or detects an alteration in environmental conditions.

Receptor Site: Specific protein-binding site with which a chemical mediator or neurotransmitter combines to exert its effect.

Reciprocal Innervation: Inhibition of motor neurons activating those muscles whose contraction would oppose the intended movement (e.g., inhibition of flexor motor neurons during extensor motor neuron activation).

Recommended Daily Allowance (RDA): Daily intake of nutrients considered sufficient to prevent nutritional insufficiency in most healthy persons.

Reduced Hemoglobin: See *deoxyhemoglobin*.

Reflex: Involuntary response when a stimulus is linked with a response and mediated by a reflex arch composed of neural and/or hormonal elements.

Reflex Arc: Components that mediate a reflex; composed of a receptor, afferent pathway, integrating center, efferent pathway, and effector.

Refractory Period: Time during which an excitable membrane does not respond to a stimulus.

Absolute Refractory Period: Time during which an excitable membrane is unable to generate another action potential in response to any stimulus.

Relative Refractory Period: Time during which an excitable membrane will produce an action potential only in response to stimuli of greater strength than the usual threshold strength.

Releasing Hormones: Hormones secreted by the hypothalamus that control the release of hormones by the anterior pituitary.

Renin: Enzyme secreted by the kidneys that acts on angiotensinogen in the blood to form angiotensin I.

Repolarization: Return of the value of the transmembrane potential to its resting state.

Residual Volume: Volume of air remaining in the lungs after maximal expiration.

Resistance Vessels: Vessels that offer the greatest frictional resistance to blood flow (arterioles).

Respiratory Acidosis: Acidosis resulting from the failure of the lungs to eliminate CO_2 as rapidly as it is produced (hypoventilation).

Respiratory Alkalosis: Alkalosis resulting from the elimination of CO_2 from the lungs faster than it is produced (hyperventilation).

Respiratory "Pump": Effect of the changing intrathoracic and intra-abdominal pressures associated with breathing on the venous return to the heart.

Respiratory Quotient (RQ): Ratio of CO_2 produced to oxygen consumed during metabolism.

Resting Membrane Potential: Voltage differences across a plasma membrane between the inside and outside of a resting cell.

Rh Factor: Group of antigens that may (Rh positive) or may not (Rh negative) be present on the plasma membrane of RBCs.

Rhinorrhea: Thin, watery discharge from nose; suspect CSF leakage in scenario of head injury, basal skull fracture, and/or dural tear.

Rostral-to-Caudal: Head-to-toe.

Saltatory Conduction: Conduction that occurs along myelinated axons in which the myelin sheath is interrupted by the nodes of Ranvier and the action potential skips from node to node, enhancing the rapidity of impulse conduction.

Saturated Fatty Acid: Fatty acid whose carbon atoms are all linked by single covalent bonds.

Saturation: Degree to which binding sites are occupied by specific molecules; if all sites are occupied, the binding sites are fully saturated; adding more of the substance will not increase its concentration.

Secretin: Hormone secreted by cells in the upper part of the small intestine; stimulates pancreas to secrete bicarbonate into the small intestine; bicarbonate neutralizes the acid chyme entering the duodenum.

Semipermeable Membrane: Membrane permeable to some substances but impermeable to other substances.

Serotonin: Chemical mediator with potent vasoconstrictor effects present in platelets, gastrointestinal mucosa, and mast cells; a monoamine neurotransmitter thought to be involved in neuromechanisms associated with sensory perception and sleep.

Serum: Blood plasma from which fibrinogen has been removed as a result of clotting.

Shift to the Left: Increase in band neutrophils indicative of acute infection.

Shunt:

Right-to-Left Shunt: Mixing of deoxygenated blood with oxygenated blood; passage of blood from right to left side of the heart.

Left-to-Right Shunt: Mixing of oxygenated blood with deoxygenated blood; passage of blood from left to right side of the heart.

Skeletal Muscle "Pump": Pumping action of contracting skeletal muscles, especially in the lower extremities, that assists venous return to the heart.

Sliding Filament Theory: Process of muscle contraction wherein shortening occurs as a result of the sliding of thick (myosin) and thin (actin) filaments past each other.

Sodium Inactivation: Closing of sodium channels in the plasma membrane at the peak of an action potential when the membrane is depolarized.

Solubility Coefficient: Refers to the extent that molecules of gas are physically and chemically attracted to water molecules.

Solute: Molecules dissolved in a liquid.

Solution: Liquid containing dissolved molecules or ions.

Solvent: Liquid in which molecules or ions are dissolved.

Somatomedin: Group of growth-stimulating hormones released primarily from the liver in response to growth hormone.

Somatosensory (Somesthetic) Cortex: Strip of cerebral cortex in the parietal lobe where nerve fibers transmitting somatic (i.e., pertaining to the body) sensations (i.e., touch, temperature, vibration) synapse. It provides a representation of senses from various segments of the body.

Somatostatin: Hormone that inhibits release of somatotropin (growth hormone) and thyroid-stimulating hormone (TSH) from the anterior pituitary. This hormone is also secreted by D cells of the pancreatic islets of Langerhans and stomach, inhibiting secretion of insulin and gastrin.

Specificity: Ability of a protein-binding site to react with one type, or a limited type, of structurally related molecules.

Spinal Cord Syndrome: Incomplete spinal cord injuries having different patterns of neurologic dysfunction.

Spinal Shock (Neurogenic Shock): Sudden complete transection of the spinal cord, causing immediate loss of motor, sensory, reflex, and autonomic function below the level of the injury; spinal shock may also occur in incomplete transection of the cord.

Starling's Law of the Heart: States that, within limits, an increase in the end-diastolic volume of the heart (i.e., increasing stretch of muscle fibers) increases the force of cardiac contraction.

Stimulus: Any change in the environment detectable by a receptor (sensory).

Stroke Volume: Volume of blood ejected by a ventricle during each beat of the heart.

Submucosa: Connective tissue layer underlying the mucosa in the walls of the stomach and intestines.

Substrate: Reactant in an enzyme-mediated reaction.

Suppressor T Cells: Class of T lymphocytes that inhibit antibody production and cytotoxic T-cell function.

Surface Tension: Unequal attractive forces at the surface of a liquid in contact with a gas or another liquid, wherein the attraction of the molecules to each other results in a net force that acts to reduce the surface area.

Surfactant: Phospholipid agent produced by type II pneumocytes that markedly reduces surface tension within the alveoli. This reduces the tendency of the alveoli to collapse, thereby minimizing atelectasis.

Sympathetic Nervous System: Division of autonomic nervous system whose preganglionic fibers leave the thoracolumbar region of the spinal cord; most of the postganglionic neurons release the neurotransmitter norepinephrine.

Sympathetic Trunk: One of a pair of chains of interconnected sympathetic ganglia that lie on either side of the vertebral column.

Sympathomimetic: Drug that produces effects similar to those of the sympathetic nervous system.

Synapse (Chemical): Anatomically specialized junction between two neurons where the electrical activity in one neuron (presynaptic) influences the excitability of the second neuron (postsynaptic) by a chemical neurotransmitter.

Synaptic Cleft: Narrow extracellular space separating the presynaptic and postsynaptic neurons at a chemical synapse.

Synergistic: Enhancement of the activity of one molecule by the activity of another, producing an effect that neither could produce alone; or the total effect may be greater than the summation of each substance functioning by itself.

Systemic (Peripheral) Vascular Resistance: Resistance to blood flow offered by the systemic vasculature, including, in particular, that offered by the arterioles and metarterioles.

Systole: Period when the ventricles of the heart are contracting.

Systolic Pressure: Maximum arterial blood pressure reached during the cardiac cycle.

T Cells (T Lymphocytes): Lymphocytes derived from precursors in the thymus (see also *cytotoxic T cells, helper T cells,* and *suppressor T cells*).

Thick Filaments: Filaments in muscle cells consisting of myosin molecules.

Thin Filaments: Filaments in muscle cells consisting of actin, troponin, and tropomyosin molecules.

Third Spacing: Shift of fluid from intravascular space to transcellular spaces (e.g., ascites).

Thoroughfare Channel: Capillary that connects arterioles and venules directly and from which capillaries branch to make up the capillary bed.

Threshold (Renal): Plasma levels at which a substance begins to appear in the urine.

Threshold (Threshold Potential): Membrane potential to which an excitable membrane must be depolarized to initiate an action potential.

Threshold Stimulus: Stimulus capable of depolarizing the membrane to threshold potential.

Thrombin: Enzyme that catalyzes the conversion of fibrinogen to fibrin.

Thrombosis: Formation, presence, or development of a blood clot (thrombus) that obstructs a blood vessel, partially or completely, or occurs in a cavity of the heart.

Thyroglobulin: Large iodine-containing protein synthesized by the thyroid gland and stored in its colloid substance to which thyroid hormones bind and are stored.

Thyroid Hormone: Hormones synthesized and secreted by the thyroid gland; include thyroxine (T_4) and triiodothyronine (T_3); these hormones increase the metabolic rate of most cells.

Thyroid-Stimulating Hormone (TSH; Thyrotropin): Hormone secreted by the anterior pituitary that induces its target gland, the thyroid gland, to secrete thyroid hormones.

Thyrotropin-Releasing Hormone (TRH): Hormone released by hypothalamus that stimulates thyrotropin (TSH) by the anterior pituitary.

Tidal Volume: Volume of air entering and leaving the lungs during a single spontaneous breath.

Tight Junction: Type of junction formed between adjacent epithelial cells in some tissues that restricts diffusion of molecules across a layer of epithelial cells by way of the extracellular space between cells (e.g., blood-brain barrier, in which two adjacent ependymal cells are fused together).

Tissue Thromboplastin: Extravascular enzyme capable of initiating the extrinsic clotting cascade leading to the formation of a fibrin clot.

Total Lung Capacity: Equal to the sum of the vital capacity plus the residual volume.

Tract: Large bundle of myelinated nerve fibers in the central nervous system (brain and spinal cord).

Transudation: Passage of fluid or solute through a membrane as a result of hydrostatic and osmotic pressure gradients.

Transverse Tubule (T Tubule): Tubule extending from the sarcolemma (i.e., the delicate membrane surrounding the muscle fiber) into the fiber interior; conducts action potentials into the muscle fibers.

Tremor: Involuntary, quivering type movement of a part or parts of the body associated with alternate contractions of opposing muscles.

Flapping: Coarse tremor seen in outstretched arm or hand and associated with hepatic coma and other diseases that cause encephalopathy (asterixis).

Intention: Tremor when voluntary movement is attempted.

Resting: Presence of tremor at rest, but absent or diminished when movement is attempted.

Tropomyosin: Regulatory protein associated with the actin filament that is capable of reversibly covering the binding sites on actin, thereby preventing myosin heads from binding to actin to form cross-bridges.

Troponin: Regulatory protein that attaches to both actin and tropomyosin.

Tubular Reabsorption: Transfer of substances from lumen of kidney tubule to the peritubular capillaries.

Tubular Secretion: Transfer of substances from the peritubular capillaries to the lumen of the renal tubules.

Ultrafiltrate: Fluid that is essentially protein free; formed by plasma as it is forced through capillary walls by a pressure gradient.

Unsaturated Fatty Acid: Fatty acid containing one or more double bonds.

Uremia: Complex multisystem alterations that occur when the level of kidney function can no longer support the internal milieu.

Valsalva's Maneuver: Maneuver wherein an attempt is made to exhale forcibly against a closed glottis, thereby increasing intrathoracic pressures; this, in turn, decreases venous return to the heart; associated vagal stimulation results in slowing of the heart rate.

Vapor Pressure: Pressure exerted by water molecules as they escape from the fluid surface.

Vasoconstriction: Decrease in diameter of blood vessels caused by vascular smooth muscle contraction.

Vasodilation: Increase in diameter of blood vessels caused by vascular smooth muscle relaxation.

Velocity: Rate of fluid movement per unit time, expressed as mL/sec.

Venous Capacitance: Ability of veins to accommodate large volume increases without large increases in pressure.

Venous Return: Volume of blood filling the ventricles during diastole; preload.

Ventilation: Bulk flow exchange of air between atmosphere and alveoli.

Alveolar Minute Ventilation: Equal to the number of breaths per minute (i.e., the respiratory rate) times the tidal volume minus the anatomic dead-space volume (i.e., alveolar volume).

Minute Ventilation: Total volume of gas inspired each minute; equal to the respiratory rate times the tidal volume.

Ventilatory Dyscoordination: Disruption of the orderly sequence of contraction of muscles of inspiration and expiration associated with extreme weakness or fatigue.

Ventilation-Perfusion Ratio ($\dot{V}/\dot{Q}$): Reflects the relationship between alveolar ventilation and pulmonary capillary blood flow. (Normally the ratio is about 0.8.)

Ventral: Anterior, toward the front.

Villi: Projections of the highly folded surface of the mucosal lining of the small intestine; increases surface area for digestive and absorptive activities.

Viscosity: Property of a fluid that makes it resist flow, caused by the frictional interactions between its molecules.

Vital Capacity: Volume of gas that is maximally expired following a maximal inspiration.

Vitiligo: Appearance upon otherwise normal skin of loss of pigment with white skin patches of varied sizes, frequently symmetrically distributed.

Voltage: Measure of the potential of separate electric charges to do work, expressed in volts.

Water Intoxication: State of excess water and sodium retention.

Weak Acid: Acid whose molecules do not completely ionize to form H^+ when dissolved in water.

Work of Breathing: Energy or work required to expand the lungs and thorax to provide for a given volume of ventilation; effort generated by the contraction of expiratory musculature.

Index

Note: Page numbers followed by f indicate figures; page numbers followed by t indicate tables.

ISBN 0-8036-0025-9

90000>

EAN

9 780803 600256